"Adorn the Halls"

History of the Art Collection at Thomas Jefferson University

Julie S. Berkowitz

Published by Thomas Jefferson University, Philadelphia, Pennsylvania

ISBN 0-9674384-1-1
Library of Congress Catalog Card Number 99-73843

Edited by Malcolm Clendenin
Photographs by Rick Echelmeyer
Design, type composition, printing, and binding by
William T. Cooke Publishing, Inc., Devon, Pennsylvania

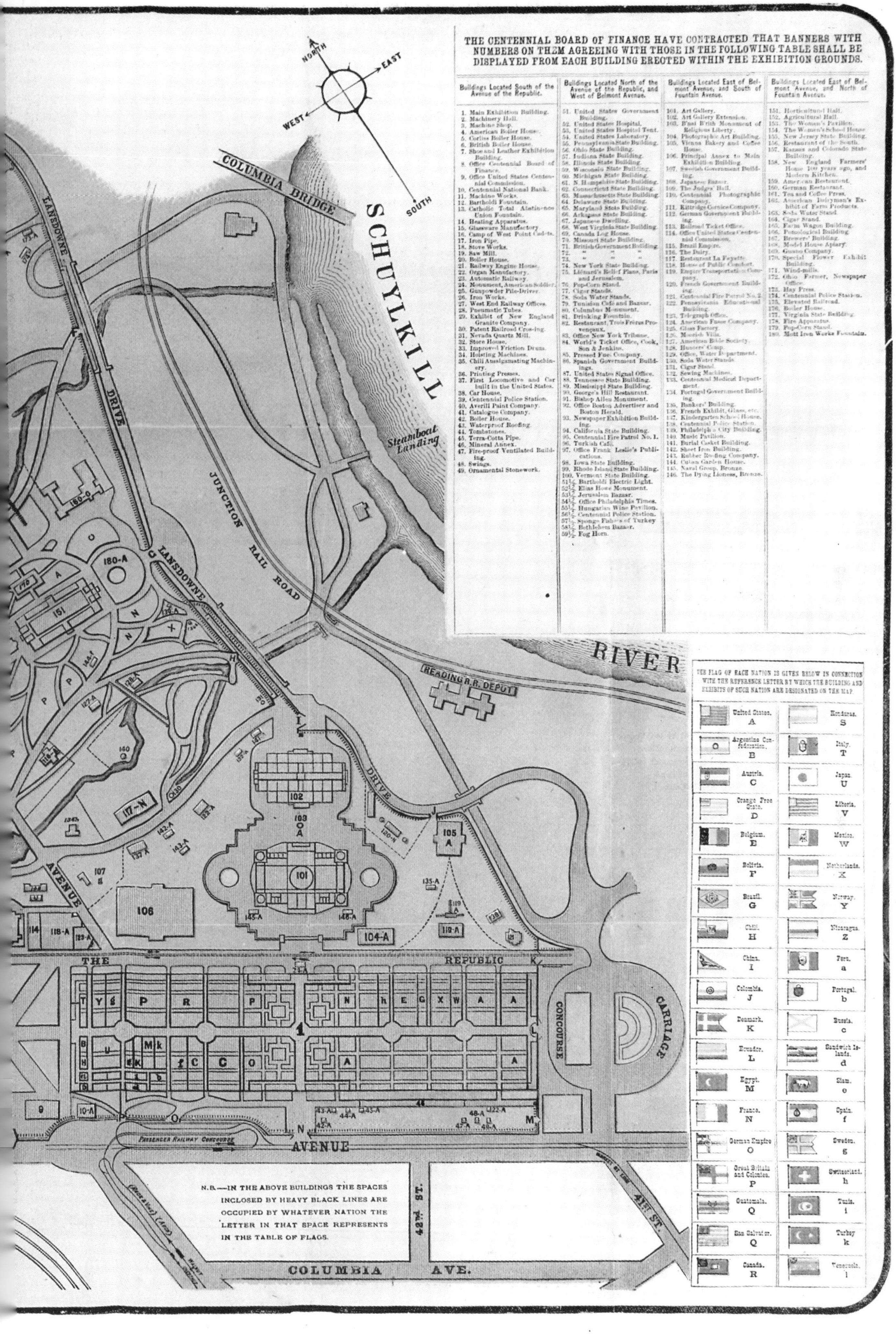

THE CENTENNIAL BOARD OF FINANCE HAVE CONTRACTED THAT BANNERS WITH NUMBERS ON THEM AGREEING WITH THOSE IN THE FOLLOWING TABLE SHALL BE DISPLAYED FROM EACH BUILDING ERECTED WITHIN THE EXHIBITION GROUNDS.

Buildings Located South of the Avenue of the Republic.	Buildings Located North of the Avenue of the Republic, and West of Belmont Avenue.	Buildings Located East of Belmont Avenue, and South of Fountain Avenue.	Buildings Located East of Belmont Avenue, and North of Fountain Avenue.
1. Main Exhibition Building.	51. United States Government Building.	101. Art Gallery.	151. Horticultural Hall.
2. Machinery Hall.	52. United States Hospital.	102. Art Gallery Extension.	152. Agricultural Hall.
3. Machine Shop.	53. United States Hospital Tent.	103. B'nai B'rith Monument of Religious Liberty.	153. The Women's Pavilion.
4. American Boiler House.	54. United States Laboratory.	104. Photographic Art Building.	154. The Women's School House
5. Corliss Boiler House.	55. Pennsylvania State Building.	105. Vienna Bakery and Coffee House.	155. New Jersey State Building.
6. British Boiler House.	56. Ohio State Building.	106. Principal Annex to Main Exhibition Building.	156. Restaurant of the South.
7. Shoe and Leather Exhibition Building.	57. Indiana State Building.	107. Swedish Government Building.	157. Kansas and Colorado State Building.
8. Office Centennial Board of Finance.	58. Illinois State Building.	108. Japanese Bazaar.	158. New England Farmers' Home 100 years ago, and Modern Kitchen.
9. Office United States Centennial Commission.	59. Wisconsin State Building.	109. The Judges' Hall.	159. American Restaurant.
10. Centennial National Bank.	60. Michigan State Building.	110. Centennial Photographic Company.	160. German Restaurant.
11. Machine Works.	61. N. Hampshire State Building.	111. Kittredge Cornice Company.	161. Tea and Coffee Press.
12. Bartholdi Fountain.	62. Connecticut State Building.	112. German Government Building.	162. American Dairyman's Exhibit of Farm Products.
13. Catholic Total Abstinence Union Fountain.	63. Massachusetts State Building.	113. Railroad Ticket Office.	163. Soda Water Stand.
14. Heating Apparatus.	64. Delaware State Building.	114. Offices United States Centennial Commission.	164. Cigar Stand.
15. Glassware Manufactory.	65. Maryland State Building.	115. Brazil Empire.	165. Farm Wagon Building.
16. Camp of West Point Cadets.	66. Arkansas State Building.	116. The Dairy.	166. Pomological Building.
17. Iron Pipe.	67. Japanese Dwelling.	117. Restaurant La Fayette.	167. Brewers' Building.
18. Stove Works.	68. West Virginia State Building.	118. House of Public Comfort.	168. Model House Apiary.
19. Saw Mill.	69. Canada Log House.	119. Empire Transportation Company.	169. Guano Company.
20. Boiler House.	70. Missouri State Building.	120. French Government Building.	170. Special Flower Exhibit Building.
21. Railway Engine House.	71. British Government Building.	121. Centennial Fire Patrol No. 2.	171. Wind-mills.
22. Organ Manufactory.	72. " " "	122. Pennsylvania Educational Building.	172. Ohio Farmer, Newspaper Office.
23. Automatic Railway.	73. " " "	123. Telegraph Office.	173. Hay Press.
24. Monument, American Soldier.	74. New York State Building.	124. American Fusee Company.	174. Centennial Police Station.
25. Gunpowder Pile-Driver.	75. Léonard's Relief Plans, Paris and Jerusalem.	125. Glass Factory.	175. Elevated Railroad.
26. Iron Works.	76. Pop-Corn Stand.	126. Moorish Villa.	176. Boiler House.
27. West End Railway Offices.	77. Cigar Stands.	127. American Bible Society.	177. Virginia State Building.
28. Pneumatic Tubes.	78. Soda Water Stands.	128. Hunters' Camp.	178. Fire Apparatus.
29. Exhibit of New England Granite Company.	79. Tunisian Café and Bazaar.	129. Office, Water Department.	179. Pop-Corn Stand.
30. Patent Railroad Crossing.	80. Columbus Monument.	130. Soda Water Stands.	180. Mott Iron Works Fountain.
31. Nevada Quartz Mill.	81. Drinking Fountain.	131. Cigar Stand.	
32. Store House.	82. Restaurant, Trois Frères Provençaux.	132. Sewing Machines.	
33. Improved Friction Drum.	83. Office New York Tribune.	133. Centennial Medical Department.	
34. Hoisting Machines.	84. World's Ticket Office, Cook, Son & Jenkins.	134. Portugal Government Building.	
35. Chili Amalgamating Machinery.	85. Pressed Fuel Company.	135. Bankers' Building.	
36. Printing Presses.	86. Spanish Government Buildings.	136. French Exhibit, Glass, etc.	
37. First Locomotive and Car built in the United States.	87. United States Signal Office.	137. Kindergarten School House.	
38. Car House.	88. Tennessee State Building.	138. Centennial Police Station.	
39. Centennial Police Station.	89. Mississippi State Building.	139. Philadelphia City Building.	
40. Averill Paint Company.	90. George's Hill Restaurant.	140. Music Pavilion.	
41. Catalogue Company.	91. Bishop Allen Monument.	141. Burial Casket Building.	
42. Boiler House.	92. Office Boston Advertiser and Boston Herald.	142. Sheet Iron Building.	
43. Waterproof Roofing.	93. Newspaper Exhibition Building.	143. Rubber Roofing Company.	
44. Tombstones.	94. California State Building.	144. Cuban Garden House.	
45. Terra-Cotta Pipe.	95. Centennial Fire Patrol No. 1.	145. Naval Group, Bronze.	
46. Mineral Annex.	96. Turkish Café.	146. The Dying Lioness, Bronze.	
47. Fire-proof Ventilated Building.	97. Office Frank Leslie's Publications.		
48. Swings.	98. Iowa State Building.		
49. Ornamental Stonework.	99. Rhode Island State Building.		
	100. Vermont State Building.		
	51½. Bartholdi Electric Light.		
	52½. Elias Howe Monument.		
	53½. Jerusalem Bazaar.		
	54½. Office Philadelphia Times.		
	55½. Hungarian Wine Pavilion.		
	56½. Centennial Police Station.		
	57½. Sponge Fishers of Turkey		
	58½. Bethlehem Bazaar.		
	59½. Fog Horn.		

THE FLAG OF EACH NATION IS GIVEN BELOW IN CONNECTION WITH THE REFERENCE LETTER BY WHICH THE BUILDING AND EXHIBITS OF SUCH NATION ARE DESIGNATED ON THE MAP.

United States. A	Honduras. S
Argentine Confederation. B	Italy. T
Austria. C	Japan. U
Orange Free State. D	Liberia. V
Belgium. E	Mexico. W
Bolivia. F	Netherlands. X
Brazil. G	Norway. Y
Chili. H	Nicaragua. Z
China. I	Peru. a
Colombia. J	Portugal. b
Denmark. K	Russia. c
Ecuador. L	Sandwich Islands. d
Egypt. M	Siam. e
France. N	Spain. f
German Empire O	Sweden. g
Great Britain and Colonies. P	Switzerland. h
Guatemala. Q	Tunis. i
San Salvador. Q	Turkey k
Canada. R	Venezuela. l

"ADORN THE HALLS"

History of the Art Collection at Thomas Jefferson University

This book is dedicated to Dr. Frederick B. Wagner Jr.,
for his generosity in sharing an encyclopedic
knowledge of and passion for Jefferson history,
and for his collegial encouragement of my work.

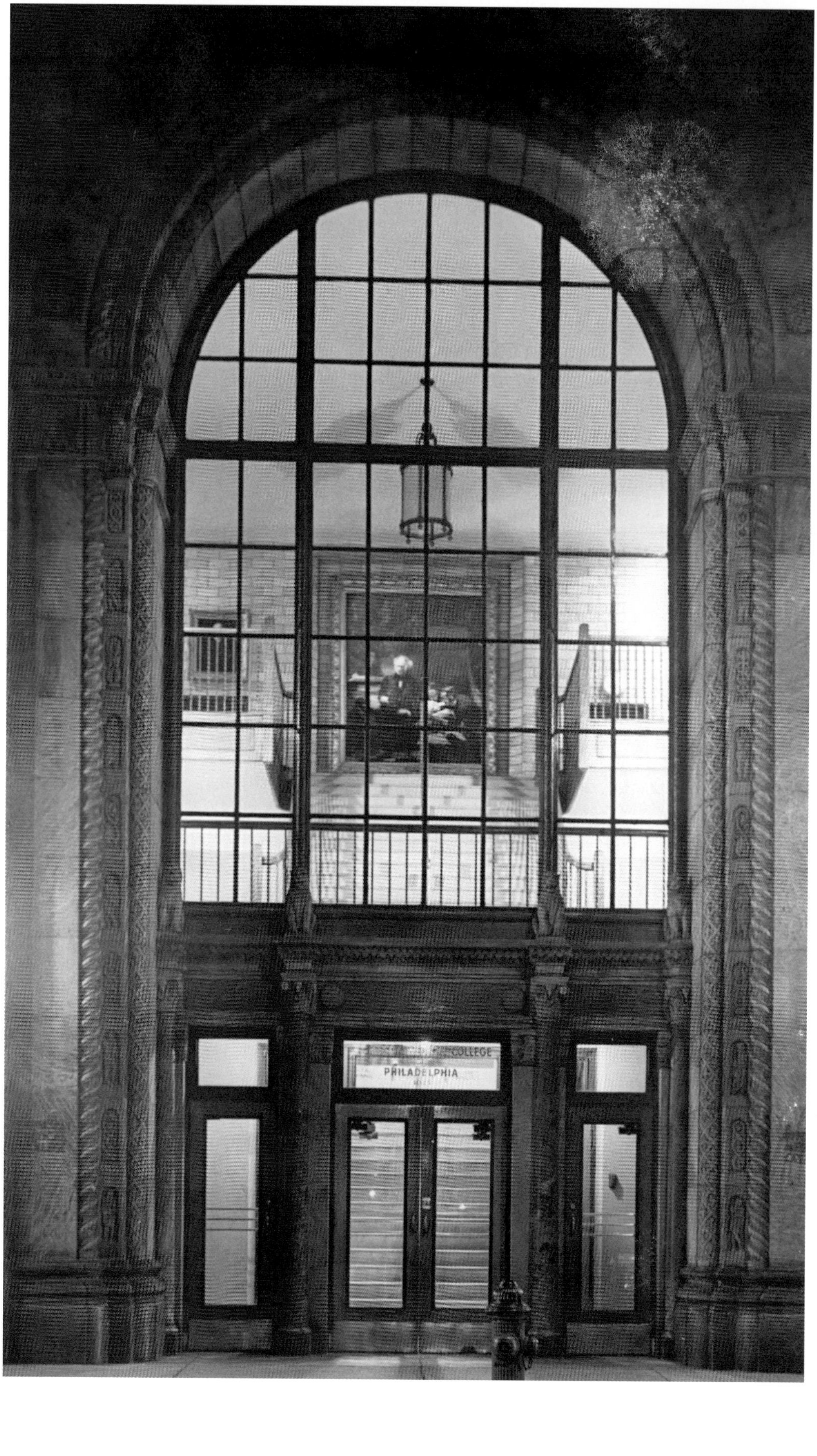

The Gross Clinic
on Stairway Landing,
College Building
(ca. 1940-60)

CONTENTS

Color plates are inserted between pages 288 and 289.

Biographical information about each artist is provided the first time one of his works is discussed, but not with each additional work. To find this information, use the index of artists.

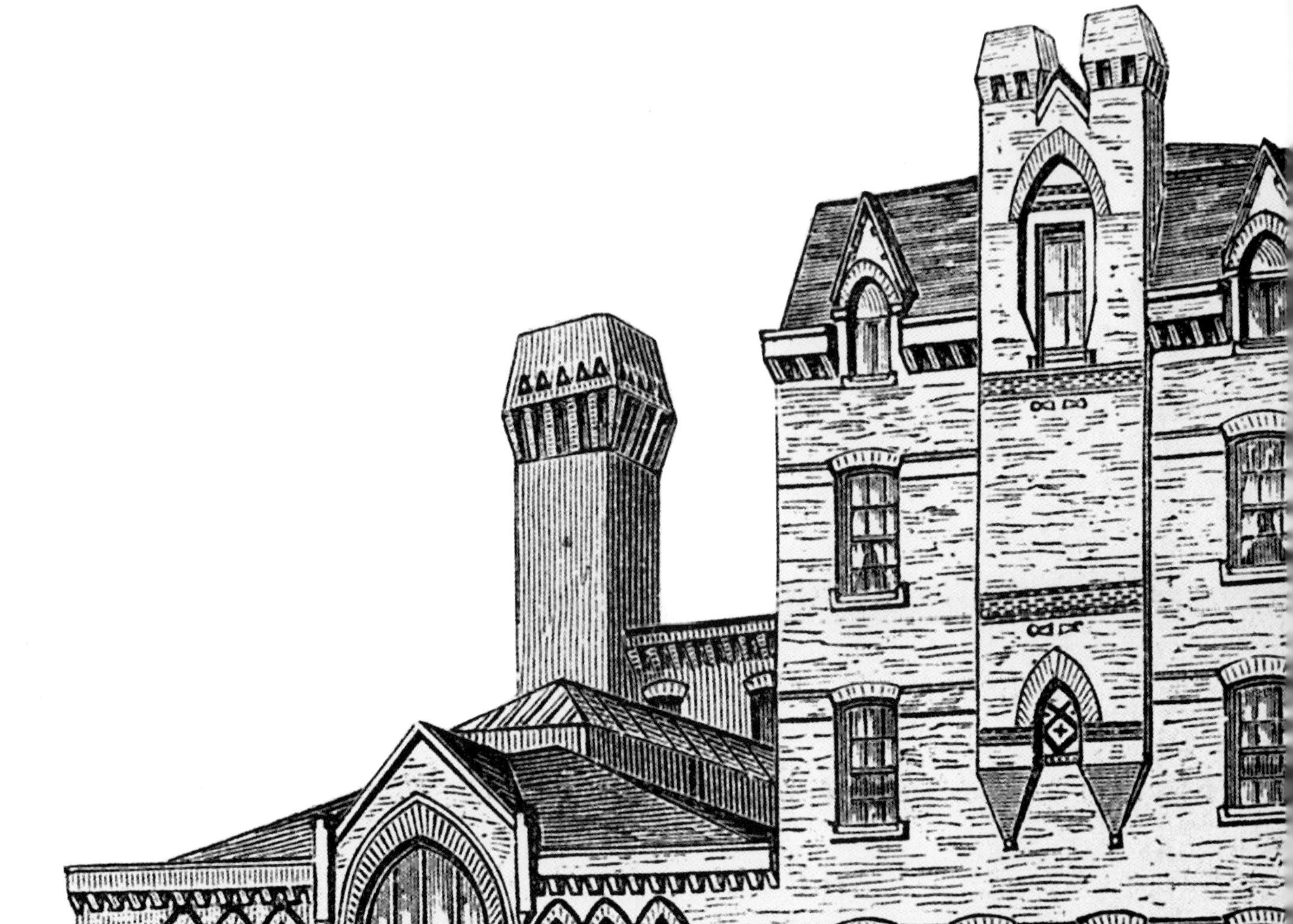
JEFFERSON=MEDICAL=COLLEGE=HOSPITAL=

FOREWORD

Thomas Jefferson University has a discerning appreciation of its artistic as well as scientific heritage. The university takes immense pride in its collection of painted and sculpted portraits, art works on paper, rare books, and decorative arts. These are on display throughout the campus in libraries, auditoriums, offices, conference areas, and reception rooms.

When the decision was made to sponsor a book about the history of the collection, it was readily apparent that an outside author would have to be found. Many at Jefferson knew the work of Julie Berkowitz, then a museum educator at the Philadelphia Museum of Art. She had recently written a fine catalogue on the portrait collection at the College of Physicians of Philadelphia.

We were not disappointed. Soon after her arrival at Jefferson she was searching an administrative storage room and serendipitously found the original medical college charter, an 1824 document that had mysteriously disappeared. Later she established that the torso of a marble *Athena* located in a hospital lobby had been sculpted in ancient Rome. Another exciting discovery was a rare collotype of *The Gross Clinic* inscribed by the artist Thomas Eakins to a Jefferson anatomy professor. Eventually she found hundreds of other objects, especially art works on paper.

Julie Berkowitz's growing excitement about the extent of the collection and her determination to document and preserve the objects have been admired by her many colleagues. Through articles, lectures, exhibits, and participation on the university's art committee, she has generously shared her knowledge with the Thomas Jefferson University family, and made us even more appreciative of the links between art and science and history.

Paul C. Brucker, M.D., President
Thomas Jefferson University

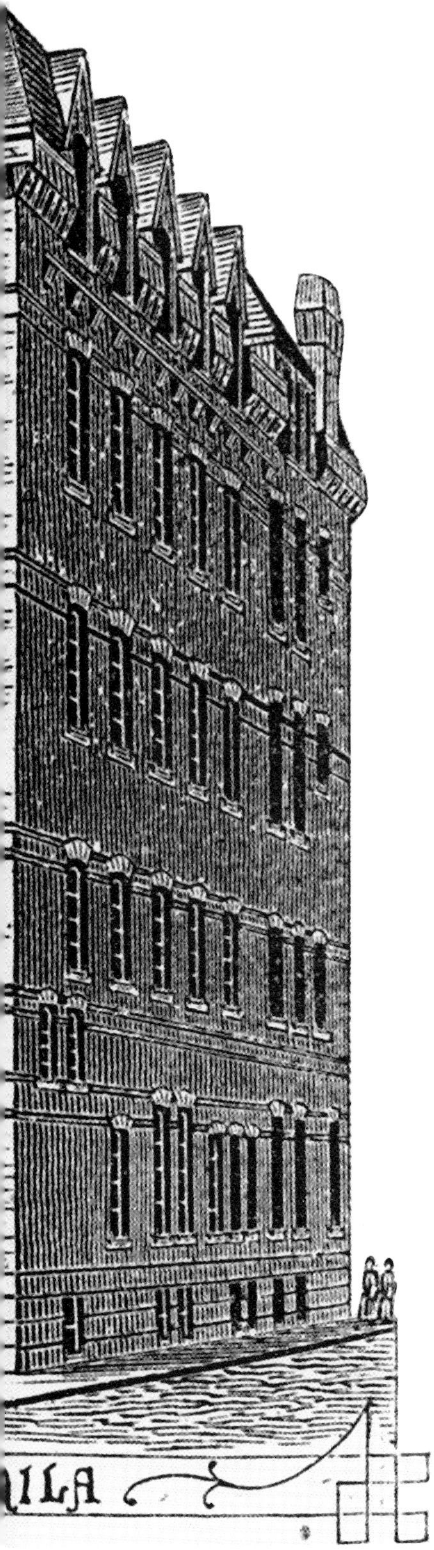

1877 Hospital from 1877 *Annual Announcement*

PREFACE

On March 11, 1871 Samuel D. Gross, M.D., the internationally celebrated surgeon and author, entreated fellow Jefferson alumni to "adorn the halls" with portraits of those who had "devoted their lives to the service of the school," and thus "inspire the pupil with ambition to excel in great and noble works." This clarion call to emulate European medical and scientific institutions by memorializing their great men was taken up almost immediately.

One hundred and twenty-five years later, Thomas Jefferson University is still securing portraits, accepting art donations and bequests, and exhibiting art works effectively. By manifesting an appreciation for the power of art to teach, inspire, and enlighten, the university continues to honor Gross's profound idea. The consciousness of succeeding generations of Jeffersonians, who undergo daily the intense pressures of professional study and practice, has been uplifted by an abundant display of visual arts.

Individual art objects considered collectively can construct a pictorial history of and describe the spirit of the institution, even though every

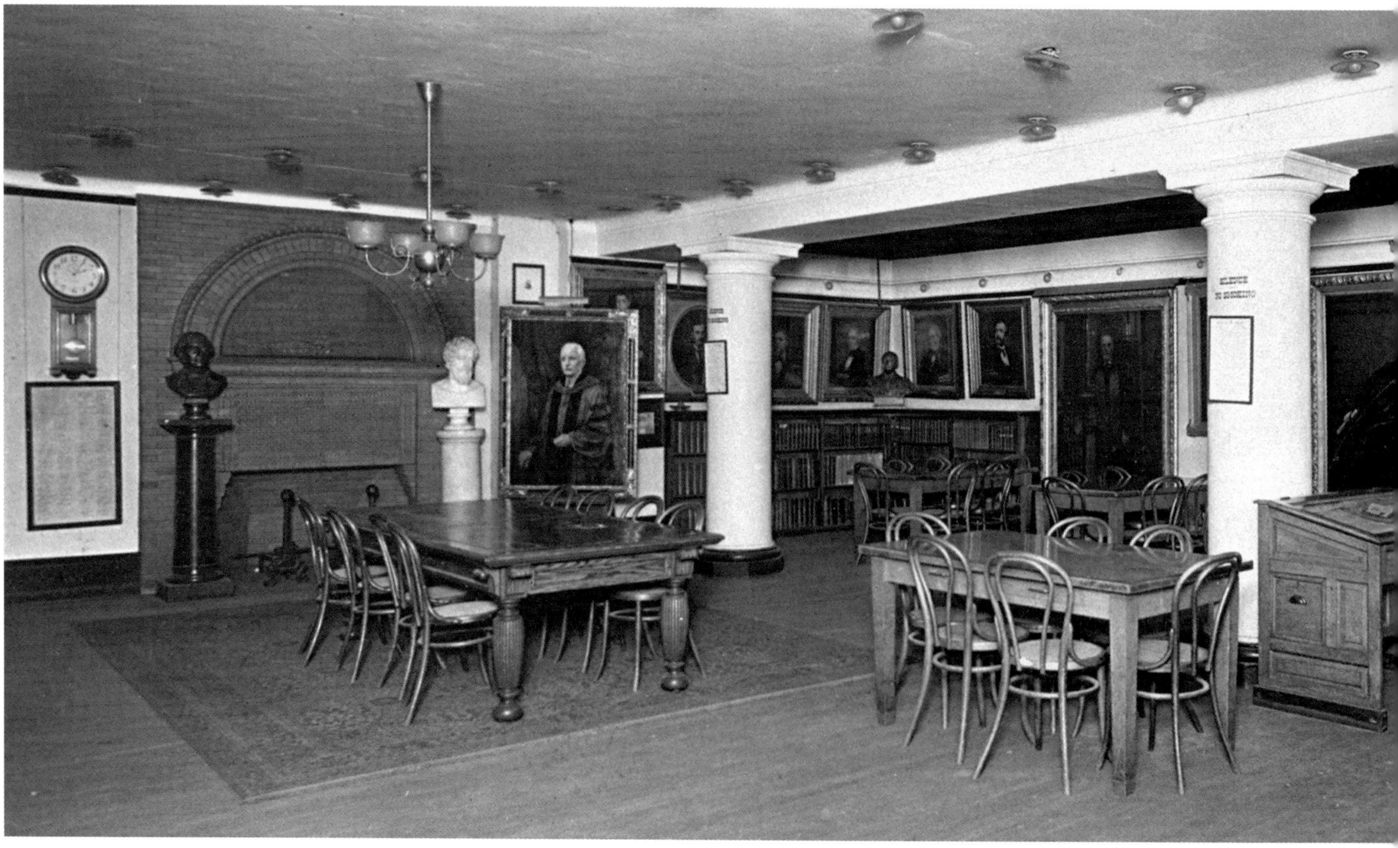

Library of 1898 College Building

worthy individual is not represented by an image. The Jefferson collection is diverse enough to trace a meaningful history of public portrait trends in late-nineteenth- and twentieth-century Philadelphia.

Research on the collection was daunting because there was little standard documentation on art objects and artists. Therefore, I read virtually all historic and contemporary published materials (student yearbooks and alumni bulletins; college announcements and catalogues; and college, hospital, and library annual reports); and unpublished materials (minutes of meetings of the board of trustees, executive faculty, and alumni association; insurance lists, appraisals, and other financial records; conservation reports; and related correspondence).

By exploring both public spaces and obscure, private storage areas throughout the campus, sifting through the rich repository of then uncatalogued art works on paper in the university archives, and conducting interviews with "old-timers" and others, I was able to piece together the history of the collection. My work was abetted by the cooperation of dozens of Jefferson faculty and staff. I am grateful for the university's patience while I assembled the materials into usable forms, and for the funds provided for documentary photography and object conservation.

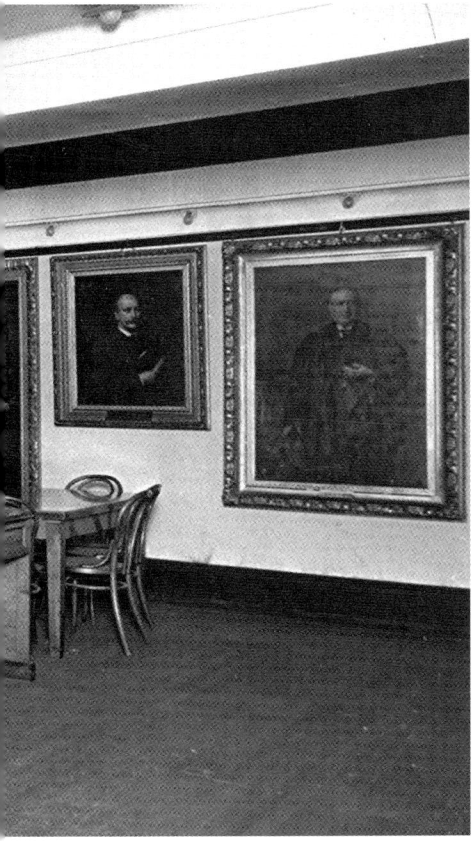

My goals were to 1) show the unexpectedly wide range of art in a nonmuseum institution; 2) describe the evolution of Jefferson's proprietary attitudes toward the art; 3) depict the stewardship of the celebrated *Gross Clinic*, and contribute new information about the painting's history and Thomas Eakins's relationships with the medical profession; 4) describe my research processes for the benefit of other students and scholars of art, medical, and Philadelphia history; and 5) encourage, by example, other historic public institutions to search their own corporate "attics" for forgotten or unrecognized art objects.

The writing of this book was concluded in January 1998. Regrettably, I could not include the most recent faculty portraits and other additions to the collection in the interim before publication.

DONORS TO THE PUBLICATION OF THIS BOOK

Warm thanks to the many individuals whose generosity made this book possible:

Arthur Allen, Ph.D.

Mr. & Mrs. Gustave G. Amsterdam

Leonard Apt, M.D.

Benjamin Bacharach, M.D.

S. Jack Bascove, M.D.

Henry D. Berkowitz, M.D.

Lewis W. Bluemle Jr., M.D./The Connelly Foundation

Mrs. William W. Bodine

Dr. & Mrs. Paul A. Bowers – *In memory of Mary Russell Laffey*

Doris E. Bowman, R.N.

Edward C. Bradley, S.J., M.D.

Robert L. Brent, M.D., Ph.D.

Paul C. Brucker, M.D.

W. W. Keen Butcher & Madeleine K. Butcher

Clara A. Callahan, M.D.

Gary G. Carpenter, M.D.

Dr. & Mrs. Herbert E. Cohn

Joe Henry Coley, M.D.

Samuel S. Conly Jr., M.D.

Julius M. Coon, M.D.

Dr. & Mrs. Douglas T. Corwin

Dr. & Mrs. Jerome M. Cotler – *In memory of Dr. Cotler's parents, Mitchell and Elizabeth Cotler*

Leslie Crabtree

Nancy S. Czarnecki, M.D.

William E. Delaney III, M.D.

Edward C. Driscoll

Sandra Eglin – *In memory of Meyer Eglin*

Richard A. Ellis, M.D.

Allan J. Erslev, M.D.

Dr. & Mrs. Sanford Fitzig

Lenore Forsted, Esq.

Dr. & Mrs. Abol H. Fotouhi

Elmer H. Funk Jr., M.D.

Joanna Griffith Gabel – *In memory of Reynold S. Griffith, M.D.*

John J. Gartland, M.D.

Canzio E. Giuliucci, M.D.

Warren P. Goldburgh, M.D.

Dr. & Mrs. Joseph S. Gonnella

Frank D. Gray Jr., M.D. & Frieda Gray, M.D.

The Samuel D. Gross Archives Fund

Lebron Hardie

Dr. & Mrs. William V. Harrer

Armason Harrison

Mrs. Benjamin F. Haskell

David S. Haskell, M.D.

Jean R. Haskell

John R. Healy, M.D.

William I. Heine, M.D. – *In memory of Eleanor Schneider*

Walter Herman, M.D.

Polly Hill & Mary Louisa B. Hill

Joseph Hodge, M.D.

Dr. & Mrs. John H. Hodges

W. W. Keen James

Dr. & Mrs. Ronald P. Jensh

Matthew E. Johnson, M.D.

Louis G. Kareha, M.D.

Sandra P. Kenton

Margaret Keyes – *In memory of Baldwin L. Keyes, M.D.*

Audrey Knowles

Robert T. Lentz

Daniel Lieberman, M.D.

Charles Lee Liggett, M.D.

Mr. & Mrs. Robert D. Linck – *In memory of Mrs. Frank Binswanger Sr.*

William Lincoff, M.D.

John N. Lindquist, M.D.

Dr. & Mrs. Herbert A. Luscombe

Elaine D. Mackowiak, Ph.D.

John S. Madara, M.D.

Phillip J. Marone, M.D.

Edward H. McGehee, M.D.

The John P. McGovern History of Medicine Fund

Fred D. McWilliams, M.D.

Elinor S. Medoff

Thomas D. Michael, M.D.

Bernard J. Miller, M.D.

John E. Mills, M.D.

Mr. & Mrs. James F. Monteith

Bruce B. Montgomery, M.D.

Mr. & Mrs. Kenneth W. Moore

Gino Mori, M.D.

Michael A. Naidoff, M.D. & Stephanie W. Naidoff, Esq.

Richard L. Nemiroff, M.D.

L. Roy Newman, M.D.

A. Edward O'Hara, M.D.

George R. Pechstein, M.D.

Henry Pechstein, M.D.

Abraham Perlman, M.D.

Mr. & Mrs. Robert A. Peterson

Dr. & Mrs. Marvin Podolnick

George Popp, M.D.

H. Phelps Potter, M.D.

Theresa M. Powers – *In memory of her parents, Mr. & Mrs. William H. Powers*

Susannah F. Prindle

James J. Rafter, M.D.

Nancy Freeman Horwitz Regalado

Mrs. Hobart A. Reimann

Dr. & Mrs. Joseph F. Rodgers

Dr. & Mrs. Francis E. Rosato

Harold Rovner, M.D.

Sheldon Rudansky, M.D.

Edward J. Saltzman, M.D.

Joseph Sataloff, M.D.

J. Woodrow Savacool, M.D.

Russell W. Schaedler, M.D.

Edward A. Schauer, M.D.

Nathan S. Schlezinger, M.D.

Joan E. Schott – *In honor of Dr. Frederick B. Wagner Jr.'s 80th birthday*

Erwin R. Smarr, M.D.

Harry L. Smith Jr., Ph.D.

Nathan M. Smukler, M.D.

Dr. & Mrs. Stanton N. Smullens

Mrs. Francis J. Sweeney Jr.

Dr. & Mrs. John Y. Templeton III

Henry J. Teufen, M.D.

Troy L. Thompson II, M.D.

Juan E. Veve, M.D.

George B. Voigt, M.D.

Dr. & Mrs. Frederick B. Wagner Jr. – *In memory of Ruth Coley, Judith Connelly Delouvrier, Esther Wagner Doto, John N. Lindquist, M.D., Thomas B. Mervine, M.D., Nicholas R. Varano, M.D., Ruth Escott Wagner, Mrs. William Wagner*

Dr. & Mrs. Burton L. Wellenbach

The Burton L. Wellenbach Portrait Fund

Richard M. Whittington, M.D.

George J. Willauer Jr., Ph.D.

C. Wilmer Wirts Jr., M.D.

Robert I. Wise, M.D.

The Women's Board of Thomas Jefferson University Hospital

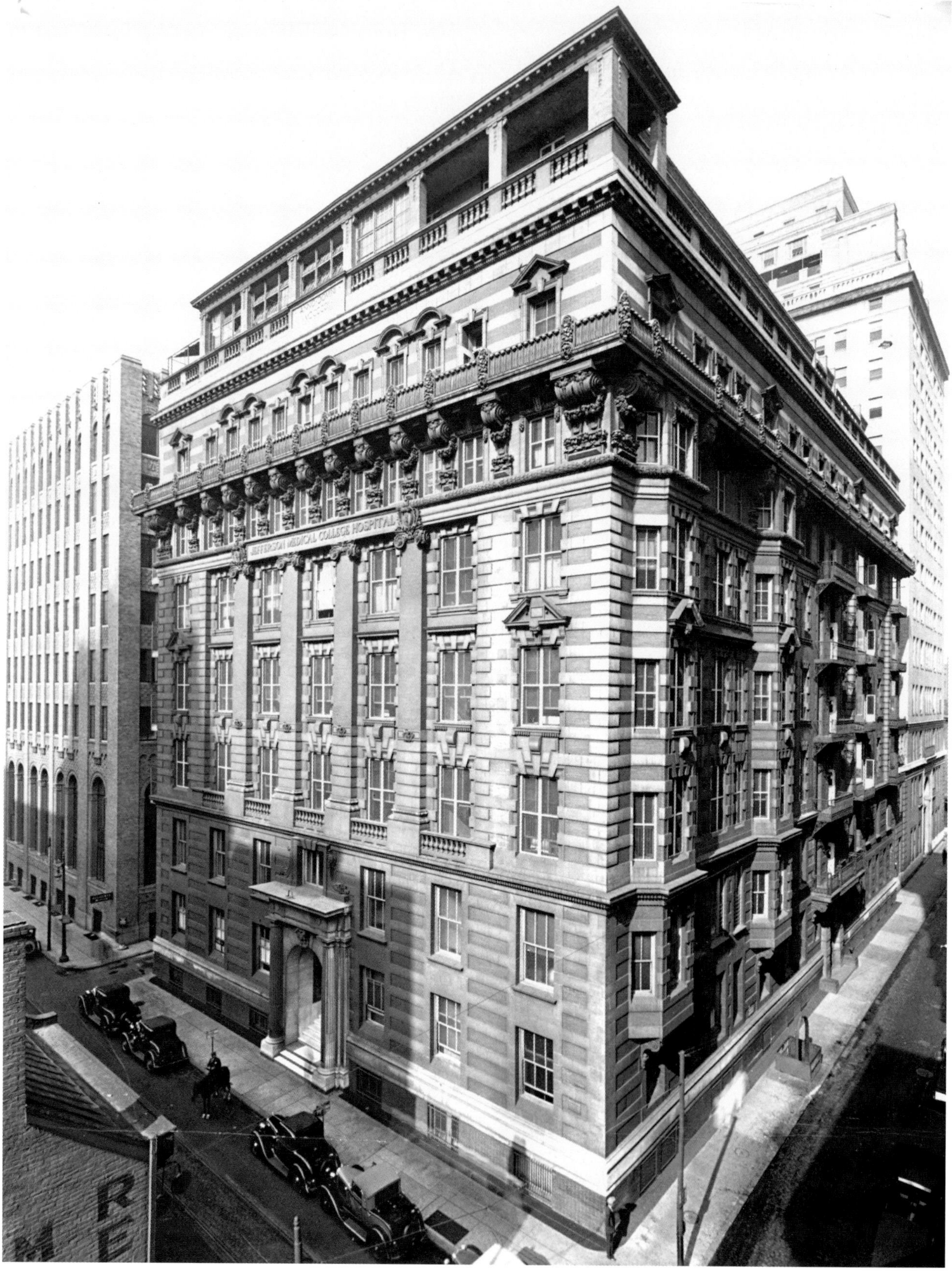

1907 "Old Main" Hospital

ACKNOWLEDGMENTS

I am enormously grateful to two presidents of Thomas Jefferson University: Dr. Lewis W. Bluemle Jr. for initiating the art book project and Dr. Paul C. Brucker for his continuing support of the endeavor.

Malcolm Clendenin contributed indispensable talent and unflagging energy toward achieving this book through his sensitive yet rigorous editing of my manuscript abetted by his knowledge of art and architectural history. Rick Echelmeyer admirably photographed the diverse objects of the Jefferson art collection.

I also owe special thanks to Darrel Sewell and Doug Paschall for access to Lloyd Goodrich's Thomas Eakins papers at the Philadelphia Museum of Art; to Cheryl Leibold for access to archival materials at the Pennsylvania Academy of the Fine Arts; and to Jeanette M. Toohey, formerly of the Academy, for assistance in identifying some photographic and printmaking processes.

Finally, I extend sincere thanks to members of the university art committee chaired by Russell W. Schaedler, M.D. and many additional colleagues at Jefferson and elsewhere whose contributions helped me to research, conserve, and organize the art collection, and to realize this book:

Lawrence Abrams, Ed.D.
Arlene M. Adair
Martha A. Anderson
Benjamin Bacharach, M.D.
Julie Baker
Beth Bensman
Grace Bishko
Mark Bockrath
David Borodin
Eloise B. Bowers
Christopher D. Braster
Robert L. Brent, M.D., Ph.D.
Carmhiel J. Brown
Clarissa Carnell
Gary G. Carpenter, M.D.
Anthony Ciambella
Cynthia J. T. Clendenin
Joe Henry Coley, M.D.
Frank Colgan
Jerome M. Cotler, M.D.
Thomas F. Cresswell
George Curran
Carol Lynn Daly
Keith Davis

Samuel Davis
William E. Delaney III, M.D.
Susan Duhl
Sandra Eglin
Shelly D. Elliott
Gina Erdreich
Benjamin Evans
Rebecca Fabiano
Catherine M. Farrell
Phyllis M. Fisher
Dan Flanagan
Lenore Forsted, Esq.
Victoria A. Fullam
Tamsen Fuller
Elmer H. Funk Jr., M.D.
Joanna Griffith Gabel
Rosamunde Ginsburg
Jean C. Givey
Joseph S. Gonnella, M.D.
Shirley Gray
Ryck Guyre
Ruth Hadik
Randolph Haines
Gisele V. Hamilton
William V. Harrer, M.D.
Armason Harrison
Terrance M. Harvey
Howard A. Haynes
Joy L. Hlavka
Ursula Hobson
Janet Hoefling
Alexander Horn
Joan Hughes
Joanna S. Hynes
W. W. Keen James
Hal Jones
Ellen B. Kahn
Sandra P. Kenton
Ceil Kinney
Fred Koszewnik
Marie Kraus
Mary R. Laffey
Robert T. Lentz
David C. Levin, M.D.
Helen A. Levins
Thomas J. Lewis
Annette & Robert E. Linck
John N. Lindquist, M.D.
Andrew Lins
Joan Longo
James D. Mahoney
Robert J. Mandle, Ph.D.
Sal Marandola
Gerald J. Marks, M.D.
Doris Martin
Luann C. Marziani
Holly Maxson
George McCardle
Claire McCurdy
Faith J. McDowell
Francis J. McGovern
Randy McLaughlin
Patricia S. McMorrow
Melissa Meighen
Susan S. Miller
Marian Mitchell
Mary B. Monteith
Joan Moore
Kenneth W. Moore
Rodney B. Murray, Ph.D.

Elaine Nader
Michael A. Naidoff, M.D.
Stephanie W. Naidoff, Esq.
Peter A. Nelson
Robert Neroni
Eneida Nieves
Richard Palmer
George R. Pechstein, M.D.
Kathleen Perillo, Esq.
Robert A. Peterson
Ellen Phillips
John Phillips
JoAnne Poinsard
Theresa M. Powers
Nancy Quaile
Maryanne Quinn
Andrew J. Ramsay, Ph.D.
Nancy Roberts
Judith A. Robins
Adrienne Rodgers
Trudy Rosato
Gayle C. Rowan
Frederick Ruccius
Lorraine T. Sacchetti
Joseph Sataloff, M.D.
Robert T. Sataloff, M.D.
J. Woodrow Savacool, M.D.
Richard J. Schmid
Joan E. Schott
Martha Small
SaraKay Smullens
Stanton N. Smullens, M.D.
Lyn Sobolewski
Kurt Solmssen
Thomas Sommerville
Earl J. Spangenberg
Darryl Stanley
Connie Stinson
Dave Super
Steven Tatti
Edward W. Tawyea
Tony Tigro
Catherine Tomeo
Carol A. Trent
Mark Tucker
Don Walker
Vincent T. Walsh
Edward Watson
Clifford K. Weber, Esq.
Ruth A. Weintraub
Burton L. Wellenbach, M.D.
Suzanne Wheeling
Sylvia Yount
Florence D. Zeller
Diana Zinnato
Gloria Zoski

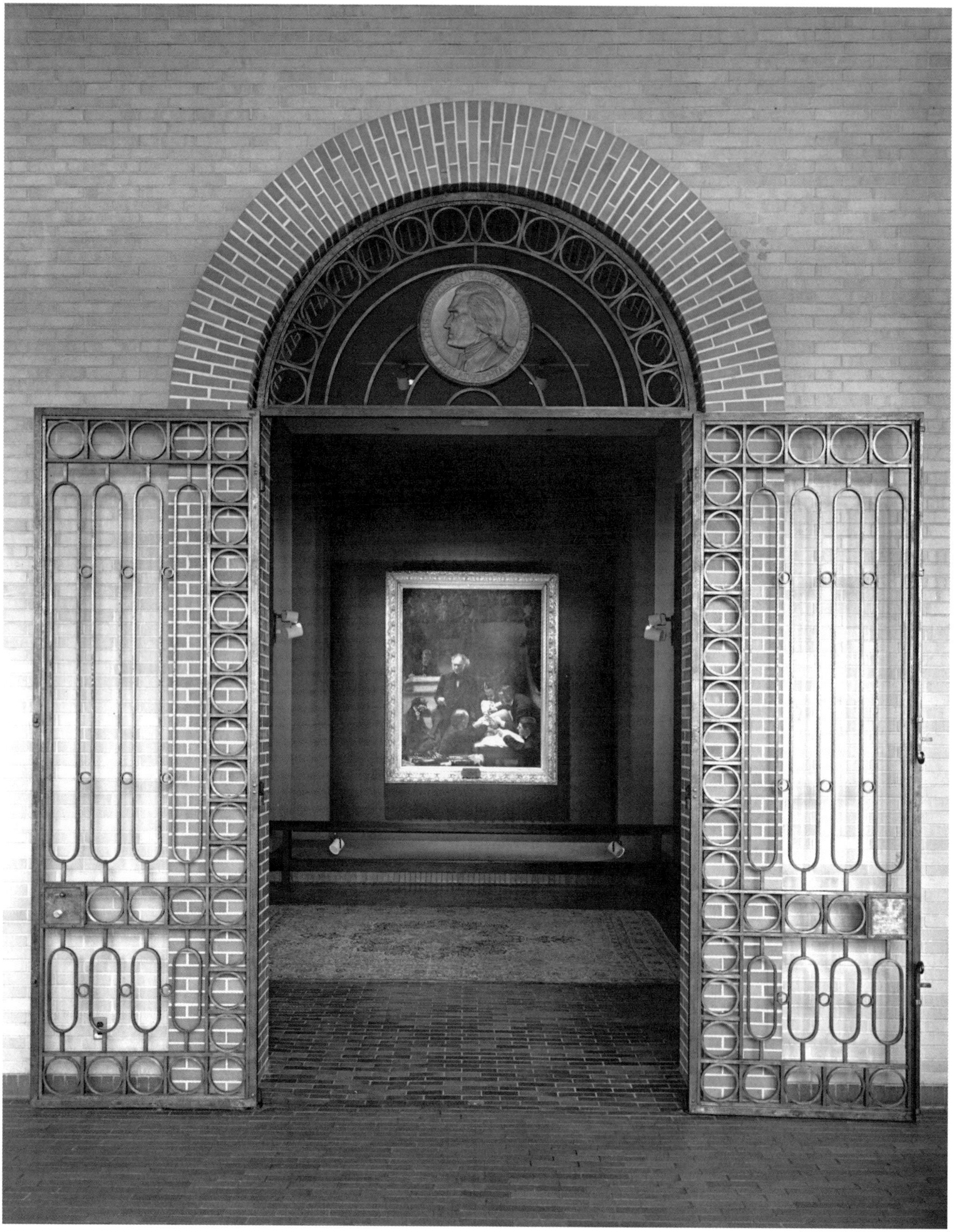

The Gross Clinic in the Eakins Gallery

The Collection as a Whole

Contents of the Collection

When I first arrived at Thomas Jefferson University in 1988 as a part-time consultant appointed to write a book about the art collection, I presumed that the objects would consist almost exclusively of portraits of the institution's celebrated faculty members painted or sculpted by local artists. A year later as the full-time university art historian with some preliminary research accomplished, I was determined to discover how and why the medical center had acquired such an unexpectedly diverse art collection created by a wide range of American and European artists.

By January 1998 Thomas Jefferson University's art collection included 284 paintings and forty-three sculptures. Eighty-five percent of the paintings and seventy-nine percent of the sculptures are portraits. The great majority of individual sitters are Jefferson physicians, although there are also portraits of European physicians as well as nonmedical figures. In addition there are several important medical group portraits. Other categories of paintings include landscapes, genre scenes, architecture, and some abstractions.

The vast majority of art works date from the last half of the nineteenth century to the present. The oldest by far is a full-length, marble statue of Athena whose torso was carved around the second century A.D.

An eclectic group of decorative arts includes antique American and European furniture; silver presentation cups and trays; gold, silver, and bronze medals and coins; gold-headed and carved canes; ivory-handled surgical instruments; gold and jewelled badges; antique oriental carpets and silk wall hangings; a collection of Chinese jade figures and animals; a stained glass window triptych; and some Russian, Middle Eastern, and European metal objects. With some notable exceptions, the majority of decorative arts date from the nineteenth and twentieth centuries.

A small but representative sample selected from over one thousand art works on paper includes original prints, drawings, and vintage photographs. Subjects range from portraits and caricatures of European and Jefferson individuals and groups to embellished military and medical certificates, and from images of Jefferson architecture to European cityscapes. This account of the art collection also includes about two dozen selections from the more than four thousand richly illustrated, rare medical books in the library's special collections.

Finally, many of Jefferson's historic and modern buildings that were designed by leading Philadelphia architects are described in the context of the chronological survey.

Who's Who among Artists at Jefferson

There are a total of 165 known and twenty-seven unidentified artists represented in Jefferson's collection of sculptures and paintings. Artists range from the internationally celebrated to those of local repute. With some striking modern exceptions, the most acclaimed artists created their works in the late nineteenth and first half of the twentieth century. Most exhibited frequently in museum exhibitions and world's fairs in America and abroad. Some taught at prominent American art schools or gave classes privately. Still others developed a favorable reputation through the celebrity of their portrait sitters, and/or their obliging compliance with their sitters' requirements.

Many of these artists are still admired today, and their works have entered the permanent collections of museums and attract vigorous bidding at auctions. There are also lesser-known portraitists whose works are rarely displayed in public any longer, but whose portraits are still greatly esteemed by their owners and descendants.

There are 105 known portrait painters in the collection, and over a third of them have contributed two or more works. There are also portraits by seventeen unidentified painters.

Among the Jefferson-related portrait painters, the earliest distinguished artist is Jacob Eichholtz whose "grand manner" portraits of John Eberle, M.D. and his wife, Salome Eberle, were painted in 1827 and 1831, respectively. The outstanding mid-nineteenth-century painter is Thomas Sully whose romantic depiction of Thomas D. Mütter, M.D. was painted circa 1842.

The first artist to receive multiple commissions from Jefferson Medical College was Samuel B. Waugh. Though little known today, Waugh was a sought-after portraitist in the late nineteenth century and influential in the Philadelphia art establishment. Between 1872 and 1880 he was commissioned to paint five traditional, bust-length portraits of distinguished Jefferson faculty members, including Samuel D. Gross, M.D. A sixth Waugh portrait of the surgeon's wife, Louisa Weissell Gross, was donated to Jefferson by a descendant in 1986.

Ever since Samuel B. Waugh produced his standard likenesses in the 1870s, numerous other fashionable artists have received multiple commissions from Jefferson faculty members. One concludes that the initial depictions were pleasing to the portrait sitters, their families, and the institution, and having "caught on" these artists secured successive commissions, until a newer artist supplanted them in popularity to start a fresh fashion.

Thomas Eakins, however, was an exception to the rule. He was younger than Waugh and far less successful in obtaining portrait commissions than Waugh and other rivals. Although the Jefferson collection includes two early portraits by Eakins—the 1874 portrait of Benjamin H. Rand, M.D. in his study and the celebrated 1875 portrait of Samuel D. Gross, M.D. in his surgical clinic—both were created at the artist's own initiative. Only the portrait of William S. Forbes, M.D. was commissioned by the college, late in the artist's career in 1905. Ironically, Waugh is considered merely competent today, while Eakins is viewed by many scholars as the preeminent American portraitist and a giant figure in American painting.

Other outstanding late-nineteenth-century and early-twentieth-century painters working in the grand manner include William Merritt Chase, Robert W. Vonnoh, Adolphe Borie, and Bernard Uhle all of whom contributed single works; Julian Story who painted two portraits; and George W. Pettit who painted four (including two of Dr. Samuel W. Gross). Of this distinguished group, perhaps Chase is best remembered today, especially for his colorful life as artist, teacher, and socialite.

Other prominent artists who contributed similarly polished and refined portraits in the first three decades of the twentieth century are Henry R. Rittenberg with two paintings and a third attributed to him, and Hugh H. Breckenridge with two paintings. In the twenties and thirties Robert S. Susan painted two portraits, and William T. Thomson contributed eleven portraits of prominent Jefferson faculty, including three different interpretations of the famed surgeon John Chalmers DaCosta, M.D. Almost as numerous are the eight portraits painted by Benedict A. Osnis in the 1930s, in addition to his three charcoal portrait drawings. The collection also includes four landscapes of rural Bucks County, Pennsylvania painted by Walter E. Baum.

Other artists whose works date from the 1930s and 1940s include Leopold G. Seyffert and Alice Kent Stoddard with two works each; Daniel Garber and illustrator Dean Cornwell with one each; and Lazar Raditz with two early works of 1911 and two from the 1930s. In the 1940s and early 1950s Cameron Burnside contributed five portraits of Jefferson faculty, a portrait of his wife, Irene, and a Jefferson Medical College Hospital operating scene. Maurice Molarsky painted three portraits between 1929 and 1947.

Prominent mid-twentieth-century artists include Sir Gerald F. Kelly, Gerald L. Brockhurst, and Julius T. Bloch with one work each, and John C. Johansen who provided six portraits in the 1950s. Roy C. Nuse painted four portraits in the forties and fifties, Roy F. Spreter painted two portraits in 1961, and Paul Froelich contributed a portrait in 1962. Favored in the 1970s were Molly Guion with five portraits, and Furman J. Finck and José F. Marcote with two each. Between 1968 and 1983 Robert O. Skemp painted eleven portraits. The most favored painter in this period was Alden M. Wicks who completed seventeen portraits of Jefferson medical and nursing faculty members between 1959 and 1985.

Noted contemporary portraitists are James W. ("Bo") Bartlett III, Ned Bittinger, Paul DuSold, Stephen S. Kennedy, Russell W. Recchion, Frank H. Mason, and Charles H. Cecil with one each; William A. Smith and Mark E. Skolsky with two each; Dean M. Larson with three; and Nelson Shanks with five. Dean L. Paules's total of nineteen portraits has surpassed the previous record of Alden M. Wicks's seventeen portraits, and Paules painted his works in an astonishing ten-year period.

Leading trends of the 1980s and 1990s are the formal, elegantly polished characterizations by Shanks, Bartlett, Skolsky, Kennedy, Bittinger, Cecil, and Recchion; the more informal, loosely brushed portrayals by Larson,

DuSold, Mason, and Smith; and the ultra-detailed, illusionistic likenesses by Paules.

Among the thirty-nine sculptors in Jefferson's collection, eight are unidentified. Mid-nineteenth-century sculptors with national reputations include Horatio Stone, M.D. and George E. Ewing. Famous late-nineteenth-century and early-twentieth-century sculptors include William Ordway Partridge, Alexander Stirling Calder, Samuel A. Murray, and H. Daniel Webster. Best known today of this group is Calder whose standing, full-length bronze statue of Samuel D. Gross, M.D. located in the Scott Plaza was commissioned jointly by the Jefferson Medical College alumni association and the American Surgical Association in 1897.

Rudulph Evans was active in the first half of the twentieth century, and Agnes Yarnall in mid-century. Lloyd Lillie's full-length bronze statue of Thomas Jefferson was originally created in 1975 and a special cast was made for Thomas Jefferson University in 1987. Henry W. Mitchell's cherished bronze monuments on the Jefferson campus include the *Winged Ox* of 1975 and the *William W. Bodine Jr. Fountain* ("The Otter Fountain") of 1978-79.

Of all the sculptors, only Henry Mitchell and Samuel Murray have contributed two works. The collection also includes Joseph Obermeier's three identical plaster busts of Samuel D. Gross, M.D., casts after a marble original located at the College of Physicians of Philadelphia.

Other nonportrait sculptors vary widely from the American artist John Rogers, whose popular, diminutive plaster groups like the *Charity Patient* were manufactured by the thousands, to the Italian Scipione Tadolini, whose neoclassical, marble figure of the *Greek Slave* is conceived on a monumental scale.

Geographical distribution of artists is another factor in the profile of a collection. Philadelphia has been an artistic center for fine arts and crafts since the eighteenth century. Even today the city supports four major professional art schools including the country's oldest, the Pennsylvania Academy of the Fine Arts, founded in 1804. Therefore, one might expect the great majority of portrait sitters, as well as other art donors, to have patronized Philadelphia artists.

However, the statistics are surprising. Only about half the painters represented in the art collection forged their careers in Philadelphia, whether they created portraits of Jefferson-related sitters or contributed any other subject. The number drops to forty percent in the case of sculptors.

There were always Philadelphians, including some represented in the Jefferson collection, who preferred the cachet of selecting a notable portrait artist from New York or occasionally other cities. This was especially true in the late nineteenth and early twentieth centuries. Furthermore, several portrait sitters in recent decades have utilized the services of portrait consultants, agents for artists residing in several cities.

Also, it should be remembered that many of the portraits and other paintings and sculptures did not emanate from the university, but were gifts or bequests from alumni and other donors living in other cities or from local residents who had acquired works created elsewhere.

In addition to American artists, the collection includes several donations of European portrait and nonportrait art works. The best-known foreign artists are the English portrait painters Sir Gerald F. Kelly and Gerald L. Brockhurst; French sculptors Paul Dubois and Jean-Baptiste Pigalle; and Italian sculptor Scipione Tadolini.

Another surprising feature about the collection is the relatively large number of women portrait artists, most of whom were from Philadelphia. Seventeen percent of the known portrait painters and eight percent of the known portrait sculptors are female. With the notable exception of Susan Macdowell Eakins (1851-1938) and a few contemporary twentieth-century artists, most women represented in the Jefferson collection forged their careers around the middle of the twentieth century, including painters Alice Kent Stoddard and Agnes Allen, and sculptor Agnes Yarnall.

Four artist-physicians with art works in the collection include the professional sculptor Horatio Stone, M.D., and Jeffersonians Robert M. Lukens, M.D., Martin E. Rehfuss, M.D., and Hobart A. Reimann, M.D. Unfortunately, the collection contains no examples by other Jefferson physicians who were also accomplished amateur artists: Drs. Chevalier Jackson, John H. Gibbon Jr., Thaddeus L. Montgomery, and Solomon Solis-Cohen.

Noted earlier American and European artists of works on paper include photographers John Plumbe Jr., Frederick Gutekunst, and William H. Rau; and printmakers Jacobus Houbraken, Thomas Rowlandson and Augustus Pugin, John Sartain, Albert Rosenthal, Erwin F. Faber, and Sir Frank Brangwyn. More recent printmakers include Grant Wood, Alfred Bendiner, Salvador Dali, Man Ray, Lowell B. Nesbitt, and Wolf Kahn.

Well known European illustrators of medical books

from the sixteenth through the eighteenth centuries include Albrecht Dürer, Hans Burgkmair the Elder, Jost Amman, Jan Wandelaar, and Jan Stephan van Calcar.

Introduction to the Survey of Paintings and Sculptures

It is instructive to highlight the general characteristics of the painting and sculpture collection before the detailed individual entries that follow. Two basic questions regarding iconography will be explored. First, do the portraits depict actual scholarly or medical motifs to distinguish them from contemporary generic portraits of business, society, or other professional people? Second, do the portraits and scenes with visual references to the academic position or working environment of their subjects include specific Jefferson settings and/or materials?

Allowing for the changes in prevailing taste and styles over the last 125 years, there were other factors to be considered before drawing conclusions about the iconography of the Jefferson collection. Portraits intended for public display are often more formal and didactic in conception, style, and mood than private portraits. Specifics about pose, length of figure, costume, background, attributes, and dimensions are negotiated among the interested parties: sitter, artist, and institution. Decisions are often dependent upon funds available, availability of subject and artist for sittings, impending deadlines for portrait presentation, intended installation location, and of course, personality and character of the subject.

Generally speaking, because of their medium and support paintings have greater potential than sculptures for extensive descriptive material. Depending on the circumstances of the commission and the taste and requirements of the sitter, an artist can include an almost unlimited number of attributes and/or costume elements that describe the sitter's occupation or character. A painter can potentially place his subject in a room or setting that suggests his profession or rank. A painter can depict the subject either "posing" or actively engaged in his work or other activity.

Portrait subjects wearing conservative business attire can suggest their station in life through the cut and style of the clothing, and details like wrist watches or watch fobs, club crests, shirt or necktie jewelry, and rings, but these elements alone give no hint of their occupations. In contrast, ceremonial academic robes allude to the professorial rank of their sitters, and white medical coats or nursing uniforms state the profession of their sitters quite specifically.

Painting Survey: Characteristics of Individual Subjects and their Portraits

The vast majority of portraits in the Jefferson collection depict subjects who lived during the period represented by the existence of the institution, and many portraits of earlier sitters were posthumous works created during this same time period.

There are multiple painted portraits of eleven important subjects closely related to the history of Jefferson Medical College, including four each of Drs. Samuel D. Gross and John C. DaCosta; two each of Drs. Samuel W. Gross, Willis F. Manges, Thomas McCrae, Randle C. Rosenberger, Charles M. Gruber, and Robert L. Brent; and two each of trustees William Potter, Alba B. Johnson, and Daniel Baugh. There are also three portraits of the institution's namesake, Thomas Jefferson.

The following twelve sitters are rendered in both painted and sculpted images: Jefferson physicians and/or alumni Drs. George McClellan, Joseph Pancoast, Samuel D. Gross, Silas Weir Mitchell, Chevalier Jackson, Ross V. Patterson, Martin E. Rehfuss, and Joseph S. Gonnella; as well as Louis Pasteur, William Harvey, Thomas Jefferson, and Mary R. Cardeza, a Jefferson benefactor.

The overwhelming majority of the Jefferson-related, individual portrait sitters have received advanced academic training. Seventy-five percent have earned M.D. or Sc.D. degrees; another eight percent have earned Ph.D. degrees; and three percent have earned combined M.D./Ph.D. or M.D./Sc.D. degrees. The Reverend Ezra Stiles Ely, an early benefactor of the college, earned a Doctor of Divinity degree, and "Father Doctor" Edward C. Bradley is a Jesuit priest as well as a medical doctor. A few other Jefferson sitters have earned R.N. degrees and/or master's degrees in education and library science. The preceding list does not include numerous portrait subjects who have been awarded honorary degrees.

There are three physicians and three nurses included among the fifteen Jefferson-related female portrait subjects. Other women sitters include Jefferson benefactors, women's board members, wives of trustees and physicians, and the wife of an artist.

The Jefferson collection includes dual portraits of many related sitters, including the following married couples: Dr. and Mrs. Samuel D. Gross, Dr. and Mrs. John Eberle, Dr. and Mrs. Edward L. Bauer, and Dr. and Mrs. Robert L. Brent; as well as trustee Percival E. Foerderer and Mrs. Foerderer.

Portraits of physician fathers and sons include Drs. Joseph Pancoast and William H. Pancoast; Samuel D. Gross and Samuel W. Gross, John K. Mitchell and S. Weir Mitchell; and John H. Gibbon and John H. Gibbon Jr. An example of grandfather and grandson physicians are the George McClellans. Uncle and nephew physicians are Drs. Edward E. Montgomery and Thaddeus L. Montgomery. A related trio consists of brother physicians, Drs. Jacob da Silva Solis-Cohen and Solomon Solis-Cohen, and Solomon's son, trustee D. Hays Solis-Cohen.

An unusual pair of related sitters is Katherine Ashman Howell depicted in an oil painting as an engaging young child, and Katherine Ashman Veech Howell, her captivating mother depicted in a pastel. Although not previously associated with Thomas Jefferson University, the former became a Jefferson benefactor in 1990, and both paintings were included in her generous bequest.

Ninety-three percent of the total number of individual portrait sitters have associations with Thomas Jefferson University, as members of the medical, administrative, trustee, or volunteer staffs, as benefactors, or as their spouses. Almost half of the Jeffersonians are alumni of the medical college or nursing school. The positions and medical specialties of faculty portrait subjects are fairly evenly distributed among the various clinical fields and basic sciences.

Important non-Jefferson painting subjects include modern copies after celebrated oil originals, such as the *Anatomy Lesson of Dr. Tulp* by Rembrandt van Rijn and *Andreas Vesalius Dissecting* by Edouard-J.-C. Hamman. The collection also includes a copy after an important portrait of Benjamin Franklin by Joseph Siffred Duplessis, and copies after three celebrated portraits of Thomas Jefferson by Gilbert Stuart, Charles Willson Peale, and Rembrandt Peale.

Of the individual portraits of Jeffersonians, forty-three percent are bust or half length, fifty-two percent are two-thirds or three-quarters length, and five percent are full length. Fifty-seven percent of male Jefferson sitters wear business suits; another seven percent wear more informal attire ranging from sport jackets and slacks, to bare shirtsleeves, to a velvet lounging jacket. One sitter wears clerical garb and another wears a military uniform.

Close to one-third of the male sitters are garbed in scholarly or medical attire: nineteen percent wear academic robes and ten percent wear white lab coats. Another sitter wears a surgical scrub suit, and two others combine a lab coat over a scrub suit. Gregory C. Kane, M.D. is shown wearing a white medical coat and examining a patient. The most uncommon depiction is the portrait of surgeon Herbert E. Cohn, M.D. in which the central figure of Dr. Cohn wearing business attire is surrounded by vignettes showing him at work dressed variously in a surgical scrub suit or white medical coat.

The women physicians and nurses are attired in tailored daytime dresses or suits, except one who wears a nursing uniform. Two-thirds of the nonprofessional women sitters wear day dresses or suits, while the remainder wear evening attire. Many of the latter costumes are accessorized with jewelry, fans, gloves, shawls, hair ornaments, or hats. The most flamboyantly dressed is Irene Burnside, wife of artist Cameron Burnside, even though she wears daytime apparel.

The portrait of Clara Melville, R.N., directress of nurses from 1915 to 1937, demonstrates how a costume can affirm the sitter's personality. Nurse Melville's starched uniform and cap, combined with her rigid posture and sober expression, render her appearance so formidable that the artist has softened the effect by adding a vase of flowers on a nearby table.

More than sixty percent of the portraits employ either atmospheric backgrounds alone (the dark or neutral tones that suggest the immediate space surrounding the sitter), or a depiction of the sitter's chair, table, desk, or bookcase added to the atmospheric background. Several others employ background drapery alone or drapery with furniture or columns for a similar effect. About one-fifth deepen the space by suggesting a generic office or study with furniture or at least a partial view of a panelled wall or wallpaper along with furniture. Three portraits are situated outdoors and several include views toward a distant landscape.

Often the sitter's occupation can be inferred even when the background is nonspecific. For example, in three-fifths of the portraits with atmospheric or drapery backgrounds their sitters wear an academic gown trimmed in green velvet (which signifies an M.D. degree) or a white doctor's coat (often with the subject's name and department embroidered on the pocket), thus establishing them as professors or physician-scientists.

In many other portraits with atmospheric backgrounds and furniture and in which subjects are garbed in business suits, medical objects such as legible medical textbook titles, stethoscopes, microscopes, test tubes, or X-rays are seen. Less obvious are examples where the sitters wear jewelry with the university or medical college insignia or lapel pins of Alpha Omega Alpha, the medical honor society. A few other portraits show a plaque with the university logo, an architectural rendering of a Jefferson building, or an inscription naming the institution.

Numerous portraits with atmospheric or generic office backgrounds suggest the scholarly pursuits of their sitters in a more general way by scattering on desk or tabletops objects such as books, pamphlets, papers, writing materials, files, certificates, legal documents, maps, globes, computers, or slide projectors. The implication of scholarly or intellectual pursuits is also achieved in multiple portraits by the presence of reading glasses held in the hand or in jacket pockets, or by cigarettes, cigars, and especially pipes. The presence of smoking materials to suggest contemplation was once a prevalent artistic device (before the Surgeon General's report on the hazards of smoking).

A special message is intended in those historical portraits which include classical columns. Columns are a traditional artistic device denoting "the measure of man" and alluding to classical erudition, moral rectitude, and elevated social rank. Usually the symbolic columns are accompanied by swags of drapery, curtains, and/or "high style" furniture, suggesting the high social status of the sitter.

The "grand manner" pendant portraits of Dr. and Mrs. Eberle incorporate several of these devices. Both sitters are fashionably dressed and situated in a room with elegant furniture, drapery, and a column, and a view toward a distant landscape. Most likely the view is generic, but it implies land ownership and wealth.

Close to one-quarter of individual portrait sitters are shown actually at work or at least posing in their working environment with appropriate materials nearby. In descending order of frequency the subjects are shown reading, writing or performing other desk work, lecturing, performing laboratory work, interpreting X-rays, and in various clinical activities such as operating, examining a patient, and in the case of Chevalier Jackson, M.D., examining a foreign object removed from a patient's tracheobronchial tubes.

Some interesting examples combine several of the above elements. Depicted in their white doctor coats are Edward H. McGehee, M.D. posed in his patient examining room which contains a stethoscope, otoscope, ophthalmoscope, and a sphygmomanometer; and Emanuel Rubin, M.D. seated in his office which displays some antique microscopes from his own collection and an image from the celebrated *Fabrica* of Andreas Vesalius, the great sixteenth-century anatomist and author. In contrast, Richard G. Berry, M.D. is informally garbed in rolled-up shirtsleeves, but he poses in his neuropathology laboratory displaying human brain specimens on a tray and in jars, awaiting examination and photography.

Many portraits of professors lecturing contain legible scientific formulas or anatomical diagrams, usually in the form of charts or blackboard drawings and text. The most unusual portrait that includes a legible book or journal title is Dean Paules's portrait of Joseph S. Gonnella, M.D.: the dean holds a copy of Dr. Frederick B. Wagner Jr.'s history book of 1989, *Thomas Jefferson University: Tradition and Heritage*, on whose cover *The Gross Clinic* is faithfully reproduced in miniature. Several protagonists from *The Gross Clinic* are also symbolically present in Charles H. Cecil's recent portrait of Francis E. Rosato, M.D., the Samuel D. Gross Professor of Surgery.

Almost one-tenth of individual portraits depict specific Jefferson locations including X-ray rooms, lecture rooms, laboratories, and examining rooms. In the recently acquired pendant portraits of Dr. and Mrs. Robert L. Brent each subject poses in the morning room of the A. I. duPont mansion at the Wilmington campus of the duPont Institute children's hospital.

Examples of other unique Jefferson material can be found in the portrait of Joe Henry Coley, M.D. by Dean Paules which includes a framed reproduction of the facade of the Daniel Baugh Institute of Anatomy, a pastel painting by Hobart Reimann, M.D.; the portrait of President Lewis W. Bluemle Jr., M.D., by Nelson Shanks which includes a small model of the life-sized bronze sculpture of Thomas Jefferson by Lloyd Lillie; and the portrait of Joseph F. Rodgers, M.D. by Dean Paules which includes a framed reproduction of the entrance of the College Building, an oil painting by Ben Eisenstat.

Six nonportrait paintings related to Jefferson Medical College include two architectural subjects, three clinical scenes, and one historical pastiche of Jefferson Hospital nursing uniforms. These art works are a further indication of the institution's consciousness of its history as expressed in the visual arts.

Survey of Group Portraits

Group portraits present different objectives and challenges to both artists and sitters. Often these works use architecture or landscape to describe the setting more completely than do individual portraits, and they manifest meaningful interaction and communication among the figures.

The Gross Clinic is by far the most complex and largest of the twelve group portraits, measuring ninety-six inches high by seventy-eight inches wide. It is also the most descriptive of the medical activity being performed, with Dr. Gross and his surgical team of assistants being observed by dozens of students seated above the operating arena. The amphitheater depicted by Thomas Eakins is the only extant visual record of the upper lecture room of Medical Hall which was used from 1828 until 1877 when the "pit" was transferred to the newly opened hospital.

The majority of other group portraits in Jefferson's collection are from the similar genre of a professor teaching. Most often the setting is an amphitheater, sometimes the students are visible, and occasionally assistants or a patient is included.

In contrast with *The Gross Clinic*, Eakins's portrait of William S. Forbes, M.D. moves the protagonist to the foreground, reduces the number of students, and makes the architectural space shallower. Dr. Forbes is shown lecturing on anatomy in an amphitheater used from 1877 to 1922 in the first detached Jefferson Medical College Hospital. A similar viewpoint is depicted in Cameron Burnside's portrait of Hobart A. Reimann, M.D., teaching in Jefferson's third clinical amphitheater in the Thompson Annex, used from 1924 to 1966. Here the professor stands at a lectern in the foreground and an assistant leans against the curving amphitheater wall below rows of students.

Variations of professors teaching in the amphitheater in the presence of students include Alden M. Wicks's depiction of Bernard J. Alpers, M.D. lecturing next to a blackboard; Benedict A. Osnis's portrait of Thomas McCrae, M.D. standing at the head of a patient's bed; and Richard B. Farley's portrait of John C. DaCosta, M.D. sitting next to an assistant. In Roy C. Nuse's classroom portrait of George A. Ulrich, M.D. the obstetrician stands at a lectern in front of an anatomical chart of a female pelvis, and a nurse walks across the lecture room behind him. No students are visible here.

The instruction scene moves outdoors in Dean Cornwell's *Osler at Old Blockley*. In a dappled sunlit park adjacent to the former city hospital, Dr. William Osler discusses a patient's condition with young physicians while other patients are seen nearby convalescing in the fresh air.

Two other group scenes include Woiciech von Kossak's *Mary Cardeza as a Nurse*, in which the uniformed young American nurse attends a wounded soldier in a field hospital during World War I; and Lazar Raditz's formal and elegant society portrait of Daniel Baugh posing with his two young grandsons.

Sculpture Survey: Characteristics of the Works

When compared with paintings, the Jefferson sculpture collection is unexpectedly diverse with regard to age, media, and subject, even though it represents only fourteen percent of the total collection. All works are sculpted in the round except for five bas-reliefs. More than half of the forty-three works date between 1850 and 1925, a period when representational portrait sculpture was very popular in America.

Sculptures range in size and media from two diminutive plaster or bronze figurative groups and a small bronze full-length portrait, to six monumental bronze or marble, full-length, life-sized statues. The remainder of the sculpted portraits are bust length or head and shoulders. Five of the twenty different portrait sitters are represented by more than one sculpture: Samuel D. Gross, M.D. (five), George McClellan, M.D. (three), Chevalier Jackson, M.D. (two), and Hippocrates (two); there are also three freestanding sculptures and two architectural reliefs of Thomas Jefferson.

Among the nonportrait sculptures are an allegorical World War I relief, two bronze monuments depicting animals, and an expansive wood, steel, and enamel abstraction.

The vast majority of portrait subjects are physicians. Of this group more than half are Jefferson Medical College alumni, and more than half have been associated with the college as faculty members, deans, or benefactors. The most famous of the earlier portrait subjects are Joseph Pancoast and Samuel D. Gross, both surgeons and anatomists; J. Marion Sims, the "Father of American Gynecology"; S. Weir Mitchell, pioneer neurologist and novelist; and Carlos Finlay, discoverer of the yellow fever vector.

The only female portrait subjects are Mary Cardeza and an unidentified Jamaican woman. Other non-Jeffersonians include Hippocrates, William Harvey,

Louis Pasteur, and ironically, President Thomas Jefferson.

Besides the authentically ancient statue of *Athena*, several other sculptures are in an antique mode. The *Greek Slave* is a nineteenth-century marble, semi-nude figure in chains whose generic pose stems from Greek and Roman statues of Aphrodite and Venus. Direct modern copies of famous ancient art works are *Hippocrates* and the *Spinario* (or "Thorn Extractor"). The statue of *Mercury* also harkens back to an antique subject.

When modern subjects are garbed in the drapery folds of togas, such as the busts of Samuel D. Gross, M.D. by Joseph Obermeier and Thomas Jefferson by Rudulph Evans, and the commemorative World War I bas-relief figure by Doyle, the attire suggests lofty and idealized associations with past civic great events and worthy individuals. Another example of an ancient motif is Carl Conrad's coin-like, bas-relief portrait of Abraham Coles, M.D., featuring a swag of laurel leaves below the subject's head.

In contrast, several other subjects such as Mary Cardeza and physicians William Harvey, George McClellan, J. Marion Sims, Joseph Pancoast, and Ross V. Patterson are depicted with chest area too minimal to indicate any detail of costume or decoration. Likewise when subjects are attired in contemporary street clothes, like Carlos Finlay, the costume gives no hint of their profession.

There are several sculptures that include scholarly or specifically medical references. Two busts of physicians wearing academic robes are S. Weir Mitchell, M.D. by William Ordway Partridge and James C. Wilson, M.D. by Samuel A. Murray. In Dr. Chevalier Jackson's bust by Maurine Ligon the subject wears an operating gown and hat, and a mask hanging from his neck. In Samuel D. Gross's day surgeons operated in their street clothes, as shown in Alexander Calder's life-sized bronze statue, but here Gross holds a scalpel exactly as in the Eakins portrait.

Two other portraits with medical references include the busts of Ross V. Patterson, M.D. by Giuseppe Donato with a caduceus carved on the base, and that of Francis X. Dercum, M.D. by Carl A. Heber with a quotation from his own medical writing inscribed on the base.

The only sculpture that refers to a specific Jefferson setting with doctors at work is a small diorama of *The Gross Clinic*, a visual aid in three dimensions to elucidate to Eakins Gallery visitors the foreshortened posture of the painting's patient, and the relative positions of the assisting surgeons around the operating table. A generic medical scene is John Rogers's *Charity Patient* which depicts an elderly physician preparing some medicine for a poor young mother holding a sick infant.

Impetus for and Momentum in Collecting Art, 1870-1930

Although Jefferson Medical College was founded in 1824, a chronological survey of existing art works and a careful reading of internal documents indicate that no acquisitions were made in its initial half-century. The first stated policy for collecting portrait art was recorded in 1871. Significantly, the impetus came from one of Jefferson's most illustrious faculty members, Samuel D. Gross, M.D., the internationally celebrated surgeon, anatomist, teacher, author, and administrator.

The occasion used to introduce an art policy occurred on March 11, 1871 at the first anniversary commemorating the founding of the Jefferson Medical College alumni association. As founder and president, Dr. Gross delivered a stirring address describing his ideal of a great American medical school "far in advance of anything we have at present in this country."

Acknowledging that some of his far-reaching reforms could only be achieved through action of a congress of leading American medical schools, Gross listed more immediately attainable goals, the last of which was an earnest plea to learn the history of the college. He contrasted the absence of portraits and statues of great men in most American learned institutions with the presence in European schools of such "memorials of the dead as among the proudest trophies of art, adorning the halls of the academy and university, the amphitheater of the medical school, and the vestibule of the hospital, recalling the features of illustrious teachers, and inspiring the pupil with ambition to excel in great and noble works." He implored the alumni association to "adorn the College with memorials of this kind."[1]

He made strikingly similar remarks in his autobiography, recounting an experience at a dinner of the British Medical Association held in the hall of Christ Church College, Oxford University, in 1868.[2] In response to a toast complimenting the American delegation, Gross said, "I felt...as if every portrait in the large and majestic room were watching me and saying, 'Hear! hear! hear!' and felt as if ten centuries were looking down upon that grand and learned assembly." He deplored the fact that Philadelphia, so distinguished for its scientific, charitable, and literary institutions, lacked such inspiring monuments.

Primary and secondary sources attest to the alumni association's rapid response to Gross's entreaty. The minutes of an April 16, 1875 meeting of its executive committee stated that Dr. Samuel W. Gross moved to appoint a committee to "confer with the families of the earlier professors of the College with a view of procuring their portraits." In subsequent meetings in 1876 "progress" was reported by the new Committee on Portraits of Earlier Professors. By then the college had acquired the Samuel B. Waugh oil portraits of Drs. Joseph Pancoast, Robley Dunglison, and Samuel D. Gross.

Minutes of the 1880s describe the embryonic beginnings of new portrait traditions. On October 19, 1882 a committee of three was appointed to procure busts of Professors Joseph Pancoast, M.D. and Samuel D. Gross, M.D. and "to see what steps are necessary for their deposit in the amphitheater of the College." On February 19, 1883 it was resolved that the Committee on Busts be continued and instructed to invite Gross, still president of the alumni association, to present the bust of the late Professor Pancoast to the trustees of the college on graduation day the following April.

In a history of Jefferson Medical College written in 1904 by alumnus George M. Gould, M.D., the author stated that soon after the completion of the 1877 hospital, "friends of the institution began the commendable work of adorning the walls with gifts of paintings, portraits, busts and other desirable decorations...of interesting historical significance or a memorial to some prominent character in the life of the College."[3] He singled out the marble busts of J. Marion Sims, M.D. and George McClellan, M.D. (founder of the college) which overlooked the arena of the clinical amphitheater; and eight oil portraits, some of which were moved from the hospital to Medical Hall, the new Jefferson Medical College Building which opened in 1898.

Gould added that "hundreds of portraits" (probably an exaggerated number of works that were predominantly prints and photographs) and other interior adornments and furnishings were acquired directly and indirectly through the alumni association. They were placed in the halls, offices, reception rooms, library, classrooms, and "even remote corners" of the hospital, laboratory, and Medical Hall.

Minutes of the March 28, 1910 board of trustees meeting stated that appreciation of the faculty should be sent to trustee Daniel Baugh and Dr. H. R. M. Landis for their loyalty and generosity in presenting to the college the "very excellent collection of likenesses" of faculty and distinguished alumni. Most likely trustee Baugh and alumnus Landis were members of a committee that handled portrait acceptances and installations.

By 1915, the college's collection of twenty-four oil portraits was of sufficient interest to be the subject of a ten-page article by librarian Charles Frankenberger in the November 1915 *Jeffersonian*, a monthly student publication. Frankenberger praised the "fine and valuable" collection as a whole: "Not only are these paintings interesting to the medical profession, and especially to Jefferson Alumni and students, because of their subjects, but to the world of art as well, for their artistic excellence." Paraphrasing Dr. Samuel D. Gross, he continued, "The presence of these paintings constitutes a reminder of past achievements and in them is to be found a stimulus to endeavor on the part of the students."

Frankenberger mentioned that during the previous summer the entire collection was completely "renovated" by an expert restorer, T. H. Stevenson, who had studied his craft in London and worked on collections at prestigious institutions in Philadelphia and Washington, D.C. It was Mr. Stevenson who described the portraits in the article and who made mostly laudatory or occasionally disparaging comments about their quality. The paintings were esteemed enough to inaugurate a conservation program, but unfortunately no records exist detailing the actual treatments.

The January 1916 *Jeffersonian* referred to Frankenberger's article and explained that it was written at the behest of Dean Ross V. Patterson, M.D. The dean felt that "the artistic value and excellence of the collection of paintings in the possession of the College possibly has not been fully appreciated before." The paintings mentioned were located in the library, lecture rooms, and trustees' room.

In 1930 the trustees approved a formal resolution establishing guidelines for the acceptance, quality, and display of oil portraits. The minutes of November 17, 1930 stated:

> WHEREAS, the Jefferson Medical College of Philadelphia has a collection of portraits of distinguished artistic merit, the display of which may be properly considered as an inspiration to students, Faculty and guests using the building, and
>
> WHEREAS, it is of great importance that the quality of the collection as a whole, and the individual pictures

> in the collection be not impaired by overcrowding or by the hanging of inferior portraits, NOW THEREFORE BE IT
>
> RESOLVED that it is the view of the Board of Trustees that except in unusual circumstances the only portraits to be accepted by Jefferson should be portraits of members living or dead of either the Faculty or of the Board of Trustees, and
>
> FURTHER RESOLVED, that no portrait shall be accepted unless in the opinion of the Board of Trustees its quality as a work of art is consistent with the quality of the paintings now owned and hung.

In addition to thirty-nine oil paintings the collection also included two pastel portraits in 1930. A striking omission from the trustees' resolution regarding "works of art" is any mention of sculpture, only "portraits," "pictures," or "paintings." By 1930 Jefferson also owned eighteen sculpted busts or full-length figures, three bas-reliefs, and two architectural rondels.

An explanation of this attitude may be that during some historical periods painting has been considered a "higher" medium than sculpture in the hierarchy of art media. Ironically, though, in the late nineteenth and early twentieth centuries, portrait busts were very popular, and large-scale public sculptural monuments were still being erected in many cities to the acclaim of critics and the general public.

Institutional Responsibility for Art, 1930 to the Present

Scanty surviving records indicate that probably the dean's office, the hospital, and the art/archives committees of the alumni association and the trustees all had some responsibility for the art collection through the 1940s. Inevitably, overlapping and lack of coordination occurred.

Therefore, in 1950 board president Vice Admiral James L. Kauffman appointed the library committee of the executive faculty to take on the responsibility for decorating, lighting, and arranging portraits in the College Building's auditorium, McClellan Hall. Minutes from 1952 and 1953 show increased responsibility for surveying the total collection and then rehanging portraits among the various buildings, thereby avoiding any "hard feelings among partisans, families and friends" as a result of the reshuffling. This committee also coordinated with the alumni association in planning the portrait presentations and for portrait exhibitions of faculty members during commencement week.

Despite effective supervision of art activities under the chairmanship of Dr. Thaddeus L. Montgomery, library committee minutes expressed discomfiture with spending library funds for these art projects and with differences of opinion regarding the hanging of new portraits. As early as September 29, 1952 the committee asked to be relieved of its portrait responsibilities as "probably not an integral part of its duties."

At the May 25, 1953 meeting of the college's executive faculty, Professor Kenneth Goodner, Ph.D. submitted a resolution to create a special committee to exert better control over art policies regarding choice of portrait subjects, artists, and acceptability standards. This was prompted by a recently presented portrait which had aroused considerable negative criticism. The resolution was approved, and the first executive faculty portrait committee included the chairman, Dean George A. Bennett, M.D., and faculty members Drs. Goodner, J. Earl Thomas, and William H. Perkins. Subsequent chairmen were Drs. Perkins, John B. Montgomery, Peter A. Herbut, and Andrew J. Ramsay.

By 1959 the collection had expanded to ninety-nine portraits and the new portrait committee had undertaken the manufacture of bronze plaques with information about the subjects, and occasionally, the artists, to accompany the pictures. Chairman Perkins decried the present arrangement in McClellan Hall as "atrociously bad."

Instead, he decided that portraits of living teachers should be hung in lecture rooms, while portraits of founders, trustees, deans, and deceased faculty members should be hung in McClellan Hall. He added, *sotto voce,* that "less well done or less important personages could be removed to the vault." He added that "no art gallery hangs all of its possessions and that is what vaults are for."

Minutes and correspondence show that the portrait subcommittee functioned smoothly throughout its existence until the final meeting of the executive faculty on June 3, 1969. The committee had paid particular attention to matters of insurance, conservation, and approval for selection of artists and finished portraits.

In July 1969 Jefferson Medical College became one of four components of the newly formed Thomas Jefferson University. Art responsibilities were taken over by the committee on academic protocol of the executive faculty. The new committee chairman was Dr. Andrew J. Ramsay, an accomplished photographer who had introduced an audiovisual center in the department of anatomy, and was responsible for the first photographic survey of the art collection.

In 1971 President Herbut decided that matters of art were still too decentralized and should be made the business of the entire university, so he created the Thomas Jefferson University committee on art "to be responsible to the president." Its first chairman was Dr. Ramsay. The chairmanship passed to Robert J. Mandle, Ph.D. in 1972 and Russell W. Schaedler, M.D. in 1986. President Lewis W. Bluemle Jr., M.D. and his successor Paul C. Brucker, M.D. have been members of the committee, along with other members representing the medical and corporate staffs.

Since 1971 the art committee has continued to monitor all art matters at the university, sometimes coordinating with the art committees of the Jefferson Medical College senior class and the alumni association. In 1983 President Bluemle created a new committee "charged to set and apply standards for additions" to the collection, for maintaining both the high quality of the art work and appropriate worthiness of the portrait sitter. Chaired by Burton L. Wellenbach, M.D., the university committee on portrait standards functions as an "independent but coordinated arm of the university committee on art."

In the ebb and flow of art committee deliberations, some concerns seem eternal. Contemporary art committees still wrestle with similar issues that were addressed in the trustees' resolution of 1930: criteria for selection of portrait subjects, standards for quality of portraits, and appropriateness of hanging locations. Other ongoing concerns of the committee include conservation, security, climate control, and lighting, as well as the consideration of requests for loans of art works. A contemporary issue centers around the rights and reproduction of Jefferson art works on the Internet, World Wide Web, and CD-ROMs, a concern and challenge shared by all art institutions.

Responsibilities for the art collection extend beyond the acquisition and display of portraits. The university art historian coordinates fine arts appraisals, conservation, and photography of the collection, supervises loans to and from major museums, aids in accepting donations and bequests of art works, manages the sale of reproduction rights and photographic materials to medical and art publishers, and performs other curatorial, registration, and business-related matters in coordination with the university's legal, development, insurance, and finance departments, as well as the art committee. Other duties performed by the art historian are creating and managing centralized artist and object paper files and a computer collection management database; and writing articles and delivering slide lectures and gallery talks about the Jefferson art collection.

Fine Arts Insurance, and the Concept of One-of-a-Kind

Another indication of an institution's appreciation of art assets is its attitude toward fine arts insurance. Such insurance records can reveal valuable information about a collection that was not formally documented according to even minimal museum standards until recently. The earliest extant records at Jefferson Medical College date from December 1929: a three-way correspondence between Dean Ross V. Patterson, M.D., Board Chairman Robert P. Hooper, and Henry M. Gratz, President of the Girard Fire and Marine Insurance Company.

Patterson noted that there were thirty-seven paintings in the College Building and two in the Daniel Baugh Institute of Anatomy Building. All had been "placed in the hands of Edward Side [a hospital administrator] and put in first-class order at an expense of Five Thousand Dollars," i.e. restored, and returned to the library, corridors, and elsewhere in the College Building.

Mr. Side was asked to estimate the value of each painting in order to prepare an itemized schedule. In addition to the appraisal, the insurance company requested information on the title, artist, date acquired, and value paid, whenever possible. Unfortunately, this useful art list has not been located.

One letter inquired whether the paintings should be protected from "ordinary damage," adding, "We have had some trouble of this kind, when some one maliciously slashed one of the pictures with a knife." The collection was soon insured against fire, theft, water, and "all other damage."

Although the dean readily agreed to the necessity for insurance, he wanted to keep costs down, noting that all portraits had been given to the institution and represented "no investments whatever on its part. Their value is entirely historical and sentimental. They cannot be replaced if destroyed." He contrasted Jefferson's position with that of a picture dealer or art collector who would suffer an actual monetary loss from destruction of his art works and also loss of potential profit from sales.

In a curious contradiction he later advised that the

collection be photographed, saying, "in the event of the destruction or loss of any one of the pictures, a painter could make some sort of reproduction which would satisfy the sentimental requirements." This thought ignores the historical or real artistic value of the original painting by suggesting that it could be replaced by a secondhand copy. It shows that above all he valued the likeness of the portrait subject over the uniqueness of the original work of art. One wonders whether this was a prevailing view among nonmuseum institutions with art collections.

Interestingly, Patterson singled out only five portraits that "might be considered works of art—the Eakins paintings, the Van Dyke [*sic*], and the Sully." His admiration for the three Eakins portraits is understandably well-advised. The portrait head of Thomas D. Mütter, M.D. by Thomas Sully is a charming picture, though of modest scale. However, the so-called portrait of William Harvey allegedly painted by Anthony Van Dyck was sorely misattributed, as the painting neither resembles known portraits of Harvey nor even approaches the style of Van Dyck. Here the donor's claim of subject and artist was apparently accepted by the institution without seeking a concurring opinion from any art scholar.

The dean's knowledge of art was misinformed in another way. In assessing the worthwhile portraits, he ignored excellent paintings by other artists with national and international reputations, such as William Merritt Chase, Robert W. Vonnoh, Adolphe Borie, Hugh H. Breckenridge, Lazar Raditz, Bernard Uhle, and others. The dean, too, overlooked all the sculptures as valuable works of art.

The oil portrait tradition has steadfastly continued despite intermittent misgivings about expenses and availability of exhibition space, and the university has not turned to smaller and less costly photographic portraits for honoring its esteemed personages. A special account was established by the university's president in 1987 to reserve ten percent of portrait fund subscriptions for defraying the costs of future conservation.

Since 1980 the university has averaged three to four new Jefferson-related oil portraits annually, the actual numbers ranging from one new portrait in 1988 to a high of seven in 1982 and 1990. The camaraderie engendered in choosing portrait subjects and artists, and the impressive ceremonial traditions displayed in the portrait presentations have come to embody the special Jefferson spirit both towards its honored faculty and administrators and towards its valued art collection.

Acquisition by Donation and a Collection by Chance

Explicit in the above-mentioned art collection policies is the knowledge that most works have been donations to the university, either outright gifts or paid for by subscription by a group of donors, except for the class portraits. Jefferson has never had a policy of collecting specific artists, images of specific physicians or other medical subjects, or specific periods in the history of art or medicine.

The institution has rarely purchased art directly from artists, dealers, or at auction in order to enhance its collection. Exceptions are outdoor public sculptures and fountains: for new works the university has dealt directly with the artist who has won a juried competition; for preexisting works the university has negotiated with a donor.

Jefferson does not impose the choice of artist for new portrait commissions. The portrait honoree chooses his own artist, and may seek suggestions from the organizing portrait committee or the university art committee, if desired. Gifts and bequests of portraits and other fine and decorative art works are usually accepted gratefully, and the university is typically more interested in the person depicted in the portrait and in the generosity of the donor, rather than in standard museum acquisition criteria.

Therefore, the collection is broadly eclectic because it was never conceived of as a whole entity. Art works have arrived from multiple sources, one by one, and been funneled through different channels. Over generations the collection has become richly diverse, reflecting the tastes and attitudes of its donors and portrait subjects. Thomas Jefferson University has developed a reputation for appreciating art and displaying its collection with respect and good taste.

What, then, ties the collection together? The obvious general theme is *ars medica*, portraits of physicians and other medical thematic material. Another unifying factor is that the majority of donors have connections to the institution, so that their gifts are generally relevant to the history of or the medical/cultural mission of the university.

Samuel D. Gross, M.D. would be gratified to know that currently portraits and other art works "adorn the halls" of almost all campus buildings. Gross would be pleased at the generally high quality of the art, but he would probably *not* be astonished at the sources of the donations of painted and sculpted portraits.

The donor category with the longest tradition and most numerous examples is the senior class of Jefferson Medical College. Since 1924 the graduating class has commissioned a portrait of its most inspiring faculty or medical college member, the one who best exemplifies excellence in teaching and patient care. Until the 1950s only department chairmen were eligible for the class portrait. Since then any worthy faculty member or administrator may be considered. To be selected by vote of the senior class is still considered a high honor. Class gifts account for thirty-six percent of all the painted portraits in the collection.

The next most numerous category is friends and colleagues of the portrait subject. When combined with specific Jefferson Medical College departments whose members are also colleagues, this category accounts for twenty-four percent of painted portraits.

Portrait sitters themselves, their families, or descendants have contributed fifteen percent of the total number of painted portraits. Another generous donor category is the Jefferson Medical College alumni association and/or individual alumni who account for seven percent of donations. Other significant donor categories are the board of trustees, artists or artists' families, and the hospital women's board.

In many cases donor categories overlap. For example, Thomas Eakins's portrait of Benjamin H. Rand, M.D. was given to Jefferson Medical College by the professor who was an alumnus, faculty member, and dean, as well as the portrait subject. The portrait of President William W. Bodine Jr. was donated by faculty, trustees, and friends. An unusually circuitous donation path was followed by the bronze bust of J. Marion Sims, M.D. It was given by the subject's family to the Jefferson Hospital surgical staff which requested that the alumni association present it to the college trustees who would then install it in the 1877 hospital.

The Class Portrait: A Case Study

Although there were intermittent student portrait commissions in the late nineteenth and early twentieth centuries, the Jefferson Medical College class portrait did not become an ingrained annual tradition until 1924. This tradition has been interrupted only once, when the choice of portrait honoree of the class of 1956 was rejected by the college's administration for political reasons, and students opted instead to donate an intercom system for the medical clinic.

There have been some variations on the general rule. The class of 1932 gave its traditional faculty portrait that year and then an additional historical portrait in 1985. In 1944 during World War II Jefferson Medical College graduated January and September classes, and both classes donated a portrait. There were also two portrait donations in 1951: the traditional class portrait, and the other from the class of 1917 which decided to memorialize Dean William H. Perkins, M.D. In 1953 a depiction of the honoree was so roundly criticized that a second portrait was commissioned from a different artist. Ironically, today the university is pleased to own both versions.

Class portraits are still a source of pride among the alumni, and during graduation weekend the class portraits of the twenty-fifth and fiftieth reunion classes are displayed prominently in Jefferson Alumni Hall. One can't help wondering if Jefferson's longstanding class portrait tradition is unique among American health care institutions, or among all American universities, for that matter.

The class of 1861 was the first to commission a portrait. The occasion was the retirement of the professor of obstetrics, Charles D. Meigs, M.D., and the portrait was given to him personally as a gift. A copy of this original portrait painted by Samuel B. Waugh in 1872 was donated to Jefferson Medical College by Meigs's son, John Forsyth Meigs, M.D., in 1880.

Subsequent class portraits of professors were accepted by and hung at the college, including those of James A. Meigs, M.D. by the class of 1879-80; William H. Pancoast, M.D. by the class of 1886; Samuel W. Gross, M.D. by the class of 1890; Roberts Bartholow, M.D. by the class of 1892; William W. Keen Jr., M.D. by the class of 1901; and William S. Forbes, M.D. by the classes of 1905-08 and "junior alumni" in 1905.

According to Jefferson lore, the class of 1924 decided to honor its beloved professor, John Chalmers DaCosta, M.D. with a portrait. Since the modest contributions of five dollars per student were not enough to pay expenses, the organizers raised funds by challenging the University of Pennsylvania School of Medicine to a basketball game. Even though they lost the game played in front of medical students and nurses on the Penn campus, Jefferson students earned enough extra money to pay the artist, Richard Blossom Farley, and a framemaker.

In recent decades escalating costs for class portraits have been subsidized by the medical college. However, most artists reduce their customary fees for the opportunity to enhance their reputation by inclusion in the noteworthy Jefferson portrait collection.

Portrait presentations at Jefferson are not the abbreviated, perfunctory events found at many similar institutions, but instead may include half a dozen speakers and incorporate very personal and heartwarming rituals. For example, in 1992 the class portrait honoree was Clara A. Callahan, M.D., then a clinical associate professor of pediatrics and assistant dean for student affairs. She is shown in the photograph with artist Stephen S. Kennedy (second from right), and the class portrait committee chairmen, Amy E. Martin and James J. McKeith.

At the unveiling ceremony in McClellan Hall opening remarks were made by the senior class portrait committee cochair, followed by a biographical sketch touchingly recounted by the chairman of pediatrics, Robert L. Brent, M.D., Ph.D. Accompanied by slides dating back to the subject's childhood, even one as flutist in her high school band, Dr. Brent emphasized Dr. Callahan's personal as well as academic and professional accomplishments.

He said "she is a joy to work with" because of her dependability, dedication, and accessibility to those important in her life: students, colleagues, family, friends, and patients and their families. He quoted Jefferson Medical College Dean Joseph S. Gonnella, M.D. and others saying that Dr. Callahan "displays both compassion and courage," and that "she is an excellent role model for students."

Dr. Callahan displayed her modest but radiantly enthusiastic disposition in remarks following the unveiling of the portrait, saying "this was truly the best day of my life." The portrait was received for Jefferson Medical College by Dean Gonnella, and accepted on behalf of the Thomas Jefferson University board of trustees by President Paul C. Brucker, M.D. Both men praised the class of 1992 for their selection of Dr. Callahan.

Then the portrait artist was recognized and asked to stand for a round of applause. Finally the other cochair of the class portrait committee thanked Frederick B. Wagner Jr., M.D., the University Historian and the Grace Revere Osler Professor Emeritus of Surgery, for his lively organ recital preceding the ceremony, and invited the audience of more than 150 guests for refreshments in the Eakins Lounge. As is custom-

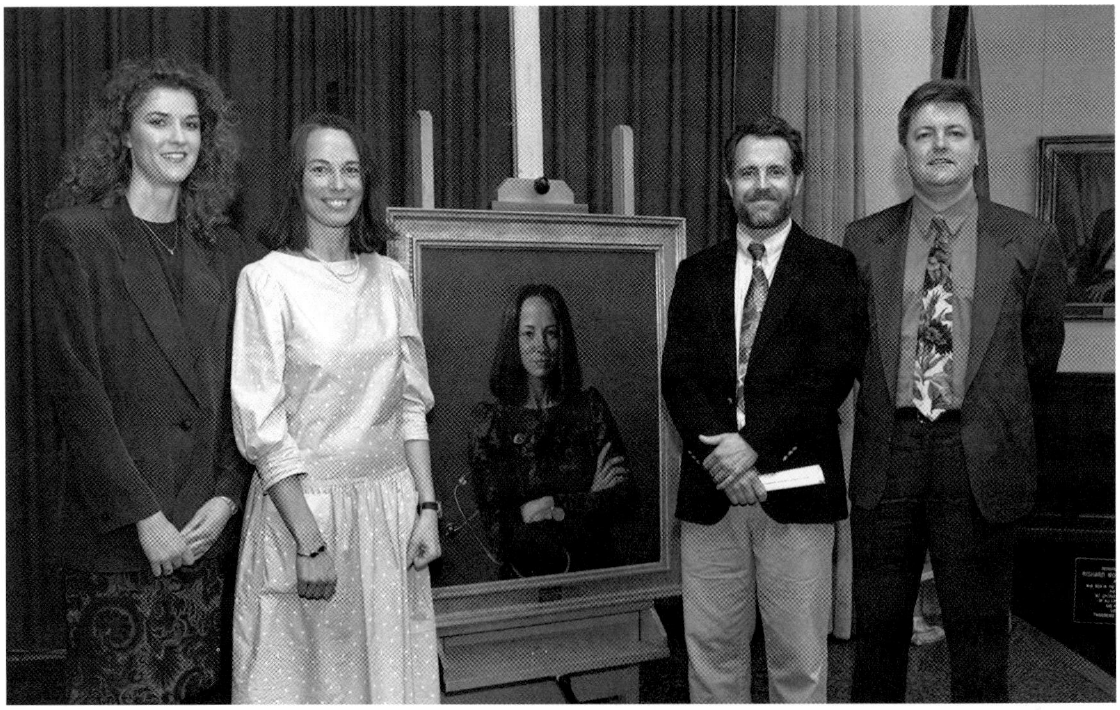

Clara A. Callahan, M.D. at her Portrait Presentation Ceremony (Photograph by Robert Neroni)

ary, the portrait was displayed for three months in the ground floor lobby of Jefferson Alumni Hall for maximum exposure to students and faculty, and then relocated to a place that is relevant to the sitter's specific professional activity.

The Placement of Art

Virtually all of the paintings and sculptures in the Jefferson collection are on permanent display on the Jefferson campus, except for two portraits on loan off-site and a few works in storage. With the exception of the three Thomas Eakins portraits, the statue of Athena, and the Susan Eakins portrait which are located in the Eakins Gallery, all other paintings and sculptures are distributed throughout the campus in eleven different buildings. Some decorative arts and a small selection of art works on paper are also widely disbursed; the remainder are housed in the university's archives.

University art committee chairmen still acknowledge that the placement of portraits can be a political as well as artistic decision. The current guiding principle is to place portraits of physicians in the building most appropriate to their professional work. For example, the portraits of most recent basic science professors and researchers are situated in Jefferson Alumni Hall near the location of their offices and laboratories, or in the Bluemle Life Sciences Building.

Most portraits of recent clinicians are located in the Herbut Auditorium of the College Building, in the Scott Library Building, or in various departmental offices. The majority of portraits in McClellan Hall are of department chairmen from the late nineteenth to the mid-twentieth centuries.

Many of the most outstanding historic portraits of physicians and administrators are located in reception areas and offices of the university president, the dean of the medical college, and a few clinical departments; in the university's library and its auditoriums; and in public corridors and stairwell landings near classroom and conference areas in the College and Curtis Buildings.

Public Outdoor Art at Jefferson

Jefferson is justifiably proud of its five outdoor art works, four of which are visible and accessible to the general public as well as its own personnel. Two full-length, standing bronze sculptures situated out-of-doors were acquired through the university's own initiative. Alexander Calder's statue of Gross is located in Scott Plaza, a landscaped, city-park-like area, behind the Scott building. Lloyd Lillie's statue of Thomas Jefferson is set in a niche adjacent to a small fountain in the landscaped west atrium of Jefferson Alumni Hall.

The three other outdoor works resulted from Jefferson's participation in the Philadelphia Redevelopment Authority's Fine Arts Program. Philadelphia was the first major American city to establish a program for acquiring works of contemporary public art, and since 1959 one percent of all construction costs must be spent on the acquisition of fine arts in urban renewal areas and in new public buildings. The Philadelphia model has been widely copied by other American cities.

Regulations require that the artist chosen must be a practicing professional of recognized ability. The work must be permanent and original, created specifically for the site. Media and type can vary from mural painting to sculpture to works made of glass, mosaic, fiber, light, water, or other materials. Plans and execution are subject to approval by the Redevelopment Authority's Fine Arts Committee. For guidance through the art selection process, the redeveloper must employ a recognized visual arts professional as consultant and/or a panel of visual arts professionals. In multiple building projects funds can be pooled to allow for "more significant art projects."

The selection process for choosing artists and their proposals often includes a competition. Henry Mitchell's bronze *Winged Ox*, Jefferson's first such commission in 1975, was judged by a jury to be the most appropriate sculpture entry for the site. A winged ox (the attribute of St. Luke, patron saint of physicians and painters) crowns a sixteen-and-a-half-foot column containing a spiral inscription of the names of fifty great physicians in the history of medicine. The sculpture is adjacent to the busy corner of Tenth and Walnut Streets, between the Scott Library-Administration Building and the Orlowitz Residence Hall.

Jefferson's second "one percent" art work also resulted from a juried competition won by Mitchell. The *Bodine Fountain* was dedicated in 1979, honoring William W. Bodine Jr., former president of the university, then chairman of the board of trustees. Animating Scott Plaza, the fountain includes five bronze otters swimming and playing on rocks in an octagonal pool. As with the *Winged Ox* funds were combined from construction costs of two buildings, in this case the nearby Barringer Residence Hall and the university parking garage.

The *Roundabout*, Jefferson's third "one percent" public art display, also incorporates flowing water. It is an expansively complex entrance park to the Bluemle Life Sciences Building at Tenth and Locust Streets, dedicated in 1992. Installation artist Alice Adams has combined a terraced granite water wall, flagstone paths, trees, shrubbery, and gardens to evoke elements of Jefferson's home at Monticello. Adjacent door frames and stairways recall neighborhood row houses of eighteenth-century Philadelphia.

Regular Exhibitions by Jefferson Artists

During the last two and one-half decades there has been an unusual amount of art activity at Jefferson, considering its health care mission. Since 1968 the Jefferson Medical College faculty wives club has sponsored an annual art exhibit in Jefferson Alumni Hall, a nonjuried show of original art work open to "the Jefferson family," i.e. faculty, students, alumni, employees, and their families. Other shows of archival materials are displayed in the library from time to time.

In 1992 a new art tradition began under the initiative of Robert A. Peterson, then the senior vice president for administration and finance: one-person shows by members of the Jefferson family held in a gallery space on the administrative sixth floor of the Scott Building. These popular exhibitions remain on view for several months, and to date have included pastels, watercolors, prints, drawings, photographs, and mixed media. Subjects have ranged from realistic western landscapes, eastern tidal and shore areas and baseball scenes, to dreamlike figural arrangements and reworked childhood drawings. Other shows in this gallery have occasionally included non-Jeffersonian art works recently donated to the university.

The Gross Clinic as Institutional Symbol

One celebrated art work, *The Gross Clinic*, is preeminent in Jefferson's collection. It is rare that a single work is so paramount that it helps to define a public institution, even an art museum. Thomas Eakins's *Gross Clinic* has been a continuing factor in delineating the internal and external perception of Thomas Jefferson University. Long recognized by art scholars and the general public as one of the great masterpieces of American art, it has also evolved into an institutional icon at Jefferson.

Originally painted to celebrate the surgeon's international renown and for display at the art exhibition of the 1876 Philadelphia Centennial, this strikingly heroic art work still symbolizes great achievements at Jefferson, both past and present. The image is used most effectively by the university to call attention to a wide variety of medical endeavors, in its various publications, postcards, note cards, and a poster. The painting is a "must" on campus tours for all visiting dignitaries and for prospective and new students, faculty, and employees.

Beyond its artistic merit as a medical history painting and portrait, it has established its own presence in the spiritual consciousness of the institution by recalling the values that led to its creation. The painting itself has become a part of Jefferson's history and its acclaim and positive reflection on the institution have long been a source of great pride.

For example, the painting was lent to the Philadelphia Museum of Art's *Diamond Jubilee Exhibition* held November 1950 to February 1951. Correspondence and articles show that Jefferson faculty, students, and administrators were extremely gratified that the painting received third place in a "public popularity" poll taken among the eighty-eight thousand visitors to the exhibition. (The first place choice was Peter Paul Rubens's *Flight of Lot and his Family from Sodom*, and second place was El Greco's familiar *View of Toledo*.)

One other example among many occurred in 1964 when the Pennsylvania Senate passed a resolution to include a reproduction of the painting in the *Pennsylvania Manual*, an official compendium of state information. The resolution stated that the world-famous painting "would indeed be an appropriate symbolic tribute to the greatness of our Seats of Learning of the Healing Arts generally, and that of Jefferson Medical College in particular."

The university has long demonstrated an abiding interest in the career, reputation, and medical connections of artist Thomas Eakins. Under the auspices of the faculty wives club of Jefferson Medical College, Lloyd Goodrich, author of the first definitive monograph on Thomas Eakins, delivered a public lecture on Eakins and *The Gross Clinic* on January 21, 1970. Goodrich was then advisory director to the Whitney Museum of American Art, and the Eakins portrait was scheduled to be exhibited at the Whitney and at the Metropolitan Museum of

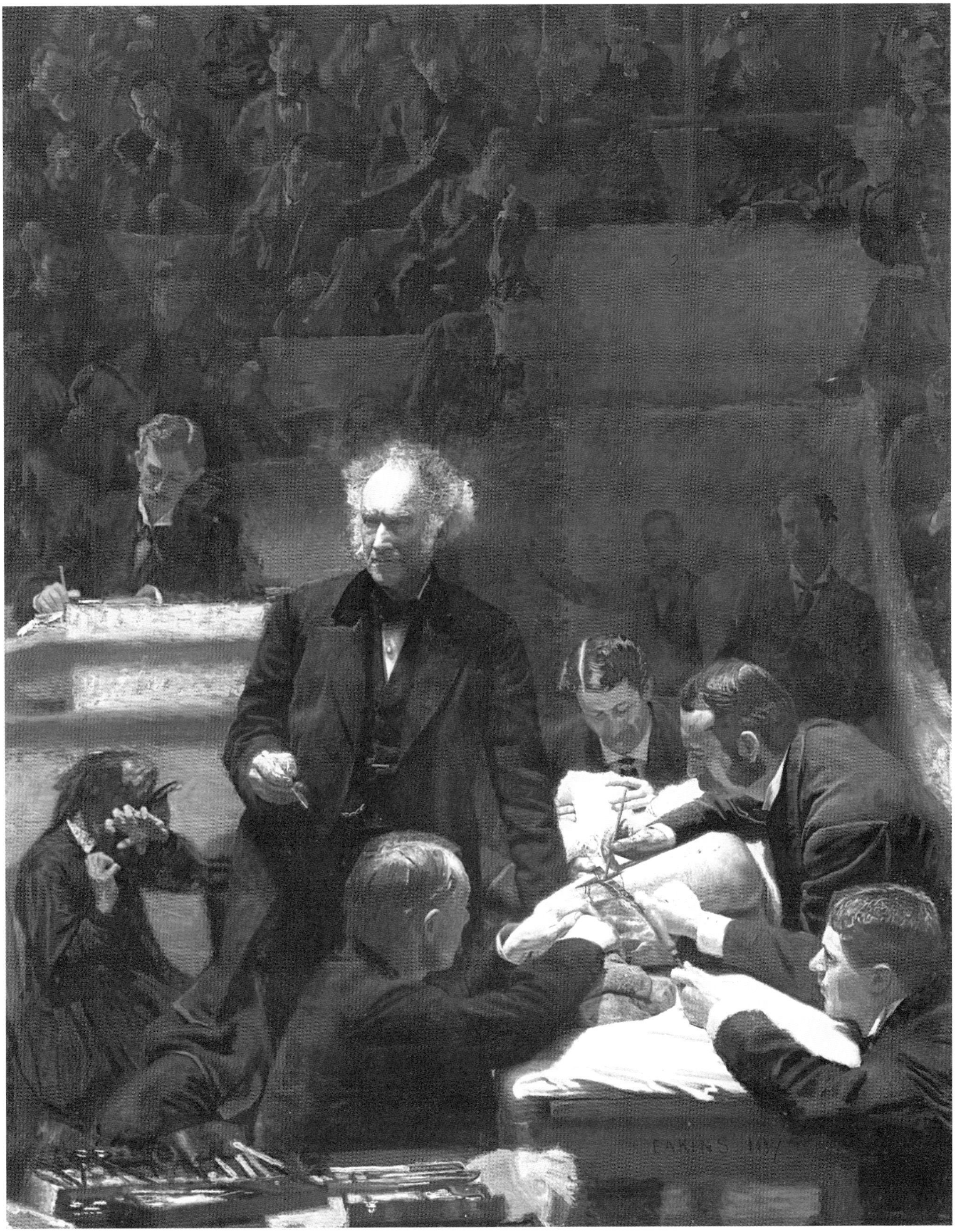

The Gross Clinic

Art later that year.

When the painting returned from the New York exhibitions it was reinstalled in the new Basic Sciences/Commons Building (later called Jefferson Alumni Hall). To celebrate the event a benefit reception and exhibition was cosponsored by the university and the Thomas Eakins House Restoration Committee on March 21, 1971. The featured speaker at the reception was Evan H. Turner, Ph.D., director of the Philadelphia Museum of Art. The museum planned to administer the nearby Eakins house and studio as a community art center after the run-down dwelling was refurbished. The house had been purchased by an anonymous donor who was an Eakins devotee and friend of the artist's wife. He gave the house to the city on the condition that it be converted into an art center and repository of Eakins memorabilia.

As one fund-raising device the Eakins House Restoration Committee issued a special limited edition, silver, commemorative medal of Thomas Eakins, designed

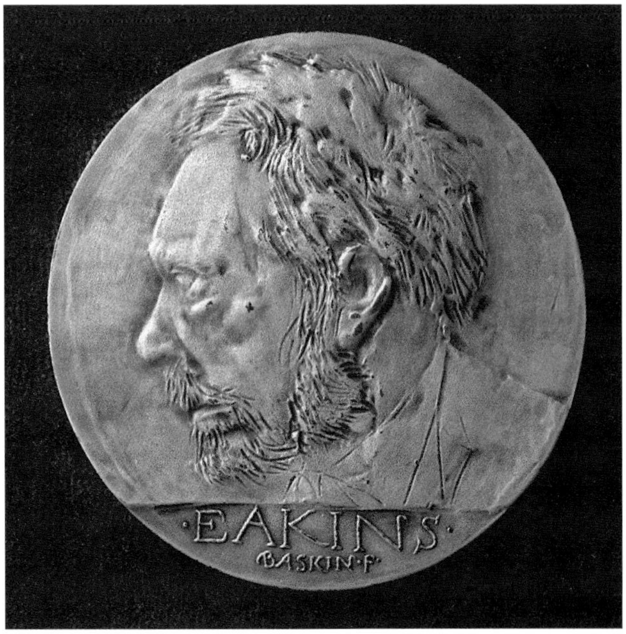

Medallic Portrait of Thomas Eakins by Leonard Baskin[4]

gratis by American artist Leonard Baskin, and produced without charge by the Franklin Mint. The portrait is a head and shoulders profile depiction of the shaggy-haired, middle-aged artist looking defiant.

Baskin, an internationally known sculptor, painter, and graphic artist, was a member of the Eakins House Restoration Committee. Winner of a Guggenheim Foundation fellowship, Baskin was a professor of art at Smith College (1953-74), a member of the National Institute of Arts and Letters, and founder of the Gehenna Press, designer and publisher of fine arts books and broadsides.

Jefferson administrators have steadfastly believed that *The Gross Clinic* must remain permanently on its college campus in Philadelphia, to be displayed in the context of Gross's life and career. Therefore, they have rejected intermittent proposals from museums, dealers, collectors, and donors to buy the painting or borrow it on long-term loan. There has only been one serious, but short-lived consideration of an offer to buy the painting in the mid-1970s.

A few years after that particular offer was soundly rejected, the alumni association formed the Gross Portrait Committee to plan a celebration for the centennial of the painting's acquisition in 1878. Soon the committee's emphasis changed from a celebration of the acquisition to an improvement in the aesthetic display of the painting and the effectiveness of lighting and security. After careful reflection it was decided to assemble in one room *The Gross Clinic* and the two other Eakins portraits of Professors Forbes and Rand. This resulted in the creation of a new gallery which was dedicated April 23, 1982, with a noted Eakins scholar, Professor Elizabeth Johns, Ph.D., as the special guest speaker.

Significantly, the Eakins Gallery is named after the artist, rather than the more customary practice of naming special rooms in honor of a donor, institutional leader, or role model. Thanks to generous contributions from the Connelly Foundation, the William Penn Foundation, and the Jefferson Medical College alumni association, an elegant and imposing gallery was created to house Jefferson's three Eakins portraits.

Because of the gallery's high ceilings and spacious proportions, subdued decor and lighting, and the placement of paintings behind platforms and railings, visitors sense immediately the special treatment afforded these three important art works. Adjoining the gallery is the Eakins Lounge, a reception area where guests can glimpse *The Gross Clinic* through impressive wrought iron gates. To accommodate visitors the gallery is opened upon request seven days a week and is free of charge.

The Eakins Gallery is testimony to the institution's appreciation of the inspirational value of great art. Besides being a constant presence in the thoughts of Jeffersonians, the painting also attracts a steady stream of outside visitors to the gallery. Many art lovers have traveled to Philadelphia from other states and foreign countries specifically to view the works of Thomas Eakins, and the culmination of such a pilgrimage is almost always *The Gross Clinic.*

Art Works as Ambassadors: Collaborations with Other Cultural Institutions

There are some who question whether a health care institution like Thomas Jefferson University is an appropriate repository for an important art collection. One standard of measurement is the institution's relations with sister educational and cultural organizations.

Jefferson has long been a generous lender of art works to special exhibitions at world's fairs, museums, and other cultural centers. A few outstanding instances are listed below, and all loans are detailed in subsequent individual entries.

In 1887 Jefferson lent five works to the *Centennial Celebration: Loan Collection of Portraits* at the College of Physicians of Philadelphia, including Eakins's portrait of Dr. Benjamin H. Rand and Samuel B. Waugh's portraits of Drs. Samuel D. Gross, James A. Meigs, Joseph Pancoast, and Robley Dunglison. A century later in 1989 Jefferson lent *The Gross Clinic* to another centennial art exhibition of a medical institution, this time honoring the Johns Hopkins Medical Institutions which held its celebratory exhibition at the Walters Art Gallery in Baltimore.

Jefferson participated in two other significant medical art exhibitions: *The Art of Philadelphia Medicine* at the Philadelphia Museum of Art in 1965, to which it lent the three Eakins portraits and the portraits of John Eberle, M.D. and Thomas D. Mütter, M.D., as well as a case of surgical instruments used by nineteenth-century Jefferson surgeons; and *The Art of Healing: Medicine and Science in American Art* at the Birmingham Museum of Art in 1981, to which it again lent the three Eakins portraits and also the portraits of Samuel D. Gross, M.D. by Samuel B. Waugh and Richard G. Berry, M.D. by José Marcote.

On three occasions Jefferson has borrowed Eakins medical portraits from other medical and art institutions. In 1971 Pennsylvania Hospital lent its Eakins portrait of Jacob Mendez DaCosta, M.D. for the Eakins House Restoration benefit held at Jefferson. In 1982 Jefferson borrowed the Eakins portrait of William Thomson, M.D. from the College of Physicians of Philadelphia while *The Gross Clinic* traveled to the Philadelphia Museum of Art and the Museum of Fine Arts, Boston for the exhibition *Thomas Eakins: Artist of Philadelphia*. In 1983 Jefferson borrowed the Eakins portrait of James W. Holland, M.D. (known as *The Dean's Roll Call*) from the Museum of Fine Arts, Boston while *The Gross Clinic* traveled to the Museum of Fine Arts, the Corcoran Gallery of Art in Washington, D.C., and the Grand Palais in Paris for the landmark exhibition *A New World: Masterpieces of American Painting*.

Jefferson has also collaborated with cultural organizations in other ways. For example, in 1985 Jefferson held two public lectures and an exhibition in collaboration with the Philadelphia Museum of Art's *Ars Medica* exhibition, joining with twenty other Philadelphia-area medical institutions which also sponsored special events.

In 1992 Jefferson hosted an exhibition on the career of anatomist William S. Forbes, M.D. in collaboration with the Pennsylvania Academy of the Fine Arts exhibition *Thomas Eakins Rediscovered*. Forbes's role in pioneering legislation to make unclaimed cadavers available for medical education was analogous to Eakins's equally firm insistence on the study of the human body in art education. Addressing the theme of freedom of expression, both exhibitions were part of a citywide celebration of the bicentennial of the Bill of Rights.

In 1993 Jefferson received national prominence resulting from unprecedented collaborations among the university, the National Portrait Gallery, the National Archives, and the University of Virginia. In April *The Gross Clinic* traveled to Washington as a featured painting in a major commemorative exhibition, *American Art at the 1893 World's Fair: Revisiting the White City*, cosponsored by the National Portrait Gallery and the National Museum of American Art, Smithsonian Institution.

In a direct exchange for *The Gross Clinic*, Jefferson hosted its own special show, *Six Notable Philadelphians from the National Portrait Gallery*, including portraits of artist Mary Cassatt painted by Edgar Degas; painter Charles Willson Peale in a self-portrait; his artist son Rubens Peale, painted by his brother Rembrandt Peale; writer and critic Talcott Williams, painted by Thomas Eakins; actress Juliana Westray Wood, painted by Rembrandt Peale; and her husband, impresario William Burke Wood, painted by an unidentified artist.

The exhibition was timed to become an integral part of the university's celebration of the 250th anniversary of the birth of Thomas Jefferson on April 13. It was one of several related events on campus including a keynote lecture by Brown University professor of history and Pulitzer Prize-winning author, Gordon S. Wood, Ph.D., and an archival exhibit, *Robley Dunglison, Personal Physician to Thomas Jefferson*. This exhibit was loaned to the University of Virginia which sent a reciprocal exhibition on the history of the university and the president. Thomas Jefferson University also helped sponsor walking tour brochures highlighting programs at all Philadelphia sites relating to the president.

In another important outreach effort, the university contributed to the conservation of Thomas Jefferson's correspondence with the U.S. Congress for a display in Washington, *"A Splendid Misery": Challenges of Thomas Jefferson's Presidency*, created by the Center for Legislative Archives of the National Archives. Facsimiles of these documents were exhibited at the visitors' center at Independence National Historic Park in Philadelphia, in a show that opened July 4. The university also funded educational packets about the important issues discussed in Jefferson's letters for distribution to high school students and teachers throughout Pennsylvania, New Jersey, and Delaware.

There are other means of attracting attention to Thomas Jefferson University's cultural heritage. The university has readily granted reproduction rights of its art works to the many American and foreign publishers of medical and art books and journals requesting such images. Jefferson has also been proud to allow videotaping of *The Gross Clinic* for several scholarly television programs on American art and culture and on the career of Thomas Eakins. Finally, the university offers slide and gallery talks about the collection and also provides written materials.

From early on Jefferson has realized that lending its art works as ambassadors of the university to the local, national, or international art community has the benefit of revealing another facet of the institution's identity. Making the collection accessible to a wider public demonstrates the university's willingness to share its art treasures and confirms the institution's pride in its cultural history and traditions.

---

1. Samuel D. Gross, M.D., *An Address Delivered before the Alumni Association of the Jefferson Medical College of Philadelphia at its First Anniversary* (Philadelphia: Collins, 1871), 28-29.
2. Gross, *Autobiography of Samuel D. Gross, M.D.*, ed. Samuel W. Gross, M.D. and A. Haller Gross, 2 vols. (Philadelphia: George Barrie, 1887), 1:320.
3. George M. Gould, M.D., *The Jefferson Medical College of Philadelphia: A History*, 2 vols. (New York: Lewis Publishing Co., 1904), 1:331.
4. *PORTRAIT OF THOMAS EAKINS* (1844-1916)
By Leonard Baskin (b. 1922)
Silver medal
1972
2 1/2 in. diameter
Signed obverse lower center: "BASKIN F"
Inscription obverse: "EAKINS"
Inscription reverse: "TO/COMMEMORATE/THE RESTORATION/OF THE HOUSE AND/STUDIO OF THOMAS EAKINS/1972"
Given in 1973 by JMC alumni association
Accession number: 1973+e.M.01

Opposite: W. W. Keen Jr., M.D. in His Clinic (1904)

Historical Survey

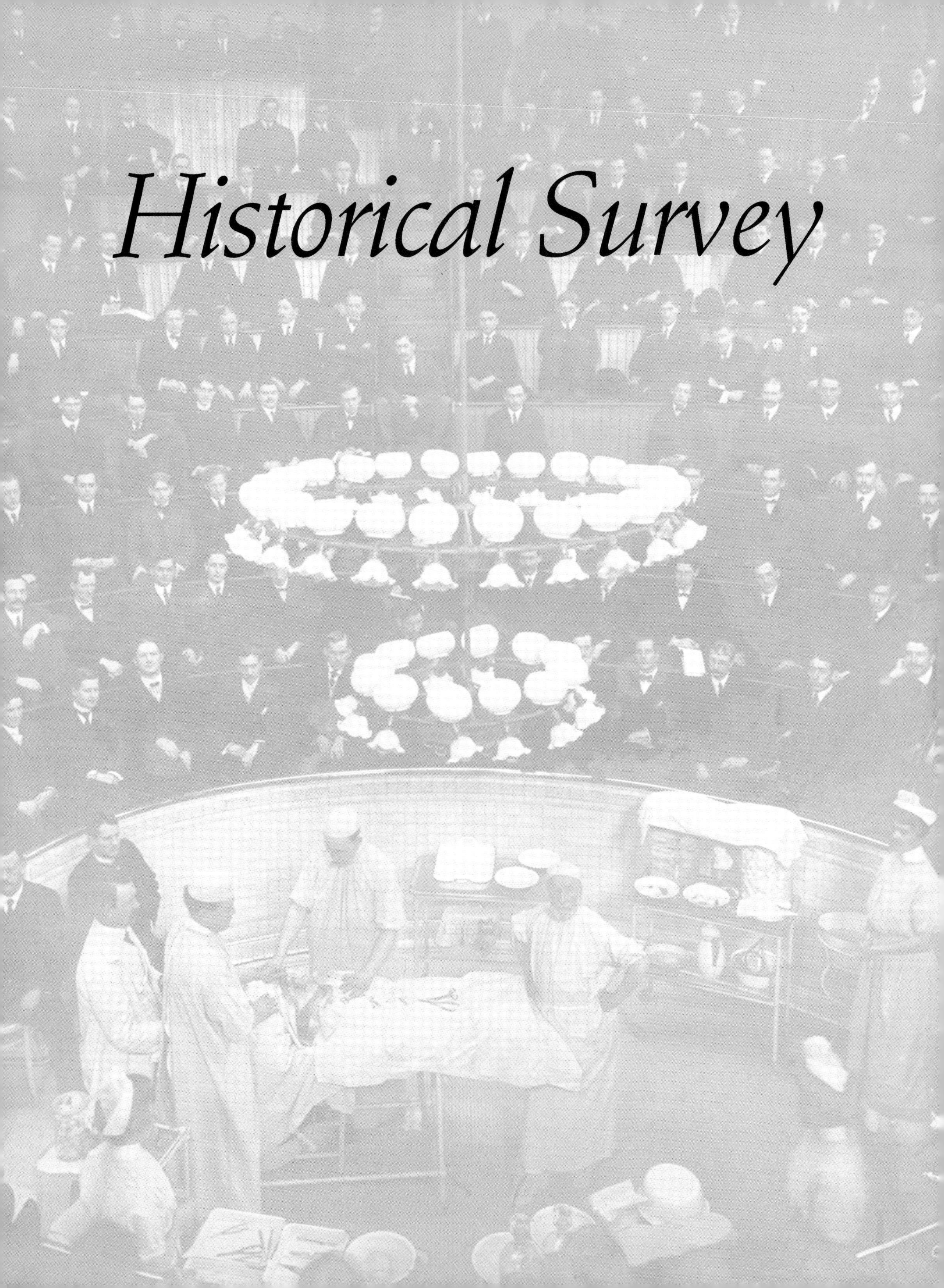

CHAPTER 1

The Early Years (1824-40)

The Jefferson art collection is fortunate to have acquired fine arts and artifacts related to most of its early professors and benefactors. These period paintings, sculptures, prints, furniture, and documents illuminate the early history of the institution. Their presence indicates an early predilection for collecting, preserving, and exhibiting such images and memorabilia.

Jefferson Medical College of Philadelphia was originally established as the medical department of Jefferson College, a small liberal arts college located in Canonsburg in western Pennsylvania. The charter for Jefferson Medical College was granted by the Pennsylvania state legislature in 1824. Dr. George McClellan is the physician most closely associated with the earliest history of the school.

McClellan was born in Woodstock, Connecticut in 1796 and educated at the Woodstock Academy where his father was principal. After graduation from Yale College he immediately began the study of medicine in the office of Dr. Thomas Hubbard in Pomfret, Connecticut. In 1817 he came to Philadelphia as a private pupil of Dr. John Syng Dorsey, a professor of materia medica and anatomy in the medical department of the University of Pennsylvania. McClellan enrolled at the university where he graduated in 1819, and while a resident medical student at the Philadelphia Almshouse he is said to have worked tirelessly day and night in the dissecting room. McClellan elected to remain in Philadelphia and with his indomitable energy and talent was soon known as a bold surgeon.

Because of his great intelligence, a vivacious and agreeable manner, and a desire to transmit his extraordinary knowledge, he began to deliver lectures on anatomy and surgery privately. The lecture room was next to his office in his home at Walnut and Swanwick Streets (the latter ran between Sixth and Seventh Streets), directly north of Potter's Field (now Washington Square). The success of these lectures soon prompted a move to larger quarters to accommodate an increasing number of students.

He found space at the nearby home of the noted artist Rembrandt Peale (1778-1860), who had fitted out his home at Swanwick and George (now Sansom) Streets with a picture gallery known as The Apollodorian. With promotional objectives similar to those of McClellan's school, Peale had raised the roof of his stable and added skylights for public display (with entrance fee) of his portraits, landscapes, and history paintings in order to show his skills in different genres to prospective clients.

To increase the range of subjects offered in his popular lectures at the rear of Peale's gallery, McClellan became associated with Dr. John Eberle who delivered the lectures on materia medica and practice. During this period McClellan had become an ardent advocate and acknowledged leader in the movement to form a second medical college in Philadelphia, and his reputation as a superior teacher helped to consolidate and strengthen the drive for a second school.

Although the University of Pennsylvania had blocked all previous attempts to win approval from the Pennsylvania state legislature to grant a charter for a new medical school, George McClellan with colleagues John Eberle, M.D., Joseph Klapp, M.D., and Jacob Green, devised an ingenious strategy to circumvent this barrier. In 1824 they convinced the trustees at Jefferson College to create a medical school in Philadelphia, with them as its first professors. The charter was granted by the legislature on October 30, 1824.

However, the University of Pennsylvania and its allies in the state legislature challenged the right of Jefferson to award diplomas to its graduates. Drs. McClellan and Eberle made several trips to the capital, Harrisburg, to lobby in favor of a bill to enable Jefferson to grant medical degrees and to create a board of trustees in Philadelphia. McClellan never lost his determination, and when he learned that the bill was coming up for a final vote on April 7, 1826 he enlisted the aid of a powerful legislator to speak on its behalf. Throwing caution to the wind, McClellan drove a horse and buggy all day and night to attend this session when the bill finally passed. In 1838 the charter was revised to separate Jefferson Medical College in Philadelphia from Jefferson College in Canonsburg, allowing the medical school's trustees to be financially independent and to acquire property.

Forty-five years after McClellan's lobbying Professor Samuel D. Gross, M.D. delivered a first anniversary address to the alumni association of Jefferson Medical

College, saying that McClellan more than anyone else was the "master-spirit" and the "main agent" in the founding of the college; that he was "boundless in ambition, and untiring in energy and perseverance, [and] the word failure found no place in his vocabulary."

But by the session of 1838-39 the thriving school was beset by faculty dissension over policy and fees and rebellion against McClellan's now dictatorial and sometimes erratic domination. The board of trustees thereby dissolved the faculty. Most members requested reappointment, but not Dr. McClellan, and he was not reelected. Though mortified by this rejection, the resourceful McClellan was successful in 1839 in starting another new school which lasted almost two decades: the Medical Department of Pennsylvania College at Gettysburg. Again quarrels arose and in 1843 McClellan resigned his professorship and spent the rest of his career in clinical practice. He died suddenly in 1847 at the age of fifty-one.

Thomas Jefferson University is fortunate to own several contemporary images in a variety of media of founder George McClellan, M.D., as well as personal objects owned by him. Depictions include a mid-nineteenth-century daguerreotype, three marble busts, several portrait engravings, as well as a modern oil painting (copied from a lithograph after an original photograph). Artifacts include written notes on arguments in favor of chartering the Jefferson Medical College, class lecture notes, correspondence, his personal calling card, his University of Pennsylvania medical school diploma, and a magnificent mahogany secretary-desk.

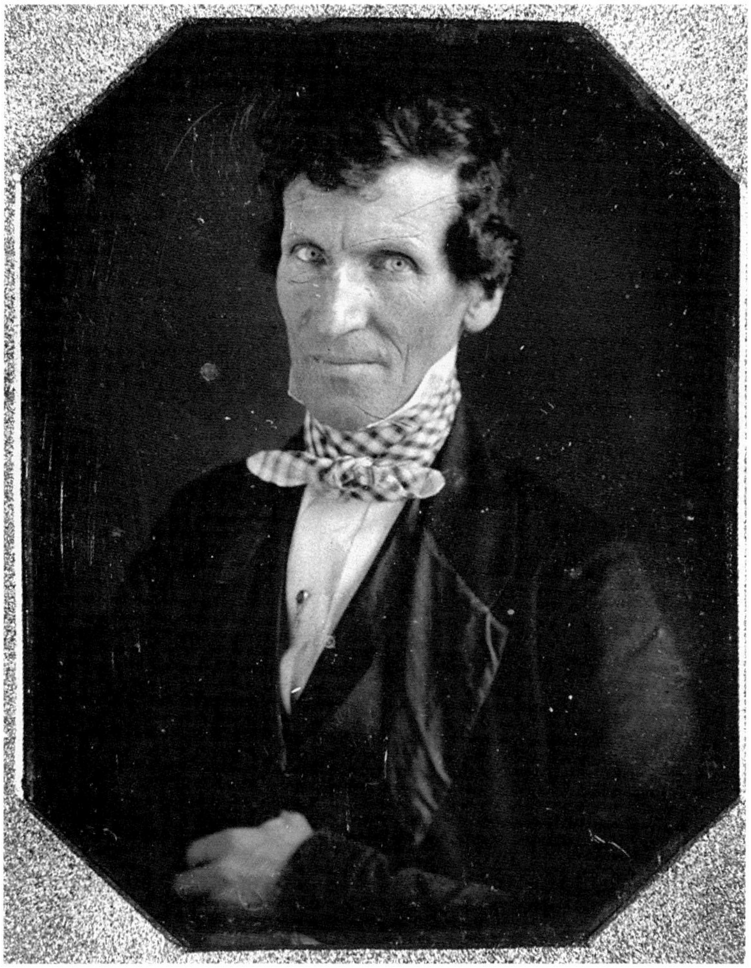

Portrait of George McClellan

GEORGE McCLELLAN, M.D. (1796-1847)
By firm of John Plumbe Jr. (active 1840-47)

Daguerreotype
1844-47
3 1/8 x 2 3/4 in.

Inscription: leather case stamped: "PLUMBE/ MANUFACTURER/NY"

Given after 1870 by unknown donor
Accession number: 1870+f.Ph.03

In a daguerreotype made by the firm of John Plumbe Jr., McClellan is shown bust length with arms placed in front of his body. He glances out of the corner of his eyes with a lively expression. A notable feature of his attire is the jaunty checkered neckwear ending with an unusually long and thin bow.

As was customary with daguerreotypes, the photograph is displayed in its own handsome leather case with a decorative imprint. The lid of the maroon case is stamped "Plumbe Manufacturer NY." The inside is lined in padded red silk (velvet started to replace silk linings around 1843).[1] The case's interior mat of sheet brass is octagonal, a shape popular in the 1840s.

The daguerreotype of Dr. McClellan is a rare vintage photograph in remarkably good condition, considering its fragile material and age. The daguerreotype process itself, one of the earliest forms of photography, was not invented until 1839. The university's undated photograph must have been made no later than 1847, the year Dr. McClellan died and the year that John Plumbe sold his galleries, and no earlier than 1844 when Plumbe began manufacturing his own cases in New York.

The daguerreotype process involved the exposure of a copper plate coated with a thin sheet of highly polished silver to the action of iodine vapor which made the silver surface sensitive to light. When the plate was placed in the camera it was exposed to the action of light. After exposure the latent image was developed by mercury vapor, plunged into cold water to harden the surface, and submerged into a solution of common salt and hot water to dissolve the particles of silver iodine not affected by the light. The resulting image was mounted under glass. The earliest daguerreotypes required outdoor light and posing times as long as fifteen minutes, but advances were very quickly made in lighting and posing specifications.

John Plumbe Jr., one of the first Americans to establish a reputation as a daguerreotypist, was as energetic, inventive, ambitious, and sometimes erratic as Dr. George McClellan. Born in Wales in 1809, Plumbe emigrated to the United States with his family in 1821 and by age twenty-three was superintendent of a southern railroad. He soon won notoriety as one of the first persons to advocate a transcontinental railroad. Toward this goal he organized citizens' meetings, wrote extensively in the newspapers, and petitioned Congress which awarded him two thousand dollars for a survey in Wisconsin.

It is not known where Plumbe learned the new photographic art, but he turned to the technique in order to earn a livelihood while promoting his railroad interests in the east. His daguerreotype career began in Boston in late 1840, and in a few months he was known there as a "professor of photography;" having opened a studio called the United States Photographic Institute. By 1841 he was distributing wholesale daguerreotype materials and was giving instructions in Boston. He had his own case manufactory in New York from 1844 to 1847.[2]

Plumbe opened a second gallery in Philadelphia at 173 Chestnut Street in late 1841. By mid-1843 he had galleries (called "depots") in New York, Baltimore, Albany, and Saratoga Springs. Soon thereafter his chain of photographic galleries could also be found in Washington, New Orleans, St. Louis, Newport, Louisville, Cincinnati, Dubuque, Iowa, Portland, Maine, and Norfolk and Petersburg, Virginia; and abroad in Paris and Liverpool. The portraits made in each branch were stamped with Plumbe's name on the mat or on the case, regardless of the identity of the actual photographer.

In late 1842 John Plumbe bought the patent rights for coloring daguerreotypes by electrolysis from the inventor. The entrepreneurial Plumbe also solved the problem of providing patrons with multiple copies of their photograph by employing artists to copy the original daguerreotype by means of lithography, a technique he called "Plumbeotype." Many of his celebrity portraits were featured in his publication, the *National Plumbeotype Gallery*. John Plumbe was very proud of having won eight medals and other awards from the American, Mechanic's, and Franklin Institutes for "the most Splendid Coloured Daguerreotypes" and "best Apparatus."

Because of his constant travel, too rapid expansion of his enterprises, and the alleged dishonesty of some of his gallery agents, Plumbe met financial disaster in 1847 and had to sell his galleries to meet the demands of his creditors. After this failure he joined the hopeful throngs in the gold rush of 1849 but his California venture was not successful. He became despondent and died in 1857 by his own hand at his brother's home in Dubuque.

Portrait of George McClellan

GEORGE McCLELLAN, M.D.
Attributed to Hugh Cannon (ca. 1814-ca. 1864)

Marble
Ca. 1840-60
22 7/8 x 13 3/4 x 10 1/4 in.

Given in 1877 by John H. Brinton, M.D. who had received it from his aunt, Mrs. John Grigg, sister of the subject
Accession number: 1877+e.S.01

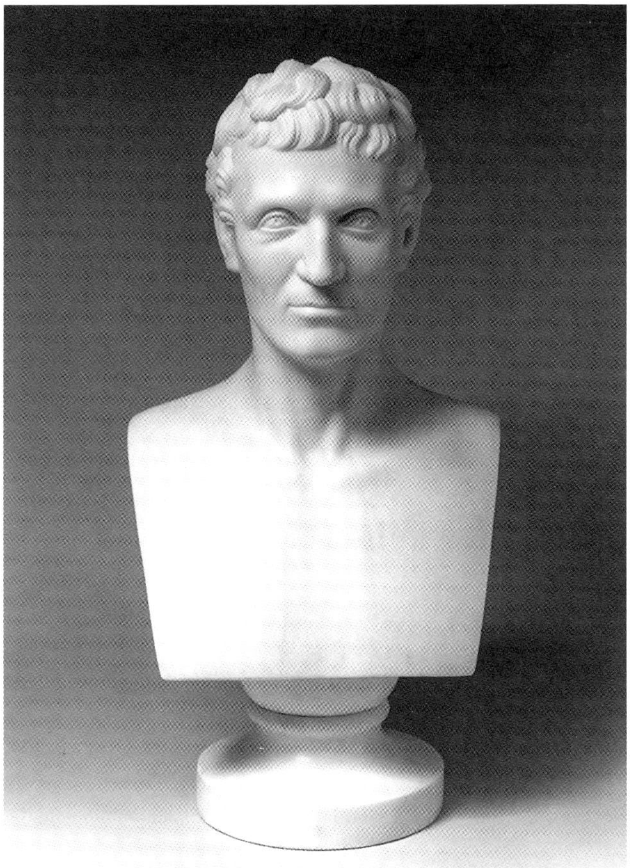

The Jefferson board of trustees minutes of March 9, 1877 record a letter from Dr. John H. Brinton about presenting an "original marble bust by Cannon" of Dr. George McClellan. Brinton received the bust from his aunt, Mrs. John Grigg, a sister of Dr. McClellan. Nancy McClellan Grigg stated that the "most proper" place for the bust's "preservation" was "beneath the roof of the renowned Institution of which he was the founder."

The trustees promptly placed the unsigned portrait bust in a prominent position on a shelf over the south entrance doors of the amphitheater of the first Jefferson hospital of 1877. It is shown still in place in a turn-of-the-century photograph of a hospital clinic in the amphitheater, and its location is confirmed in Dr. George Gould's *The Jefferson Medical College of Philadelphia: A History* (1904).

An 1881 *Report of the Trustees of the Jefferson Medical College of Philadelphia to the Contributors to the Jefferson Medical College Hospital* also documents that in March 1877, Mrs. N. M. Grigg presented the original marble bust by Cannon and that the bust, "with an appropriate inscription," had by 1881 been placed over the arena of the clinical amphitheater. The bust has no inscription today, but the identification might have been attached to the supporting shelf, not carved into the figure or its integral base.

Except for a pronounced aquiline nose, the image of McClellan conforms to the typical nineteenth-century, neoclassical style in which the sitter's features are idealized. This is especially true in the regularized, thick curls of hair (recalling Roman emperors), and in the absence of any signs of age on the figure's smoothly polished face. The shoulders are squared off and the corners of the chest are angular.

Hugh Cannon was in Philadelphia for two years before McClellan departed, so there was adequate time for him to have depicted the physician from life, or even later from a photograph. The Jefferson sculpture is not similar stylistically to a Cannon self-portrait at the Pennsylvania Academy of the Fine Arts. There are only a few extant sculptures by Hugh Cannon, so making a firm attribution is difficult without further research of other works.

Scholars differ as to whether Cannon was born in Ireland or Pennsylvania, and no information is yet available about his early days. He was listed in Philadelphia city directories variously as a marble mason, carver, sculptor, and agent between 1837 and 1863. Sculptures were commonly unsigned in this period.

Hugh Cannon exhibited works intermittently at the Artists' Fund Society and annuals at the Pennsylvania Academy of the Fine Arts in Philadelphia, and at the Apollo Association in New York. Documented portrait subjects include Chief Justice Marshall, Henry Clay, Edwin Forrest, Nicholas Biddle, Daniel W. Coxe, and a self-portrait.

The two other unsigned busts of Dr. McClellan are similar in size, style, and probable date of origin. They have sloping shoulders and rounded corners of the chest, unlike the more angular bust pictured in the amphitheater. Neither could be the bust mentioned in Dr. Brinton's letter.

Portrait of George McClellan

GEORGE McCLELLAN, M.D.
By unknown artist

Marble
Mid-nineteenth century
15 7/8 x 10 x 7 1/2 in.

Given in 1929 by Mrs. McClellan, a descendant of the subject
Accession number: 1929+e.S.01

Portrait of George McClellan

GEORGE McCLELLAN, M.D.
By unknown artist

Marble
Mid-nineteenth century
19 1/2 x 14 1/8 x 9 3/8 in.

Given before 1925 by JMC alumni association
Accession number: 1925+b.S.01

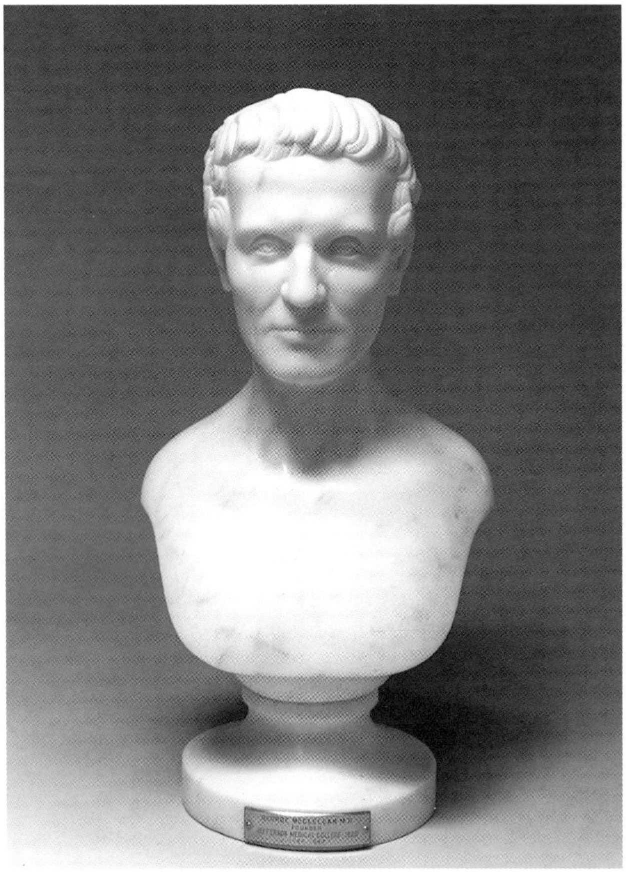

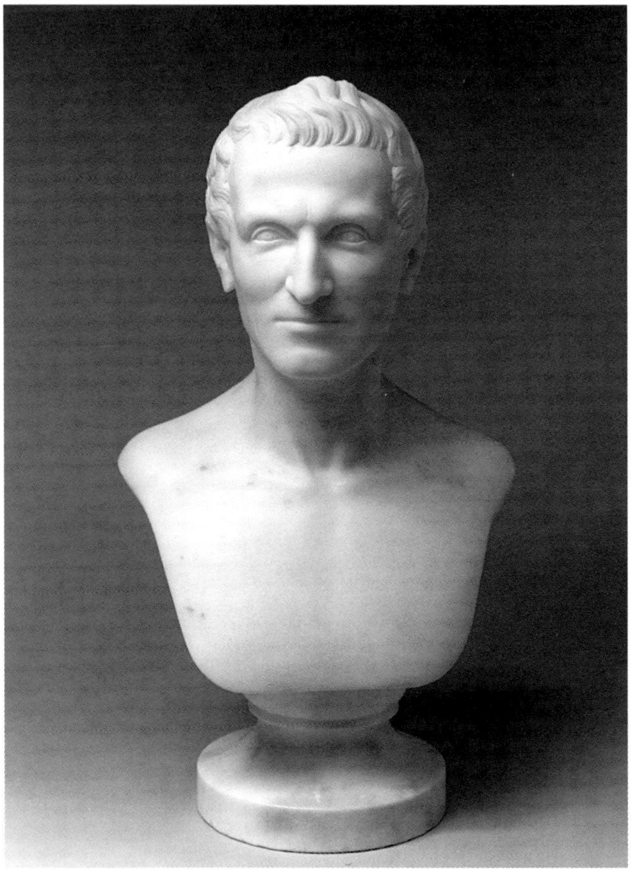

The *Jefferson Medical College Alumni Bulletin* of January 1930 announced that a McClellan bust, "worked in Italian marble," had recently been presented by Dean Ross V. Patterson, M.D., to whom it was given by a "Mrs. McClellan," with no further information provided. This is probably a second bust seen in a 1975 photograph of Dean William F. Kellow, M.D.'s office.

In an informal history of the alumni association written in the mid-1920s, Dean Patterson stated that among other "adornments" the alumni association had given a bust of McClellan, implying that this donation was early in the history of the association (founded in 1870). This must be the third bust of McClellan which in 1955 was moved for a time to the stage of McClellan Hall in the College Building.

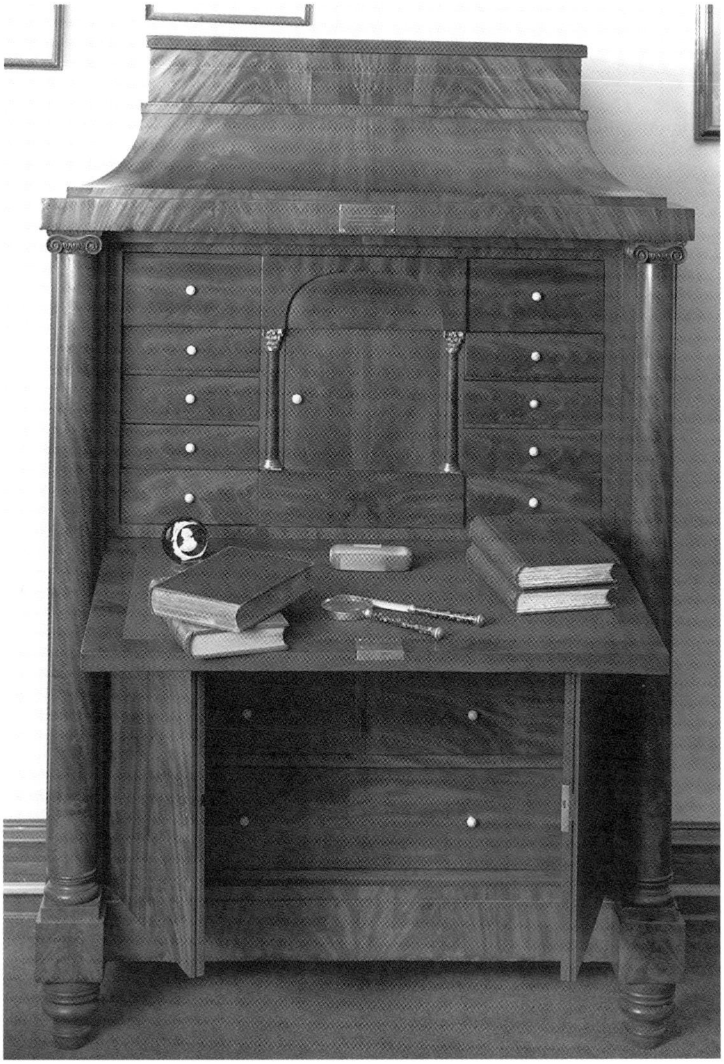

Secretary-Desk

(See color plate)

SECRETARY-DESK
By unknown American craftsman

Mahogany, with white pine secondary wood
1820-40
63 x 41 5/8 x 21 in.

Given ca. 1938 by bequest of Dean Ross V. Patterson, M.D.
Accession number: 1938+c.DA.01

One of the most important pieces of furniture in the Jefferson collection is a handsome secretary-desk thought to have been owned by George McClellan, M.D. It is in the American classical style, a simplified and pared-down version of the French Empire style in which veneered surfaces substituted for extensively carved embellishment.

The "McClellan desk" is veneered with matched, crotch-grain mahogany, and has a removable steep cornice. It is fitted with a single shallow drawer at the top and supported upon a pair of freestanding Ionic columns above compressed turnip feet. The columns flank a straight front which is hinged with a fall-front writing board. One of the books now displayed on the writing board is *Principles and Practice of Surgery*, a posthumous work of 1848 edited by Dr. McClellan's son, John H. Brinton McClellan, M.D.

The desk's interior has ten drawers with ivory pulls flanking a central section of a protruding cornice drawer raised on engaged Corinthian half-columns with brass capitals and bases, flanking a door opening to a single shelf. Below the writing board is a pair of cabinet doors opening to a flush interior of four graduated drawers with ivory pulls.

Information about the provenance of the desk comes from an unsigned report dated January 30, 1946 addressed to Dean William H. Perkins, M.D. listing articles in the Jefferson library formerly in the home of Dean Ross V. Patterson, M.D., including "Doctor McClellan's Desk (now in the Museum)" and a small case of McClellan's dissecting instruments. Dr. Patterson never married, and he bequeathed these objects and his estate to Jefferson at his death in 1938. Almost assuredly the desk was given to Dean Patterson by the widow of Dr. George McClellan, grandson of the founder.[3]

Jefferson Medical College at the Tivoli Theater

JEFFERSON MEDICAL COLLEGE
AT THE TIVOLI THEATER
Building by unknown architect

Photograph
By unknown photographer
Ca. 1900
Image size: 4 1/4 x 3 1/4 in.
Sheet size: 10 1/4 x 8 in.

Given after 1900 by unknown donor
Accession number: 1900+f.Ph.14

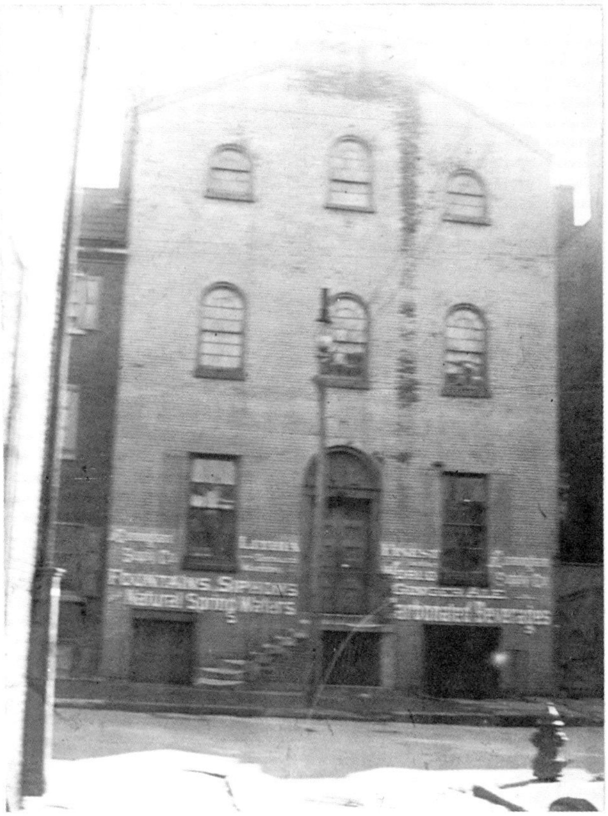

In 1825 Dr. George McClellan and his colleagues rented a building at 518-520 Prune Street (now Locust Walk) for Jefferson Medical College's first meeting place. Originally a cotton factory, in 1820 the premises had been converted to a theater, known first as the Winter Tivoli Theater and then the City Theater. It is said that Edwin Forrest appeared there as a young actor and that the beloved song "Home Sweet Home" was first performed in America there. After the medical school vacated the building in 1829, the old structure was used for various manufacturing purposes until destroyed by fire in the 1920s. The architect of the original building is unknown.

In this vintage, turn-of-the-century photograph one can read blurred signs on the wall advertising the Cunningham Supply Company, a bottler of ginger ale and other beverages, and a manufacturer of siphons and fountains. The facade of the utilitarian brick building has a low peaked roof, an arched fanlight entrance and arched windows on the second and third floors, and rectangular windows on the raised first floor.

Professor John Chalmers DaCosta, M.D., a distinguished surgeon who was interested in Jefferson history, remembered the largely unwholesome neighborhood surrounding the original medical college:

> Directly across the street from the college was the Walnut Street Prison for criminals and debtors, one of the rules of which was that the yard must be "kept free from cows, hogs, dogs, and fowls." On the east the college looked out directly on the burial ground of the Free Quakers...To the west...was the potter's field... Directly back of the college was an ale house, and a block or two away were several churches. Crime and misery in front, death on either hand, and manifold consolations in the rear![4]

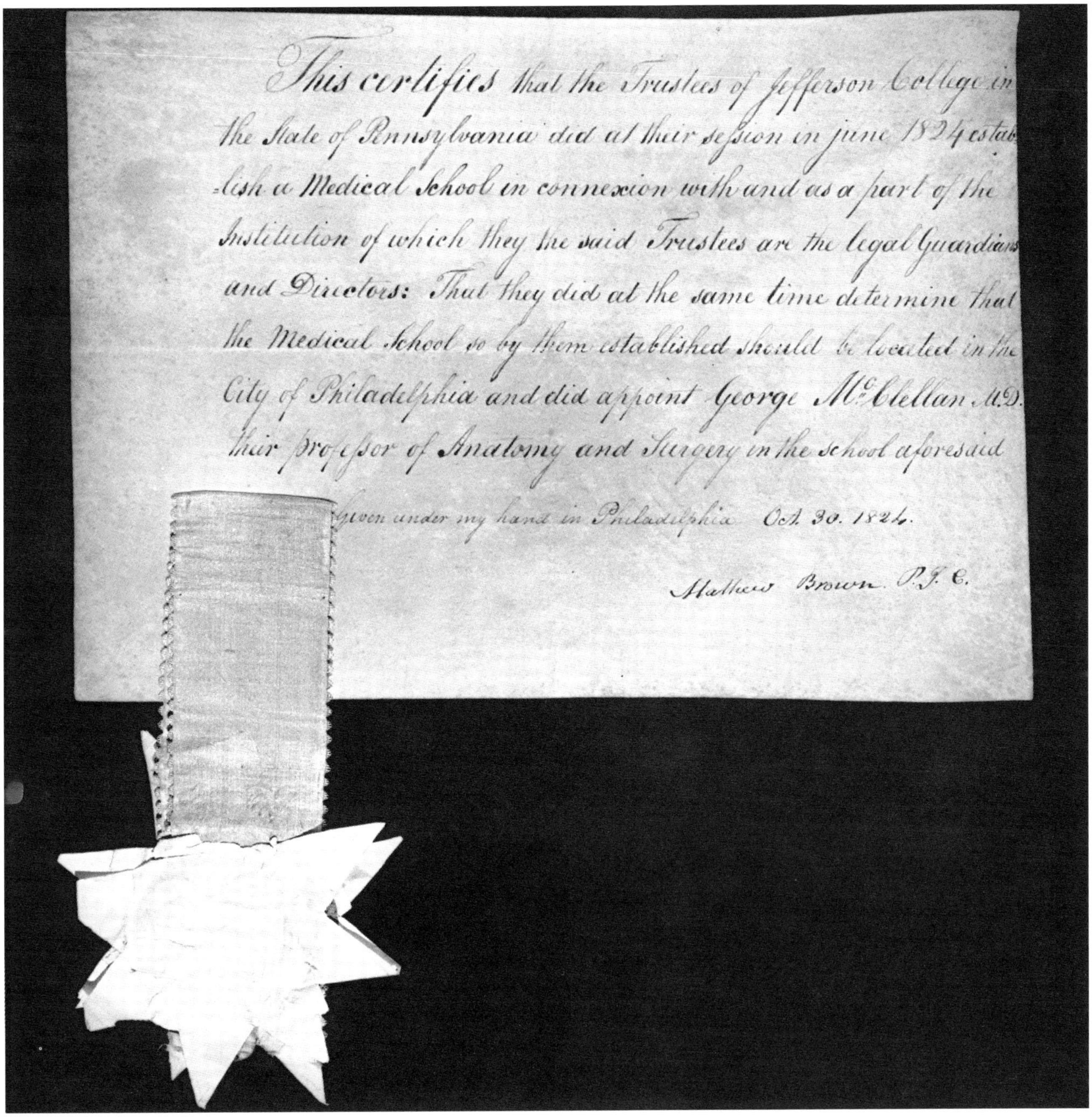
This certifies that the Trustees of Jefferson College in the State of Pennsylvania did at their session in june 1824 establish a Medical School in connexion with and as a part of the Institution of which they the said Trustees are the legal Guardians and Directors: That they did at the same time determine that the Medical School so by them established should be located in the City of Philadelphia and did appoint George M^c^Clellan M.D. their professor of Anatomy and Surgery in the school aforesaid

Given under my hand in Philadelphia Oct. 30. 1824.

Mathew Brown P.J.C.

Certificate of Jefferson Medical College

CERTIFICATE OF JEFFERSON MEDICAL COLLEGE

Ink on parchment, fabric ribbon, paper/wax/resin seal
1824
6 3/4 x 9 3/4 in.

Signed and dated: "Oct. 30. 1824./ Mathew Brown. P.J.C."

Given probably after 1880 by unknown donor
Accession number: 1880+f.Ms.01

The discovery of the only known copy of Jefferson Medical College's "birth certificate" was mysteriously connected with the physician Atkinson Pelham, a member of Jefferson Medical College's first class of 1826. The document lay hidden away for decades, and had long been searched for at Thomas Jefferson University and at Washington and Jefferson University (formerly Jefferson College). It was found serendipitously in 1989 in Dean Joseph S. Gonnella, M.D.'s "vault," a large, cabinet-lined storage closet.

I had invited the former University Librarian, Robert

T. Lentz, M.S., to accompany me in an investigation of the vault, in the hope of finding art objects or art-related documentary materials, such as insurance appraisals or records of donations. In the midst of a survey of the room's contents, most of which were dust-covered records of little interest to us, I noticed a decorative old frame on the uppermost shelf of the last cabinet to be inspected. Upon examining it, Mr. Lentz almost fell off his ladder from excitement when he realized he was holding "the" certificate.

After our initial exhilaration over the find subsided, we enlisted the service of a paper conservator to preserve the document. When the frame and its backing were removed, we were surprised to find a mounted photograph of about 1880 of William H. Pancoast, M.D. with a group of anatomy students gathered around a dissected cadaver. Evidently the photograph had previously been displayed in this frame and the certificate was folded in four to fit the frame and to be stored away for safekeeping. Then long forgotten!

The 1824 document was written in iron gall ink and is still extremely legible, probably because of storage away from the deleterious effects of daylight. The signature of Mathew Brown and date seem to be executed by a different hand than the text; Mathew (usually "Matthew") Brown was then the president of Jefferson College. Typically for this period, the document text crowds against the far right edge of the parchment skin.

A paper seal is adhered to a sky-blue fabric ribbon which is laced through two parallel slits in the lower left corner of the parchment. The embossed seal was created by applying two eight-pointed paper stars to either side of a warm wax/resin wafer at the end of the doubled ribbon. A two-sided matrix was used to impress the seal design. The fragile points of the paper stars were badly creased, folded, and torn. The document itself was creased, stained, and covered with surface grime. The conservation process included surface cleaning, humidification, and flattening and reinforcing of the creases.

The document reads:

> This certifies that the Trustees of Jefferson College in/the State of Pennsylvania did at their session in june 1824 estab/lish a Medical School in connexion with and as a part of the/Institution of which they the said Trustees are the legal Guardians/and Directors: That they did at the same time determine that/the Medical School so by them established should be located in the/City of Philadelphia and did appoint George McClellan M.D./their professor of Anatomy and Surgery in the school aforesaid.
>
> Given under my hand in Philadelphia Oct. 30.1824.
> Mathew Brown. P.J.C.

On the reverse side of the certificate is the name "Atkinson Pelham" written twice in ink and once in pencil. It is not known how this document came to be in the possession of alumnus Atkinson Pelham, M.D. (1797-1880) or why he signed it. After graduation from Jefferson Medical College Dr. Pelham established a practice first in North Carolina and then in Alexandria, Alabama where he also owned a thousand-acre plantation on land purchased from his father-in-law, William McGehee. Coincidentally, a contemporary Jeffersonian, Edward H. McGehee, M.D., originally of Mobile, Alabama and an alumnus of the class of 1945, is a direct descendant of Dr. Atkinson Pelham's mother.

In February 1912 Dr. George McClellan, grandson of the first George McClellan, gave a banquet talk to various college societies about his grandfather's contributions to the founding of Jefferson Medical College. When talking about events at the session of the Pennsylvania legislature in 1824 in which the college was established, he said, "I am glad...to show you this all-important bit of parchment which my grandfather brought back with him and which is the first charter of the college. It is dated October 30, 1824." It is not known whether this is the same document once in the possession of Dr. Atkinson Pelham; there may have been more than one copy of the certificate.

The birth certificate now hangs in the office of the dean of Jefferson Medical College. Almost exact replicas using authentic period materials were crafted in 1990 for the offices of Jefferson's president and the board of trustees.

Portraits of Dr. John Eberle and Mrs. John Eberle

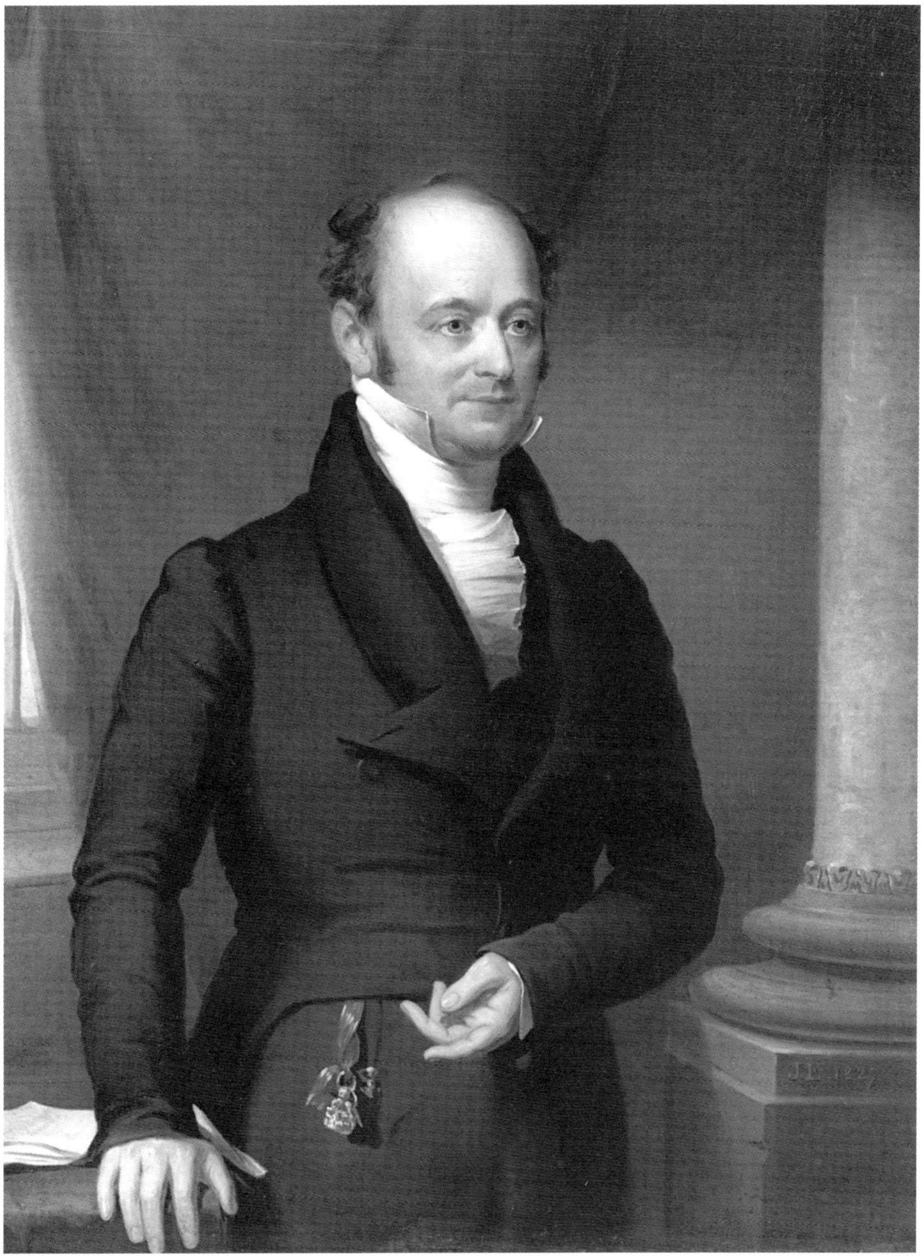

JOHN EBERLE, M.D.
(1787-1838)
By Jacob Eichholtz
(1776-1842)
(See color plate)
Oil on canvas mounted on masonite
1827
43 1/4 x 33 in.

Signed and dated lower right: "J.E. 1827"
Exhibition: Philadelphia, *The Art of Philadelphia Medicine,* Philadelphia Museum of Art, 1965

Given in 1950 by Charles Eberle Piety, great-grandson of the subject
Accession number: 1950+e.P.01

Dr. John Eberle was a co-founder of Jefferson Medical College and a distinguished professor, author, and editor. However, his career at Jefferson Medical College was even more short-lived than that of Dr. George McClellan and it was correspondingly troubled.

John Eberle's parents were German immigrants who established a farm in Lancaster where his father worked as a blacksmith. The industrious boy was an avid reader who mastered three foreign languages. He began his study of medicine with a local country doctor. He moved to Philadelphia and received an M.D. from the University of Pennsylvania in 1809 and entered the office of Dr. Joseph Klapp, his preceptor. After a brief attempt at establishing a medical practice in Lancaster, he settled in Philadelphia in the late teens. There he founded and edited the *American Medical Recorder* and soon published a two-volume book, *Treatise on the Materia Medica and Therapeutics* (1823).

After the founding of Jefferson Medical College in 1824 Eberle was first professor of the theory and practice of medicine and midwifery and then of materia medica, and served as dean from 1827 to 1828. He was a meticulous and scholarly, if monotonous, lecturer, and was admired by his students for his erudition. Because revenues from the college failed to support his growing family, in 1831 Dr. Eberle moved to Cincinnati to join the faculty of the newly merged Medical College of Ohio and the medical department of Miami University.

There Eberle founded and edited the *Western Medical Gazette* with Dr. Daniel Drake, also a former professor at Jefferson Medical College. Ensuing faculty quarrels and uncertain finances in Ohio forced Eberle to move again in 1837, this time to Transylvania University in Lexington, Kentucky where he became an editor of the *Transylvania Journal of Medicine*. Eberle had long suffered from a chronic abdominal disorder, and already careworn and ill he died prematurely at the age of fifty in 1838. Tragically he left his wife and eight children in an impecunious state.

Dr. John Eberle's considerable fame rested on the clarity and originality of his textbooks and editorial skills, rather than on his clinical practice or teaching. Like his text on therapeutics, many other books went through multiple editions including: *Notes of Lectures on the Theory and Practice of Medicine Delivered in the Jefferson Medical College* (1827), *A Treatise on the Practice of Medicine* (1830), and *A Treatise on the Diseases and Physical Education of Children* (1833).

While residing in Philadelphia Dr. Eberle commissioned Jacob Eichholtz to paint his own portrait in 1827 and that of his wife in 1831, a period when he was evidently confident about his circumstances. The companion pictures share elements common to "grand manner" portraits which made middle-class American sitters resemble English aristocracy in their manners and dress. Both elegantly dressed subjects are situated in a generic room boasting architectural columns and swags of maroon drapery. Mrs. Eberle's portrait has a glimpse of landscape in the distance, a conventional suggestion of property ownership.

Socially, Eberle is said to have been of melancholy temperament, retiring, and embarrassed by his lingering German accent. He was of short and "dumpy" stature, and earned the nickname of the "German tripod" for his usual stance of standing with legs far apart and leaning on a table with his right hand, as depicted in Eichholtz's portrait. The doctor's expression is somber and his partially turned figure gazes into the distance. But he appears proud to point toward an elaborate gold watch fob hanging below his waist and toward a pile of lecture notes or manuscript papers on the table.

SALOME (MRS. JOHN) EBERLE
By Jacob Eichholtz

Oil on canvas mounted on masonite
1831
43 1/4 x 33 1/4 in.

Given in 1951 by Charles Eberle Piety, great-grandson of the subject
Accession number: 1951+e.P.01

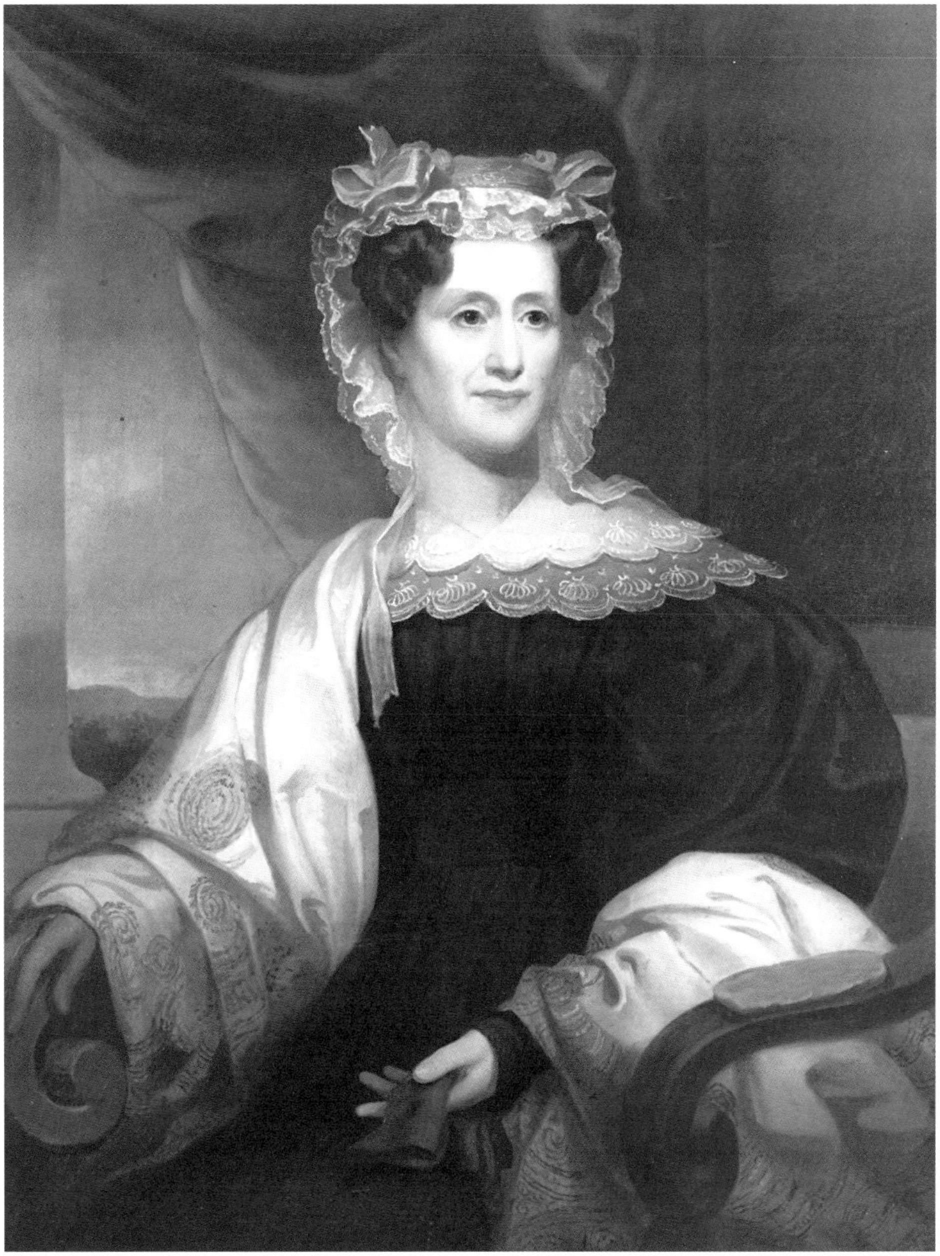

Exuding a suitably confident expression, Salome Eberle sits in a fine period armchair, turning her body to display her elaborate costume to best advantage. Her black Empire dress with puffed sleeves is set off by a scalloped collar of ruffled white organdy and an organdy and ribbon headpiece. Her white satin stole is decorated with colored, circular paisley patterns. Her gloved right hand grasps the curving chair arm, and she holds the other gray glove in her left hand.

Records show that Dr. Eberle paid sixty dollars for both portraits.[5] Probably they were in his family's possession for over a century until their donation in 1950 and 1951 by Dr. Eberle's great-grandson, Charles Eberle Piety of Terre Haute, Indiana.

Dr. John Eberle and painter Jacob Eichholtz were not only contemporaries, but both had spent their formative years in Lancaster, Pennsylvania and both were of German descent. However, Eberle was able to pursue his career undeviatingly, while circumstances forced Eichholtz to delay a full-time career as an artist.

The painter never enjoyed the advantages of a formal education and was largely self-taught, but he demonstrated a similar determination to succeed. His only early art instruction was from a local sign painter, and Eichholtz established a business as an expert coppersmith in 1802. "Haunted" by his more "agreeable" love of painting, he devoted some time to painting portraits of local clients and studying the work and writings of established artists.

In return for using his studio while in Lancaster, the celebrated artist Thomas Sully gave Eichholtz some of his half-worn brushes as well as instruction and encouragement in 1809. Eichholtz boldly paid a visit to the renowned Boston painter Gilbert Stuart and showed Stuart his own portrait of Nicholas Biddle, president of the United States Bank. Accounts differ as to whether Stuart's criticism was harsh or heartening, but by 1812 Eichholtz turned exclusively to painting as a career.

Eichholtz's portraits emulated the compositions of fashionable painters of the day, especially Sully and Stuart, while maintaining his own essentially linear style with its emphasis on detail.

Early in his painting career Eichholtz led an itinerant life, traveling to Philadelphia, Harrisburg, and Baltimore to seek portrait commissions. Starting in 1823 he set up his studio in Philadelphia and was successful in gaining portrait commissions from sitters prominent in society, business, and the professions. He exhibited his work at the Society of American Artists from 1811 to 1814 and almost annually at the Pennsylvania Academy of the Fine Arts from 1823 until 1842. In 1831 he returned to Lancaster where he bought a house for his large family, but traveled frequently to Philadelphia for commissions until his death in 1842.

Portrait of Jacob Green

JACOB GREEN, M.D. (hon.) (1790-1841)
By John Sartain (1808-97)

Mezzotint, etching, engraving
Before 1858
Image size: 4 3/4 x 3 7/8 in.
Plate size: 6 5/8 x 5 1/2 in.
Sheet size: 10 3/4 x 8 1/8 in.

Inscriptions below image: "Painted by H. Bridport." and "Engraved & Printed by J. Sartain."; facsimile signature "Jacob Green"; "PROFESSOR OF CHEMISTRY IN JEFFERSON MEDICAL COLLEGE PHILADELPHIA."

From the "Murray Scrapbook," given in 1974-75 by Mrs. John A. Murray, R.N. (JMC Nursing 1928), widow of John A. Murray, M.D. (JMC 1931)
Accession number: 1974-1975.Pr.03

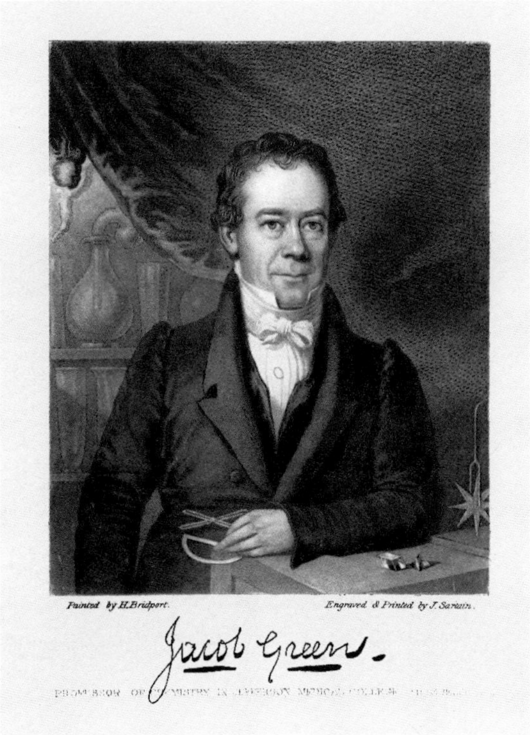

Jacob Green was the first professor of chemistry at Jefferson Medical College. His career at Jefferson was the longest of any of the four founders.

Born in Philadelphia in 1790, he was the youngest son of Ashbel Green, president of the College of New Jersey (later Princeton). Jacob Green was interested in science from boyhood and earned undergraduate degrees at the University of Pennsylvania (1807) and Rutgers (1812). After a brief period of practicing law in Philadelphia, he accepted a professorship in chemistry, natural history, and experimental philosophy at Princeton in 1818, remaining for four years.

Soon after his appointment as the first professor of chemistry at Jefferson, it is said that "Old Jaky" was beloved by his students and colleagues. His *Text-book of Chemical Philosophy on the Basis of Dr. Turner's Elements of Chemistry* was published in 1829. The mild-mannered professor weathered the "turbulent storms" of Jefferson's earliest decades and remained until his death in 1841 at age fifty.

Green received honorary A.M. degrees from Rutgers and Princeton, honorary M.D. and LL.D. degrees from Jefferson, and an honorary M.D. from Yale.

In the mezzotint by John Sartain, Professor Green is shown half length, resting his forearm against a table and looking out toward the viewer. He stands in front of a curtain which reveals several glass flasks on shelves, and the setting also includes prisms and various measuring devices.

John Sartain's undated engraving after an original oil painting by Hugh Bridport was published in Dr. James F. Gayley's 1858 book, *A History of the Jefferson Medical College of Philadelphia*. The painting's date is unknown, but even if it were taken from life, the engraving could have been posthumous, so therefore the book's publication date, not the sitter's dates, is a *terminus ante quem* for the Sartain print.

Hugh Bridport (1794-ca. 1869) was born in London and studied at the Royal Academy there. He came to Philadelphia about 1816 and opened a drawing academy with his brother. He conducted an architectural drawing school with architect John Haviland (1792-1852), and engraved all the plates for Haviland's book *The Builder's Assistant* (1818). Besides teaching drawing, Bridport painted portraits and miniatures and also practiced engraving and lithography. He exhibited regularly at the Pennsylvania Academy of the Fine Arts, where he was made an academician in 1824, and at the Artists' Fund Society. He was an original member of the Franklin Institute.

Also a native of London, John Sartain was an engraver and a painter of portraits and miniatures who emigrated to Philadelphia in 1830. For the next two decades he was an illustrator for and publisher of magazines, including one for which he had controlling interest and which he renamed *Sartain's Magazine*. He was considered the leading mezzotint engraver in the United States. After 1850 he did general engraving including banknote work and also some portrait painting.

John Sartain was a formidable power in Philadelphia's art institutions such as the Pennsylvania Academy of the Fine Arts, the Artists' Fund Society, and the Philadelphia School of Design for Women. He was named chief of the fine arts bureau for the Philadelphia Centennial Exposition (see chapter four), and also was American representative for several international art exhibitions. His autobiography, *The Reminiscences of a Very Old Man, 1808-1897*, was published posthumously.

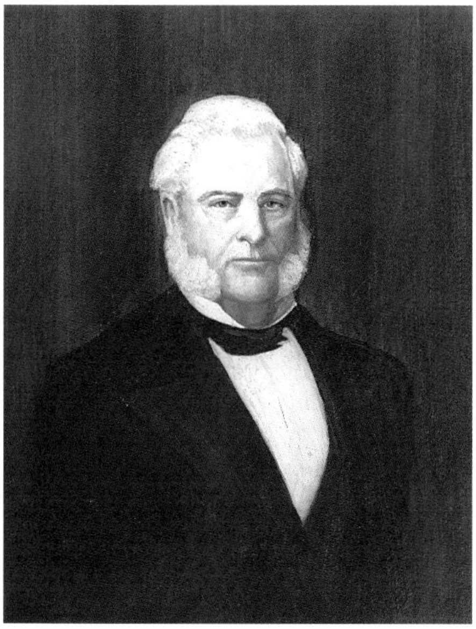

Portrait of Nathan L. Hatfield

NATHAN LEWIS HATFIELD, M.D. (1804-87)
By Agnes Allen (b. 1897)

Oil on canvas
1935
30 1/2 x 25 in.

Signed and dated on reverse of canvas: "DR. N.L. HATFIELD/painted by AGNES ALLEN MARCH, 1935"

Given between 1935 and 1946 by unknown donor
Accession number: 1935-1946.P.01

Dr. Nathan L. Hatfield was a member of the first graduating class of Jefferson Medical College. He was never a member of the Jefferson faculty, but was named chairman of the organizing committee of the college's alumni association and served as its president in 1874 and 1875.

After Nathan L. Hatfield had attended two courses of lectures in medicine at the University of Pennsylvania he transferred to Jefferson Medical College where he graduated in 1826. He oversaw a large and lucrative private practice and was active in local medical societies. He served as president of the City Board of Health and vice president of the Pennsylvania State Medical Society, and was a manager of the Northern Dispensary of Philadelphia and chairman of its committee on physicians.

Dr. Hatfield was a fellow of the College of Physicians of Philadelphia for fifty-two years. In 1917 the Nathan Lewis Hatfield Lectureship was established at the college in his memory by the physician's sons, Walter and Henry. The Nathan Lewis Hatfield Professorship in Urology was established at Jefferson Medical College by bequest of Henry Reed Hatfield in 1946.

In 1935 Agnes Allen painted a posthumous portrait

of Dr. Hatfield, taken after an unknown image. The physician is shown bust length, turned slightly to the right and looking out solemnly toward the viewer. His face is encircled by thick white hair and mutton-chop whiskers. Unfortunately, the painting's surface has been badly eroded over the years.

Agnes Allen was a native Philadelphian who received a bachelor's degree in fine arts at the University of Pennsylvania, and also studied at the Pennsylvania Academy of the Fine Arts and at the Barnes Foundation. She exhibited widely in the forties and fifties and received awards from the Pennsylvania Academy (1947) and the National League of American Pen Women (1948, 1953, and 1955).

Allen was commissioned by many public institutions and private clubs to paint portraits and to make copies of earlier ones. Her paintings can be found in the following Philadelphia collections: the University of Pennsylvania, the Insurance Company of North America, the Mutual Assurance Company, the Drexel Institute, the Westminster Theological Seminary, and the Episcopal Academy, as well as murals at the Mask and Wig Club. She is also represented at the Yale University Law School in New Haven, the American Psychiatric Association in Washington, D.C., and Cooper Hospital in Camden, New Jersey.

Portrait of Ezra S. Ely

EZRA STILES ELY, D.D. (1786-1861)
By unknown artist

Oil on canvas
Ca. 1825-35
15 x 13 in.

Given in 1961 by Francis A. Ely, M.D., grandson of the subject (presented in his behalf by Tom B. Throckmorton, M.D., JMC 1909)
Accession number: 1961+e.P.04

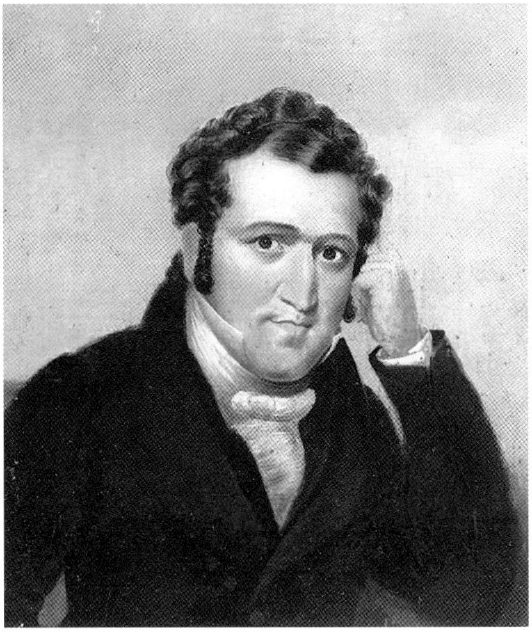

The newly established Jefferson Medical College was so successful in attracting students that the faculty sought larger and more appropriate headquarters soon after the founding. Hampered by a lack of endowment, college expansion was accomplished only through the generosity of the Reverend Dr. Ezra Stiles Ely, who was one of ten "additional trustees" elected by the trustees at Canonsburg in 1826 for the purpose of governing the fledgling medical school in Philadelphia. He would serve as secretary of the medical college's board for many years.

In 1827 a property was secured and the following year a building erected on the west side of Tenth Street, between what are now Sansom and Moravian Streets. The college leased this building from the Reverend Ely, and ultimately purchased it in 1870. The Medical Hall was renovated and enlarged several times and used until 1898 when the college moved to Tenth and Walnut Streets. The original site of Medical Hall is now occupied by the Jefferson Medical College Hospital of 1907.

Reverend Ely was born in Lebanon, Connecticut in 1786. Like his father he was a graduate of Yale College and an ordained Presbyterian minister. His missionary work as chaplain of the New York City Hospital and Almshouse is described in his book, *Visits of Mercy*. In 1814 he was installed as minister of the Old Pine Street Church in Philadelphia. He was a well known contributor to the literature on polemic theology and also left in manuscript form a *History of the Churches of Philadelphia*.

In contrast to his upright religious and civic activities, another side of his character is revealed in his ruinous financial entanglements in the business world. The panic of 1837 depressed the value of thousands of acres of land he had purchased in Missouri where he planned to establish a college and seminary, and Ely was accused by creditors there of fraud. When finally cleared of this charge he returned to Philadelphia with his second wife and became minister of the Presbyterian Church of the Northern Liberties. But more trouble awaited him.

The widower of his ward, Mary Ann Ely Miles, sued Reverend Ely for indebtedness to her. This claim and twenty-two others against Ely were subsequently settled with his creditors and he was discharged from further liability, but his memoir discloses a fear of ending his days at hard labor in Philadelphia's Eastern Penitentiary. Fortunately Ely's financial misadventures had no lasting effect on the reputation of Jefferson Medical College and he was elected president pro tempore of the board of trustees succeeding the aged Ashbel Green. Among Ely's twelve children were two physicians, a minister, and a notorious Parisian courtesan.

In the small oil portrait Reverend Ely is shown bust length and facing forward, seated at a table with his head resting on his left hand. He gazes directly toward the viewer with questioning eyes and pursed lips. The painting shows evidence of having been cut down from a larger size, and is probably unfinished because pencil marks are still discernible and unpainted primed canvas is noticeable around the sitter's head.

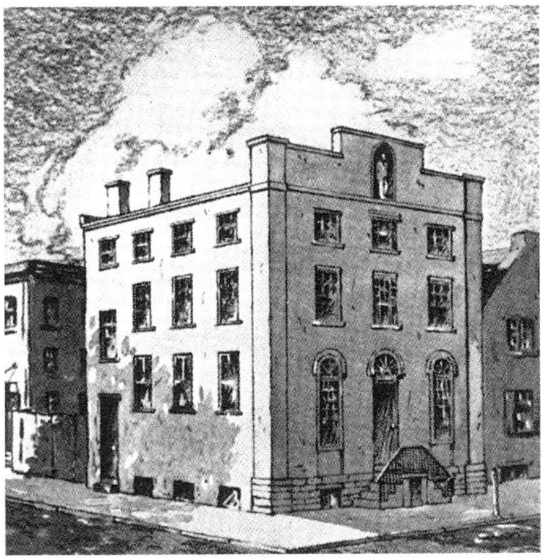

Medical Hall of Jefferson Medical College (Ely Building)

ELY BUILDING
Building by unknown architect

Modern reproduction of a published print, source unknown
1828-39 (original image)
5 x 4 in.

Given after 1900 by unknown donor
Accession number: 1900+f.Ph.18

By August 1828 the cornerstone was laid for Jefferson's new Medical Hall at Tenth and Sansom Streets. Designed by an unknown architect, the original stucco over brick building was two and one-half stories high over a raised basement. The dimensions of the modest building were fifty-one feet wide by fifty-seven feet deep.

A modern reproduction of an unidentified published print of the building's facade shows a double-sided staircase with railing which reached the entrance fronting on Tenth Street; there was also a rear entrance. Tall, narrow windows with arched fanlights on the first floor were surmounted by two rows of rectangular windows. Over the low attic story was a horizontal false front with a central niche hiding the flat roof. Nothing is known about the statue in the niche. Medical Hall remained as depicted in the photograph until the renovations of 1839.

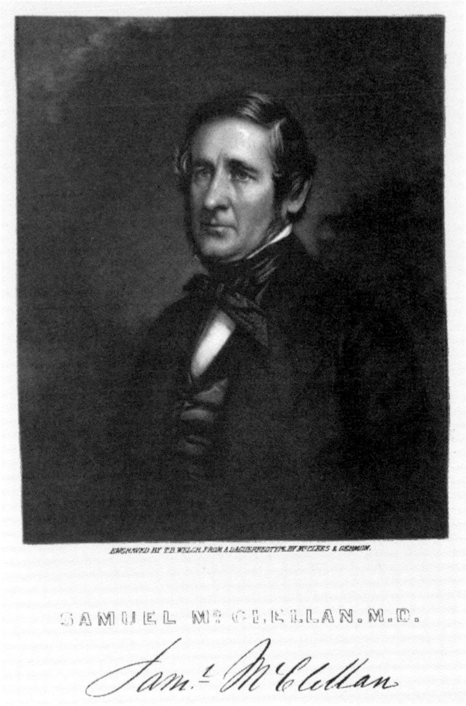

Portrait of Samuel McClellan

SAMUEL McCLELLAN, M.D. (1800-54)
By Thomas B. Welch (1814-74)

Mezzotint, etching, engraving
Ca. 1847-61
Image size: 5 3/8 x 4 1/2 in.
Plate size: 9 1/2 x 7 in.
Sheet size: 13 x 10 in.

Inscriptions below image: "ENGRAVED BY T.B. WELCH FROM A DAGUERREOTYPE BY McCLEES & GERMON"; "SAMUEL McCLELLAN. M.D."; facsimile signature "Saml McClellan"

Given after 1870 by unknown donor
Accession number: 1870+f.Pr.09a

As noted above, Jefferson Medical College experienced several years of instability in the late 1820s and 1830s when faculty members were "removed" and confusion ruled while chairmanships rotated. This uncertain period is exemplified in the career of Samuel McClellan, M.D., the younger brother of Dr. George McClellan.

Born in Woodstock, Connecticut in 1800, Samuel McClellan began to study anatomy with a local physician. In 1820 he entered his brother's office in Philadelphia. He took further medical training at the Almshouse, Pennsylvania Hospital, and the University of Pennsylvania, and then earned a medical degree from Yale School of Medicine (1823). After traveling for several years with a naturalist in Mexico, McClellan returned to Philadelphia and joined the faculty at Jefferson Medical College.

He rose rapidly from assistant demonstrator of anatomy in 1828 to professor in 1830. Forced to yield the anatomy chair to Granville S. Pattison, M.D. in 1831, McClellan was named chair of institutes of medicine, medical jurisprudence, and midwifery. In 1836 the first two of these departments became a separate chair given to Robley Dunglison, M.D.; McClellan then held the chair of obstetrics and diseases of women from 1836 to 1839. He also had served as dean from 1830 to 1834. Although he was reelected to the chair of obstetrics when the faculty was dissolved in 1839, he chose to resign. Dr. McClellan devoted the last twenty years of his life to the relative seclusion of private practice.

The mezzotint image of Samuel McClellan, M.D. is a three-quarters view that resembles a standard photograph with no background setting. The sitter's face is described in solidly rendered forms for a sculptural effect. His expression is bland and neutral, befitting the personality described in James F. Gayley's history of Jefferson Medical College as a "quiet, unassuming man, who rather shrank from than sought the applause of the world."

The source of Thomas B. Welch's mezzotint of Dr. McClellan is a daguerreotype by the firm of McClees and Germon. James Earle McClees (1821-87) and Washington Lafayette Germon (1823-78) were American daguerreotypists in partnership from about 1846 to 1855. They began working with paper printing techniques in 1851. Their firm won awards from the Franklin Institute and the American Institute in 1847 and 1848. The Jefferson archives also has several mezzotints of Dr. Samuel McClellan by John Sartain (one hand-colored).

James McClees had learned the daguerreotype process from Montgomery P. Simons in 1844 and continued working in this trade until the late 1850s. In 1856 he won a bronze medal from the American Institute for the best photographic view. He was a pioneer in stereo views and made many scenes of Washington, D.C. from about 1854 to 1861. After 1869 McClees sold his business and became a dealer in paintings, frames, and mirrors.

Washington L. Germon was an engraver of banknotes and business cards in 1845 and joined James E. McClees the following year. He exhibited daguerreotypes, talbotypes, and crystalotypes intermittently at the Institute of American Manufactures. Germon specialized in studio portraiture after 1856 and was listed as an artist in city directories from 1856 to 1859.

Thomas B. Welch, engraver and portrait painter, was born in Charleston, South Carolina in 1814. After an apprenticeship with engraver and publisher James B. Longacre (1794-1869) in Philadelphia he spent most of his career in that city. Welch formed a partnership with Adam B. Walter, although he executed many mezzotint and stipple engravings in his own name. Welch exhibited portraits in various media at the Pennsylvania Academy of the Fine Arts and the Artists' Fund Society and also at New York's American Academy of Fine Arts and the Apollo Association. About 1861 he abandoned engraving and went abroad to paint. He died in Paris in 1874.

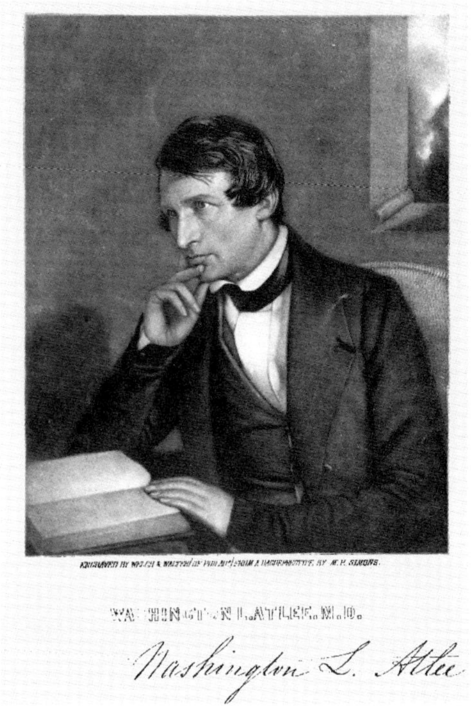

Portrait of Washington L. Atlee

WASHINGTON LEMUEL ATLEE, M.D. (1808-78)
By firm of Welch & Walter (active 1840-48)

Mezzotint, etching, engraving
1845-48
Image size: 5 x 4 in.
Sheet size: 8 x 5 3/4 in.

Inscriptions below image: "ENGRAVED BY WELCH & WALTER/ OF PHILAD^A./FROM A DAGUERREOTYPE BY M.P. SIMONS."; "WASHINGTON L.ATLEE.M.D."; facsimile signature "Washington L. Atlee"; "Professor of Medical Chemistry./IN THE MEDICAL DEPARTMENT OF PENNSYLVANIA COLLEGE."

Given after 1874 by unknown donor
Accession number: 1874+f.Pr.02

Washington L. Atlee, M.D. was another early graduate of Jefferson Medical College. He became a prominent gynecologist and is remembered today for establishing ovariotomy as a legitimate practice.

Born in Lancaster, Pennsylvania in 1808, he began the study of medicine with his brother John. Washington Atlee moved to Philadelphia and became a private pupil in the office of Dr. George McClellan. He graduated from Jefferson Medical College in 1829. After ten years of private practice in Lancaster he joined the faculty at the University of Pennsylvania in 1845 as professor of medical chemistry, remaining until 1853.

Before leaving Lancaster he had performed two ovariotomies with his brother. In 1845 he collected statistics on 101 ovariotomies and published the results in the *American Journal of the Medical Sciences*. Initially denounced by prominent colleagues for this procedure, Dr. Washington Atlee was even called "dangerous" by his vehement opponents. Eventually he was vindicated and honored by the profession.

His extensive experience was summarized with the publication *General and Differential Diagnosis of Ovarian Tumors, with Special Reference to the Operation of Ovariotomy* (1873), and by 1878 he had completed 387 ovariotomies. In 1853 he had reported on myomectomy for uterine fibroids in *The Surgical Treatment of Certain Fibrous Tumors of the Uterus, heretofore considered beyond the Resources of Art.*

A leader in medical administration, Atlee was a founder of the American Gynecological Society, president of the Philadelphia County Medical Society and the Pennsylvania State Medical Society, and vice president of the American Medical Association.

The portrait engraving of Dr. Atlee by the firm of Welch and Walter shows the thoughtful subject seated at his desk with chin on hand, contemplating an idea while glancing away from his open book. There is a hint of landscape through an open window in the upper right corner.

The print can be securely dated by information provided in the inscription and by the scant information known about the Welch and Walter partnership. Atlee was professor at the University of Pennsylvania from 1845 to 1853, and Thomas B. Welch and Adam B. Walter were partners from about 1840 to 1848, therefore the print dates from 1845-48.

Mezzotint and stipple engraver Adam B. Walter (1820-75) was a native Philadelphian who apprenticed with Thomas B. Welch in 1835 and later became his partner. He is best known for book illustrations.

Montgomery P. Simons (1817-77) was a Philadelphia daguerreotypist who took the original photograph of Washington L. Atlee, M.D. He is recorded as an active photographer from 1845 to 1875, and exhibited daguerreotypes at the Institute of American Manufactures from 1845 to 1848. Simons lived in Richmond, Virginia from 1853 to 1856 and then returned to Philadelphia. He manufactured miniature photographic cases and won a patent in 1843 for coloring daguerreotypes.

Simons is the author of several photographic manuals including *Plain Instructions for Coloring Photographs* (1857), *Photography in a Nut Shell* (1858), and *Secrets of Ivorytyping Revealed* (1860). When he died in 1877 he left an impressive collection of photographs of distinguished sitters. After his death Mrs. Simons continued operation of his studio.

Portrait of J. Marion Sims

JAMES MARION SIMS, M.D.
(1813-83)
By Paul Dubois (1829-1905)

Bronze
1876
16 7/8 x 9 x 9 in.

Signed lower right: "P. DUBOIS/Paris 1876"
Inscriptions: on integral base "Dr. MARION SIMS"; on rear "GRUET. J^{NE}. F^{DEUR}."

Given in 1880 by the Jefferson Medical College Hospital Surgical Staff, which had just received it from Dr. Sims's family
Accession number: 1880+e.S.01

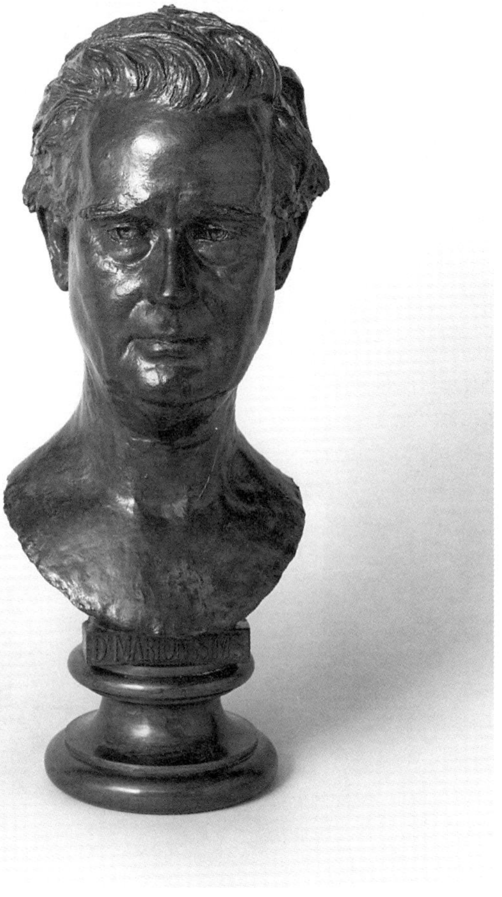

Dr. J. Marion Sims was one of the most distinguished early graduates of Jefferson Medical College. His reputation as the "Father of Gynecology" is a source of pride to his alma mater, although he pursued his career elsewhere and never held any academic position.

Sims was born in Lancaster County, South Carolina in 1813, the son of the local sheriff. He graduated from South Carolina College in 1832. After a three-month course of lectures at the new Medical College of South Carolina he entered the Jefferson Medical College and graduated in 1835.

By 1840 he had established a large and lucrative surgical practice in Montgomery, Alabama. In 1852 he published his cure for vesico-vaginal fistula, previously considered incurable. He had developed his technique after many years of research when he gave shelter and free treatment to women suffering from this condition in his private hospital. While perfecting this procedure he invented the silver wire suture and the duck-bill speculum which established his fame. In 1845 Sims had discovered the knee-chest position, later modified to the lateral Sims position for gynecological examination. He also excelled in operation for abscess of the liver, tumors of the jaw, cholecystotomy, gunshot wounds of the abdomen, and other conditions.

Two years after moving to New York in 1853, Dr. Sims established the first Woman's Hospital in this country, acting as its surgeon-in-chief. A native southerner, he spent the Civil War years in Europe, practicing and consulting in England, France, Germany, and Italy. He demonstrated his techniques to many of Europe's most celebrated surgeons, and recipients of his operative prowess included the nobility as well as charity patients.

In 1870 during the Franco-Prussian War Sims organized and became surgeon-in-chief of the Anglo-American Ambulance Corps. His professional service was so appreciated that the French Republic conferred upon him the Order of Knight of the Legion of Honor. He also received decorations from the governments of Portugal, Spain, Belgium, and Italy, and was made an honorary member of many learned societies. For the next decade until his death in 1883 he lived and worked alternately in Europe and America.

Sims was elected president of the American Medical Association in 1875, and in 1880 president of the American Gynecologic Society of which he was a founder. His most important literary contribution was *Clinical Notes on Uterine Surgery* (1866). His autobiography, *The Story of My Life*, was edited by his son, H. Marion Sims, M.D., and published posthumously in 1884. In 1955 the J. Marion Sims Obstetrical and Gynecological Society was established in his honor by Jefferson Medical College senior students.

A lasting contribution by Dr. Sims was not realized until after his death. A special hospital for female cancer patients which he had long advocated was opened in 1887. The Astor Pavilion for Women at the New York Cancer Hospital is now known as the Memorial-Sloan Kettering Cancer Center.

The bronze bust of Dr. Sims by Paul Dubois was the second sculpture to enter the Jefferson collection, after that of Dr. George McClellan; both were "conspicuously placed" in the surgical amphitheater of the 1877 hospital. The March 15, 1880 *College and Clinical Record* reported that the Jefferson Medical College alumni association tendered a vote of thanks to the surgical staff of the hospital for their "energy, enterprise, and liberality, in obtaining this memorial." Alumni president Samuel D. Gross, M.D. added that the gift was appreciated "not only for its intrinsic worth as a work of art, but also on account of the eminent services to science" rendered by Sims, "one of the most distinguished alumni of Jefferson College." The bust was later relocated to the library of the 1898 College Building.

Dr. Richard J. Levis, who presented the bust to the trustees on behalf of the surgical staff "in order that it might be placed in a prominent position in the new hospital," said it was a copy of a bronze bust made for Dr. Sims by "one of the first artists in Paris." Four years later, Dr. H. Marion Sims, son of J. Marion Sims, presented a similar bust to the New York Academy of Medicine. Other busts of Sims were presented to the Woman's Hospital in New York, Harvard Medical School, and the Royal Society of Medicine in London. In 1894 a full-length bronze statue of Dr. Sims was unveiled in New York; others adorn the capitol grounds of Columbia, South Carolina and Montgomery, Alabama.

Sims was sixty-three years old when sculptor Paul Dubois modeled the naturalistically conceived head. The doctor's most arresting features are the angular jaw line, clenched lips, thick, overhanging eyebrows, and shock of wavy hair. His wide-set eyes look slightly to the side, as though he were deep in thought.

Paul Dubois was a distinguished French painter and sculptor, best known as a portraitist. He had first studied the law, but soon changed his vocation and studied painting in the atelier of Fernand Toussaint and then was admitted to the École des Beaux-Arts. He was a consistent medal winner at the Paris Salon from 1865 though the 1880s. Besides contemporary portraits, he also executed many monuments of religious and historical personages.

In 1876 Dubois was made a member of the Institut National. Between 1867 and 1896 he was successively

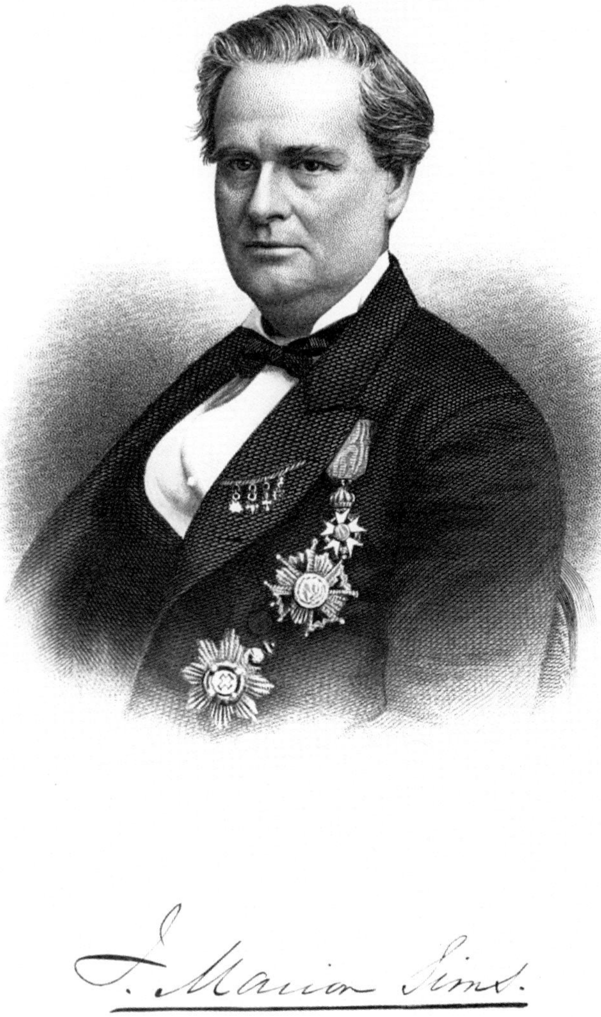

Portrait of J. Marion Sims

JAMES MARION SIMS, M.D.
By Henry Bryan Hall Jr. (active second half nineteenth century)

Engraving, etching, stipple
Ca. 1865-70
Image size: 4 x 3 1/2 in.
Sheet size: 10 x 6 3/4 in.

Inscriptions below image: "H. B. Hall, Jr."; facsimile signature "J. Marion Sims."

Given in 1946 by Mrs. William Rockwell of River Hebert, Nova Scotia (probably related to William Rockwell, M.D., JMC 1886)
Accession number: 1946+e.Pr.01

made a knight, officer, commander, and grand-cross of the Legion of Honor. He also pursued a career in art administration, first as conservator of the Musée du Luxembourg and then as director of the École des Beaux-Arts. His sculptures of French notables can be found in museums throughout the country.

Another well known image of Dr. J. Marion Sims was created by engraver Henry B. Hall Jr. The bust-length portrait is a beautifully rendered depiction of surface textures: the thick hair of head and eyebrows, fleshy jowls, patterned suit coat, and jewel-like decorations. The sitter's direct glance adds to the attractiveness of the image. Hall's perfection of the stipple technique produced an exceptionally rounded, three-dimensional figure whose forms are delicately carved out in light and shadow.

A native of London, Henry B. Hall Jr. emigrated to New York in 1850. Hall apprenticed with his father, Henry Bryan Hall, a well known portrait engraver and painter, and also with Charles Knight in London in 1858, after which he returned to New York. Henry Jr. served in the American Civil War and engraved many portraits of generals and officers. Besides portraits he also engraved historical subjects and copies after famous paintings. After the Civil War he joined his brothers, Charles Bryan Hall and Alfred Bryan Hall, in their father's successful engraving and publishing business. Henry Jr. retired in 1899.

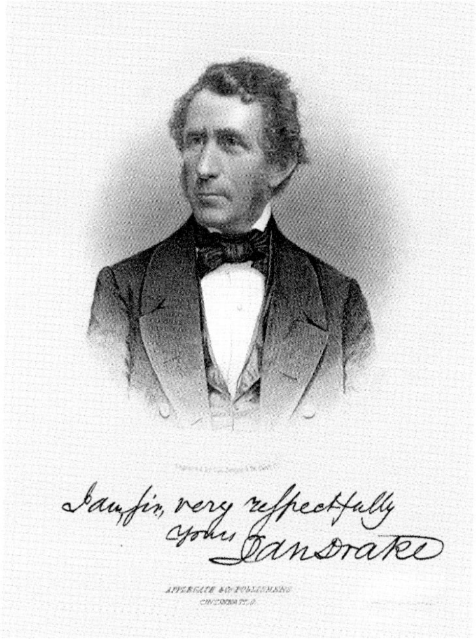

Portrait of Daniel Drake

DANIEL DRAKE, M.D. (1785-1852)
By C. A. Jewett & Co. (active 1850s)

Engraving, mezzotint, etching
Ca. 1853-57
Image size: 5 x 4 3/4 in.
Plate size: 7 1/2 x 5 1/2 in.
Sheet size: 8 1/4 x 6 3/4 in.

Inscriptions below image: "Engraved by C. A. Jewett & Co. Cinnti O."; facsimile signature "I am, Sir, very respectfully/ yours/Dan Drake"; "APPLEGATE & CO. PUBLISHERS/ CINCINNATI, O."; "Middleton, Wallace & Co. Printers."

Given after 1870 by unknown donor
Accession number: 1870+f.Pr.04b

Dr. Daniel Drake was a peripatetic physician, medical administrator, and author, with fleeting ties to new medical institutions in Ohio and Kentucky. He also served briefly on the early Jefferson Medical College faculty as professor of the theory and practice of medicine.

Daniel Drake was born in 1785 in Plainsfield, New Jersey and reared in a log cabin in May's Lick, Kentucky. In 1800 he began his study of medicine with Dr. William Goforth Jr. in Cincinnati. After receiving a medical degree from the University of Pennsylvania in 1816, he held the chair of materia medica at Transylvania University in Lexington, Kentucky. His plans for establishing the Medical College of Ohio in Cincinnati were successful by 1819, but in 1821 misunderstandings among faculty members arose and he was expelled. He returned to Transylvania University where he stayed until 1827.

In 1830 Drake returned to Philadelphia and made a very favorable impression as professor of theory and practice of medicine at Jefferson Medical College, but stayed only one year. He left Jefferson to organize a medical faculty at Miami University in Oxford, Ohio, taking Dr. John Eberle with him, as noted earlier. However, this new school merged with the Medical College of Ohio before the formal opening, and after one session Drake retired to private practice for a short time.

In 1835 his next endeavor was to organize the Medical Department of Cincinnati College (where one of his colleagues was Samuel D. Gross, M.D.). When this school closed after four years Drake moved to the University of Louisville where he was professor of clinical medicine and pathological anatomy, and then chair of the practice of medicine. He resigned in 1849 and returned to the Medical College of Ohio but resigned after one year. Remarkably, he returned to Louisville and then back to Ohio again in the next two years.

Dr. Daniel Drake was a voluminous author and editor. He edited the *Western Journal of the Medical and Physical Sciences* from 1827 to 1836. He is most celebrated for his comprehensive research published in *A Systematic Treatise, Historical, Etiological, and Practical, on the Principal Diseases of the Interior Valley of North America, as they appear in the Caucasian, African, Indian and Esquimaux Varieties of its Population*. This large-scale work was profusely illustrated with maps, charts, and plates and published in two volumes in 1850 and 1854.

The posthumous engraved portrait of Dr. Daniel Drake by the firm of C. A. Jewett and Company gives little hint of the subject's powerful personality because his head is turned and his eyes averted. The image appeared in Dr. James F. Gayley's *A History of the Jefferson Medical College of Philadelphia* (1858). Gayley described the eloquent and popular Drake as "winning and attractive, full of force, energy, and expression, riveting the attention of the dull intellect, captivating and charming the refined and cultivated. His success was complete." Gayley commented on Drake's "remarkably regular" features, especially his eyes of "wonderful power and penetration." His dress and living style were plain, his habits "eminently social," and his physical and mental endurance "extraordinary."

Charles A. Jewett was born in 1816 in Lancaster, Massachusetts and began engraving in New York City about 1838. From 1850 to at least 1857 he worked in Cincinnati where the Charles A. Jewett Company was established in 1853. Jewett returned to New York in 1860 and died in that city in 1878.

Portrait of John Revere

JOHN REVERE, M.D. (1787-1847)
By John Sartain (1808-97)

Mezzotint, etching, engraving
Ca. 1831-41
Image size: 4 3/4 x 3 3/4 in.
Plate size: 7 x 5 1/2 in.
Sheet size: 10 x 7 1/4 in.

Inscriptions below image: "Painted by H. Bridport" and "Engraved & Printed by J. Sartain"; facsimile signature "J. Revere M.D"; "PROFESSOR OF THE THEORY AND PRACTICE OF PHYSICK IN JEFFERSON MEDICAL COLLEGE/PHILADELPHIA"

From the "Murray Scrapbook," given in 1974-75 by Mrs. John A. Murray, R.N. (JMC Nursing 1928), widow of John A. Murray, M.D. (JMC 1931)
Accession number: 1974-1975.Pr.06

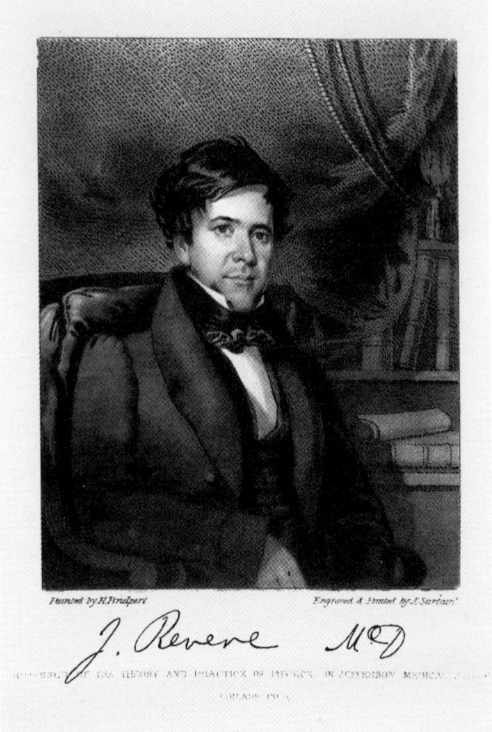

John Revere, M.D. was an able professor of medicine at Jefferson Medical College, filling the chair vacated by Dr. Daniel Drake. He subsequently departed with Dr. Granville S. Pattison for the University of New York.

John Revere was born in Boston in 1787, the son of Paul Revere, the celebrated Revolutionary War patriot and noted silversmith. After graduating from Harvard College in 1807 Revere studied medicine first with James Jackson, M.D. in Boston, then received a medical degree from the University of Edinburgh in 1811. After practicing in Boston and Baltimore, he was named professor of the theory and practice of medicine at Jefferson Medical College in 1831. He had translated François Magendie's *A Summary of Physiology* from the French in 1822 and while in Philadelphia he was editor of the *Medical Record*.

Revere served Jefferson Medical College with distinction for a decade and was highly ranked among teachers of medicine for his scholarship and lecturing skills. He was also admired for his amiability and courtesy. He served as Jefferson's dean from 1839 until 1841 when he left for the University of New York to fill the chair of the theory and practice of medicine. The family name Revere reentered Jefferson history when Dr. John Revere's grandniece, Grace Linzee Revere, became the wife of Dr. Samuel W. Gross in 1876.

The setting of John Sartain's undated mezzotint portrait of Dr. Revere resembles the artist's image of Dr. Jacob Green: a half-length figure seated in front of a swag of drapery. Here the curtain is tied back to reveal book-laden shelves instead of scientific instruments. The professor looks directly out toward the observer with a serious expression. The source for Sartain's print was a painting by Hugh Bridport.

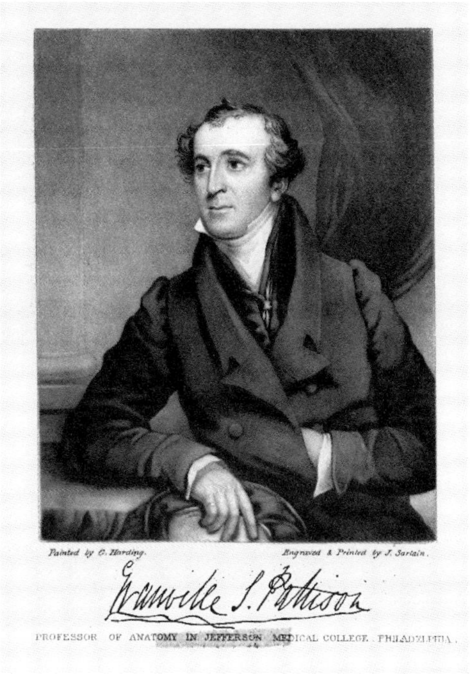

Portrait of Granville S. Pattison

GRANVILLE SHARPE PATTISON, M.D. (1792-1851)
By John Sartain (1808-97)

Mezzotint, etching, engraving
1831-41
Image size: 4 3/4 x 3 3/4 in.
Plate size: 7 1/2 x 6 1/8 in.
Sheet size: 10 1/2 x 8 1/4 in.

Inscriptions below image: "Painted by C. Harding." and "Engraved & Printed by J. Sartain."; facsimile signature "Granville S. Pattison"; "PROFESSOR OF ANATOMY IN JEFFERSON MEDICAL COLLEGE, PHILADELPHIA."

From the "Murray Scrapbook," given in 1974-75 by Mrs. John A. Murray, R.N. (JMC Nursing 1928), widow of John A. Murray, M.D. (JMC 1931)
Accession number: 1974-1975.Pr.05

For a decade Dr. Granville Sharpe Pattison was professor of anatomy at Jefferson Medical College. He was widely respected as a teacher of visceral and surgical anatomy.

Granville S. Pattison was born in 1792 in Glasgow, Scotland where he first studied medicine in the office of Dr. Allan Burns, a celebrated anatomist. After working for Burns as a demonstrator of anatomy, Pattison was appointed lecturer in anatomy, physiology, and surgery at the Andersonian Institution in Glasgow; later he emigrated to America.

From 1819 to 1820 he gave private anatomy lessons in Philadelphia, and was disappointed not to receive the promised chair of anatomy at the University of Pennsylvania. Known as the "vivacious and pugnacious Scot," Pattison quarreled with Dr. Nathaniel Chapman who had originally opposed his appointment to the University of Pennsylvania. This culminated in a duel in 1822 between Pattison and Chapman's brother-in-law, General Thomas Cadwalader. The general received a disabling wound in his "pistol arm" but the physician was uninjured.

From 1820 to 1826 Pattison was chair of anatomy, physiology, and surgery at the University of Maryland, then left for an appointment as professor of anatomy at the University of London. He returned to America in 1831 when named professor of anatomy at Jefferson Medical College where he received the M.D. degree. He remained until 1841 when he left for yet another position as chair of anatomy at the University of New York. He stayed there for a decade until his death in 1851.

Pattison was highly regarded as a teacher of anatomy at Jefferson, and for enlarging the anatomical rooms and founding the museum. Author of *Experimental Observations on the Operation of Lithotomy* (1820), Pattison was a translator of anatomy treatises and editor of the *American Medical Recorder* and the *Register and Library of Medical and Chirurgical Science*.

The undated mezzotint of Dr. Granville S. Pattison by John Sartain is taken after an original painting by Chester Harding. Something of Pattison's cockiness is suggested by the sitter's haughty expression and Napoleonic pose of hand thrust inside his suit coat. Background elements are a column and swag of drapery, the standard features implying erudition and high social status.

Painter and miniaturist Chester Harding (1792-1866) was born in Conway, New Hampshire. His career was even more peripatetic than that of Dr. Pattison. He started out as a sign painter in Pittsburgh and subsequently lived or worked in Kentucky, St. Louis, Washington, D.C., Boston, Springfield, and Northampton, Massachusetts, Richmond, Baltimore, New Orleans, and Canada. From 1823 to 1826 Harding also enjoyed a three-year sojourn in London where he was a fashionable success. He was made an honorary professional member of the National Academy in 1828.

Portrait of Robley Dunglison

ROBLEY DUNGLISON, M.D. (1798-1869)
By Alexander Hay Ritchie (1822-95)

Mezzotint, engraving, etching
1846
Image size: 5 x 4 in.
Plate size: 9 x 6 in.
Sheet size: 14 1/2 x 11 1/2 in.

Inscriptions below image: "ENGRAVED BY A.H.RITCHIE FROM A DAGUERREOTYPE BY M.P.SIMONS"; "ROBLEY DUNGLISON.M.D."; facsimile signature "Robley Dunglison"; "Professor of Institutes of Medicine/In THE JEFFERSON MEDICAL COLLEGE OF PHILADELPHIA"; "Entered according to Act of Congress in the Year 1846 by V.F.Harrison Philad[a]. Published by V.F.Harrison, N[o] 27 S[o]. 8th. S[t]."

Given in 1942 by Olcott H. Parker
Accession number: 1942+e.Pr.02

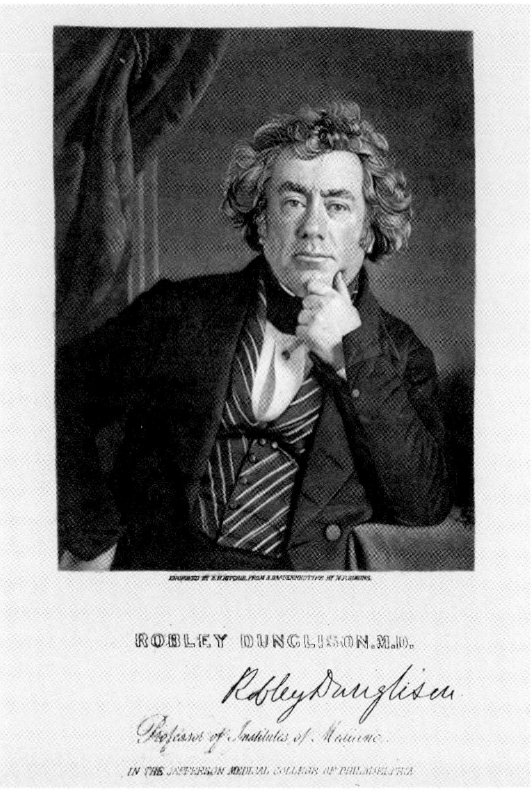

Dr. Robley Dunglison was Jefferson's first truly outstanding and loyal faculty member. He served the institution with distinction as chair of the institutes of medicine for thirty-two years starting in 1836. A prominent author, editor, and educator, he is considered by many scholars to be the "Father of Physiology."

Robley Dunglison was born in Keswick, England in 1798, the son of a wool manufacturer. He began to study medicine under a village physician before taking courses in Edinburgh, Paris, and London. Licensed by the Royal College of Surgeons and the Society of Apothecaries in London, he opened a private practice in 1819. He received his medical degree from the University of Erlangen circa 1824 and then became accoucheur to the Eastern Dispensary in London. He was also an editor of the *London Medical Repository* and the *Medical Intelligencer.*

Late in 1824 Dunglison left his obstetrical practice in London to accept an invitation from Thomas Jefferson, then rector of the University of Virginia, to fill a comprehensive chair of anatomy, physiology, materia medica, and pharmacy at that institution. Dunglison developed a close relationship with and became personal physician to Thomas Jefferson, and attended the former president during his final days in 1826. Robley Dunglison left Virginia to become professor of materia medica and jurisprudence at the University of Maryland in 1833.

In 1836 the acclaimed physician was persuaded by Professor Granville S. Pattison, M.D. to join the faculty at Jefferson Medical College as chair of the institutes of medicine and medical jurisprudence. Warned that he would encounter faculty jealousy and dissension Dunglison remained determinedly independent during the tumultuous formative years at Jefferson Medical College.

During the period of acrimony over policies and fees George McClellan, M.D., Samuel McClellan, M.D., and Samuel Colhoun, M.D. (the latter, professor of materia medica and dean) were often pitted against Granville S. Pattison, M.D., John Revere, M.D., and Jacob Green. By 1839 dissension among the faculty erupted into public declarations, especially by Dr. George McClellan who castigated the newly powerful board and denigrated the medical school.

Largely as a result of Dr. Robley Dunglison's letter appealing to the faculty to submit to the authority of the board and to "promote harmony of action," the board declared all chairs vacant and called for reorganization. Drs. George McClellan and Samuel Colhoun (neither reelected) and Samuel McClellan (reelected) departed abruptly. The faculty was further decimated by the death of Jacob Green and the resignations of Drs. Revere and Pattison, all occurring in 1841.

Robley Dunglison, M.D. was a renowned member of Jefferson's newly restructured "Famous Faculty of 1841" which straightaway instituted a period of growth and harmony in the school. Dunglison gave up his practice and devoted his efforts entirely to academic work. He is generally known as America's first full-time physiologist. Partly because of his effective peacemaking efforts he acceded to the deanship in 1854, a position he held until 1868.

Dunglison established his literary reputation with an almost encyclopedic range of subjects, and many of his texts went through multiple editions and became standards in their fields. Among his outstanding works are: *Human Physiology* (1832), *A New Dictionary of Medical Science and Literature* (1833), *Elements of Hygiene* (1835), *General Therapeutics, or Principles of Medical Practice* (1836), *New Remedies: the Method of Preparing and Administering Them* (1839), and *Practice of Medicine, or A Treatise on Special Pathology and Therapeutics* (1842). His medical dictionary went through an astonishing twenty-three editions and sold fifty-five thousand copies during his lifetime. Dunglison was also a founder and editor of the *American Medical Library and Intelligencer*.

Among the many tributes to Dr. Dunglison were his honorary LL.D. degrees from Jefferson College (1852) and Jefferson Medical College (1853). At the time of his retirement in 1868 he was elected emeritus professor. The physician died of congestive heart failure the following year.

In the early 1980s his grave site at Philadelphia's Laurel Hill Cemetery was found in disarray by Frederick B. Wagner Jr., M.D., Thomas Jefferson University's Grace Revere Osler Professor Emeritus of Surgery and University Historian. Distressed by the seeming disrespect toward the memory of an outstanding Jeffersonian, Dr. Wagner spearheaded a successful effort to restore the tombstone and plot and to erect a commemorative headstone.

The mezzotint portrait of Dr. Dunglison by Alexander H. Ritchie shows the subject seated with his chin resting on his left hand and looking thoughtfully toward the viewer. The print with its conventional pose and drapery background were taken after a daguerreotype by M. P. Simons. Most interesting are the subject's fashionable costume with its diagonally striped vest, and the detailed rendering of his full head of curly hair.

Printmaker Alexander H. Ritchie was born in 1822 in Glasgow, Scotland. He studied drawing with Sir William Allan in Edinburgh and emigrated to America in 1841. He settled in New York about 1847 and established a thriving engraving business there. He was best known as an engraver of portraits in mezzotint. He also painted in oils and started to exhibit at the National Academy of Design in 1848; he was elected an academician in 1871. Alexander Ritchie died in New Haven, Connecticut in 1895.

Dr. Robley Dunglison was held in such high esteem by his colleagues that on April 16, 1875 the executive committee of the alumni association ordered a posthumous portrait to be painted and presented to the trustees of the college at the next commencement. The

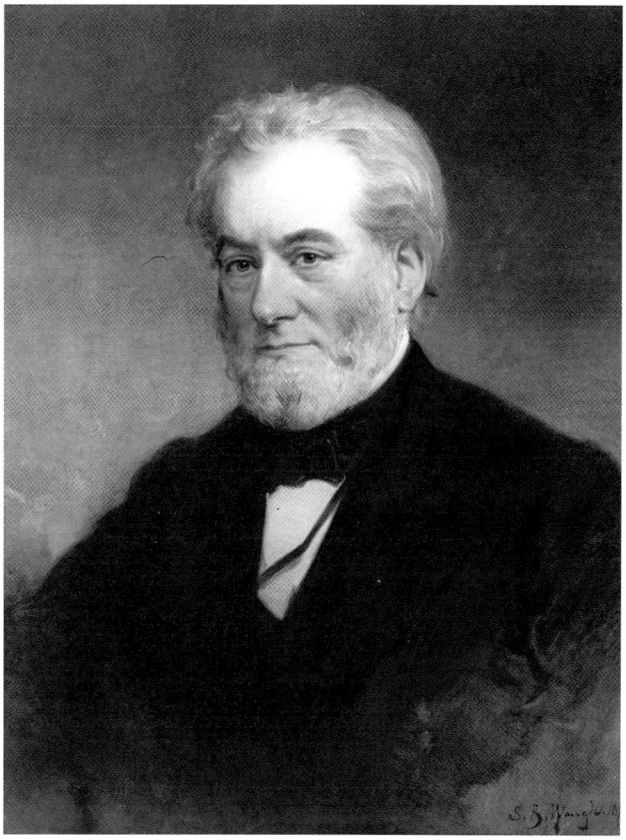

Portrait of Robley Dunglison

ROBLEY DUNGLISON, M.D.
By Samuel Bell Waugh (1814-85)

Oil on canvas mounted on wooden board
1876
30 x 25 in.

Exhibition: Philadelphia, *Centennial Celebration Loan Collection of Portraits,* College of Physicians of Philadelphia, 1887

Given in 1876 by JMC alumni association
Accession number: 1876+e.P.01

portrait presentation was made by Dr. Addinell Hewson substituting for Dr. Samuel W. Gross who was originally given this honor.

Dr. Hewson's handwritten speech is still preserved in the Jefferson archives. He described Dr. Dunglison as "not only one of the firmest pillars but...the chief corner stone on which renown of this school has heretofore rested," and that it was "natural" that the members of the alumni association should be "impatient" to have his portrait placed in the "college gallery." He also mentioned that although several previous portraits of Dr. Dunglison had been painted, his friends and family concurred that the Waugh portrait "has no superior." The painting was originally installed in the amphitheater of the 1877 hospital and then relocated with a group of other portraits of distinguished faculty members to the library of the 1898 College Building.

Dr. John H. Brinton's memoir about the Jefferson faculty of 1841 in the March 15, 1880 issue of *The College and Clinical Record* described Dunglison's keen observation, judicial temperament, and commanding and fluent speech in extemporaneous lectures delivered with "Johnsonian" diction that always captured the undivided attention of his class. In Waugh's portrait the physician is shown bust length, facing slightly left, and with his head tilted. His rather bland facial expression does not really embody Brinton's vivid characterization.

The source for Waugh's portrait may be an undated *carte-de-visite* photograph of Dr. Robley Dunglison in the Jefferson archives (or a similar one taken late in life). The physician's head tilt, hair and beard style, and costume elements including neckwear and diagonal strap holding his pince-nez are very similar, although the figure in the photo is three-quarters length and includes the subject's hands.

The Dunglison depiction was the fourth of five portraits commissioned by Jefferson Medical College from painter Samuel Bell Waugh, late in his career between 1872 and 1880. A popular portrait and landscape painter, Waugh was born in 1814 in Mercer, Pennsylvania. As a young man he traveled abroad studying the old masters and archaeological ruins and spent eight years in Italy. In 1841 the largely self-taught artist returned to America and made his residence mainly in Philadelphia.

During the 1840s he exhibited numerous Italian scenes at the American Art Union and at the National Academy of Design in New York. He was widely known for panoramic views of Italy one of which was first exhibited in Philadelphia in 1849. He was a prolific exhibitor at the Pennsylvania Academy of the Fine Arts between 1842 and 1869 and served a term as president of the Artists Fund Society. In the 1840s Waugh was made an associate member and then an honorary professional member of the National Academy of Design.

Other artistic members of Samuel B. Waugh's family include his wife, Mary Eliza Young Waugh (a miniaturist); his daughter, Ida Waugh (a figure painter); his son, Frederick Judd Waugh (a marine painter); and his nephew, Henry W. Waugh (a landscape, panorama, and scenery painter).

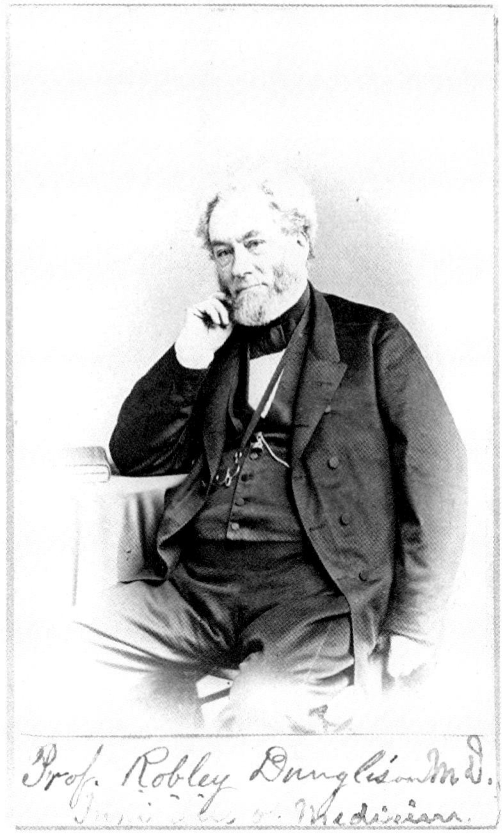

Portrait of Robley Dunglison

ROBLEY DUNGLISON, M.D.
By unknown photographer

Carte-de-visite
Ca. 1859-69
Image size: 3 5/8 x 2 1/2 in.
Mount size: 4 x 2 1/2 in.

Inscription in ink below image: "Prof. Robley Dunglison M.D./Institutes of Medicine"

Given after 1870 by unknown donor
Accession number: 1870+f.Ph.06

Cartes-de-visite, or card photographs, originated in 1857 when the Duke of Parma directed his court photographer to make small photographs mounted on his calling cards. The fad soon spread to Paris and London, and by 1859 to the United States. Small, inexpensive, and produced in quantity, *cartes-de-visite* mounted on cards soon supplanted daguerreotypes and ambrotypes. By 1860 their popularity reached new heights and they were eagerly collected and displayed in the first picture albums.

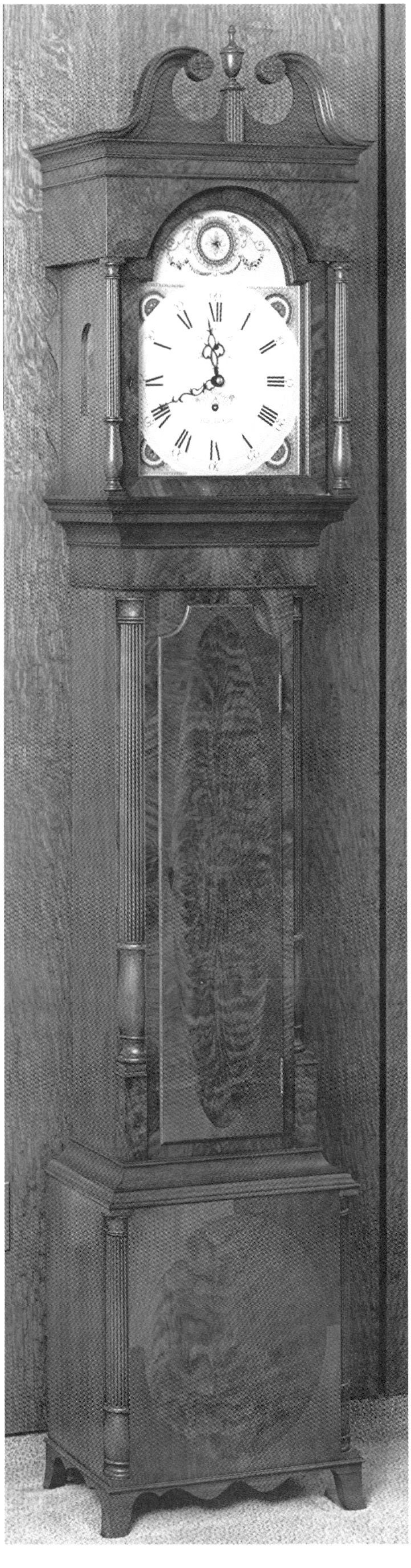

Replica of Jefferson-Dunglison Tall Case Clock

REPLICA OF JEFFERSON-DUNGLISON TALL CASE CLOCK
By the Franklin Mint

Mahogany
1978
93 1/2 x 20 x 11 3/4 in.

Inscription on face: "Thos. VOIGHT./PHILAD^{A}."

Given in 1981 by an anonymous donor
Accession number: 1981+e.DA.01

In gratitude for Dr. Robley Dunglison's medical services, Martha Randolph, the daughter of Thomas Jefferson, gave the physician a tall case clock that had been by the president's bed from 1815 until his death in 1826. The clock was inherited by the physician's son, William Leadam Dunglison, and his widow presented the clock to the Historical Society of Pennsylvania in 1894 according to his wishes.[6] Since about 1993 the clock has been on long-term loan to Monticello.

Dr. Dunglison recollected the president's fondness for and usage of the clock and the circumstances of his own possession of it:

> Its rate of going is marked on the inside of the case in the handwriting of Mr. Jefferson; and the days of the week, as reached by the weight of the clock, day after day, are indicated, the clock going eight days, and being wound up on the Sundays. Isolated...often in the recess of his own study, the precise day of the week might readily escape him, and this was a convenient method of reminding him thereof.
>
> I had no knowledge of the intention of Mrs. Randolph to bestow this clock on me; but had determined to possess it, if it went at a reasonable rate, at the sale [of the president's furniture]. When put up...I bade 150; and it was knocked down to Mr. Trist [an executor of the president's will] for one hundred and fifty-five dollars. I immediately went up to Mr. Trist, apologizing for having opposed unwittingly the desire of the family to possess the clock, when he told me I might make my mind easy, as he had been commissioned by them to buy it, in order that they might present it to me.[7]

The special clock was made for Jefferson "for astronomical purposes" because he had inadvertently missed an eclipse in 1811. It was made with no striking mechanism because he had another clock in his bedroom that chimed every thirty minutes. The tall case clock was ordered in 1811, but did not arrive at Monticello until 1815, due to difficulty in transportation by ship because of bad weather and a British blockade during the War of 1812.

The original clock was made by Thomas Voight, the son of Henry Voight (1738-1814), a leading Philadelphia clock and watch maker and chief coiner to the United States Mint. Thomas Voight maintained a clock shop in Philadelphia from 1811 to 1836, and his fame rests primarily on the Jefferson-Dunglison clock and the "Ohio Clock" in the Capitol building in Washington, D.C.

The replica of the Federal-style clock is from a limited edition made for the Franklin Mint's Heirloom Furniture division, with the mahogany cabinetry by the Colonial Manufacturing Company of Zeeland, Michigan, and the works by Jacques of Germany.

The cabinet is crowned by a swan's neck cresting ending in rosettes and flanking a fluted urn finial. The plain frieze is raised on freestanding reeded columns above vase-turned bottom sections. The waisted trunk is fitted with a pendulum door veneered with matched crotched grain mahogany, flanked by engaged quarter-columns on vase-turned bottom sections. The base section has similar elements and is raised on diminutive splayed bracket feet. The original height of eight feet, two inches was scaled down to accommodate the lower ceilings of modern buildings.

The face is painted white with a black chapter ring with Roman numerals. It is flanked by gold and polychrome spandrels with half rosettes, corresponding to the full rosette in the lunette, and with no moon phases. The reproduction clock has an eight-day movement with brass weights, a brass pendulum, and Westminster chimes.

Portrait of Caspar Wistar

CASPAR WISTAR, M.D. (1761-1818)
Attributed to Hannah Mee Horner (active mid-twentieth century)

Oil on canvas
Mid-twentieth century
37 x 31 in.

Given in 1986 by Elizabeth M. Wistar, descendant of the subject
Accession number: 1986+e.P.04

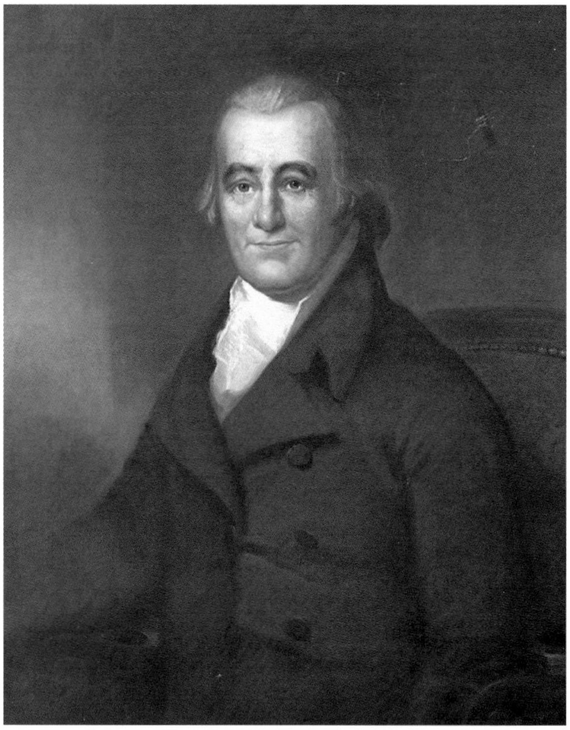

Portraits of Dr. Caspar Wistar and Dr. Philip Syng Physick, important early Philadelphia physicians, are included in Jefferson's art collection even though these physicians forged their careers elsewhere. But in both cases there are connections with Jefferson Medical College.

Dr. Wistar was a prominent anatomist who died in 1818, six years before Jefferson Medical College was even established. He was largely instrumental in accomplishing the union of the medical school of the University of the State of Pennsylvania with its rival, the College of Philadelphia, resulting in the school of medicine of the University of Pennsylvania in 1792.

Born in 1761 in Philadelphia, Caspar Wistar was inspired to become a physician while helping to tend the wounded during the Battle of Germantown. He studied medicine privately with Dr. John Redman and attended lectures at the medical school of the University of the State of Pennsylvania where he received a bachelor of medicine degree in 1782. Four years later he earned a doctor of medicine degree at the University of Edinburgh.

Upon his return to Philadelphia he set up a highly successful practice with the assistance of Dr. John Jones. Early academic positions were as physician to the Philadelphia Dispensary and professor of chemistry and physiology at the College of Philadelphia. He was physician to the Pennsylvania Hospital from 1793 to 1810. In 1792 he was appointed adjunct professor of anatomy, midwifery, and surgery at the University of Pennsylvania, then in 1808 professor of anatomy, a post he held until his death in 1818.

An animated and distinguished teacher, Dr. Wistar made his most significant literary contribution with *A System of Anatomy for the Use of Students of Medicine* (1811-14), the first comprehensive treatise on the subject written and published in America. Some early faculty members of Jefferson Medical College must have known Dr. Wistar when studying anatomy at the university.

Dr. Wistar was a man of far-ranging intellectual, civic, and social interests. His family established an institute to house his private collection of anatomical models, specimens, and drawings in the early 1890s. From the very beginning the institute was equipped with research laboratories and facilities to study comparative anatomy and experimental biology. The renowned Wistar Institute of Anatomy and Biology, though located on the campus of the University of Pennsylvania, is the oldest independent biomedical research center in the country. Among the many internationally celebrated investigators who made significant discoveries at Wistar are current Jeffersonians, Drs. Carlo M. Croce and Hilary Koprowski.

Dr. Wistar succeeded Thomas Jefferson as president of the American Philosophical Society in 1815 and he succeeded Dr. Benjamin Rush as president of the Society for the Abolition of Slavery in 1813. Saturday night "Wistar parties" at his home gathered together members of the American Philosophical Society with visiting dignitaries, and these parties were perpetuated as a Philadelphia tradition after his death.

The unsigned portrait of Caspar Wistar was attributed to Hannah M. Horner in correspondence from the counsel representing the executors of the donor's estate. Today Miss Horner is best remembered as a painting restorer who worked on the collections of many Philadelphia institutions including Jefferson Medical College. Horner's mid-twentieth-century work is probably a copy after one of three original depictions of Wistar by Bass Otis (1784-1861) or after numerous painted and printed copies of the Otis portraits.[8]

The half-length portrait shows the subject seated and turned slightly to the left, looking straight toward the observer. His characteristic thick and dark eyebrows, bumpy nose, thin lips, and square jaw, as well as the sloping shoulder line are faithfully rendered by the copyist. It is probable that the sitter's sallow complexion with its greenish overtones is a result of deterioration of the pigment.

Jefferson acquired the portrait in 1986 by donation from Elizabeth M. Wistar, a descendant of the physician. Interestingly, the wife of Joseph L. Eastwick (a former Jefferson trustee elected in 1943) is also a direct descendant of Dr. Wistar.

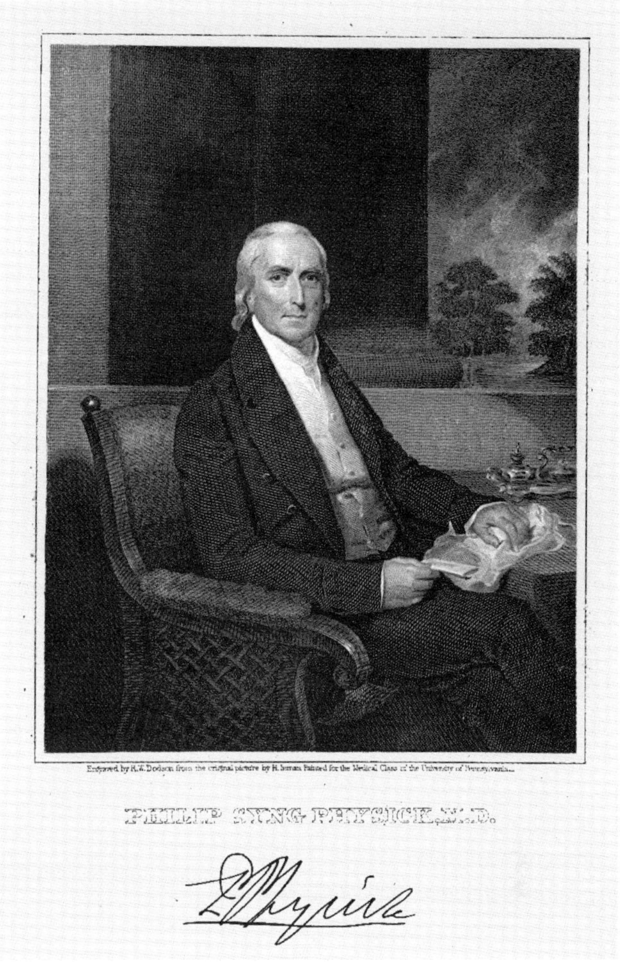

Portrait of Philip S. Physick

PHILIP SYNG PHYSICK, M.D. (1768-1837)
By Richard W. Dodson (1812-67)

Engraving, etching, stipple
Ca. 1838
Image size: 5 x 3 7/8 in.
Sheet size: 9 7/8 x 6 1/2 in.

Inscriptions below image: "Engraved by R.W. Dodson from the original picture by H. Inman. Painted for the Medical Class of the University of Pennsylvania"; "PHILIP SYNG PHYSICK, M.D."; facsimile signature "P S Physick"

Given after 1900 by unknown donor
Accession number: 1900+f.Pr.23

Another prominent early Philadelphia physician is Dr. Philip Syng Physick, known as the "Father of American Surgery" during his lifetime. Born in Philadelphia in 1768 to a distinguished family, he was descended from the famous silversmiths, Philip Syng Sr. (1676-1739) and Philip Syng Jr. (1703-89). His father, Edmund Physick, managed the colonial interests of the Penn family in America.

Philip Syng Physick graduated from the University of the State of Pennsylvania in 1785 and earned an M.A. from the university in 1788. He took a three-year preceptorship with Dr. Adam Kuhn before moving to London to study with Dr. John Hunter, the celebrated anatomist and surgeon. He lived in Hunter's home and his gracious host arranged an appointment for Physick as house surgeon to St. George's Hospital. He received his M.D. degree from the University of Edinburgh in 1792.

That same year Dr. Physick returned to Philadelphia where he gradually established a successful office practice. During the great yellow fever epidemic of 1793 Physick was attending surgeon at Bush Hill, a charity hospital, and he supported the controversial bloodletting treatment espoused by Dr. Benjamin Rush. Physick also performed numerous autopsies and helped to popularize the procedure.

In 1794 he was appointed to the staffs of the Pennsylvania Hospital and the Philadelphia Almshouse. He began to deliver lectures on surgery at the University of Pennsylvania and in 1805 Physick was appointed to the first separate chair of surgery at the University of Pennsylvania. His lectures were said to have been models of clarity, his surgery was conservative and practical, and he made many advances in surgical technique and devised technical improvements of surgical instruments.

He relinquished the chair of surgery in 1819 and was appointed to the chair of anatomy, a post he held until 1831 when he was made emeritus professor. Among other societies he was a member of the Academy of Medicine of France and was posthumously named an honorary fellow of the Royal Medical and Chirurgical Society of London.

Dr. Physick had contact with several professors from Jefferson Medical College: he recommended that Dr. W. P. C. Barton (later professor of material medica and dean) be given an appointment as surgeon in the U.S. Navy; and he was the teacher of Drs. George McClellan and John B. Biddle at the University of Pennsylvania.

Physick was the subject of a biographical sketch by Dr. Samuel D. Gross who praised his "marked ability," but pointedly added that his designation as "Father of American Surgery" was due to the fact that "he had the field of surgery to himself" in the first quarter of the nineteenth century. Gross faulted Physick's excessive use of venesection, intolerance of others' theories, and lack of written records.[9]

The image of Physick is a small engraving by Richard W. Dodson after an original oil painting by Henry Inman (1801-46) commissioned by medical students at the University of Pennsylvania in 1836. There are oil copies of the Inman painting at the College of Physicians of Philadelphia and at the Pennsylvania Hospital.

The "grand manner" composition shows the lean physician seated erectly in an upholstered armchair. His legs are crossed and his body is turned three-quarters to the right next to a table. He holds a folded paper in his right hand and a handkerchief in his left hand. A silver tray with an inkwell is on the table. Behind the figure is a low stone parapet, the base and partial shaft of columns, and a view toward distant trees, river, and clouds.

The physician has dark eyes, an aquiline nose, and long, powdered hair. He turns his head to look intently toward the viewer. In his autobiography Dr. Gross described Physick's "remarkable-looking" visage as "strikingly handsome, but pallid...as if it had been chiselled out of marble."

Printmaker Richard W. Dodson was born in 1812, a native of Cambridge, Maryland. He was a pupil of Philadelphia engraver James B. Longacre (1794-1869). He spent his professional career in Philadelphia and was a specialist in portrait engraving and book illustration. Dodson made some of the finest portraits, including the image of Dr. Physick, published in *The National Portrait Gallery of Distinguished Americans* (1838) by James B. Longacre and James Herring (1794-1867). The Jefferson collection also includes another engraved portrait of Dr. Physick by Asher B. Durand (1796-1886).

1. Beaumont Newhall, *The Daguerreotype in America*, 3d rev. ed. (New York: Dover Publications, 1976), 128.

2. For the most complete biographical information on John Plumbe see Floyd Rinhart and Marion Rinhart, *The American Daguerreotype* (Athens, Ga.: University of Georgia Press, 1981), 65-75, 405-06. The authors also say that Plumbe manufactured cameras, miniature cases, and possibly mats and plates over the period 1841 to 1847, but do not mention in what location.

3. I am grateful to Dan Flanagan, archives technician at Thomas Jefferson University, for showing me an article in the *Philadelphia Record* of May 11, 1930 about the mystery of the Cooke skull (see entry on the younger Dr. George McClellan). The article says that the famous theatrical prop was owned by the elder Dr. George McClellan who passed it to his son Dr. John Hill Brinton McClellan, who in turn passed it to his son, the younger Dr. George McClellan. In 1928 the latter's widow bequeathed the skull along with "certain papers and belongings of her husband which also had belonged to the founder of Jefferson Medical College" to Dr. Ross V. Patterson.

Dr. Patterson was the physician for both Dr. McClellan and Mrs. McClellan, according to Frederick B. Wagner Jr., M.D. and J. Woodrow Savacool, M.D., ed., *Jefferson Medical College of Thomas Jefferson University: Legend and Lore* (Devon, Pa.: William T. Cooke Publishing, 1996), 648.

4. John Chalmers DaCosta, M.D., *Selections from the Papers and Speeches of John Chalmers DaCosta, M.D., LL.D.* (Philadelphia: W. B. Saunders Co., 1931), 326.

5. Rebecca J. Beal, *Jacob Eichholtz 1776-1842: Portrait Painter of Pennsylvania* (Philadelphia: Historical Society of Pennsylvania, 1969), 54.

6. Frederick B. Wagner Jr., M.D., "The Jefferson-Dunglison Grandfather Clock," offprint from the *Transactions and Studies of the College of Physicians of Philadelphia* 3 (June 1981): 156.

7. Samuel X. Radbill, M.D., ed., "The Autobiographical Ana of Robley Dunglison, M.D.," *Transactions of the American Philosophical Society* 53 (Dec. 1963): 34-35.

8. For information on the various Bass Otis original portraits and copies, see Anthony N. B. Garvan and Carol A. Wojtowicz, *Catalogue of the Green Tree Collection* (Philadelphia: The Mutual Assurance Co., 1977), 57-58.

9. Samuel D. Gross, M.D., *Autobiography of Samuel D. Gross, M.D.*, ed. Samuel W. Gross, M.D. and A. Haller Gross, 2 vols. (Philadelphia: George Barrie, 1887), 2:240-46.

CHAPTER 2

Mid-nineteenth-century Period of Growth

In 1841 the Board of Trustees set the formidable task of reorganizing the faculty and reestablishing the faltering reputation of Jefferson Medical College. By shifting chairs and recruiting new members, the trustees formed a prestigious faculty whose members worked harmoniously and progressively together for fifteen years. Collectively these seven professors achieved a leading position for the college. The Jefferson art collection includes multiple images of all these professors, of which a few have been selected to show the range of media and artists.

Over the years the Jefferson archives has received dozens of class admission tickets as well as lecture notes, catalogues, published addresses, diplomas, photographs, and other memorabilia formerly in the possession of nineteenth-century medical students.

Jefferson Medical College's Famous Faculty of 1841

THE FAMOUS FACULTY OF 1841
By Robert Whitechurch (1814-ca. 1880) & Bartas P. Newman (b. ca. 1824)

Engraving, etching, stipple
1855
Image size: 21 1/8 x 16 5/8 in.
Sheet size: 24 x 18 in.

Inscriptions below image: "Entered according to Act of Congress in the year 1855 by Joseph M. Wilson in the Clerk's Office of the Dist. Court of the U.S. for the Eastern Dist. of PA."; "This Engraving of the PROFESSORS OF JEFFERSON MEDICAL COLLEGE OF PHILADELPHIA is Respectfully/Dedicated to the Alumni by/JOSEPH M. WILSON, PUBLISHER./Southwest Corner of Ninth & Arch Streets: Philadelphia/Engraved by R. Whitechurch & B. P. Newnam *[sic]* at J. M. Butler's establishment: 84 Chestnut St. Philad[a]."

Given after 1970 by J. D. Williford, grandson of Dr. Robert A. Fleming (JMC 1857)
Accession number: 1970+f.Pr.01

An outstanding engraving of the "Famous Faculty of 1841" includes images of the following professors, from left to right: Thomas D. Mütter, M.D. (surgery), Joseph Pancoast, M.D. (anatomy), Robert M. Huston, M.D. (materia medica and therapeutics, also dean), Robley Dunglison, M.D. (institutes of medicine and medical jurisprudence), John K. Mitchell, M.D. (medicine), Franklin Bache, M.D. (chemistry), and Charles D. Meigs, M.D. (obstetrics and diseases of women and children).

Reflecting on the faculty of 1841 in an address to the Jefferson alumni association, John H. Brinton, M.D., a later professor of the practice of surgery and clinical surgery, characterized the years 1841 to 1856 as the "period of the true rise and healthy growth of the school."[1] He said, "Many of those great advances in teaching were then effected which gave the stamp to the school...Chief among these was the origination of the great system of Collegiate Clinics." In addition to medical and surgical clinics at Jefferson, the students were transported twice a week in "large omnibuses hired for the purpose" to lectures at Pennsylvania Hospital and Blockley Almshouse. Even recognizing the importance of college art works, Brinton said that the professors "look down upon us to-night from canvas and from marble pedestal."

The Jefferson archives is fortunate to possess three copies of the large-scale, decorative engraving of the "Famous Faculty of 1841," and a fourth copy in which the image of Dr. Mütter was replaced with that of Dr. Samuel D. Gross who succeeded him in 1856. In addition, the archives has individual sheets with the same images which also illustrated James F. Gayley's *History of the Jefferson Medical College of Philadelphia* (1858).

Each bust-length figure is surrounded by a rope molding which contains the subject's name. Intertwining the images are ornamental arrangements of plants including grape and other flowering vines and cornstalks. At the bottom center are fruit-filled cornucopias flanking a shield bearing a caduceus. Above the central image of Dr. Dunglison is a medallion with the profile bust of Thomas Jefferson, and below Dunglison is a rendering of Jefferson Medical College's Ely Building. The Jefferson medallion is one of the earliest examples of what would become the official college and university logotype.

One of the artists was Robert Whitechurch, a native of London who emigrated to Philadelphia in 1848. He worked as a portrait engraver until about 1872 when he moved to Washington and worked as a banknote engraver for the Treasury Department. Little is known about the life of the second-named engraver, Bartas P. Newman, except that he was a native Philadelphian. Apparently both men were employed by the firm of J. M. Butler.

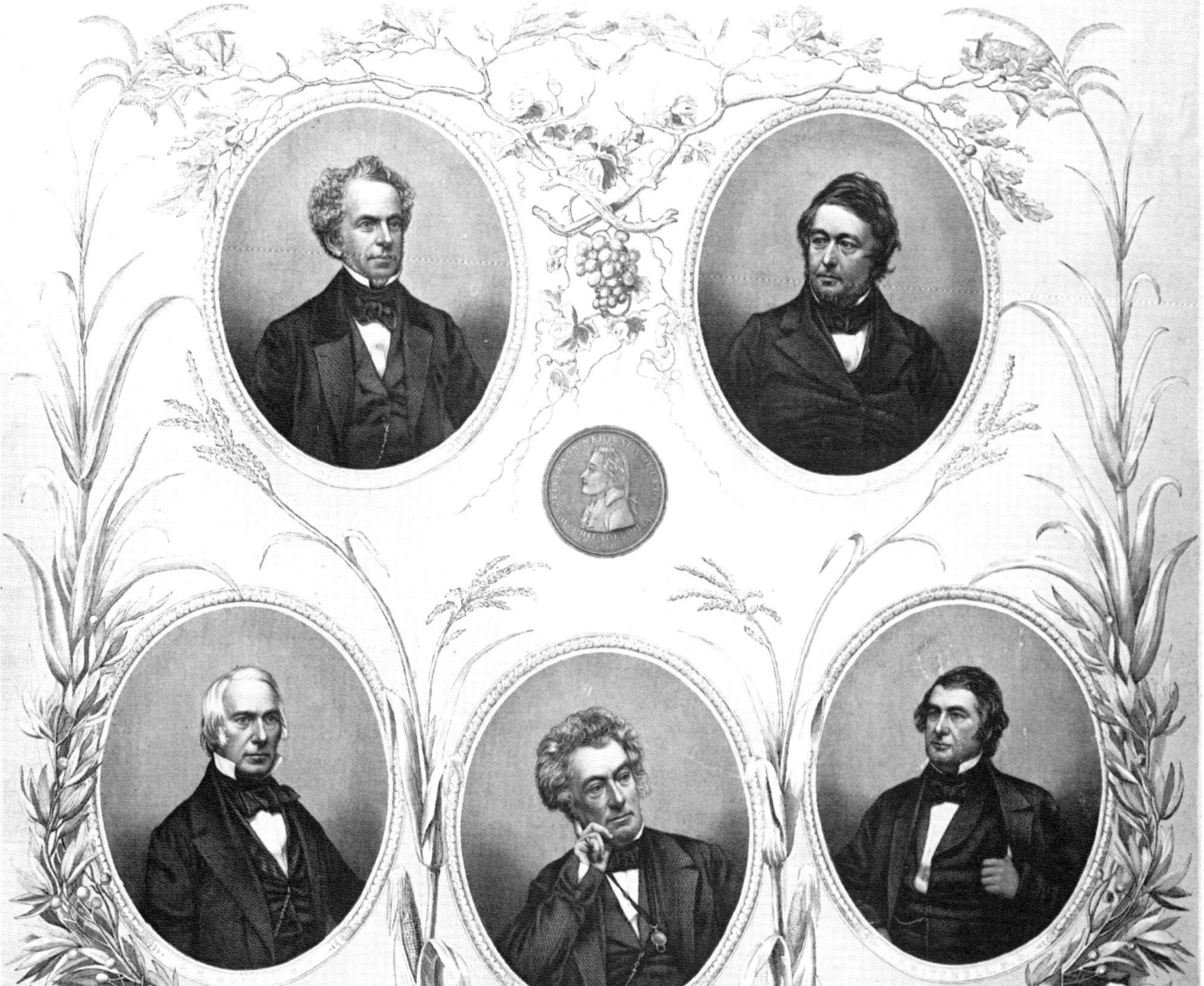

Portrait of Thomas D. Mütter

(See color plate)

THOMAS DENT MÜTTER, M.D. (1811-59)
By Thomas Sully (1783-1872)

Oil on canvas mounted on wood
Ca. 1842
33 1/2 x 29 1/2 in.

Exhibition: Philadelphia, *The Art of Philadelphia Medicine,* Philadelphia Museum of Art, Sept. 15-Dec. 7, 1965

Given in 1881 by Miss Clara P. Alsop, a relative of Mrs. Thomas D. Mütter

Accession number: 1881+e.P.01

Dr. Thomas Dent Mütter was professor of surgery at Jefferson Medical College from 1841 until 1856. He is best remembered for his collection of anatomical and pathological specimens, now located at the College of Physicians of Philadelphia.

Thomas Mütter was born in 1811 in Richmond, Virginia to parents whose forbears rendered distinguished service during the Revolutionary War. Orphaned at age eight, Mütter was sent to Hampden-Sydney College in Virginia by a guardian. He received his medical degree from the University of Pennsylvania in 1831 and spent the following year studying in European clinics. In Paris he encountered some of the most advanced and distinguished surgeons in the world, and there he developed a special interest in plastic and orthopaedic surgery.

Upon his return to Philadelphia in 1832 Mütter established a practice and began his teaching career with private instruction and then as assistant lecturer at the Philadelphia Medical Institute, a summer school. In 1841 he received an appointment at Jefferson Medical College as professor of the principles and practice of surgery.

Mütter was a careful and adroit surgeon, best known

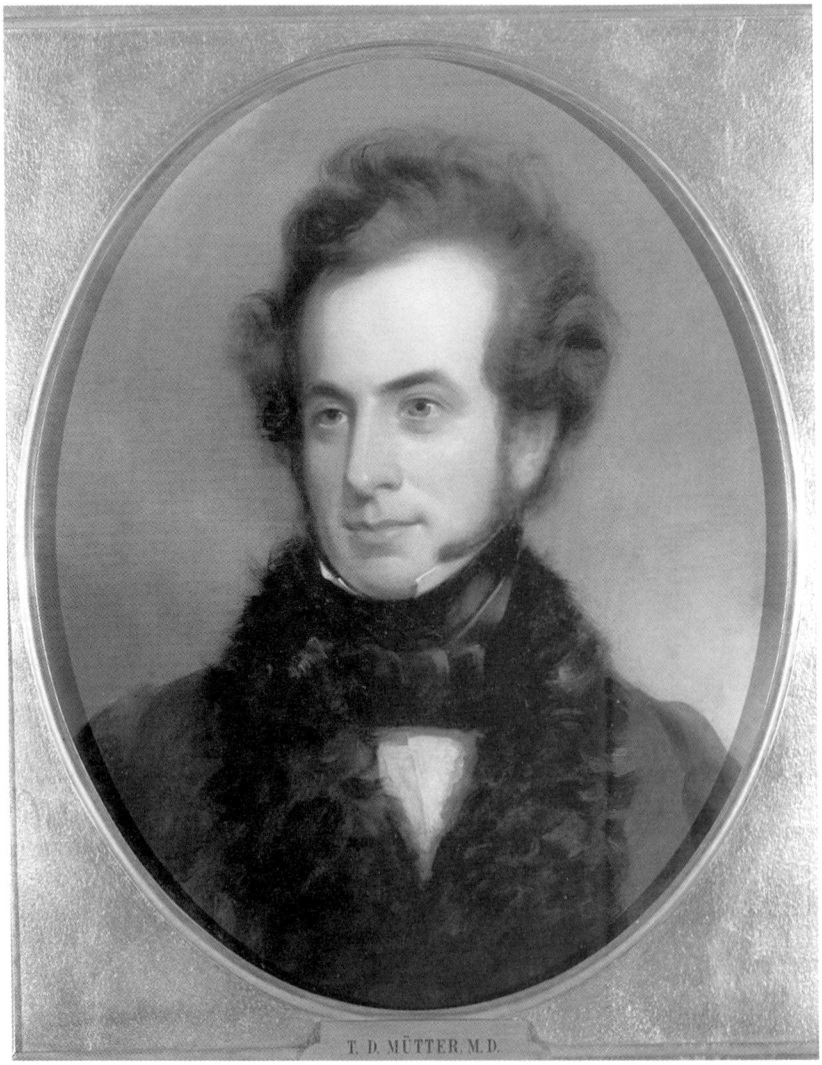

for operations for clubfoot, cleft palate, and the repair of traumatic deformities resulting from burns or injuries. He was the first Philadelphia surgeon to employ ethyl ether for anesthesia. His eloquent lectures were much admired by students because of his skillful use of illustrative materials such diagrams, models, and specimens. When a lung ailment forced him to retire in 1856, Mütter was immediately elected emeritus professor. He died three years later at the early age of forty-eight.

Though not a prolific writer, Mütter was the author of *A Lecture on Loxarthrus, or Club Foot* (1839) and was editor of Robert Liston's *Lectures on the Operations of Surgery* (1846). He bequeathed his private museum of anatomical and pathological specimens to the College of Physicians of Philadelphia, with a gift of thirty thousand dollars for its maintenance and for the establishment of a named lectureship. The Mütter Museum and lectureship at the college still perpetuate the donor's name.

Dr. John H. Brinton remembered Mütter's appearance from his student days at Jefferson: he was "small in stature, delicately framed, with a clear, blue eye, high forehead, and hair prematurely gray." He was a charming lecturer with a "wonderfully musical voice" that could be distinctly heard by the audience, and possessed the marvelous gift of "stamping a fact, a theory, a discipline, indelibly on the student's mind."

The small, oval oil portrait of Dr. Thomas D. Mütter is a bust-length romantic depiction emphasizing the subject's thick, tousled hair, ruddy cheeks, limpid eyes, and sensuous mouth, all accentuated by a coquettish turn of the head. The texture of his fur-collared coat is as loosely brushed as his facial features and hair. Highlights in his eyes and nose and on the edge of his standup collar suggest a pervasive vivacity. The atmospheric background is a dusty pink color with bluish shadows. In this case the painted depiction accords perfectly with verbal descriptions of the subject.

Because of one important document there was some uncertainty as to the artist of this unsigned portrait in the past. The November 23, 1881 minutes of the board of trustees meeting state that Dr. John H. Brinton presented to the hospital committee a communication he had received from Miss Clara P. Alsop announcing the gift of an "original portrait by Lambdin of the late Professor Thomas D. Mütter" and that a record of this gift was made in the minutes of the hospital. Neither the hospital minutes nor Miss Alsop's communication still exist to confirm that the artist actually named was Lambdin. James Reid Lambdin (1807-89) came to Philadelphia to study with Thomas Sully in 1823, but never achieved his teacher's popularity.

However, all later college records attribute the work to Thomas Sully; for example, Charles Frankenberger's 1915 article about Jefferson's portrait collection referred to the Mütter portrait as a "very valuable picture" by Sully painted about 1841 or 1842. Three contemporary curators of American art and painting conservators who have studied the painting reject the Lambdin attribution and award the portrait to Thomas Sully on both stylistic and technical grounds.

However, the portrait is not listed in *Thomas Sully's Register of Portraits 1801-1871*. Although the artist did record over twenty-five hundred portraits during his seven-decade career, Sully scholars have noted that the artist's list is incomplete. But interestingly, number 1245 in the *Register* is a "head" of Mrs. Mütter painted in 1842, with Sully's annotation, "a subscriber to my low price $50." Numerous examples in the *Register* show that Sully frequently painted several family members, especially husband and wife or parents and children, at around the same date. In the Jefferson collection's oval portrait, Mütter's hair is still dark and he looks young and dashing, quite possibly about thirty-one years, the age he would have been in 1842. Almost assuredly Sully painted a pair of portraits for Dr. and Mrs. Mütter.

The donor, Miss Clara P. Alsop, was from Middletown, Connecticut, as was Dr. Mütter's wife, the former Mary Alsop. It is not known how Clara and Mary Alsop were related. Dr. and Mrs. Mütter had been visiting the South to escape the harsh Philadelphia winter when Dr. Mütter died suddenly in Charleston, South Carolina in 1859. His young widow made arrangements for his burial in Middletown.

Thomas Sully was born at Horncastle, England, the son of actors who emigrated to America in 1792, settling in Richmond, Virginia, then Charleston, South Carolina. His earliest instructors, including his elder brother Lawrence, were miniature painters. The brothers moved to Norfolk in 1801 where Thomas Sully painted his first works. Lawrence died in 1804 and after two years of assuming responsibility for his brother's widow and three children, Thomas married his sister-in-law. He moved the family to New York and was successful almost immediately in receiving portrait commissions.

He himself commissioned a portrait from artist John Trumbull (1756-1843) to observe his technique first-hand; he also observed Gilbert Stuart (1755-1828) at work and received criticism from the master in Boston. In 1808 the Sullys settled in Philadelphia where the painter was kept busy, but like Dr. Mütter, the artist was advised to complete his training in Europe. Sully followed Stuart's advice to study with Benjamin West (1738-1820) in London. West, in turn, directed him to Sir Thomas Lawrence (1769-1830), Britain's leading portraitist, whose style greatly influenced the young American.

In 1810 Sully returned to Philadelphia where he soon became the city's most fashionable portrait painter. Over his very long career he developed into the country's leading portraitist of sitters from all the principal American cities. Sully's works were stylish, sentimental, and pleasing to patrons, and often displayed his knowledge of earlier masters. His most famous portrait subjects were Queen Victoria, the Marquis de Lafayette, actress Fanny Kemble, actor George Frederick Cooke dressed for the role of Richard III, as well as many American patriots and members of society. He also painted historical pictures and landscapes.

In 1812 Thomas Sully was elected an academician of the Pennsylvania Academy of the Fine Arts. Though he served as a director there for fifteen years, he refused an offer to become its president. He also ran a thriving commercial gallery for twenty-eight years with a partner, James Earle. Sully's *Hints to Young Painters and the Process of Portrait Painting* was published posthumously in 1873, almost two decades after it was written. He died in 1872 in his ninetieth year. Thomas Sully retrospective exhibitions have been held at the Pennsylvania Academy of the Fine Arts (1922) and at the National Portrait Gallery (1983).

Portrait of Joseph Pancoast

JOSEPH PANCOAST, M.D. (1805-82)
By Samuel Bell Waugh (1814-85)

Oil on canvas mounted on wood
1872
30 1/4 x 25 1/4 in.

Signed and dated lower right: "S. B. Waugh 1872"
Exhibition: Philadelphia, *Centennial Celebration Loan Collection of Portraits,* College of Physicians of Philadelphia, 1887

Given in 1874 by JMC faculty and alumni association
Accession number: 1874+e.P.01

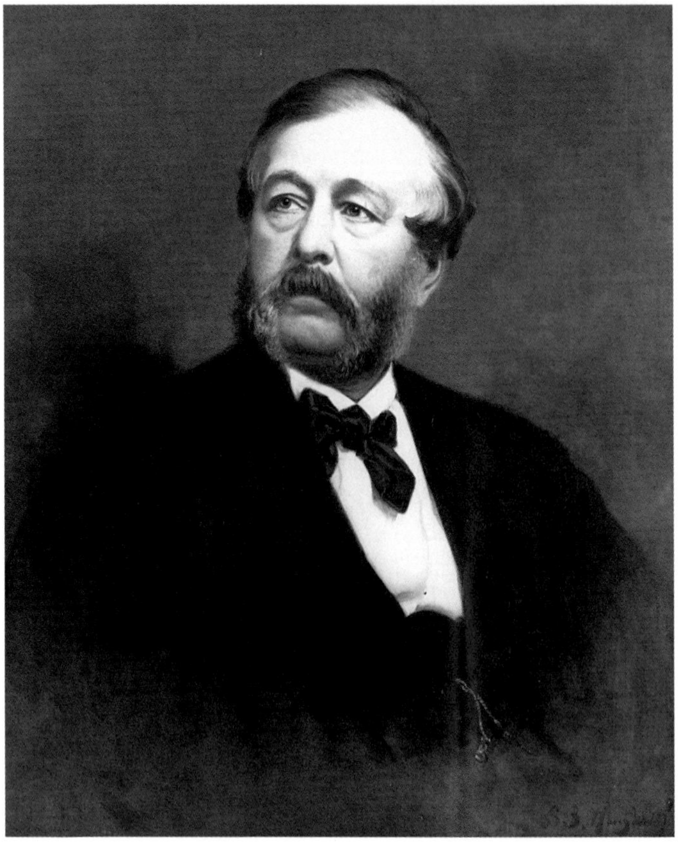

Dr. Joseph Pancoast was a distinguished and beloved professor of surgery and anatomy at Jefferson Medical College. He served the school for thirty-five years.

Born in Burlington, New Jersey in 1805, Joseph Pancoast descended from forbears who came to America with William Penn. He graduated from the Medical Department of the University of Pennsylvania in 1828, and began a surgical practice soon thereafter. By 1831 Dr. Pancoast was teaching classes in practical anatomy at the Philadelphia School of Anatomy and was appointed physician to the Philadelphia Hospital.

In 1839 he succeeded George McClellan, M.D. as professor of surgery at Jefferson Medical College. When the school was reorganized in 1841, Dr. Joseph Pancoast was shifted from the surgery chair to the chair of general, descriptive, and surgical anatomy. A Jefferson Medical College alumnus of 1846 recalled Pancoast's "untiring enthusiasm, with which he united with Professor Mütter to establish and sustain the surgical clinic of the college...[and] the originality and brilliancy of their operations [which] established the Jefferson Clinic as a fixed institution, far leading those of any other school."[2] Dr. Joseph Pancoast worked just as harmoniously with Dr. Thomas Mütter's successor, Samuel D. Gross, M.D.

Dr. Gross was lavish in his praise of Dr. Pancoast's skills, saying that he

> knew how to infuse life into the cadaver; how to wake up the bones and muscles and nerves and viscera, and make them respond to the diagnosis and treatment of disease and accident. His knowledge of topographical anatomy was profound, and few surgeons ever wielded a knife more gracefully, more boldly, or with greater accuracy and skill.[3]

Dr. Joseph Pancoast devised many original surgical procedures and instruments, including a hooked needle for cataract surgery, a hollow ivory tube to puncture obstructed lachrymal ducts, and an original "plow and groove" for rhinoplastic operations. He achieved the first surgical repair of exstrophy of the bladder; invented an abdominal tourniquet for compression of the aorta during hip and thigh amputations; and for empyema of the chest he innovated the practice of raising a semicircular flap of the integuments over the ribs through which he punctured the pleura and inserted a catheter for drainage.

Dr. Pancoast's chief literary works were his textbook, *Treatise on Operative Surgery* (1844), and a revised edition of Caspar Wistar's *System of Anatomy for the Use of Students of Medicine* (1842-43). In addition to editing several learned works, Pancoast was a frequent contributor to the *American Journal of Medical Sciences*, the *American Medical Intelligencer*, and the *Medical Examiner*.

Dr. Joseph Pancoast was also surgeon to the Pennsylvania Hospital from 1854 to 1864, and a member of the American Philosophical Society. Upon his retirement from Jefferson in 1874 he was elected emeritus professor. As his last official act Dr. Pancoast was given the honor of making the formal opening address of the new Jefferson Medical College Hospital in 1877.

Samuel B. Waugh's depiction of Pancoast is one of the artist's stronger efforts. The torso of the bust-length figure faces right slightly, while his head turns to the left. His eyes look up with an engaging glance into the near distance, perhaps to acknowledge a visitor. His ample girth fills the whole width of the canvas and his necktie is slightly askew. The pose and details of his features—roundness of his face, circles under his eyes, details of mustache, sideburns and beard, and emphatic curve of hair at his temples—bear a close resemblance to several prints and *cartes-de-visite* of the physician in the Jefferson art collection.

The portrait was presented to the trustees on behalf of the alumni association at the commencement of 1874. A trustees report of 1881 on contributions to the Jefferson Medical College Hospital states that the portrait had been installed in the amphitheater. A photo of about 1929 shows that the portrait was moved to the library's "portrait gallery" in the 1898 College Building.

Portrait of Joseph Pancoast

JOSEPH PANCOAST, M.D.
By George Edwin Ewing (1828-84)

Marble
1882-83
21 3/4 x 14 1/4 X 11 in.

Signed on back of right shoulder: "EWING Fec[t]"
Inscription on beveled edge of base: "PROF. JOSEPH PANCOAST.M.D./DECEASED MARCH 7TH 1882./PRESENTED BY/PROF. W[M] H. PANCOAST.M.D."

Given in 1883 by Dr. William H. Pancoast, son of the subject
Accession number: 1883+e.S.01

A marble sculpture and a bronze medal of Dr. Joseph Pancoast are less naturalistic and more idealized in style than the oil portrait by Samuel B. Waugh.

The imposing marble bust was created by George E. Ewing and presented by Dr. William H. Pancoast in 1883. While the sculptor has retained Dr. Joseph Pancoast's idiosyncratic hair, beard, and sideburns connected to a long mustache, he has lengthened the physician's rotund face into an ideal oval, straightened and slimmed his nose, and brought forward his receding chin. The narrowed eyes and knitted brows impart a sterner expression than in the painting. In characteristic neoclassical style the sitter's chest is not described anatomically but serves as the bust's integral base.

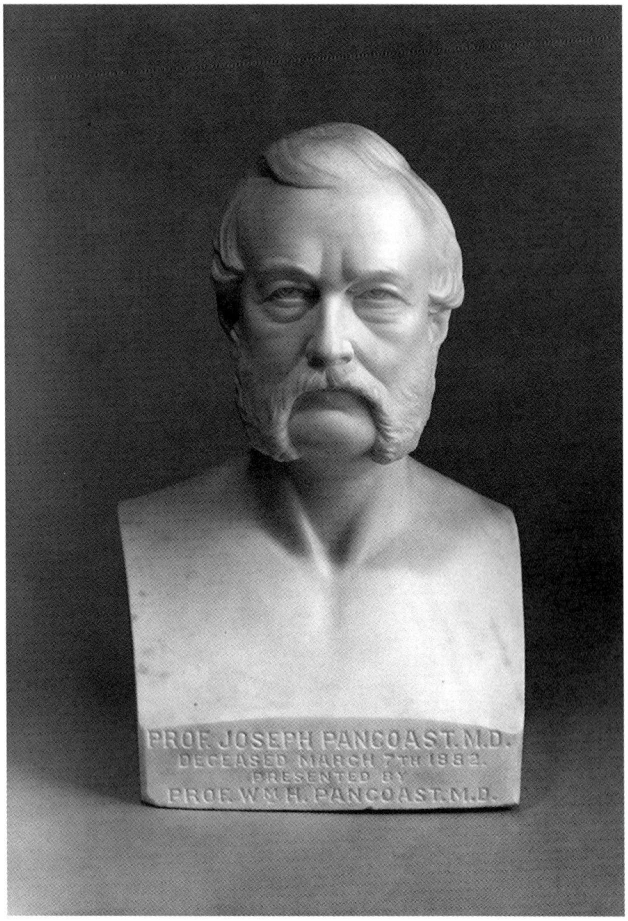

The sculpture bears a very close resemblance to an unsigned marble bust of Pancoast, of slightly different dimensions, at the College of Physicians of Philadelphia. That bust was also presented by Dr. William H. Pancoast, in 1887.

Ewing's sculpture of Dr. Joseph Pancoast caused quite a stir upon its arrival at Jefferson. In an emotional acceptance of the art work on March 31, 1883, Dr. Samuel D. Gross, president of the alumni association, said, "The fame of Professor Pancoast needs no marble for its preservation, but as the years roll on it will grow brighter and brighter, shedding a perpetual halo around this institution, which has been so highly honored and so signally benefitted by his services." In his *Autobiography* Gross paid further tribute to his friend and colleague of twenty years, saying that receiving the bust from Pancoast's son was an occasion that "almost unnerved me for the performance of this sad duty."

The bust was unveiled and presented to the trustees at the Jefferson Medical College commencement on April 2, 1883. At the presentation Dr. Addinell Hewson, vice president of the alumni association, requested that it be kept "where it may always be seen in intimate association with the special field of his labors, and by those who are peculiarly bound to admire and to emulate his example. It is not only a fine work of art, but a faithful likeness." The bust was placed in the surgical amphitheater.

Sculptor George E. Ewing was born in 1828 in Birmingham, England and forged his career in Great Britain, New York, and Philadelphia. He was best known for sculptures and medallions of literary and theatrical personalities such as William Shakespeare, Robert Burns, Ellen Terry, and Henry Irving. He also received commissions from the Duke and Duchess of Wales and the Duchess of Sutherland, among other members of the nobility, and exhibited works at the Royal Academy of London. Ewing worked in Philadelphia for the last three years of his life, but was much less successful in the United States than abroad, despite the help of theatrical patrons. He became despondent and died by his own hand in a New York hotel in 1884.

A bronze medal of Dr. Joseph Pancoast was struck at the United States Mint in Philadelphia in 1870, "issued on no other basis than an admiration for this man by Director of the Mint James Pollack."[4]

Portrait of Robert M. Huston

ROBERT MENDENHALL HUSTON, M.D. (1795-1864)
By unknown artist, after Thomas Buchanan Read

Oil on canvas mounted on wood
Before 1882
30 1/4 x 25 in.

Given in 1882 by Dr. Charles Huston (JMC 1842), son of the subject
Accession number: 1882+e.P.01

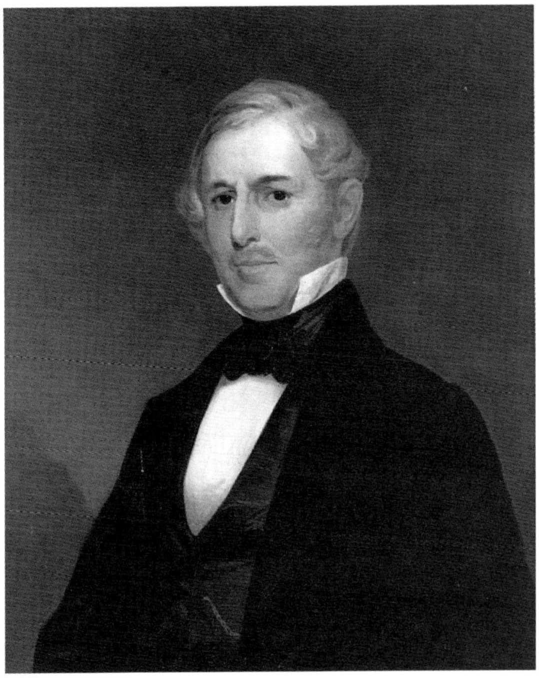

Professor Robert M. Huston's chair was also reassigned during the Jefferson Medical College faculty reorganization of 1841, from obstetrics to materia medica and therapeutics. He served for a time as dean during the "golden years."

Robert Huston was born in 1795 in Abingdon, Virginia and graduated from the Medical Department of the University of Pennsylvania in 1825. After serving in the War of 1812 as assistant surgeon in the army, he began the practice of medicine in Philadelphia.

In 1838 Dr. Huston was appointed chair of obstetrics, and then in 1841 moved to the chair of materia medica and therapeutics. He remained in the latter post until his retirement in 1857 when he was named emeritus professor. As dean from 1841 until 1854, he was credited with improving the financial affairs of the college. Huston edited the American edition of Fleetwood Churchill's *On the Theory and Practice of Midwifery* (1843) and was coeditor of the *Medical Examiner*.

In his address on the "Famous Faculty of 1841" Dr. John H. Brinton described Dr. Huston as "cool-headed and clearsighted" and "a constant toiler" whose most compelling trait was "perfect simplicity." The half-length portrait depicts the subject turned slightly to the left and wearing a neutral, even lifeless expression. The subject's vacuous expression is not necessarily excused by the fact that it is a copy and not a life portrait; it has much less vitality than another copy in the Jefferson archives: an engraving by Alexander H. Ritchie after a daguerreotype by Montgomery P. Simons.

The oil portrait's provenance is established by the March 29, 1882 minutes of the board of trustees in which a letter from Dr. Robert Huston's son, Charles Huston, M.D., stated that in accordance with the request of Professor John H. Brinton, the Huston family had presented a copy of a portrait by "T. Buchanan Reed" [*sic*, actually Thomas Buchanan Read].

Born in 1822, Read was a portrait and historical painter, sculptor, illustrator, and poet. He worked in Cincinnati and Boston before moving to Philadelphia in 1846, where he stayed until 1850 when he went abroad to live in Rome and Florence. He died in 1872. The original Read portrait of Dr. Robert Huston, from which the present one was copied, must have been made in the late 1840s when the artist resided in Philadelphia.

One unconvincing document in the Jefferson records that tenuously ascribes the Huston portrait to Jacob Eichholtz must be totally discounted on historical and stylistic grounds.

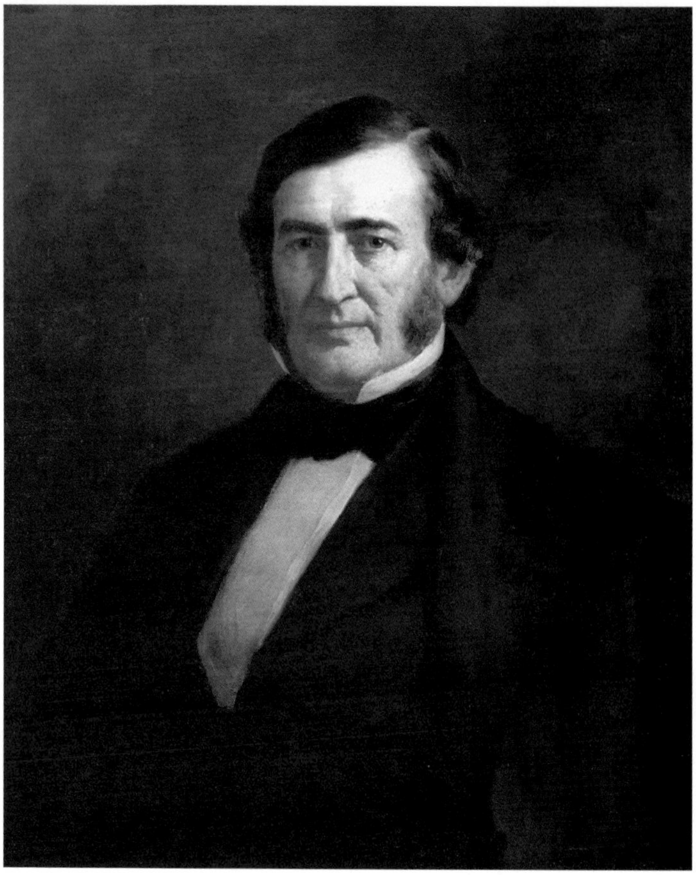

Portrait of John K. Mitchell

JOHN KEARSLEY MITCHELL, M.D.
(1793-1858)
By unknown artist

Oil on canvas mounted on wood
Before 1883
30 x 25 in.

Given in 1883 by Dr. S. Weir Mitchell, son of the subject
Accession number: 1883+e.P.01

Dr. John Kearsley Mitchell was appointed chair of the practice of medicine at Jefferson Medical College in 1841, succeeding Dr. John K. Revere. He was much respected and beloved by the students.

Mitchell was born in 1793 in Shepherdstown, Virginia to a notable medical family. He was the son and grandson of Scottish physicians, and would be the father and grandfather of physicians. He received an undergraduate degree from the University of Edinburgh, and then a medical degree from the University of Pennsylvania in 1819. After three years as ship's surgeon on voyages to China and the East Indies, Mitchell settled in Philadelphia and established a medical practice there.

In 1822 he was appointed lecturer in medical chemistry at the Philadelphia Medical Institute, and then professor of chemistry at the Franklin Institute. In 1841 he became chair of the practice of medicine at Jefferson Medical College, and held that position until his death in 1858. He also served on the medical staffs of the Pennsylvania Hospital and the Philadelphia City Hospital.

Mitchell's writings include papers on the osmosis of fluids and gases, an apparatus to solidify gaseous carbonic acid, the spinal origin of rheumatism, the use of nitrate of silver in typhoid fever, the parasitic etiology of malaria and other epidemical fevers, and the toxic effects of arsenic. He also invented a spine car for cases of vertebral disease. In addition to writings on philosophy and social matters, Mitchell published a volume of poetry.

Dr. John H. Brinton wrote that Dr. Mitchell was "open handed and hospitable, a charming companion," genial yet dignified. His lectures were terse but powerfully illustrated, spiced with anecdote and lively wit, making a "favorable impression on the class, an impression strengthened by their personal love for their teacher." In appearance he was "tall and portly, with a gentle, polished bearing."

In the half-length portrait Mitchell is turned slightly

to the left. His expansive torso fills the entire width of the canvas. His face is depicted in detailed, three-dimensional volume, and the expression suggests an engaging and kindly disposition.

The acquisition of the unsigned portrait was recorded in the June 11, 1883 minutes of the board of trustees meeting, in which appreciation was expressed to the donor, the subject's son S. Weir Mitchell, M.D. (JMC 1850). The artist's name is not mentioned in the minutes, very likely because it was a copy.

Charles Frankenberger's article of 1915 about the Jefferson art collection names George W. Pettit as the artist, but the painting does not stylistically resemble other signed Pettits in the Jefferson collection. In fact, the portrait bears a strong resemblance in pose, costume, and expression to an engraving in the Jefferson collection made in 1846 by Welch and Walter after a daguerreotype by Montgomery P. Simons. It is more likely that the oil copy was after the engraving or after the original daguerreotype.

Portrait of Franklin Bache

FRANKLIN BACHE, M.D. (1792-1864)
By Frederick Gutekunst (1831-1917)

Photograph
1860-64
Image size: 3 1/2 x 2 1/4 in.
Card size: 4 x 2 3/8 in.

Stamped on back of card: "F. Gutekunst/704 & 706 Arch St./Philadelphia"

Given after 1870 by unknown donor
Accession number: 1870+f.Ph.02

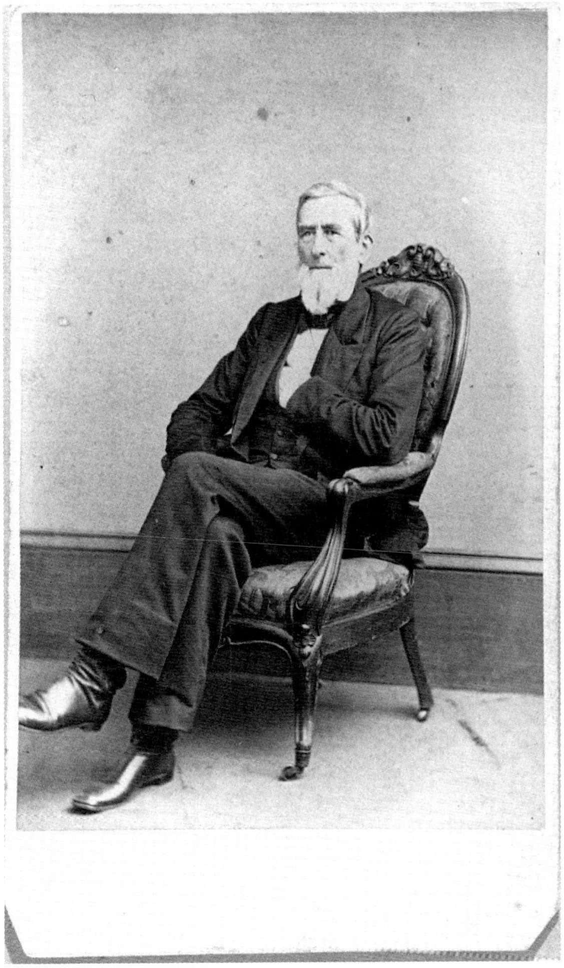

Dr. Franklin Bache was elected to the chemistry chair at Jefferson Medical College in 1841, succeeding Dr. Jacob Green. Bache was greatly esteemed for his literary work as author and editor.

Franklin Bache was the great-grandson of Benjamin Franklin whose only daughter, Sarah, was married to Richard Bache, an English gentleman from Lancashire. Franklin Bache was born in 1792 in Philadelphia. Educated at the University of Pennsylvania he received an undergraduate degree in 1810 and a medical degree in 1814. He began his study of medicine as a private pupil of Dr. Benjamin Rush and his son, Dr. James Rush.

Bache established a practice in Philadelphia after three years of service as a surgeon in the army during the War of 1812. Before his appointment as chair of chemistry at Jefferson in 1841 he filled the following posts: physician to the Walnut Street Prison and the Eastern Penitentiary, and professor of chemistry both at the Franklin Institute and the Philadelphia College of Pharmacy. He remained at Jefferson from 1841 until his death in 1864.

Dr. Franklin Bache's greatest medical contributions were literary. His *System of Chemistry for the Use of Students of Medicine* was published in 1819. He participated in four revisions of the *United States Phar-*

macopoeia; served as coeditor with Dr. George B. Wood of eleven editions of the *Dispensatory of the United States of America*; and wrote articles for and coedited the *North American Medical and Surgical Journal*. Seventy-nine thousand copies of the *Dispensatory* were sold during Bache's lifetime.

Dr. Bache was elected president of the American Philosophical Society, vice president of the College of Physicians of Philadelphia, and an honorary member of the Imperial Academy of Naturalists in Moscow.

The small, undated *carte-de-visite* photograph of Dr. Bache by Frederick Gutekunst dates between 1860 when the format was first popularized in the United States and 1864 when Bache died. The subject is shown sitting erectly but stiffly in an armchair in the photographer's studio. His legs are crossed and his left hand is tucked into his vest, a stock gesture. His white hair is thick and his beard is extraordinarily long and pointed.

The subject's taciturn countenance recalls Dr. John H. Brinton's description of Bache's lecture room accuracy: "His speech was measured and slow, devoid of metaphor, free from all blemish...He was a man of absolute precision and this quality he carried into all his relations in life."

The Jefferson archival collection also has a close-up photograph of Dr. Bache by Frederick Gutekunst taken about the same time, showing the physician with a similarly steely and determined expression. In an earlier engraving of 1846 by Alexander H. Ritchie after a daguerreotype by Montgomery P. Simons, the subject has dark hair and is clean-shaven.

Frederick Gutekunst was one of the most popular and successful of the nineteenth-century portrait photographers. Born in Philadelphia in 1831, he was the son of a German cabinetmaker. Always scientifically inclined, Gutekunst experimented with chemistry and electricity while employed by a druggist after a "common school" education. As a young man he conceived the idea of making copper electrotypes from daguerreotypes, although this method was of little commercial value.

Perhaps more than any other contemporary photographer, he was sought after by the country's most notable celebrities including presidents, generals, princes of the church, actors, writers, statesmen, and business tycoons. He personally directed his photographic gallery for over sixty years, from 1856 to 1917. He purchased the U.S. rights to the phototype in 1878. He reportedly had the largest collection of celebrity cabinet-sized portrait photographs.

Frederick Gutekunst was awarded many medals, honors, and gifts for his work. An obituary in the Philadelphia *Evening Bulletin* reported that his famous panoramic picture of the Philadelphia Exposition of 1876, purportedly the largest photograph ever made, was so acclaimed that he received a pair of gold-lined bronze vases from the Mikado of Japan, a gold medal from King Victor Emmanuel of Italy, and a decoration from Emperor Francis Joseph of Austria.

Portrait of Charles D. Meigs

CHARLES DELUCENA MEIGS, M.D. (1792-1869)
By Samuel Bell Waugh (1814-85)

Oil on canvas mounted on wood
Ca. 1872-79
30 x 25 in.

Signed and dated lower right: "S. B. Waugh 187-" (last digit indecipherable)

Given in 1880 by Dr. John Forsyth Meigs, son of the subject
Accession number: 1880+e.P.01

Dr. Charles D. Meigs was professor of obstetrics and the diseases of women and children for two decades starting in 1841. A leader in American obstetrics, he was vigorously opposed to several contemporary theories and practices.

Charles Meigs was born in St. George, Bermuda in 1792. His family moved first to New Haven, Connecticut in 1796 when his father was appointed professor of mathematics and natural philosophy at Yale College, and then to Athens, Georgia in 1801 when his father became president of the University of Georgia.

After a classical education, young Meigs graduated from the University of Georgia in 1809, and began to study medicine with a local doctor. After receiving a medical degree from the University of Pennsylvania in 1817, he practiced briefly in Augusta and then returned to Philadelphia. He became one of the first editors of *The North American Medical and Surgical Journal.* He lectured on midwifery from 1830 to 1835 at the Philadelphia Association for Medical Instruction.

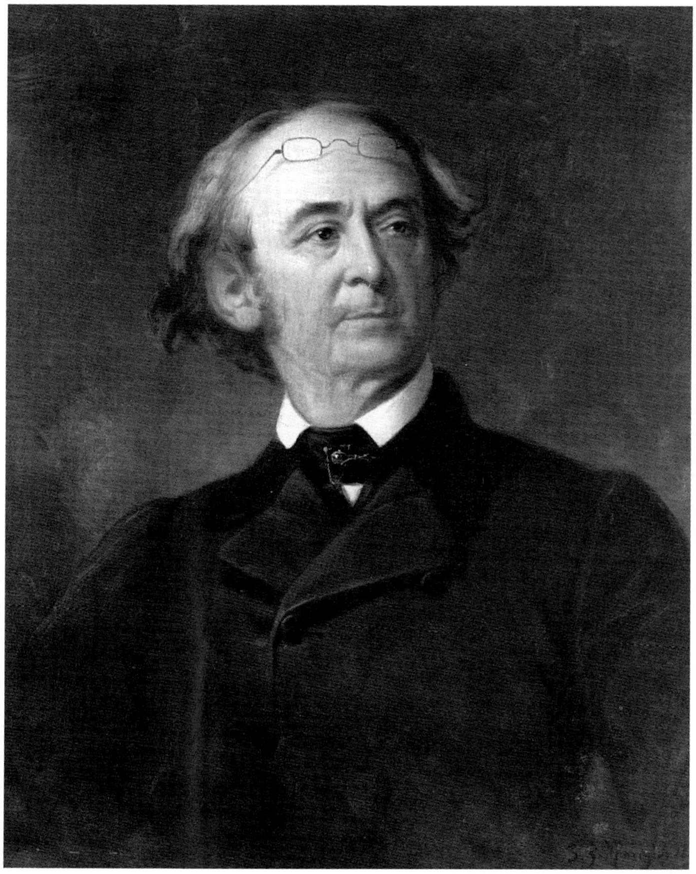

In 1837 Dr. Meigs was appointed by the College of Physicians of Philadelphia to chair a committee of midwifery that would make a report to the trustees of the Preston Retreat who were charged with the responsibility of establishing a "lying-in hospital for poor white women of Philadelphia and Delaware Counties." In 1841 Meigs was appointed to the chair of obstetrics and diseases of women and children at Jefferson Medical College, a post he held until his resignation in 1860 when he was made emeritus professor.

In 1831 Dr. Meigs translated Alfred Velpeau's *Elementary Treatise on Midwifery*, and in 1838 published his own work, *The Philadelphia Practice of Midwifery*. Some of his other contributions to the literature include: *Females and their Diseases* (1848), *Obstetrics: the Science and the Art* (1849), *Certain Diseases of Young Children* (1850), and *On the Nature, Signs, and Treatment of Childbed Fevers* (1854).

Meigs repeatedly drew attention to pulmonary embolism as a cause of sudden death in childbirth. He was contentiously opposed to the use of anesthesia in childbirth and to ovariotomy and Caesarian section. Meigs was worsted in the debate with Dr. Oliver Wendell Holmes and others on the contagiousness of puerperal fever.

In his address about the Jefferson faculty of 1841 Dr. John H. Brinton described Meigs's "zealous" manner in the classroom as "all earnestness, and immovable in his own convictions, and [he] sought to make all share them with him." But he was an engaging teacher and his lecture style had "strange charm, at times poetic, at times charged with quaint humor." Meigs was an accomplished watercolorist, even making his own illustrations for his *Acute and Chronic Diseases of the Neck of the Uterus* (1854).

In a bust-length portrait by Samuel B. Waugh the physician's body is posed frontally. His head is turned sharply to the right as though someone or something has just captured his attention. His wispy brown hair trails into the portrait's neutral atmospheric background. His pursed lips and knitted brows give him a somber expression. Wire reading glasses perched on his high-domed forehead must have been a customary practice: a contemporary *carte-de-visite* in the Jefferson archives shows Meigs with his spectacles in the same position.

The bust-length portrait in the Jefferson collection is Waugh's own copy of the half-length portrait of Dr. Meigs he had painted in 1860. The faltering and uncertain beginnings of Jefferson's portrait tradition are demonstrated by a query and editorial reply in the January 15, 1880 issue of the *College and Clinical Record.* A "graduate of the class of 1856" asked:

> What has become of the portrait of the late Professor Charles D. Meigs, which was painted for the Class and presented to the trustees of the College many years ago? Why is it not placed on the wall of the hospital lecture-room with the portraits of the other professors? The portrait is now in the possession of Dr. John Forsyth Meigs...son of the old professor, who based his claims to it on the ground that it was a personal gift from the class to his father. Many of the graduates...and members of the Board of Trustees have expressed surprise at its absence...believing...that it was painted for the College. The distinguished artist, S. B. Waugh...has always been under the latter impression. Dr. Mitchell H. Picot...who acted as spokesman of the Class on the occasion of the presentation, writes to say that it was a personal token of affection from them to Professor Meigs, not to the College. We hope that...the portrait, either original or copied, may by donation or purchase find a place alongside the other professors of the past.

Another answer to the query was printed in the February 16 issue:

> I was a member of the graduating class of 1861, which made the presentation, and I know that the portrait was painted and presented to Prof. Meigs as a token of personal esteem and affection, and Prof. Meigs received the painting himself in one of his own happy little speeches...He was much moved by that memorial of the class's love, especially as it was to be the last year of his service.

The editor added information that the Jefferson trustees had just accepted a copy of Waugh's original portrait of Meigs from his son, Dr. John Forsyth Meigs. This is confirmed in the board's minutes of the March 12, 1880 meeting, stating that an excellent "duplicate" portrait had been received and "placed in the clinical amphitheater of the Hospital by the side of his colleague, Dr. Dunglison."

It must have been an error to identify the writer of the first query as "Graduate of 1856," or else his reference to "the Class" does not refer to his own. All other documents connect the portrait with the class of 1861. It makes sense that the portrait was commissioned and painted to honor Meigs in 1860 when he was making plans to retire. He was persuaded to remain one more session because his successor was in poor health, so therefore, the portrait was presented upon his retirement in February 1861.

The original portrait remained with the Meigs family until 1975 when it was donated by Dr. John Wister Meigs, great-great-grandson of Dr. Charles D. Meigs, to the College of Physicians of Philadelphia. In the larger portrait Meigs is shown standing, but details of his pose and costume are the same as in the Jefferson portrait.

The Jefferson copy is signed and dated "S. B. Waugh 187-" (last digit is indecipherable). Charles Frankenberger stated that Waugh painted this copy in 1872, but if it was intended for Jefferson Medical College, one wonders why there was a delay in presenting it until 1880. It might well have been painted in the late 1870s.

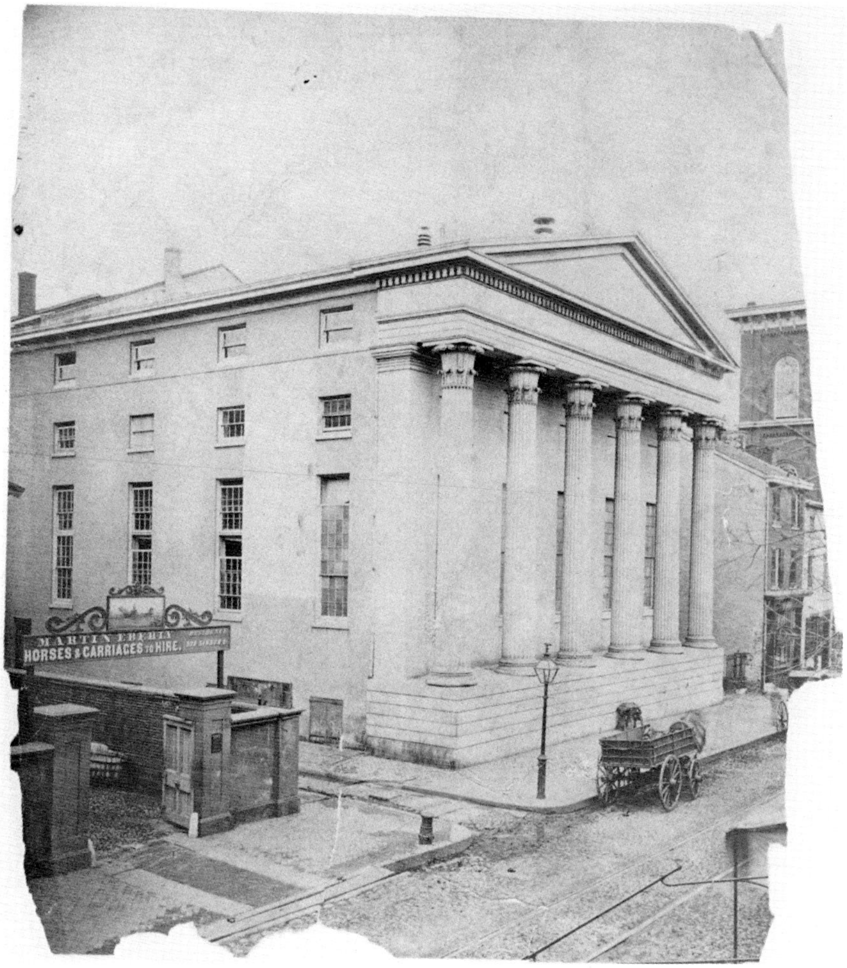

Jefferson Medical College (Ely Building)

ELY BUILDING RENOVATIONS
By Napoleon LeBrun (1821-1901)
1846

Photograph
By unknown photographer
Ca. 1870
7 1/8 x 6 1/2 in.

Given after 1900 by unknown donor
Accession number: 1900+f.Ph.12

Even before the appointment of the "Famous Faculty of 1841" the 1828 Medical Hall was deemed no longer adequate, due to increasing enrollment and revision of the charter to establish Jefferson Medical College as a separate institution. The trustees decided to renovate rather than relocate, and in 1838 hired Thomas Ustick Walter (1804-87) to remodel the building. From its earliest history Jefferson has commissioned many of the most prominent Philadelphia architects practicing in the nineteenth and twentieth centuries.

Unfortunately, no images of this first renovation are extant. But written descriptions say that Thomas U. Walter's plan included two "capacious" lecture rooms that seated 450 students and "private apartments" for professors and the janitor in the front of the building. In the rear were two large halls for dissecting rooms and for the anatomical museum which contained wet and dry preparations, models made of wood, wax, and plaster, and paintings and engravings.

Thomas Walter, who studied under William Strickland (1788-1854), is best remembered for his design of Founder's Hall of Girard College in Philadelphia, and for the wings and dome of the United States Capitol in Washington, D.C.

College expansion continued with the rental in 1844 of neighborhood rooms for postoperative patients and others too sick for home treatment. By 1846 it was decided to remodel Medical Hall again. This time architect Napoleon LeBrun was hired and the work was accomplished between May and September of that same year. This renovation was considered satisfactory until 1879.

The *Annual Announcement of Jefferson Medical College of Philadelphia* for the session 1846-47 included a detailed description of Napoleon LeBrun's improvements, and on the title page featured an engraving of the College Building for the first time. The remodeled facade was in the Roman temple form with a six-columned portico featuring Corinthian columns, pediment, and entablature. LeBrun rebuilt the north wall so that the main building was now fifty-nine feet wide. Staircases were removed from the main building so as to increase the capacity of the two lecture rooms which were now wider and longer. The six hundred seats in the upper lecture room were arranged in an octagonal form, with the effect of an amphitheater in which the lecturer stood in the center.

An adjoining lot fronting on Tenth Street, seventeen feet wide and nearly one hundred feet deep, was purchased and used as the student entrance with an iron railing and gateway. At the rear of this lot a new building thirty-six feet deep was erected. It contained staircases which connected to various rooms in the main building. The new building contained a private dissecting room, two patient rooms, a faculty room, and a janitor's room.

Napoleon LeBrun was born in Philadelphia in 1821, the son of a French diplomat. After training under Thomas U. Walter, his reputation was established in Philadelphia with the design for the Cathedral of Saints Peter and Paul in 1841. Six years later he gained experience with musical auditoriums by his enlargement of the Musical Fund Society, and in 1855 he won a competition to design Philadelphia's Academy of Music. After the Civil War he moved to New York where he designed structures for the city's fire department. LeBrun served two terms as president of the New York chapter of the American Institute of Architects and eighteen years as a member of the State Board of Architectural Examiners. He died in 1901.

The Jefferson collection is fortunate to have several vintage photographs and engravings of the Ely Building in most stages of its renovations. Among them is a cabinet-sized photograph that appears to be an enlargement of a *carte-de-visite* taken by Frederick Gutekunst and dated 1870. The Ely Building is shown in the context of its surrounding neighborhood with such elements as the gas lamp on the corner, the horse-drawn wagon, the trolley tracks, and Martin Eberly's establishment with "Horses & Carriages to Hire."

Jefferson Medical College (Ely Building)

ELY BUILDING RENOVATIONS
By Napoleon LeBrun
1846

Engraving, etching
By Richard G. Harrison (active mid-nineteenth century)
Ca. 1846-65
Image size: 3 1/4 x 8 1/2 in.
Sheet size: 5 x 11 in.

Signed lower center: "R.G. Harrison sc"
Inscription below image: "JEFFERSON MEDICAL COLLEGE"

Given after 1900 by unknown donor
Accession number: 1900+f.Pr.02

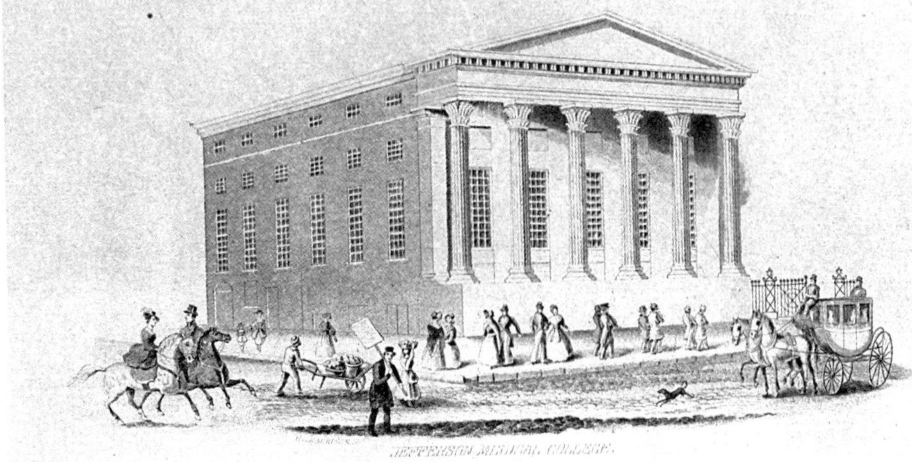

An image of the LeBrun renovation of the Ely Building was made in a different style by Richard G. Harrison. The stylized and delicate engraving is a horizontal view that accentuates urban life on the cobblestone street fronting the building. One sees fashionably dressed couples strolling or horseback riding, workers carrying a shovel or pushing a wheelbarrow loaded with baskets of produce, an elegant horse-drawn carriage with coachman and footman, and a frisky dog. The building looks like a flat stage set behind actors.

The undated engraving is signed Richard G. Harrison, but it is not known if the artist is the father or son by the same name. Both worked in Philadelphia and came from a noted family of engravers.

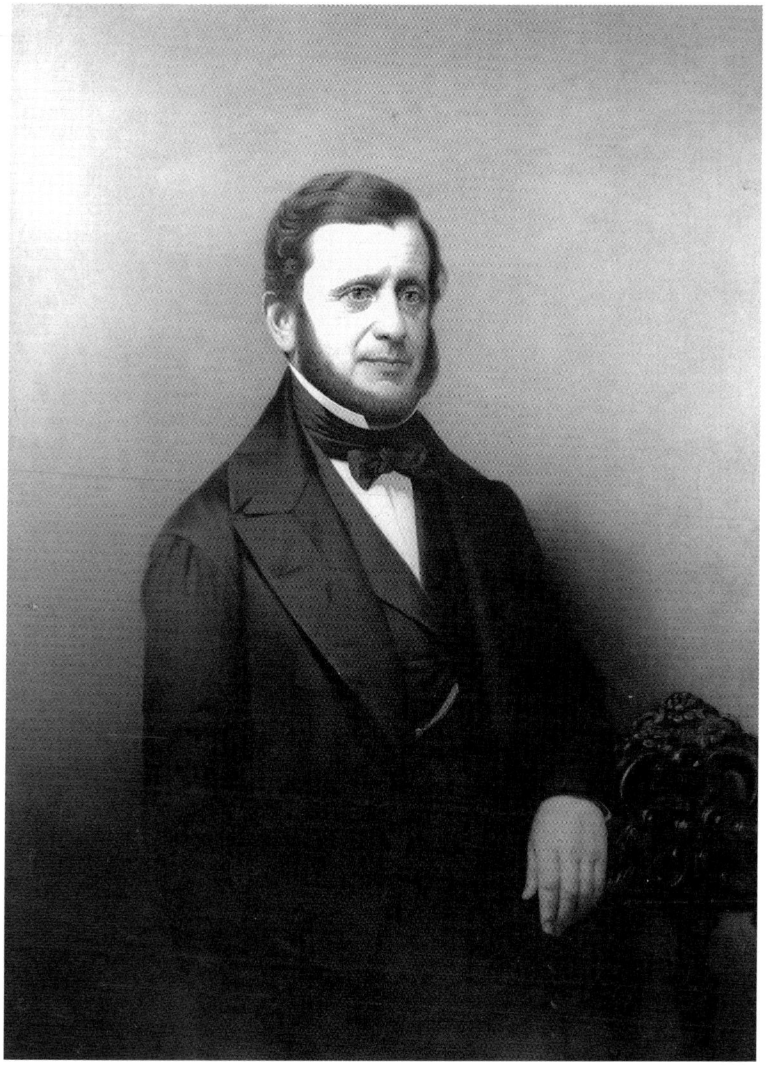

Portrait of J. Altamont Phillips

J. ALTAMONT PHILLIPS (d. 1863)
By unknown artist

Oil on canvas
Mid-nineteenth century
44 1/2 x 34 in.

Given in 1913 by Mrs. J. Bunford Samuel, daughter of the subject
Accession number: 1913+e.P.01

J. Altamont Phillips served as a trustee of Jefferson Medical College from 1859 to 1863, the year of his death. In 1913 his daughter, Mrs. J. Bunford Samuel, presented his portrait to the college, and the painting was installed in the trustees' room.

The elegantly dressed subject is shown two-thirds length and life-sized. He stands facing to the right, and his left arm rests on an ornate Renaissance Revival chair back. His oval face is framed by thick brown wavy hair, sideburns, and beard. His large blue eyes gaze thoughtfully into the distance. The picture's meticulously painted surface is smooth and glassy with no visible brush strokes. Details of facial features, hair, watch chain, and chair carving are rendered with great precision.

The undated and unsigned, mid-nineteenth-century portrait is of high quality, although much restored. It appears to have been painted by a European artist or by an American trained on the Continent, possibly France.

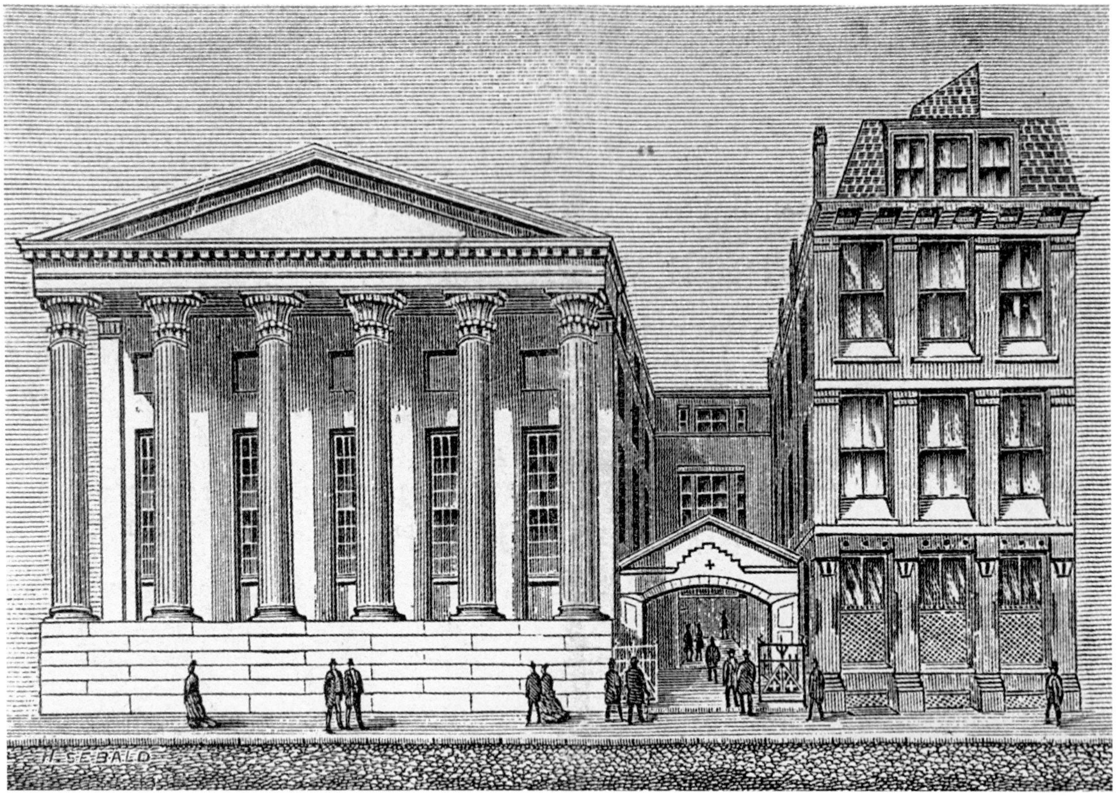

Ely Building and New Laboratory Building

ELY BUILDING
Renovated 1846 by Napoleon LeBrun
LABORATORY BUILDING
By Frank Furness (1839-1912)
1879
Depicted in the *Fifty-fifth Annual Announcement of the Jefferson Medical College of Philadelphia, Session of 1879-80*

Engraving
By H. Sebald (active mid-nineteenth century)
1879
Image size: 2 5/8 x 3 3/4 in.
Sheet size: 8 3/8 x 5 3/4 in.

Signed lower left: "H. SEBALD"

Printed for Jefferson Medical College, 1879
Accession number: 1879+e.Pr.01

The title page of Jefferson Medical College's 1879-80 *Annual Announcement* shows Napoleon LeBrun's 1846 renovation of the Ely Building and the new Laboratory Building by Frank Furness who had also designed Jefferson's first hospital built in 1877.

The *Announcement* states that the Laboratory Building contained a room for operative and minor surgery, and had spacious laboratories for practical chemistry, practical microscopy, and practical physiology. The architectural drawing depicts a narrow, three-story building surmounted by a mansard roof, typical of the work of architect Frank Furness. Though the Laboratory is just a bit taller than the adjacent College Building, its strong vertical elements of windows and pilasters make the new building seem to dominate the earlier one.

Frank Furness was born in 1839 in Philadelphia, the son of a Unitarian minister. He studied architecture first in the office of John Fraser (ca. 1825-1903?) in Philadelphia, then in the atelier of Richard Morris Hunt (1827-95) in New York. Morris had studied in Paris and was well versed in contemporary French and English design. Furness served in the Civil War during which he won the Medal of Honor. After returning to Philadelphia he formed a partnership with John Fraser and George W. Hewitt (1841-1916/17) which lasted from 1867 to 1871. He practiced just with Hewitt from 1871 to 1875, and then alone from 1875 to 1881. His last partner was Allen Evans with whom he practiced from 1881 to 1895. Frank Furness died in 1912.

Furness's notable buildings in the Philadelphia area included the Pennsylvania Academy of the Fine Arts, the Zoological Gardens, the Church of the Holy Apostles (later Shilow Baptist Church), the Rodeph Shalom Synagogue, the First Unitarian Church and Parish House, the Jewish Hospital (later Einstein Medical Center), the Provident Life and Trust Company, the Library of the University of Pennsylvania (later the art and architecture library known as the "Furness Building"), the Bryn Mawr Hotel (later the Baldwin School), the Merion Cricket Club, and the Undine Barge Club.

Furness was both admired and castigated for his originality and exuberant expressiveness in design, profuse ornamentation, and combinations of materials and color. Regrettably, many of his buildings were later demolished, but Frank Furness shaped the look of Victorian Philadelphia more than any other architect.

The architectural drawing in the *College Announcement* was signed by H. Sebald. Most likely the artist is Hugo Sebald or Hobarth Sebald, both of whom were engravers working in Philadelphia in the mid-nineteenth century.

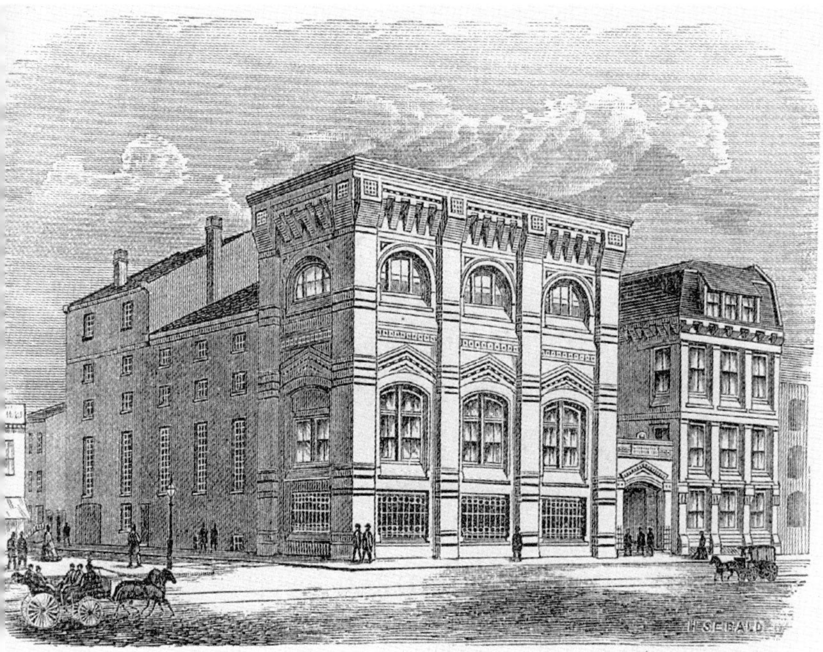

Ely Building Renovations and the Laboratory Building

ELY BUILDING RENOVATIONS
By James Hamilton Windrim (1840-1919)
1881
LABORATORY BUILDING
By Frank Furness
1879
Depicted in the *Fifty-seventh Annual Announcement of the Jefferson Medical College of Philadelphia, Session of 1881-82*

Engraving
By H. Sebald (active mid-nineteenth century)
1881
Image size: 2 3/4 x 3 3/4 in.
Sheet size: 9 1/4 x 5 3/4 in.

Signed lower right: "H. SEBALD"

Printed for Jefferson Medical College, 1881
Accession number: 1881+e.Pr.01

The Jefferson Medical College *Annual Announcement* of 1881-82 discussed the fact that increased class size had made "additional accommodations absolutely necessary" for the Ely Building. The renovation was accomplished by architect James H. Windrim.

Napoleon LeBrun's columnar porch was removed, and a new facade erected so that the interior was extended to the property line on every floor. An additional story was added in the front and rear, but the side walls were left intact. The upper and lower lecture rooms were enlarged and more commodious dissecting rooms were constructed. New rooms for practical obstetrics and for microscopy, and a laboratory for pathological histology and morbid anatomy were provided. The "extensive" anatomical, surgical, and pathological museum was located in this building.

James H. Windrim's new facade was clearly divided into three bays, with an eclectic mixture of Gothic and Roman arches separated by flat vertical elements, all surmounted by a Florentine overhang at the top with projecting eaves and brackets. The new construction was harmonious with the style of Frank Furness's Laboratory Building.

Born in Philadelphia in 1840, James H. Windrim was a member of the first graduating class of Girard College in 1856. He maintained a lifelong association with the college, and in 1871 he was appointed architect to the Girard Estate and subsequently designed and superintended the erection of many buildings there.

His earliest professional experiences were as a carpenter's assistant in West Chester, Pennsylvania and as a draftsman for a stonemason who built John Notman's (1810-65) Holy Trinity Episcopal Church in Philadelphia. In the early 1860s the Pennsylvania Railroad chose Windrim to design its Union Depot in Pittsburgh. Upon his return to Philadelphia in 1867 he won a competition to design the Masonic Temple, still an exciting city landmark today with its numerous halls in diverse Oriental, Middle Eastern, and Western styles.

Other notable architectural works in Philadelphia by James H. Windrim are the Academy of Natural Sciences, the Agricultural Hall at the 1876 Centennial Exposition, the First Regiment Armory, and the Civil War Memorial Gateway. He also designed the Pennsylvania State Library in Harrisburg, Pennsylvania. From 1889 to 1891 he served as the supervising architect of the U.S. Treasury in Washington, D.C., and from 1891 to 1895 he was director of public works for the City of Philadelphia. By 1892 Windrim's son, John Torrey Windrim (1866-1934), had joined the firm and from then on it is difficult to separate their work.

Jefferson Medical College Hospital

JEFFERSON MEDICAL COLLEGE HOSPITAL
By Frank Furness (1839-1912) and George W. Hewitt (1841-1916/17)
1877
Depicted in the *Fifty-third Annual Announcement of the Jefferson Medical College of Philadelphia, Session of 1877-78*

Engraving
By unknown artist
1877
Image size: 3 3/4 x 5 in.
Sheet size: 9 1/4 x 6 3/4 in.

Inscription: "JEFFERSON MEDICAL COLLEGE HOSPITAL PHILA"

Printed for Jefferson Medical College, 1877
Accession number: 1877+e.Pr.03

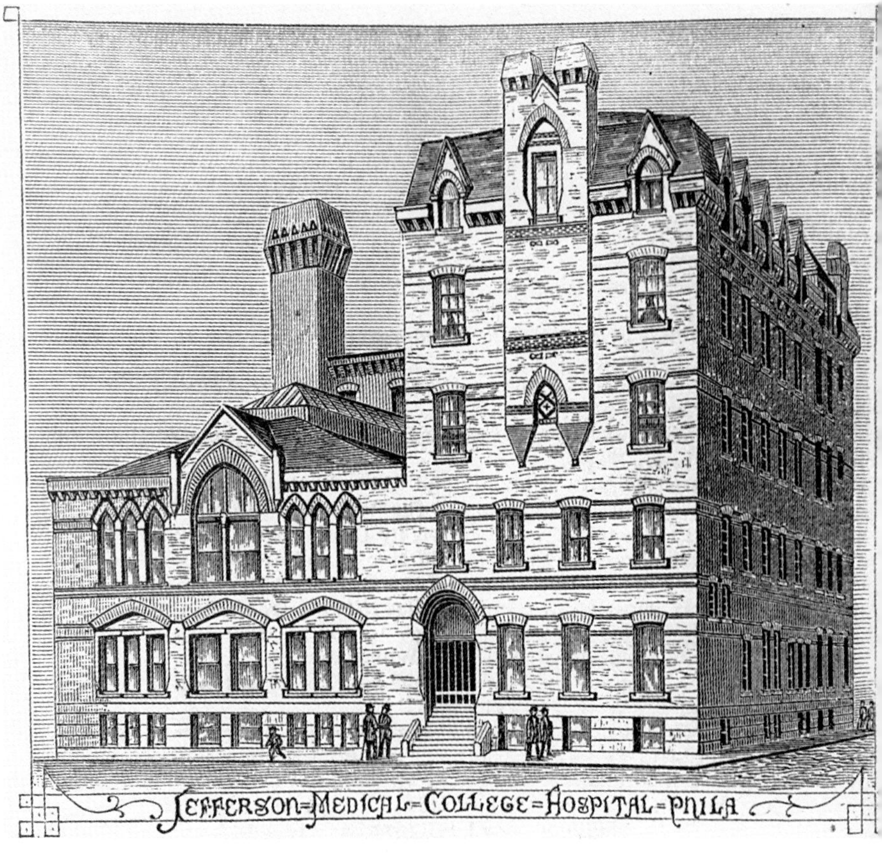

In Dr. John H. Brinton's address to new students in 1895 the physician recalled the early college clinics and patient facilities before Jefferson's first hospital was built in 1877:

> In the early days of the clinics, I mean after 1841, patients who had undergone serious operations were sent to their homes in carriages, under the charge of a clinical clerk. A little later, about 1843 or 1844, one or two rooms were rented from a stove-maker, over his shop, at the S.W. corner of Tenth and Sansom Streets, and thither grave cases operated upon before the class were conveyed and treated. After a while these accommodations proved insufficient to meet the wants of the growing clinics, and in 1849 or '50, a floor and a half or two floors were rented over a bottling establishment, then standing on the ground now occupied by the laboratories of the College. In the course of a few years, additional room having become necessary, this building was remodelled, and a very comfortable sort of miniature hospital was arranged, capable of accommodating fourteen or fifteen patients. This opened directly into the College building, and the fireproof door through which patients were carried from the clinical amphitheatre to their beds is...familiar...This small hospital served its purpose from 1843 until the 7th of September, 1877, when the new Jefferson College Hospital was officially opened by the Trustees of the College for clinical purposes.

In the early 1870s there had been strong support from trustees, faculty, and alumni for a more adequate clinical facility in a separate building. A lot was purchased on Sansom Street between Tenth and Eleventh, west of Medical Hall. Five leading local architects were invited to submit plans, specifications, and estimates: John McArthur, the firm of Frank Furness and George W. Hewitt, James H. Windrim, Joseph M. Wilson, and Thomas W. Richards. All but Windrim offered a plan and, in addition, there was one unsolicited plan from Alonso B. Jones. The competition was won by Furness and Hewitt. Final costs of $186,000 were paid for by contributions from alumni, trustees, faculty, the state legislature, and a public appeal. The hospital was opened formally on September 17, 1877.

The Victorian Gothic brick structure had two main components of two and five stories. The shed-roofed, two-story structure on the left housed the clinical amphitheater which could seat six hundred people. The basement of the five-story structure on the right held the kitchens, laundry, and storerooms. On the first floor were the entrance and public lobby, offices, apothecary, and surgical preparation rooms. The second floor housed the clinics, and the third and fourth floors held two wards each. On the fifth floor were ten private rooms, a matron's room, and three rooms for resident physicians. Altogether the hospital could accommodate 125 patients.

The 1877-78 *Annual Announcement* praised the new hospital lavishly: "The amphitheatre...is probably the largest and most convenient in the United States...The most approved appliances for heating, ventilation, etc., have been provided, and, in architectural construction, and all desirable conveniences, this hospital will be found at least equal to any American clinical hospital."

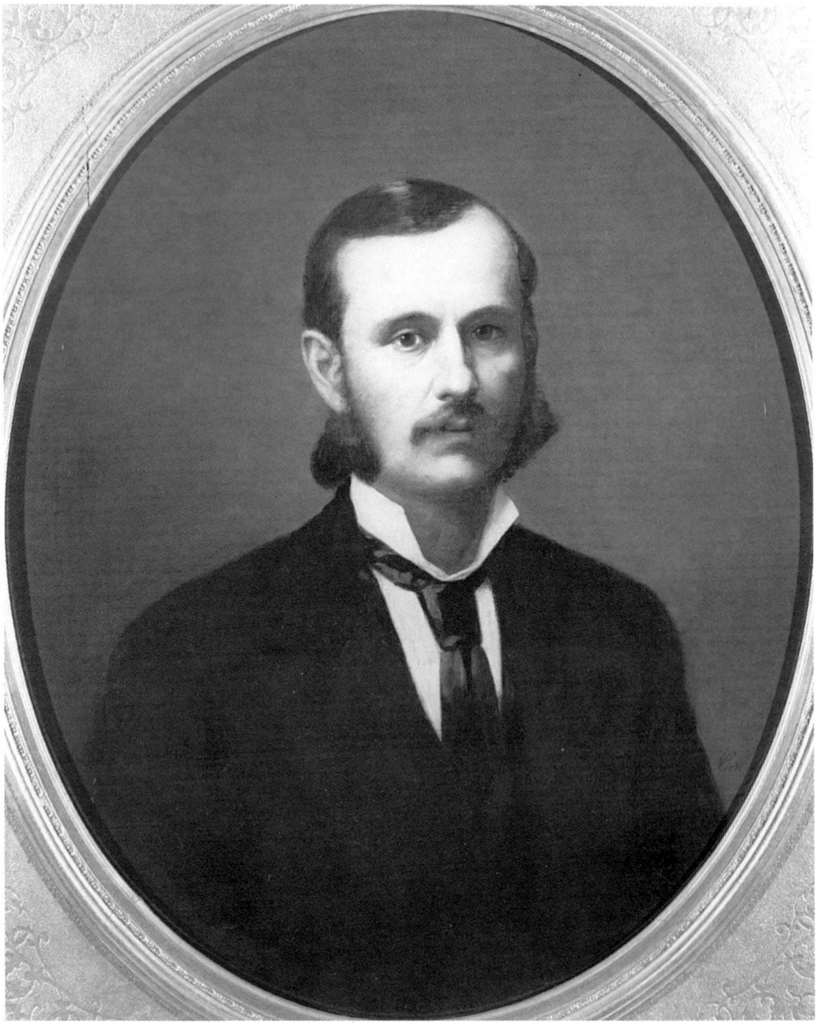

Portrait of Francis F. Maury

FRANCIS FONTAINE MAURY, M.D. (1840-79)
Attributed to Carl Lindemann (active second half nineteenth century)

Oil on canvas
Ca. 1875
30 x 25 in.

Signed and dated center right, but partially obscured: "Carl Li/18"

Given in 1879 by J. Robb Maury, brother of the subject

Accession number: 1879+e.P.02

One of the most active alumni engaged in fund-raising for the hospital was Dr. Francis Fontaine Maury. The surgeon was successful in approaching the state legislature for an appropriation of a hundred thousand dollars in matching funds.

Francis F. Maury was born in 1840 in Danville, Kentucky, the son of an Episcopal clergyman. He attended Centre College in Danville and took a course of lectures at the University of Virginia before graduating from Jefferson Medical College in 1862. He settled in Philadelphia and served as acting assistant surgeon in the U.S. Army at the South Street General Hospital in Philadelphia.

Dr. Maury became clinical assistant to Professor Samuel D. Gross in 1863 and the following year chief of Gross's surgical clinic, and surgeon to Jefferson Medical College Hospital. He started delivering lectures on dermatology in 1866. He had been appointed chief surgeon to the Philadelphia Hospital in 1865.

Dr. Francis F. Maury performed the first American gastrotomy in 1869 and was considered expert in the most advanced surgery of his day, including lithotomy, exstrophy of the bladder, and extirpation of the thyroid, among other procedures. He achieved the first recovery following amputation of the hip joint in America. With Dr. Louis Duhring he edited the *Photographic Review of Medicine and Surgery* from 1870 to 1872. Dr. Maury was a member of the American Dermatological Association and the Pathological Society of Philadelphia, among other societies. Tragically this rising star in surgery died of tuberculosis in 1879 at the age of thirty-nine.

Minutes of the July 7, 1879 meeting of the Jefferson Medical College Hospital medical staff report that Dr. Samuel W. Gross said he could obtain a life-sized crayon portrait of Dr. Maury at a cost of fifty-five dollars, and it was moved that he order such a portrait. The following October Gross announced a substitution: a portrait of F. F. Maury had been presented to the hospital by his brother, J. Robb Maury.

In the oval, bust-length portrait Dr. Maury is turned slightly to the right. He exudes a kind of sensuousness with his large, soulful brown eyes, full lips, slick dark hair, and slight tilt of the head, although his facial expression is studiously neutral. The surface of the painting is very smoothly brushed and polished. The artist has achieved a spotlighted glow to his skin with beautifully rendered coloring and shadows.

In an otherwise straightforward and factual biography in *The Dictionary of American Medical Biography* (1928) Maury's personality is described as follows: "He was an impressive lecturer, and gay and attractive to young men; but unfortunately held the utterly lax moral code common in his day." Maury died two weeks after his wife had died suddenly of acute peritonitis, leaving their two young children orphaned.

An 1881 trustees report listing donations to the new hospital mentioned that the portrait was placed in the "private operating room." In a turn-of-the-century photograph Maury's portrait is shown in the library reading room of the 1898 College Building.

There is some confusion about the identity of the portrait's artist and its date, but it does not look like a posthumous likeness. The signature and date on the painting are partially hidden by the frame. The fragmentary inscription reads, "Carl Li.../18..." Charles Frankenberger's 1915 article about the Jefferson art collection stated that the artist was "Carl Linderman" and the portrait was painted in 1875.

Since no documents have been found to date about such an artist, the painter could have been Carl F. Lindemann, an artist from Philadelphia who exhibited three portraits at the art exposition of the 1876 Philadelphia Centennial.

Jefferson Medical College Faculty of the 1865-66 Session

JEFFERSON MEDICAL COLLEGE FACULTY OF THE 1865-66 SESSION
By Frederick Gutekunst (1831-1917)

Nine photographs arranged on a board with a calling card
1865-66
Individual photograph size: 4 x 2 1/2 in.
Board size: 11 1/2 x 19 in.

All photographs stamped on back: "F. GUTEKUNST"

Given before 1930 by D. Clark Huffman, M.D. (JMC 1866)
Accession number: 1930+b.Ph.01

Around 1865 a Jefferson Medical College student, D. Clark Huffman of McKeesport, Pennsylvania, arranged nine autographed *cartes-de-visite* of his professors on a large board and placed his own calling card in the center. The photo of Benjamin Howard Rand, M.D. was dated November 3, 1865, and the photo of William H. Pancoast, M.D. was inscribed "Very Truly Your/Friend & Teacher." All of the photographs were taken by Frederick Gutekunst.

The only professors still remaining in 1865 from the "Famous Faculty of 1841" were Drs. Robley Dunglison and Joseph Pancoast. New faculty included (from left to right): Ellerslie Wallace, M.D. who succeeded Dr. Charles D. Meigs as chair of obstetrics; Samuel D. Gross, M.D. who succeeded Dr. Thomas D. Mütter as

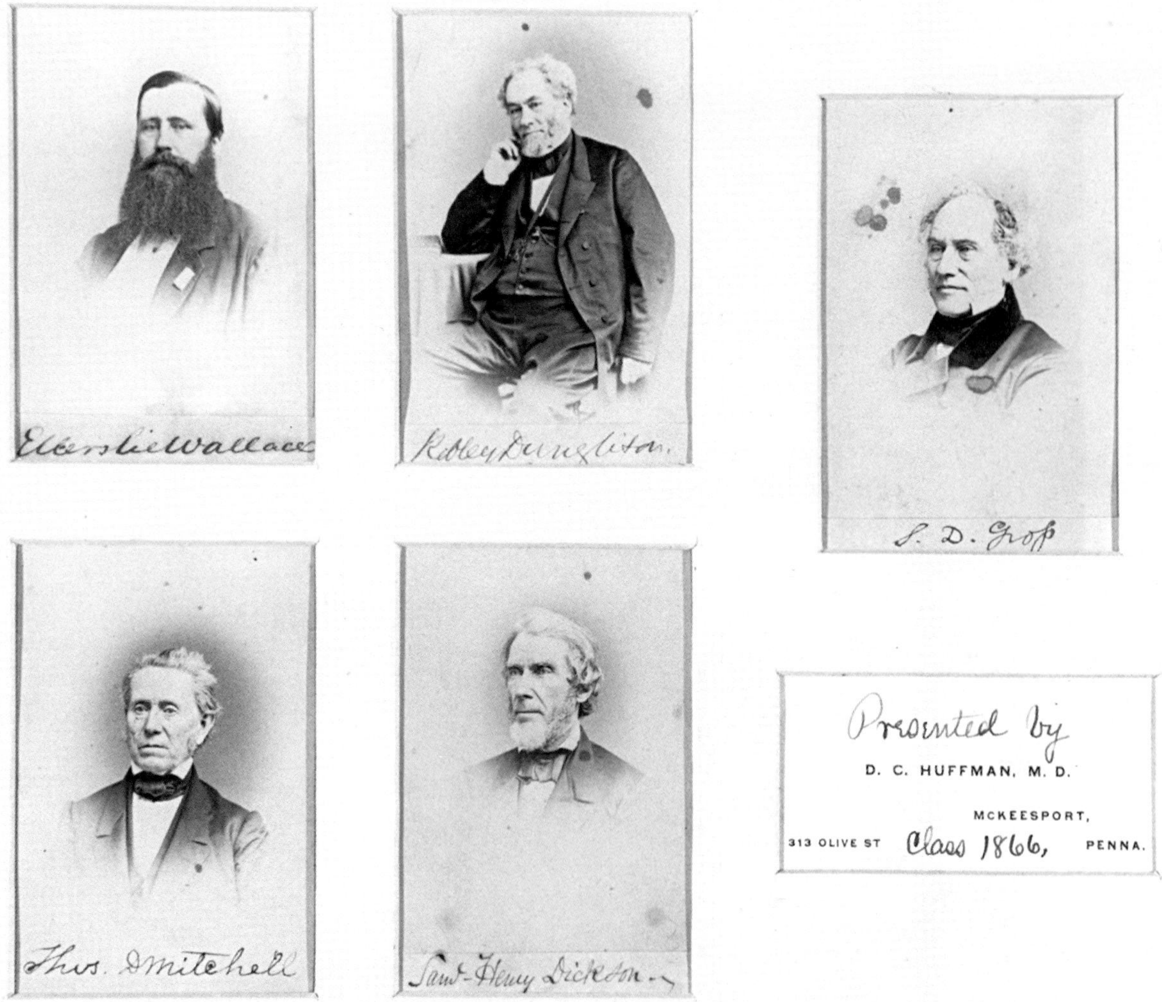

chair of surgery; John B. Biddle, M.D. who succeeded Dr. Thomas Mitchell as chair of materia medica; Thomas D. Mitchell, M.D. who succeeded Dr. Robert M. Huston as chair of materia medica and therapeutics; Samuel H. Dickson, M.D. who succeeded Dr. John K. Mitchell as chair of medicine; Benjamin H. Rand, M.D. who succeeded Dr. Franklin Bache as chair of chemistry; and William H. Pancoast, M.D. who was appointed demonstrator of anatomy.

Of this distinguished faculty only Drs. Dickson, Mitchell, and Wallace will be discussed here because all the others are represented by an oil painting and/or sculpture in the Jefferson collection. In addition, most are represented by other vintage photographs or prints in the collection which are also cherished by contemporary Jeffersonians who want to recall the appearance of their professional forbears.

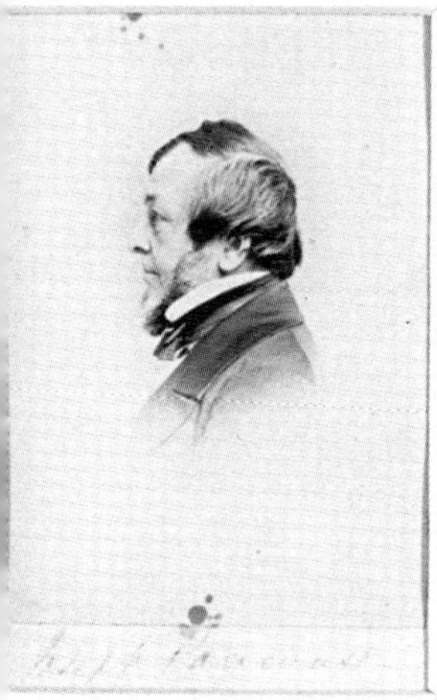

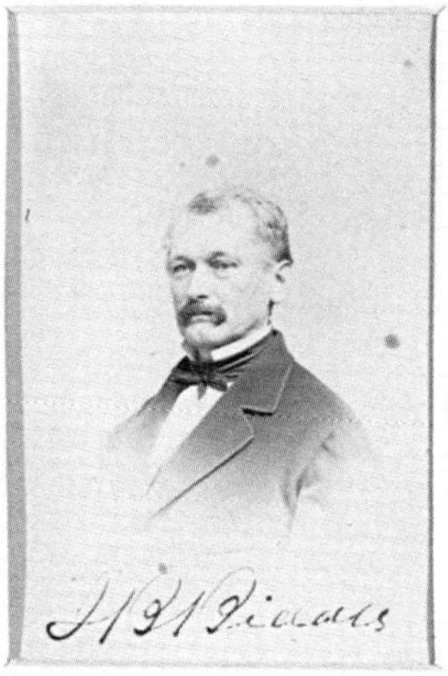

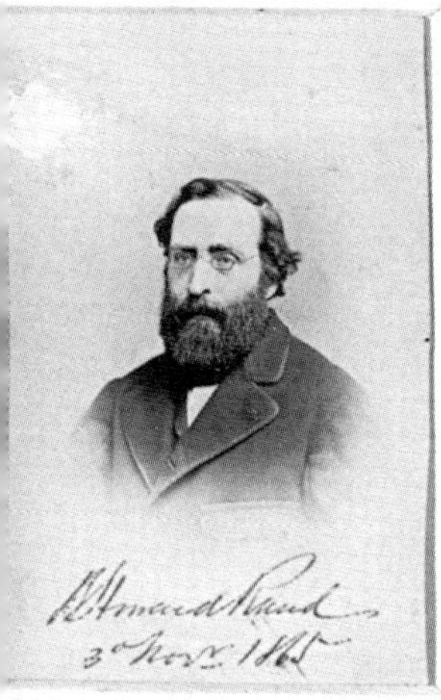

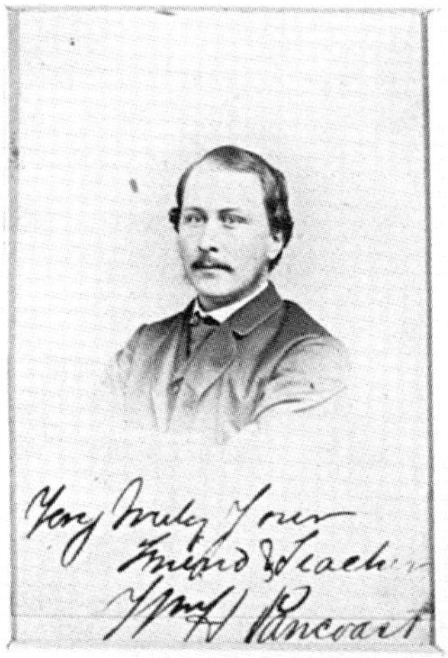

Samuel H. Dickson was born in Charleston, South Carolina in 1798. He graduated from Yale College in 1814 and the Medical Department of the University of Pennsylvania in 1819. Except for three years as professor of the theory and practice of medicine at the University of the City of New York (1847-50), his early career starting in 1824 was spent in his native city. He had a consultation practice and was professor of the institutes and practice of medicine at the Medical College of South Carolina, of which he was a founder.

Dickson was called to Jefferson Medical College to fill the chair of practice in 1858, and remained in that position until his death in 1872. He also served briefly as Jefferson's ninth dean from 1868 to 1869. His *Manual of Pathology and Practice of Medicine* (1850) was considered a standard in its day. Dr. Dickson received an honorary LL.D. degree from the University of New York in 1851.

Like Dr. Dickson, Dr. Thomas Duché Mitchell was called to Jefferson at an advanced age. Born in 1791, Mitchell was a native Philadelphian who graduated from the Medical Department of the University of Pennsylvania in 1812. That same year he was appointed professor of vegetable and animal physiology at St. John's Lutheran College. In the 1820s he practiced medicine near Philadelphia, and in 1826 he established the Total Abstinence Society.

In 1831 Mitchell was appointed professor of chemistry at the Medical College of Ohio. Four years later he became chair of materia medica and chemistry at Transylvania University in Lexington, Kentucky. He returned to Philadelphia in 1847 to accept the chair of the practice of medicine at the recently organized Philadelphia College of Medicine. He finally arrived at Jefferson Medical College as chair of materia medica in 1857 and remained there until his death in 1865.

Mitchell's outstanding contribution to medical literature was *Materia Medica and Therapeutics* (1850). He was coeditor with Dr. John Eberle of the *Western Medical Gazette* and was also editor of the *Journal of Medical and Associate Sciences*. He received an honorary A.M. degree from Princeton College in 1830.

Dr. Ellerslie Wallace performed a much longer service to Jefferson Medical College than either Dr. Dickson or Dr. Mitchell. Wallace was born in 1818 in Philadelphia. He was of Scottish and English ancestry and said to be descended from Robert Bruce. Dr. Ellerslie Wallace was educated at Bristol College, and studied medicine first with his brother, Joshua, a demonstrator of anatomy at Jefferson Medical College, and then graduated from the college in 1843.

Dr. Wallace spent three years as an intern at Pennsylvania Hospital. In 1846 he replaced his brother in Jefferson's anatomy department, until called to the chair of obstetrics in 1862 where he remained until 1883. He also served as dean from 1879 to 1883, succeeding Dr. John B. Biddle. Professor Wallace's powerful physique, cogent lectures, and attentiveness to his students added to his popularity as a teacher during his decades at Jefferson.

Portrait of John B. Biddle

JOHN BARCLAY BIDDLE, M.D. (1815-79)
By Samuel Bell Waugh (1814-85)

Oil on canvas
30 x 25 in.
1880

Signed and dated lower right: "S. B. Waugh, 1880"

Given in 1880 by JMC alumni association
Accession number: 1880+e.P.02

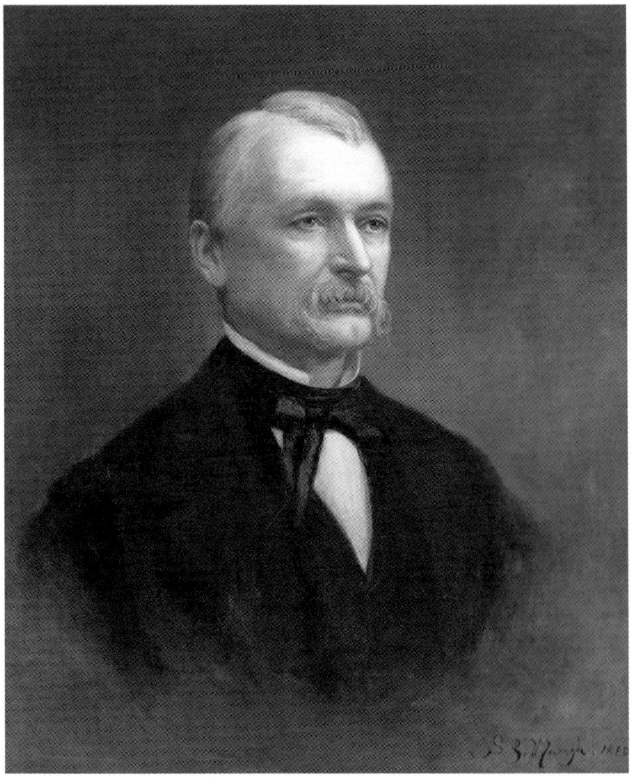

Dr. John B. Biddle was another esteemed member of the mid-nineteenth-century faculty. As dean he was a strong supporter of the establishment of the first Jefferson hospital in 1877.

John Biddle was born in Philadelphia in 1815, a descendant of William Biddle who emigrated to America before William Penn. John Biddle graduated from St. Mary's College in Baltimore about 1833. After a brief period of studying the law, he decided on a career in medicine and entered the Philadelphia office of Dr. Nathaniel Chapman, a relative by marriage. Biddle's graduation from the Medical Department of the University of Pennsylvania in 1836 was followed by a year of study in Paris.

Of an entrepreneurial bent, Dr. John Biddle was a founder and editor in 1838 of *The Medical Examiner*, a journal that merged in 1844 with the *North American Medico-Chirurgical Review*. In 1846 he joined a group of young physicians to found the Franklin Medical College of Philadelphia, a short-lived enterprise. Next he held the chair of materia medica in the Pennsylvania Medical College, a branch of Gettysburg College.

Finally, in 1865 Dr. Biddle was elected to the chair of materia medica and therapeutics at Jefferson Medical College, and held that position until his death in 1879. He also served as Jefferson's eleventh dean from 1873 until 1879, succeeding Dr. Benjamin H. Rand. Biddle was a founder in 1876 and the first president of the Association of American Medical Colleges. His best known literary work was *Review of the Materia Medica for the Use of Students* (1852), an authoritative text that went through eight editions during his lifetime.

Dr. John Biddle was an esteemed teacher and trusted advisor to medical students. When he died in 1879 the senior class sent to his funeral service a vacant chair made of flowers, to stand at the foot of his coffin "in testimony of their affection, and of sorrow for their loss."[5]

The bust-length portrait of Dr. Biddle was the fifth and last portrait by Samuel B. Waugh for Jefferson Medical College. The painting was commissioned by the alumni association in 1880, the year after the subject's death.

Dr. Biddle's head is turned slightly to the right and he looks straight ahead with a neutral expression. His regular features were often described as "patrician." As customary with Waugh, the sitter's head is described with three-dimensional volume, while the torso is flat and fades into the atmospheric background. The portrait was installed with those of other distinguished faculty in the amphitheater of the new hospital.

Portrait of William H. Pancoast

WILLIAM HENRY PANCOAST, M.D. (1835-97)
By Bernard Uhle (also called Albrecht Bernhard Uhle) (1847-1930)

Oil on canvas mounted on wood
1886
36 1/2 x 29 1/4 in.

Signed and dated lower left: "B. Uhle 1886"

Given by JMC class of 1886
Accession number: 1886+e.P.01

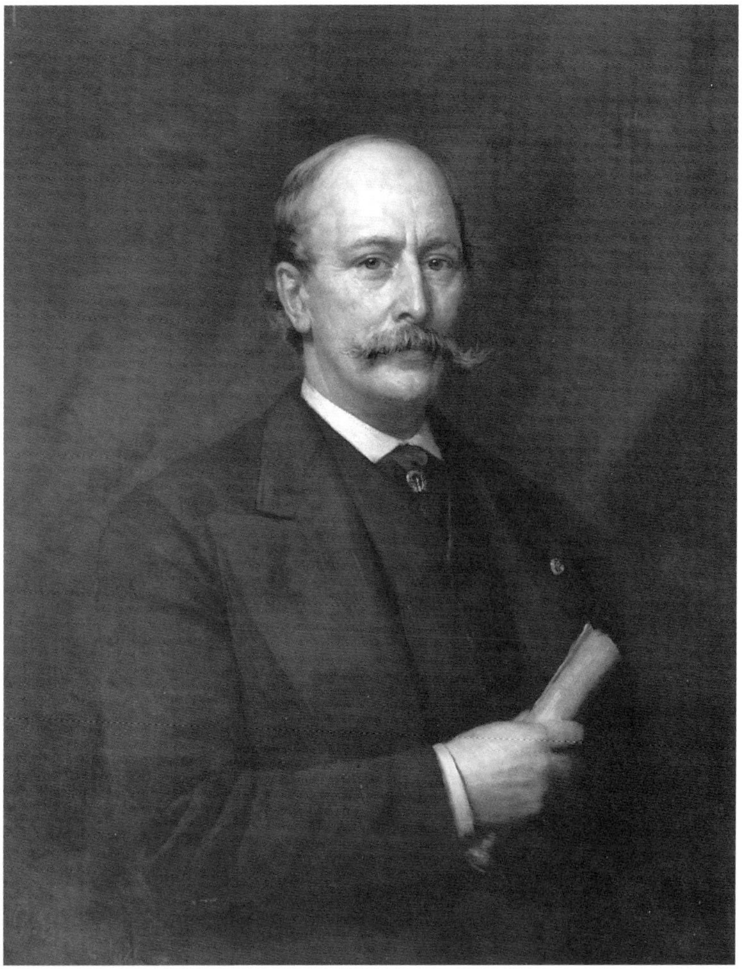

Dr. William H. Pancoast succeeded his father, Joseph Pancoast, M.D., as a distinguished Jefferson Medical College surgeon and anatomist. The younger Pancoast was a faculty member for twenty-four years.

He was born in 1835 in Philadelphia, and an alumnus of Haverford College (1853) and Jefferson Medical College (1856). Further study took him to London, Paris, Vienna, and Berlin for the next two and one-half years. Upon his return to Philadelphia Dr. William Pancoast established a reputation as a skilled diagnostician and surgeon. He instituted a large surgical clinic at Charity Hospital where he was visiting surgeon from 1859 to 1869, and then consulting surgeon. During the Civil War he was surgeon-in-chief and second officer in charge at the Military Hospital in Philadelphia.

In 1862 Dr. William Pancoast was appointed demonstrator of anatomy at Jefferson Medical College, aiding in his father's department while he served in the war. In 1866 he introduced a very successful course in visceral and surgical anatomy in Jefferson's special summer course, even attracting students from other medical schools.

When Dr. Joseph Pancoast resigned as professor of anatomy in 1873, nine candidates including Dr. William Pancoast were nominated to succeed him, but none received a majority vote after seventeen ballots. The elder Pancoast was persuaded to continue until April 1874 when his son finally won the majority and was appointed to the anatomy chair.

Dr. William H. Pancoast resigned his Jefferson professorship in 1886 to become the chair of combined departments of anatomy and surgery at the Medico-chirurgical College of Philadelphia, an institution he helped to found and where he remained until his death in 1897. He was an active member of many societies and served as vice president of the American Medical Association in 1884.

A portrait of Dr. William Pancoast by Bernard Uhle was commissioned by the senior class upon his retirement from his duties at Jefferson. The presentation ceremony took place at the annual meeting of the alumni association on April 1, 1886 in the lower lecture room of the Ely Building:

> Dr. Alston H. Bickers, of the class of 1886, made the presentation address, speaking with feeling and in a way that drew forth a vigorous expression of applause from his classmates...He said that the picture was given as a mark of esteem and gratitude to a beloved preceptor, who had by his learning and skill relieved the study of anatomy of dryness and monotony. Dr. Pancoast, in reply, said that he appreciated the action of the class the more because the presentation of the portrait of a living professor was unprecedented.[6]

Documents show that the class requested and was granted approval from the trustees to place the portrait in a "conspicuous position" on the walls of the clinic room of the hospital. One wonders whether Dr. Pancoast's comment was quoted accurately or if he were misinformed, because there had been several prior examples of portrait presentations of living professors, including that of his own father. Dr. William Pancoast might have been thinking of the posthumous portrait of Dr. James A. Meigs that had been presented by the class of 1879-80.

Uhle's half-length portrait of Pancoast shows him as a vigorous, stylishly dressed, confident gentleman. He holds a rolled-up paper in his right hand. His attractive features are distinguished by a long nose, high cheekbones, luxuriant mustache, and square jaw. The portrait's surface is smoothly brushed except for the sitter's face whose planes and volumes are depicted with mottled strokes. The artist's vigorous paint style accords with the strength and energy of the subject's demeanor.

The portrait was painted during the artist's most successful period when he was in constant demand as a portrait painter in Philadelphia. Born in 1847 in Chemnitz, Saxony, Bernard Uhle was brought to the United States at age four. Like his portrait subject, the artist followed in his father's footsteps in his career choice and also received a first-rate education here and abroad.

Bernard Uhle first studied art with the elder Uhle, then at the Pennsylvania Academy of the Fine Arts. He concentrated on photography until he went abroad to train at the Munich Academy from 1875 to 1877, and then briefly in Italy. After opening a portrait studio in Philadelphia from 1877 to 1879, he made a second trip to Europe to study the old masters in Munich and Paris.

The painter became a well known exhibitor in European salons and galleries. While in Germany he received a gold medal from King Ludwig for the best figure study of the year, *The Moor*. It is said that Uhle refused an invitation from the Bavarian king to become court painter, in order to be near his elderly mother in Philadelphia.

Bernard Uhle had portrait commissions from many of Philadelphia's most eminent business, professional, and society figures, including Drs. Alfred Stillé, David Hayes Agnew, Richard A. F. Penrose, and Joseph Leidy, as well as Colonel John G. Lankenau, Mayor Edwin H. Fitler, Mrs. Alexander Van Rensselaer, and Mrs. Edward Biddle.

The once acclaimed artist ended his life tragically as a mysterious recluse who died of starvation. Contemporary newspaper accounts described Uhle's self-imposed seclusion after his wife divorced him in 1893. He never again saw his wife, and a daughter born soon after the divorce never met her father until shortly before his death. At age eighty-two the despondent artist was found with nine cats, destitute, starving, and "ill from exposure." Though his house had been sold for taxes he had lived there for two more years "defying rent-collectors and constables."

After being discovered Uhle was taken to Lankenau Hospital where he died a few months later in April 1930. Among his effects authorities discovered more than one hundred paintings, meticulous ledgers, scrapbooks of clippings, and diaries in his house. Ironically, the paintings were auctioned off for only $3,130, about one-tenth of his annual income from sales decades earlier, yet nevertheless a sum that could have ameliorated his miserable squalor.

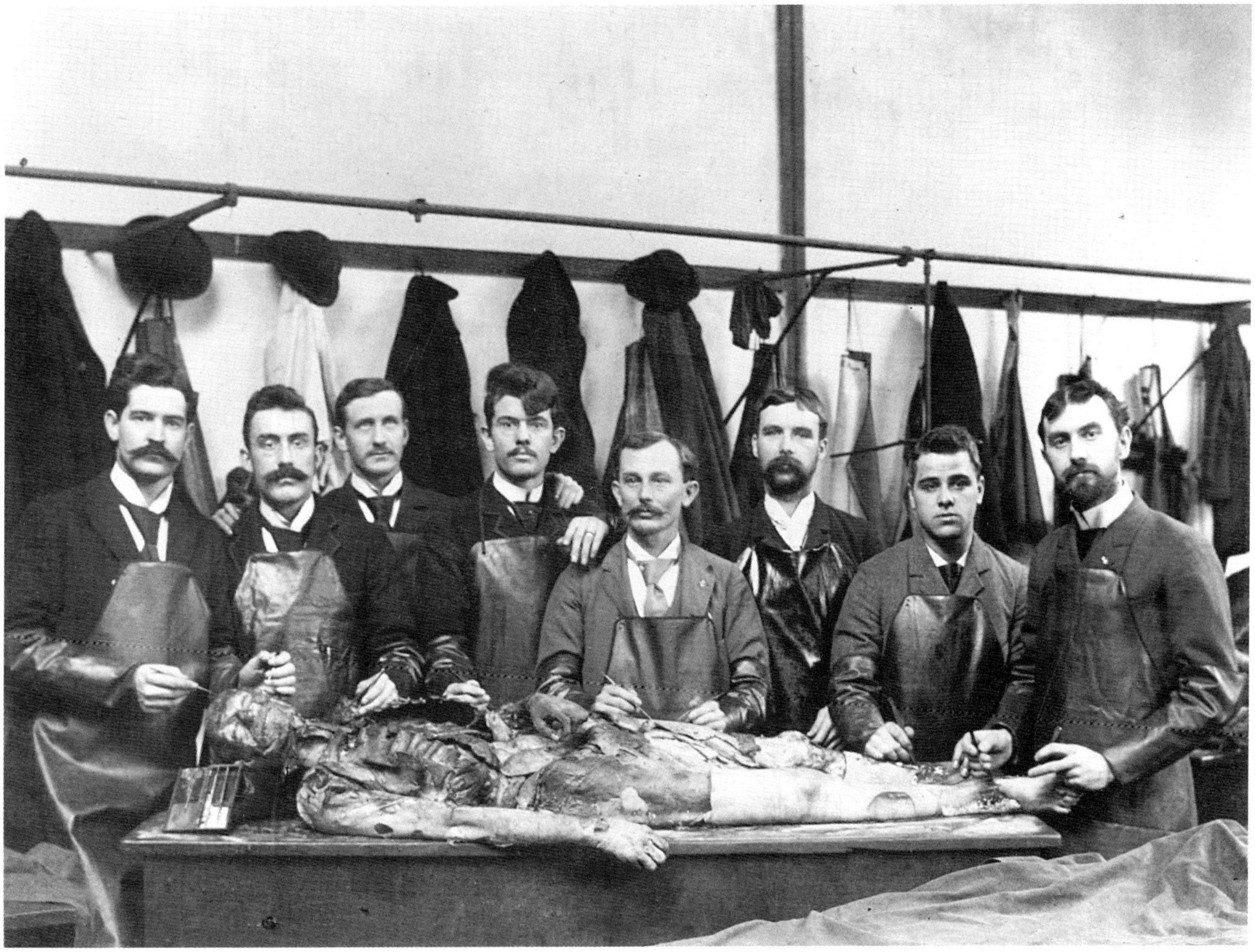

Dr. William H. Pancoast's Anatomy Dissection Laboratory

DR. WILLIAM H. PANCOAST'S ANATOMY DISSECTION LABORATORY
By unknown photographer

Photograph mounted on card
1862-74
Image size: 6 x 8 in.
Card size: 10 x 12 in.

Given after 1874 by unknown donor
Accession number: 1874+f.Ph.02

A cabinet-sized, vintage photograph of Dr. William Pancoast's anatomy dissection laboratory was found underneath the long-lost Jefferson Medical College certificate when it was discovered in 1989. It is not known who owned the photograph originally or when it was coupled with the certificate under its late-nineteenth-century frame.

Judging from Dr. Pancoast's youthful appearance resembling another photograph in the Jefferson collection identifying him as "Demonstrator of Anatomy," the anatomy laboratory photo must have been taken between 1862 and 1874, before he was made professor.

Pancoast is the shortest figure, standing in the center of a group of students in his laboratory. They are posed familiarly and collegially behind a partially dissected cadaver which is stretched out on a table with its head up on a block. The students wear aprons over their suits, and self-consciously position their scalpels on the body for the camera. Their coats and hats hang on pegs on the rear wall. Unsettling to a lay viewer, the cadaver's flayed face seems to be grimacing while the students look quite unruffled.

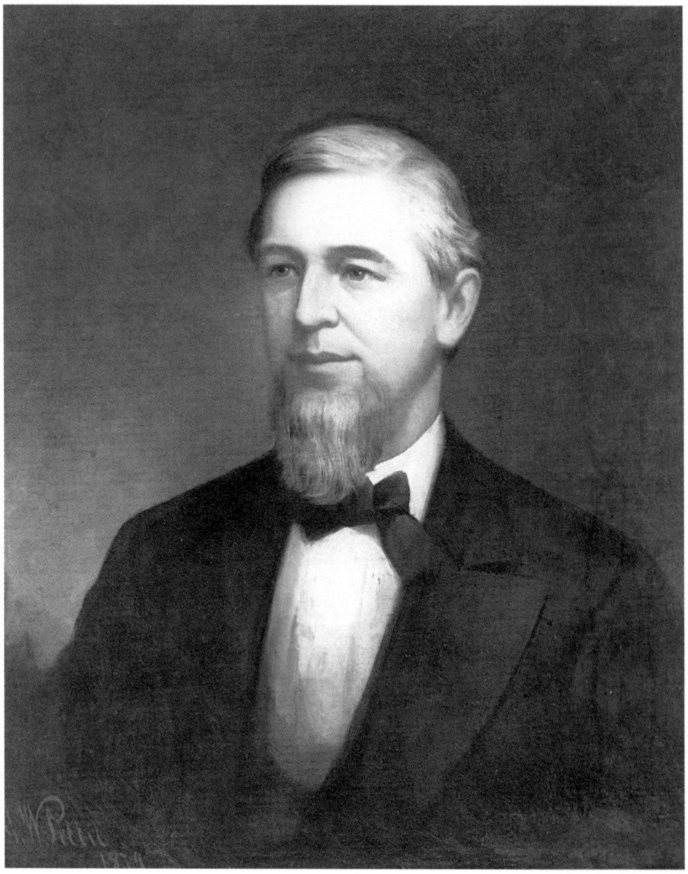

Portrait of James A. Meigs

JAMES AITKEN MEIGS, M.D. (1829-79)
By George W. Pettit (d. 1910)

Oil on canvas mounted on wood
1879
30 1/4 x 25 in.

Signed and dated lower left: "G. W. Pettit/1879"

Given by JMC class of 1879-80
Accession number: 1879+e.P.01

Another prominent, mid-nineteenth-century Jefferson Medical College faculty member was James A. Meigs, M.D., successor to Dr. Robley Dunglison. Meigs was also a noted ethnologist.

A native Philadelphian, James A. Meigs was born in 1829. He took a preceptorship with Drs. Francis G. Smith and Joshua M. Allen and graduated from Jefferson Medical College in 1851, after which he began a medical practice. In 1854 he was appointed a lecturer in climatology and physiology at the Franklin Institute, and in 1856 was named librarian and chairman in anthropology at the Academy of Natural Sciences. He became a well known ethnologist who contributed several articles on the cranial characteristics of the races of man, and a catalogue of the Academy's collection of human crania.

In 1857 he was made chair of the institutes of medicine at the Philadelphia College of Medicine, and in 1859 professor of physiology at the Medical Department of the Pennsylvania College, and consulting physician and lecturer at the Philadelphia Hospital. In 1866 he was invited to conduct a spring course of lectures on the physiology and pathology of the blood and circulation at Jefferson Medical College. In 1868 Meigs was appointed chair of the institutes of medicine and medical jurisprudence at Jefferson. He was also physician to the Howard and Pennsylvania Hospitals. His untimely death occurred in 1879 at age fifty-one.

Dr. James A. Meigs was a leading medical educator, and under his auspices a course in practical microscopy was inaugurated. His department of institutes of medicine was among the first to use live animals for demonstrations before the class, facilitated by the use of anesthesia. This technique was strenuously opposed by the antivivisectionists.

Dr. Meigs edited an American edition of *Kirke's Manual of Physiology* (1857) and prepared the first American edition of William B. Carpenter's *The Microscope and Its Revelations* (1856). His own handsome binocular microscope with accessories was bequeathed to the Academy of Natural Sciences. He was a member of numerous medical and learned societies, including anthropological and ethnological societies in Paris and London.

Dr. James A. Meigs was a favorite with both students and patients, always sympathetic and with time to offer encouraging words. His death came "like a thunderbolt from a clear sky" to his legions of friends and associates.

In 1880 eight Jefferson alumni from the classes of 1879 and 1880 established the J. Aitken Meigs Medical Association with the stated purpose to "continue and strengthen the bonds of friendship formed during student life and promote that social and intellectual condition becoming the profession." Still in existence today, the Meigs Medical Association retains a limited membership of distinguished Philadelphia physicians from various local medical institutions, and is considered one of the oldest medical associations of its type in continuous existence.

The classes of 1879 and 1880 also presented to the college a posthumous portrait by George W. Pettit to memorialize Dr. Meigs's "sterling worth, force of character and profound learning." According to the January 15, 1880 *College and Clinical Record*, the class spokesman at the presentation said, "Considering the scanty material from which Mr. Pettit...was obliged to work, the conscientious fidelity which he has manifested in his labor, and the eminent success which he has obtained...I tender him our sincere thanks." The president of the board of trustees further commented, "The portrait does credit to the artist, and brings back a smile of approbation to his class; it shall have place on the college wall, by the side of other distinguished professors."

The bust-length portrait was originally hung in the amphitheater of the new hospital and later was moved to the library of the 1898 College Building. Although the depiction by Pettit resembles photographs of the subject's features and distinctively long and narrow beard, the portrait lacks the physician's engaging collegiality and vigor as described by his admirers.

The 1887 *Catalogue of the Loan Collection of Portraits: College of Physicians of Philadelphia* lists a portrait of James A. Meigs owned by Jefferson Medical College. However, the artist's name is given as "Waugh," presumably Samuel B. Waugh. Since there is no extant document showing that Jefferson Medical College owned a second portrait of Dr. James A. Meigs by Waugh or anyone else, most likely it was the Pettit portrait that was exhibited.

George W. Pettit was a native of England. He is known to have resided in Philadelphia and exhibited portraits and subject pictures at the Pennsylvania Academy of the Fine Arts between 1862 and 1887.

Participation in the Civil War by Jefferson Faculty

Philadelphia was an important medical center during the Civil War, the next largest after Washington, D.C. There were fifteen military hospitals in the Philadelphia area by 1864, and most of the city's prominent physicians served the Union cause either as volunteers, regular army, or contract physicians. Jefferson Medical College faculty and alumni who made major contributions to Civil War medicine for the Union included Drs. John H. Brinton, Richard J. Levis, and Jonathan Letterman. Other Jeffersonians, like Drs. Hunter H. McGuire and Robert Battey, were equally devoted to the Confederacy.

Dr. Richard J. Levis (1827-90) was a Jefferson alumnus, class of 1848. He was a noted general and ophthalmic surgeon who was surgeon-in-chief to two United States military hospitals in Philadelphia. Dr. Jonathan Letterman (1824-72) graduated with the class of 1849. He rose to the position of medical director of the Army of the Potomac. He is best remembered for devising an ambulance corps for rapid evacuation of the wounded from the battlefield, and for reorganizing medical service in the field and in military hospitals.

Unfortunately, the Jefferson art collection contains no original images of Drs. Levis or Letterman. The portraits of some other Jefferson physicians active in the Civil War will be discussed in following chapters, including Drs. Samuel D. Gross, Samuel W. Gross, and William Williams Keen.

Portrait of John H. Brinton

JOHN HILL BRINTON, M.D. (1832-1907)
By Frederick Gutekunst (1831-1917)

Photograph mounted on card
Ca. 1880-90
Image size: 5 3/4 x 4 1/4 in.
Card size: 6 1/2 x 4 1/4 in.

Stamped on card: "F. GUTEKUNST PHILADELPHIA"

Given after 1907 by unknown donor
Accession number: 1907+f.Ph.01

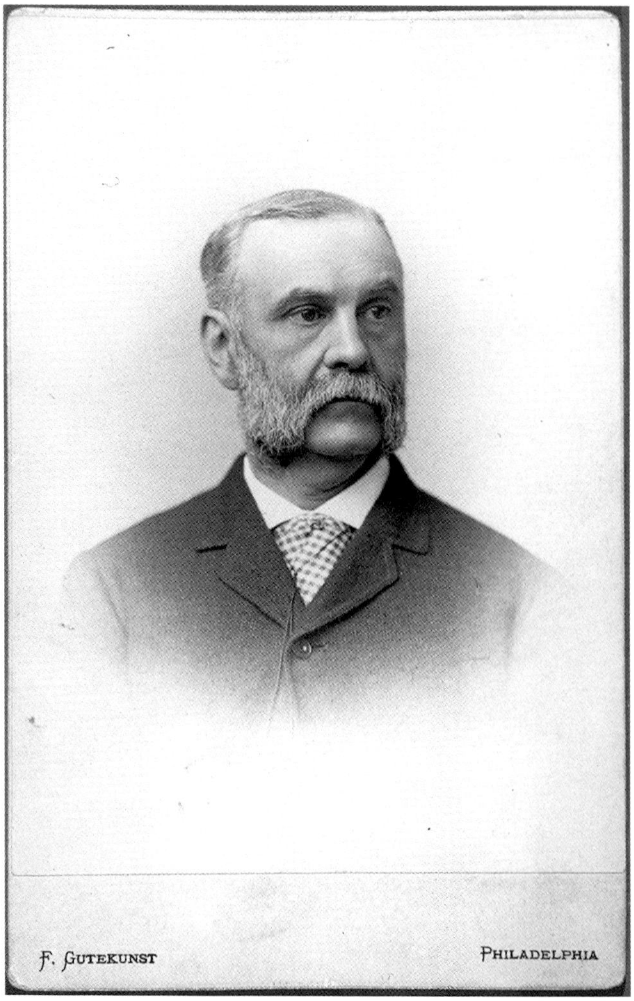

Dr. John H. Brinton had a most diverse Civil War career. He was also a distinguished surgeon and cochair of the department of surgery at Jefferson Medical College from 1882 to 1906.

Born in 1832, John H. Brinton was a native Philadelphian and a nephew of Dr. George McClellan, the founder of Jefferson Medical College. Unusually well educated for his day, Brinton received a bachelor's degree (1850) and master's degree (1853) from the University of Pennsylvania, an M.D. degree from Jefferson in 1852, and further clinical training in Paris and Vienna in 1853. He later received an honorary LL.D. degree from the University of Pennsylvania in 1901.

Upon his return to Philadelphia from Europe Brinton established a medical practice, taught anatomy and surgery at the Philadelphia School of Anatomy and the

Summer Association of the second Philadelphia Association for Medical Instruction, and was appointed to the staff of St. Joseph's Hospital.

In August 1861 he was commissioned a brigade surgeon of volunteers. He reported to the Department of the West, came under the command of General Ulysses S. Grant, and was soon named acting medical director of the Cairo District of Illinois. Dismayed by the inexperience of his military personnel, he organized the Army Medical and Surgical Society of Cairo to bolster their preparedness.

In 1862 Dr. Brinton was made medical director of the Army of Tennessee and accompanied General Grant in campaigns at Forts Henry and Donelson, and at the Battle of Shiloh. Brinton was inspector and director of patient evacuation at the battles of Antietam, Fredericksburg, Chancellorsville, and Gettysburg. He was medical director in the field during the Missouri campaign, director of general hospitals at Nashville, and acting medical director of the Army of the Cumberland.

In 1862 Brinton was transferred to the office of the Surgeon General in Washington and the headquarters of the Army of the Potomac. During his two years in Washington, he helped prepare the three-volume *Surgical History of the War of the Rebellion* (published 1870-77) to which he contributed the article on gunshot wounds. Additionally, his assignment to collect and arrange "all specimens of morbid anatomy which may have accumulated since the commencement of the rebellion in the various United States hospitals, or which may have been retained by any of the medical officers in the army" resulted in the establishment of the United States Army Medical Museum (later the Armed Forces Institute of Pathology). While visiting headquarters in the field and various hospitals he collected data and illustrations for a catalogue, as well as specimens for the museum. Brinton was the museum's first director. His proposal for an Army Medical School finally came to fruition years later in 1893.

After the war Dr. Brinton continued his surgical career in Philadelphia. In 1866 he was appointed a lecturer on operative surgery in the summer course at Jefferson Medical College, in 1867 surgeon to the Philadelphia Hospital, and in 1877 surgeon to the new Jefferson Hospital where he served as president of the staff for five years. In 1882 Drs. John H. Brinton and Samuel W. Gross were chosen as cochairs of the department of surgery, succeeding Dr. Samuel D. Gross. Brinton was made professor of the practice of surgery and clinical surgery, while Gross was made professor of the principles of surgery and clinical surgery. Brinton remained in his post until 1906 when he was named emeritus professor, the year before his death.

Dr. John H. Brinton aided Dr. Samuel D. Gross in the founding of the Philadelphia Academy of Surgery and the American Surgical Association. He also helped to found the Jefferson Medical College alumni association, and actively solicited alumni for the establishment of the first Jefferson Hospital. Cultivated and congenial, Dr. Brinton was a member of numerous social and learned societies. His *Personal Memoirs of John H. Brinton, Major and Surgeon, U.S.V., 1861-1865* was published posthumously in 1914.

The head-and-shoulders cabinet photograph by Frederick Gutekunst shows Dr. Brinton with a gray mustache and mutton-chop whiskers. A loose card inside the mount states that this photograph was taken to "accompany the document of his appointment as Brigade Surgeon in the Civil War." However this identification must be inaccurate, because other contemporary photographs from the 1860s and a later 1876 portrait by his friend Thomas Eakins show the physician looking more youthful with dark hair and a fuller, pointed beard, so this photograph must have been taken at a later date.[7]

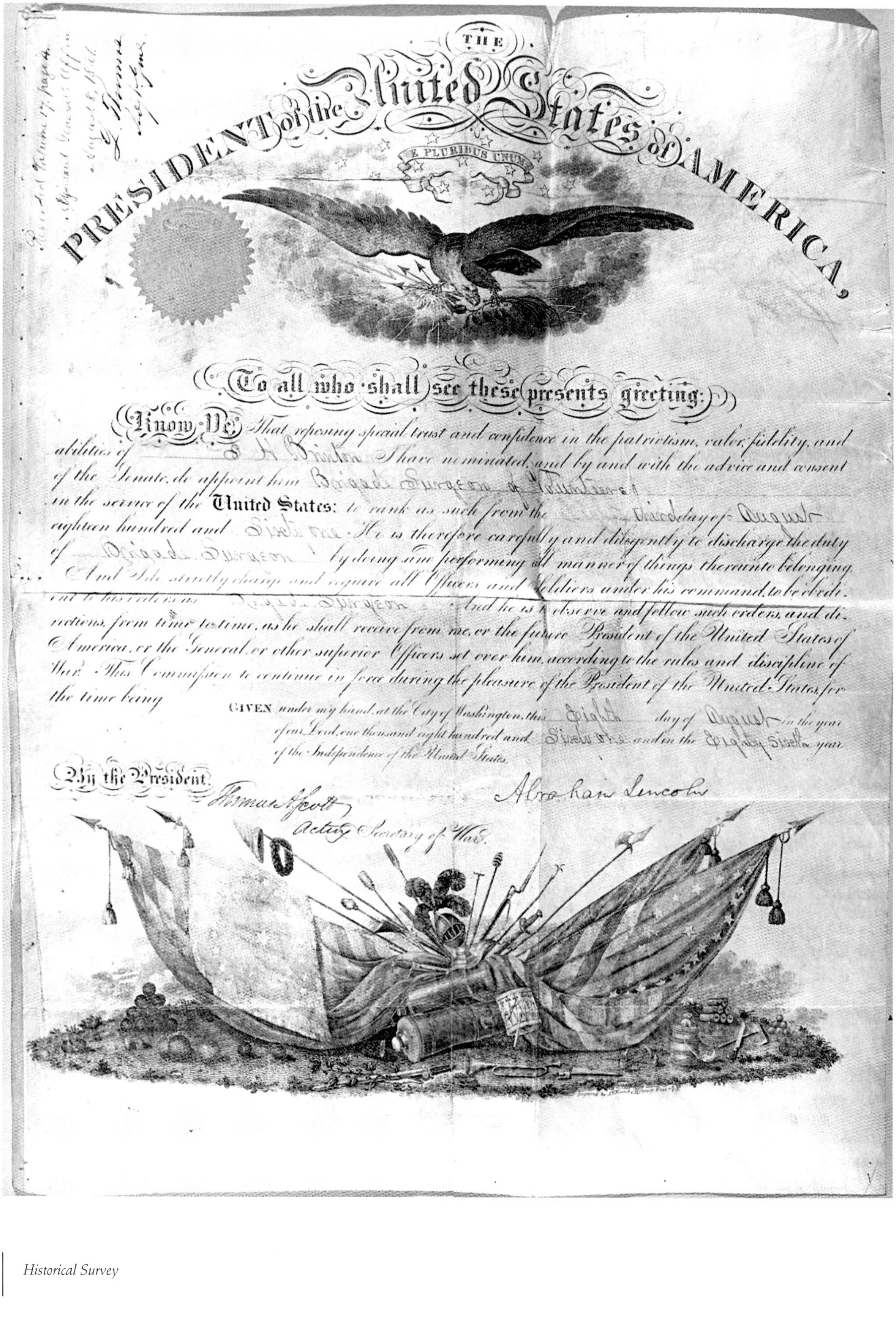

Recorded Volume 1? page 4
Adjutant General's Office
August 8, 1861
L. Thomas
Adjt. Genl.

THE PRESIDENT of the United States of AMERICA,

E PLURIBUS UNUM

To all who shall see these presents greeting:

Know Ye, That reposing special trust and confidence in the patriotism, valor, fidelity, and abilities of J. H. Brinton I have nominated, and by and with the advice and consent of the Senate, do appoint him Brigade Surgeon of Volunteers in the service of the United States: to rank as such from the third day of August eighteen hundred and Sixty one. He is therefore carefully and diligently to discharge the duty of Brigade Surgeon by doing and performing all manner of things thereunto belonging. And I do strictly charge and require all Officers and Soldiers under his command to be obedient to his orders as Brigade Surgeon. And he is to observe and follow such orders, and directions, from time to time, as he shall receive from me, or the future President of the United States of America, or the General, or other superior Officers set over him, according to the rules and discipline of War. This Commission to continue in force during the pleasure of the President of the United States for the time being.

GIVEN under my hand, at the City of Washington, this Eighth day of August in the year of our Lord, one thousand eight hundred and Sixty one and in the Eighty Sixth year of the Independence of the United States.

By the President.

Abraham Lincoln

Thomas A Scott
Acting Secretary of War.

John H. Brinton's Certificate of Commission as Brigade Surgeon of Volunteers

CERTIFICATE OF COMMISSION AS BRIGADE SURGEON OF VOLUNTEERS
By John Peter Van Ness Throop (1794-ca. 1861) and Orramel Hinckley Throop (b. 1798)

Engraving on vellum, with ink
Inscribed August 8, 1861
17 1/4 x 13 1/2 in.

Signed lower right: "Engraved by J. V. N. and O. H. Throop Wash^{n}. City."

Given after 1907 by unknown donor
Accession number: 1907+f.Pr.01

Dr. John H. Brinton's certificate of commission as brigade surgeon of volunteers was bound into the first of three volumes of his wartime correspondence donated to the Jefferson archives. These volumes contain orders and communications from Generals Grant, Rosecrans, McPherson, and Sheridan, letters from the surgeon general, and Brinton's own correspondence to his family. It is not known if Brinton himself placed the certificate into the book, or if this was done at a later time. At present the vellum document is faded and stained and in fragile condition, with many deep creases. The commission was signed personally by President Abraham Lincoln.

Decorating the upper portion of the document is an eagle with spread wings and claws grasping bolts of lightning encircled by clouds. Above the eagle is the inscription "THE/PRESIDENT of the United States of AMERICA." Below is a banner containing the words "E. PLURIBUS UNUM." Another decoration under the central text is an elaborate trophy arrangement featuring flags, cannon balls, powder barrels and charges, swords, bayonets, hatchets, plumed helmets, and bugles.

The stirring full text of the document is as follows (with handwritten words underlined):

> To all who shall see these presents greeting:/Know ye, That reposing special trust and confidence in the patriotism, valor, fidelity and/abilities of <u>J. H. Brinton</u> I have nominated, and by and with the advice and consent/of the Senate do appoint him <u>Brigade Surgeon of Volunteers</u> in the service of the United States: to rank as such from the <u>Third</u> day of <u>August</u>/eighteen hundred and <u>Sixty-one</u>. He is therefore carefully and diligently to discharge the duty/of <u>Brigade Surgeon</u> by doing and performing all manner of things thereunto belonging.
>
> And I do strictly charge and require all Officers and Soldiers under his command to be obedi/ent to his orders as <u>Brigade Surgeon</u>. And he is to observe and follow such orders, and di-/rections, from time to time, as he shall receive from me, or the future President of the United States of/America, or the General, or other superior Officers set over him, according to the rules and discipline of/War. This Commission to continue in force during the pleasure of the President of the United States for/the time being.
>
> GIVEN under my hand in the City of Washington, this <u>Eighth</u> day of <u>August</u> in the year/of our Lord, one thousand eight hundred and <u>Sixty-one</u> and in the <u>Eighty-sixth</u> year/of the Independence of the United States.
>
> By the President [signed] <u>Abraham Lincoln</u>
>
> [signed] Thomas A. Scott/<u>Acting</u> Secretary of War.

Additional handwritten text in script in the upper right corner reads, "Recorded Volume 17, page 4./Adjutant General's Office/August 8, 1861./J. Thomas/Adj. Genl."

The document's engravers were John P. V. N. Throop and Orramel H. Throop, brothers from Oxford, New York. J. P. V. N. Throop worked for New York and Baltimore publishers, then settled in Washington about 1830 and worked there until his death. O. H. Throop is known to have worked in New York and New Orleans.

The Jefferson archives has another Civil War military commission signed by Abraham Lincoln, that of Dr. Joseph Turner Van Pelt who graduated with the class of 1854.

Major General George B. McClellan on the Battlefield of Antietam

GEORGE BRINTON McCLELLAN (1826-85)
By Adam B. Walter (1820-75) after painting by Christian Schussele (1824/26-79)

Colored mezzotint, engraving
1863
Image size: 24 x 18 1/2 in.
Plate size: 28 x 21 1/2 in.
Sheet size: 30 1/2 x 24 1/2 in.

Painting signed and dated lower left: "C. Schussele/1863"
Inscriptions below image: "Painted by Schussele";
"PUBLISHED BY WM. SMITH.PRINT SELLER. 702 SO. THIRD ST. PHIL^A."; "Eng. by A.B. Walter";/"MAJ. GEN. GEO. B. M^c.CLELLAN./ON THE BATTLEFIELD OF ANTIETAM/To the Army of the Potomac this picture of their Old Commander is respectfully dedicated by the Publisher/Entered according to act of Congress by John Dainty in the Clerk's Office of the District Court of the Eastern District of Pennsylvania in the year 1863."

Given in 1993 by Dr. Russell W. Schaedler (JMC 1953), the Plimpton-Pugh Professor of Microbiology at JMC
Accession number: 1993+e.Pr.01

George Brinton McClellan was a major general in the Civil War. He was the son of Jefferson Medical College founder Dr. George McClellan, and the first cousin of Dr. John Hill Brinton.

George Brinton McClellan was the second ranked graduate of the class of 1846 at West Point. He served with the Engineers in Mexico, returned to West Point to teach practical military engineering, then worked in railway surveying in the West and Southwest, reaching the rank of first lieutenant of engineers. He also was assigned to study the European military system, then resigned his commission to serve as a high official in the Illinois Central Railroad and the Ohio and Mississippi Railroad.

His first service in the Civil War was as major general of Ohio Volunteers, followed by an appointment in the regular army as major general in command of the Department of Ohio, which included the states of Ohio, Indiana, Illinois, and parts of Pennsylvania and Virginia. He was credited with separating western Virginia territory from the Confederacy, and for this success was dubbed "Little Mac: the Young Napoleon." He was given command of the Division of the Potomac whose demoralized troops he reorganized and infused with new discipline and energy, and when General Scott retired McClellan became general-in-chief of the Army of the Potomac.

Although his troops suffered unexpected reverses at the hands of General Robert E. Lee outside of Richmond, McClellan attributed his defeat to a lack of support from Washington and to the fact that his army was outnumbered. His next order was simply to prepare for the defense of Washington, but General Lee was moving not toward Washington but toward the upper crossings of the Potomac, so McClellan assumed personal command of an advance. Although the Confederate troops were much scattered and McClellan had superior numbers, he hesitated too long and attacked Lee piecemeal instead of simultaneously. Instead of McClellan cutting Lee's sole line of retreat and intercepting his army, Lee avoided destruction at the battles of South Mountain and the Antietam and accomplished a withdrawal of his army across the Potomac.

Because of his conduct of the Antietam campaign McClellan was ordered to turn over his command and to proceed to Trenton to await orders, but he was never again employed in the field. In 1864 McClellan ran as the Democratic presidential candidate but was overwhelmingly defeated at the polls by Abraham Lincoln. He was later elected for one term as governor of New Jersey.

In Adam B. Walter's copy of a painting by Christian Schussele of Major General McClellan, the equestrian commander is silhouetted against the smoky sky of the battlefield. Holding his reins, field glasses, and cap, he views the scene around him calmly and resolutely. In contrast, his horse froths at the mouth and paws the ground which is covered in straw and broken tree limbs. The horse's navy-blue blanket is embroidered with a gold eagle and stars, matching the colors and insignia of the general's uniform. In the right corner is a section of cannon, a loose wheel, and a cannon ball.

Gesticulating soldiers on horseback and on foot, one waving his cap in a salute to the general, are in the left and center middle ground. A group surrounding a cannon is on the far right. There are just a few wisps of blue showing through the smoky gray sky. Although the bloody carnage is not depicted, one wonders if McClellan was meditating on the horrendous casualties: nearly five thousand killed and twelve thousand wounded.

Although this beleaguered general was soon to be relieved of his command, he nonetheless was regarded affectionately by the enlisted men. The Battle of the Antietam took place in 1862, and Schussele's painting was made the following year. The print after Schussele's painting was made by Adam B. Walter in 1863, presumably to circulate and popularize the image. The print has an inscription dedicating the image of the "Old Commander" to the Army of the Potomac.

Christian Schussele was born in Alsace, France. He studied in Strasbourg and Paris, and worked in the latter city as a chromolithographer before coming to Philadelphia in 1848. Although he established a reputation for chromolithography in this country as well, he much preferred painting, notably portraits and history subjects. He exhibited his work at the Pennsylvania Academy of the Fine Arts regularly from 1851 to 1869.

Schussele was active in Philadelphia art institutions, as a member of the Philadelphia Sketch Club, president of the Artists' Fund Society, and president of the Pennsylvania Academy of the Fine Arts' academicians. In 1868 he became superintendent of the Academy's school and professor of painting and drawing, remaining there until his death in 1879. Many other paintings by Schussele were engraved by John Sartain.

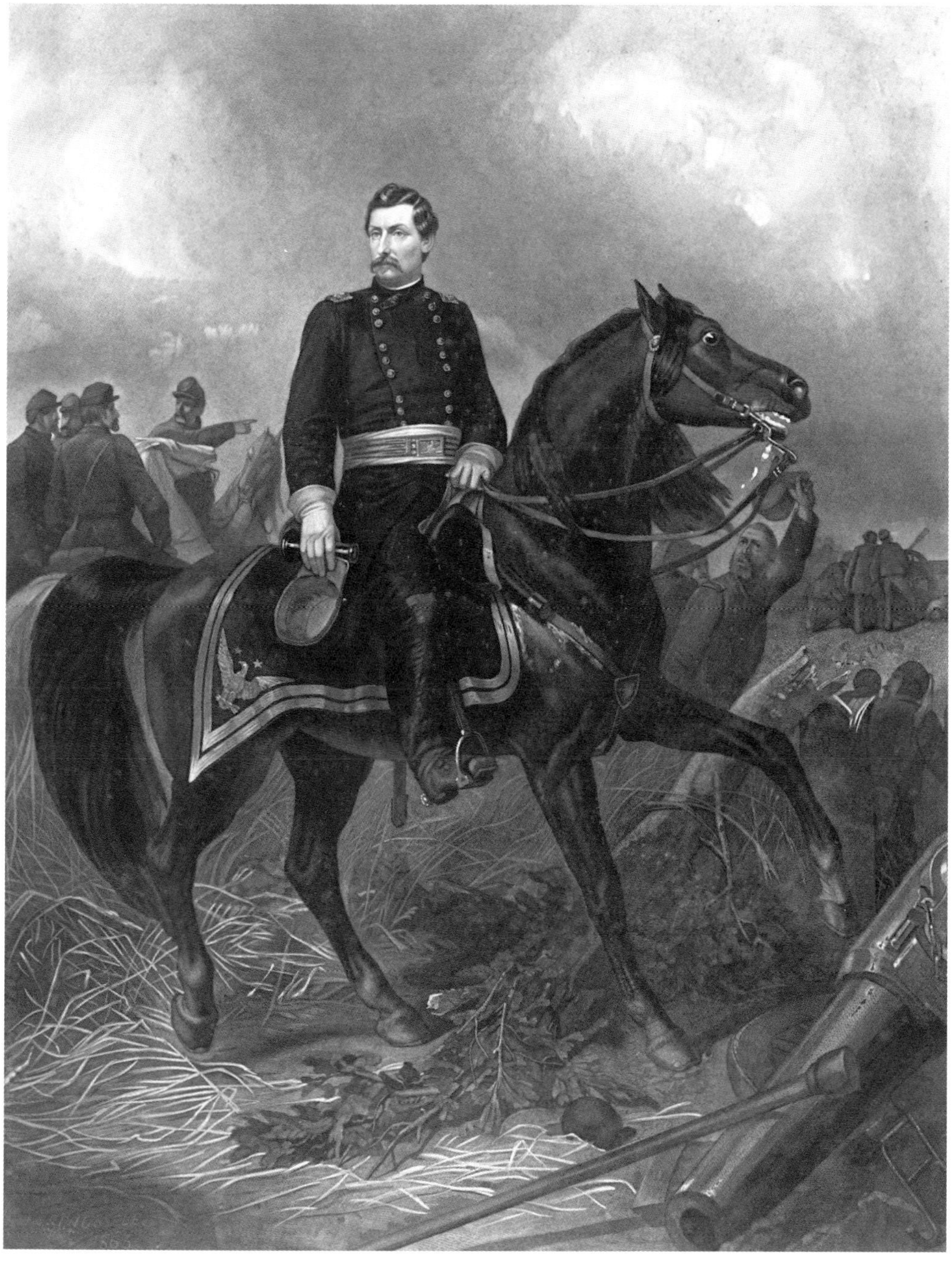

Portrait of Gilbert L. Parker

GILBERT LAFAYETTE PARKER, M.D. (1822-1915)
By Max Rosenthal (1833-1919)

Oil on canvas
1907
39 1/2 x 30 in.

Signed and dated lower right: "Max Rosenthal/1907"
Exhibition: American Art Society, 1907

Purchased in 1953 by Mrs. Gilbert S. Parker, the subject's daughter-in-law, and her daughter, Katherine, from Frances Rosenthal, daughter of artist Max Rosenthal; purchased in 1953 by Elizabeth Theodorides, granddaughter of the subject, and given by her in 1995
Accession number: 1995+e.P.02

Dr. Gilbert Lafayette Parker was a decorated officer in the Civil War. He graduated from Jefferson Medical College after his wartime service in 1874, and maintained a large private practice in Philadelphia for more than thirty years.

Gilbert L. Parker was born in 1832 in Harrisburg, Pennsylvania and was educated at the Partridge Military Academy there. Family records recount that in his early days Parker traded with the Indians in Nebraska in the company of Bartram Snyder, a descendant of John Bartram, a colonial Philadelphia naturalist.

At the outset of the Civil War Gilbert Parker returned to Philadelphia and enlisted as a first lieutenant in Company D, Twenty-eighth Regiment of Infantry, Pennsylvania Volunteers. In 1863 he was appointed captain and assistant quartermaster for the Army of the Potomac, and then captain and quartermaster at Savannah, Georgia. For "meritorious service" in maneuvering 420 wagons on a foraging expedition from Atlanta to Flat Rock he was made a brevet major of the U.S. Volunteers. Later he was made brevet lieutenant colonel for "energetic service" in campaigns in Georgia and the Carolinas. For a year after the war he settled up accounts under his jurisdiction in Vicksburg, Mississippi.

Family members wrote that his exploits included having his horse shot from under him in the battle at Gettysburg, and riding up Missionary Ridge and Lookout Mountain with Abraham Lincoln. Parker was also present at Antietam, Chancellorsville, Chattanooga, Kenesaw Mountain, the Siege of Atlanta, the March to the Sea, the Siege of Savannah, and the Campaign of the Carolinas.

As a brevet lieutenant colonel Gilbert L. Parker was made a member of the Loyal Legion. The legion's insignia appears on a lapel pin Parker wore in his 1907 portrait by Max Rosenthal.

In the two-thirds-length portrait the subject is seated and facing partly to the left. His head is turned to look straight ahead toward the viewer. The most distinguishing feature is his long and unkempt gray beard, mustache, and sideburns which conceal his mouth. The physician holds his pince-nez in one hand and a small pamphlet in the other. His shirt cuffs seem unusually large, and curiously, his black business attire includes a western-style hat although he is situated indoors. Behind the sitter is a maroon curtain hung in a curving diagonal to reveal a distant sky with scudding clouds.

The portrait exudes the palpable presence of the figure, especially his face and hands. He seems to occupy the space with three-dimensional solidity. The elderly physician's expressive pale blue eyes seem sad and weary, as though meditating on past experiences. The portrait was exhibited at the American Art Society where it won a silver medal in 1907.

Dr. and Mrs. Gilbert Lafayette Parker were the parents of a daughter, Annie, and two sons, Gilbert Sunderland Parker, a curator at the Pennsylvania Academy of the Fine Arts, and Ernest Lee Parker, a painting appraiser and restorer and also a curator at the Academy. Family records state that the painting was never owned by the family until its purchase in 1953 for $150. The portrait was acquired from artist Max Rosenthal's daughter, Frances, by Gilbert S. Parker's wife, Anna Bley Parker, and their daughter, Katherine. The picture was sold almost immediately (for the purchase price) to the daughter of Ernest L. Parker, Elizabeth Theodorides. In 1995 she donated the portrait to Thomas Jefferson University.[8]

The Parkers were friends and neighbors of the Eakins family on Philadelphia's Mount Vernon Street, and Gilbert S. Parker was the organizer of the Thomas Eakins memorial exhibition at the Academy in 1917. In 1910 Thomas Eakins had painted portraits of Dr. Gilbert L. Parker and his wife, as well as their two sons.

Max Rosenthal was born in Turck, in Russian Poland, in 1833. He went to Paris to study drawing and painting, as well as lithography with the Alsatian artist Martin Thurwanger (d.1890). He emigrated to Philadelphia in 1849 and continued his studies at the Pennsylvania Academy. His duty as an artist during the Civil War was to follow the Army of the Republic and make sketches for the U.S. Military Commission.

Max Rosenthal and several brothers established a

lithographic firm in Philadelphia which became famous for decorative chromolithographic advertisements, trade cards, architectural studies, and book illustration. Max Rosenthal retired from the family firm in 1884, and turned to etching, mezzotint, and oil painting. He received a bronze medal from the Louisiana Purchase Exposition in 1904, and an award from the World's Columbian Exposition in 1893 for engraved portraits of prominent historical figures which he had made with his son, Albert. More than three hundred of these portraits were purchased for the Smithsonian Institution. Among other societies Max Rosenthal was elected a fellow of the Royal Academy of England.

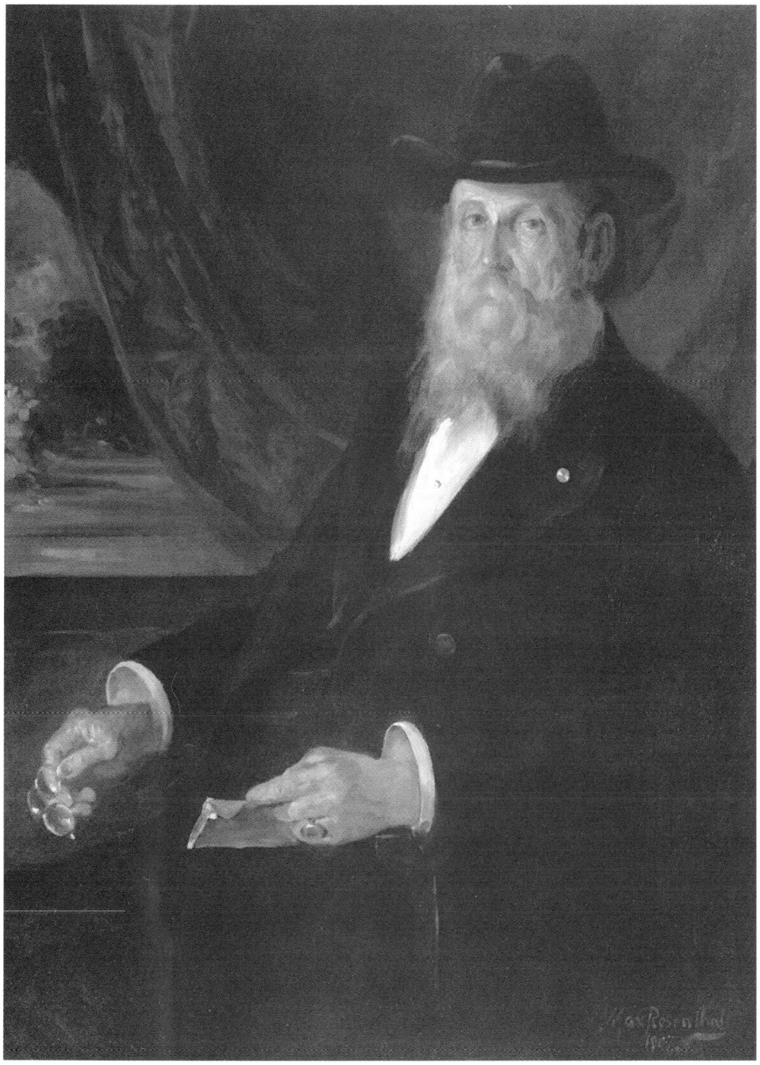

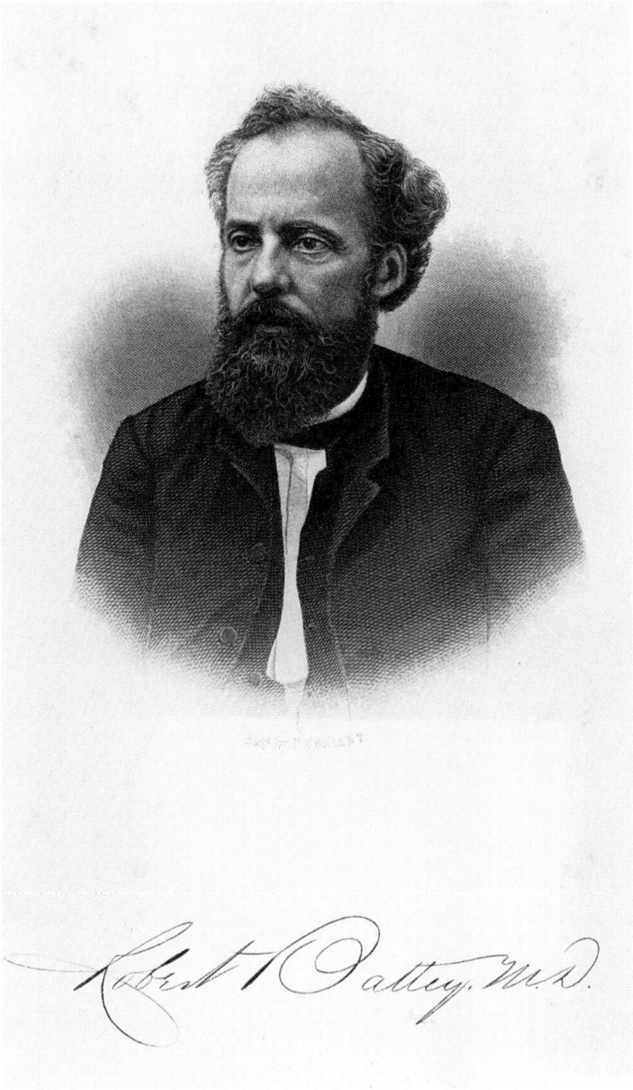

Portrait of Robert Battey

ROBERT BATTEY, M.D. (1828-95)
By Robert O'Brien (active mid-nineteenth century)

Steel engraving, stipple
Ca. 1870-80
Image size: 3 3/4 x 3 1/4 in.
Sheet size: 9 1/2 x 5 7/8 in.

Signed below image: "Eng[d]. by R. O'Brien. N.Y."
Facsimile signature: "Robert Battey, M.D."

Given after 1895 by unknown donor
Accession number: 1895+f.Pr.03

The Confederacy also had outspoken loyalists at Jefferson Medical College. In fact, sixty-two percent of the members of the class of 1859-60 were from southern and border states. Emotions were so polarized by events leading up to the Civil War, that in December 1859 over two hundred students were led by the southerner Dr. Hunter H. McGuire (1835-1900), a popular anatomy quizmaster for Dr. Joseph Pancoast, to resign from Jefferson and transfer to the Medical College of Virginia in Richmond or other hospitable cities in the South.

McGuire became the medical director of the Army of the Shenandoah under the command of General "Stonewall" Jackson who requested that McGuire be assigned to him as brigade surgeon. He also served under Generals Ewell and Early and was with General Lee at Appomattox. Dr. McGuire became chair of surgery at the Medical College of Virginia and was president of the American Surgical Association and the American Medical Association. Apparently after the war there were no hard feelings among Jefferson faculty because Dr. McGuire was invited to lecture in the amphitheater of the new Jefferson hospital in 1877 and was awarded an LL.D. degree in 1888. Although the Jefferson collection has no original image of Dr. Hunter McGuire, it is fortunate to have an engraving of Dr. Robert Battey, another distinguished southerner who volunteered his services for the Confederacy.

Robert Battey was born in 1828 in Augusta, Georgia. He graduated from the Philadelphia College of Pharmacy in 1856 and from Jefferson Medical College the following year. After several years of postgraduate study in Paris, he opened a practice in Rome, Georgia and volunteered his services at the outbreak of the Civil War. He was commissioned a surgeon of the Nineteenth

Regiment of Georgia Volunteers, served as senior surgeon of Archer's Brigade, and was surgeon-in-charge for several military hospitals.

An eminent gynecologist of his day in Rome, Georgia, he was the surgeon-in-charge of the Gynecological Infirmary and consulting surgeon and business manager of the Martha Battey Hospital; Dr. Battey was the benefactor of the latter institution and named it for his wife. From 1873 to 1875 he was professor of obstetrics at the Atlanta Medical College, and served briefly as editor of the *Atlanta Medical and Surgical Journal*.

In 1872 Dr. Robert Battey originated the operation of oophorectomy known as "Battey's operation," a procedure now in disrepute for treating sexual and other maladies. He also devised an improved operation for vesicovaginal fistula, and was the originator of iodized phenol.

Dr. Battey served a term as president of the American Gynecological Society and of the Georgia Medical Association. He was a fellow of the Obstetrical Society of Edinburgh and of the British Gynecological Society. He was highly regarded at Jefferson Medical College which awarded him an LL.D. degree in 1891. The October 1913 *Jeffersonian* reported that an effort was being made to procure a "lasting memorial of another of her illustrious sons," but apparently such an oil portrait or marble bust was never commissioned.

The engraver of Dr. Robert Battey's portrait was Robert O'Brien who is known to have worked in New York during the 1850s and 1860s. His bust-length portrait of Dr. Battey depicts a man of steely determination and exactitude. In a profile of Battey in the January 1915 *Jeffersonian* the doctor's bluntness was illustrated by the following story: "Once, at a gathering of celebrated surgeons in Philadelphia, a young doctor boasted that he had spent fifteen thousand dollars for his surgical instruments. Dr. Battey remarked that he always carried ten and tried to keep them clean, *and he held up his hands and counted his fingers one by one.*"

Civil War American Flag

CIVIL WAR AMERICAN FLAG
Manufactured by William G. Mintzer

Bunting, rope, brass
1859-61
77 x 46 1/2 in.

Inscription stamped on upper border: "WM. G. MINTZER/MAKER PHILADA."

Given after 1865 by unknown donor
Accession number: 1865-1900.DA.01

The Civil War was one of the most patriotic and partisan periods in American history, and flags flew from most public buildings, shops, and manufacturing plants, as well as many private residences. A Union flag lay unnoticed until 1997 in the office of Robert A. Peterson, then Thomas Jefferson University's senior vice president for administration and finance and chief financial officer. He had received it from a previous administrator whose office was down the hall, but neither knew the flag's provenance.

However, a clue was provided by a note accompanying the flag stating that "it was flown on Mssrs. Howell and Smith's store, Philadelphia, during the early part of the rebellion, 1861" and that "William G. Steel was a partner in that firm." *McElroy's Philadelphia City Directory* of the early 1860s listed Howell, Smith, and Company as a white goods firm at 503 Market Street, and added that the firm had two other partners including William G. Steel. It is likely that the flag was given by a relative of Mr. Steel, as there were three alumni named Steel who attended Jefferson Medical College after the Civil War.

The flag is stamped with the name of the manufacturer, William G. Mintzer. Located at 131 North Third Street in Philadelphia from 1839 to 1869, Mintzer's firm specialized

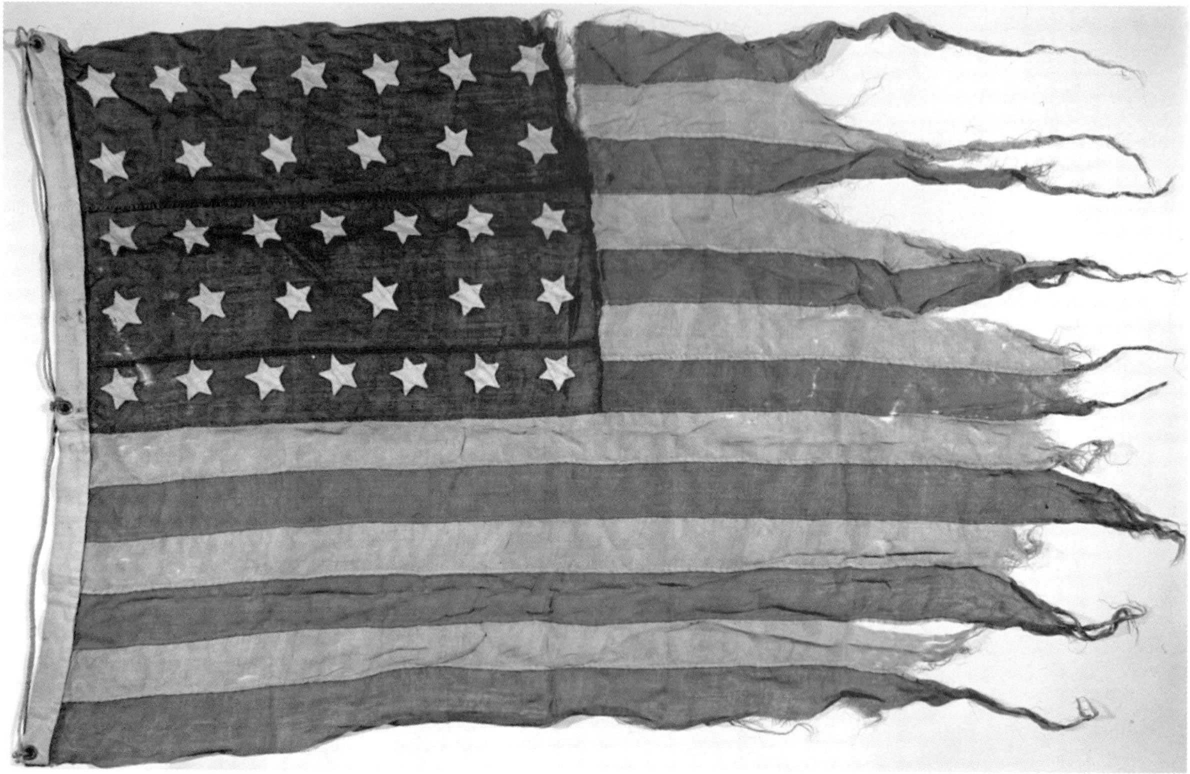

in military goods, coach lace, fly nets, lodge regalia, fringes, and militia buttons. The Mintzer firm was only a few blocks from Howell, Smith, and Company.

The machine-made flag is made of bunting with rope and brass grommets for hanging. The blue canton has thirty-three stars arranged in straight rows horizontally, but in a scattered pattern vertically. The flag must have been made when the country had thirty-three states between July 4, 1859 and July 6, 1861. Judging from its tattered condition, it was probably used throughout the Civil War period.

Portrait of Abraham Lincoln

ABRAHAM LINCOLN (1809-65)
By Joseph K. Davison's Sons

Bronze medal
3 in. diameter

Signed below left shoulder: "COPYRIGHT DAVISON'S SONS PHILA"
Inscription obverse: "WITH MALICE TOWARD NONE WITH CHARITY FOR ALL/1809 1909"
Inscription reverse: "THIS MEDAL/WAS STRUCK FOR/THE GRAND ARMY/OF THE REPUBLIC/IN COMMEMORATION/OF THE/100TH ANNIVERSARY/OF THE BIRTH OF/ABRAHAM LINCOLN"

Given after 1909 by unknown donor
Accession number: 1909+f.M.02

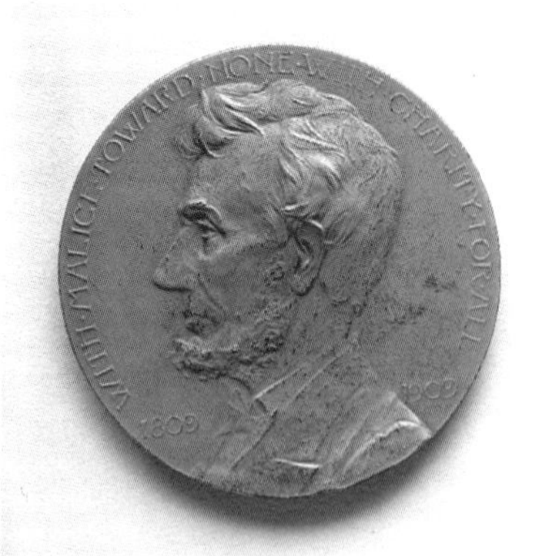

A bronze medal commemorating the hundredth anniversary of the birth of Abraham Lincoln was presented by an unknown donor. The medal was struck in 1909 for the Grand Army of the Republic by the Philadelphia medallic firm, Joseph K. Davison's Sons. The obverse shows a profile view of the bearded president facing left, with the famous aphorism, "With malice toward none, with charity for all." The commemorative inscription on the reverse is surrounded by a wreath of laurel.

Some Nineteenth- and Mid-twentieth-century Images and Memorabilia of Doctors at Work, Students, and Patients

The Thomas Jefferson University archives contain memorabilia and images of some famous mid-nineteenth-century, non-Jefferson physicians like Dr. William T. G. Morton; little known Jefferson alumni who pursued different career paths, among them James F. Noyes, M.D., an urban surgeon, and Buchan Richards, M.D., a country doctor; and some unidentified students. The collection also contains images in various media of anonymous physicians and patients who were emblematic of their respective periods.

William T. G. Morton Administering Anesthesia

WILLIAM THOMAS GREEN MORTON (1819-68)
By George R. Hall (b. 1818)

Engraving, etching, stipple
After 1854
Image size: 4 1/8 x 3 1/4 in.
Sheet size: 9 1/4 x 6 1/8 in.

Inscriptions below image: "Eng^{d}. by G.R. Hall"; "W^{m}. T. G. MORTON, M.D. SURGEON DENTIST, BOSTON, ADMINISTERING ETHER/PREPARATORY TO PERFORMING THE OPERATION BY WHICH HE FIRST DISCOVERED AND/DEMONSTRATED THE MARVELOUS ANAESTHETIC POWERS OF ETHER IN SURGERY."

Given after 1900 by unknown donor
Accession number: 1900+f.Pr.10

Considerable controversy still exists over the credit for the first use of ether anesthesia, but most medical historians recognize Dr. Crawford W. Long, a rural physician in Jefferson, Georgia who used it for minor procedures in 1842. Failing to realize the significance of his breakthrough, Long did not widely publish his work until after a public demonstration in 1846 by William T. G. Morton in Boston.

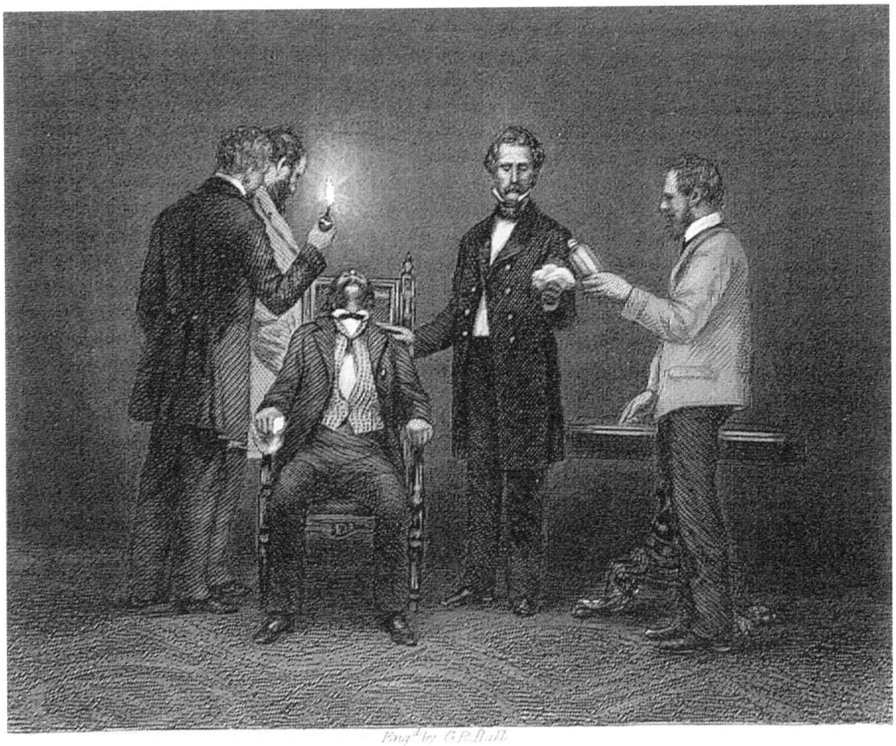

Eng^{d} by G.R.Hall

Born in 1819 in Charlton, Massachusetts, Morton had studied at the College of Dental Surgery in Baltimore in 1840. After opening a dental practice in Farmington, Connecticut he sought ways to lessen the pain of dental surgery. Morton was briefly a partner of Connecticut dentist Horace Wells who had used nitrous oxide in the extraction of teeth in 1844. Wells's demonstration of inhalation anesthesia at the Massachusetts General Hospital in January 1844 failed, and he was labeled "swindler" and his technique "humbug."

William T. G. Morton resettled in Boston where he studied with Dr. Charles T. Jackson who was experimenting with sulfuric ether as a painkiller. Morton successfully used this substance for a tooth extraction on September 30, 1846 and developed a spherical container for the administration of the anesthetic. He then persuaded Professor of Surgery John Collins Warren, M.D. to allow another demonstration of ether anesthesia at Harvard Medical School.

With Dr. Warren as surgeon and Morton as anesthetist, a successful operation for removing a tumor from a patient's jaw took place on October 16, 1846 in the same surgical amphitheater as Wells's fiasco. When the patient awoke and testified that he felt no pain, Dr. Warren uttered his famous words about the dawn of a new era in surgery: "Gentlemen, this is not humbug, no, this is not humbug." Only two months later at Jefferson Medical College, Dr. Thomas D. Mütter became the first Philadelphia surgeon to administer anesthesia, for a case removing a tumor from the cheek.

However, there was initial resistance by many in the medical profession, and there were bitter legal fights over the patent rights between Morton and other pioneer claimants to the discovery including Drs. Jackson and Wells. Although Morton eventually received testimonials and prizes for full credit from various medical societies, and an M.D. degree from Washington University in Baltimore (1849), he staggered from one failed business to another. He died in 1868 at the age of forty-nine leaving his family in abject poverty.

An undated engraving by George R. Hall does not depict Morton's dramatic demonstration at Massachusetts General Hospital where the ether was administered through a glass apparatus with two openings for a rubber tube used as a mouthpiece, but instead shows an earlier technique. Morton prepares to soak ether into some folded fabric which will be held over the mouth and nose of the patient, who is seated in an armchair with his head held back awaiting oral surgery.

English engraver George R. Hall studied in London with his brother, Henry B. Hall Sr. (1808-84). George Hall first worked as an engraver in London and Leipzig, and then in 1854 joined his brother in New York where he worked for banknote and publishing houses. This print might have been a book illustration originally.

James F. Noyes's Certificate of Attending the Practice at Pennsylvania Hospital

CERTIFICATE OF JAMES FANNING NOYES, M.D. (1817-96)
Designed by William Strickland (1788-1854) and engraved by Samuel Seymour (active 1796-1823)

Etching, engraving, ink on parchment
Designed 1811, inscribed to James F. Noyes in 1850
Image size: 9 3/4 x 16 1/2 in.
Image plate size: 11 1/2 x 17 3/4 in.
Text plate size: 8 3/4 x 17 1/2 in.
Sheet size: 21 1/4 x 18 1/2 in.

Signed below image lower left: "W^{m}. Strickland F.S.A. del^{t}."
Signed below image lower right: "Saml. Seymour A.A. Sculp^{t}."
Inscription above image: "SOUTH FRONT OF THE PENNSYLVANIA HOSPITAL"
Inscription below image: "This building by the bounty of Government and of many private Persons was piously founded for the Relief of the Sick and Miserable Anno 1755."
Inscription on certificate: "WE The attending Managers Physician and Surgeon OF THE/PENNSYLVANIA HOSPITAL,/Do Certify that J. F. Noyes, M.D. Student of Medicine/of Waterville, Maine hath attended the practice the PHYSICIANS/and SURGEONS of the said HOSPITAL for two years/In Testimony whereof We have respectively set our Names to this/Certificate and caused the Seal of the Hospital to be thereunto affixed this/Twenty-third day of February in the Year of our Lord 1850./James.../Med. Board Managers/Geo. B. Wood Physician/Geo. W. Norris Surgeon"
Followed by signatures of managers, physician, and surgeon

Given after 1900 by unknown donor
Accession number: 1900+f.Pr.28

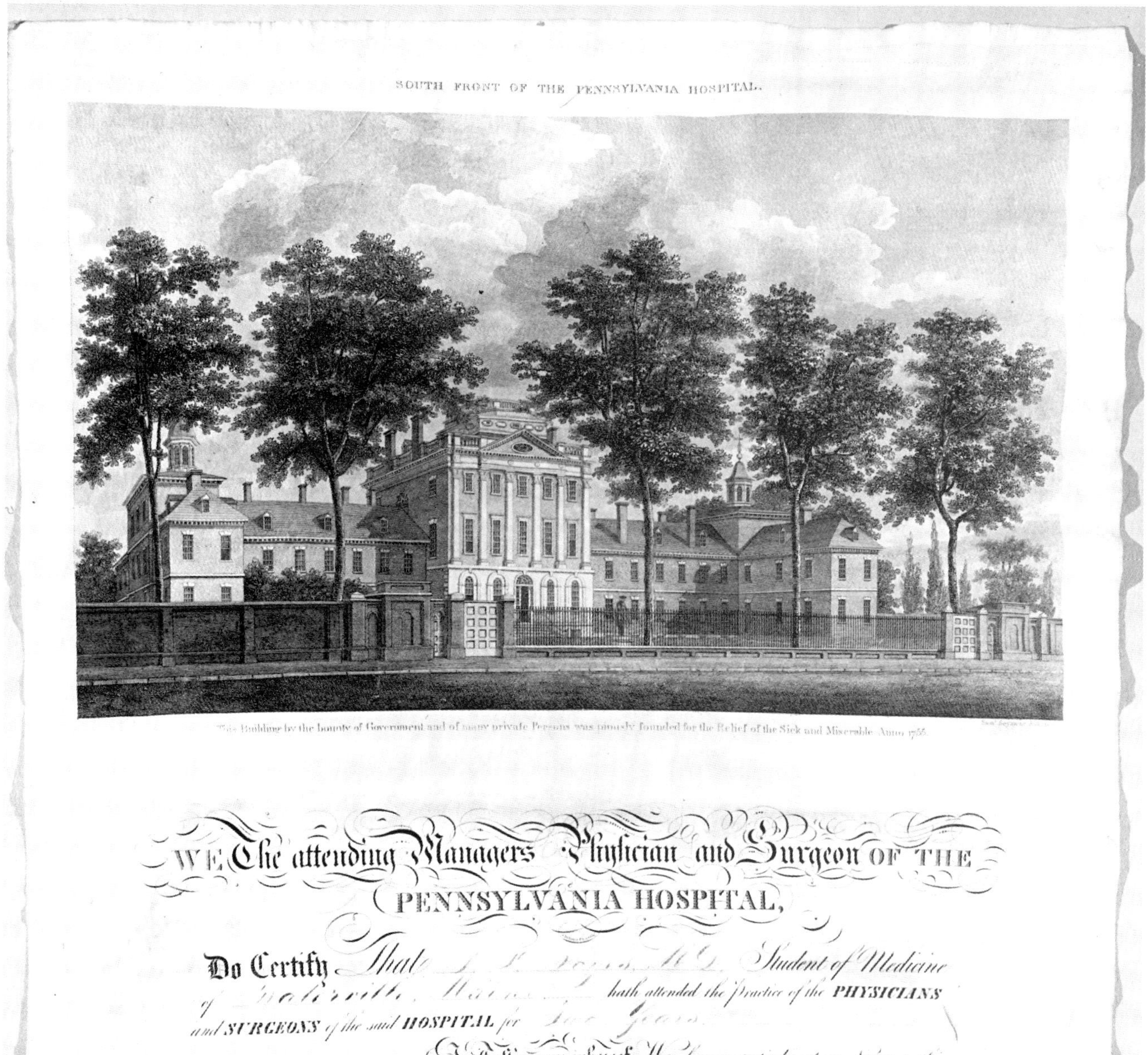
SOUTH FRONT OF THE PENNSYLVANIA HOSPITAL.

This Building by the bounty of Government and of many private Persons was piously founded for the Relief of the Sick and Miserable Anno 1755.

WE The attending Managers Physician and Surgeon OF THE PENNSYLVANIA HOSPITAL,

Do Certify That [illegible] M.D. Student of Medicine of [illegible] hath attended the practice of the PHYSICIANS and SURGEONS of the said HOSPITAL for [illegible]

In Testimony whereof We have respectively set our Names to this Certificate and caused the Seal of the Hospital to be thereunto affixed this [illegible] day of [illegible] in the Year of our Lord [illegible]

[illegible] Managers

Geo B. Wood Physician

Geo W. Norris Surgeon

Dr. James F. Noyes was born in 1817 in Kingston, Rhode Island, and began his study of medicine with a private physician in Waterville, Maine. After studying at Harvard Medical School in 1842, he graduated from Jefferson Medical College in 1846 with the largest class to date. He practiced first in Waterville and Cincinnati and then continued his study of ophthalmology abroad in Berlin and Paris. Noyes settled permanently in Detroit in 1863 and began an active clinical and academic career. He was professor of ophthalmology and otology at Detroit Medical College from 1869 to 1879 and practiced aural and ophthalmic surgery at several local hospitals. He was a founder and president of the Detroit Academy of Medicine.

By 1850, the year his name was inscribed on the decorative certificate, Dr. James Noyes had just completed two years of attending at the Pennsylvania Hospital. The hospital, the nation's first, was founded in 1751 by a group of public-spirited citizens led by Benjamin Franklin and Dr. Thomas Bond. The hospital was completed in three stages—the east portion facing Eighth Street in 1756; the west portion facing Ninth Street in 1796; and the central portion, pictured in the certificate, about 1800 to 1805.

The circumstances surrounding the creation of this famous print have been recorded. On February 25, 1811 the board of managers voted to have a view of Pennsylvania Hospital taken and an engraving made to be used for a certificate for the students and a similar plate for every "Contributor of Ten Pounds and upwards."

At the meeting of March 25, 1811 the managers approved the drawing of the south front of the hospital made by William Strickland, for which he was paid twenty-five dollars. For some unknown reason Strickland did not engrave the drawing but Samuel Seymour was hired to do that work. A third artisan, John Vallance, engraved the text. The latter two were paid four hundred dollars for their work and for their supplies. The engraving on the contributors' plate was later done by John Exilius.[9]

The Pennsylvania Hospital etching is rendered in delicate, feathery strokes, but its architectural features are manifest. Of greatest interest is the Georgian central section topped with a skylighted dome which surmounts the surgical amphitheater. A full-length lead statue of William Penn, donated by his grandson John Penn, is visible behind the iron gate and to the right of the entrance. Five large shade trees grace the property.

The son of a carpenter, designer William Strickland was born in New Jersey in 1788 and reared in Philadelphia. In 1803 he apprenticed with Benjamin H. Latrobe (1764-1820), considered the leading architect in the country. Before winning the commission to design the Second Bank of the United States in Philadelphia, Strickland worked as a surveyor, engraver, and painter, as well as an architect. Designing in several different styles for buildings in Philadelphia, he was most celebrated for the United States Naval Asylum, the Merchants' Exchange, St. Stephen's Episcopal Church, and the steeple of Independence Hall.

The versatile Strickland also worked as an engineer. He was a member of the American Philosophical Society, a director of the Pennsylvania Academy of the Fine Arts, recording secretary of the Franklin Institute, and a member of the Royal Institution of Civil Engineers. William Strickland's last great work was the Tennessee State Capitol. He died in Nashville in 1854 and his body is interred beneath the Capitol's north portico.

Engraver Samuel Seymour was born in England. It is not known when he arrived in America, but he resided in Philadelphia at least by 1796. He studied engraving and painting with artist William Birch (1755-1834). He was best known as an engraver of certificates and book illustrations, and for his engravings after work by William Birch and his son Thomas Birch (1779-1851). Seymour was a draftsman for Stephen Long's expedition to the Rocky Mountains in the early 1820s, and his sketches are among the earliest illustrations of the western United States.

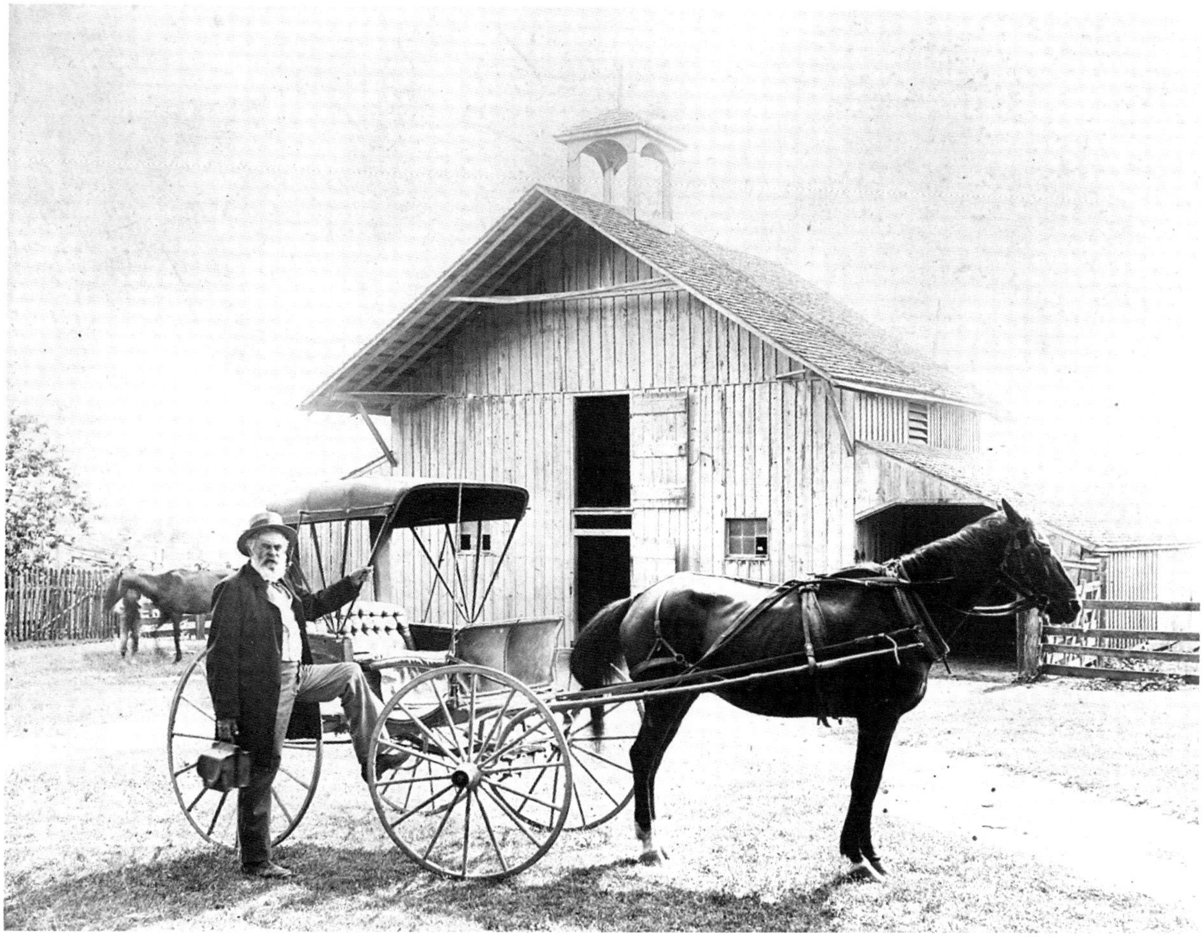

Portrait of Buchan Richards

BUCHAN RICHARDS, M.D.
By American View Co.

Photograph mounted on card
Ca. 1880-90
Photo size: 7 1/8 x 9 1/4 in.
Card size: 10 x 12 in.

Inscription on mount: "PHOTO BY AMERICAN VIEW COMPANY CHARLOTTE, N.C."

Given in 1984 by the estate of C. Gardiner Johnson, a descendant of the subject
Accession number: 1984+e.Ph.01

Buchan Richards was a classmate of James Noyes in the Jefferson Medical College class of 1846. Virginia is listed as his place of residence in early college records.

In the photograph he personifies the quintessential late-nineteenth-century country doctor boarding his horse-drawn buggy. Since Dr. Richards is carrying a leather saddle kit medical bag, he is probably commencing or returning from a house call. Patients were customarily seen at home rather than in a hospital or the physician's office.

Though graced with a white beard, the doctor looks youthfully energetic and a bit impatient about posing for this photograph. He has turned his body to face the camera while his left leg is already poised to board the buggy. The setting is a farm, complete with a barn and fences surrounding the adjoining pasture.

The photograph was a donation from the estate of C. Gardiner Johnson, a descendant of the physician.[10] Mr. Johnson also bequeathed to Thomas Jefferson University the mortgage to Tuckoman Farm in West Point, Virginia. It may be too sentimental to assume that the property shown in the photograph is the family farm, and not the farm of a patient he was visiting.

Portrait of Unidentified Jefferson Medical College Student

UNIDENTIFIED STUDENT
By unknown photographer

Hand-colored ambrotype
Ca. 1854-65
Image size: 3 1/4 x 2 3/4 in.
Case size: 3 5/8 x 3 1/4 in.

Given after 1900 by unknown donor
Accession number: 1900+f.Ph.21

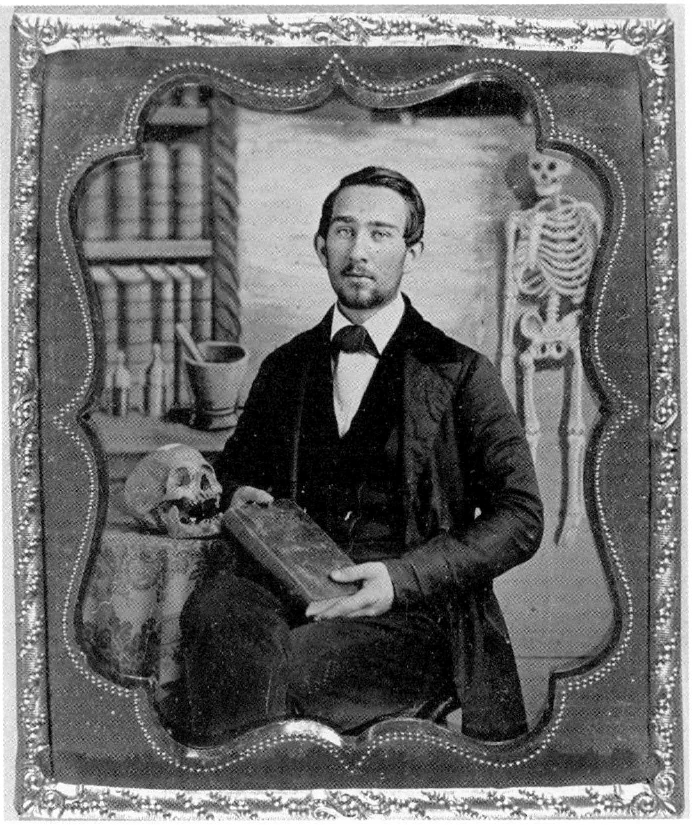

This photograph of a mid-nineteenth-century student at Jefferson Medical College is one example among many that have been donated to the archives.

The unidentified student is posed in an elaborate setting that describes his field of study unquestionably. He holds a book in both hands and his left arm rests next to a skull on a tabletop. A mortar and pestle are placed on a shelf in front of a bookcase. To top it off, a small skeleton is suspended nearby. The young man looks so earnest that one supposes he was a dedicated student.

The image contains some sparing use of color which was applied by hand: pink in the sitter's cheeks and pale green on the tablecloth. The photograph is surrounded by a brass sheet mat cut in a continuous volute shape. The ambrotype and mat are housed in their original brown leather case which is embossed with a floral design on the outer lid. The case is lined in orange velvet.

Rival photographic processes were being invented with great rapidity throughout the nineteenth century, and the ambrotype process was first patented in 1854. Like the daguerreotypes which they largely supplanted, ambrotypes were one-of-a-kind images, and were fitted into similar miniature cases. The ambrotype process was in vogue only until the middle 1860s, though still made occasionally until about 1880.

Unlike the earlier daguerreotype method of printing on a silvered copper plate, ambrotypes were positive images secured on glass plates by the wet collodion process. Resembling negatives, the images appeared as positives only when seen by reflected light against dark background supports such as dark glass or clear glass backed with black velvet or black varnish.

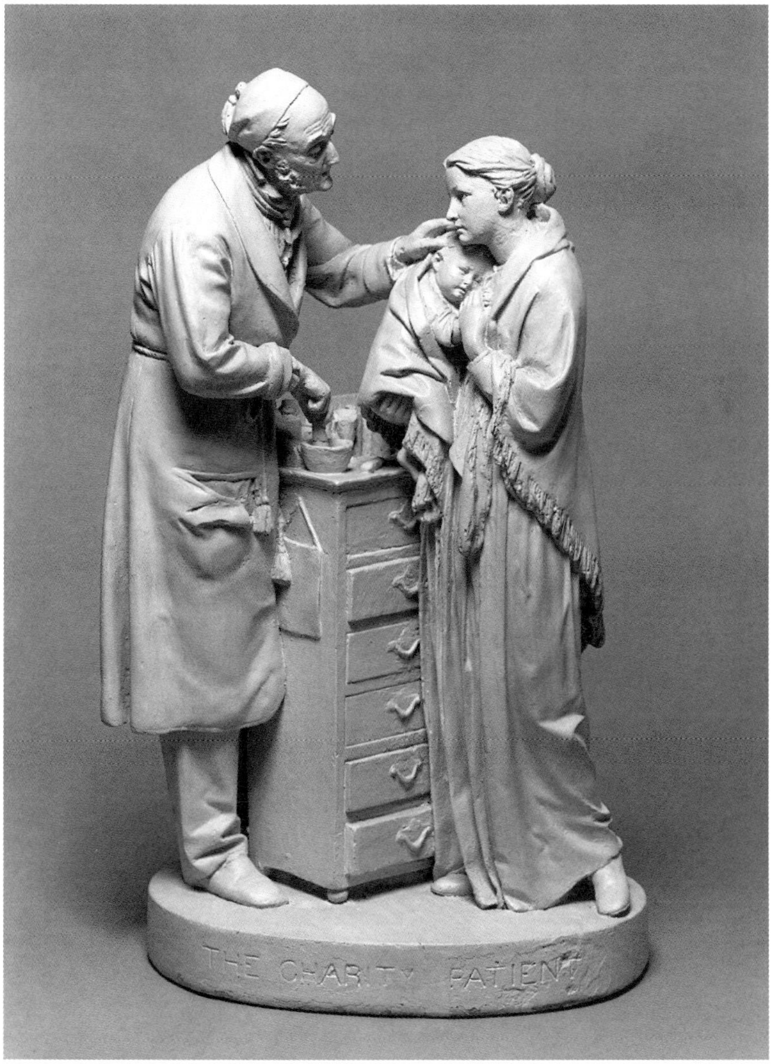

The Charity Patient

THE CHARITY PATIENT
By John Rogers (1829-1904)

Painted plaster
1866
22 x 13 5/8 x 8 1/2 in.

Dated center back: "PATENTED/DEC. 4/1866"
Inscription on center of integral base: "THE CHARITY PATIENT"

Given in 1981 by Dorothy Rue
Accession number: 1981+e.S.01

The physician as a kindly, healing figure began to appear in genre paintings, oil portraits, and sculptures in mid-nineteenth-century American art. A wonderful example of this type is a small plaster group, *The Charity Patient*, by American sculptor John Rogers.

This sentimental work shows an elderly doctor preparing medicine with one hand, and touching the head of a sick infant held by its mother. The figures are separated by a chest laden with jars, bottles, and a spatula.

The doctor's solicitous gesture comforts the child who is wrapped in a blanket and nestled on her mother's breast. The beautiful young mother wears a fringed shawl over her gown and looks anxiously and respectfully toward the doctor. In contrast, the elderly doctor's body is stooped with age and the gaunt features of his wrinkled face are almost hawklike. Garbed in a long robe and cap, he has perhaps been awakened in the middle of the night to tend to an emergency.

The social message of the sculpture is further emphasized by the prominent placement of the title on the integral base: "THE CHARITY PATIENT." This work and its sequel, *Fetching the Doctor*, were among John Rogers's most popular groups, and were prized decorations in physicians' offices throughout the country.

John Rogers created a uniquely American group of mid-nineteenth-century sculptures that treated the everyday scenes of contemporary life. Born in Salem, Massachusetts in 1829, he grew up in a Boston family descended from merchants and scholars, but then in reduced circumstances. Even while working in machine shops in Manchester, New Hampshire and Hannibal, Missouri, Rogers began to model little clay figures as a pastime. When he realized that his diminutive groups were pleasing, he decided to become a sculptor and went to study in Paris and Rome.

After returning to America in 1859, he settled in Chicago where he worked with the city surveyor. In his spare time he sculpted a little group entitled *The Checker Player*, and it scored a fabulous success at a fund-raising fair where it sold for seventy-five dollars. Rogers then conceived the idea of mass-producing plaster copies of sculptures to be sold at reasonable prices.

He moved to New York and set up an attic studio over Broadway. He entered three genre groups in the 1860 National Academy of Design exhibition where they attracted considerable attention. His abolitionist Civil War groups and subsequent genre subjects made his name and fortune. Soon his studio employed twenty artisans to manufacture the copies.

Rogers began to issue illustrated catalogues, and new subjects were eagerly awaited. To meet popular demand as many as ten thousand copies of particular favorites were produced, most selling for ten to fifteen dollars. Though mass-produced, "Rogers groups" are beautifully modeled and with just enough detail to tell a narrative with warmth, wit, or pathos. Most are paeans to a simple and virtuous American way of life. For decades it seemed that almost every middle-class American parlor proudly displayed a Rogers group. The sculptor died in 1904.

Family Doctor

FAMILY DOCTOR
By Grant Wood (1892-1942)

Lithograph
1941
Image size: 10 x 12 in.
Sheet size: 12 1/4 x 17 1/2 in.

Signed in pencil below image lower right: "Grant Wood"
Inscribed in pencil below image lower left: "Family Doctor"
Exhibition: Birmingham, Ala., *The Art of Healing: Medicine and Science in American Art,* Birmingham Museum of Art, 1981

Given after 1941 by unknown donor
Accession number: 1941+f.Pr.01

Although Grant Wood made his famous image, *Family Doctor*, seventy-five years after John Rogers's *Charity Patient*, both portray similar sentiments. But Wood's lithograph reduces the elements to the barest essentials, and his physician is even more anonymous and quite abstract.

All one sees of the doctor are his hands and part of his jacket cuffs and necktie. His strong and capable hands hold the most common medical instruments: a thermometer and a stethoscope. A pocket watch lies on the table under his hands. Somehow, one senses the physician's dedication and kindness to his patients without even seeing them.

Perhaps one feels the actual presence of the family doctor because his hands are life-sized and rendered in solid and three-dimensional forms. Also, the tonal quality of the lithograph with its careful description of textures of flesh, rubber, glass, metal, wood, and fabric, and the play of light and shade add to the sense of realism. The title of the print ensures that every observer gets the point.

It is said that Wood used his own physician as a model for the *Family Doctor*. A few years earlier he had made a print called *General Practitioner*, one of a series of illustrations for Sinclair Lewis's *Main Street*, in which the two hands depicted are of a doctor taking the pulse of a patient.[11]

Attached to the back of the lithograph was a printed label from Abbott Laboratories, the Chicago pharmaceutical firm, expressing pleasure in presenting "with

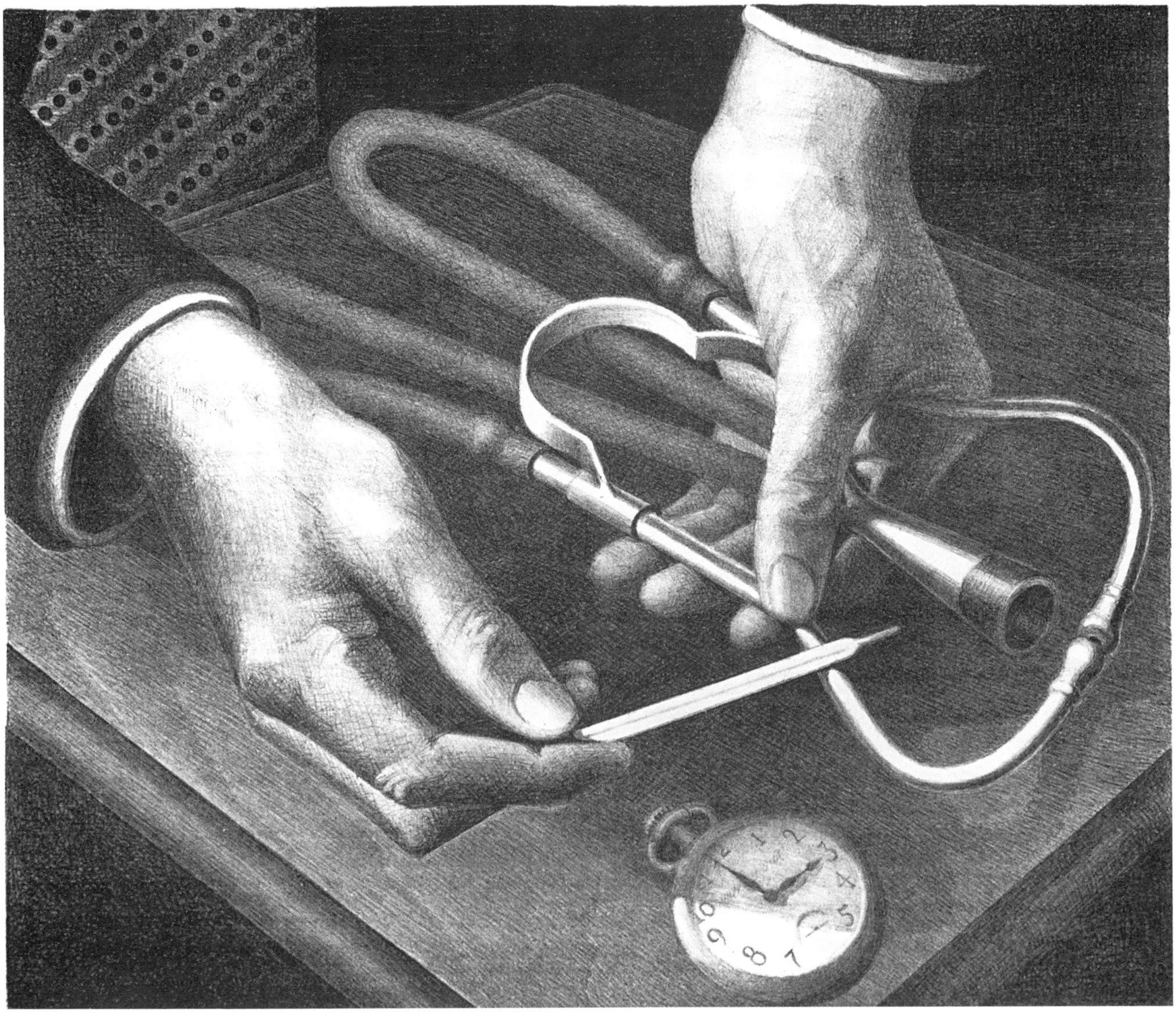

cordial greetings this signed original lithograph by Grant Wood, executed as a tribute to the skill and artistry of members of the medical profession." The unnumbered print must have been issued in large quantities, and probably this example decorated the office of a Jefferson physician who then left it to the college.

Grant Wood was the famed portrayer of midwestern rural American life in the early twentieth century. Among his most famous oil paintings are the brilliantly ironic *American Gothic* (Art Institute of Chicago) and *Daughters of Revolution* (Cincinnati Art Museum), and the fantasy landscape *Stone City* (Joslyn Art Museum, Omaha, Nebraska).

Born in 1892 in Anamosa, Iowa, Wood studied at the Art Institute of Chicago, the Minneapolis Handicraft Guild, and Iowa State University. In the 1920s he took a sabbatical from teaching school in Cedar Rapids, Iowa to study in Paris at the Académie Julian and to experiment briefly with modernist European styles. Upon receiving a commission for a stained glass window for the Veterans Memorial Building in Cedar Rapids in 1927, he traveled to Munich to study glass design. While in Germany he admired and adopted the precise clarity of traditional northern European oil painting. Folk art was another influence on his style.

Grant Wood was the director of WPA projects in Iowa and taught at the University of Iowa from 1934. In 1937 he started making lithographs for commercial patrons, such as the Associated American Artists, to help pay off accumulated debts. Four years later *Family Doctor* was produced in quantity. The famed regionalist artist died in 1942.

The Common Cold

THE COMMON COLD
By Alfred Bendiner (1899-1964)

Lithograph
1942
Image size: 12 1/2 x 14 1/2 in.
Sheet size: ca. 19 3/4 x 21 1/4 in.

Signed in pencil on the image lower right: "Alfr Bendiner"
Inscription in pencil on the image lower left: "The Common Cold"
Exhibition: Philadelphia, *Alfred Bendiner: Lithographs,* Philadelphia Museum of Art, Jan. 21-Mar. 4, 1965

Given in 1983 by Gertrude Haskell, widow of Dr. Benjamin Haskell, JMC Clinical Professor of Surgery (Proctology)[12]
Accession number: 1983+e.Pr.01

It is not known whether Philadelphia artist Alfred Bendiner was aware of Grant Wood's famous *Family Doctor*, but Bendiner's *Common Cold* made the following year depicts a patient who could have tested the patience of any dedicated family practitioner. Unlike the solemn and spare style of Grant Wood, Alfred Bendiner's broad caricature depicts the sickroom clutter of a sulking patient, satirizing a hypochondriac with the most prosaic of ailments, the common cold.

The dozing patient is swaddled in a sweater under his bedcovers and rests his head on plumped-up pillows. His hands are folded on his stomach and his eyes are closed under his glasses. He is surrounded by medicine bottles, tissue boxes, an atomizer, an ice pack, and a bed tray with food. The patient has unsuccessfully tried to divert his own attention with books, newspapers, magazines, radio, telephone, and a backgammon board. His companion is a faithful Dalmatian who rests his head and front paws on the patient's raised knees and looks on inquiringly.

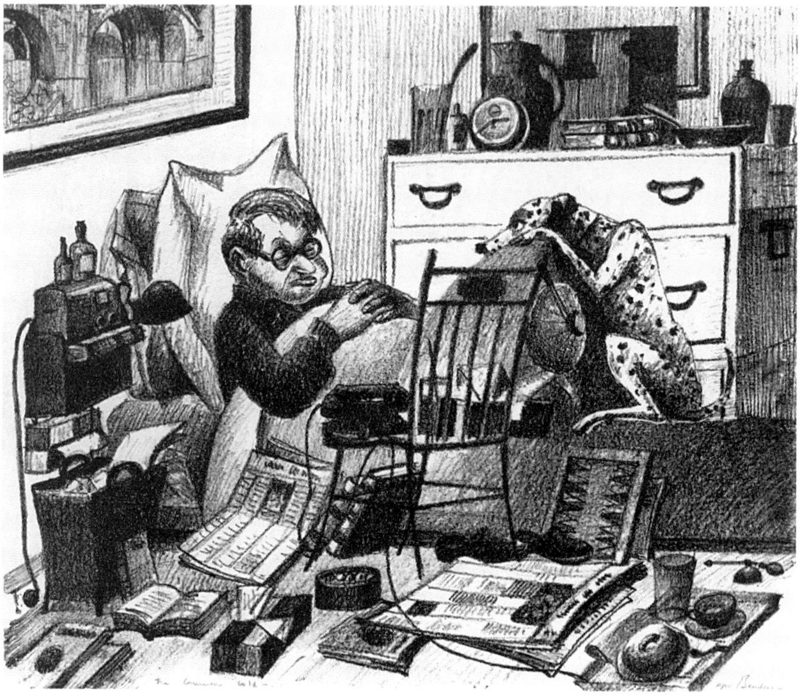

Multitalented Alfred Bendiner was an architect, caricaturist, watercolorist, muralist, printmaker, and writer. He was born in 1899 in Pittsburgh, but his family soon moved to Philadelphia. He graduated from the Pennsylvania Museum School of Industrial Arts and served in the U.S. Army during World War I. He received a bachelor's degree in architecture (1922) and a master's degree in architecture (1927) from the University of Pennsylvania, and also studied at the American Academy in Rome. He worked as a draftsman for the Paul Cret architecture firm in Philadelphia, and served as an artist for University of Pennsylvania archeological expeditions to Iraq in 1937 and to Guatemala in 1960.

Among other professional societies Alfred Bendiner was a fellow of the Royal Society of Arts. His prints are included in museums and universities throughout the United States and in Paris, Florence, Oslo, and elsewhere. He conducted research for the American Philosophical Society and the Jewish Publication Society. He wrote and illustrated articles for numerous newspapers and magazines, and created the illustrated books *Music to My Eyes* (1952), *Bendiner's Philadelphia* (1964), and *Translated from the Hungarian* (1967), the latter a posthumous "autobiography."

One-man shows of Alfred Bendiner's work were held at the American Institute of Architects in Washington, D.C., the New York Architectural League, and Art Associations in Newport, Rhode Island and Concord, Massachusetts; and in Philadelphia at the Pennsylvania Academy of the Fine Arts, the Academy of Music, and the Philadelphia Art Alliance. A traveling show of his art was sent to Portugal, Spain, France, and Italy by the U.S. Information Service.

It is evident that the nineteenth-century works in the Jefferson art collection considered so far are modest in character and scale. In addition to small documentary and portrait photographs and prints, the majority of oil paintings and sculptures are confined to head and shoulders or bust-length depictions, with a few notable exceptions like the portraits of Dr. and Mrs. John Eberle by Jacob Eichholtz. Stylistically and compositionally they are quite conventional, even though many are skillfully, even beautifully rendered. The next two chapters will treat the portraits of Thomas Eakins, a much bolder, more original, and more ambitious artist.

---

1. John H. Brinton, M.D., "The Faculty of 1841," *The College and Clinical Record* (Jefferson Medical College) 1 (Mar. 15, 1880): 33-42. Brinton's address commemorating the Jefferson Medical College alumni association's tenth anniversary was delivered on March 11, 1880.
2. Daniel Leasure, M.D., "A Tribute to the Late Professor Joseph Pancoast," *The College and Clinical Record* 3 (May 15, 1882): 107.
3. Samuel D. Gross, M.D., *Autobiography of Samuel D. Gross, M.D.*, ed. Samuel W. Gross, M.D. and A. Haller Gross, 2 vols. (Philadelphia: George Barrie, 1887), 2:420.
4. R. W. Julian, *Medals of the United States Mint* (El Cajon, Calif.: Token and Medal Society, 1977), 217. One Pancoast medal was presented to the college in 1913 by George McClellan, M.D., grandson of the founder, and two others were presented in 1985 by Elmer H. Funk Jr., M.D. (JMC 1947).
5. E. B. Gardette, M.D., "Memoir of John Barclay Biddle, M.D.," *Transactions and Studies of the College of Physicians of Philadelphia*, ser. 3, 4 (1879): lxxx.
6. "College News and Miscellany: Alumni Association of Jefferson Medical College," *The College and Clinical Record* 7 (May 1, 1886): 104.
7. The Eakins portrait is at the National Portrait Gallery, Washington, D.C., on loan from the National Museum of Health and Medicine of the Armed Forces Institute of Pathology.
8. The donation of the portrait was accompanied by documents, photographs, and written records concerning Dr. Gilbert L. Parker's Civil War military career.
9. Thomas G. Morton, M.D., *The History of the Pennsylvania Hospital 1751-1895* (Philadelphia: Times Printing House, 1895), 328-30.
10. C. Gardiner Johnson also gave other photographs, some manuscript financial records, an oil portrait of Dr. Buchan Richards (unfortunately, irreparably damaged), and the actual saddle bag seen in the photograph.
11. William H. Gerdts, *The Art of Healing: Medicine and Science in American Art* (Birmingham, Ala.: Birmingham Museum of Art, 1981), 101-02.
12. In 1983 Mrs. Benjamin Haskell also presented another Alfred Bendiner print, *Flat Foot Floogie*, as well as other pictures.

CHAPTER 3

Thomas Eakins as a Scientist and His Relationship with Jefferson Medical College

Imposing portraits of three eminent Jefferson Medical College professors are celebrated in a special gallery named in honor of the artist Thomas Eakins. A contemporary visitor to the Eakins Gallery might assume that he was the official portraitist for Jefferson Medical College in the late nineteenth and very early twentieth centuries. Ironically, while he is so esteemed and cherished today, during his lifetime the controversial painter was repeatedly passed over for Jefferson portrait commissions in favor of Samuel B. Waugh, George W. Pettit, and other competent but conventional artists scarcely known today.

However, by his own request Thomas Eakins did depict two members of the faculty, Drs. Benjamin H. Rand and Samuel D. Gross, whose portraits became part of the Jefferson collection. A third portrait in the collection is of Dr. William S. Forbes, commissioned by Jefferson Medical College in 1905 near the end of the careers of both sitter and artist.

Many distinguished art scholars now laud Thomas Eakins as America's greatest portraitist and one of its preeminent artists in any genre. Art historians have researched and placed into their cultural contexts the biographical details and guiding motivations of his life, the depth of his artistic training, and the legacy of his demanding standards and rigorous scientific preparation as an art educator. The influence of European artists and traditions on Eakins, his uncompromising personality, tensions between realism and artifice in his work, and his overt and underlying themes have all been extensively interpreted.[1]

Therefore, this account will explore Thomas Eakins's professional relationships with Jefferson Medical College faculty and present relevant new information about his father's work; and describe the physical history of, and the public and institutional attitudes toward Jefferson's three portraits, especially *The Gross Clinic*.

I will trace Thomas Eakins's lifelong, passionate interest in human anatomy as the basis for his art; describe the medical environment in institutions where he pursued training in and teaching of anatomy, especially the Pennsylvania Academy of the Fine Arts and Jefferson Medical College; discuss his admiration for physicians and other scientists; and summarize his own contributions to the scientific community. As will be seen, portraits of leading intellectuals formed a significant portion of his total output.

In addition, my delineation of a medical institution's perspective of ownership of three important portraits may contribute to Eakins scholarship from a viewpoint not often considered. The documentary record shows that although Jefferson Medical College did not favor Eakins with multiple commissions (nor did any other institution), it revealed pride of ownership and admiration for the artist from the time it first acquired one of his works in 1877, long before he was at all fashionable. Late-nineteenth- and twentieth-century attitudes have been culled from contemporary minutes of Jefferson Medical College meetings of trustees, alumni, and faculty; annual reports and ledgers; catalogues, announcements, and yearbooks of the college; lectures and addresses; medical journals and books; memoranda and correspondence; and period photographs of portraits *in situ*.

Thomas Eakins: Student and Teacher, Expert Anatomist

Thomas Cowperthwait Eakins was born in Philadelphia in 1844 and except for study and travel in Europe in the 1860s passed his whole life in that city. His scenes of sporting and leisure activities and his portraits of men and women of achievement are his testimonial to and celebration of late-nineteenth-century and early-twentieth-century Philadelphia.

His father, Benjamin Eakins (1818-99), was a well known professional calligrapher and writing master widely admired for his superb technique and methodical teaching standards. Mr. Eakins very likely gave the son his first drawing lessons, and always encouraged his desire to become a professional artist with both financial and moral support. The Eakins family lived in comfortable circumstances and was well acquainted with many of the city's best known painters and graphic artists.

An 1861 graduate of Central High School, Thomas Eakins placed in the upper level of his class and received a grade of one hundred in drawing all four years.[2] Among the school's requirements was a considerable amount of science: four years of natural history including zoology, anatomy, and physiology, and three years of chemistry and physics.[3] Four years of classes in drawing and writing included penmanship, outline drawing, drawing from solid objects, mechanical and perspective drawing, and ornamental lettering. Problems in the construction of complex geometric shapes led to the representation of machines and architecture. Advanced figure drawing was taught exclusively from casts of sculpture, not from the live model.[4]

The curriculum was so rigorous that the school awarded the bachelor's degree, and in Eakins's time students could go directly from Central to medical or other professional school. In an assessment of Eakins's high school education, noted Eakins scholar Elizabeth Johns wrote,

> Eakins' intellectual heritage from Central High School—a way of thinking, a faith that this method applied to all pursuits, and a deep respect for intellectual achievement—informed his entire career as a painter...Like the emerging anthropologists, psychologists, and sociologists of his time who investigated man with the objectivity other scientists trained on the rest of the natural world, Eakins applied himself to portraiture to study the intellect and spirit of man.[5]

After graduation from Central High School Eakins applied unsuccessfully for the post of drawing master at the school, and worked briefly helping his father engross documents and teach penmanship. At the same time he enrolled at the Pennsylvania Academy of the Fine Arts where he drew from antique casts, attended lectures on anatomy, and took life classes (drawing or painting from the live model). For formal instruction in painting and sculpture, lessons were arranged on a private basis with established artists.

Artistic anatomy was the only course taught by a regular instructor at the Academy. From 1856 to 1870 this post was filled by Dr. Amos R. Thomas (1826-95), a graduate of both the Syracuse Medical College and Penn Medical College (later Penn Medical University). Thomas was a demonstrator and then professor of anatomy from 1854 to 1862 at the latter school. He also taught artistic anatomy at the Philadelphia School of Design for Women (now Moore College of Art and Design). Sometime during this period Thomas converted to homeopathy and in 1867 was made professor of anatomy at Philadelphia's Hahnemann Medical College and then dean there.[6]

Dr. Thomas's synopsis of his artistic anatomy course at the Academy written a few months before the first session in the autumn of 1856, stated that he planned to deliver twenty lectures to cover the skeletal, muscular, adipose, areolar, and nervous systems, and the anatomy of expression. Materials included cadavers, live models, and skeletons.[7] At least some of his lectures for the art students were delivered at the amphitheater of the Penn Medical University at Ninth and Arch Streets.

Eakins scholar Elizabeth Milroy stated that Dr. Thomas had to discontinue dissection from his curriculum in 1860 for "unspecified reasons." She added, "The study of gross anatomy had long been a recognized adjunct to life drawing and many European as well as American art schools encouraged students to attend medical school courses."[8] Milroy conjectured that Dr. Thomas might have suggested anatomy lectures at Jefferson Medical College to Academy students seeking more in-depth study of anatomy.

One may wonder why Eakins specifically chose Jefferson Medical College to study anatomy. Actually, his choices were few during the Civil War years. Most of Philadelphia's private medical schools and schools of anatomy either closed or foundered during this period. For example, classes were suspended at Penn Medical University after the session of 1862-63 until the session of 1874-75. Even the leading medical schools, Jefferson Medical College and the Medical Department of the University of Pennsylvania, experienced difficult times with the loss of southern students and faculty and with so many professors serving in war hospitals or in the army.

Another Eakins scholar, Ellwood C. Parry III, offered a practical reason for Eakins's choice stating that Jefferson Medical College was "but a short walk" down the street from the Pennsylvania Academy then at Tenth and Chestnut Streets.[9] However, he could also have selected the Medical Department of the University of Pennsylvania. It was not until the mid-1870s that the University of Pennsylvania gradually moved from Ninth between Market and Chestnut Streets to a new site twenty-five blocks west across the river. The Medical Department began sessions in West Philadelphia in 1874, the same year that the new Hospital of the University of Pennsylvania was dedicated.[10]

I think it most likely that Eakins chose to study anatomy at Jefferson Medical College because of the presence of Dr. Joseph Pancoast. The artist would probably have heard about the fifty-nine-year-old professor's reputation as a beloved teacher, prolific author, and inventive surgeon, noted for his stirring and learned addresses and lectures on anatomy.

A striking contrast to Dr. Pancoast in 1864 was the professor of anatomy at the University of Pennsylvania, Dr. Joseph Leidy, then aged forty-one. He had been appointed professor in 1853, and had already contributed to the literature in several natural science fields and would eventually become one of America's greatest naturalists. But unlike most anatomists of his day, he was not a practicing surgeon; and he was not regarded by his students as an accomplished orator, and "in his anatomic teaching...did not display his best gifts."[11]

In addition to the presence of the estimable Dr. Pancoast (and Dr. Benjamin H. Rand, see below) a further incentive for Eakins to attend Jefferson Medical College was his own father's connections to the institution. I have discovered a Jefferson Medical College ledger showing that from 1846 to 1878 Benjamin Eakins was paid for inscribing diplomas with the names of Jefferson graduates for the annual March commencement ceremonies.[12]

Through his decades of service Benjamin Eakins was surely acquainted with several Jefferson deans and faculty members. In a manuscript diary in the Jefferson archives Dean Robley Dunglison, M.D. described activities in his office and made several references to Mr. Eakins, including a typical notation of February 10, 1859: "Directed the Janitor to have the diplomas sent up to the President of the College—Judge King for his signatures. Saw Mr. Eakins, and arranged with him in regard to the filling up of the Diplomas so that there may be as little detention as possible."

Jefferson Medical College Anatomy Admission Ticket

ANATOMY ADMISSION TICKET
(obverse, earlier ticket)
Engraving, ink on card
1864
Card size: 3 1/2 x 5 in.

Inscription: "JEFFERSON MEDICAL COLLEGE/'Optimi Consultores Mortui'/Practical/Anatomy/By Joseph Pancoast, M.D./Admit Mr. T. C. Eaken" *[sic]*

Courtesy Collection Archives, Charles Bregler material. Hirshhorn Museum and Sculpture Garden, Smithsonian Institution. Photograph by Lee Stalsworth

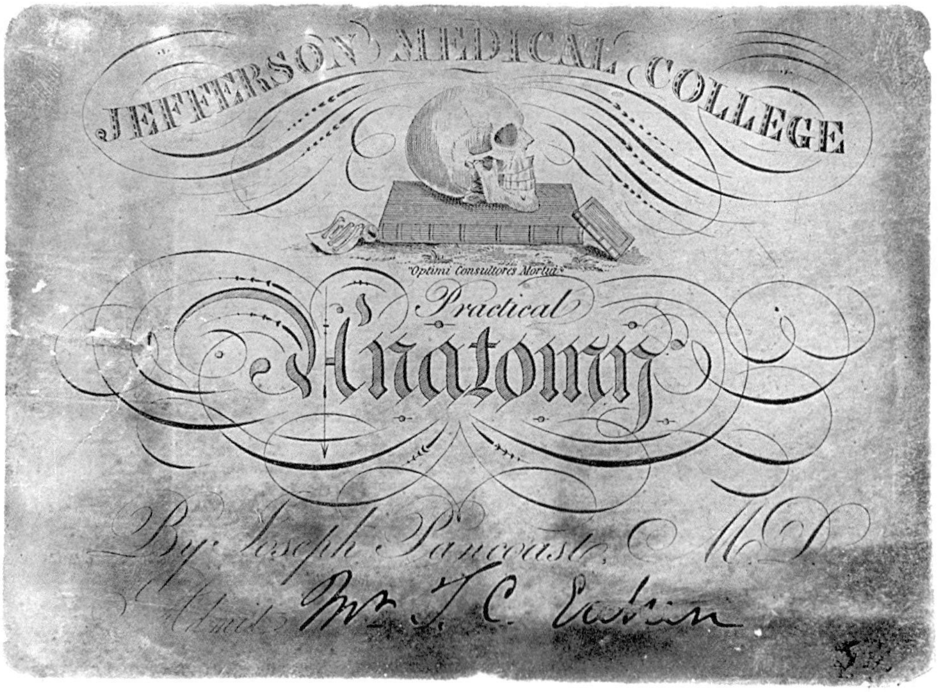

ANATOMY ADMISSION TICKET (reverse, earlier ticket)
Ink on card
1864
Card size: 3 1/2 x 5 in.

Inscription: "Session 1864 & 65-/Wm H. Pancoast M.D./ Demonstrator"

As a nonmatriculating student Thomas Eakins's name does not appear on the official Jefferson Medical College register, but his earlier and later tickets of admission to anatomy courses are preserved in the Charles Bregler material in the collection archives of the Hirshhorn Museum and Sculpture Garden. Like most medical schools at this time Jefferson was a proprietary institution, and student fees were distributed by the dean directly to the professor of anatomy.

The first of the tickets identifies the professor as Dr. Joseph Pancoast and the student as "Mr. T. C. Eaken" [*sic*]. The reverse of the card is clearly dated the session of 1864 and 1865, and Dr. William H. Pancoast is named as the demonstrator. The ticket's authenticity is confirmed by identical tickets in the Jefferson archives issued to medical students for the 1864-65 winter session. These other cards are the same size, same orange color, and inscribed in a handwriting that appears the same as the Hirshhorn ticket issued to Thomas Eakins.

The *Jefferson Medical College Annual Announcement* for 1864-65 stated that the winter anatomy session would commence on October 10 and terminate on the last day of February. The dissecting rooms would open on October 1, under the direction of the professor of anatomy and the demonstrator. Dr. Joseph Pancoast was listed as the professor of general, descriptive, and surgical anatomy, and he held that position from 1841 through the 1873-74 session. His son, Dr. William H. Pancoast, listed as the demonstrator of anatomy, retained that position from the session of 1863-64 until April 1874 when he succeeded his father as the professor of anatomy.

Eakins would have been eligible to attend the anatomical dissections and also the clinics of Dr. Samuel D. Gross, the professor of the institutes and practice of surgery. The *Announcement* describes the "clinical riches" that students including Thomas Eakins could avail themselves of, in addition to the formal lectures:

The General Dispensary of the College, which the students...have the exclusive privilege of attending gratuitously, will be in active operation in September. The College Clinic, connected with this, affords admirable opportunities for the student to learn the practical parts of his profession, and the proper application of the principles which he is taught from the various chairs. The clinic is richly supplied with medical and surgical cases, and throughout the session it forms a prominent, and in the estimation of the Faculty, a most important element of the educational course. The patient is examined, prescribed for, and if a surgical operation is needed, it is performed before the class...The hours of attendance at the clinic of the College are so arranged as to permit the students to attend, every Wednesday and Saturday, the clinics held at the Pennsylvania Hospital and the Philadelphia Hospital.

Dr. Joseph Pancoast's introductory lecture to the anatomy course for the 1849-50 session may suggest what Eakins took in when he attended in 1864-65. Pancoast's philosophical address discussed the "most perfect" construction of the human body in terms of both mechanical practicality and spirituality:

> We prefer to look at the structure of man, directly in reference to its uses. To carry out a course of anatomical instruction on this basis...to display the parts as they actually exist, and particularize carefully their medical and surgical relations, will be my aim...inasmuch as it makes the subject more plain and easy, and is in full accordance with the practical tendency of the times...
>
> You have a machine laid before you, for investigation and management, more perfect in its construction...than anything that has ever entered into the heart of man to wish for, or the mind of man to conceive; a machine, moreover, of God's own construction, and made to serve as the habitation of that divine essence which was breathed into it with the breath of life, and which is held in durance for a while in the material body.

Jefferson Medical College Anatomy Admission Ticket

ANATOMY ADMISSION TICKET (obverse, later ticket)
Engraving, ink on card
Ca. 1874
Card size: 3 5/8 x 5 1/16 in.

Inscription: "'Optimi Consultores Mortui.'/Anatomy/BY/Wm. H Pancoast M.D./For Thos. C. Eakins./1864 & 65"

Courtesy Collection Archives, Charles Bregler material. Hirshhorn Museum and Sculpture Garden, Smithsonian Institution. Photograph by Lee Stalsworth

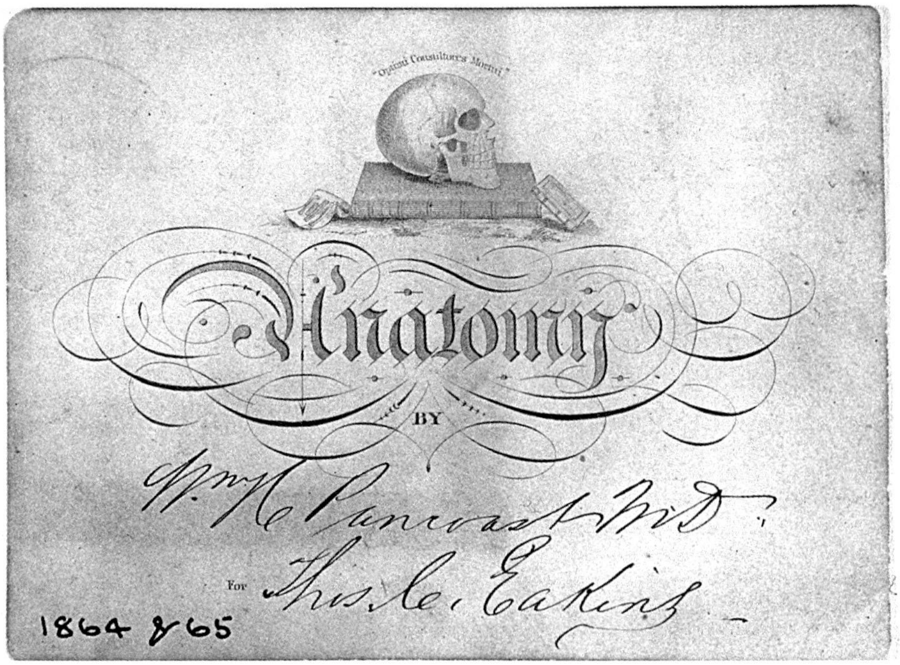

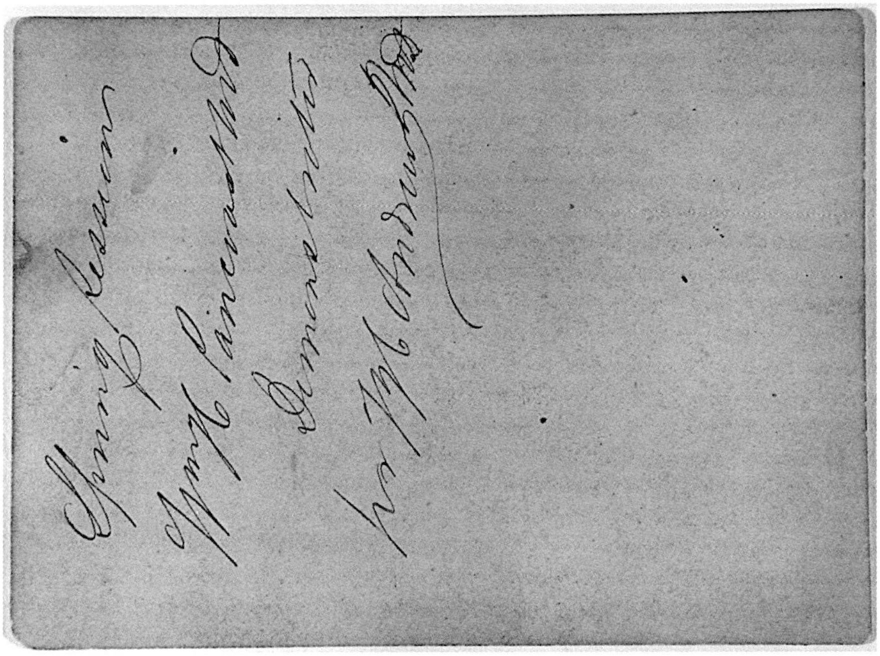

ANATOMY ADMISSION TICKET
(reverse, later ticket)
Ink on card
Ca. 1874
Card size: 3 5/8 x 5 1/16 in.

Inscription: "Spring Session/Wm H Pancoast MD/Demonstrator/per T H Andrews MD"

For lack of documentary evidence about much of Eakins's activities in the early 1870s, several scholars have been understandably confused about the exact date of the artist's enrollment for a second course in anatomy at Jefferson Medical College. Some suggest that he attended in the early 1870s. Of those who state the year 1874 none has heretofore offered evidence. Several have omitted any reference to a second course in the 1870s. Lloyd Goodrich states the dates 1873 and 1874.[13]

A second anatomy ticket of admission also owned by the Hirshhorn Museum identifies the instructor on the front of the card as Dr. William H. Pancoast and the student as "Thos. C. Eakins." The date "1864 & 65" was written in ink decades later by someone not affiliated with Jefferson Medical College.[14] The reverse of the card identifies the course as the "Spring Session," with "Wm H Pancoast MD/Demonstrator/per T H Andrews MD."

The dates 1864 and 1865 cannot be correct because of the physicians mentioned: Drs. William H. Pancoast and Thomas Hollingsworth Andrews were not yet colleagues. Dr. Andrews graduated from Jefferson Medical College in 1864 and was named demonstrator of surgery in 1873.

The session of 1873-74 was a transitional year. In both the college's *Announcement* and *Catalogue* of 1873-74 Dr. William H. Pancoast is listed as demonstrator of anatomy for the regular winter session (October through March), but as lecturer in visceral and surgical anatomy in the supplementary summer course (April through June). In various Jefferson documents the terms "summer" and "spring" are used interchangeably for these supplementary sessions from April through June.

Unfortunately the name of the demonstrator of anatomy for the summer course is not listed, but presumably it was Dr. Andrews. The reason is that in the following winter session of 1874-75 both *Catalogue* and *Announcement* list Dr. Joseph Pancoast as emeritus professor and Dr. William Pancoast as the professor of general, descriptive, and surgical anatomy, with Dr. Thomas H. Andrews as demonstrator of anatomy. Dr. William Pancoast did not lecture in the summer session of 1875; probably Dr. Andrews was given this primary assignment because he was the demonstrator during the regular winter session.

Therefore, the evidence points to the 1874 spring session as the time when Thomas Eakins took a second course at Jefferson Medical College: visceral and surgical anatomy. Professor Samuel D. Gross was the lecturer on clinical surgery in the 1874 spring session, and Dr. John H. Brinton was listed as lecturer on operative surgery.

After attending the Pennsylvania Academy of the Fine Arts and between his two anatomy courses at Jefferson Medical College, Thomas Eakins studied abroad. He embarked for Paris in September 1866, in the hopes of receiving the highest quality art education. His application for admission to the École des Beaux-Arts, the prestigious state-run academy, was finally accepted after a determined campaign on his part.

Eakins was also very pleased to enter the atelier of the celebrated realist painter Jean-Léon Gérôme (1824-1904), a popular teacher at the École whose students drew the figure first from plaster casts and then from the live model. The teacher encouraged his students to take supplementary instruction in human and comparative anatomy, including dissection at the École. It is not known whether Eakins sat for anatomy examinations.[15] It is thought that he took advantage of opportunities to dissect and attend surgical clinics at the Paris hospitals and the École de Médecine.[16]

During Gérôme's absences from Paris Eakins studied clay modeling with the sculptor Augustin Dumont (1801-84) and figure painting with the independent portraitist Léon Bonnat (1833/34-1922). In a letter to his father dated October/November 1867, Eakins wrote, "It has been my good fortune to have spoken personally with some of the greatest men in the world known in Europe and America alike," and significantly, he listed Dr. Joseph Pancoast among them, the only physician mentioned.[17] While abroad Eakins visited numerous museums throughout France, Italy, Germany, Belgium, and Spain. He returned home in July 1870.

During his first few years back in Philadelphia he sent work to Gérôme for criticism, and began to exhibit paintings at the Union League of Philadelphia in 1871, at the American Society of Painters in Water Colors in New York in 1874, and at the Paris Salon in 1875. He had some modest sales during this period. In the 1870s and early 1880s his subjects were portraits and domestic scenes of close family and friends, nostalgic "old-fashioned" themes, and sporting scenes of coaching, hunting, sailing, and rowing.

Eakins's lengthy period of artistic training was followed by two decades of teaching at many different schools. He began his career conducting life classes at the Philadelphia Sketch Club without pay from 1874 to 1876.

By 1876 Eakins became an instructor at the Pennsylvania Academy of the Fine Arts which had suspended classes for six years during construction of its new building at Broad and Cherry Streets. He became an unpaid assistant to the aging professor of painting and drawing, Christian Schussele (1824-79), by teaching his evening life classes. Eakins was also unremunerated for his service as chief demonstrator in Dr. William W. Keen's course of artistic anatomy. In 1877 Schussele was admonished to discontinue delegating his evening duties.

In 1877 a group of disgruntled Academy students who formed the Art Students' Union persuaded Eakins to serve as an unpaid instructor for additional life study classes. The same year a petition from women students at the Academy requested an evening life class with Eakins as the instructor, but he was not yet reinstated. The petition was presented by Susan Macdowell, a leader among the students who would become Eakins's wife in 1884.

A few months later the board rescinded a previous resolution to allow Schussele assistance. By the fall of 1878 the Academy formally named Eakins as assistant professor of painting and the chief demonstrator of artistic anatomy. Upon Schussele's death the following fall, Eakins was promoted to professor of drawing and painting, and for the first time received a salary (six hundred dollars a year, half of Schussele's salary). He now had full charge of the classes on drawing from ancient art works and drawing from live models.

In 1882 he was appointed director of the Academy and drew up a plan to reorganize the school. Though following the Academy's traditional figure-based curriculum (itself based on the French method), Eakins shortened the period of drawing from casts of antique sculptures and encouraged his students to paint from the live model as soon as possible. His more rigorous curriculum was concerned with "pure art education" for all students including amateurs and those entering the commercial arts. It included human and animal anatomy, modeling the human figure in clay, portraiture, photography, and perspective. He strove to encourage the students' independence and visited the classroom only once or twice a week.[18] In Eakins's words, "The course of study is believed to be more thorough than that of any other existing school. Its basis is the nude human figure."[19]

Eakins's arrival at the Pennsylvania Academy of the Fine Arts in 1876 coincided with the appointment of Dr. William W. Keen as the professor of artistic anatomy there. Keen remained in his Academy post through the session of 1889-90. From 1878 to 1882 he was also professor of the anatomy of animal forms as applied to decorative art at the Pennsylvania Museum School of Industrial Art. Keen was to become a distinguished surgeon at Jefferson.

Prior to his post at the Academy Keen had been lecturer in pathological anatomy at Jefferson Medical College from 1866 to 1875 and director of the Philadelphia School of Anatomy during the same period. At the latter school he had lectured each year on descriptive and surgical anatomy and operative surgery, and had given three courses on clinical or surface anatomy and two courses on artistic anatomy.[20]

Keen's first session on artistic anatomy at the Academy consisted of thirty lectures. The introductory lecture emphasized the importance of anatomy to art; this was followed by eight lectures on the skeleton, twelve and one-half on muscles, one each on the nose and ear, one and one-half on the eye, two on the skin and subcutaneous fat and veins, one on hair and postural expression, and two on the influence of sex on the development of the body. In addition to dissection, Dr. Keen utilized skeletons, plaster casts, drawings, and a live model whose muscles were "called into play" with dumbbells, weights, rings, and a galvanic battery, the latter especially for facial muscles.[21]

Keen developed an innovative teaching technique of hanging the cadaver upright by two iron hooks inserted into trephine openings in the sides of the skull, so that cadaver, skeleton, and living model were all in the same vertical position, and "no mental transposition from a cadaver lying horizontal on a table to a skeleton and living model in the vertical position was necessary."[22]

Always fascinated with teaching methods, Keen delivered a paper, "On the Systematic Use of the Living Model in Teaching Anatomy," at the International Medical Congress in London in 1881. Lamenting the absence of a satisfactory textbook on artistic anatomy, he began a manuscript on this subject but found little time to complete the book due to his burgeoning surgical practice.

In his *Memoirs* Keen described the benefits of teaching artistic anatomy:

> These excursions into artistic and decorative anatomy were very delightful by-products...of my anatomical work. They broadened my conception of the uses and value of anatomy and brought me into intimate personal acquaintance with both officers and students in these two institutions. Not a few of my old pupils, especially in the Academy, have become distinguished painters, sculptors, and illustrators.

Keen's annual reports to the Pennsylvania Academy made frequent mention of Thomas Eakins's assistance. In his first annual report of 1876-77 Dr. Keen expressed "very deep obligation" to Eakins and some students for their dissections of the "subjects"; and for Eakins's dissections and casts of the muscles of the dog and cat. Keen also asked authorization for Eakins to have casts made of his dissections of the horse and sheep.[23]

Keen's report for 1877-78 praised Eakins for superintending the dissections, and complimented Eakins and some students for preparing the muscles of the face in the horse, dog, and sheep with illustrative diagrams for the comparative anatomy of expression. He mentioned that they also marked on one side of the human and horse skeletons the exact origin and insertion of each muscle.

For 1878-79 Keen reported that his course had expanded to thirty-seven lectures for "more thorough study" of the bones, muscles, and proportions. In accordance with instructions from the board, Keen appointed Eakins as chief demonstrator and six students as assistant demonstrators. Keen's report praised Eakins's "extremely valuable casts showing not only the surface of dissections but also the cross sections of the muscles," and said that gelatin molds would be made of the casts for easy reproduction and availability to students.

Keen's annual report of 1879-80 mentioned that Eakins had been promoted to professor of painting, and so was replaced as chief demonstrator of artistic anatomy. The number of lectures was reduced to thirty-four but the course was substantially the same.

Keen's last extant annual report of 1880-81 stated that the course was a repetition of former years, except in one respect. Bowing to the suggestion of the committee on instruction, he "omitted the lectures to the male and female life classes on the sexual differences of form. It was feared that it might give rise to unfavorable criticism and I very gladly yielded to the judgment of the Committee." In subsequent years Academy *Circulars* stated that Keen's course consisted of about thirty-five lectures, the last of which was devoted to proportions.

From the beginning of his tenure Keen proposed and implemented the formation of a library of richly illustrated books and periodicals devoted to anatomy. At the same time Eakins was assembling a photographic collection of male and female nudes for use by Academy students. Some photos were of professional models, others of male and female students, and a few even of himself.

Partly because of Eakins's innovations, his teaching career at the Academy was marked by continuous friction with school authorities. He was resentful that his actual salary was less than had been promised. And he was stung that the Academy vehemently seconded criticisms of his curriculum and methods, such as lack of emphasis on composition, aesthetics, art history, decorative arts, or landscape painting.

In a largely complimentary article of 1879 about the Academy's curriculum compared with art schools in New York, literary and art critic William C. Brownell questioned whether the exhaustive study of anatomy could result in the habit of "looking for anatomy and nothing else," whether students would "acquire a habit of looking solely at structure and neglect both character and color and all the other elements of art not less important than structure, which depend so much on intuitive perception and so little on exact knowledge."[24]

In reply to this criticism Eakins said, "We turn out no physicians and surgeons. About the philosophy of aesthetics, to be sure, we do not greatly concern ourselves, but we are considerably concerned about learning how to paint." Eakins acknowledged that dissection is "disagreeable" work, adding, "No one dissects to quicken his eye for, or his delight in beauty. He dissects simply to increase his knowledge of how beautiful objects are put together to the end that he may be able to imitate them."

This latter thought does seem to echo Dr. Joseph Pancoast's ideas on the essence of anatomical structure, and a few Eakins scholars have noted that anatomical study at the Pennsylvania Academy approached or even surpassed that of some contemporary medical schools. However, Dr. Keen agreed with Eakins about not "turning out" physicians or surgeons, and asserted strongly in Brownell's article that the object of his lectures is "not a study of pure anatomy, but of anatomy in relation to form; not to make anatomists but artists."

A more sensational and delicate issue that disturbed the Academy's directors was internal and external criticism about Eakins's lack of propriety in his own behavior and moral judgment. On the one hand Eakins was justly proud of the Academy's facilities for women art students: separate life classes and dissection sessions, and joint attendance with male students for anatomy lectures. On the other hand Eakins's uninhibited attitude toward study of the human body exceeded the tolerance of Victorian society in Philadelphia.

Some of Eakins's male and female students willingly posed for each other in the nude in their homes or in his studio, and allowed themselves to be photographed by him and his assistants. Eakins was criticized for posing male and female models next to each other in the life classes. In his private studio he himself disrobed in order to explain the movement of the pelvis to a promising female student, and is said to have asked female students to pose nude for him.

The board of directors reacted to mounting criticism about his coarse behavior and alleged lack of morality from some female students and their parents as well as criticism about his narrow curriculum from a group of younger rival associates who were former students. They wanted to include more courses in drawing, pictorial composition, and watercolor. In February 1886 the board demanded his resignation when he allegedly defied Academy regulations by removing the loincloth from a male model in front of female students.[25]

Almost immediately following this crushing dismissal and after student petitions demanding his rehiring were ignored, some of Eakins's advanced pupils established a new private school, the Art Students League of Philadelphia, and asked Eakins to develop the curriculum and take charge there. Eakins served devotedly with no pay at the club-like school until it closed in 1893.

Eakins's subsequent teaching was confined to lectures in artistic anatomy, and his persistence in using completely nude models caused predictable confrontations with administrators at other schools as well. He was expelled from the Philadelphia Sketch Club the same year as his dismissal from the Academy. In 1895 he was abruptly dismissed during his first season at Philadelphia's Drexel Institute amid a hail of adverse publicity about sexual improprieties.

However, he lectured on anatomy without incident at several other schools: the Art Students Guild of the Brooklyn Art Association (1881-85), the Art Students League of New York (1885-89), the National Academy of Design (1888-95), the Women's Art School of the Cooper Union, New York (1891-98), and the Art Students' Guild in Washington, D.C. (mid-1890s).[26]

Eakins retained a lifelong devotion to anatomy as the underlying basis for his art. His student and long-term disciple and friend, Charles Bregler, wrote,

> His knowledge of the human and animal anatomy was profound, and equal to that of a surgeon. This was acquired by years of study in the most unpleasant and gruesome way possible namely in the dissecting rooms of a Medical College. He had only contemp *[sic]* for those who try to acquire this knowledge in any other way. I quote his words on this subject,
>
> To learn anatomy out of a book is like learning to paint out of a book. It's a waste of time.[27]

Some Eakins acquaintances and art scholars have speculated about whether Eakins considered becoming a physician. Lloyd Goodrich traces that notion to Cecilia Beaux, a successful turn-of-the-century portrait artist and teacher, who wrote, "He is said to have hesitated in his youth in the choice of a profession. Should he be a surgeon or an artist? He decided on the latter."[28] In 1931 Goodrich asked Susan Macdowell Eakins, the artist's widow, if this were true and she replied, "He was so serious about study that he very likely contemplated both professions." Goodrich could find no confirmation of Beaux's statement elsewhere.[29]

In a trenchant description of her husband Susan Eakins painted him as being "so simple, so unwilling to work for admiration, never a Club man or society man" but one who was "welcomed by men of science. Dr. Gross admitted him in his Clinic. He saw that the young Eakins interest was to learn."[30]

Eakins's scientific legacy was not confined to preparing anatomic materials and teaching artistic anatomy. He also made a thorough study of perspective and lectured on that subject at the Pennsylvania Academy and several other art schools. His unpublished manuscript on linear perspective (notes for formal lectures) is located at the Philadelphia Museum of Art, and several of his preparatory perspectival drawings are still extant.[31]

On at least two other important occasions Eakins was accepted as a peer by Philadelphia's scientific community and treated with great respect. In 1884 Eakins was appointed to a commission that supervised the pioneering "stop-action," serial locomotion studies of humans and animals conducted by the photographer Eadweard Muybridge on the hospital grounds at the University of Pennsylvania. The commission chairman was Edward H. Coates, chairman of the Academy's committee on instruction, and the other seven members were Penn faculty members in medicine, anatomy, engineering, and physics.

Muybridge had first been invited to lecture at several locations in Philadelphia by Fairman Rogers, a former professor of engineering at the University of Pennsylvania and a director there and at the Pennsylvania Academy, as well as a sportsman and photographer. In 1879 Rogers had commissioned Eakins to depict his handsome coach drawn by horses in motion, *The Fairman Rogers Four-in-hand* (Philadelphia Museum of Art).

The Muybridge photos of human figures moving down a track were taken with a battery of twenty-four cameras each of which made exposures from a different viewpoint as well as cameras from the side making diagonal shots. At the same time the commission financed a shed for Eakins to experiment with his own apparatus; he used a single camera of his own design to create multiple exposure images of athletes in motion on one plate, an adaptation from a method developed by a French photographer, Étienne-Jules Marey (1830-1904).

The original Muybridge publication of 1887 was a sumptuously illustrated, eleven-volume, folio edition of the work on animal locomotion. The following year the university published a more modest but scholarly version called *Animal Locomotion: The Muybridge Work at the University of Pennsylvania: The Method and the Result,* with essays about technical processes and analyses written by several professors. The treatise by Dr. William Marks, a professor of engineering, included a description of Eakins's methods and apparatus prepared by the artist.

Because of his expertise in equine anatomy which he had been investigating for almost twenty years, in 1894 Eakins was invited to deliver a lecture to the members of Philadelphia's Academy of Natural Sciences entitled "The Differential Action of Certain Muscles Passing More Than One Joint."[32] In preparation for the published version, he received assistance from physiologist Dr. Harrison Allen, a colleague from the Muybridge Commission.[33] In the article Eakins noted his dissatisfaction with standard accounts of the muscular action in equine locomotion in which the muscles were classified as flexors and extensors, working and resting alternately.

In his years of dissection and photographic observation of the horse, he had discovered that the flexors and extensors were "in strong action at the same time." Although Eakins began his illustrated lecture with the remark, "It is not without diffidence that I, a painter, venture to communicate with a scientific body upon a scientific subject," he ended with confidence describing his own artistic viewpoint,

> On the lines of the mighty and simple strains dominating the movement, and felt intuitively and studied out by him, the master artist groups, with full intention, his muscular forms. No detail contradicts. His men and animals live. Such is the work of three or four modern artists. Such was the work of many an old Greek sculptor.

After his forced resignation from the Academy, in the summer of 1887 Eakins spent ten weeks among cowboys on a ranch in the Dakota Territory to recover from emotional exhaustion. Most Eakins scholars attribute this "rest treatment" to the recommendation by one or both of his friends, Dr. S. Weir Mitchell, an eminent Philadelphia neurologist (and Jefferson graduate of 1850), and Dr. Horatio C. Wood, professor of nervous diseases at the University of Pennsylvania, and part owner of the B-T Ranch. Always an outdoor enthusiast, Eakins partook fully in this immersion in nature. He returned to Philadelphia refreshed and inspired.

After 1886 Eakins concentrated mainly on portraiture but few of these were commissioned works; in most cases he asked the sitters to pose for him. Unlike rival portrait painters Eakins eschewed socially prominent and political subjects, in favor of men and women of scientific, intellectual, artistic, religious, or athletic accomplishment.

Because of his expertise in artistic anatomy of humans and animals, in experimental photography, optical perspective, and other elements of science, and his acquaintance with professional men at Jefferson Medical College and elsewhere, it is not surprising that he depicted so many physicians and other scientists.[34] Today one may regret that Jefferson Medical College never attempted to acquire portraits of its numerous other alumni or faculty painted by Eakins, but a program of collecting works by particular artists was never its mission.

Thomas Eakins's portraits often show the subjects at work or in their working environment. His figures display muscular or psychological energy or tension when concentrating on a task or even when resting but deep in thought. The artist's mastery of the underlying skeletal and muscular structure is so complete that his figures exude an almost palpable sculptural presence in space.

Even though he felt comfortable with his chosen sitters, the resulting portraits were often displeasing to the subjects and their families or institutions. Not only were Eakins's sitters never flattered or idealized, sometimes they were deliberately aged, as comparisons with contemporary photographs attest. Many appear somber, withdrawn, tense, preoccupied, or resigned, sometimes vulnerable, and they rarely make eye contact with the viewer. Young female sitters, especially, were offended because the penetrating delineation of their character often came at the expense of physical grace or conventional ideals of beauty.

Eakins's objective was to probe his sitters' permanent, innate character and spirit by means of posture, gesture, and expression rather than to imitate their outward appearance at a specific moment in time. Their prevailing mood of introspection bespeaks intelligence, creativity, and seriousness of purpose, qualities that modern viewers find appealing. The poet Walt Whitman was unusual for valuing his own portrait, saying that it "fulfills its purpose, sets me down in correct style without feathers, without fuss of any sort. I like the picture always—it never fades or weakens."

Even though many critics, sitters, and the general public considered Eakins personally unconventional and coarse and his painting style too harsh and unyielding, it would be erroneous to assume that his career was totally unsuccessful and that he had no supporters. Although several paintings were rejected by exhibition juries, and those exhibited were usually ignored or criticized, and many paintings were never approved by their intended owners, he still received some significant acceptance by the art establishment.

Many of his works *were* accepted at the most prestigious museum exhibitions and international expositions where he was awarded several prizes. At the Chicago Exposition of 1893 he won a bronze medal for ten paintings including *The Gross Clinic*. In 1900 he won an honorable mention at the Exposition Universelle in Paris. In 1901 he won a gold medal at the Pan-American Exposition in Buffalo. In 1904 he served on the Philadelphia advisory committee for the Louisiana Purchase Exposition in St. Louis where *The Gross Clinic* won a gold medal. The same year he won the Temple Gold Medal at the Pennsylvania Academy of the Fine Arts. In 1905 he won the Thomas R. Proctor Prize at the National Academy of Design. In 1907 he won a gold medal at the American Art Society of Philadelphia.

In 1907 he also won a medal of the second class at the Carnegie Institute where he served on the juries of awards five times for the institute's international exhibitions. In 1902 he had been made a full academician of the National Academy of Design. He actually declined his election in 1908 to the National Institute of Arts and Letters (writing caustically to the treasurer that he could not afford the five dollar membership fee). His only one-man show occurred at Philadelphia's Earle's Galleries in 1896.

Near the end of his life critics began to single him out as a leading American realist painter, and art collector Dr. Albert Barnes of Philadelphia was victorious among rival collectors vying for his portrait of Dr. D. Hayes Agnew. Moreover, from the outset of his career he had a small but fervent band of admirers and defenders among art students, fellow artists, and a few critics, and the constant support of many family members, especially his father and his wife.

Posthumous recognition was almost immediate. The year after his death in 1916 a memorial exhibition was initiated by the Metropolitan Museum of Art in New York and then shown at the Pennsylvania Academy of the Fine Arts. In the next two decades his reputation slowly ascended and museums and collectors began to buy his paintings.

Susan Eakins fervently hoped to establish her husband's reputation in Philadelphia, the city of his birth. In 1930 she and Mary Adeline Williams, family friend and companion, made a magnificent gift of fifty oil paintings and other works remaining in their possession to be installed in a special gallery in the recently built Pennsylvania Museum (later the Philadelphia Museum of Art). That donation and significant later additions of art works and manuscripts, combined with the outstanding portrait and archival collections at Thomas Jefferson University, the Pennsylvania Academy of the Fine Arts, and Saint Charles Borromeo Seminary, have made Philadelphia a center for Eakins scholars and admirers ever since.

Happily, there is no evidence that either Jefferson Medical College or the three Jefferson professors depicted by Eakins were dissatisfied with their depictions. Quite the contrary. The portraits of Drs. Benjamin H. Rand, Samuel D. Gross, and William S. Forbes were installed at important locations at the medical school soon after their completion and have always been esteemed by the institution.

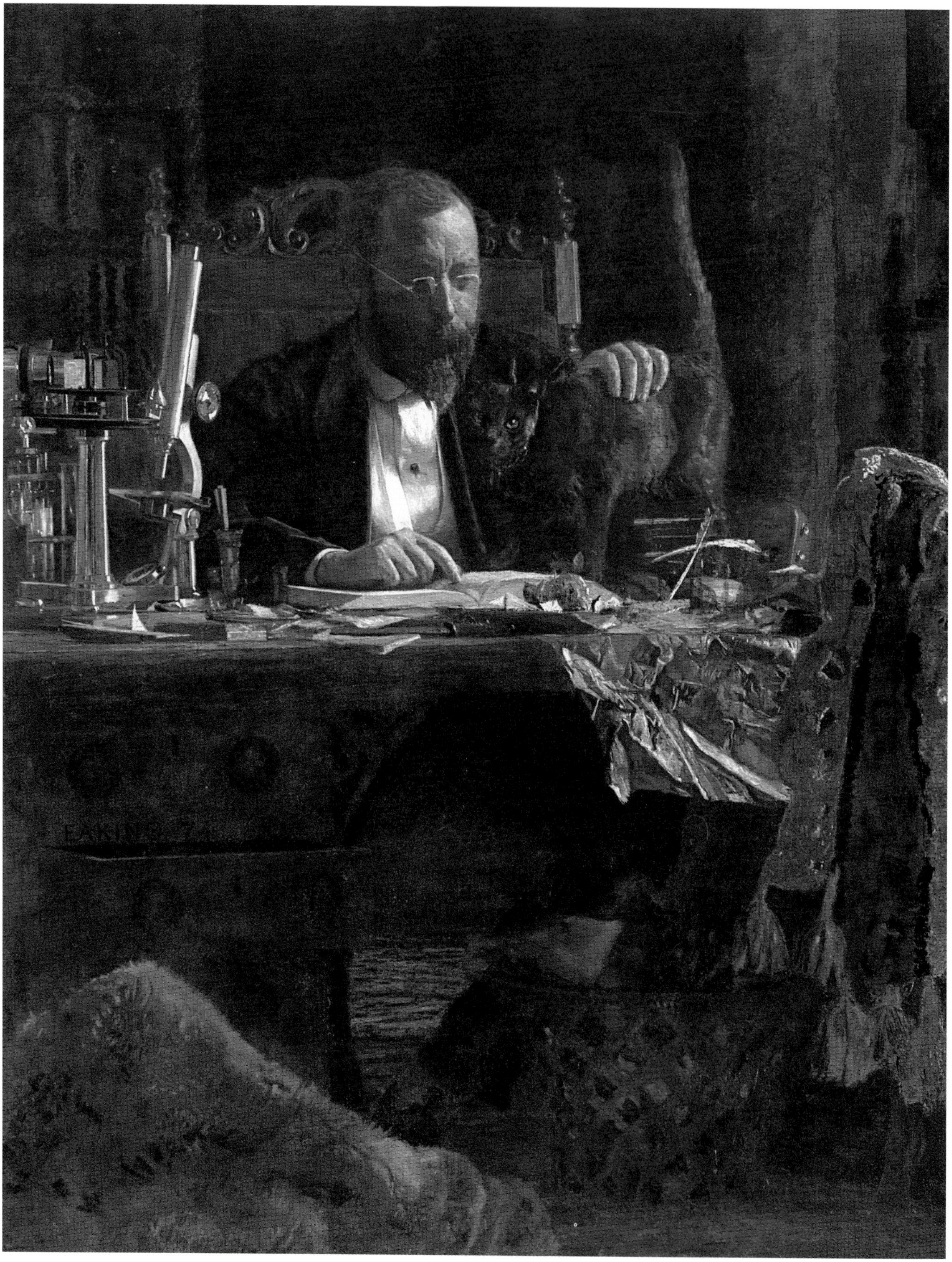

Portrait of Benjamin H. Rand[35]

(See color plate)

BENJAMIN HOWARD RAND, M.D. (1827-83)
By Thomas Eakins (1844-1916)

Oil on canvas
1874
60 x 48 in.

Signed and dated center left: "Eakins 74"

Exhibitions: Philadelphia, Centennial International Exposition, May 10-Nov. 10, 1876; Philadelphia, *Centennial Celebration: Loan Collection of Portraits*, College of Physicians of Philadelphia, 1887; New York, *Loan Exhibition of the Works of Thomas Eakins*, Metropolitan Museum of Art, Nov. 5-Dec. 3, 1917; Philadelphia, *Memorial Exhibition of the Works of the Late Thomas Eakins*, Pennsylvania Academy of the Fine Arts, Dec. 23, 1917-Jan. 13, 1918; Philadelphia, *Thomas Eakins 1844-1916*, Pennsylvania Museum of Art, Mar. 5-Apr. 16, 1930; Philadelphia, *150th Anniversary Exhibition*, Pennsylvania Academy of the Fine Arts, Jan. 15-Mar. 13, 1955; Toronto, *American Painting 1865-1905*, Art Gallery of Toronto (Jan. 6-Feb. 5, 1961), Winnipeg Art Gallery Association (Feb. 17-Mar. 12, 1961), Vancouver Art Gallery (Mar. 29-Apr. 23, 1961), and Whitney Museum of American Art (May 17-June 18, 1961); Philadelphia, *The Art of Philadelphia Medicine*, Philadelphia Museum of Art, Sept. 15-Dec. 7, 1965; New York, *The American Vision: Paintings 1825-1875*, Public Education Association at M. Knoedler & Co., Oct. 8-Nov. 2, 1968[36]; Philadelphia, summer loan, Philadelphia Museum of Art, June 15-Aug. 30, 1969; New York, *Thomas Eakins Retrospective Exhibition*, Whitney Museum of American Art, Sept. 22-Nov. 21, 1970; Birmingham, Ala., *The Art of Healing: Medicine and Science in American Art*, Birmingham Museum of Art, 1981; Collegeville, Pennsylvania, *Inaugural Exhibit: A Selection of American Art*, Fetterolf House at Ursinus College, Sept. 26-Oct. 5, 1986; London, *Thomas Eakins (1844-1916) and the Heart of American Life*, National Portrait Gallery, Oct. 8, 1993-Jan. 23, 1994

Given in 1877 by the subject
Accession number: 1877+e.P.01

Benjamin Howard Rand, M.D. was the artist's first sitter outside his circle of family and close friends, and first in a long series of portraits of physicians and scientists. As in the two other large-scale, full-length portraits of Jefferson professors, Dr. Rand is shown at work with attributes that identify his professional specialty and allude to his intellectual prowess.

Subject and artist had been acquainted since Eakins's student days at Philadelphia's Central High School where Rand was the chair of chemistry from 1859 to 1864 and of which he also was an alumnus. Rand held similar posts at the Franklin Institute (1850-64), the Medical Department of Pennsylvania College (1859-61), and the Philadelphia College of Medicine (1854-58).

Benjamin Howard Rand was born in 1827 in Philadelphia. He began his medical studies in 1843 with Dr. Robert M. Huston, and graduated from Jefferson Medical College in 1848 after serving as clinical assistant to Drs. Thomas Mütter and Joseph Pancoast. Rand succeeded Dr. Franklin Bache as professor of chemistry at Jefferson Medical College in 1864.

Board of trustees minutes show that Dr. Rand was in competition with several distinguished chemists for the post, and finally reached a majority vote on the tenth ballot. He was evidently deemed very effective because he was appointed dean of the medical school just five years later. He served as dean until 1873 and held the chemistry chair until his resignation in 1877.

Rand contributed numerous articles to scientific journals and also edited Samuel L. Metcalf's third edition of *Caloric: Its Agencies on the Phenomena of Nature* (1859). Original textbooks written by Rand include *An Outline of Medical Chemistry for the Use of Students* (1855) and *Elements of Medical Chemistry* (1867). Dr. Rand was a member of the American Medical Association and the American Philosophical Society, a fellow of the College of Physicians of Philadelphia, and an active member and secretary (1852-64) of the Academy of Natural Sciences.

Jefferson medical students valued Rand's emphasis on applied rather than theoretical chemistry in the practice of medicine, and found his lectures practical and instructive. This pragmatic approach, not unlike Eakins's teaching "how to paint" rather than "the philosophy of aesthetics," is evident in his textbooks in which the sections on chemistry of the elements and organic chemistry highlight their medical effects. Rand's teaching also stressed the professional and social responsibilities students should assume when they become physicians. In a commencement address of 1866, he cautioned the new graduates who were in the "flush of youth, full of hope and ambition, eager to plunge into the battle of life" to abide by the following duties:

> 1. To yourselves—Avoid sloth and procrastination. At first you will not be overwhelmed with patients or with fees; still you may spend your hours, not in card-playing, dissipation, or worse still, politics, but in the

> study of the more exact portions of your profession, which the necessarily condensed character of your teaching heretofore has touched but lightly...
>
> 2. To the sick—You owe all the skill, gentleness, assiduity, and patience of which you are possessed. If a patient suffer by your neglect, or ignorance, or rudeness, or petulance, you are criminal...
>
> 3. To your professional brethren—The Code of Ethics adopted by our profession is sadly misunderstood by the public...It draws the line between a profession and a trade, and he who is not willing to be guided by its precepts has no place in our ranks; he had better seek some more easy and profitable, though less honorable vocation...
>
> 4. To the public—You are enjoined by the same Code 'to be ever vigilant for the welfare of the community,' to give freely all information likely to promote public health, and the ends of justice; in time of pestilence to face the danger and to continue your labours for the alleviation of the suffering even at the hazard of your own lives.[37]

Rand's untimely retirement in 1877 at age fifty-one was caused by an unfortunate accident and he died six years later. Bouts of pneumonia interfered with his teaching after he had accidentally inhaled arseniuretted hydrogen (a colorless, extremely poisonous gas) during a medicolegal investigation.[38] Thereafter he remained almost housebound until his death at which time the executive committee of Jefferson's alumni association noted that the organization had "sustained a loss of one of its sincere friends and most active and faithful members." An obituary noted that Dean Rand had been "kind and obliging to the students, always sympathizing with their troubles, and ready to listen and to advise."

As noted, Professor Rand began his career at Jefferson Medical College in 1864 when Thomas Eakins first studied anatomy there, and it is possible that the chemist influenced his choice of medical school. The young painter asked Rand to sit for his portrait in 1874 when he was enrolled for a second anatomy course at Jefferson. Several scholars have conjectured about Eakins's choice of the estimable Professor Benjamin H. Rand as his first public portrait subject.

Ellwood C. Parry III pointed out that in 1874 Eakins would have been aware that Jefferson's alumni association was beginning its tradition of commissioning portraits.[39] Starting in the early 1870s, Jefferson had begun to commission and collect paintings of illustrious professors at the urging of Dr. Samuel D. Gross. William H. Gerdts developed this line of thought, noting Eakins's admiration for Rand and that "he wanted to create a notable portrait that would advertise his talents" and secure other commissions.[40]

Elizabeth Johns has contributed information in two other areas. One was a more personal connection between Eakins and Rand in their mutual interest and participation in the popular sport of rowing. Eakins and many of his friends at Central High School had taken up rowing, and Benjamin H. Rand was for a time president of Philadelphia's Undine Barge Club where Eakins was likely a member.[41] Johns also suggested a second connection: that Dr. Rand might have asked Eakins to arrange for the purchase of a French fossil collection for Philadelphia's Academy of Natural Sciences while he was studying art in Paris.[42]

I have investigated another personal connection between artist and sitter: the profession of their fathers. Both were well known writing masters in Philadelphia. Benjamin Eakins (1818-99) engrossed diplomas for local schools and colleges and inscribed other documents such as deeds and marriage certificates. He taught writing at several local private schools, including Friends' Central School for fifty-one years, from 1845 to 1896.[43] An influence on his son can be seen in the handsome lettering, the numerous figures who are writing, and the plethora of writing materials in many Eakins paintings, including those at Jefferson.[44]

Benjamin Howard Rand the elder (1792-1862), also a professional calligrapher, taught penmanship for more than twenty-five years, and published several popular books on the subject.[45] It is not known whether the two writing masters knew each other personally, but it is almost certain that their sons knew of their fathers' common profession.

A contemporary Jefferson Medical College ledger shows that both writing masters were employed to "fill in" student diplomas. Benjamin Rand did this briefly from 1843 to 1845. Benjamin Eakins succeeded him the following year and remained until 1878.[46] Considering the family connections with Jefferson Medical College and especially Thomas Eakins's familiarity with Dr. Benjamin H. Rand, it is not surprising that he chose the chemistry professor for his first public portrait. Aged thirty and optimistic about his future as a portrait painter in 1874, Eakins was confident enough to portray the distinguished physician boldly, unconventionally, and with kindly humor.

The professor is shown working at a desk in his home study. Presumably he posed in Eakins's studio, for he is seated in an upholstered Jacobean Revival armchair with an elaborately carved cresting rail. This chair was purchased for the Eakins household and appears in about a dozen portraits.[47]

Rand is positioned in the middle ground, seated frontally on the far side of an expansive partner's desk which bisects the composition horizontally. A more traditional composition would have placed the scholar in front of or next to his desk in the foreground, and he would be partially turned to make eye contact with the viewer.

As painted by Eakins, he reticent, sober-faced scholar is so absorbed in private thoughts that he ignores the viewer and gazes downward. The mood of absolute concentration is expressed solely by his knitted brows. His mouth is hidden by his full beard and his eyes are obscured by the narrow, rectangular lenses of his wire-rimmed spectacles. For comparison see the contemporary photograph where he looks serious but more relaxed. The *carte-de-visite* was donated by a student who had attended Rand's chemistry lectures in 1875 and 1876.

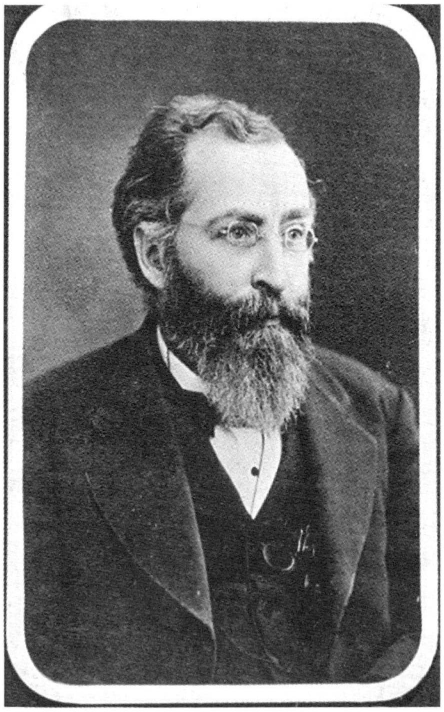

Portrait of Benjamin H. Rand

BENJAMIN HOWARD RAND, M.D.
By unknown photographer

Photograph
Ca. 1876
3 7/8 x 2 1/2 in.

Given after 1940 by family of Thomas M. Throckmorton, M.D. (JMC 1877)
Accession number: 1940+f.Ph.04

In Eakins's portrayal Dr. Rand uses his finger to keep his place in a passage in an open book. His left hand rests awkwardly on the arched back of a gray cat which insouciantly rests a front paw at almost the same place, interrupting Dr. Rand's reading. The fall of the cat's foot contrasts with Rand's careful gesture. At first glance it is difficult to detect this congenial house pet because of the dark coloration. Eventually its upright tail, proprietary stance, bright red collar, and direct outward stare engage one's attention. Its sinuousness and luxuriant fur are a counterpoint to the cerebral pursuits of the professor.

The chemist's self-effacing posture and locale prompt most viewers to scrutinize the desktop first. Its surface is crowded with a gleaming array of objects, ranging from the scientific and academic to the personal and domestic. Brightly highlighted brass instruments on the left include a compound microscope and a spectroscope. Behind is a wooden rack with test tubes, and to the right of this group, a red, graduated, pharmaceutical cylinder with a spatula. A letter opener (or knife) parallels the edge of the desk over the kneehole, and reading materials and quills are strewn about left and center.

On the far right is a bright pink rose, and a sheet of crinkled, cool-white tissue paper that hangs over the edge of the desk. Blurred forms behind appear to be a perpetual calendar and some fruit. In the right foreground is a brilliant pink, tasseled afghan or shawl draped over the back of a chair. Below the desk is a red-figured oriental rug and wicker trash basket, and on the left a fur rug in a pyramidal heap, and an open desk drawer.

The murky interior space is very shallow and largely undescribed architecturally, except for a bookcase in the left rear and curtains on the right. The prevailing dark neutral tones are punctuated by daylight entering the room on a raking angle from the right, highlighting Rand's face and spectacles, his shirt front, and the desktop objects. This spotlighting effect, coupled with the dominant brown tones of the furnishings, produces a warm glow that suffuses the painting.

Bright red accents, therefore, come as a surprise, and are scattered so as to encourage the viewer's eye to circle the whole painting. Red or bright pink are found on the graduated cylinder, the cat's collar, the flower, the afghan, and the oriental carpet. There is a touch of green, the complementary color, in the curtains.

The physician's attire and some nearby objects suggest nonacademic, social pursuits. He has removed his necktie, and his highlighted white shirt is wrinkled. Do the white vest and the flower suggest a recent return from some special evening occasion, and do the shawl and the flower suggest the unseen presence of a woman? Eakins does not overtly provide the answers. In 1869 Rand had married Mary M. Washington, great-granddaughter of Fairfax Washington. The physician had been a widower for fifteen years following the death of his first wife, Hannah M. Kershaw, after only one year of marriage.[48]

In this initial major portrait by Eakins there are two rather disconcerting elements. First, the sitter is upstaged by his own attributes. The magnificently painted still life cluttering his desk on the left draws

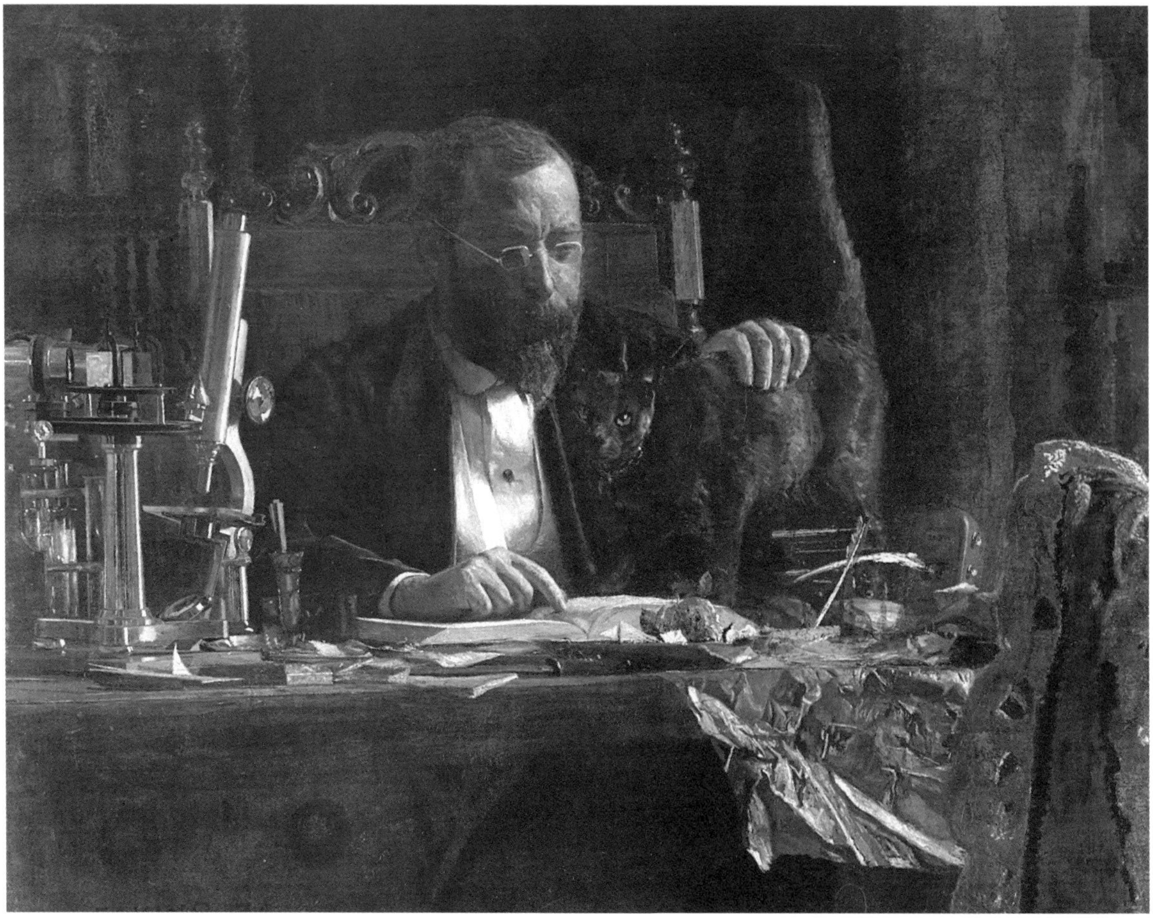

Detail: Dr. Rand, the Cat, and Desktop

attention away from Professor Rand, the nominal subject. Many of the objects on the right side of the desk are included gratuitously with no visible means of explanation. The shawl and fur rug in the foreground are overly prominent distractions. Possibly the effect of the subject's secondary position behind the desk and the arrangement of sensuous objects before him was both an intended comment on Rand's self-effacing personality, and also a manifestation of the young artist's desire to create a showpiece demonstrating his ability to render an impressive variety of textures and shapes.

Nevertheless one is disconcerted by the unconvincing rendering of the portion of Professor Rand's body seen under the desk. His legs and feet are barely discernible and do not seem aligned properly with his upper body.

The portrait of Dr. Rand was exhibited at the Centennial's international art exhibition, along with two other oils, *Elizabeth at the Piano* and *The Chess Players*, and two watercolors. While expressing general disappointment with the American paintings, one local critic

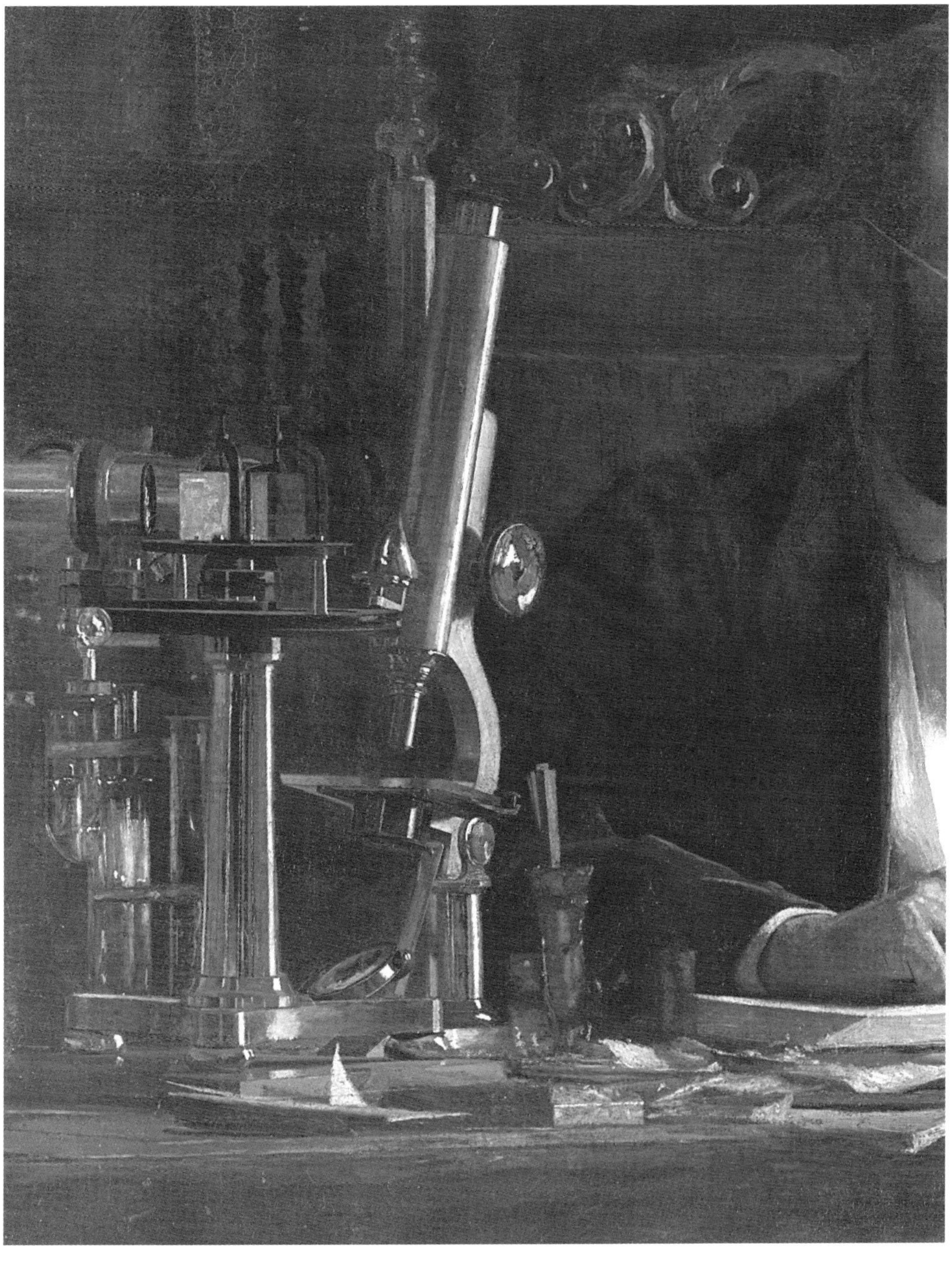

Detail: Left Side of the Desk

praised Eakins's oils particularly and called the depiction of Rand "a portrait which is made a picture by the many accessories introduced and which is one of the best contributions to the section."[49]

A second review was written by Eakins's friend William Clark, head of the Philadelphia Sketch Club and a newspaper critic as well as a former student at the Pennsylvania Academy of the Fine Arts. One of the few discerning contemporary critics who appreciated Eakins's work, Clark gave a balanced evaluation of the strengths and weaknesses of the Rand portrait:

> Dr. Rand who is shown seated behind his library table—upon which are scattered a number of articles such as a microscope, books, papers, etc.—with one hand petting a Maltese cat, and with a finger of the other following the lines on a page in the book before him. The composition in this last-named picture is rather too elaborate for a portrait, and the eye is confused by the multitude of objects that are introduced. The picture is carefully and consistently worked out, however, and although it lacks the simplicity that is desirable in a portrait, it is an admirable example of genuinely artistic workmanship...Unfortunately, both of these pictures [the Rand and Elizabeth portraits] are in too low a key for their best qualities to be easily discerned in the badly-lighted galleries in which they are hung. It can be seen at a glance, however, that the artist has attempted something more than the mere making of recognizable likeness, and has aimed to make his portraits pictures in every sense of the word.[50]

Professor Rand expressed pride that his portrait was included in the Centennial's art exhibition and showed a sense of urgency in donating the work to Jefferson Medical College. Minutes of an April 27, 1877 board of directors meeting included the professor's letter of resignation dated April 14, 1877, and a second letter dated one week later offering his portrait to the college. He wrote, "I am not able to leave the house else should have called upon you before this, to state that my portrait by Eakins lately on exhibition at Memorial Hall, is at the disposal of the Board of Trustees."

In response Jefferson's board of trustees immediately resolved "that the portrait tendered by Dr. Rand be received with thanks." The minutes of the May 1 meeting mentioned another communication from Rand stating that "as soon as it was decided where his portrait was to be hung he would send it." The matter was referred to the president of the board who decided on the location.

An 1881 board of trustees report on donations mentioned that the portrait had been hanging in the reception room of the Jefferson Medical College Hospital. Librarian Charles Frankenberger reported in 1915 that the Rand portrait was hanging in the west lecture room of the 1898 College Building, in the same room with *The Gross Clinic*.[51] Before the Rand portrait was moved to the Eakins Gallery in Jefferson Alumni Hall in 1982, it was installed for more than five decades in the stairwell leading to the second floor landing of the 1929 College Building, in the vicinity of portraits of some of Jefferson's most prominent professors, deans, and trustees; *The Gross Clinic* was the focal point of Jeffersonians ascending to the second floor landing. Each of these subsequent locations was a conspicuous, public area where the Eakins portraits would have been highly visible to all passersby.

Professor Rand was a popular figure who would probably have been pleased to know that successive generations of Thomas Jefferson University students, professors, and staff have admired Eakins's insightful portrayal of him. These viewers respond affectionately to the wry humor of the cat and the controlled clutter of disparate objects on the desk. They identify with the preoccupied and reticent professor as a familiar type, hard at work even in the privacy of his home. Thomas Eakins lost an enthusiastic supporter early in his painting career when Dr. Benjamin H. Rand became incapacitated and died.

In certain ways Eakins's portrait of Dr. Rand prefigures his portrait of Dr. Samuel D. Gross: its large scale, innovative composition, restricted neutral palette accented by one bright color, and dramatic highlights and contrasts of light and dark. When Eakins first undertook the group portrait known as *The Gross Clinic*, few would have prophesied that it would eventually become his most acclaimed masterpiece, as will be discussed in the following chapter.

To understand the magnitude of Eakins's accomplishment it is important to place the work and the artist's canny choice of Dr. Gross as portrait subject in the context of the professor's teaching and clinical career and his contributions to American surgery; and to compare the work with Jefferson's other, official portraits of this acclaimed professor and his family.

The Life and Career of Samuel D. Gross, M.D.

Dr. Samuel D. Gross, sometimes referred to as the "Emperor" or "Nestor" of American surgery, was born in 1805 into modest circumstances on a farm near Easton, Pennsylvania. His family spoke the Pennsylvania German dialect common in that area, and Gross did not learn "correct" German or even English until he was an adolescent. In his *Autobiography* Gross said he was a "natural-born" doctor whose desire to enter the field of medicine "seized" him before the age of six.[52]

As was customary in Gross's era, he began the study of medicine as a private pupil in the office of a practicing physician. After trying three different preceptors, he realized that his prior education at the local one-room school had been inadequate to the task. To obtain a more classical education he studied first at the Wilkes Barre Academy in Pennsylvania and then at the Lawrenceville High School in New Jersey, concentrating on Latin, Greek, mathematics, geography, and English grammar. Two years later he reentered the office of one of his original preceptors, Dr. Joseph K. Swift of Easton, before entering medical school.

Although Dr. Swift provided Gross with letters of recommendation to faculty members at his alma mater, the University of Pennsylvania, instead the young student sought out Dr. George McClellan who accepted him as a private pupil for two years. In 1828 Gross received his medical degree with the third class to graduate from Jefferson Medical College.

After struggling to make a living as a surgeon in Philadelphia, in 1830 he returned to Easton where he was more successful. During those lean years he filled any spare time by translating foreign medical texts into English, and by anatomic dissection and animal experimentation, even transporting a cadaver by buggy all the way from Philadelphia by himself. His first treatise, *The Anatomy, Physiology, and Diseases of the Bones and Joints*, was published in 1830.

His first academic appointments were at the Medical College of Ohio at Cincinnati as demonstrator of anatomy (1833-35) and at the Medical Department of Cincinnati College as chair of pathological anatomy (1835-39), remaining at the latter school until it closed. While in Cincinnati he published his first important text, *Elements of Pathological Anatomy* (1839), a pioneering, systematic work that went through three editions.

In 1840 Dr. Gross accepted the professorship of surgery at the Louisville Medical Institute (later the University of Louisville). His next sixteen years (except for one year at the University of the City of New York) were spent very productively in Louisville. There he published on such diverse subjects as: wounds of the intestines; diseases and injuries of the urinary bladder, prostate gland, and urethra; operations for malignant diseases; foreign bodies in the air passages; lithotomy; ovariotomy; aneurysm; and gunshot wounds.

Although Dr. Samuel D. Gross held the University of Pennsylvania in the highest esteem, he declined their offer to be a candidate for chair of surgery, and instead accepted the professorship at Jefferson Medical College in 1856 at the age of fifty-one, succeeding Dr. Thomas Mütter. During his twenty-six-year tenure as professor of the institutes and practice of surgery, Gross was revered as an operator and teacher, internationally celebrated as an author, and widely respected as a founder and member of local, national, and international medical societies.

Dr. Gross made many contributions to surgical technique and instrumentation, although few are still associated with his name because of modification or obsolescence. He was the first to treat ganglia of the hand or foot by subcutaneous division of the cyst; to use adhesive plaster for skin traction in treating fractures of the lower extremities; to perform high amputation in senile gangrene; to suture divided nerves and tendons; to operate directly for hernia by suturing the pillars of the external ring; to do laparotomy for rupture of the bladder; and to wire the ends of the bones in dislocations of the sternoclavicular and acromioclavicular joints.

He invented an instrument for extraction of foreign bodies from the air passages; a special catheter for draining urine mixed with blood; forceps for arterial compression to arrest hemorrhage from deep-seated vessels; and a tourniquet for arterial compression of vessels of the extremities during amputations.

Considering his prodigious surgical and teaching responsibilities, Gross's contribution to the medical literature is astounding. He appropriated early morning hours before breakfast and late evenings for study and writing whenever possible, and even composed in his carriage on the way to visit patients.[53] The first edition of his most famous work, *System of Surgery*, appeared in 1859. This text eventually went through six editions, the last in 1882, and was translated into several foreign languages, spreading his fame throughout the world. He wrote *A Manual of Military Surgery* at the beginning of the Civil War in

1861 at the government's request.

In 1861 he also edited a biographical work, *Lives of Eminent American Physicians and Surgeons of the Nineteenth Century*. For the U.S. Centennial he wrote the history of American surgery for "A Century of American Medicine, 1776-1876," published in the *American Journal of Medical Sciences*. In addition to textbooks, Gross's literary contributions included almost one thousand published medical articles, case histories, addresses, biographies, and introductory lectures.

Although he has been the subject of numerous biographies and memoirs from his own day to the present, the most enduring description of his life and career is his autobiography, edited by his sons, Dr. Samuel Weissell Gross and Albert Haller Gross, and published in 1887, three years after his death. He wrote the "sketch" of his life for the gratification of his children and grandchildren, and for members of his profession for the sake of "stimulating the ambition of whose who may come after me to work for the advancement of science and the amelioration of human suffering." He hoped that his devotion to medical science may "exert a salutary influence upon the conduct of young physicians, and thus to inspire them with a desire to excel in good deeds."[54]

Gross also exerted a profound influence in the establishment and leadership of professional societies ranging from the local to the international.[55] On the local level, Dr. Gross was a founder and president of the Kentucky State Medical Society, the Jefferson Medical College alumni association, the Philadelphia Pathological Society, and the Philadelphia Academy of Surgery; and was president of the Pennsylvania State Medical Society.

On the national scene he was president of the American Medical Association, the American Philosophical Society, and the American Academy of Sciences; and a founder and president of the American Surgical Association. Internationally, Gross was president of the World Medical Congress in 1876; and a member of the Imperial Medical Society of Vienna, the Medical Society of Christiana of Norway, the Royal Medical and Chirurgical Society of London, the Medical Society of Vienna, the Medical Society of London, the Medico-chirurgical Society of Edinburgh, the British Medical Association, and the Royal Society of Medicine of Belgium.

Aside from the public display of his portraits, honors accorded Gross's memory in Philadelphia include the Samuel D. Gross Room and Endowed Library at the College of Physicians of Philadelphia, and the Gross Prize of the Philadelphia Academy of Surgery. At Jefferson Medical College, the Gross Professorship of Surgery was endowed in 1910 by the professor's daughter, Maria Gross Horwitz. Jefferson's Department of Surgery created the Samuel D. Gross Distinguished Service Award in 1979 and dedicated the Gross Conference Room in 1982.

Gross's honorary degrees from American and European universities include the LL.D. from Jefferson College, Canonsburg, Pennsylvania (1861); the D.C.L. from Oxford University (1872); and LL.D. degrees from Cambridge University (1880), Edinburgh University (1884), and the University of Pennsylvania (1884).

In 1882 at age seventy-seven Gross resigned from the chair of surgery and was named emeritus professor. He died of congestive heart failure in 1884 and his desire to be cremated was honored, his ashes being placed in the family grave at Woodlands Cemetery in Philadelphia.

Gross had declared that when he died he could wish no better epitaph than "A teacher of Principles." He felt that medicine and surgery are so closely allied as to be indivisible, writing, "The principles of surgery are the principles of medicine, or, in other words, the principles of the art of healing."[56]

Accordingly, the opening seven weeks of his lecture course on surgery were devoted to a discussion of principles including inflammation and its consequences, syphilis, struma, tumors, and wounds. The rest of the course was devoted to diseases and injuries of particular regions and tissues. He confined himself to "matters of fact," not to "hypothesis, conjecture, or speculation."

Dr. Gross took the long view in his approach to educating medical students, impressing them with both advances and discarded ideas in the history of medicine, and giving credit to those professional forbears who deserved it. In "Then and Now," an introductory address in 1867 of which new medical students specially requested printed copies, Gross ranged over the entire body of medical and surgical knowledge of that day compared with what had been known four decades earlier when Jefferson Medical College was founded.[57] He singled out anatomy and histology for having almost entirely "attained [the] highest degree of perfection," and for their important effect upon the knowledge of physiology and pathology.

In his discussion of surgical procedures and instrumentation, he considered at some length the recent publicity on the subperiosteal resection of entire bones, or of portions of their shafts and even of joints, "the operation being founded upon the well-known agency exerted by the periosteum in the regeneration of osseous tissue." He said that he had "in all the numerous operations that I have performed during the last thirty years for the removal of dead bone [the procedure shown in *The Gross Clinic*] scrupulously respected this envelope," and presumed that "there is not an enlightened surgeon anywhere who has not pursued a similar plan of treatment."

Gross's exhortations about seriousness of purpose and personal conduct were also directed toward newly minted physicians at the 1868 commencement ceremonies: "I am no oracle, but if I were consulted as to the means by which a young physician, emulous of distinction, could obtain the greatest and most honorable fame, my response would be, 'By steady, unswerving devotion to his profession, by boundless industry, and by a profound love for his species.'"

He told the students how a physician's presence can dispel a patient's "gloomy cares and unpleasant forebodings":

> The sorrows of the sick-room are often materially lightened by the agreeable manners of the medical attendant...A genial smile, a kind word, a gentle pressure of the hand, a timely anecdote, are often much more effective remedies than quinine and opium, nay even than milk-punch and beef-essence, so fashionable at the present day in the treatment of disease and injury.
>
> You need not be told that, while you are expected to be men of science, and refined, cultivated, high-toned gentlemen, you are also to be earnest working physicians, watching and caring for the sick...The interests of your patients will be paramount to every other duty; nothing must be left to chance; nothing must be regarded as too trivial or insignificant when life is trembling in the balance.[58]

Images of Dr. Samuel D. Gross and His Family

There are more original images of Dr. Samuel D. Gross in the Thomas Jefferson University art collection than of any other professor since Dr. George McClellan: four paintings, two sculptures, one drawing, five prints, and eleven vintage photographs, in addition to diverse memorabilia. Not surprisingly, there are interconnections among the works since several were created posthumously and relied on earlier sources. The university is also gratified to possess portraits of the professor's beloved wife, Louisa Weissell Gross, and their son, Samuel W. Gross, M.D.

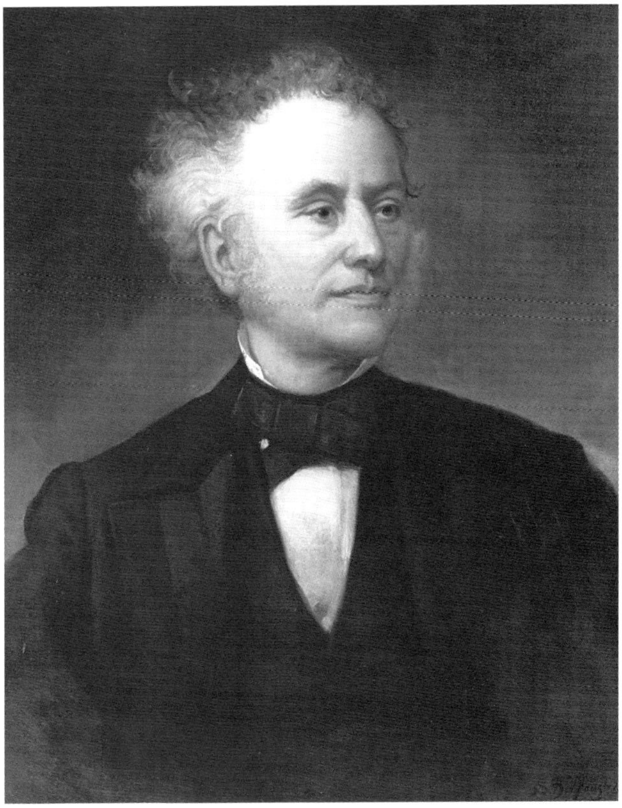

Portrait of Samuel D. Gross

SAMUEL DAVID GROSS, M.D. (1805-84)
By Samuel Bell Waugh (1814-85)

Oil on canvas, mounted on wood
1874
30 x 25 in.

Signed and dated lower right: "S. B. Waugh 1874"

Given in 1875 by JMC alumni association
Exhibition: Philadelphia, *Centennial Celebration Loan Collection of Portraits*, College of Physicians of Philadelphia, 1887
Accession number: 1875+e.P.01

The first image of Dr. Samuel D. Gross owned by Jefferson Medical College is an oil portrait by Samuel B. Waugh. This painting and a sculpture of Gross by Alexander S. Calder are among the few early portraits in the Jefferson collection for which details of the commission process are extant.

Minutes of the alumni association's executive committee meeting of April 16, 1874 noted that Dr. Thomas H. Andrews moved that a committee "wait upon Prof. Gross and request him to sit for his picture, the same to be paid for by subscription."

In addition to Dr. Andrews members of the original Committee on Professor Gross's Picture included Drs. Ralph M. Townsend (JMC 1866), Richard J. Dunglison (JMC 1856), and Lemuel J. Deal (JMC 1865). Dr. James M. Barton (JMC 1868) was added the following October in place of Dr. Deal. Their primary task was to solicit subscriptions, and by the meeting of March 8, 1875 they announced that the picture "had been some time completed and paid for." Dr. William B. Atkinson (JMC 1853) was selected to present the portrait to the trustees at the March 11 commencement.

Reporting on the commencement, the *Philadelphia Evening Bulletin* noted succinctly that the portrait was "well executed and handsomely framed." Further, Dr. Gross was omnipresent at this ceremony: he not only awarded a prize for the "best report of his surgical clinic," but also delivered a stirring valedictory address. Documents state that the painting was hung in a place of honor in the amphitheater of the hospital when the building opened in 1877. Archival photographs show that later it was moved with other portraits to the library of the 1898 College Building.

Like Waugh's other commissioned portraits of Jefferson professors, this is a conventional depiction in its size, format, likeness, and paint style. Dr. Gross is shown bust length and seated frontally with his head turned slightly to the right, located in an atmospheric, neutral background. The smoothly painted surface accentuates the professor's distinctive features, even overemphasizing the windswept appearance of his naturally wavy, thick hair. His bland facial expression is not particularly revealing of any inner thoughts or character traits.

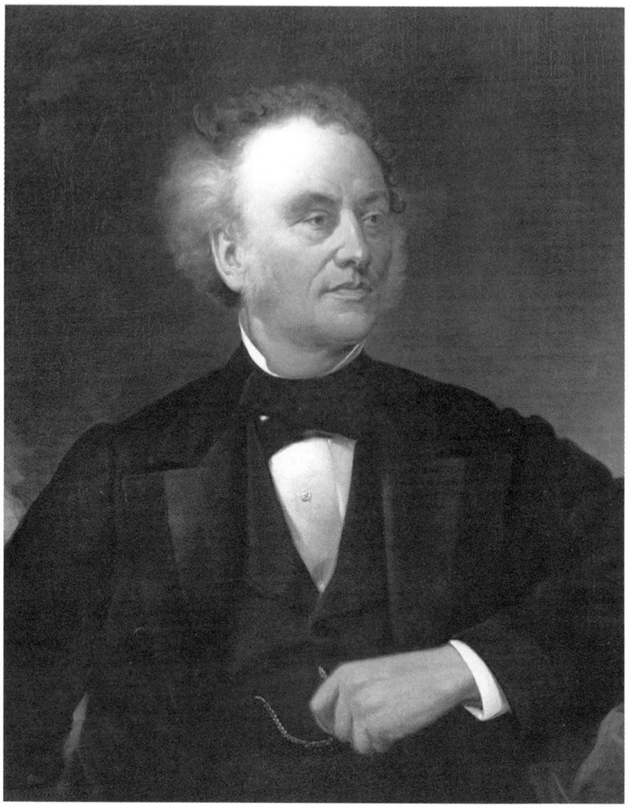

Portrait of Samuel D. Gross

SAMUEL DAVID GROSS, M.D.
Attributed to T. Dimino

Oil on canvas
Ca. 1909
36 x 29 in.

Given in 1987 by Susan Bullitt Ward, M.D. (JMC 1985), great-great-great-granddaughter of the subject
Accession number: 1987+e.P.02

This unsigned painting is an augmented copy after Samuel B. Waugh's 1874 portrait of Dr. Gross. It is almost identical to another copy of Waugh's portrait of Gross in the collection of the College of Physicians of Philadelphia.[59] This latter work is signed and dated "T. Dimino/Roma, 1909" and was presented to the College of Physicians in 1909 by Dr. Gross's children, Maria Gross Horwitz and Albert Haller Gross. Albert Gross wrote that he had two portraits of his father, that "neither does him justice," and that he would take "very great pleasure" in having a third painted for the College of Physicians.

In both oil copies Dimino changed the format from

bust length to half length, adding a more complete view of the arms and hands. Here Professor Gross's left arm leans on a table covered with red cloth, and he fingers the gold chain of his watch fob, an addition that symbolizes material attainment. Compared with Waugh's original portrait, the physician's features are somewhat flattened and the activity of the hair is more restrained.

The painting at Jefferson descended in the Gross family and was presented to the university in 1987 by Susan Bullitt Ward, M.D. (JMC 1985), the professor's great-great-great-granddaughter. She also generously donated to the Jefferson archives a family scrapbook (compiled by his daughter) containing correspondence and news clippings mainly related to Professor Gross's final illness and funeral. About her illustrious forbear, Dr. Ward said in a *Philadelphia Inquirer* article of June 7, 1985, "It wasn't until after I had been here for quite some time that I realized how big a figure he was. I've never made a big thing out of it, but I *do* feel pride." She is presently a clinical assistant professor of medicine in the division of rheumatology at Thomas Jefferson University.

Portrait of Samuel D. Gross

SAMUEL DAVID GROSS, M.D.
By Frederick Gutekunst (1831-1917)

Photograph
Ca. 1870-80
Image size: 5 5/8 x 4 1/8 in.
Card size: 6 1/2 x 4 1/4 in.

Stamped below image: "F. Gutekunst, Philadelphia"

Given after 1884 by unknown donor
Accession number: 1884+f.Ph.03

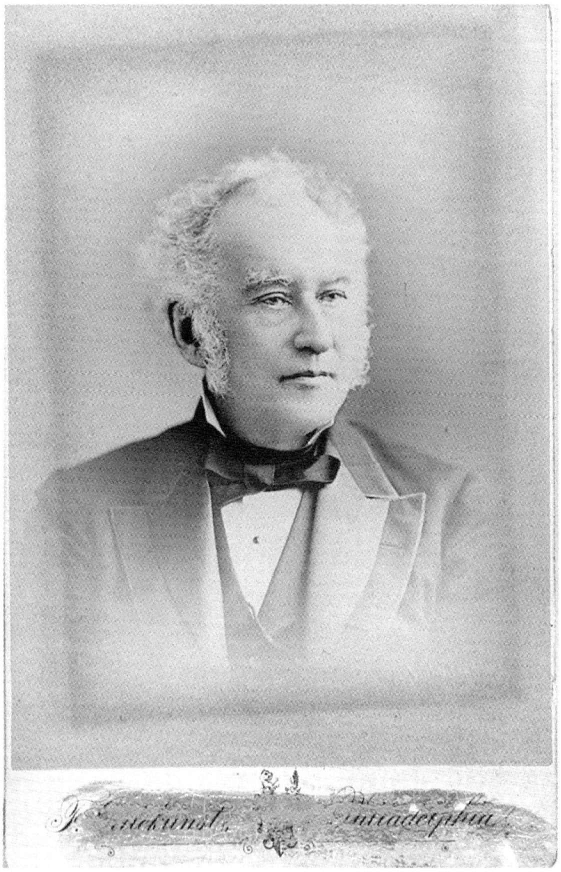

This undated cabinet-sized photo is roughly contemporaneous with Samuel B. Waugh's portrait of Dr. Gross. The pose is almost identical in photo and painting. The arrangement of the necktie, the upturned shirt collar, the suit lapels and waistcoat, and the watch chain are the same. The photo existed in many copies; this and similar ones in the Jefferson archives could have served as an aid for the Waugh portrait and for prints that followed.

Differences between the Waugh painting and the photo lie in the artist's interpretation. In the photo the professor's face is longer, his eyes more almond shaped, his mouth thinner and wider, and his wiry hair more constrained than in the painting. His shoulders are squarer and his neck thicker than in Waugh's interpretation.

Portrait of Samuel D. Gross

SAMUEL DAVID GROSS, M.D.
By Samuel Sartain (1830-1906)

Engraving, mezzotint, etching
Before 1887
Image size: 4 x 3 1/2 in.
Sheet size: 13 x 10 1/2 in.

Inscription below image: "Engraved by Samuel Sartain, Phil[a]"; followed by facsimile signature "S. D. Gross"

Given before 1887 by unknown donor
Accession number: 1887+b.Pr.01

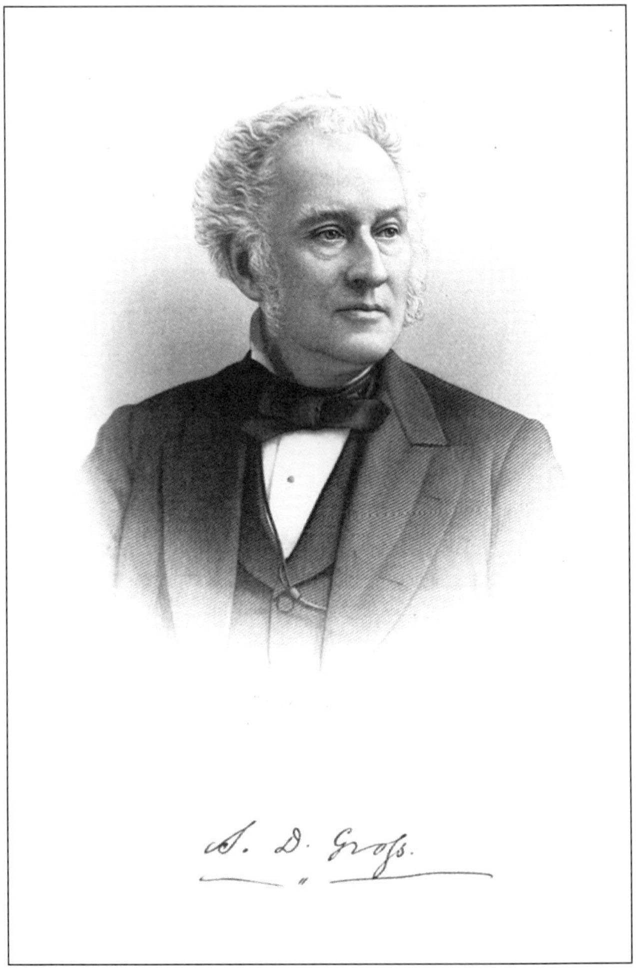

This undated print of Dr. Samuel D. Gross by Samuel Sartain relates to the oil portraits and photograph above in pose and costume. The print bears an ever closer resemblance to an unsigned steel engraving of Dr. Gross which forms the frontispiece to volume one of his autobiography. (The frontispiece to volume two is an etching after *The Gross Clinic.*) Significantly, this image was chosen by Dr. Gross's sons who edited the autobiography, while they pointedly ignored the oil painting by Samuel B. Waugh which had been displayed at Jefferson Medical College since 1875.

Samuel Sartain was a member of a distinguished Philadelphia family of engravers: the son of John Sartain and the brother of William, Emily, and Henry Sartain, all printmakers. Samuel Sartain was born in Philadelphia in 1830 and studied engraving with his father. Then he studied at the Pennsylvania Academy of the Fine Arts where he exhibited paintings and engravings between 1848 and 1866. In 1851 he founded his own firm in Philadelphia and produced engravings and mezzotints for local publishers. Later in life he served as manager and treasurer of the Franklin Institute.

Portrait of Samuel D. Gross

SAMUEL DAVID GROSS, M.D.
By Ludwig E. Faber (1855-1913)

Etching
1898
Image size: 11 3/4 x 8 in.
Plate size: 13 3/4 x 10 1/4 in.
Sheet size: 18 x 14 in.

Inscription upper left: "Published by Isaiah Price D.D.L. March 1898"; inscription lower left: "Etched by L.E. Faber"; followed by facsimile signature "S. D. Gross"
Signed in pencil below image, lower right: "L. E. Faber"

Given after 1913 by unknown donor
Accession number: 1913+f.Pr.01a

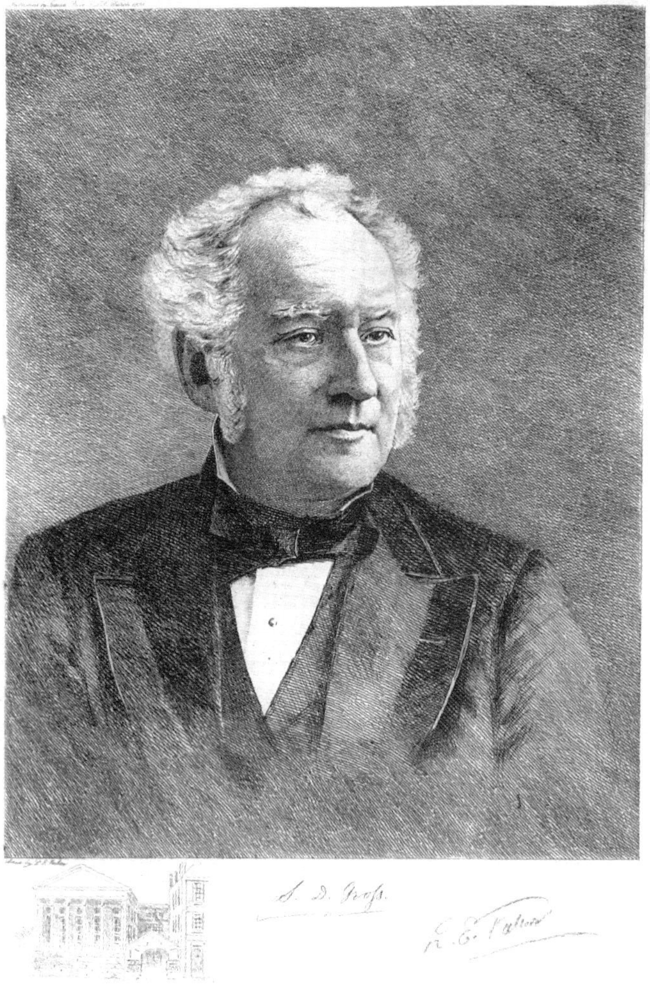

This delicately rendered etching of Dr. Samuel D. Gross by Ludwig E. Faber is another in the family of images derived in part from the Gutekunst photo discussed above, or a similar one. The features, hair style, costume, posture, and expression closely resemble the photographic source.

The artist shows a mastery of anatomic structure in depicting the face with strength and vigor. Like the Gutekunst photograph and the Sartain print, the light source for Faber's large print is from the right, dramatically spotlighting the forehead and side of the sitter's face. The feathered area at the bottom of the print mimics the faded area at the bottom of the photograph. Compared with the Sartain print, Faber's depiction is much freer and lighter in weight.

The posthumous, etched portrait was made in 1898, but was symbolically anachronistic in one respect. The remarque (vignette in the margin below) shows the Ely Building with the renovations by Napoleon LeBrun and the new Laboratory Building by Frank Furness, as they appeared only between 1879 and 1881. Since Dr. Gross served on the Jefferson faculty from 1856 to 1882, it would have been more appropriate to depict an earlier version of the Ely building or to a lesser extent the 1877 Jefferson Hospital, to suggest a locale of longer duration for the surgeon's triumphs.

Like Samuel Sartain, Ludwig E. Faber was a Philadelphia native and the son and brother of artists. Born in 1855, Faber was trained at the Pennsylvania Academy of the Fine Arts before going abroad. He studied in Paris at the Académie Julian with Benjamin Constant (1845-1902), Jules Lefebvre (1836-1912), and Tony Robert-Fleury (1837-1911), and then at the Munich Academy.

A painter and etcher, Ludwig Faber collaborated with his father, Hermann, and his brother, Erwin, to illustrate George A. Piersol's *Human Anatomy* (1907) on which they labored twelve years. The brothers also illustrated Gwilym G. Davis's *Applied Anatomy* (1910).

Ludwig Faber was a member of the Philadelphia Sketch Club, the Philadelphia Society of Etchers, the American Art Association of Paris, and the Pennsylvania Society of Miniature Painters.

Collage of Photograph of Samuel D. Gross and Surgery Admission Cards

SAMUEL DAVID GROSS, M.D.
By Lothrop (active late nineteenth century)

Vintage photograph
Ca. 1875-77
3 3/4 x 2 3/8 in.
Surgery admission cards: 3 3/8 x 4 7/8 in.
Photograph and cards mounted on paper: 14 3/4 x 6 7/8 in.

Inscriptions on cards: "Jefferson Medical College/OF/PHILADELPHIA/Lectures/ON/SURGERY./BY Samuel D. Gross M.D./Admit/T.M. Throckmorton 1875-6"; and "Jefferson Medical College/OF/PHILADELPHIA/Lectures/ON/SURGERY./BY Samuel D. Gross M.D./Admit Thos. M. Throckmorton 1876-7/Iowa"

Given after 1940 by unknown donor
Accession number: 1940+f.Ph.03

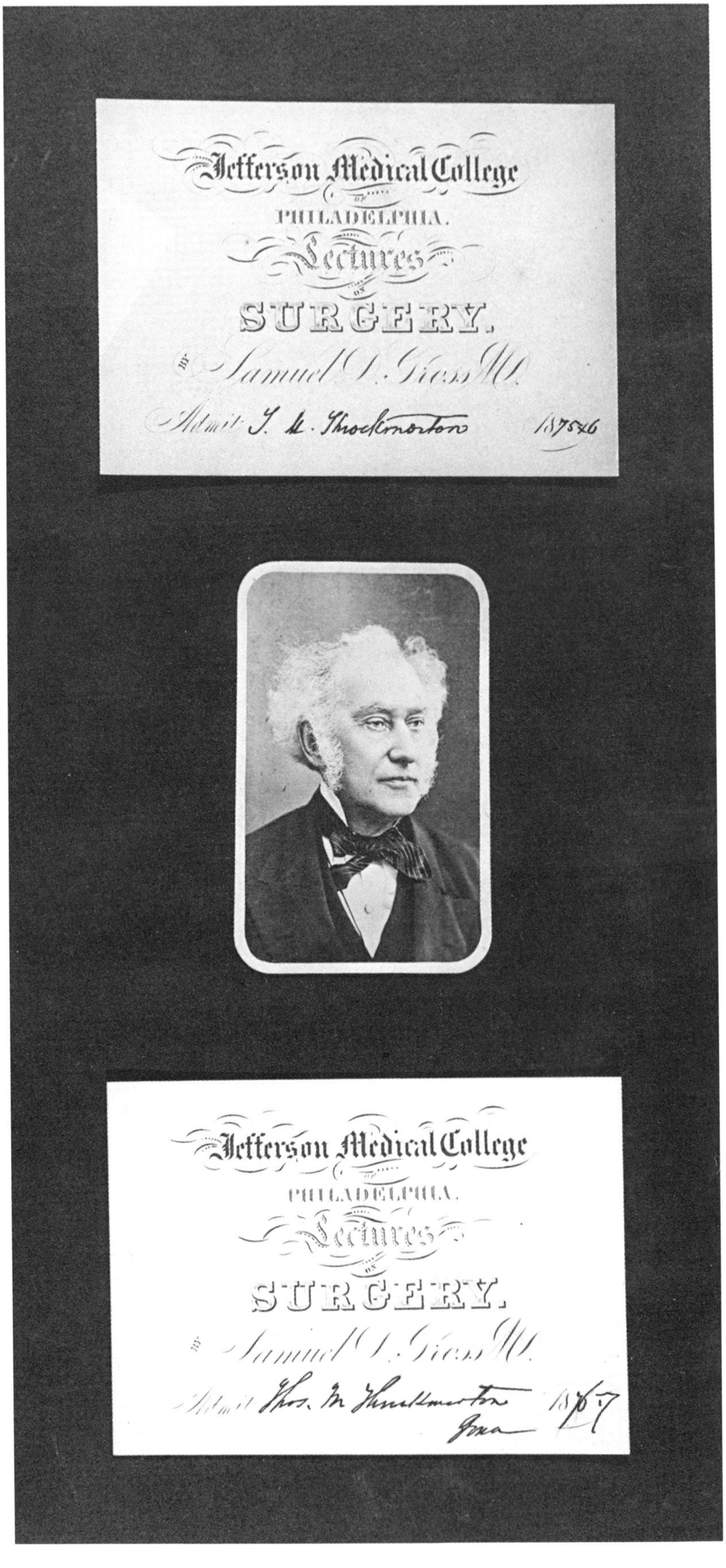

Dr. Thomas M. Throckmorton was a member of the Jefferson Medical College class of 1877, and almost certainly a relative of the donor of the Reverend Ely's portrait (who very likely also donated this collage). One imagines that the Iowa student was inspired to arrange a collage of his surgery admission cards with a contemporary photograph of Dr. Samuel D. Gross to keep alive memories of his experiences from 1875 to 1877. This photograph records Dr. Gross's appearance around the time of Samuel B. Waugh's portrait and of Thomas Eakins's *Gross Clinic*.

The Jefferson archives include a larger version of this photograph of Dr. Samuel D. Gross stamped with the name "Lothrop," a Philadelphia photographer. The larger photograph is less faded, so the surgeon's features are outlined with greater clarity. A notable variation in costume from the other images seen so far is Gross's jaunty striped bowtie, knotted asymmetrically.

Portrait of Samuel D. Gross

SAMUEL DAVID GROSS, M.D.
By Hubert F. Praeger, M.D.

Charcoal on paper
1877
20 x 16 in.

Signed and dated lower right: "H.F. Praeger/1877."

Given after 1877 by unknown donor
Accession number: 1877+f.D.01

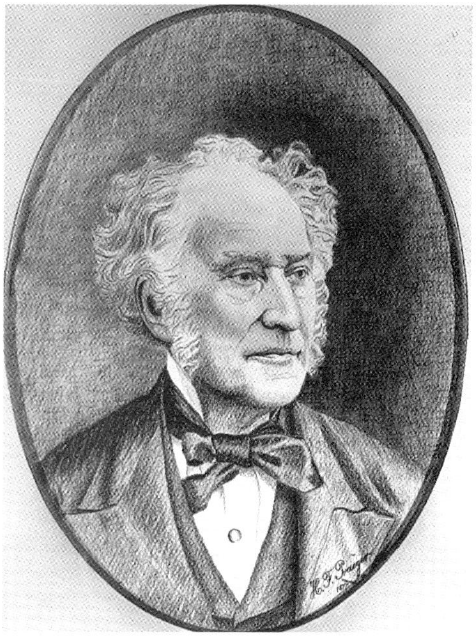

This charming and animated, if untutored, charcoal drawing of Dr. Samuel D. Gross by Hubert F. Praeger seems to be a faithful enlargement of the Lothrop photograph. The only change is that the sitter's bow tie is solid black instead of striped.

The refreshingly direct but amateurish quality steered me to the medical anthologies rather than to the art directories to learn more about the artist. The drawing is the only nineteenth-century example in the Jefferson art collection of a medical student being inspired to render such a private, artistic tribute to an honored professor. The only information retrieved so far about Dr. Praeger is that he graduated from Jefferson Medical College in 1878, and that he came originally from Sweden.

Portrait of Samuel D. Gross

SAMUEL DAVID GROSS, M.D.
By J. Obermeier (active second half nineteenth century)

Plaster
1870-80
32 1/2 x 19 5/8 x 12 7/8 in.

Signed left center of rear: "J. OBERMEIER"

Given before 1929 by unknown donor
Accession number: 1929+b.S.01

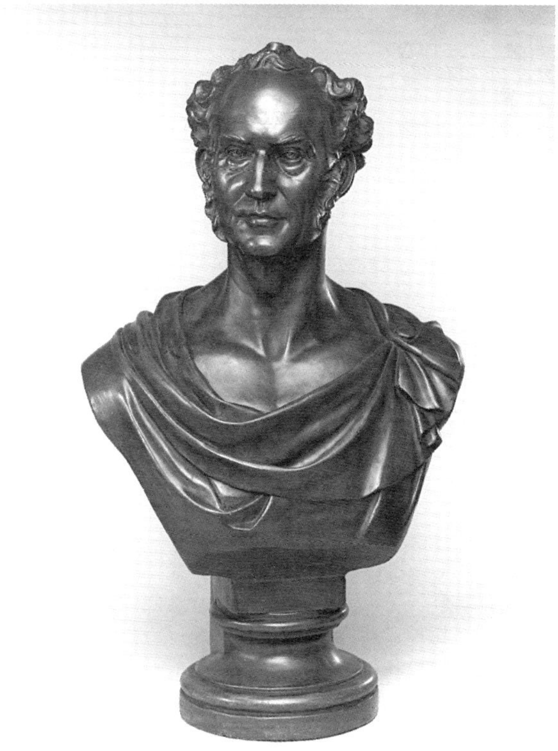

This neoclassical style sculpture of Dr. Samuel D. Gross is one of three identical plaster busts by J. Obermeier at Thomas Jefferson University. All are painted dark greenish-black to simulate bronze. They closely resemble a marble bust of Gross by Joseph Obermeier at the College of Physicians of Philadelphia, presented in 1884 by Albert Haller Gross.

The marble bust of Gross at the College of Physicians is signed "Jos. Obermeier," while the bust at

Thomas Jefferson University is signed "J. Obermeier." An artist named Joseph Obermeier exhibited at the National Academy of Design in 1867 (no address listed). A James Obermeier from Philadelphia exhibited sculptures in various media at the Pennsylvania Academy of the Fine Arts in 1868 and 1869. One wonders whether Joseph and James are the same artist, and one name was misspelled.

As early as October 19, 1882, minutes of the executive committee of Jefferson's alumni association report a motion to procure busts of Drs. Samuel D. Gross and Joseph Pancoast. The Pancoast bust was presented to the trustees the following year by Dr. Gross. Several years passed before the college acquired a bust of Gross.

The earliest record yet found is a report of the Jefferson Medical College Hospital of 1901 in which Dr. Jacob da Silva Solis-Cohen's donation of a bust of Gross was mentioned, but it is not known which of the three busts is his gift. A photograph of the alumni office in the Jefferson Medical College Building (occupied from 1898 to 1929) shows a Gross bust on top of a filing cabinet.

In Obermeier's depiction the surgeon's expression is neutral and his features are regularized and idealized, especially the aquiline nose. His eyes are upraised as if looking for divine inspiration. His chest is exposed and he wears a toga, common characteristics of neoclassical busts connecting contemporary subjects with a heroic past. The carving is very smooth and the surface is uniformly dark.

The Samuel D. Gross Monument

SAMUEL DAVID GROSS, M.D.
By Alexander Stirling Calder (1870-1945)

Bronze
1895-97
105 x 51 x 36 in.
Granite pedestal: 97 x 54 3/8 x 54 3/8 in.
Cement steps: 22 5/8 x 132 x 132 in.

Signed lower right on integral base of statue: "Calder"
Inscription lower left on integral base: "JABOEUF & BEZOUT.Fondeurs à Paris"
Inscription on pedestal: "SAMUEL D. GROSS/AMERICAN PHYSICIANS HAVE ERECTED/THIS STATUE TO COMMEMORATE THE GREAT DEEDS/OF A MAN WHO MADE SUCH AN IMPRESS/UPON AMERICAN SURGERY THAT IT HAS SERVED/TO DIGNIFY AMERICAN MEDICINE/1897"

Commissioned jointly in 1894 by the JMC alumni association and the American Surgical Association for the "people of the United States" in Washington, D.C.; relocated in 1970 to Thomas Jefferson University through the efforts of JMC alumni association
Accession number: 1970+e.S.01

In contrast to the generally negative public and critical reaction accorded Thomas Eakins's *Gross Clinic* when the immense painting was first exhibited in 1876, Alexander S. Calder's larger than life-sized bronze statue of Dr. Samuel D. Gross was treated with great anticipation and admiration two decades later. The official monument was initiated by medical peers to memorialize the professor in the nation's capital and the sculptor was selected by competition, whereas the unofficial painting had been initiated by the artist himself.

Although decades after its unveiling the sculpture passed through a period of neglect in its original site in Washington, D.C., it was resurrected with great fanfare and moved to Philadelphia in 1970. Finally, Thomas Jefferson University proudly displayed the two major depictions of Dr. Samuel D. Gross. Another boast expressed in the 1890s was that the only public full-length bronze monuments of distinguished physicians in this country were both of Jefferson alumni: the statues of Dr. J. Marion Sims in New York and of Dr. Samuel D. Gross in Washington.

Many aspects of the sculpture's history have been documented in Jefferson correspondence, board of trustees minutes, and *College and Clinical Record* accounts. It was reported in December 1891 that the American Surgical Association had recently appointed a committee to confer with friends and admirers of Dr. Gross and with the "profession at large" to initiate a movement to erect a monument to the professor in Washington, D.C. Six months later it was reported that the association did not want to limit subscribers to its own members but resolved to open the opportunity to the "entire American profession," because Gross was "of no exclusive faction, but a leading member of the whole profession."

The Jefferson Medical College alumni association actively participated in raising funds, but resolved in March 1893 to take steps to change the proposed mon-

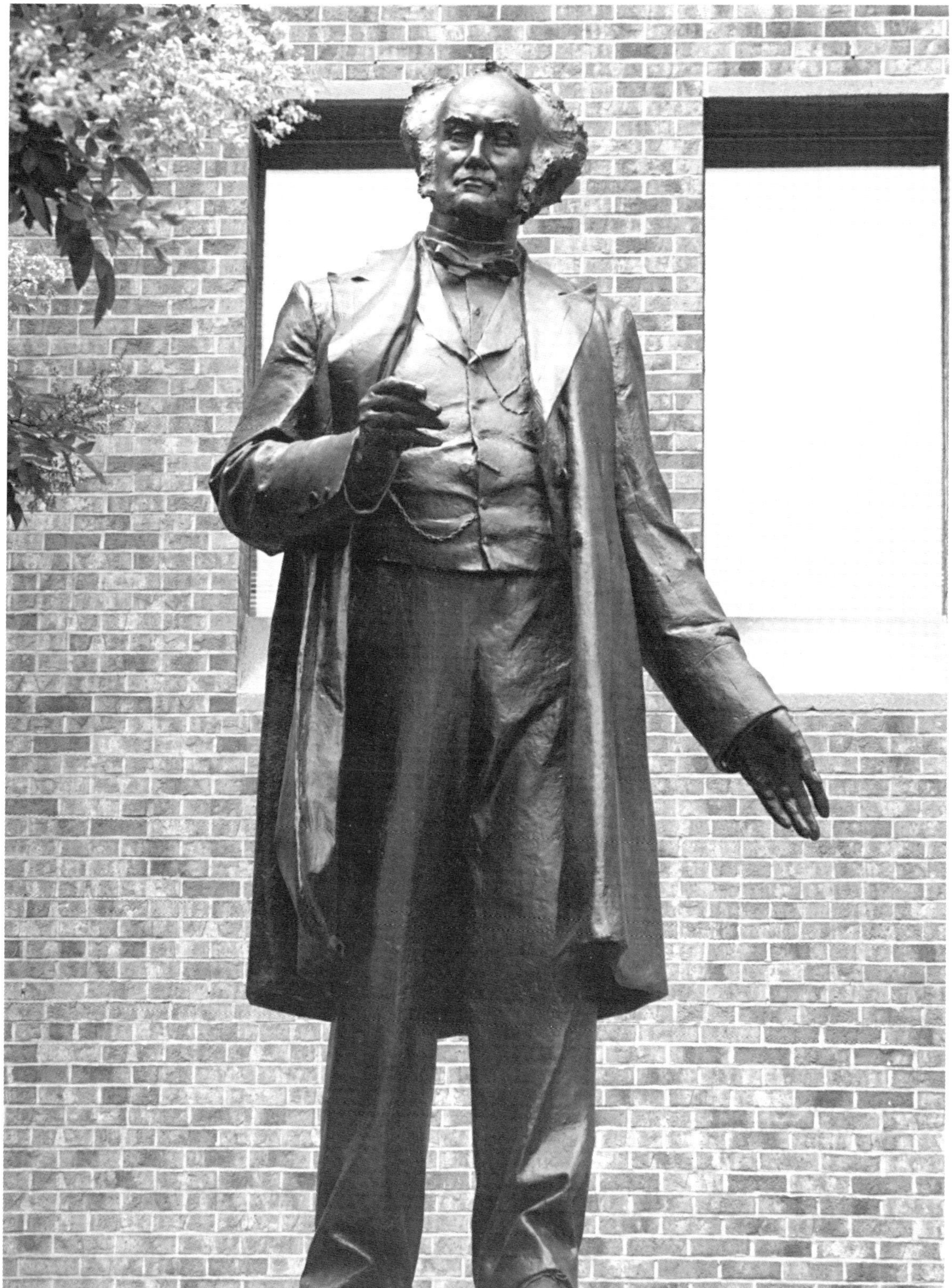

ument site from Washington to Philadelphia, "where Gross had lived and died, and by his diligent and successful work as a surgeon and teacher had made his name an honor to the medical profession." There is no further notice about an effort to change the location, so the effort must have been rejected straightaway.

By February 1895 it was clear that the credit for fund-raising and sponsorship was jointly shared by Jefferson Medical College which had raised $1521.37 and the American Surgical Association which held over six thousand dollars. In addition, the U.S. Congress agreed to appropriate fifteen hundred dollars for a granite pedestal.

A letter dated June 20, 1894 in the archives of the Pennsylvania Academy of the Fine Arts from Dr. William W. Keen, Jefferson's representative to the Gross Monument Committee, to Academy president Edward H. Coates, asked the latter for a recommendation of the "four or five best artists in the country to whom we might entrust this." The committee then invited three artists to enter a juried design competition. One unnamed sculptor withdrew, and the other two, Alexander S. Calder and Charles Grafly (1862-1929), briefly exhibited their models for the Gross memorial in special galleries during the Academy's 1894 *Annual Exhibition*, held December 17, 1894 to February 23, 1895.

The 1897 *Transactions of the American Surgical Association* recounted other details about the statue's history and reprinted the dedication speeches. The monument models were inspected by Edward H. Coates and the Pennsylvania Academy's main teacher of painting, Thomas P. Anshutz (1851-1912); famed New York sculptor Augustus Saint-Gaudens (1848-1907); Samuel D. Gross family member Dr. Orville Horwitz (grand-nephew by marriage) and son A. Haller Gross; and Dr. William W. Keen. The jury awarded the commission to Alexander Calder who subsequently modeled the statue in Paris where it was cast in bronze, and then shipped it to America where it was reportedly to be admitted duty free.

A letter of February 1897 from Dr. Keen invited all Jefferson alumni to "assist" at the unveiling of Gross's statue during the triennial meeting of the Congress of American Physicians and Surgeons in Washington on May 5 at five o'clock. At the same time Jefferson trustees were also making arrangements to be "fittingly represented," and board secretary Simon Gratz reported in May that many trustees, and "the greater part" of the faculty, demonstrators, instructors (and presumably also students) left Philadelphia at 1:12 P.M. on a special train provided through the kindness of trustee Sutherland M. Prevost, a vice president of the Pennsylvania Railroad.

The planned ceremonies for the occasion were: an opening prayer by the Reverend B. L. Whitman, president of Columbian University in Washington; presentation of the statue by Dr. Claudius H. Mastin of Mobile, Alabama, president of the American Surgical Association and initiator of the monument; unveiling by Miss Adele Horwitz of Baltimore, a granddaughter of Dr. Gross; reception of the statue on behalf of the government by Brigadier General George M. Sternberg, Surgeon General of the United States Army; and a closing address by Dr. W. W. Keen.

The May 1897 issue of *Dunglison's College and Clinical Record* gave a colorful description of the unveiling events attended by distinguished medical men from throughout the country:

> The ceremonies...will form a memorable event in the history of the medical profession of the country...The time fixed for the unveiling was 5 P.M., but throughout the greater part of the day, until within an hour or so of that time, sporadic showers fell over the city, completely drenching the drapery covering the statue and the stand erected on the Smithsonian grounds for the speakers and invited guests immediately alongside of the monument. At about 3 o'clock the joint committee...decided to remove the drapery from the statue, and, in consequence of the drenched condition of the grounds, to hold the ceremonies in the library of the Army Medical Museum... It was a brilliant tribute to a great surgeon.

Toward the end of Dr. W. W. Keen's emotional dedicatory address he noted that Washington's squares, parks, and circles were filled with statues of deserving statesmen and warriors, but that these men were not the "sole possessors of bravery." He recalled that Gross's hometown of Easton had sent the young surgeon to New York in July 1832 to assess the cholera epidemic there, in dread of this plague spreading to Pennsylvania. He had stayed a week visiting hospitals and charnel houses. Keen urged greater public recognition of men of science who have won victories of peace: "scores of courageous physicians ready to sacrifice their lives for their fellowmen with no blare of trumpets, no roar of cannon, no cheer of troops, no plaudits of the press! No battlefield ever saw greater heroes; no country braver men!"

As has been seen, the conception and erection of the Gross monument was truly a national effort. The impressive but derivative bronze portrait of Dr. Samuel D.

Gross was completed when Alexander Stirling Calder was twenty-seven years old, and his mature work still lay in the future. This public work helped to launch his career.

Interestingly, in his diary Calder referred to only one competitor for the commission, his friend Charles Grafly. Calder praised Eakins's depiction of Professor Gross and mentioned the painter's use of photographs (no longer extant), saying that Eakins had painted Gross's clinic before and "had made some very fine photographs of Dr. Gross for his own use." By appointment the two sculptors called on Eakins at his home on a Sunday in 1894 to "obtain the use" of the painter's negatives. He continued, "Eakins came into the parlor to greet us with a monkey on his shoulder. Perfectly unself-conscious, he was apt to be careless of formalities."[60]

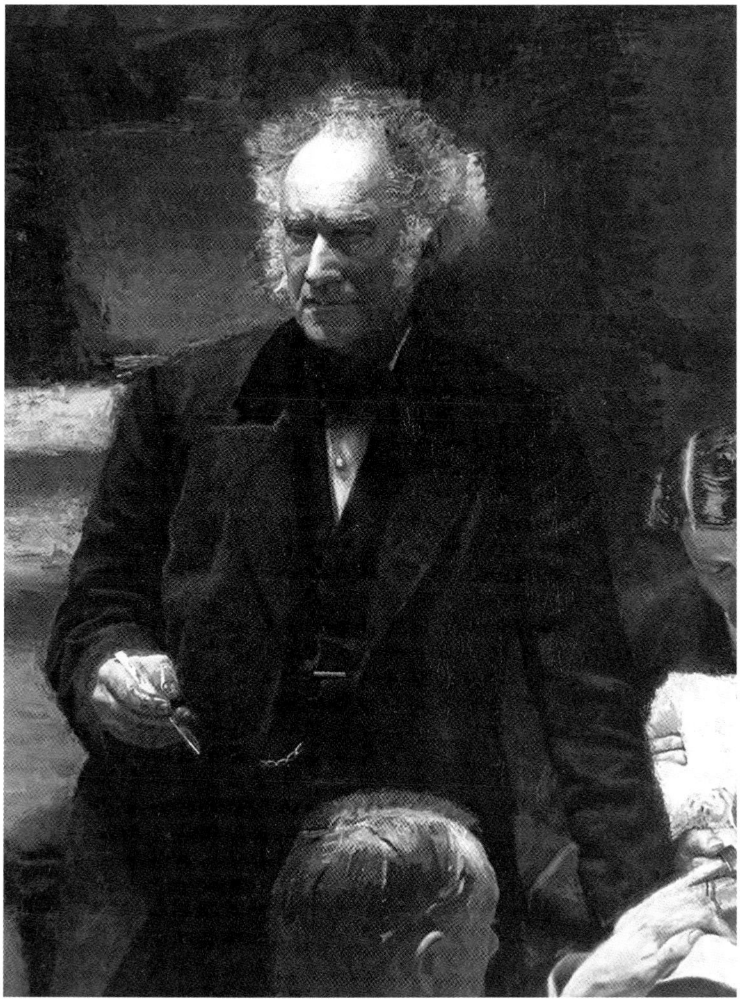

Detail: Figure of Dr. Samuel D. Gross from *The Gross Clinic*

Larger than life-sized atop a monumental granite pedestal, Calder's imposing sculpted figure is stiff and stolid compared with Eakins's naturalistic figure in *The Gross Clinic*, yet is clearly derived from the painting in details of costume and pose, even the scalpel in the surgeon's right hand. Slight variations from the painting can be found in the statue's left arm which is bent more, the right forearm which is raised a bit, and the position of the head which is frontal and tilted slightly. In the statue the physician's jaw is squarer, his features are regularized, and his hair protrudes like frozen triangles.

Alexander Stirling Calder was born in Philadelphia in 1870. He was the son of Alexander Milne Calder (1846-1923), celebrated for his extensive sculpture program for Philadelphia's City Hall, and the father of Alexander Calder (1898-1976), credited with inventing the mobile, a moving sculpture made of sheet metal and wire.

Stirling Calder entered the Pennsylvania Academy of the Fine Arts at age sixteen. Although he studied only briefly with Thomas Eakins, because that was the year of the artist's forced resignation as Academy director, Calder recalled that Eakins was then the "idol of the school, at least of that part of it that I met, the men. During rests...he often talked with us informally about methods and showed us a few simple gymnastic feats...I knew little and cared little about the controversy raging about Eakin's [*sic*] lack of decorum and shocks to prudery, not having been long enough under his tuition to succumb to his mastership and charm."[61]

Calder also described Dr. W. W. Keen's artistic anatomy course at the Academy in which senior students prepared the dissected subject for his exhibition of the muscles. He boasted that the physician praised his dissections and that he became a "sort of deputy demonstrator of anatomy." Keen's presence on the Gross monument committee might have tipped the balance in favor of Calder over Grafly.

In 1890 Calder had also studied sculpture in Paris with Henri Chapu (1833-91) at the Académie Julian and with Alexandre Falguière (1831-1900) at the École des Beaux-Arts. He returned to Philadelphia in 1892 and became assistant instructor in modeling at the Pennsylvania Academy of the Fine Arts where he served on the jury of selection and the hanging committee. He won a gold medal at the Philadelphia Art Club the following year.

By 1903 he also began teaching at the Pennsylvania School of Industrial Art. A consistent prizewinner at major exhibitions, Calder was awarded an honorable mention at the Pan-American Exposition in Buffalo in 1901, the Lippincott Prize at the Pennsylvania Academy in 1905, the grand prize at the Alaska-Yukon-Pacific Exposition in 1909, the Designer's Medal in San Francisco in 1915, and the silver medal at the Philadelphia Sesqui-centennial Exposition of 1926.

He served on the sculpture advisory committee and won a silver medal at the St. Louis Exposition in 1904. He was in charge of the sculptural decoration at the Panama-Pacific Exposition of 1915 in San Francisco where he contributed two fantastic groups: *The Nations of the West*, featuring mounted cowboys and Indians, explorers and scouts, and oxen pulling covered wagons; and *The Nations of the East*, with Arabian horsemen, desert tribesmen on camels, Asian warriors, and a bejewelled elephant.

By 1910 Calder was living in New York and teaching at the National Academy of Design and later at the Art Students League. A famous work in Manhattan is his monument of George Washington at the Washington Arch. He also continued to receive commissions in Philadelphia, notably the *Swann Memorial Fountain* at Logan Circle in 1924, and *Tragedy and Comedy*, the nearby Shakespeare memorial.

The Samuel D. Gross Monument in Washington, D.C.

By unknown photographer

Photograph
Ca. 1897
9 x 6 1/2 in.

Given after 1898 by the College of Physicians of Philadelphia which had received it from DeForest Willard, M.D., a pioneering orthopaedic surgeon from Philadelphia
Accession number: 1898+f.Ph.01

Alexander Stirling Calder would have been astonished to know of the Gross statue's subsequent fortunes. Its original location was on the mall near the old Army Medical Museum and the Surgeon General's library. That site became obsolete when the Army Medical Museum was renamed the Armed Forces Institute of Pathology and most of its collection was moved to the grounds of the Walter Reed Army Medical Center in the 1950s, and its library became part of the National Institutes of Health and moved to the National Library of Medicine in Bethesda, Maryland. The old medical museum was eventually demolished to make way for the Hirshhorn Museum and Sculpture Garden.

The effort to find and relocate the statue was initiated in 1969 by alumnus Harold L. Stewart, M.D. (JMC 1926) of Rockville, Maryland who contacted Norman J. Quinn Jr., M.D. (JMC 1948), then chairman of the Jefferson alumni association's centennial committee. In early 1970 administrators of the Armed Forces Institute escorted Dr. Quinn and Dr. John J. McKeown Jr. (JMC 1947) to inspect the abandoned statue. It had been "dismantled," but was found to be structurally sound, if badly weathered, and located on a nearby driveway.

Largely through the negotiations of Dr. Quinn and the Jefferson Medical College alumni association approval was won from the Department of the Army and the Armed Forces Institute of Pathology to relocate the sculpture in Philadelphia. But arrangements became more complicated. It even took a Congressional bill to "de-commission" the statue, because the original commission had stipulated that it was to be erected in Washington; and it was also necessary to win the concurrence of the District of Columbia parks, planning, and fine arts commissions.

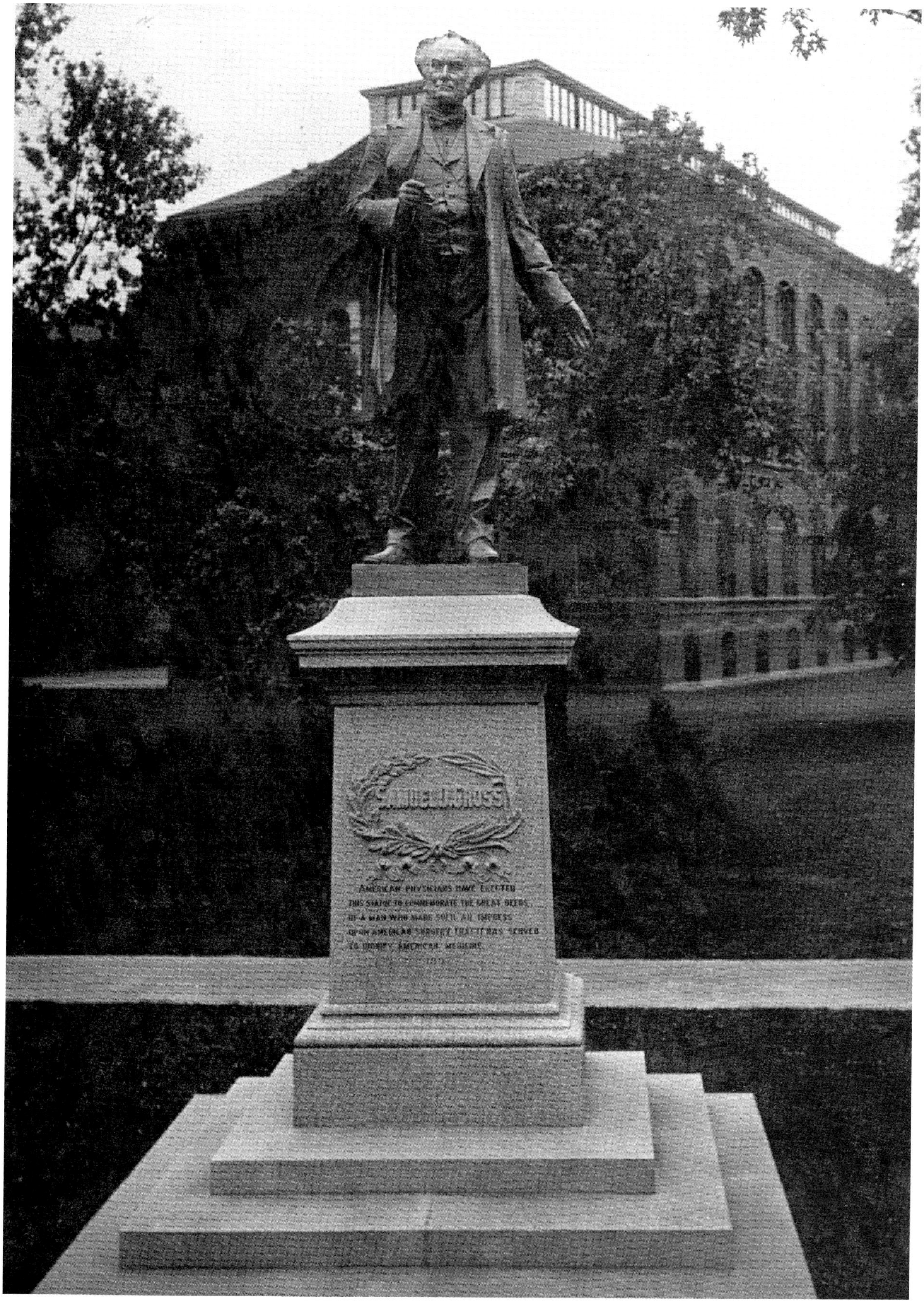
SAMUEL D. GROSS
AMERICAN PHYSICIANS HAVE ERECTED
TO DIGNIFY AMERICAN MEDICINE

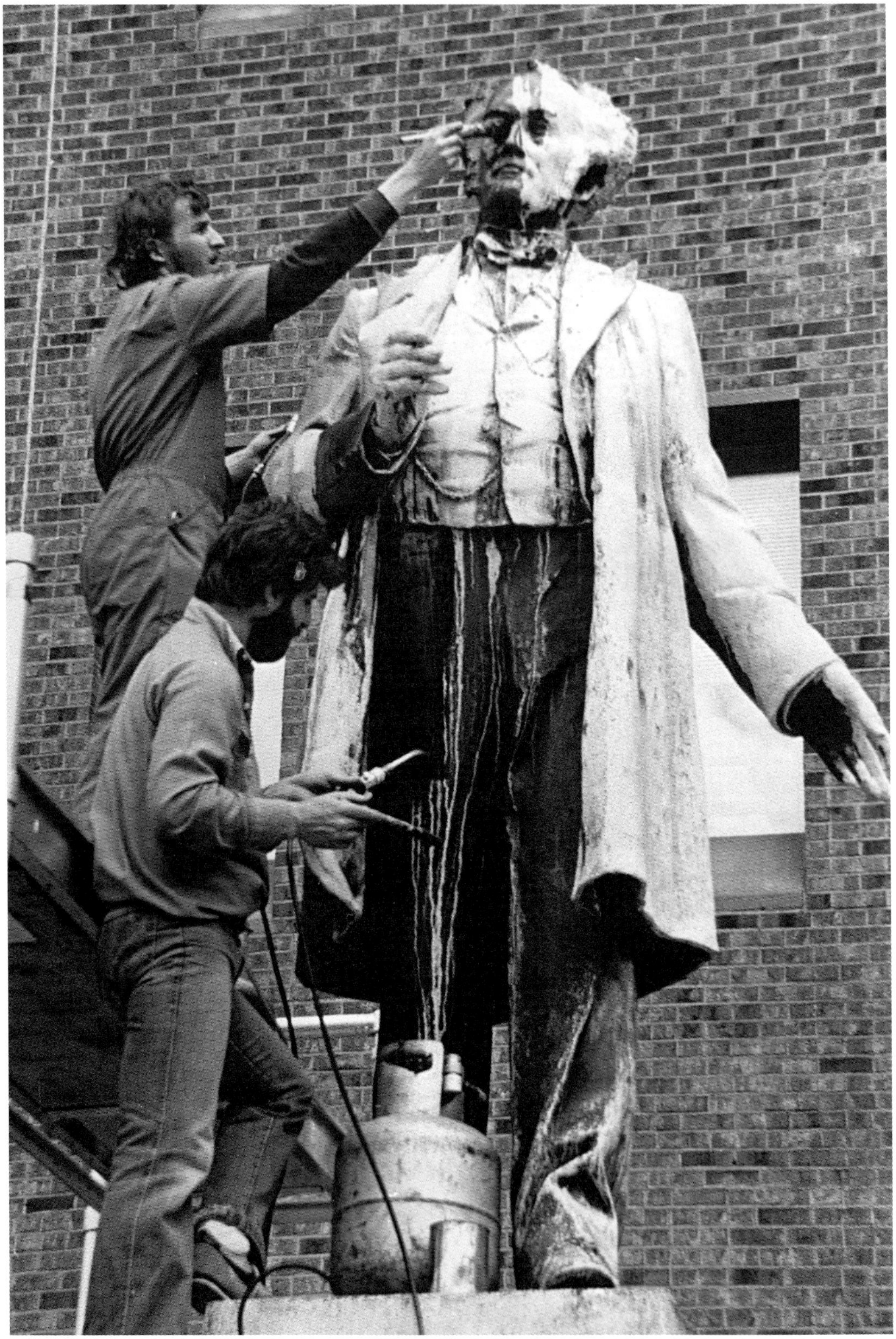

Conservation Work on the *Gross Monument*

On April 4, 1970 the *Samuel D. Gross Monument* was brought to Philadelphia where it underwent thorough cleaning and conservation at the university's Scott Plaza. The festive rededication ceremony on May 1 was a major event in commemorating the centennial of the Jefferson Medical College alumni association.

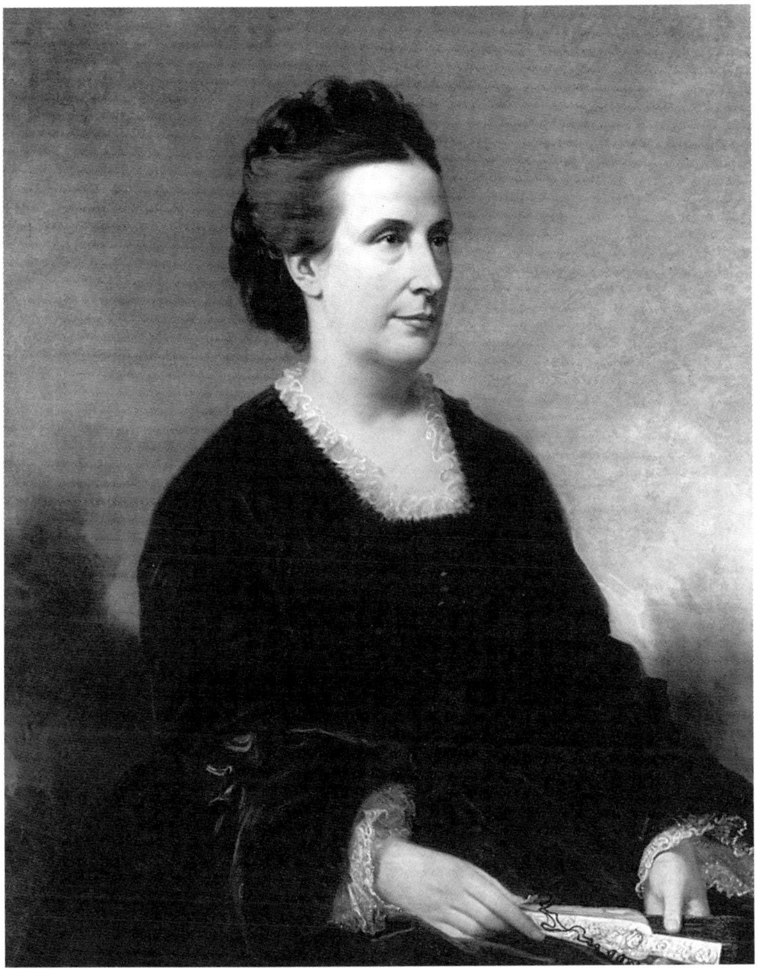

Portrait of Louisa Weissell (Mrs. Samuel D.) Gross

LOUISA WEISSELL GROSS (1807-76)
By Samuel Bell Waugh (1814-85)

Oil on canvas
1872
36 x 29 in.

Signed and dated lower left: "S.B. Waugh 1872"

Given in 1986 by Orville H. Bullitt Jr., Ph.D. and family; Dr. Bullitt was a great-great-grandson of Dr. Samuel D. Gross and a TJU trustee until recently

Accession number: 1986+e.P.01

Dr. Samuel D. Gross referred to Louisa Weissell Gross as his "crown and jewel of a wife." A long, affectionate description of his wife and their family can be found in his autobiography.[62]

He wrote that Louisa Ann Weissell was born in 1807 near London during a visit of her parents to England. A refined and cultured young woman, she became acquainted with S. D. Gross in 1827 when he was a student at Jefferson Medical College and they were married the following year. Gross acknowledged that they were both poor, so their "affection was therefore of a pure and unselfish character." He noted that "few men have ever been so blessed in their matrimonial relations." They had been married for almost forty-eight years when she died in 1876. Her headstone at Philadelphia's Woodlands Cemetery bears the simple inscription, "A NOBLE, CHRISTIAN WOMAN." Gross wrote these tender and respectful words about their mutual devotion:

> The attachment formed in our young days gradually increased in intensity as we advanced in years, and burned with a steady flame until my wife expired in my arms, mingling thus her last breath with mine. I know of nothing more touching than the sight of a young and loving wife encouraging her husband in his efforts to earn a livelihood for his family, and watching his rising fame...She was contented with her lot, and sympathized in all my movements, labors, and aspirations. I never knew her to be guilty of one selfish act. Her ambition always was to accommodate herself to circumstances...Unlike many of the women around her, she never lived above her means or her husband's income...
>
> Her musical talents, her remarkable intelligence, her fine conversational powers, and her genial disposition drew around her a coterie of friends, always as welcome as they were improved and gratified, and made her one of the most attractive women in the social circle whom I have ever known...Although she was fond of fashionable society, she never allowed herself to be influenced by its exactions, or to be drawn aside by its allurements...
>
> With my wife religion was not a mere sentiment; it was a positive reality...Reared in the Episcopal Church...she was a scrupulous observer of its rites and ceremonies, and a devout believer in the truth of its doctrines...
>
> I know she loved me with an intense ardor. I need not add how fondly I was attached to her, and how constantly I strove to augment her happiness...As a mother she was in every respect quite as exemplary; warm-hearted, generous, indulgent, and yet exacting, with an eye constantly alive to the moral and religious training of her children.

Samuel B. Waugh's portrait of Mrs. Gross was painted in 1872, two years before he painted the portrait of her husband, so the two works were not planned as pendants. Perhaps Waugh was commissioned to portray Dr. Gross by Jefferson's alumni association because the professor liked the earlier depiction of his wife.

Louisa Weissell Gross is shown two-thirds length, seated facing the right, holding a closed fan in her lap. Her thick, dark brown hair is crowned with a braid on top, and she appears younger than her sixty-five years. She gazes serenely into the distance. This attractive woman wears a modest black dress trimmed with lace at the cuffs and square neckline. The decorative fan is her only embellishment since she wears no jewelry.

Portrait of Samuel W. Gross

SAMUEL WEISSELL GROSS, M.D. (1837-89)
By George W. Pettit (d. 1910)

Oil on canvas mounted on board
1890
30 x 25 in.

Signed and dated lower left: "G.W. Pettit/1890."

Given by JMC class of 1890
Accession number: 1890+e.P.01

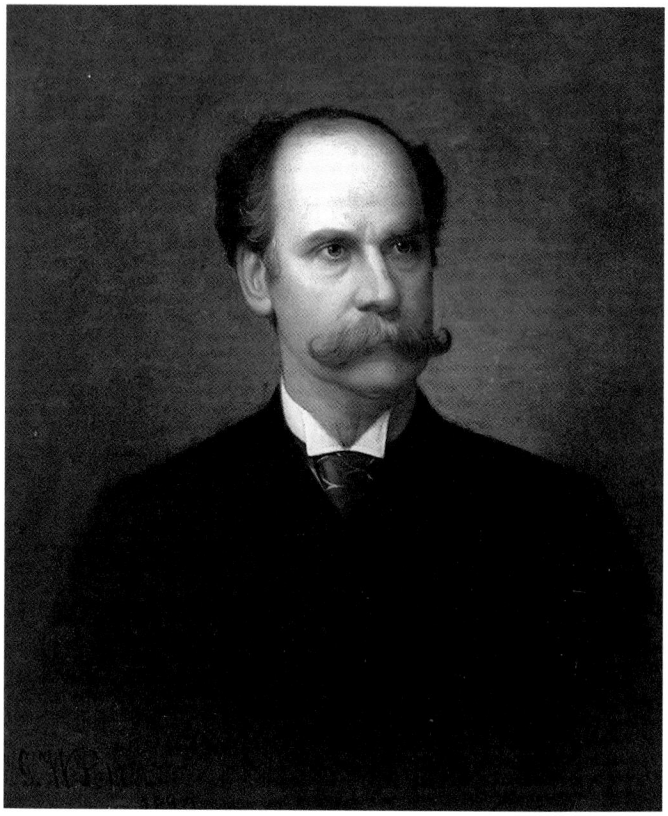

Dr. Samuel Weissell Gross followed in his father's footsteps by succeeding him as professor of surgery at Jefferson Medical College. He was one of four surviving children of Dr. Samuel D. Gross and Louisa Weissell Gross. Samuel W.'s brother, Albert Haller Gross, became a successful Philadelphia lawyer. His two accomplished sisters, Maria and Louisa, married brothers from Baltimore who were attorneys.

Dr. Samuel W. Gross was born in 1837 in Cincinnati. After graduating from Shelby College in Kentucky he began his study of medicine at the University of Louisville where his father was then professor of surgery. He received his medical degree from Jefferson Medical College in 1857 after which he began a practice in Philadelphia and helped his father edit the *North American Medico-chirurgical Review*. He served for almost four years during the Civil War as brigade surgeon with the rank of major, and was awarded the brevet of lieutenant colonel in 1865.

He returned to Philadelphia after the war and lectured on genito-urinary diseases and general surgery in Jefferson's summer courses that began in 1866. He joined the Jefferson, Howard, and Philadelphia Hospital staffs. In 1882 he was named professor of principles of surgery and clinical surgery at Jefferson (surgery was "divided" with two chairs following the resignation of his father as professor of surgery).

Dr. S. W. Gross was well deserving of this exalted post according to his colleagues. Dr. John Chalmers DaCosta said that "only a singularly notable man could have escaped being dwarfed into insignificance by his father's transcendent reputation."[63] In another essay about S. W. Gross, DaCosta wrote, "He was not only learned in surgery and in literature of surgery, but also in pathology, in fact, he personally sectioned and examined all the tumors he removed. He was a teacher of the very first order, even a greater one, I believe, than his illustrious father. He was a formidable person and we, his assistants, had a proper dread of him."[64]

Dr. S. W. Gross was the first American surgeon to advocate extensive operations for cancer of the breast and shares with Dr. William S. Halsted and others the modern radical operation for cure. His Civil War experiences in combatting hemorrhage taught him that veins, like arteries, could be ligated with safety. He made the first comprehensive study of bone sarcoma. He was one of the first surgeons in Philadelphia to adopt antiseptic surgery.

Among his literary contributions are: *A Practical Treatise on Tumors of the Mammary Gland, Embracing Their Histology, Pathology, Diagnosis, and Treatment* (1880), and *A Practical Treatise on Impotence, Sterility, and Allied Disorders of the Male Sexual Organs* (1881). Prominent in local and national medical societies, Dr. Gross was a founder of the Philadelphia Academy of Surgery in 1879, and president of the Pathological Society of Philadelphia that same year. He was a founder of the American Genito-urinary Association and a prominent fellow of the American Surgical Association.

Dr. Samuel Weissell Gross died prematurely of pneumonia in 1889 at age fifty-two. His wife was the former Grace Linzee Revere, great-granddaughter of the colonial patriot Paul Revere. Seventeen years younger than her husband, the widow married Dr. William Osler three years later. Her will of 1928 stipulated a bequest to Jefferson Medical College to establish a lectureship in surgery in her first husband's memory, today known as the Grace Revere Osler Professorship of Surgery.

In tribute to their revered teacher the Jefferson Medical College class of 1890 presented a posthumous portrait of Dr. Samuel W. Gross at the April 1890 commencement. Their spokesman said about Professor Gross,

> And today this class, who loved him living and revere him dead, meet with mingled feelings of joy and sorrow—joy for his great deeds, tears for his untimely taking off—to pay an affectionate tribute to his memory...
>
> Take it [the portrait] and place it in the amphitheatre of the hospital, the scene of his labors and professional triumph. Place it side by side with the portraits of the great dead who have gone before, the elder Pancoast, Meigs, Mitchell, and the other Gross, kindred in blood, kindred in genius. And as...future generations of students pass through those old Halls...may they...never fail to honor his worth and do justice to his memory.[65]

The artist selected for Dr. S. W. Gross's posthumous portrait was George W. Pettit who had also painted the posthumous portrait of Dr. James A. Meigs in 1879 and would take on several others for Jefferson. Pettit's bust-length depiction of Gross facing slightly right could have been based on one of several photographs in the Jefferson archives by Frederick Gutekunst featuring the same pose.

The subject's most distinguishing features are his long oval face, high domed forehead, and luxuriantly curled mustache. Oddly, his shirt in the painting has a collar with wing tips pointed down, but pentimenti reveal an earlier version with standing collar. His collar appears in both styles in various cabinet-size photographs. It is not known if Pettit himself made the change in collar style.

The Jefferson collection has a heavily restored, close copy of the portrait, also signed and dated "G. W. Pettit/1890." This second portrait entered the Jefferson collection before 1947 from an unrecorded donor. Interestingly, the shirt collar is turned down in this copy, with no sign of alteration. There is a very similar, third portrait of Dr. S. W. Gross with standing collar at the College of Physicians of Philadelphia, a copy of Pettit's work painted by Philadelphia artist Frances van Horn Heberton and presented in 1890 by Mrs. S. W. Gross and Albert Haller Gross.

---

1. The following selected bibliography contains useful references on the life and art of Thomas Eakins:

Berger, Martin A. *Determining Manhood: Constructions of Sexuality in the Art of Thomas Eakins*. Ph.D. diss., Yale University, 1995. Ann Arbor, Mich.: University Microfilms International, 1997.

Chamberlin-Hellman, Maria J. *Thomas Eakins as a Teacher*. Ph.D. diss., Columbia University, 1981. Ann Arbor, Mich.: University Microfilms International, 1987.

Foster, Kathleen A. *Thomas Eakins Rediscovered: Charles Bregler's Thomas Eakins Collection at the Pennsylvania Academy of the Fine Arts*. New Haven: Yale University Press and the Pennsylvania Academy of the Fine Arts, 1997.

Foster, and Cheryl Leibold. *Writing about Eakins: The Manuscripts in Charles Bregler's Thomas Eakins Collection*. Philadelphia: University of Pennsylvania Press for the Pennsylvania Academy of the Fine Arts, 1989.

Fried, Michael. *Realism, Writing, Disfiguration: On Thomas Eakins and Stephen Crane*. Chicago: University of Chicago Press, 1987.

Goodrich, Lloyd. *Thomas Eakins*. 2 vols. Cambridge, Mass.: Harvard University Press for the National Gallery of Art, Washington, D.C., 1982.

Hendricks, Gordon. *The Life and Work of Thomas Eakins*. New York: Grossman Publishers, 1974.

Homer, William I. *Thomas Eakins: His Life and Art*. New York: Abbeville Press Publishers, 1992.

Homer, ed. *Eakins at Avondale and Thomas Eakins: A Personal Collection*. Chadds Ford, Pa.: Brandywine River Museum and the University of Delaware, 1980.

Johns, Elizabeth. *Thomas Eakins: The Heroism of Modern Life*. Princeton: Princeton University Press, 1983.

Lubin, David M. *Act of Portrayal: Eakins, Sargent, James*. New Haven: Yale University Press, 1985.

Milroy, Elizabeth. *Thomas Eakins' Artistic Training, 1860-1870*. Ph.D. diss.,

University of Pennsylvania, 1986. Ann Arbor, Mich.: University Microfilms International, 1988.

Rosenzweig, Phyllis D. *The Thomas Eakins Collection of the Hirshhorn Museum and Sculpture Garden*. Washington, D.C.: Smithsonian Institution Press, 1977.

Sewell, Darrel. *Thomas Eakins: Artist of Philadelphia*. Philadelphia: Philadelphia Museum of Art, 1982.

Siegl, Theodor. *The Thomas Eakins Collection: Philadelphia Museum of Art*. Philadelphia: Philadelphia Museum of Art, 1978.

Wilmerding, John, ed. *Thomas Eakins (1844-1916) and the Heart of American Life*. London: National Portrait Gallery, 1993.

2. Goodrich, *Eakins*, 1:5.

3. Johns, "'I, A PAINTER': Thomas Eakins at the ANSP," *Frontiers: Annual of the Academy of Natural Sciences of Philadelphia* 3 (1981-82): 46.

4. Milroy, 41, 44.

5. Johns, "'I, A PAINTER,'" 47-49.

6. For biographical information on Dr. Amos R. Thomas see: Howard A. Kelly, M.D. and Walter L. Burrage, M.D., *Dictionary of American Medical Biography* (New York: D. Appleton & Co., 1928), 1199; Donald C. Geist, M.D., "William Williams Keen, M.D., and the Teaching of Artistic Anatomy," *Transactions and Studies of the College of Physicians of Philadelphia* 41 (Apr. 1974): 305; Harold J. Abrahams, M.D., *Extinct Medical Schools of Nineteenth-century Philadelphia* (Philadelphia: University of Pennsylvania Press, 1966), 213; and Ronald J. Onorato, *The Pennsylvania Academy of the Fine Arts and the Development of an Academic Curriculum in the Nineteenth Century* (Ph.D. diss., Brown University, 1977) (Ann Arbor, Mich.: University Microfilms International, 1994), 62-63.

7. Manuscript dated June 6, 1856, Archives, Pennsylvania Academy of the Fine Arts.

8. Milroy, 63.

9. Ellwood C. Parry III, "*The Gross Clinic* as Anatomy Lesson and Memorial Portrait," *Art Quarterly* 32 (1969): 373, 384 n. 3.

10. George W. Corner, M.D., *Two Centuries of Medicine: A History of the School of Medicine, University of Pennsylvania* (Philadelphia: J. B. Lippincott Co., 1965), 129-38.

11. Corner, 104-05.

12. I am currently researching *The Writing Master* (Metropolitan Museum of Art), Thomas Eakins's 1882 portrait of Benjamin Eakins at work inscribing a document. From the legible marks on the painted certificate, I have concluded that it is probably a Jefferson Medical College diploma, unlike any other diploma yet encountered from schools where Benjamin Eakins is known to have worked.

13. Goodrich, 1:323 n. 123:7-8, states that both Jefferson dean Ross V. Patterson, M.D. and librarian Joseph J. Wilson wrote to him in 1931 saying that "records" (unnamed) showed that Eakins studied at Jefferson in 1873 and 1874. Contemporary Jefferson historians say that the only records available in 1931 were probably the same as today: the Jefferson student register in which students signed their own names, and various official printed materials of the college. None of these include the names of nonmatriculating students such as Thomas Eakins, nor do the archival files on the relevant Jefferson professors. Probably, it never occurred to Patterson and Wilson that Eakins could have attended class in the spring or summer of 1874 rather than the entire 1873-1874 session.

It should be remembered that Jefferson art records were spotty at best, and false information can be perpetuated. Patterson wrote about *The Gross Clinic* in the *Jefferson Medical College Alumni Bulletin* of April 1925, stating incorrectly that the painting was exhibited at the Buffalo exposition of 1901, repeating an error made by Charles Frankenberger in 1915 (see next chapter).

Interestingly, *The Gross Clinic* is shown in George M. Gould, M.D., *The Jefferson Medical College of Philadelphia: A History*, 2 vols. (New York: Lewis Publishing Co., 1904). A caption reads in part, "Reproduced by permission of Thomas Eakins, N.A., who made the painting from which it is taken, while studying anatomy as an art student in Jefferson Medical College in 1873." Gould's book, the first history of the college since a modest work of 1858 by James F. Gayley, M.D., is no longer considered totally reliable.

14. Goodrich, 1:315 n. 13:1-6, says that the date was written by Charles Bregler (Eakins's former student, disciple, friend, advisor to the artist's widow, and compiler of a collection of the artist's manuscripts and memorabilia now at the Pennsylvania Academy of the Fine Arts).

15. Milroy, 141.

16. Johns, *Thomas Eakins*, 55.

17. Milroy, 169-70, 185 n. 78.

18. Johns, "Thomas Eakins and 'Pure Art' Education," *Critical Issues in American Art: A Book of Readings*, ed. Mary Ann Calo (Boulder, Colo.: Westview Press, 1998), 171-76.

19. Goodrich, 1:187.

20. William Williams Keen, M.D., "The History of the Philadelphia School of Anatomy and its Relation to Medical Teaching," *Addresses and Other Papers* (Philadelphia: W. B. Saunders & Co., 1905), 40-67, a lecture delivered March 1, 1875 at the dissolution of the school.

21. Information about Dr. William W. Keen's course of lectures is derived in part from his five annual reports to the Pennsylvania Academy of the Fine Arts' board of directors (from the sessions 1876-77 through 1880-81), and thereafter from the Academy's *Circular of the Committee on Instruction*.

22. Keen, *Memoirs*, ed. W. W. Keen James (Doylestown, Pa.: privately printed, 1990), 40.

23. For a discussion of Eakins's anatomical drawings and casts see Foster, 98-100, 306-30, 447.

24. William C. Brownell, "The Art Schools of Philadelphia," *Scribner's Monthly*, Sept. 1879, 737-50.

25. See Homer, *Thomas Eakins*, 166-82, for further details of scandals relating to Eakins's morality.

26. Homer, *Thomas Eakins*, 190.

27. Charles Bregler, "Thomas Eakins as I Knew Him," manuscript in Charles Bregler's Thomas Eakins Collection, Archives, Pennsylvania Academy of the Fine Arts.

28. Cecilia Beaux, *Background with Figures: Autobiography of Cecilia Beaux* (Boston: Houghton Mifflin Co., 1930), 96.

29. Goodrich, 1:315 n. 13:12-14.

30. Letter of July 9, 1936 from Susan Eakins to Alton O'Steen, a music educator and acquaintance; manuscript in Charles Bregler's Thomas Eakins Collection, Archives, Pennsylvania Academy of the Fine Arts.

31. For Eakins and perspective see Siegl, 54-56, 109; Foster, passim; and Amy Beth Werbel, *Perspective in the Life and Art of Thomas Eakins* (Ph.D. diss., Yale University, 1996) (Ann Arbor, Mich.: University Microfilms International, 1998).

32. Published in *Proceedings of the Academy of Natural Sciences of Philadelphia* 46 (1894): 172-180, and also issued as a reprint that year.

33. Johns, "'I, A PAINTER,'" 45-46.

34. I am currently researching Thomas Eakins's portraits of physicians. Of his more than two hundred portraits, a significant number of sitters were physicians, many of whom he knew through his associations with Central High School, Jefferson Medical College, the University of Pennsylvania, the Academy of Natural Sciences, and elsewhere. He

painted physicians' portraits throughout his career beginning with Dr. Benjamin H. Rand in 1874, his first public portrait subject, and ending with Dr. Edward A. Spitzka, his very last portrait painted in 1913 or 1914; both were Jefferson Medical College professors.

Of Eakins's twenty-four medical portraits, almost half (eleven) sitters were Jefferson alumni (superscript 1 below) and/or faculty members (superscript 2). The Agnew and Gross clinic group portraits are treated as one each. (All but one of Gross's assistants were Jefferson alumni, though none of Agnew's was.)

Eakins's subjects who earned M.D. degrees include: *The Agnew Clinic* (including portraits of D. Hayes Agnew [also represented in a completed oil sketch], J. William White, Joseph Leidy II, Ellwood R. Kirby, and Fred H. Milliken); George F. Barker (well known as a professor of physics, but received an M.D. degree in 1863 from Albany Medical College); *The Medical Examiner* (Henry Beates Jr.); Daniel G. Brinton[1] (also an ethnologist); John H. Brinton[1,2]; Matthew H. Cryer (an oral surgeon with both medical and dental degrees); Jacob M. DaCosta[1,2]; Thomas H. Fenton; William S. Forbes[1,2]; Albert C. Getchell[1,2]; Frank L. Greenewalt; *The Gross Clinic*[1,2] (including portraits of Samuel D. Gross, Samuel W. Gross, Daniel M. Appel, Charles S. Briggs, James M. Barton, W. Joseph Hearn, and Franklin West); *The Dean's Roll Call* (James W. Holland)[1,2]; Joseph Leidy II (two versions); Charles L. Leonard; Edward J. Nolan; Gilbert L. Parker[1]; Benjamin H. Rand[1,2]; *The Oboe Player* (Benjamin Sharp); Edward A. Spitzka[2]; William Thomson[1,2] (two versions); J. William White; George B. Wood; and Horatio C. Wood.

Other scientists who sat for portraits include: William D. Marks, an engineer; Henry A. Rowland, a physicist; William P. Wilson, a biologist and museum founder; and Frank H. Cushing and Stewart Culin, ethnologists.

35. Some parts of the description of Eakins's portrait of Dr. Rand first appeared in my cover article for the *Journal of the American Medical Association* 264 (Aug. 15, 1990): 787, and in my contribution to Wilmerding, 76-78.

36. I am grateful for access to the Lloyd Goodrich and Edith Havens Goodrich, Whitney Museum of American Art, Record of Works by Thomas Eakins, Philadelphia Museum of Art, for calling my attention to this exhibition which was not documented in existing papers at Thomas Jefferson University.

37. Benjamin H. Rand, M.D., *Valedictory Address to the Graduates of the Jefferson Medical College* (Philadelphia: Collins, 1866), 6-9.

38. "Death of Professor Rand," *The College and Clinical Record* (Jefferson Medical College) 4 (March 15, 1883): 72 (reprinted from the *Philadelphia Medical Times*, Feb. 24, 1883). The accident occurred in 1875 according to Edward L. Bauer, M.D., *Doctors Made in America* (Philadelphia: J. B. Lippincott Co., 1963), 153-54.

39. Parry, 373-74.

40. William H. Gerdts, *The Art of Healing: Medicine and Science in American Art* (Birmingham, Ala.: Birmingham Museum of Art, 1981), 60.

41. Johns, *Thomas Eakins*, 23-24. Later, in footnote 20, page 54, Johns stated incorrectly that Rand retired from the faculty in 1873, so perhaps the portrait was painted as a "retirement tribute," but, in fact, Rand retired in 1877, not 1873.

42. Johns, "'I, A PAINTER,'" 47.

43. Goodrich, 1:2-3.

44. See Fried for a Freudian analysis of "writing/drawing and painting," an exploration of unresolved tensions between materiality and illusion in Eakins's art.

45. According to *Appleton's Cyclopaedia of American Biography* (New York: D. Appleton & Co., 1888), 168, Rand's books included *The American Penman, Rand's System of Penmanship, Rand's Copy-Book,* and *Appendix;* the books went through several editions and sold more than one and one-half million copies in his lifetime.

46. To give an idea of late-nineteenth-century wages, Benjamin Eakins earned between $25.62 and $84.69 for his annual services, depending on the number of graduates per year.

47. Foster, 11, 449-50. The chair is dated ca. 1860 and is included among the memorabilia in the Charles Bregler Thomas Eakins Collection at the Pennsylvania Academy of the Fine Arts.

48. See Berger, who puts a slightly different construction on the objects: "Eakins established a metaphoric and visual tension in his canvas" by setting the physician in the center of a male grouping of objects on the left and female grouping of objects on the right, on a "continuum" between the "hard/soft" and "metallic/organic" objects; and that the artist himself was the "scientist's partner along the depicted sexual continuum" (pp. 74-84).

49. *Philadelphia Evening Bulletin*, May 17, 1876.

50. William Clark, "The Centennial," *The Evening Telegraph*, June 16, 1876.

51. Charles Frankenberger, "The Collection of Portraits Belonging to the College," *The Jeffersonian* 17 (Nov. 1915): 2.

52. Samuel D. Gross, M.D., *Autobiography of Samuel D. Gross, M.D.*, ed. Samuel W. Gross, M.D. and A. Haller Gross, 2 vols. (Philadelphia: George Barrie, 1887), 1:16.

53. Gross, *Autobiography*, 1:xxv-xxvi, xxix.

54. Gross, *Autobiography*, 1:1.

55. For Gross's professional societies and honors and for his contributions to surgical technique, I am indebted to Frederick B. Wagner Jr., M.D., ed., *Thomas Jefferson University: Tradition and Heritage* (Philadelphia: Lea & Febiger, 1989), 522-24; and Wagner, "Revisit of Samuel D. Gross, M.D.," *SURGERY, Gynecology, & Obstetrics* 152 (May 1981): 663-74.

56. Gross, *Autobiography*, 1:161-62.

57. Gross, *Then and Now: A Discourse Introductory to the Forty-third Course of Lectures in the Jefferson Medical College of Philadelphia* (Philadelphia: Collins, 1867).

58. Gross, *The Live Physician: Charge to the Graduates at the Forty-third Annual Commencement of the Jefferson Medical College of Philadelphia* (Philadelphia: Collins, 1868), 4, 14-15.

59. See Julie S. Berkowitz, *The College of Physicians of Philadelphia Portrait Catalogue* (Philadelphia: College of Physicians of Philadelphia, 1984), 58-61.

60. Alexander Stirling Calder, *Thoughts of A. Stirling Calder on Art and Life* (New York: privately printed, 1947), 6.

61. Calder, 3-4.

62. Gross, *Autobiography*, 1:363-74.

63. John Chalmers DaCosta, M.D., "Character Sketch of Professor Samuel W. Gross, M.D., LL.D.," *Selections from the Papers and Speeches of John Chalmers DaCosta, M.D., LL.D.* (Philadelphia: W. B. Saunders Co., 1931), 220.

64. DaCosta, "The Last Surgical Clinic in the Old Amphitheater of the Jefferson Medical College Hospital, Held before the Senior and Junior Classes, May 10, 1922, by Professor John Chalmers DaCosta," *Selections*, 340, reprinted from the *Jefferson Medical College Alumni Bulletin* 1 (Feb. 1925).

65. *The College and Clinical Record* (Jefferson Medical College) 11 (May 1890): 119-20.

CHAPTER 4

The Gross Clinic by Thomas Eakins

THE GROSS CLINIC
By Thomas Eakins (1844-1916)

Oil on canvas
1875
96 x 78 in.
(See color plate)

Signed and dated on edge of operating table, lower right: "EAKINS 1875"
Exhibitions: Philadelphia, Haseltine's Galleries, late Apr.-early May 1876; Philadelphia, Centennial International Exhibition, May 10-Nov. 10, 1876; Philadelphia, Haseltine's Galleries, late Nov. or early Dec. 1876; New York, *Second Annual Exhibition*, Society of American Artists, Kurtz Gallery, Mar. 10-Mar. 29, 1879; Philadelphia, *Fiftieth Annual Exhibition*, Pennsylvania Academy of the Fine Arts, Apr. 28-June 2, 1879; Philadelphia, *Works of Art to be Exhibited at the World's Columbian Exposition, Chicago, 1893*, Pennsylvania Academy of the Fine Arts, Jan. 16-Feb. 4, 1893; Chicago, World's Columbian Exposition, May 1-Oct. 30, 1893; St. Louis, Louisiana Purchase Centennial International Exposition, Apr. 30-Dec. 1, 1904; New York, *Loan Exhibition of the Works of Thomas Eakins*, Metropolitan Museum of Art, Nov. 5-Dec. 3, 1917; Philadelphia, *Memorial Exhibition of the Works of the Late Thomas Eakins*, Pennsylvania Academy of the Fine Arts, Dec. 23, 1917-Jan. 13, 1918; Philadelphia, *Thomas Eakins 1844-1916*, Pennsylvania Museum of Art, ca. Mar. 5-ca. Apr. 15, 1930; Philadelphia, *Thomas Eakins Centennial Exhibition*, Philadelphia Museum of Art, Apr. 8-May 14, 1944; Philadelphia, *Diamond Jubilee Exhibition*, Philadelphia Museum of Art, Nov. 4, 1950-Feb. 11, 1951; Philadelphia, *150th Anniversary Exhibition*, Pennsylvania Academy of the Fine Arts, Jan. 15-Mar. 13, 1955; Washington, D.C., Chicago, and Philadelphia, *Thomas Eakins: A Retrospective Exhibition*, National Gallery of Art, Smithsonian Institution, Oct. 8-Nov. 12, 1961, Art Institute of Chicago, Dec. 1, 1961-Jan. 7, 1962, and Philadelphia Museum of Art, Feb. 1-Mar. 18, 1962; Philadelphia, short-term loan, Philadelphia Museum of Art, Apr. 1-Sept. 30, 1962; Philadelphia, summer loan, Philadelphia Museum of Art, July 15-Sept. 2, 1964; Philadelphia, *The Art of Philadelphia Medicine*, Sept. 15-Dec. 7, 1965; Philadelphia, summer loan, Philadelphia Museum of Art, ca. June 25-Sept. 14, 1967; Philadelphia, summer loan, Philadelphia Museum of Art, 1968; Philadelphia, summer loan, Philadelphia Museum of Art, June 15-Aug. 30, 1969; New York, *Nineteenth Century America: Painting and Sculpture*, Metropolitan Museum of Art, Apr. 16-Sept. 7, 1970; New York, *Thomas Eakins Retrospective Exhibition*, Whitney Museum of American Art, Sept. 22-Nov. 21, 1970; Philadelphia, *Philadelphia: Three Centuries of American Art*, Philadelphia Museum of Art, Apr. 11-Oct. 10, 1976; Birmingham, Ala., *The Art of Healing: Medicine and Science in American Art*, Birmingham Museum of Art, Feb. 7-Mar. 29, 1981; Philadelphia and Boston, *Thomas Eakins: Artist of Philadelphia*, Philadelphia Museum of Art, May 29-Aug. 1, 1982, and Museum of Fine Arts, Boston, Sept. 22-Nov. 28, 1982; Boston, Washington, D.C., and Paris, *A New World: Masterpieces of American Painting 1760-1910*, Museum of Fine Arts, Boston, Sept. 7-Nov. 13, 1983, Corcoran Gallery of Art, Dec. 7, 1983-Feb. 12, 1984, and Grand Palais, Mar. 16-June 11, 1984; Baltimore, *Thomas Eakins: Image of the Surgeon*, Walters Art Gallery (in commemoration of the centennial of Johns Hopkins Medicine), June 8-July 30, 1989; Washington, D.C., *Revisiting the White City: American Art at the 1893 World's Fair*, National Museum of American Art and National Portrait Gallery, Smithsonian Institution, Apr. 16-Aug. 15, 1993

Purchased February 23, 1878 and given by the Jefferson Medical College alumni association
Accession number: 1878+e.P.01

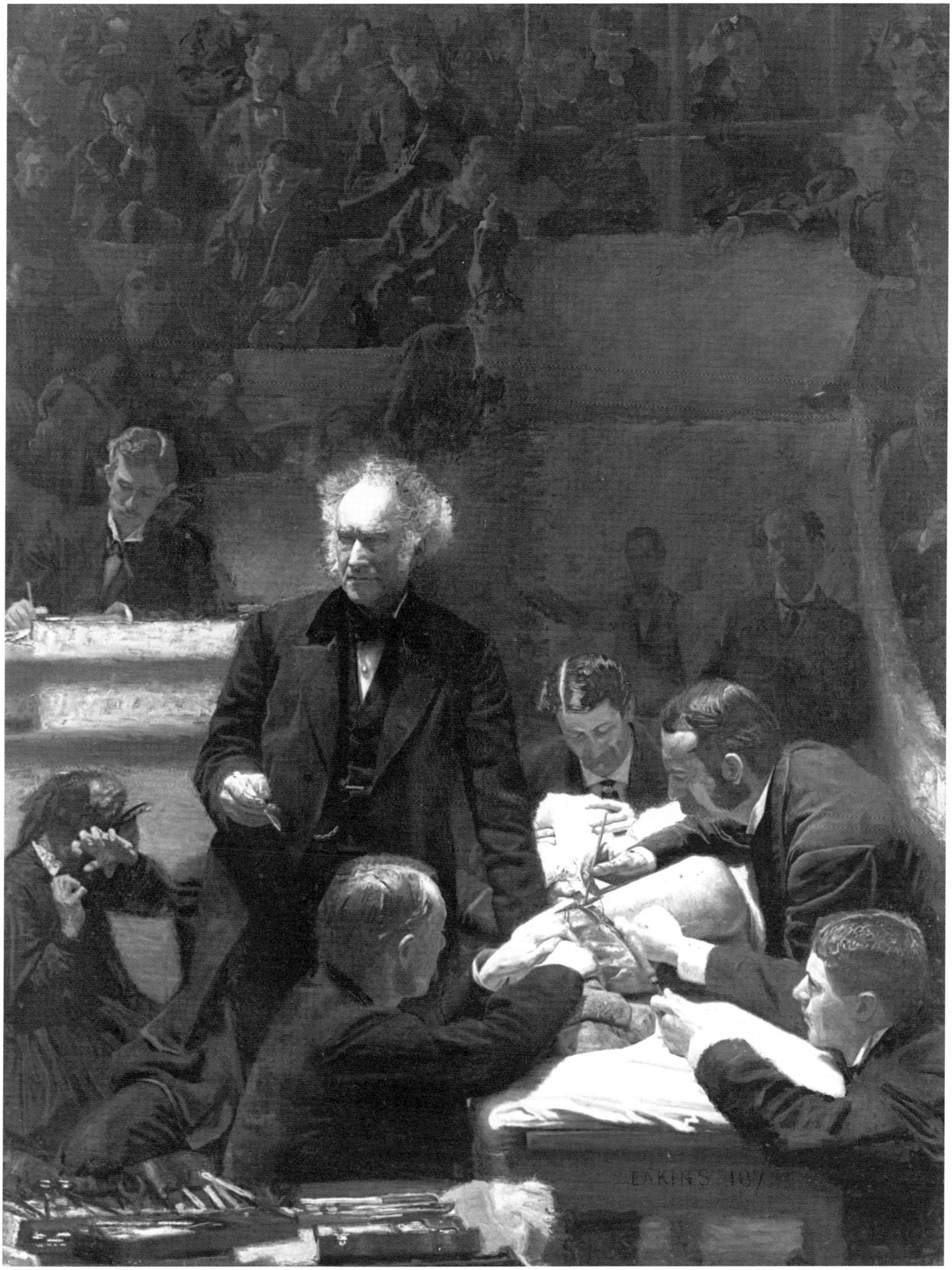
EAKINS

The Gross Clinic, Thomas Eakins's most celebrated work, was initiated solely by the artist. Thus there are no extant Jefferson Medical College documents relating to the circumstances behind its creation. Since no official planning for the painting was undertaken by the college, there was none to be noted by administrators. The first official mention of Eakins's masterpiece was a routine purchase entry on a Jefferson Medical College ledger of 1878 (see below).

Although no contemporary records have surfaced elsewhere about the origin of *The Gross Clinic*, several Eakins scholars have conjectured about the artist's objectives in conceiving and executing his ambitious painting of Dr. Samuel D. Gross. The overarching question is whether he created the work specifically for the 1876 Philadelphia Centennial art exhibition. If his primary motive was to enhance his reputation by making an important painting for the Centennial why did he choose Dr. Gross as its subject?

Ellwood C. Parry III discussed Eakins's motives in two articles in the 1960s.[1] As noted in the discussion of the portrait of Dr. Benjamin H. Rand, Eakins became aware of Jefferson's new practice of commissioning portraits of important professors and wanted to be included in the developing collection. A further incentive was to surpass Samuel B. Waugh's portrait of 1874, a bust-length figure of Dr. Gross in a conventional formal pose. I agree with Parry's view, but feel that Eakins had already demonstrated his superiority to Waugh with his large-scale portrait of Dr. Rand the year before (as well as other nonmedical portraits).

Parry also asserted that Eakins could not have failed to know about the upcoming Philadelphia Centennial art exhibition because a Committee of Philadelphia Artists had met in March 1875 to draft an "Address to the Artists of the United States" announcing this event. Furthermore, he had already submitted two pictures to the Paris Salon of 1875, so was already accustomed to showing at an international venue.

One can expand on Parry's idea that Eakins knew about the Centennial art exhibition by scrutinizing more closely the contents of the Address to Artists.[2] First, the written address was adopted at a meeting on March 27 held at the Philadelphia Sketch Club. Eakins had begun to teach evening life classes at the Sketch Club in 1874, so surely he would have heard artists excitedly discussing the prospects for their inclusion in an international art show to be held in Philadelphia.

Second, one member of the Committee of Philadelphia Artists was William J. Clark Jr. who was head of the Philadelphia Sketch Club. He must have encouraged Eakins to submit works, for Clark and Eakins were friends.[3] Clark was also a critic for Philadelphia's *Daily Evening Telegraph*, one of the few who would review Eakins's art works positively.

Third, the address issued a clarion call to artists to compete with other American departments at the Centennial in displaying the best and most characteristically American work:

> Patriotism demands that American Artists should use their utmost efforts to make the Art Department of the Exhibition fully equal in all respects to the other departments by the contribution of works which will show the advancement of art in the United States during the past hundred years, and display to the best advantage the peculiar characteristics of American art.

Fourth, the address's chauvinistic language also challenged American artists to excel over their foreign counterparts:

> As contributions to the Exhibition will undoubtedly be made by the most celebrated foreign artists, and the display of foreign works will be exceedingly rich, it is peculiarly important that American painters, sculptors, architects, engravers, and other art-workers should use every endeavor to fill the space to be assigned them with performances which will do honor to the country and to the occasion.

Fifth, the address also mentioned that the Centennial's art department would be assigned a separate building of "very elegant architectural design" and "most admirably arranged for the effective display of all descriptions of Art works." After the Centennial the building would remain as a memorial hall and be used as a "national museum," another golden opportunity for American artists.

The likelihood is that Eakins was optimistic about creating a work worthy of the 1876 Centennial. It was the first major international fair to be held in the United States, and buildings were being planned to house separate departments of art, mining and metallurgy, manufactures, education and science, machinery, agriculture, and horticulture.

Philadelphia had long been a center of medicine in America. Eakins's choice of an internationally celebrated Philadelphia surgeon using scientific instruments while operating in an amphitheater surrounded by assistants in training and neophyte students, would seem to fulfill the address's exhortations to display the best that America had to offer. As will be seen later, medical displays including American-made surgical instruments and appliances would be included in several other Centennial departments. By choosing Dr. Samuel D. Gross, Eakins could emphasize both Philadelphia's contributions to American life and the heroic nature of late-nineteenth-century American surgery.[4]

Another consideration in explaining Eakins's choice of Dr. Gross is an important medical event spawned by the Centennial, and usually treated cursorily, if at all, in the art history literature. In the winter of 1874 the Philadelphia County Medical Society appointed Dr. Samuel D. Gross chairman of a committee to devise organizational plans for an International Medical Congress to be convened in Philadelphia in September 1876.

As noted before, Eakins was studying anatomy and attending surgical clinics at Jefferson Medical College in the spring of 1874. In mingling with students and faculty he very likely heard about Gross's leadership in planning for this upcoming medical event, and also about Gross's preparation for a landmark centennial history of American surgery that would be published in 1876.[5]

It must have come to Eakins's attention that several other Jefferson Medical College faculty or prominent alumni were on this important planning committee for the congress. Alumni included the secretary Dr. William B. Atkinson (JMC 1853); the American corresponding secretary Dr. Daniel G. Brinton (JMC 1860); and the foreign corresponding secretary Dr. Richard J. Dunglison (JMC 1856). On the executive committee were Jefferson faculty members Drs. William H. Pancoast and Robert E. Rogers, and alumni Drs. Washington L. Atlee (JMC 1829), Nathan L. Hatfield (JMC 1826), and Laurence Turnbull (JMC 1845).[6]

Dr. Gross complained in his autobiography that the labors of the planning committee were "immense, involving numerous meetings, a heavy and extensive correspondence, an uncommon degree of executive ability, and a considerable outlay of money," and explained that a smaller subcommittee made the final arrangements. Shortly after the congress convened on September 4, 1876, Gross was unanimously elected president.[7]

The week-long session was attended by 442 delegates including seventy-one foreigners. In his autobiography Gross singled out for praise the meeting's "highly interesting" addresses on the progress of American medicine in the preceding one hundred years. He concluded that the congress was "undoubtedly the best meeting of a medical character ever held on this continent, whether we consider the talents, scientific attainments, and position of its members, or the amount and character of its work."

Thus, Eakins's choice to paint the famous surgeon at work would both capitalize on the artist's own experiences at Jefferson Medical College and exemplify the goals of both the Centennial and the International Medical Congress.

But Eakins's bold composition was startlingly novel. His grand-scale portrait showed a contemporary surgeon at work in the operating room, an event rarely witnessed by the lay public. Although a discussion of prototypes for Eakins's composition is beyond the scope of this book, several scholars have compared *The Gross Clinic* with other images of surgeons and anatomists at work.[8] Famous dissection paintings that Eakins could have known firsthand or from widely distributed reproductions include Rembrandt's *Anatomy Lesson of Dr. Tulp* (1632) and F.-N.-A. Feyen-Perrin's *Anatomy Lesson of Dr. Velpeau* (1864). Ironically, if Eakins had missed seeing the painting of Dr. Velpeau at the Paris Salon of 1864, he assuredly would have seen it in Philadelphia in the French section of the Centennial art exhibition. Feyen-Perrin (1826-88) had attended dissections and clinics at the Charity Hospital in Paris where Dr. Armand Velpeau was chief surgeon, and some scholars have suggested but not substantiated that Eakins might have done the same.

But Eakins's painting had important differences from these prototypes. Up to then there had been relatively few major paintings of surgeons operating on a living patient, aside from scenes of battlefield surgery. One example that Eakins could have seen is *Ambroise Paré Applying Ligatures after an Amputation* (q.v.) by another French artist, Louis Matout (1811-88). Depicting the sixteenth-century French surgeon treating wounded soldiers, this painting was installed in the amphitheater of the École de Médecine in Paris in 1864.

Because it depicts the advancement of Philadelphia medicine and clinical education, *The Gross Clinic* is in the genre of medical history painting as well as portraiture. Eakins has captured on canvas Dr. Samuel D. Gross's supreme self-confidence in the surgical arena and his total command of the diverse elements of his profession. The charismatic professor is performing several tasks simultaneously. While leading a team of junior and senior assistant surgeons in an operation, Gross has paused momentarily to explain the principles and procedures to an assembly of medical students.

It is the professor of surgery who is ultimately responsible for his patient's welfare. He is also responsible for setting an example by judgment, technique, and de-

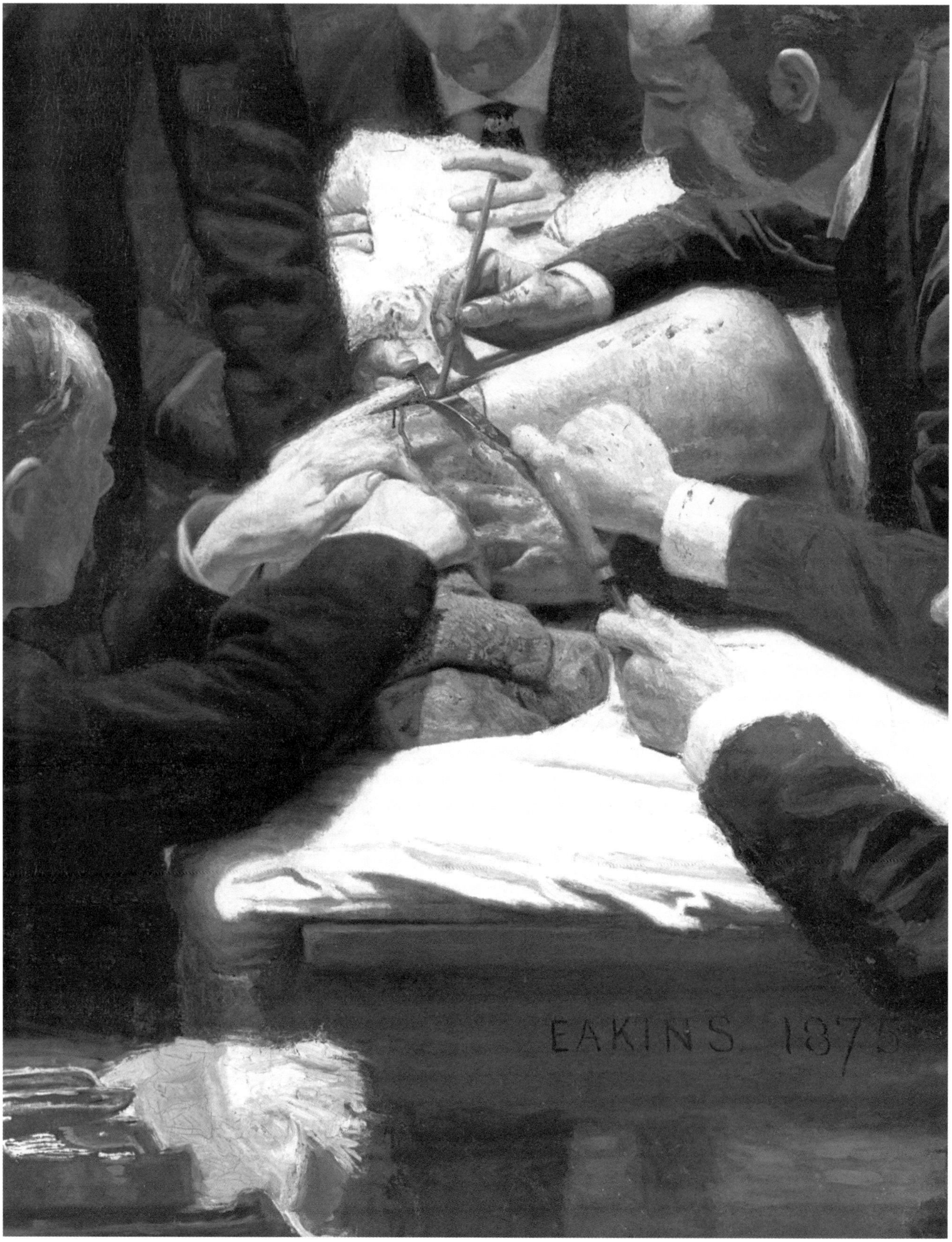

Detail: The Operative Site

portment to guide the training of and encourage participation by his surgical assistants. Further, he must educate his neophyte students about the history of the patient's disease, criteria and options for treatment, and points of surgical procedure which includes dressings and postoperative care.

Characters in the painting represent three generations of medical experience: Dr. Samuel D. Gross who is age seventy and at the pinnacle of his career, his younger surgical clinic assistants who form a hierarchy of rank among themselves, and the apprentice-like students who learn the basics from the master. Gross's instruction extended beyond the surgical arena and classroom lectures with regular reports of clinic cases to medical journals.

The graphic scene of clinical instruction takes place in an amphitheater, the upper lecture room of Jefferson Medical College's Ely Building (see chapter two). The commanding figure of Dr. Samuel D. Gross stands at the apex of a pyramidal group consisting of his surgical team, the patient, and the patient's mother. Seated to the left and behind Gross is the clinic clerk who records operative notes. In the background are students observing the proceedings from tiers of wooden benches. In the left foreground is a table with bandages and open boxes displaying trays of surgical instruments.

The adolescent male patient lies on the operating table on his right side with hips and knees bent so that his body is enigmatically foreshortened. The only exposed areas of his body are his bony buttocks and left thigh. His feet are clad in thick gray socks. His upper torso is hidden by his raised thigh and buttocks and by the arm of an assisting surgeon. His head is concealed under the anesthesia-soaked towel held by the anesthetist at the far end of the table. The patient's ailment is osteomyelitis and the purpose of the operation is to remove a segment of diseased bone from his thigh.

The cringing figure to the left of Gross has been traditionally identified as the patient's mother who, as a close relative, allegedly had the right to be present during operations on charity cases.[9] In 1875

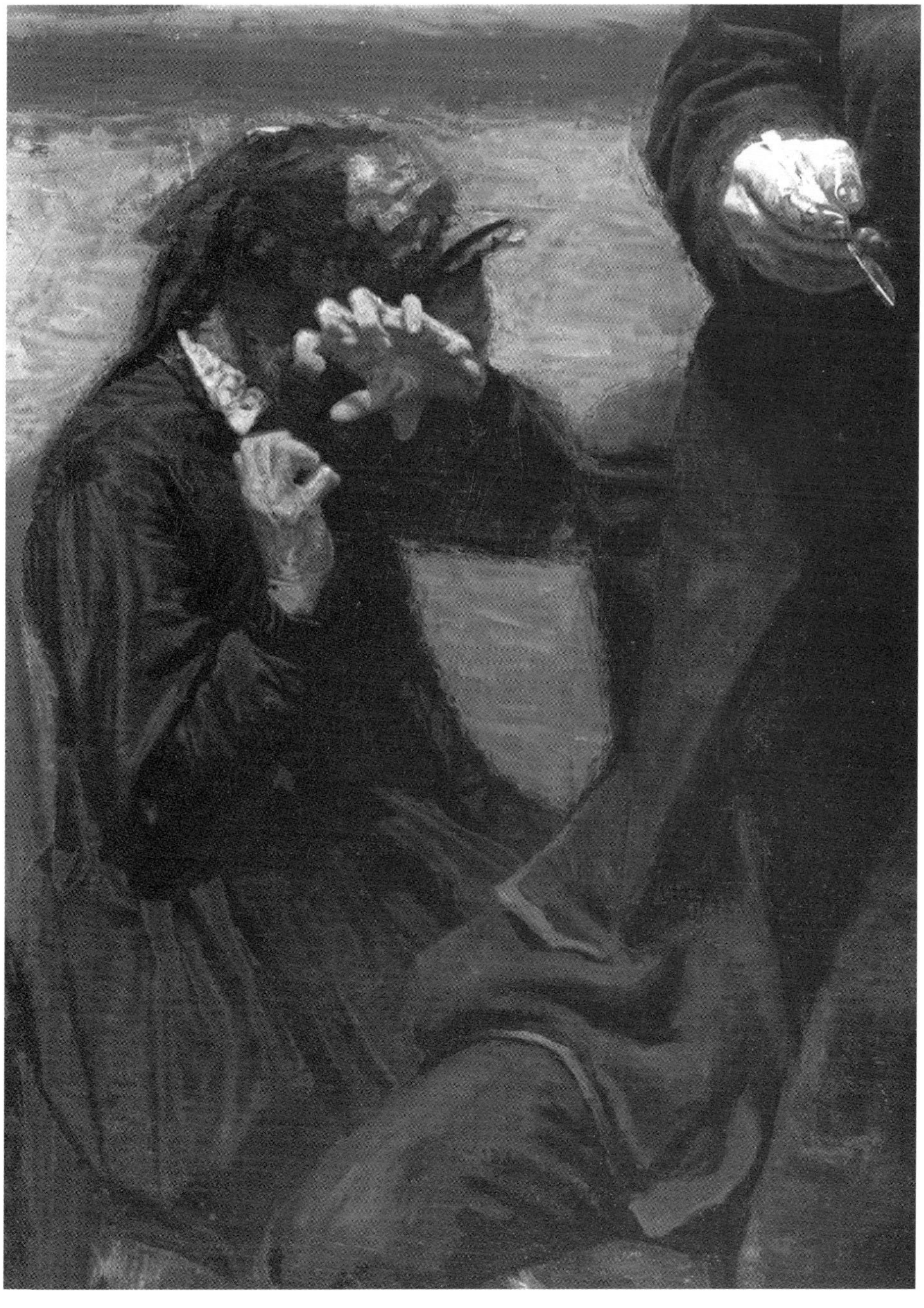

Detail: The Mother

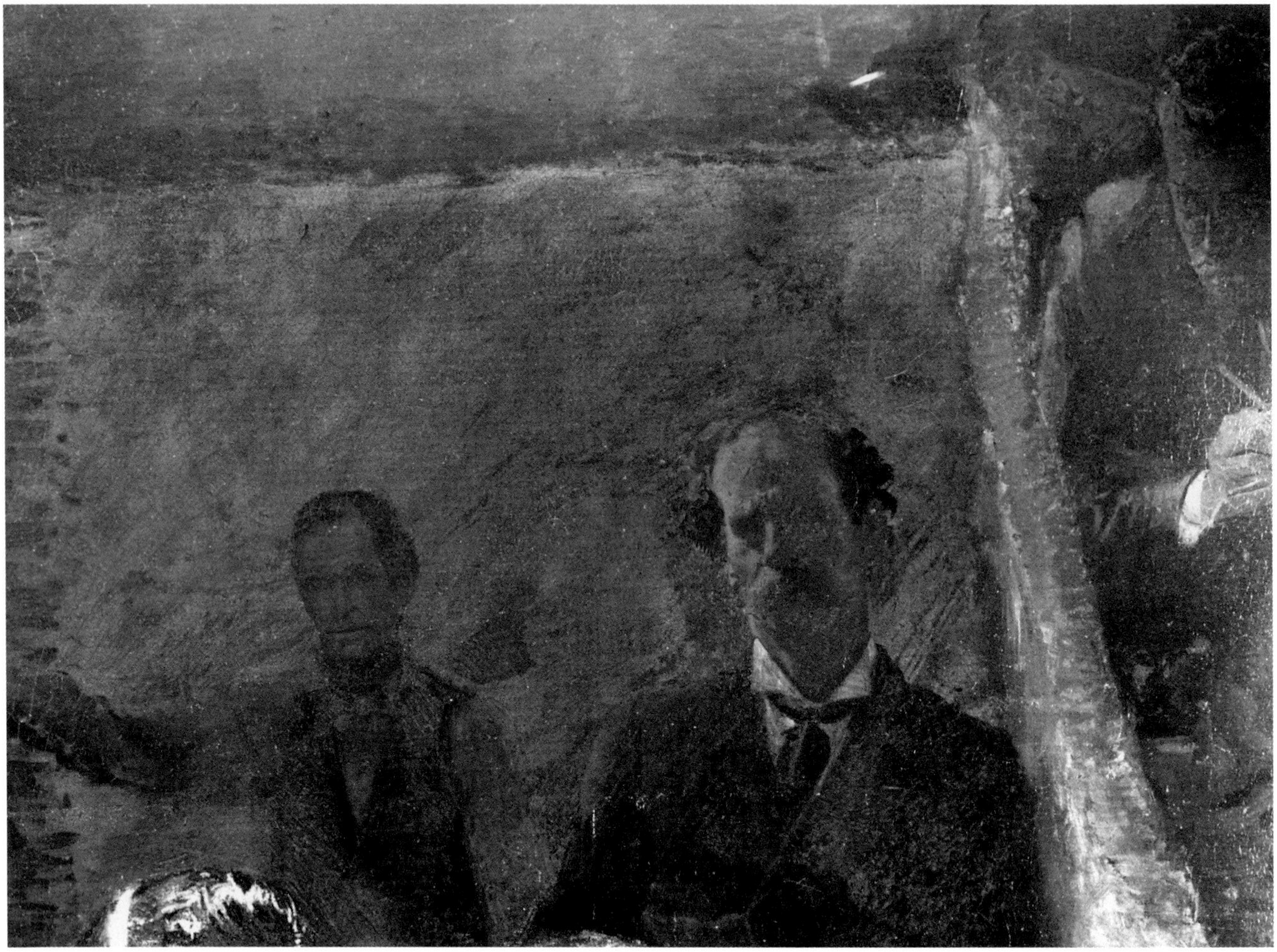

Detail: Dr. Samuel W. Gross, Hughey O'Donnell, and Thomas Eakins

there were not yet female medical students or even surgical nurses at Jefferson Medical College or most other hospitals.

Shielding her eyes from the scene, the mother is the only woman in the painting and the only figure not intensely working on or observing the operation. In contrast to all other figures whose faces are at least partially visible, her features are totally concealed by her blurred veil or scarf and her contorted hand. Her tense, agonized gesture and bony fingers are starkly juxtaposed to the relaxed, ample, and powerful hand of Gross.

As is usual in Eakins group scenes, each figure is a portrait from life. The earliest published identification of the assisting surgeons was printed beneath a reproduction of *The Gross Clinic* in Dr. George Gould's 1904

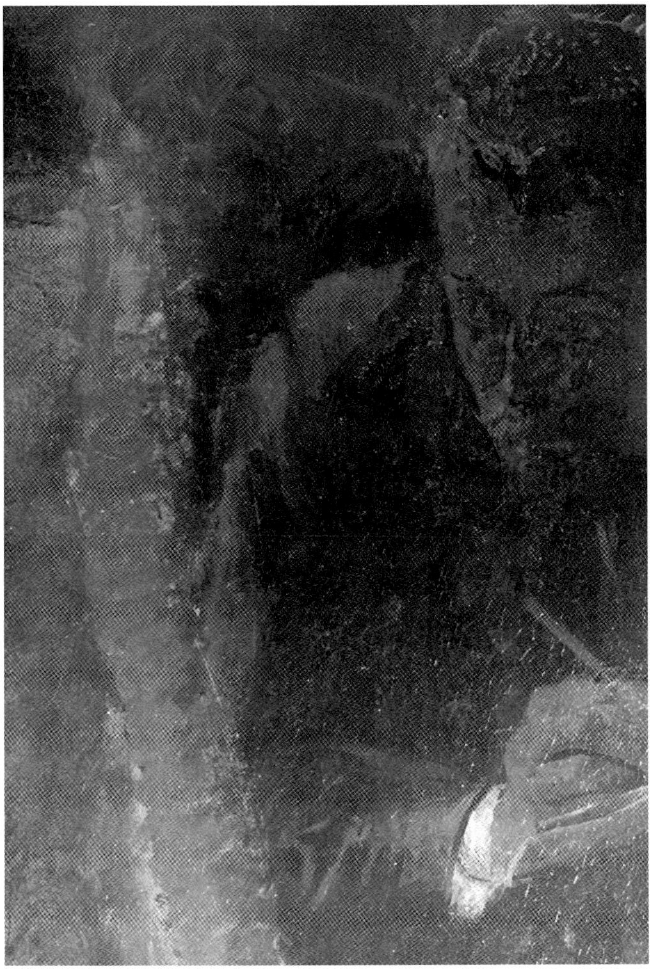

Detail: Closeup of Thomas Eakins

history of Jefferson Medical College.[10] Junior assistants are Drs. Charles S. Briggs who holds the patient's legs (lower center), and Daniel M. Appel who holds the incision open with a retractor in his right hand and holds another instrument in his left hand in a ready position (lower right). The chief of clinic is Dr. James M. Barton who bends over the patient and gently probes the incision with a tenaculum. The anesthetist is Dr. W. Joseph Hearn who is seated at the head of the table. Another unidentified assistant holding a retractor sits behind Gross and is almost totally hidden; only his left hand which holds a retractor in the incision, and the right side of his body are visible. The clinic clerk recording the proceedings at the lectern is Dr. Franklin West (center left).

The two figures standing in the adjacent tunnel are Dr. Samuel W. Gross, with his shoulder against the wall, on the right, and the orderly Hughey O'Donnell, with his arm outstretched, on the left. O'Donnell was a faithful orderly in the surgical clinic for many years. The seated figure writing or sketching to the right of the tunnel railing is thought by most Eakins scholars to be a self-portrait of the artist. An observer like the other students, his head is tilted down as he looks intently toward the operation. He is writing or sketching on a small pad.[11] Eakins had already included himself in earlier paintings of outdoor scenes, where he felt similarly comfortable in the surroundings.

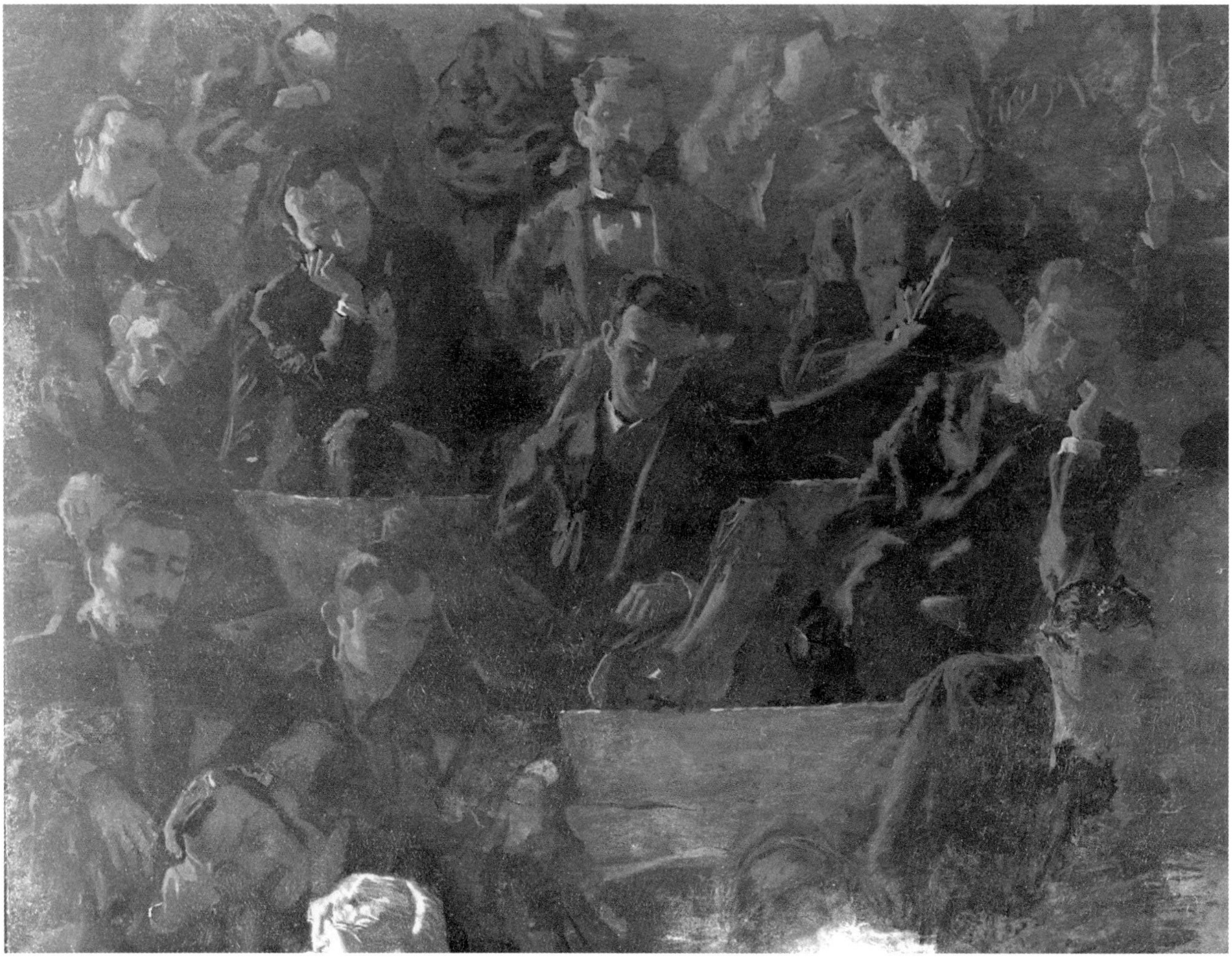

Detail: Students (left)

According to painting conservators, the dimly lit figures of students high above the surgery were thinly painted and have lost much detail over the years. They sit on the hard wooden benches in varied postures: a few leaning forward intently with chin on hand or holding on to the railing, some with legs crossed or casually raised to the chest, others slumping with fatigue or ennui. The only figure identified so far is Eakins's friend, the poet Robert C. V. Meyers, posing as a student. He is seated with chin on hand in the top row over the tunnel.

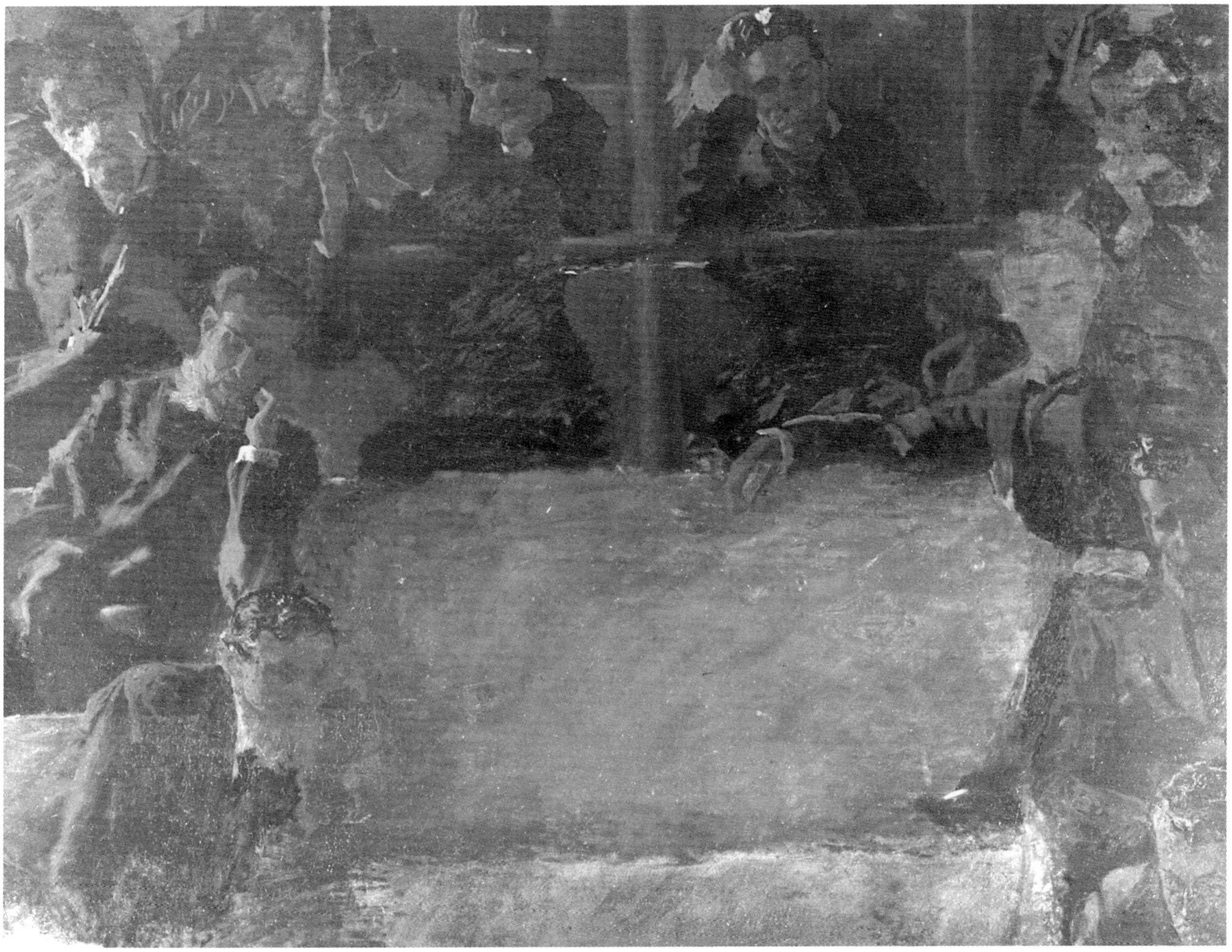

Detail: Students (right)

The painting is prevalently and relentlessly dark in tone. The students barely emerge from the murky background of the upper reaches of the amphitheater. All figures are dressed in dark everyday clothes, as was customary at the time. At first the viewer's attention is drawn to Dr. Gross with his high-domed forehead bathed in light pouring in through the overhead skylight of the upper lecture room. Before the advent of electricity surgery took place only during the brightest, midday hours.

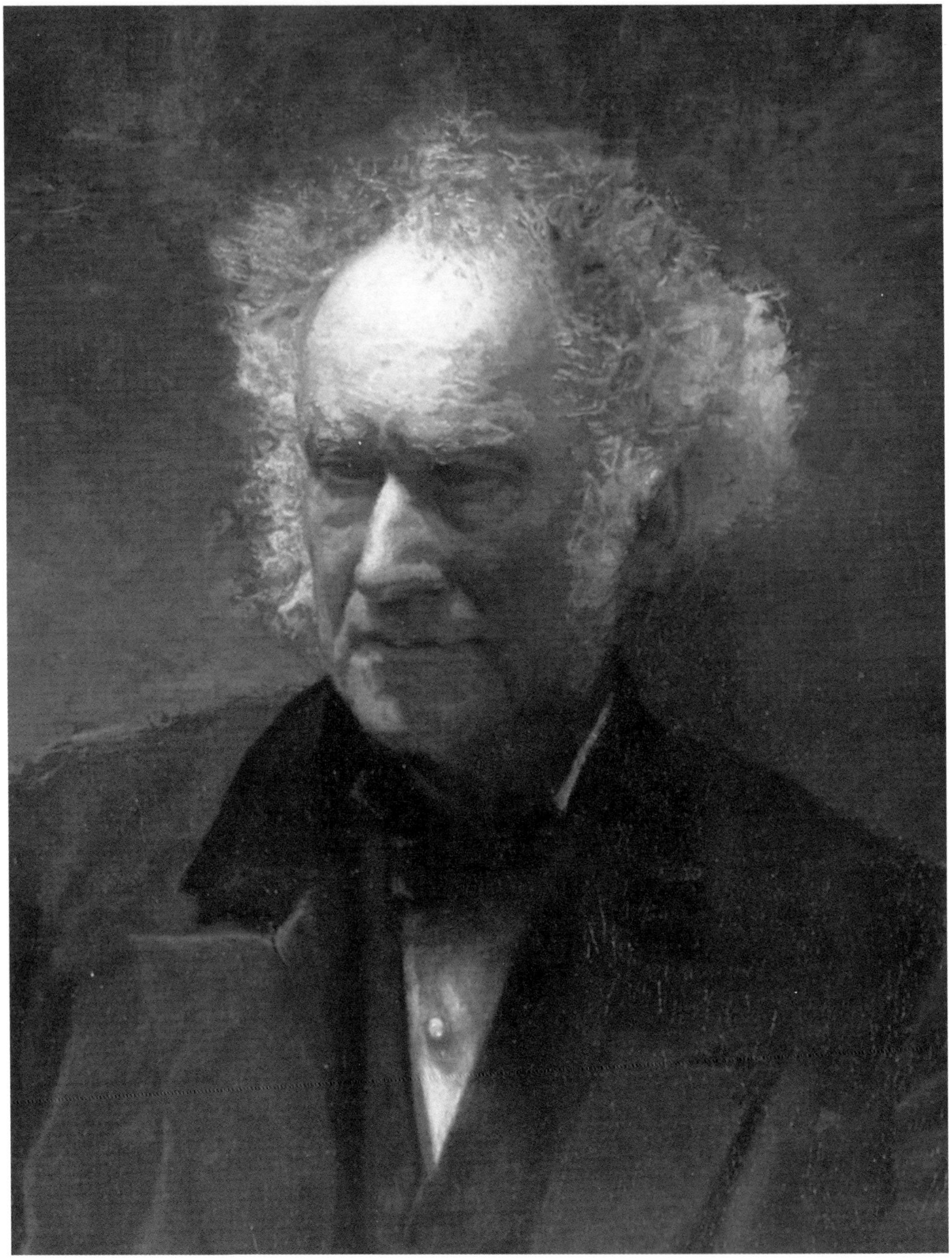

Detail: Head of Dr. Gross

The light is present both literally and symbolically to emphasize the surgeon's great intellect. His extraordinary, wiry, iron-gray hair and side whiskers form a spotlighted aura around his face. His strong, aquiline nose and firm chin are sculpturally defined by the dramatic contrasts of bright light and deep shade on his features. His sober expression exemplifies intense concentration and dedication to duty.

Dr. Gross, the only participant standing erect, is the apex of a pyramidal arrangement of seated, kneeling, and crouching foreground figures. The base is formed by the case of surgical instruments and the bottom edge of the operating table. Gross has momentarily turned away from the operative site to explain the procedure, but he is still physically connected to it. He leans the weight of his left arm on the table adjacent to the busy hands of his assistants. Gross's right hand holds his scalpel poised to resume his work.

Since the surgical team is situated at the center of the "pit," surrounded on all sides by onlookers, viewers of the painting become surrogates for the students seated opposite the visible students in the background. One feels included in the action because Eakins has omitted the railing and low wall in the foreground, a barrier that would have psychologically isolated the painted figures from the viewers. In practice, the elevated students could see very little of the procedure from their vantage point, so the professor's verbal explanation was vital to their understanding.

Most viewers shift their attention from Gross's face to his highlighted right hand holding the scalpel. His hand and instrument are stained with lustrous, wet, crimson blood. If there were any doubt, this makes it emphatically clear that Dr. Gross is a participant in, not a mere explicator of, the operation.

Then observers are attracted to the patient resting on the bright white linens of the operating table, by means of several compositional devices. The downward thrust of Gross's left arm and the scalpel are strong elements leading to the table and the patient. The anesthetist's dark hair has a wide part pointing down toward the operative site. The heads, arms, hands, and instruments of the hovering assistants all lead toward the incision. Even the fringed end of the striped fabric under the box of surgical instruments appears to flutter toward the operating table.

Fresh blood oozes from the patient's wound. More drops of blood stain the table linens, and the shirt cuffs, hands, and instruments of the assistants. This spattering of blood, the ungainly posture of the patient, and the gaping wound in his thigh are taken as a necessary matter of course by the absorbed medical professionals.

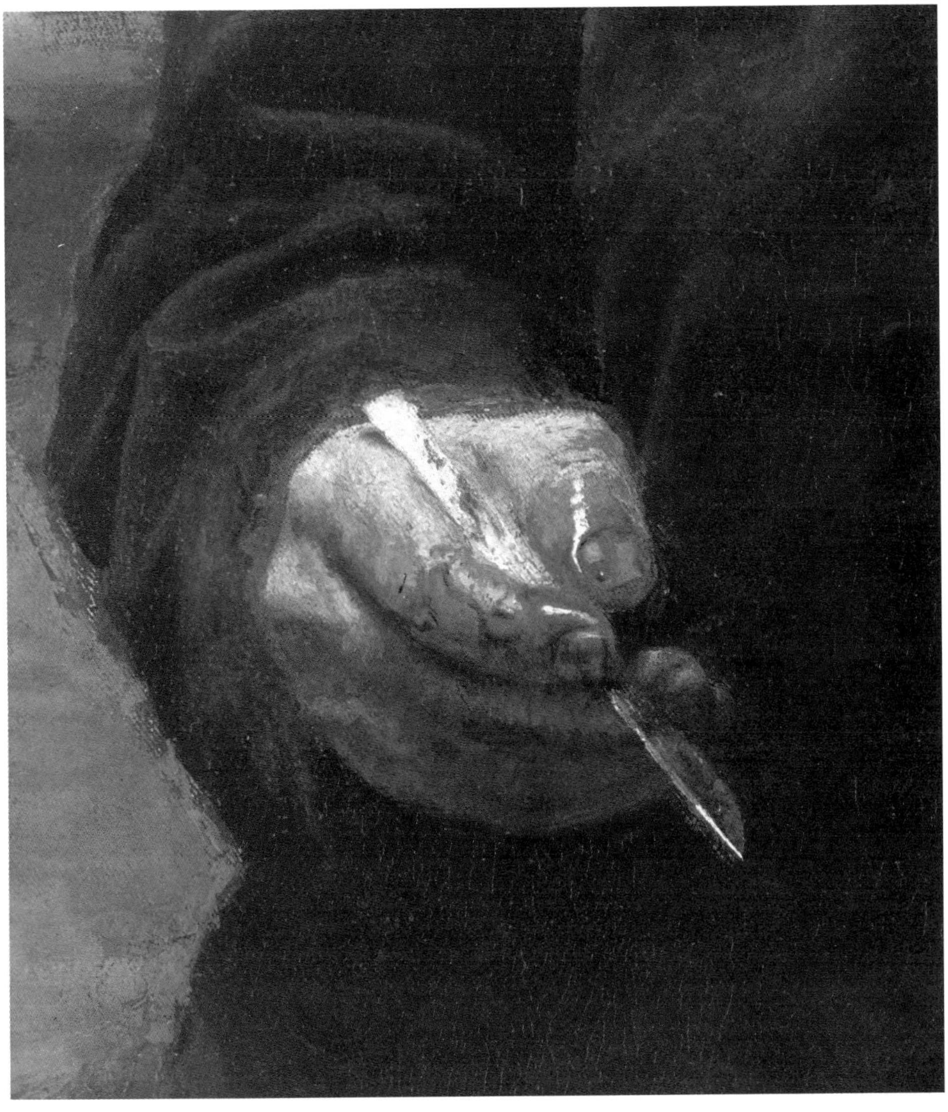

Detail: Hand of Dr. Gross

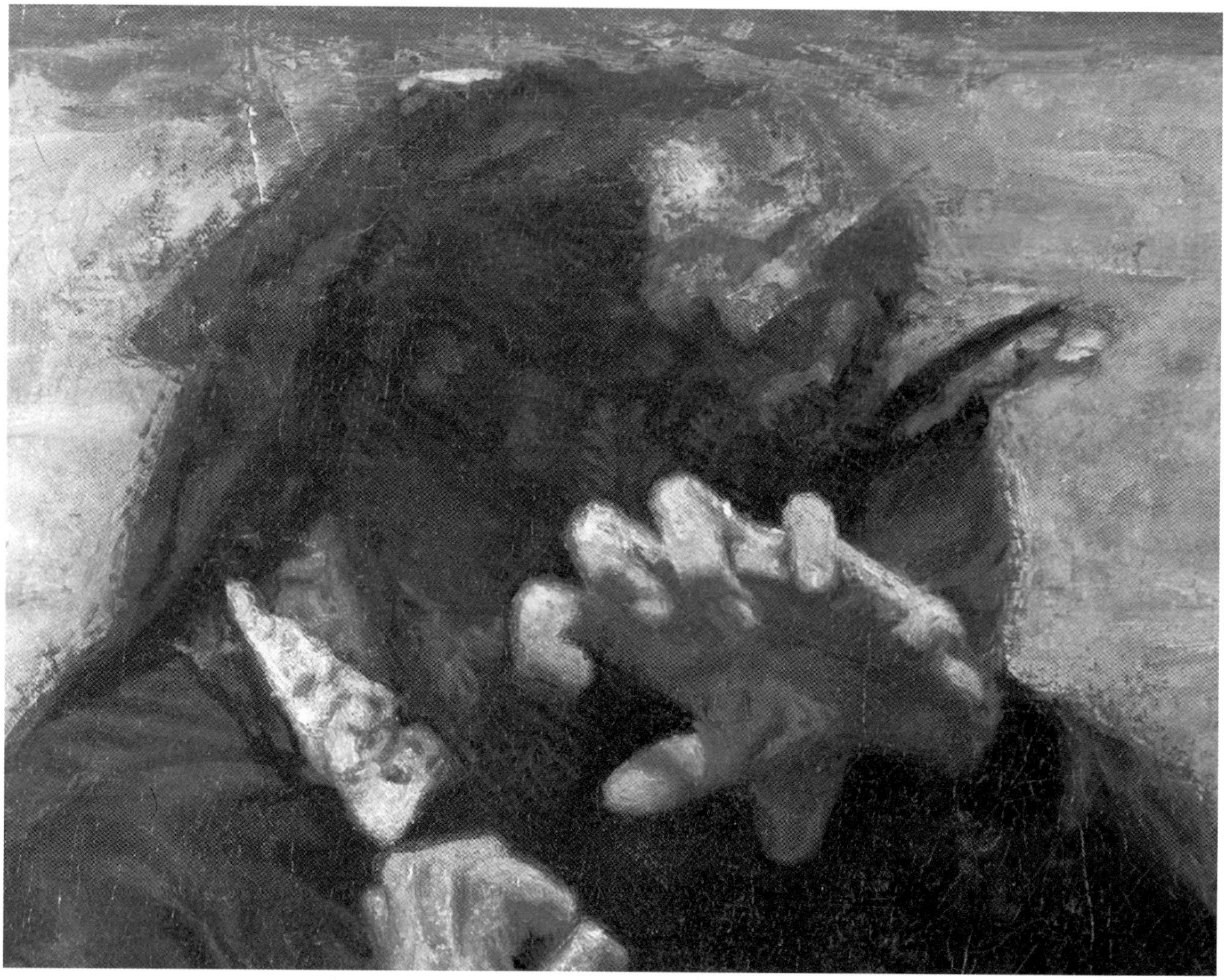

Detail: Head of the Mother

The only nonmedical person in the painting responds differently. The elderly woman is so distraught at seeing the unconscious young man undergoing the bloody procedure and hearing the unfamiliar sounds of instruments sawing, scraping, hammering, and chiseling bone, that she turns away and covers her eyes with tensely clenched, clawlike hands. Though shunted off to the side and ignored by all the participants and observers, she is nevertheless linked to them: her raised left elbow almost imperceptibly touches the right shoulder of the partially hidden assistant seated behind Dr. Gross.

Her disproportionately small, shrouded figure and agitated gesture send a strong, emotional signal that contradicts the self-assured composure of all the other characters. Though the patient's life was not at risk and the mother was certainly informed that the humane procedure would save her son's diseased leg, she looks petrified by the unfamiliar setting. Assuredly her silent suffering and cringing gesture went unnoted by the scribe's account of that day's surgical clinic. The routine operation was probably proceeding smoothly according to plan.

The requirement for the presence of a parent or close relative in the amphitheater has still not been explicitly verified, according to Gert H. Brieger, M.D., Ph.D., the William H. Welch Professor at the Johns Hopkins University, Institute of the History of Medicine.[12] Brieger expressed skepticism for the "common wisdom among art historians that in charity cases a relative of the patient was required to be present," for he was unable to find "any discussion of such a requirement for a relative's presence." On the other hand, Brieger commented that melodrama was not Eakins's "stock in trade," he was not a "frivolous reporter" and his realism permitted "no such casual intrusion," so, therefore, he must have observed such a scene. Brieger concludes that while a relative's presence was probably not stipulated, one interpretation could be that "Eakins here tried to suggest parental consent."

While the woman's cringing gesture is explicitly emotional, drama in the painting is heightened by artistic means. It occurs visually by the use of color: the monochromatic palette punctuated by bright red, and by the use of light: the prevailing darkness contrasted with spotlighted areas. It also occurs from motion and muscular tension in the participants. Dr. Gross has just turned away from the patient and his scalpel is still poised to return to the operation. The assistant surgeons are actively retracting or probing the incision, applying the anesthesia, or holding the patient's limbs. The clinic clerk is writing operative notes. Even the patient's blood is in motion, oozing from the wound and flowing or spattering onto the white linens and hands of the surgeons. Members of the audience are variously engaged, like the artist who writes or sketches, and students who are alternately eager or preoccupied.

Eakins has depicted a scene witnessed by few outside the medical establishment. According to medical historian Charles Rosenberg, middle-class patients were usually diagnosed and treated, even surgically, at their homes, or at endowed private hospitals. Prior to about 1880 no one wanted to enter a public hospital "except for that small minority of the least enterprising and lacking in self-respect." Most hospital patients were from the ranks of the working poor, and the hospital was an object of fear and an "asylum for the dependent and socially isolate." Though some of their fears were based on largely unsubstantiated rumors about unauthorized medical experimentation, cruel treatment, and desecration of bodies, still many hospital wards were in fact crowded, unclean, and badly ventilated. Before distinctions were made between the contagious and the noncontagious, many patients suffered from wound infections, dysentery, erysipelas, childbed fever, and typhus.[13]

The Gross Clinic was painted in 1875, two years before Jefferson Medical College's first official hospital was opened. A late-twentieth-century viewer only familiar with the sterile conditions of modern hospitals can hardly imagine the slow evolution that led to accommodations for patients treated in the surgical clinics of Gross's day. The following description appeared in an address delivered by Jefferson surgeon Dr. John H. Brinton in 1880:[14]

> In the early days of the [college] clinics, I mean after 1841, patients who had undergone serious operations were sent to their homes in carriages, under the charge of a clinical clerk. A little later, about 1843 or 1844, one or two rooms were rented from a stove-maker, over his shop, at the S.W. corner of Tenth and Sansom Streets, and thither grave cases operated upon before the class were conveyed and treated. After a while these accommodations proved insufficient to meet the wants of the growing clinics, and in 1849 or '50, a floor and a half or two floors were rented over a bottling establishment, then standing on the ground now occupied by the laboratories of the College. In the course of a few years, additional room having become necessary, this building was remodelled, and a very comfortable sort of miniature hospital was arranged, capable of accommodating fourteen or fifteen patients. This opened directly into the College building, and [there was a] fireproof door through which patients were carried from the clinical amphitheatre to their beds...This small hospital served its purpose from 1843 until...1877 when the new Jefferson College Hospital was officially opened.

Brinton's memoir also described patient care and resident doctors' duties:

> The kitchen stove of the family below furnished the patients' diet, a nurse at so much a week cared for them, and the clinical clerks were the resident doctors. Hard worked these latter were, too. For my part, I can remember many a night of waking and bedside watching within those narrow, cramped, and musty walls. I have sat since then at many a well-ordered table, but never have I relished dainties as I did then the savory oyster and steaming midnight cup of coffee served by the order of a crafty Faculty to ensure the wakefulness of the fagged-out watcher.

Eakins's painting is the only visual depiction extant of the Ely Building's upper lecture room. A verbal description by Dr. Albert P. Brubaker (JMC 1874) gives a student's perception of the building's superimposed lecture rooms:[15]

> The lower lecture room was dark for the most part in daytime by reason of brown walls and opaque, dirty window glass, and in the late afternoon by reason of small, feebly illuminating gas jets. At all times the atmosphere was none too fresh nor the floor too clean. The upper lecture room fortunately was bright and cheery by reason of its skylight, white walls and white wood work. The benches in both rooms were hard and lacking in polish, which made a change in position highly desirable, but not any more satisfactory.

Although the figures in *The Gross Clinic* are spotlighted from above, an observer would imagine that the room was prevalently dark, certainly not the "bright and cheery" room described by Brubaker. Since Eakins only shows four rows of students next to the tunnel and very little of the surrounding architecture, a viewer would never infer the vastness of the actual space and the distance from the operative site of those unfortunate students seated in the topmost rows. The upper lecture room in the Ely Building had been enlarged in 1846 to accommodate six hundred seats. The seats were arranged in an octagonal shape giving the effect of a curving amphitheater. The amphitheater of the 1877 hospital also held six hundred people and was circular in shape.

A physical description of the amphitheater and its accoutrements and of Dr. Samuel D. Gross's appearance and demeanor is found in an address about Dr. Gross made in 1912 by surgery professor Dr. John Chalmers DaCosta (JMC 1885). He explained that the clinic room of 1912 was not the one seen in the Eakins portrait of Gross, and that the room shown in that picture is the upstairs lecture room of the old college building on Tenth Street:[16]

> The floor of the old clinic room was of wood...To the west side...was a sink, and at this side doors opened into a passage way. The operating table was made of heavy wood, and its only motion was one of rotation on a pivot. When it was expected that much blood was going to be shed, several low open boxes of sawdust were brought in to catch some of it. Several little tables were placed around the periphery of the bull ring, and on them were put open instrument cases, marine sponges, collodion, lint, absorbent cotton, bandages, rubber and isinglass adhesive plaster, basins of water, silk ligatures, wax, silver wire, needles and sometimes cautery irons, and a charcoal brasier to heat the irons. There were also numerous suspender clips. Dr. Hearn had suggested suspender clips to catch and hold bleeding vessels, a clear anticipation of the hemostat. (Before that time, the only method of catching vessels was to pick each one up with a sharp hook known as a tenaculum, and hold it until the ligature was fastened...) If one looked into the instrument cases, he noticed that the knives had ivory handles and this fact, of course, made boiling out of the question.

Eakins omitted most of the objects listed above in order to concentrate his focus on the great surgeon and on a closeup view of assistants gathered around the patient. He included only one table with surgical materials. Although placed in the extreme foreground the two open boxes of instruments are deliberately blurred, compared with the sharply outlined figures immediately behind.

Of all those physicians trained by Gross and depicted in *The Gross Clinic*, his son Dr. Samuel W. Gross became the most famous. Two others who came to be well known surgeons were Drs. William Joseph Hearn (1842-1917) and James Morrie Barton (1846-1926).

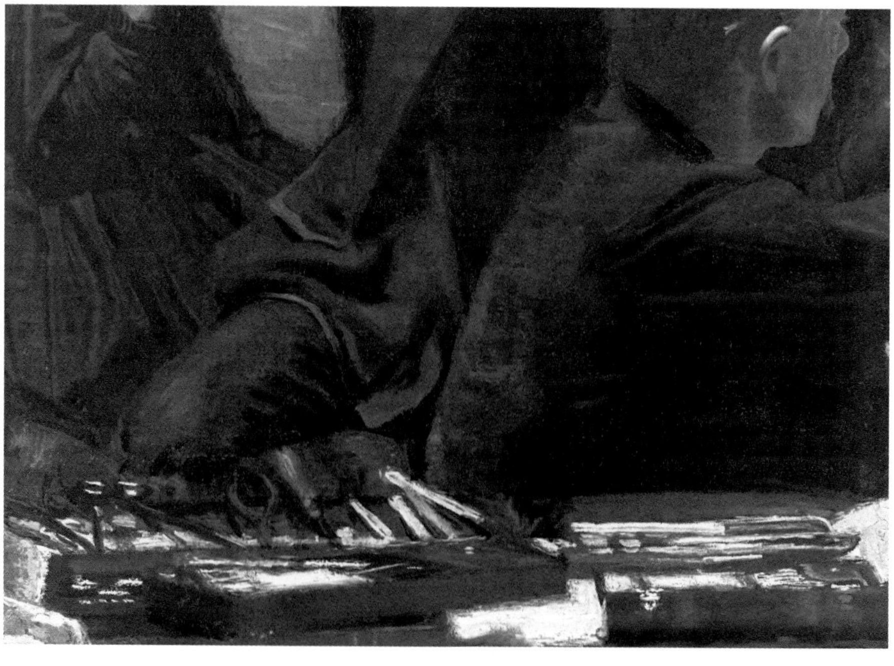

Detail: Table with Surgical Instruments

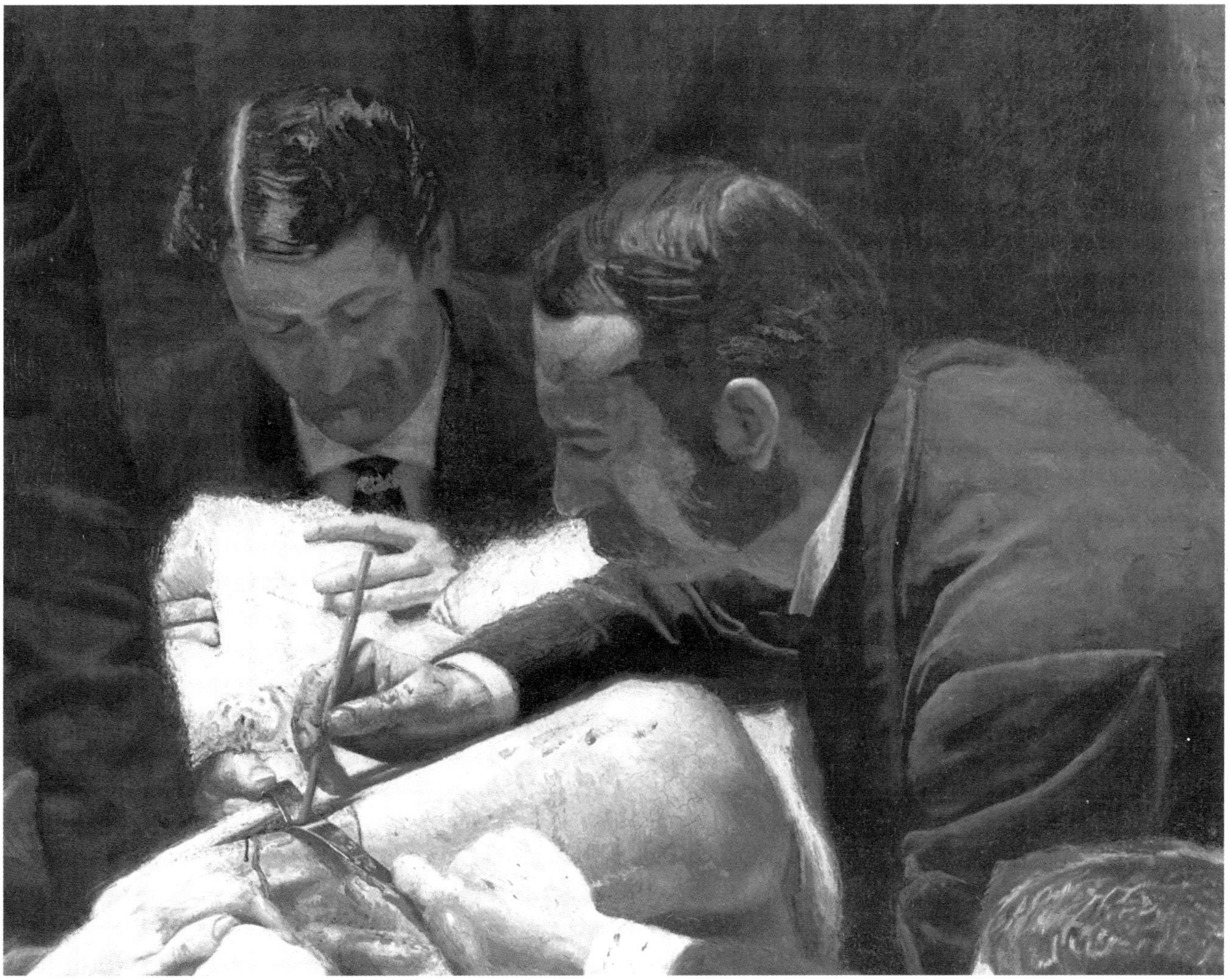

Detail: Drs. W. Joseph Hearn and James M. Barton

Dr. W. Joseph Hearn had a particularly versatile career. A native of Laurel, Delaware, he graduated from Jefferson Medical College in 1867. After practicing medicine briefly in Delaware, he returned to Philadelphia in 1870 to succeed Dr. Francis F. Maury as private assistant and anesthetizer for Dr. Samuel D. Gross. He also administered anesthesia in Dr. Joseph Pancoast's clinic for the last five years of his tenure.

Hearn was named Dr. Gross's chief of clinic when the new hospital opened in 1877, inaugurating the outpatient surgical department. In 1882 he was named surgeon to the hospital by the new professor, Dr. Samuel W. Gross. That same year he was also named surgeon to the Philadelphia Hospital, succeeding Dr. John H. Brinton.

At the Jefferson Medical College he was assistant demonstrator of anatomy (1871-79), assistant demonstrator of surgery (1879-82), and clinical professor of surgery beginning in 1894. Hearn also taught courses in dermatology and genito-urinary diseases, and was the first at Jefferson to teach a course in the microscopy and histology of tumors. He also taught operative surgery and bandaging at Dr. George McClellan's School of Anatomy.

The class of 1907 dedicated its yearbook to Dr. Hearn, and quoted Dr. W. W. Keen's oft-repeated remark to students: "I feel very much safer during a difficult operation, if I can have Prof. Hearn at my elbow and receive the benefit of his cool head and steady hand." Dr. Hearn was made emeritus clinical professor of surgery in 1910.

Hearn was one of the early surgeons to trephine and remove a portion of the motor cortex for epilepsy and to tap the lateral ventricles for hydrocephalus. His operation for diverticulum of the esophagus was the second ever performed.

The Jeffersonian of April 1902 printed a biographical sketch of Hearn noting that his "long and intimate association with that master of surgery, Samuel D. Gross, afforded him a vast experience, and one rarely equalled." The article mentioned that Hearn was depicted administering anesthesia in the "celebrated and much-cherished oil-painting by Thomas Eakins of Prof. Samuel D. Gross operating in his clinic."

Hearn's son, Dr. William Prettyman Hearn (JMC 1899), also practiced surgery and became assistant professor at Jefferson Medical College. His grandson, Dr. William P. Hearn Jr., graduated with the Jefferson class of 1935.

Dr. James M. Barton entered Jefferson Medical College in 1865 as a private student of Dr. Benjamin H. Rand and graduated three years later. After a year as resident physician at the Episcopal Hospital he served as Dr. Samuel D. Gross's chief clinical assistant for ten years starting in 1869. He helped him in office practice and in private operations, as well as attending to his practice during the professor's frequent absences from the city.

At Jefferson Medical College Barton had charge of a surgical quiz section (1869-76) and was an assistant demonstrator of anatomy (1869-74). He was made professor of surgery and surgeon to the Jefferson College Hospital in 1882. He also taught operative surgery at the Philadelphia School of Anatomy and Operative Surgery from 1874 to 1881. He served as surgeon to the Charity Hospital (1869-79) and the German Hospital (1879-86), and was made surgeon to the Philadelphia Hospital in 1889.

Barton was best known for pioneering work in abdominal surgery. He was in charge of the surgical department of the *Philadelphia Medical Times* from 1882 to 1890, and was the author of numerous reviews, translations, and articles.

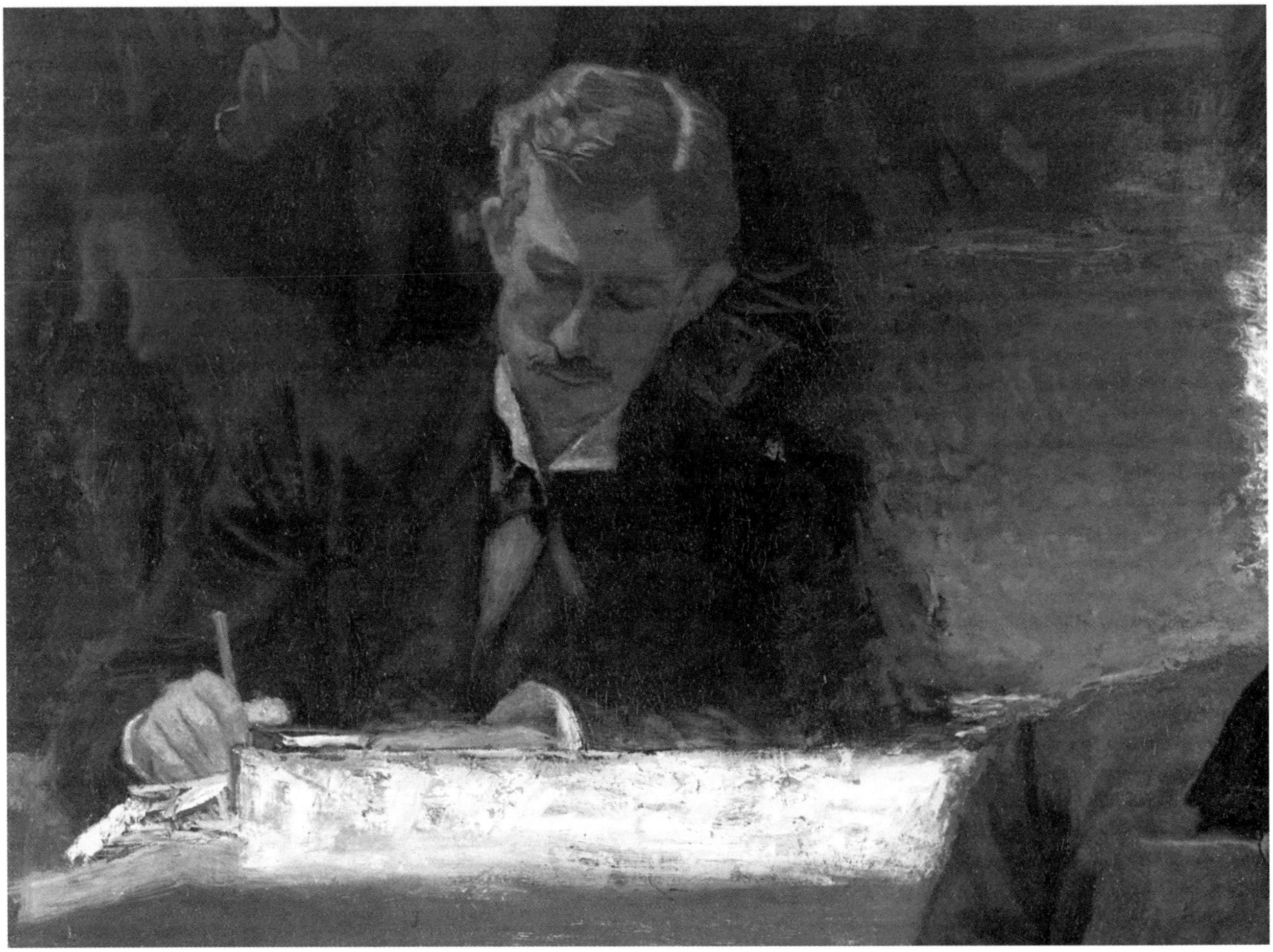

Detail: Dr. Franklin West

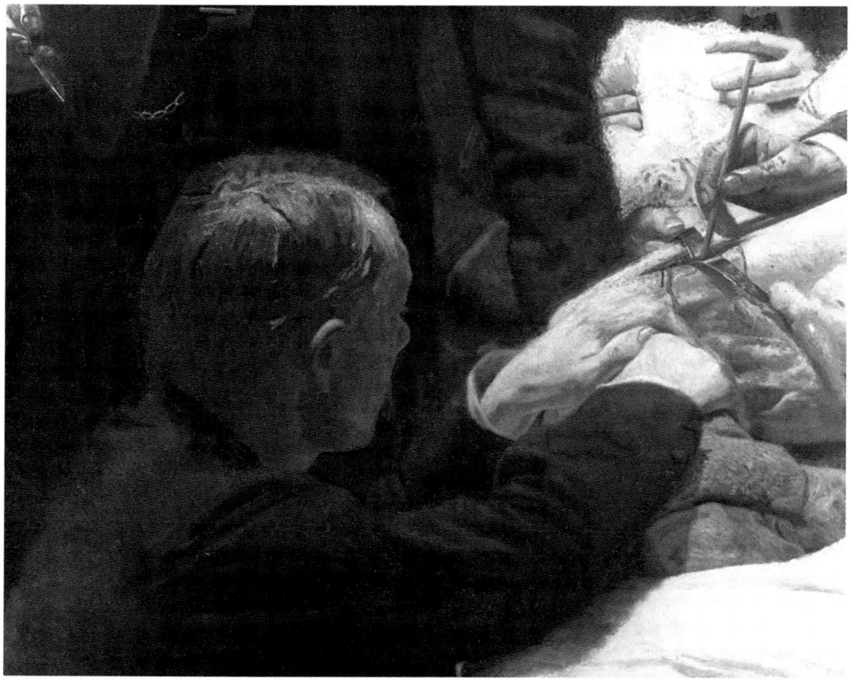

Detail: Dr. Charles S. Briggs

Dr. Franklin West (JMC 1873), the recorder in *The Gross Clinic,* became prosector to the professor of surgery and curator of the anatomical and pathological museum after his graduation. Dr. Charles S. Briggs, a surgical assistant, had been sent to study under Dr. Gross by his father, Dr. William T. Briggs, a surgeon and obstetrician in Nashville; the younger Briggs became a professor of surgery at the University of Nashville. Dr. Daniel M. Appel, a surgical assistant, was immortalized in the painting the very year he graduated from Jefferson Medical College in 1875. Of all the assistants he is literally the lowest in the painting and the farthest from Professor Gross.

The setting of *The Gross Clinic* can be more fully understood by looking at another image in the Jefferson collection.

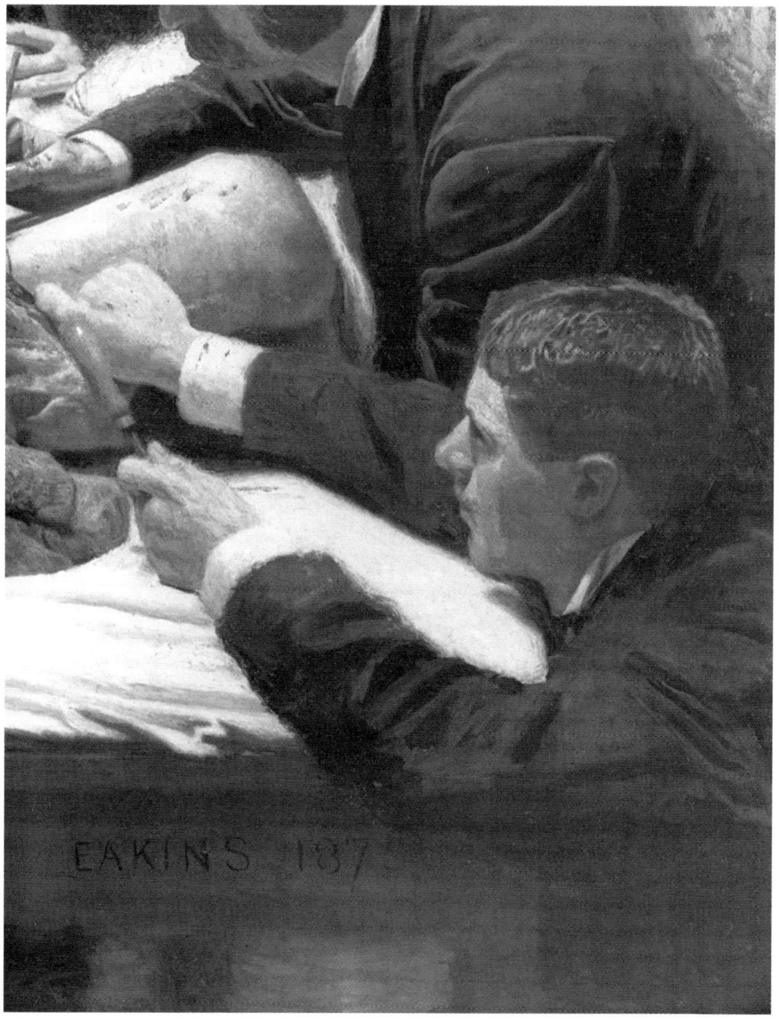

Detail: Dr. Daniel Appel

Clinic in Amphitheater of 1877 Jefferson Hospital

CLINIC IN AMPHITHEATER OF 1877 HOSPITAL
By unknown photographer

Modern copy of published photograph
Ca. 1890s
8 x 10 in.

Given by unknown donor after 1900
Accession number: 1900+f.Ph.17

This photograph depicts the amphitheater of the 1877 Jefferson Hospital in the 1890s, and gives a sense of the vast, soaring space of the room which had approximately the same dimensions as the amphitheater of the Ely Building shown in *The Gross Clinic*. The second amphitheater was located in a two-story wing attached to the new five-story hospital, and Dr. Samuel D. Gross had been given the honor of performing the first operation there.

The presence of a nurse and the style of her uniform assist in estimating the date of this medical clinic to be the 1890s. None of the figures seated on the floor around the patient has been identified. Notice the marble bust of Dr. George McClellan over the doorway.

Modern surgeons might look askance at the more public nature of surgery in Dr. Gross's day; other Jefferson faculty as well as distinguished American and foreign visitors were made welcome in the clinic. In spite of Gross's protests to the contrary, the operation *was* a kind of spectacle, with the patient as its unwitting vehicle. Inherently dramatic was the professor's formal en-

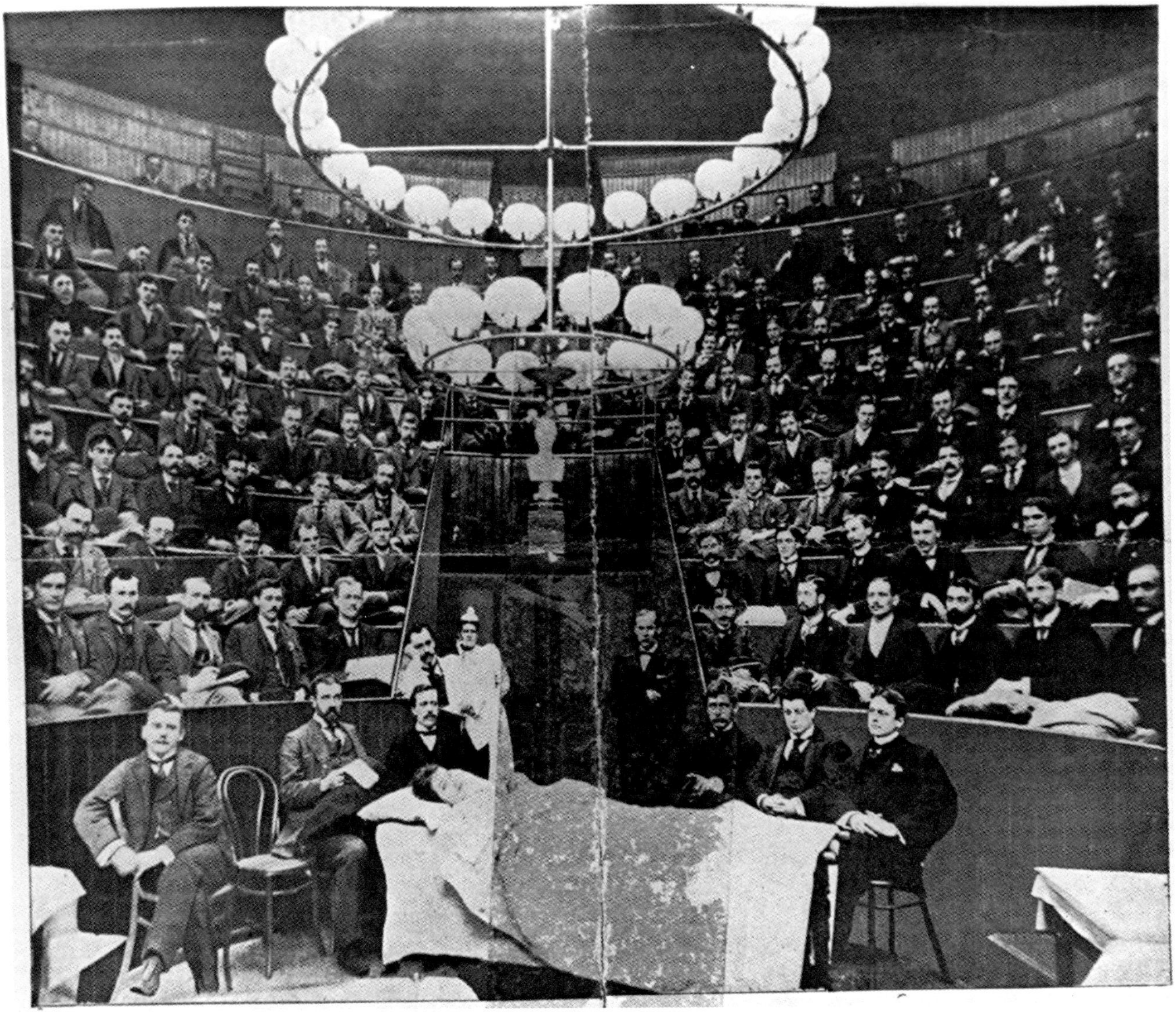

trance into the arena, followed by a physically and mentally rigorous, often lifesaving action in the center of the room. The performance could almost be likened to theater in the round, but unlike some colleagues Gross expressly forbade applause.

The following description by Dr. John Chalmers DaCosta actually referred to Gross's procedures in the 1877 amphitheater, but his customary habits corresponded to those in the earlier hall:

> Precisely at 12.30, Dr. Gross followed by his assistants, entered the arena. After them came a number of physicians from other departments, several of the surgeons of the hospital, and any visitors who happened to be present. The onlookers took seats on chairs arranged around the arena.

DaCosta recalled,

> He always made medical visitors welcome, and was accustomed to introduce them to the class. Every visiting foreign physician or surgeon came to Gross's clinic as a matter of course, felt it an honor to see him and to meet him, and was profoundly gratified at the hospitable reception that was extended to him...
>
> His entry into the lecture room was always most dignified. He strongly objected to applause, and never failed to remonstrate if it were attempted, insisting that it was particularly out of place in the hospital where the dramatic should be unknown. He never missed lectures and always entered the lecture room precisely on the hour...
>
> I can see the venerable Dr. Gross, white haired, erect and handsome, with one hand raised as he lectured just as you can see him now in the Eakins picture.

Interestingly, Eakins included no extraneous guests in *The Gross Clinic,* only the shadowy figures in the tunnel: Dr. S. W. Gross (who attended his father's clinics regularly) and Hughey O'Donnell who might have been on call. Aside from the younger Gross, there are no Jefferson faculty members or visiting American or foreign dignitaries. The presiding surgeon is plainly lecturing to the Jefferson students, not "playing" to unseen colleagues. Eakins's interpretation stresses his seriousness of purpose.

In reading DaCosta's description of Gross, even allowing for DaCosta's florid prose, one can see that Eakins has depicted Gross's character with far greater penetration and incisiveness than had Samuel B. Waugh in his portrait the year before:

> [Gross] was one of the handsomest and one of the most distinguished looking of men...He was tall and well made and moved with a dignified gait. He had a noble head, a broad high forehead, snow-white hair and small white whiskers, characteristic of gentlemen of the old school. His nose was large and significant of character. His chin was strong and his mouth, though usually firm set with a sense of his grim responsibilities and haunting cares, was prone to break into the sweetest and most gracious of smiles...His eyes were princely with courage. His forehead was royal of the truth. His voice was deep, clear and impressive and he could be distinctly heard by all even when an audience was very large. His words were admirably chosen and he usually spoke slowly which seemed to add to their force. He was the very embodiment of professional and professorial dignity and the beau ideal of a wise and learned surgeon.

DaCosta described Gross as an animated and forceful teacher who maintained that the didactic lecture tells the student what he is to *believe,* and the clinical lecture shows him what he is to *see.* They supplement each other, but neither can teach a man what to *do.* He must learn the latter as an intern, an assistant, or a practitioner. DaCosta continued,

> There never was a greater teacher of surgery...He knew exactly how to talk to capture the student's interest and to make him understand. He was animated, full of movement, profoundly interested himself in what he was doing...He was systematic, thorough, clear, absolutely convincing...He used plain English words. He often quoted his contemporaries...with kindly respect when they deserved it, but he denounced in unsparing terms, false pretence, gallery playing, questionable statistics, careless reports and anything that savored of professional dishonor...Now and then he liked to tell an anecdote in order to fix a point in the memory. He used to say: "A mere statement is a nail driven in a board. A story bends the point of the nail, and holds it fast in place."

Dr. DaCosta commented further about the clothing of Dr. Gross and his assistants and about the professor's notions of antisepsis:

> He always dressed with scrupulous care. In the college lecture room he wore a long frock coat; in the operating room, a long dark blue coat which, in accordance with the custom of the times, showed the signs of many sanguinary combats with surgical disease. The antiseptic method was just being put to trial and some years were to elapse before it was to come into general use. The assistants wore old jackets of blue cloth or duck.

DaCosta described Gross's suit as dark blue and said

that his assistants also wore blue. Was he mistaken about the color? Today all the costumes in the painting are black, except for those of Dr. Barton and the hidden surgeon whose suits have a very dark bluish-gray cast. It is not known if Eakins rendered them black or dark blue originally, but darkening of pigment over the decades would not be an unusual occurrence. Also, this painting has undergone numerous restorations without written reports, starting as early as 1915 long before painting conservation was an exacting science with rigorous standards of faithfulness to the original art work and with reversible treatments.

A more vital point is DaCosta's mention of Gross's suit showing signs of prior "sanguinary combat," followed by a mild defense of Gross for not accepting the antisepsis principle. As a matter of fact, the venerable professor was out of step with his times in this regard.

In 1867 Lord Joseph Lister had published the results of his research on antiseptic surgery in *The Lancet*: "On the Antiseptic Principle in the Practice of Surgery." Dr. Lister advocated the use of carbolic acid to kill bacteria and avert infection, for the better healing of surgical wounds; dressings and all instruments and materials that come into contact with the patient were to be sprayed with carbolic acid before use. Immediately after publication of Lister's landmark paper his thesis was hotly debated by surgeons worldwide.

But Gross was loathe to accept Lister's theory that infection could be averted by using antiseptic techniques. In the same year that *The Gross Clinic* was painted Professor Gross said, "Little, if any faith, is placed by any enlightened or experienced surgeon on this side of the Atlantic in the so-called carbolic acid treatment of Professor Lister."[17]

However, three of Dr. Gross's pupils who became eminent surgeons were among those who pioneered Listerian methods in the 1870s in Philadelphia. In 1876 Dr. W. W. Keen became the first Philadelphia surgeon to adopt Lister's principles, and Drs. J. Ewing Mears (JMC 1865) and Samuel W. Gross followed soon thereafter. As late as 1882 in the sixth edition of his *System of Surgery*, Dr. Gross remained steadfast in his view, but allowed that others *were* convinced:[18]

> When the wound is very large, as after the amputation of a limb, or the extirpation of the mammary gland, I generally cover the surface with a pledget of lint wet with olive oil or cosmoline, to prevent the contact of the air and thus diminish the chances of profuse suppuration. I have never found any appreciable benefit in such a case from the use of antiseptic dressings, although they are regarded by many surgeons as most valuable accessories.

Dr. Samuel D. Gross was among those surgeons who still staunchly regarded "laudable pus" as an inevitable step in the process of wound healing. Yet Gross advocated cleanliness on the part of the surgeon, saying, "In performing any delicate operation the hands should always be well washed as a preliminary measure, in order that no dirt or perspiration may be deposited upon the wound, and thus become a source of irritation, interfering with the reparative process." He wrote,[19]

> The surgeon and his aides should be careful, during the operation, that they do not, on the one hand, inoculate themselves with the discharges of the patient, and, on the other, that they do not communicate disease to him through their own persons, as might readily happen if they have recently been engaged in the dissection of patients dead of erysipelas, phlebitis, pyemia, or diffuse inflammation, especially of the peritoneum and of the pelvic veins of lying-in females. That there is frequently, if not generally, a virulent poison present in these affections, the influence of which may readily be disseminated by means of the hands and clothes, is fully established, and, therefore, every possible care should be taken to guard against all such contingencies...A number of cases have been recorded in which surgeons in amputating limbs and excising tumors have contracted fatal diseases by the inoculation of their hands.

In a further comment about clothes Dr. Gross urged that attendants upon the sick and wounded should keep their hands and nails perfectly clean and "never wear the same clothes in visiting their private patients that they wear in the performance of their hospital duties."[20]

The question of antiseptic surgery was vigorously debated during the first two days of the surgical section of the International Medical Congress in Philadelphia in 1876. The first day's program reviewed the medical literature and progress on the subject of germ theory since Lister's publication, with several surgeons agreeing in theory but advocating various substitutes for carbolic acid. On the second day Lister countered objections to his methods by saying that antiseptic surgery achieved better results for the patient even though a considerable increase in care and trouble was inflicted on the surgeon; it shortened the duration of treatment; and it made the treatment less costly because dressings needed to be changed less frequently.[21]

There is every indication that Dr. Samuel D. Gross and Lord Joseph Lister were on good personal terms, in spite of their disagreement on the subject of antisepsis. Lister had been made president of the surgical section of the International Medical Congress. At the culminating "grand subscription dinner" on the last evening of the congress Dr. Gross sat at the head of the central table with Lord Lister at his right side and both made hearty toasts.[22]

Dr. Gross was president of the American Surgical Society during its "Great Debate on Listerism" in 1882-83, and after further debate the society eventually embraced the concept of antiseptic surgery and awarded Lister an honorary membership.[23]

College Clinic Operating Table

COLLEGE CLINIC OPERATING TABLE
By unknown manufacturer

Walnut
Ca. 1850-55
32 2/4 x 65 1/4 x 24 1/4 in. (with leaves closed)

Inscription on bronze plaque placed by JMC class of 1916: "THIS TABLE WAS IN USE FOR MANY YEARS IN THE/JEFFERSON COLLEGE HOSPITAL/IT WAS USED BY/S. D. GROSS, J. PANCOAST, W. W. KEEN,/JOHN H. BRINTON, R. J. LEVIS, W. J. HEARN,/J. CHALMERS DA COSTA AND OTHER EMINENT SURGEONS/THIS PLATE WAS PLACED UPON IT BY THE CLASS OF 1916"

Inscription on bronze plaque placed by JMC class of 1917: "THIS TABLET/PRESENTED BY THE CLASS OF 1917/IS IN HONOR OF THE EMINENT SURGEONS WHO HAVE/USED THIS TABLE. AMONG WHOM ARE/SAMUEL D. GROSS/JOSEPH PANCOAST/SAMUEL W. GROSS/JOHN H. BRINTON/RICHARD J. LEVIS/FRANK MAURY/W. JOSEPH HEARN/W. W. KEEN/J. CHALMERS DA COSTA/THEOPHILUS PARVIN/J. EWING MEARS/NICHOLAS SENN/ROBERT F. WEIR/CHARLES B. G. DE NANCREDE/THOMAS BRYANT (OF LONDON)/LAWSON TAIT (OF BIRMINGHAM)/ARTHUR DURHAM (OF LONDON)/THOMAS ANNANDALE (OF EDINBURGH)/FR. VON ESMARCH (OF KIEL)/M. FAURE (OF PARIS)/SIR WILLIAM MAC CORMAC (OF LONDON)"

Purchased in early 1850s by Jefferson Medical College
Accession number: 1850-1855.DA.01

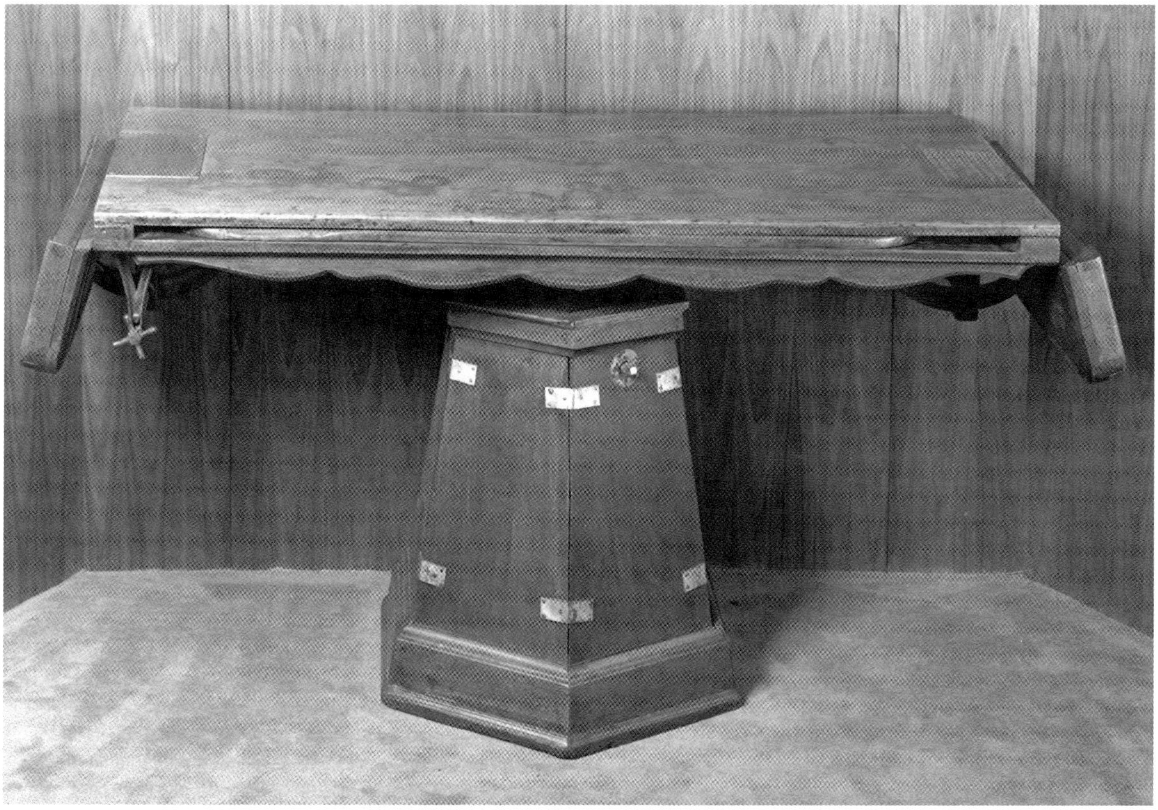

Dr. John Chalmers DaCosta's articles on Jefferson Medical College history also included a description of this operating table used by Dr. Samuel D. Gross and his contemporaries, and depicted in *The Gross Clinic*:[24]

> An old wooden table! It is not artistic or dainty but rather solid and capable. It was made for grim practical uses and not for show. It is not like a Chippendale chair, a Sheraton sideboard or a Hepplewhite table adorning a white colonial drawing room or a parlor containing a hodge-podge of furniture of various makes and ages...
>
> It is an old and scarred veteran, retired after years of active service to end its days of vivid experience in the familiar surroundings of a bull pit surrounded during certain hours by medical students...
>
> At times to look at that old table acts upon me as a magic potation and "stirs the hades of my heart." It brings before me faces and figures which have long since been gathered to infinity and puts in my ears voices which have long been stilled in the arenas of this College.

This venerated, nineteenth-century operating table is actually an ordinary-looking, American-made, utilitarian piece of furniture. Of minimal intrinsic value, the historic artifact is cherished today at Jefferson because of the eminent surgeons who operated upon it. Dr. Samuel D. Gross apparently used it throughout his Philadelphia career.

The table has a rectangular top joined in two planks, and is hinged with a short leaf at either end. The leaves are provided with an iron mechanism for adjusting their precise level. The top is sandwiched in construction to allow for a sliding leaf that fits into its interior. The top swivels upon a tall, hexagonal, plinth-form base secured with brass corner brackets. The table has a shallow apron of valence form with a molded edge.

As shown in *The Gross Clinic*, the table has an apron on the narrow end making a convenient location for Eakins's signature and date. But when the leaf hangs down on the real table, it is actually situated in front of the edge, not recessed behind it as shown in the painting. Also, the picture shows legs at the corners although the actual table has no corner legs, but is supported by a hexagonal pedestal.

The operating table stood originally in the upper lecture room of the Ely Building, and was used for surgical clinics and anatomy and obstetrical lectures. In 1877 the table was moved into the arena of the new hospital. After serving there for many years it was "gradually displaced," as some surgeons preferred more modern appliances, and then it disappeared.

DaCosta was elated to discover the table in the College Building basement where the once-prized artifact was then holding oil cans and various kinds of waste. After the "rescue" from this "appalling usage" the class of 1916 arranged for the table to be cleaned and repaired and added the first bronze tablet, followed the next year by a tablet from the class of 1917.

By now the table was regarded as an important historic artifact. Eventually it was displayed in the pathological museum of the 1898 College Building, then in the library of the 1929 College Building. In 1969 it was placed in storage until it received its permanent home in the Samuel D. Gross Conference Room which was created in 1982 by the Department of Surgery in the same building.

The Operation to Cure Osteomyelitis

The operation depicted in *The Gross Clinic* is extraction of a fragment of a sequestrum, or dead bone, that has caused an inflammatory disease called osteomyelitis in the femur, or thigh bone. It is not known whether Dr. Gross or Thomas Eakins selected the procedure to be depicted, but the choice embodies the surgeon's strong advocacy of conservative surgery.

According to Gross's description, this condition is most commonly caused by trauma such as fractures, gunshot wounds, lodging of foreign bodies in the substance of the bone, violent blows, contusions, concussion of the spongy tissue, or laceration of the endosteum by the saw in amputation of the limb; other causes are cold or sudden suppression of cutaneous perspiration operating upon a weak, delicate condition or "some peculiar taint of the system" such as syphilis, goiter, or scurvy.[25]

Excision of the sequestrum was considered a hallmark of conservative surgery compared with amputation, because in the former procedure the periosteum is left intact to help in the regenerative process of the limb which has been saved. When successful the regenerated bone forms within a few months. Although it is an "imperfect copy" at best, it "answers the purpose well enough both as its respects its length and thickness."[26]

On amputation for diseases of the bones and joints, Gross said that there was "no class of diseases in which the operation has been more frequently abused or misapplied." He added, "There can be no question that many a limb, merely temporarily crippled by remediable disease, has been ruthlessly sacrificed to ignorance and a desire for eclat...as to necrosis, pure and uncomplicated, it is difficult to conceive of a case justifying the use of the knife."[27]

Lithotomy Knife of Samuel D. Gross, M.D.

LITHOTOMY KNIFE
Manufactured by J. H. Gemrig & Son

Ivory, steel
Ca. 1800-50
6 1/4 in. long
Signed on blade: "GEMRIG"
Mahogany box with brass hinges, velvet lining
1 1/4 x 7 1/4 x 3 1/4 in.

Given in 1887 by Samuel W. Gross, M.D. to Claudius H. Mastin, M.D.; given to JMC in 1916 by William M. Mastin, M.D.

Accession number: 1916+e.DA.01-02

The archives at Thomas Jefferson University possesses instruments used by Dr. Samuel D. Gross including his own lithotomy knife and amputation set, as well as other boxes of instruments used by Gross and many of his colleagues. The lithotomy knife is the only example with an ivory handle, resembling those instruments (no longer extant) depicted in *The Gross Clinic*. Dr. Gross was well known for performing lithotomy to remove a stone from the bladder with such speed and dexterity, that the procedure only took about twenty to thirty seconds.[28]

Two paper labels in the wooden box tell how the prized object eventually came to Jefferson Medical College. One reads, "This knife, now much worn down, was used by Prof. S. D. Gross in at least forty lateral lithotomies. It was presented by me to Dr. C. H. Mastin, Oct. 7th 1887. [signed] S. W. Gross."

The other label reads, "Presented by Dr. William M. Mastin, Mobile, Alabama, to the Museum of the Jefferson Medical College, at Phila. June 1, 1916."

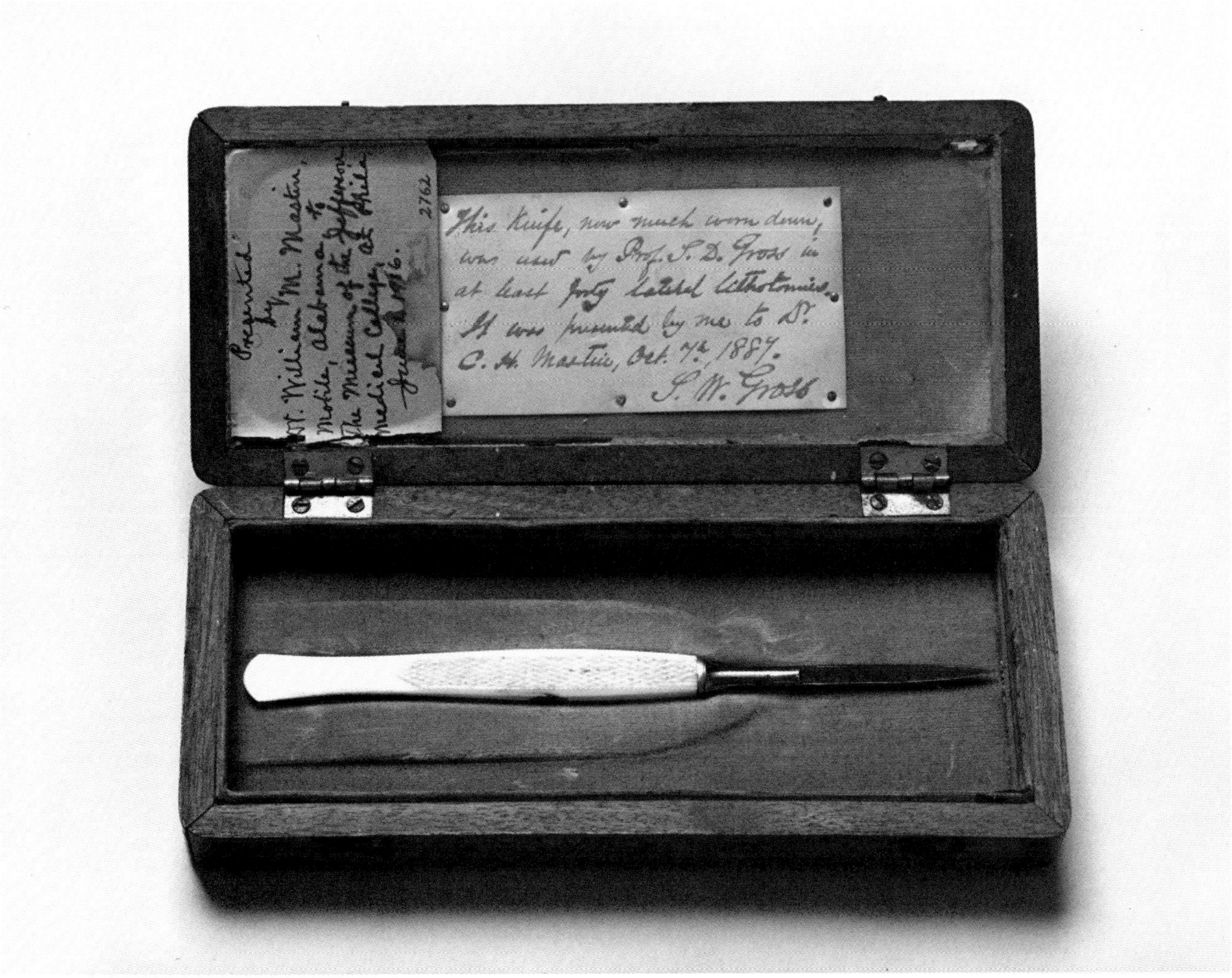

Dr. Claudius H. Mastin (1826-98) was a distinguished genito-urinary surgeon and the inventor of several instruments. In 1866 he was the first to ligate the external iliac with silver wire for aneurysm of the femoral artery in Scarpa's triangle. He received an M.D. from the University of Pennsylvania (1849), was a founder of the American Genito-urinary Association, and served as president of the American Surgical Association. Dr. Mastin hosted his friend, Dr. Samuel D. Gross, and the younger Gross at his home in Mobile, Alabama in 1880.[29] Dr. Mastin's role in initiating Alexander Calder's bronze monument to Dr. Samuel D. Gross has already been mentioned.

Viewers who are health care professionals often conjecture about the type of anesthesia being administered by Dr. Joseph H. Hearn in *The Gross Clinic*: was it chloroform or ether? Dr. Gross's preference for chloroform was stated clearly in weighing the merits of both agents in the sixth edition of his *System of Surgery*:[30]

> In the hands of certain surgeons, the use of chloroform, as an anaesthetic agent, has been attended with astonishing success. I have now administered it in all kinds of operations in several thousand cases without a single death, and in only three cases did I feel any serious alarm for the safety of the patient...
>
> I ascribe my own success in the use of chloroform to the extraordinary care with which it has been administered in my practice, to the proper selection of my cases, and to the pains which have always been taken to procure a pure article, preference having generally been given to Squibb's preparation. An assistant who is accustomed to superintend the inhalation of chloroform is far safer than an inexperienced one, and neither in hospital nor private practice should any other ever be permitted to meddle with it...
>
> The best mode of administering chloroform is to pour the fluid upon a napkin or handkerchief, previously folded into a cone or cup-shaped hollow, and held securely in the hand. Or, instead of this, a small hollow sponge may be used...
>
> The napkin, impregnated with a drachm of chloroform, is held over the mouth and nose, at a distance of about two inches, being gradually brought nearer and nearer until it is within one-fourth of that distance...
>
> At my Clinic at the Jefferson Medical College Hospital where, until recently, I employed chloroform in all my operations, no mishap from its use has ever occurred. Dr. Joseph Hearn, who has been my anaesthetizer for the last eleven years, has given it in many hundred cases, at all periods of life and under almost every variety of disease and accident without any serious occurrence.

However, in the same chapter on anesthetics, Gross conceded that he now considered ether to be "unquestionably the safest," adding that it was almost universally used in American hospitals and was preferred in private practice. But although his own confidence in the safety of chloroform was unshaken if it were properly administered, he, too, since the early 1880s restricted himself to the use of ether except in the case of children.

Dr. W. Joseph Hearn, the anesthetizer in *The Gross Clinic*, delivered a clinical lecture at the Philadelphia Hospital in 1886 entitled "The Administration of Anaesthetics," in which he said that he had been a "professional anaesthetizer" for fifteen years. He confirmed his success with chloroform and said that Professor Gross had instructed him in its use and that they never had an accident or death from it. Hearn referred to the inhaler as a towel formed into a cone, rather than a napkin or handkerchief.[31]

The Samuel D. Gross Professorship Cane

THE SAMUEL D. GROSS PROFESSORSHIP CANE
Manufactured by Simons, Bro. & Co.

Rosewood with gold fittings
1926
34 3/4 in. long

Inscription on gold plaque on handle: "CLASS OF 1926/ENDOWED IN PERPETUITY/BY/VINCENT T. MCDERMOTT, M.D./CLASS OF 1926/JEFFERSON MEDICAL COLLEGE OF PHILADELPHIA/FOUNDED 1825/SAMUEL D. GROSS CHAIR OF SURGERY"
Inscriptions on gold plaques on shaft are the names of chairmen of the department of surgery: "J. CHALMERS DA COSTA/THOMAS A. SHALLOW/JOHN H. GIBBON, JR./JOHN Y. TEMPLETON, III/HARRY S. GOLDSMITH/FRANCIS E. ROSATO"

Presented in 1926 by JMC class of 1926 to John Chalmers DaCosta, M.D. and given to JMC that year
Accession number: 1926+e.DA.01

The gold-headed cane of the Samuel D. Gross Chair of Surgery is another tribute honoring Dr. Gross. Jefferson Medical College had established this named chair, and the cane was presented by the class of 1926 to Dr. J. Chalmers DaCosta, the first to occupy the chair. In 1976 at its fiftieth reunion, the same class endowed a fund in perpetuity to add the name of each succeeding Gross professor on a separate gold plaque below Gross's name. The original idea for the cane is attributed to Vincent T. McDermott, M.D. (JMC 1926), who later endowed a fund for the gold plaques.

The handle is in a branch form, a traditional type of walking stick for more than a century. The cane is embellished with chased band borders at either end of the handle in the form of feathers or leaves. Other decorations include the Jefferson seal on the handle and a caduceus on the shaft. The hallmark of the Philadelphia manufacturer, Simons, is found on the handle: a Gothic S in a flat-topped shield.

The honors and memorials accorded by Jefferson Medical College to Dr. Gross were based not only on his surgical, teaching, and organizational skills, but also on the strong sense of medical ethics he imparted to students, as described in Dr. J. C. DaCosta's address on Gross:

> As an operator, Gross was calm, painstaking, careful, rapid, but not hurried, and always proceeding so that students might see and understand what he was doing. All the time he operated he explained...He realized to the full his grave personal responsibility, and always felt that a surgical operation was a great and solemn thing. He used to point out to the class what a wonderful and touching sign of confidence it was for a patient to allow himself to be made unconscious after giving the surgeon permission to do to him as he would, and how such confidence imposed on the surgeon an additional sense of responsibility...
>
> Before operation he studied his case with the greatest care, and thus avoided many needless operations and saved many lives, but he never refused to operate in an emergency simply because an operation was highly dangerous. He was fierce in denunciation of those who would deny the chance given by operation when the state was desperate, simply because death would spoil a surgeon's statistics...
>
> After the operation, he took personal care of the patient, assiduously watched the progress of the case, and when things were going ill, saw the sufferer frequently, and he would see the poor man in the ward as frequently as he would the rich man in a private room. It was the need that called him, not the fee. Few men of the profession have had greater opportunity to acquire wealth, but he was satisfied with a moderate fortune, because all his life the call of suffering was to him more mandatory than the jingling of the guinea...
>
> He was quick to discern young talent and eager to publically recognize and praise it, and many a young fellow, perhaps in a distant part of the country, would be cheered and delighted beyond measure after he had published some article in a medical journal to receive a letter of compliment from the first surgeon of the land.

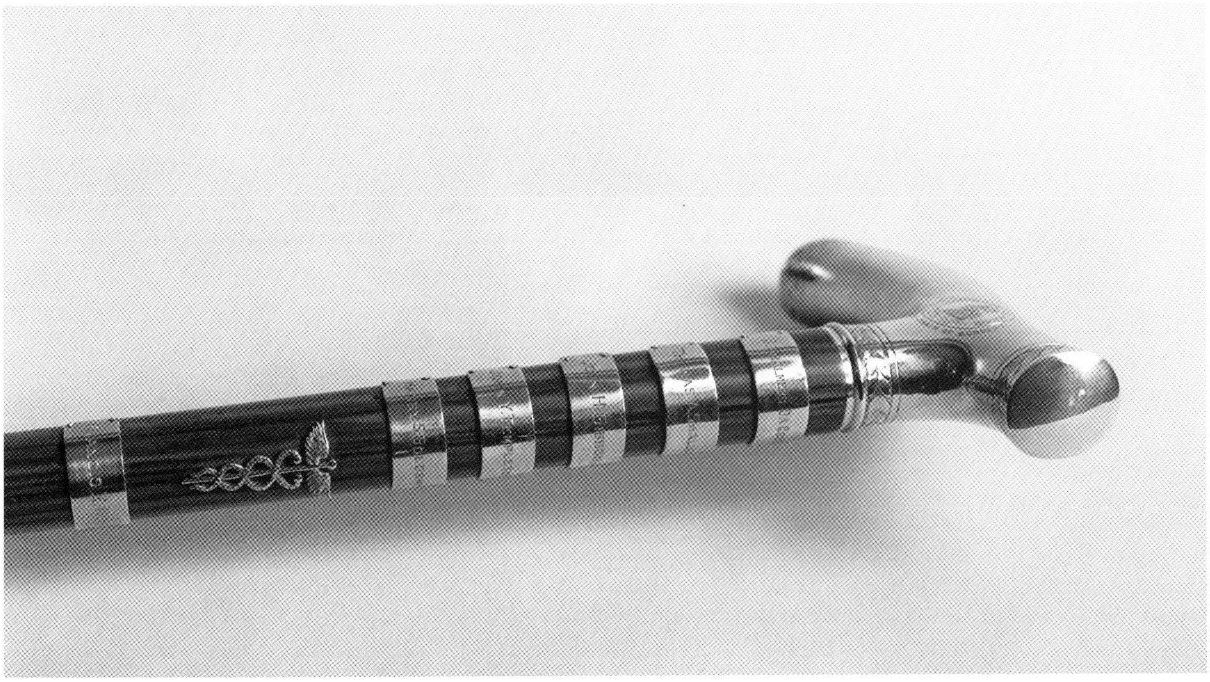

History of The Gross Clinic at Jefferson

With the exception of Dr. John Chalmers DaCosta's 1912 address on Dr. Samuel D. Gross and the 1902 biography of Dr. W. Joseph Hearn,[32] few faculty members commented in writing on *The Gross Clinic*, even though the painting had been purchased by Jefferson Medical College in 1878 and been prominently displayed. Dr. Gross himself does not remark on any of his portraits in his autobiography, although a drawing based on the Eakins painting is the frontispiece to the second volume, as already mentioned.

Yet there is ample indirect evidence that both Gross and Jefferson Medical College admired and valued *The Gross Clinic* soon after its arrival at Jefferson in 1878.

Page from Jefferson Medical College Account Book

PAGE FROM JEFFERSON MEDICAL COLLEGE ACCOUNT BOOK
Book used Oct. 1841 to April 1879
Page size: 12 1/2 x 7 1/2 in.

Accession number: 1879+f.Pr.01

There is a record of the date of purchase and amount paid to Eakins, a corroboration of the artist's comments in his Exhibition Record notebooks.[33]

The archival document is a Jefferson Medical College account book which lists the amount of two hundred dollars on February 23, 1878 for "Tho[s] Eakins, picture of surg. clinic." Some other expenses on the page include Gemrig surgical instruments and diploma printing, and prosaic necessities such as chairs, carpeting, gas fixtures, coal, paperhanging, stationery, spittoons, and insurance premiums.

Interestingly, the subject of the picture was referred to as a surgical clinic in the Jefferson ledger. In Eakins's own exhibition notebooks and elsewhere he referred to the subject as a portrait or picture of Gross, Dr. Gross, or Professor Gross. Several scholars have written about the varied titles used by the artist and in early exhibition publications.[34] However, they did not consider what it was called at Jefferson where its significance transcended the portrait of Dr. Gross to encompass the act of surgery and the clinical setting. The painting's title or description at Jefferson Medical College varied in the early years, but it often included the word "clinic" or mentioned Gross's identity as a surgeon or that he was shown operating.

The earliest reproduction of the painting in Jefferson publications was in Dr. George Gould's 1904 history of Jefferson Medical College, where it was referred to as "Dr. Samuel D. Gross Operating." *The Jeffersonian* of May 1904 wrote proudly under "College Notes" that the "large picture of the late Professor Gross, which hangs in the West Lecture room, will be on exhibit at the World's Fair." (The St. Louis fair was the second major exposition in the American Midwest, after Chicago in 1893.)

Charles Frankenberger's 1915 article on the art collection included no reproductions but began with "the masterpiece of the collection" which he called the "Clinic of Doctor Samuel D. Gross." He devoted a full page to this painting in a ten-page article.[35] The January 1916 *Jeffersonian* noted that the "Clinic of Doctor Samuel D. Gross" was relined, along with cleaning and "renovation" of the other oil paintings.

Unfortunately, no official Jefferson correspondence on loan arrangements is extant before the posthumous Eakins retrospective at the Pennsylvania Academy of the Fine Arts in 1917. At that time Dean Patterson's letter of approval referred to loans of *The Gross Clinic* and the *Portrait of Professor Benjamin Rand* and the *Portrait of William S. Forbes.*

This now familiar title must have become entrenched soon after 1917 at Jefferson, because the caption "*The Gross Clinic*" appears under a reproduction of the painting in the April 1925 *Jefferson Medical College Alumni Bulletin.*

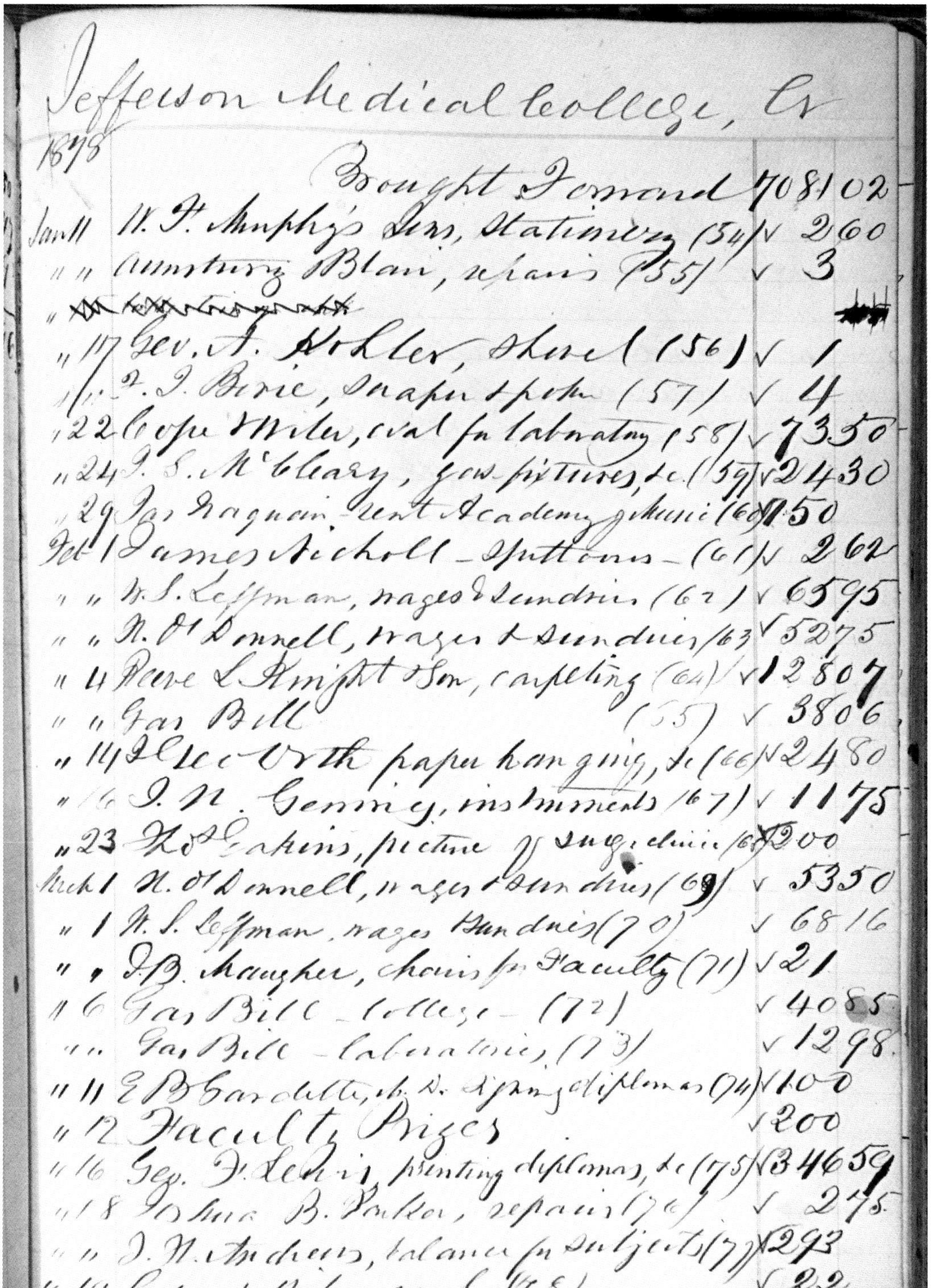

Jefferson Medical College, Cr

1878			
	Brought Forward		7081.02
Jan 11	W. F. Murphy's Sons, Stationery (54)	√	2.60
" "	Armstrong & Blair, repairs (55)	√	3
"	[struck out]		
" 17	Geo. A. Kohler, shovel (56)	√	1
" "	J. J. Bowie, soap & spoons (57)	√	4
" 22	Cope & Weiler, coal for laboratory (58)	√	73.50
" 24	J. S. McCleary, gas fixtures, &c (59)	√	24.30
" 29	Jas Maguire, rent Academy of Music (60)	√	150
Feb 1	James Nicholl — Spittoons — (61)	√	2.62
" "	W. S. Leffman, wages & sundries (62)	√	65.95
" "	N. O'Donnell, wages & sundries (63)	√	52.75
" 4	Reeve L. Knight & Son, carpeting (64)	√	128.07
" "	Gas Bill (65)	√	38.06
" 14	J. Leo Orth paper hanging, &c (66)	√	24.80
" 16	J. H. Gemrig, instruments (67)	√	11.75
" 23	Thos Eakins, picture of surg. clinic (68)	√	200
March 1	N. O'Donnell, wages & sundries (69)	√	53.50
" 1	W. S. Leffman, wages & sundries (70)	√	68.16
" "	J. B. Maugher, chairs for Faculty (71)	√	21
" 6	Gas Bill — College — (72)	√	40.85
" "	Gas Bill — laboratories (73)	√	12.98
" 11	E. B. Gardette, for Dr. signing diplomas (74)	√	100
" 12	Faculty Prizes	√	200
" 16	Geo. F. Lasher, printing diplomas, &c (75)	√	346.59
" 18	Joshua B. Parker, repairs (76)	√	2.75
" "	J. W. Andrews, balance for subjects (77)	√	293
" 19	Cope & Weiler, coal (78)	√	22
" "	C. W. Campbell, ushers, &c, commencement (79)	√	25
" "	Pa Hospital contribution	√	437.50
" 20	Insurance Premium	√	24
" "	W. S. Leffman, extra compensation (80)	√	50
	Carry Forward		9560.75

The whereabouts of *The Gross Clinic* are unknown between its exhibition at Haseltine's Gallery after the Centennial in late autumn of 1876 and its purchase by Jefferson Medical College in February 1878. Presumably it was in Eakins's studio. Various notices and two photographs in the Jefferson archives pinpoint its subsequent locations after its purchase.

Because of the painting's monumental size (framed, it measures almost 114 inches high and ninety-six inches wide) and because the institution had no formal art gallery until the 1980s, the painting has always hung in prominent, public rooms or halls in important college buildings. This demonstrates consistent awareness of the painting's importance to the institution, for less important portraits often languished in inconspicuous locations.

Surprisingly, the earliest mention of location is not a Jefferson announcement, but a Philadelphia newspaper notice of March 9, 1878, just two weeks after Jefferson purchased the painting. Under the headline of "Art and Artists," it informed readers that "Mr. Thomas Eakins, of this City, has several pictures on exhibition in New York, some with the Water Color Society and others in the exhibition of the Society of American Artists. His portrait of Dr. Gross, painted for the faculty of Jefferson College, is now in the new museum at Tenth and Sansom Streets."[36]

The original anatomical, surgical, and pathological museum in the Ely Building was created in the early 1830s. The *Annual Announcement* of 1840-41 praised the faculty's awareness of the "value of paintings, drawings, models, casts, and preparations of healthy and morbid anatomy" for illustrating surgical and anatomical lectures. Later college announcements regularly mentioned additional displays and space for the museum. A new museum occupied the entire third floor of the Laboratory Building which was constructed in the late 1870s. If the newspaper article was correct about the painting "*now*" hanging in the museum, the implication is that it had not earlier been on loan to Jefferson, as some scholars have conjectured.

In May 1884 *The College and Clinical Record* regretted to report Dr. Gross's serious illness and noted proudly that the "celebrated portrait of Prof. Samuel D. Gross, by Mr. Thomas Eakins, which was on exhibition in one of the United States Government buildings during the great Centennial Exposition of 1876, is now the property of the Faculty of Jefferson Medical College, and occupies a position on the wall of the Dean's room, on the lower floor of the College building." Perhaps this was a spacious, public reception room, rather than the dean's private office which probably could not have accommodated such a large painting.

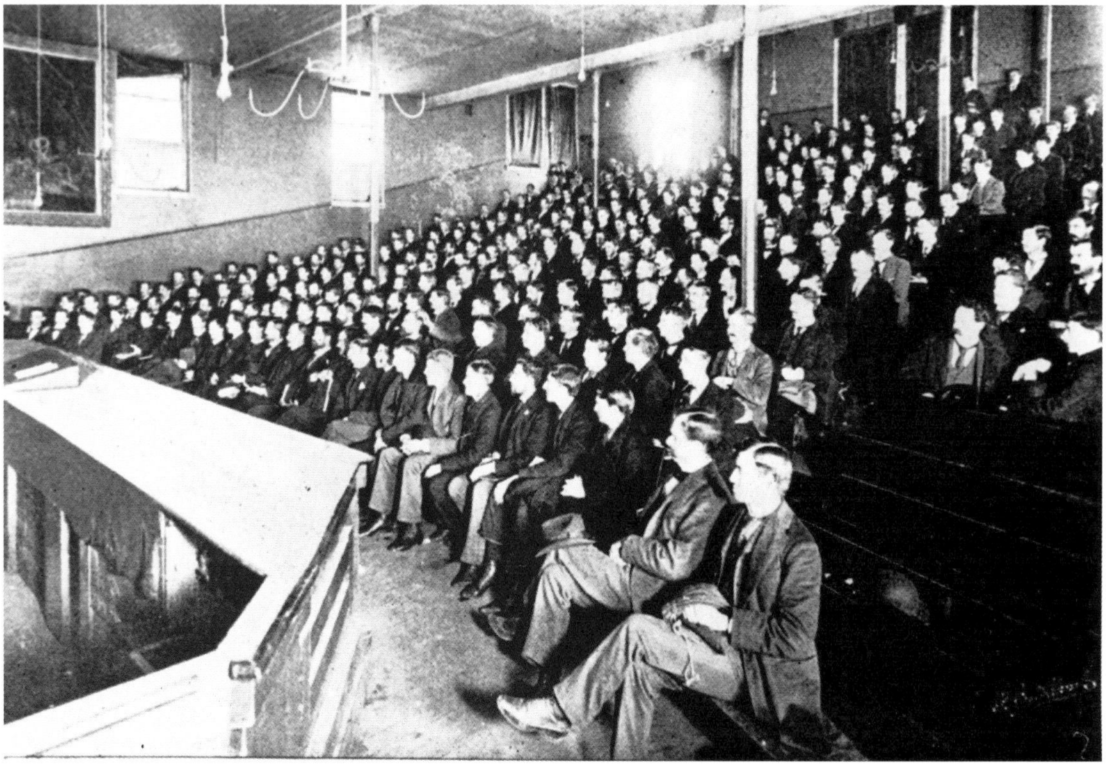

Lower Lecture Room

Lower Lecture Room, Jefferson Medical College (Ely Building)

LOWER LECTURE ROOM, ELY BUILDING
By unknown photographer

Modern photograph after unidentified publication
1884-98
8 x 10 in.

Caption: "THE LOWER LECTURE ROOM OF THE JEFFERSON MEDICAL COLLEGE"

Photograph commissioned by Jefferson Medical College
Accession number: 1898+f.Ph.02

Sometime after 1884 *The Gross Clinic* was moved to the lower lecture room of the Ely Building, as noted on the caption of the published photograph. The seats are filled with attentive students but the lecturer is not visible. Though the painting is dimly lit, its foreground figures are plainly discernible. To fit into this tight space, the picture was hung flush with the ceiling and abutted a window frame. It is unknown if other portraits were on the opposite wall.

West Lecture Room, Jefferson Medical College (1898 Building)

WEST LECTURE ROOM, 1898 BUILDING
By unknown photographer

Modern copy after original photograph
1898-1929
8 x 10 in.

Photograph commissioned by Jefferson Medical College
Accession number: 1929+f.Ph.12

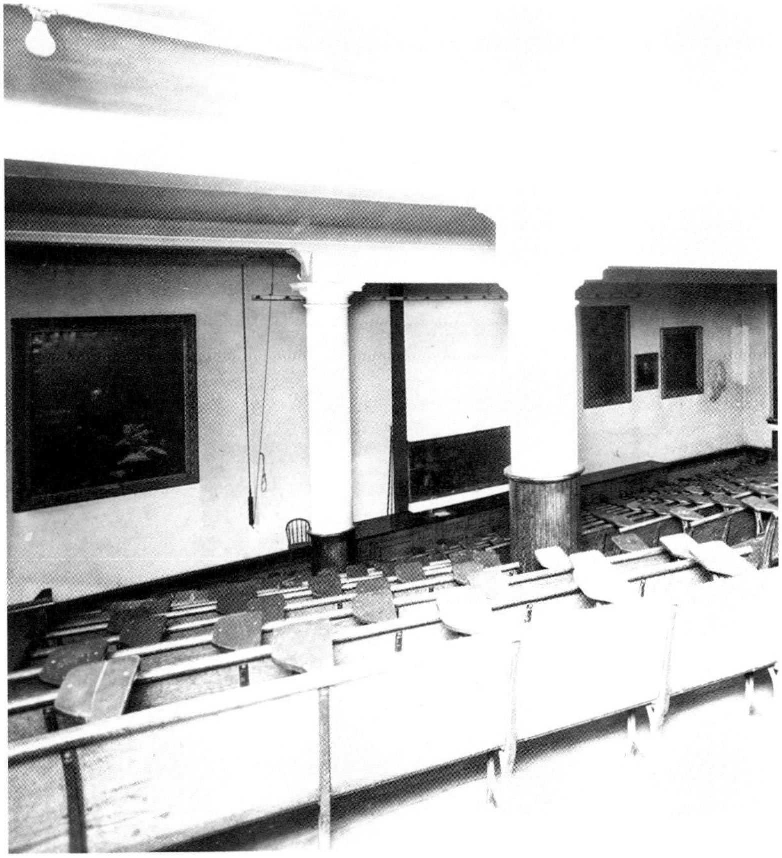

The second installation photograph of *The Gross Clinic* shows the painting hanging in the front of the west lecture room, in a wide-angle shot that has distorted the picture's proportions. Magnification shows that the other paintings to the right of the supporting column are Eakins's portraits of Drs. Benjamin H. Rand and William S. Forbes, flanking the portrait of Dr. Samuel W. Gross by George W. Pettit.

The February 1905 *Jeffersonian* announced, "The celebrated Eakin [*sic*] painting of the great surgeon, Samuel D. Gross, hanging in the west lecture room, has been recently returned from the exhibit of fine arts at the World's Fair in St. Louis, where i[t] was awarded a medal." The west lecture room was located in the new Jefferson Medical College Building which opened in 1898.

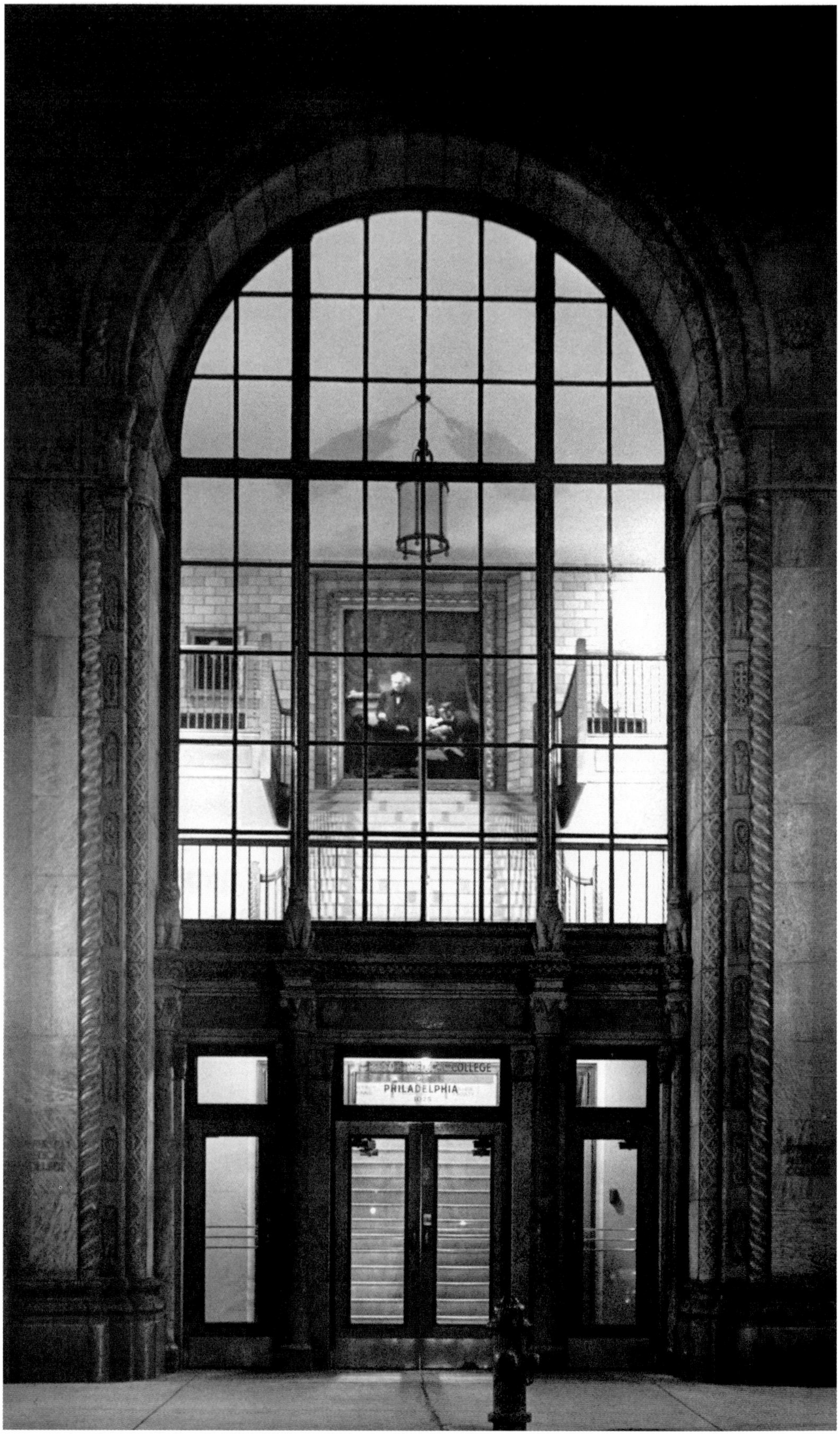
COLLEGE
PHILADELPHIA

Second Floor Landing, Jefferson Medical College (1929 Building)

SECOND FLOOR LANDING, 1929 BUILDING
Photograph
By Frank Ross
Ca. 1940-60
14 x 11 in.

Given after 1968 by unknown donor
Accession number: 1968+f.Ph.01

The painting hung in the west lecture room of the 1898 Building until the 1929 College Building was opened. The spacious interior entrance of the new building featured a wide, marble staircase flanked by portraits of Deans Ross V. Patterson, M.D. and Benjamin H. Rand, M.D. on one side and trustee Alba B. Johnson and Professor Jacob M. DaCosta, M.D. on the other. In the place of honor on the landing of the second floor stood *The Gross Clinic* between portraits of Dr. W. W. Keen and trustee and benefactor William Potter. Because of the two-story, arched, windowed entrance to the College Building, the painting was dramatically situated and visible from the sidewalk and street below.

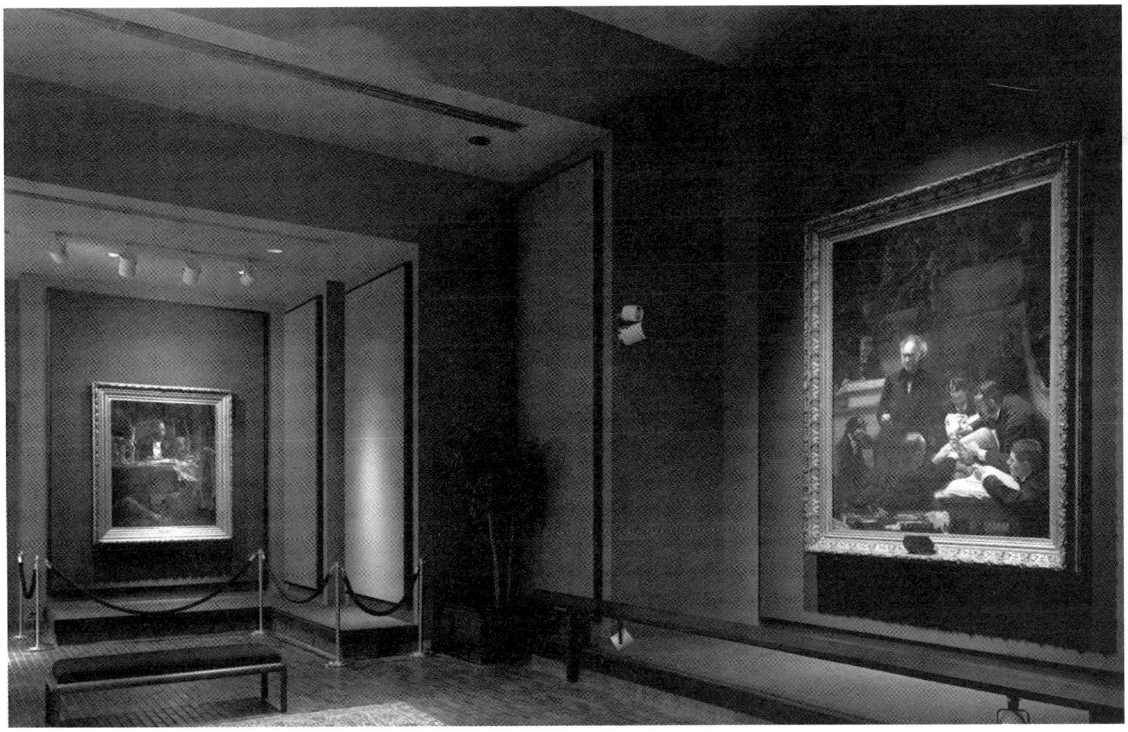

Eakins Gallery, Jefferson Alumni Hall

EAKINS GALLERY, JEFFERSON ALUMNI HALL
Photograph
1991
8 x 10 in.

Accession number: 1991+e.Ph.03

The final destination of *The Gross Clinic* was Jefferson Alumni Hall where it moved when the building opened in 1968. First it was installed next to the bookstore in a space called the Eakins Lounge. This area was disadvantageous because of reflections on the painting from windows and glass doors leading to the outdoor atrium opposite the painting and from a protective Plexiglas shield which had been placed around the painting.

The bookstore was moved to another location to make way for the Eakins Gallery, dedicated in 1982 as part of the sesquicentennial celebration of Jefferson's alumni association. The university is strongly committed to making the painting accessible to the general public, and keeps the gallery opened on a daily basis and free of charge to all visitors.

Eakins's Preparatory Methods

Portrait of Samuel D. Gross

SAMUEL DAVID GROSS, M.D. (1805-84)
By Frederick Gutekunst (1831-1917)

Phototype
1870-79
Image size: 5 1/8 x 3 5/8 in.
Sheet size: 7 3/4 x 5 3/4 in.

Signed below image: "Phototype 2. F. Gutekunst"
Inscription by Dr. Samuel D. Gross: "For my friend, Dr. Horwitz,/United States Navy,/Late Chief of Bureau."
Facsimile signature: "S. D. Gross"

Given after 1884 by unknown donor
Accession number: 1884+f.Ph.06

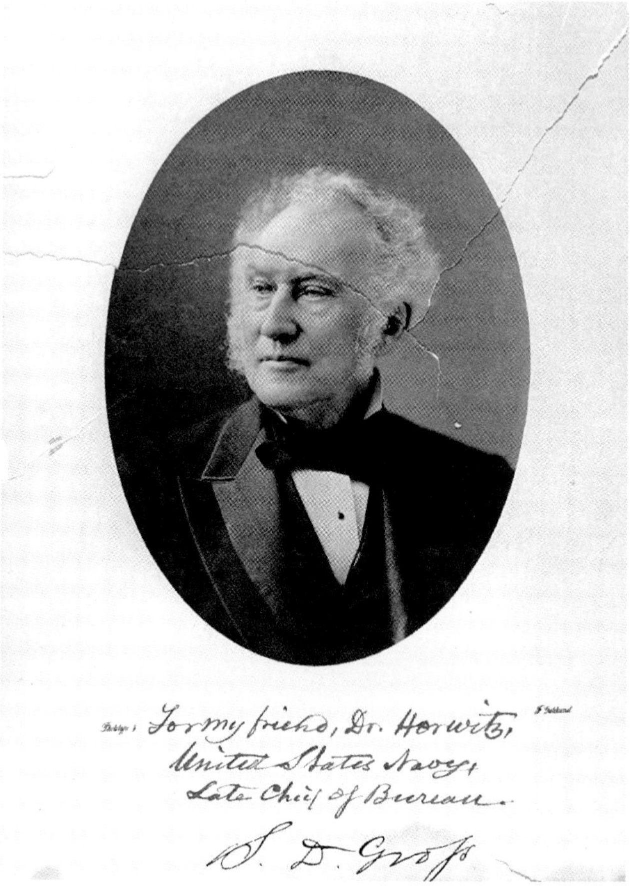

The earliest references to *The Gross Clinic* by the artist or his associates were very optimistic about the painting's prospects. According to Lloyd Goodrich two letters from Eakins to his friend Earl Shinn in the spring of 1875 are about *The Gross Clinic*. On March 26 he wrote, "I am doing far better work just now at least it is ten times better commenced"; and on April 13 he said, "What elates me more is that I have just got a new picture blocked in & it is very far better than anything I have ever done. As I spoil things less & less in finishing I have the greatest hopes of this one."[37]

In August 1875 John Sartain, who had been appointed superintendent of the Centennial's art department, wrote to his daughter Emily, "Tom Eakins is making excellent progress with his large portrait of Dr. Gross, and it bids fair to be a capital work."[38]

On August 20 Eakins wrote to his fiancée Kathrin Crowell about difficulties in arranging for portrait sittings with the busy surgeon, "I have had trouble with Dr. Gross not from any unwillingness of his, but when I wanted him most he would be away or so run down with operations that he could not find me an hour but I expect him Sunday."[39] Eakins must have pursued Gross determinedly for his widow, Susan Macdowell Eakins, told Lloyd Goodrich in 1930 that after many sittings Dr. Gross commented to her husband, "Eakins, I wish you were dead!"[40] Nevertheless, Gross's willingness to accommodate the little-known artist amid the surgeon's Herculean schedule shows that Gross respected the artist and the worthiness of his project.

The artist must still have been working on the painting, at least the background figures of students, in the fall of 1875, because in December he presented his oil sketch for the figure of Robert C. V. Meyers to his friend, and Meyers wrote on the back of the picture that the sitting had taken place on October 10.

For so complex a multifigured composition, scholars think that Eakins must have made oil studies for all the figures and a perspective drawing of the amphitheater.[41] Although a discussion of the few extant preparatory works is beyond the scope of this book, fortunately we have Mrs. Eakins's comments on the artist's working methods and his relationship with Dr. Gross. In an undated letter of about 1930 Mrs. Eakins wrote:[42]

> The picture "The Gross Clinic" painted 1875. At the Jefferson Hospital Eakins was permitted in the Clinic Room. Dr. Gross realized he was serious in his work, and gave him every opportunity to study the color, the positions of objects and general arrangements of a Clinic. Having arranged the composition on the canvas, he made studies of each person in the picture. The important figures, Dr. Gross and his assisting surgeons, requiring more finished painting, would give as many

> poses as possible, probably six poses of an hour each time in the pose of Dr. Gross, the other surgeons some what less time. The students in the background, probably one or two poses.

Although later in the letter Mrs. Gross said that Eakins "only used a photograph, when impossible to get information in the way he preferred, painting from the living, moving model," and that "he disliked working from a photograph, and absolutely refused to do so in a portrait," there is much evidence to the contrary. He used photographs as study aids for many figurative paintings and sculptures.

Eakins's photographs and negatives of Dr. Gross noted by Alexander Calder (see preceding chapter) have not been found, but the Jefferson archives has a Frederick Gutekunst phototype of Gross in a strikingly similar pose taken in the 1870s. Even the lighting on the physician's face is similar to that in *The Gross Clinic*. Judging from Dr. Gross's inscription to his friend, the Jefferson photo was taken sometime after 1869 when Dr. Phineas J. Horwitz (1822-1904) retired as chief of the Bureau of Medicine and Surgery of the Navy, and before the image was used as a frontispiece in the *College and Clinical Record* of March 15, 1880. The phototype evidences that Eakins realistically depicted a characteristic appearance of the surgeon.

In 1930 Mrs. Eakins first showed the artist's fourth floor studio in their home to Seymour Adelman, an art collector and bibliophile who became a close friend of the widow and later purchased the Eakins home as a memorial to the artist. She told him, "This is where my husband painted *The Gross Clinic*. His father prepared this studio for him when he returned home from Spain."[43] Adelman said that the room was large, high-ceilinged, and rather bare, furnished only with a table and a couple of chairs. Charles Bregler said about the studio, "This workshop as he choose [*sic*] to call it reflected the character of Eakins, it contained nothing but what was essential to a serious painter."[44]

In answer to Seymour Adelman's question about when she first saw Thomas Eakins, Susan Eakins replied that it was in 1876 when *The Gross Clinic*, which "roused a city-wide commotion," was on view at Haseltine's. Although the artist was present in the gallery, the young woman was too shy for an introduction, but she so admired the painting that she enrolled in Eakins's life classes at the Pennsylvania Academy of the Fine Arts. (See chapter eleven re a painting by Susan Eakins.)

The Importance of the Collotype of The Gross Clinic

The Gross Clinic

Collotype reproduction by Adolph Braun & Co.
1876
Image size: 11 1/8 x 9 in.
Sheet size: 17 3/8 x 15 1/4 in.

Inscription in plate, lower right: "Copyright by Eakins 1876"
Inscription in pencil below image, lower right: "To Dr. Edw. Anthony Spitzka with the/Compliments of Thomas Eakins"
Exhibition of various *Gross Clinic* collotypes during Thomas Eakins's lifetime: Philadelphia, Penn Club, Reception, Mar. 7, 1876; Philadelphia, *Forty-seventh Annual Exhibition*, Pennsylvania Academy of the Fine Arts, Apr. 24-June 5, 1876; Philadelphia, Centennial International Exhibition (in U.S. Army Post Hospital Building), May 10-Nov. 10, 1876; Philadelphia, Haseltine's Gallery, late Nov. or Dec. 1876; Philadelphia, Lindsay and Blakiston, 1878; New York, *First Exhibition*, Society of American Artists, Mar. 6-Apr. 5, 1878; New York, Art Students' League, Monthly Reception, Mar. 4, 1879; Chicago, World's Columbian Exposition, May 1-Oct. 30, 1893; Philadelphia, Earle's Galleries, from May 11, 1896; St. Louis, Louisiana Purchase Centennial International Exposition, Apr. 30-Dec. 1, 1904

Probably given before 1914 by Edward A. Spitzka, M.D., JMC chairman of general anatomy
Accession number: 1914+b.Pr.01

Soon after Eakins completed *The Gross Clinic* he arranged for high-quality reproductions of the work. Most scholars think that he sent a black-and-white, India ink wash replica painted on cardboard (now in the Metropolitan Museum of Art) to Adolph Braun and Company in Dornach, Alsace, for making copies. He made the drawing instead of relying on a photograph of the monumental and dark painting because the painting's color values could not be photographed and reproduced as effectively. Eakins said, "My drawing was made with the intention of coming out right in a photograph."[45]

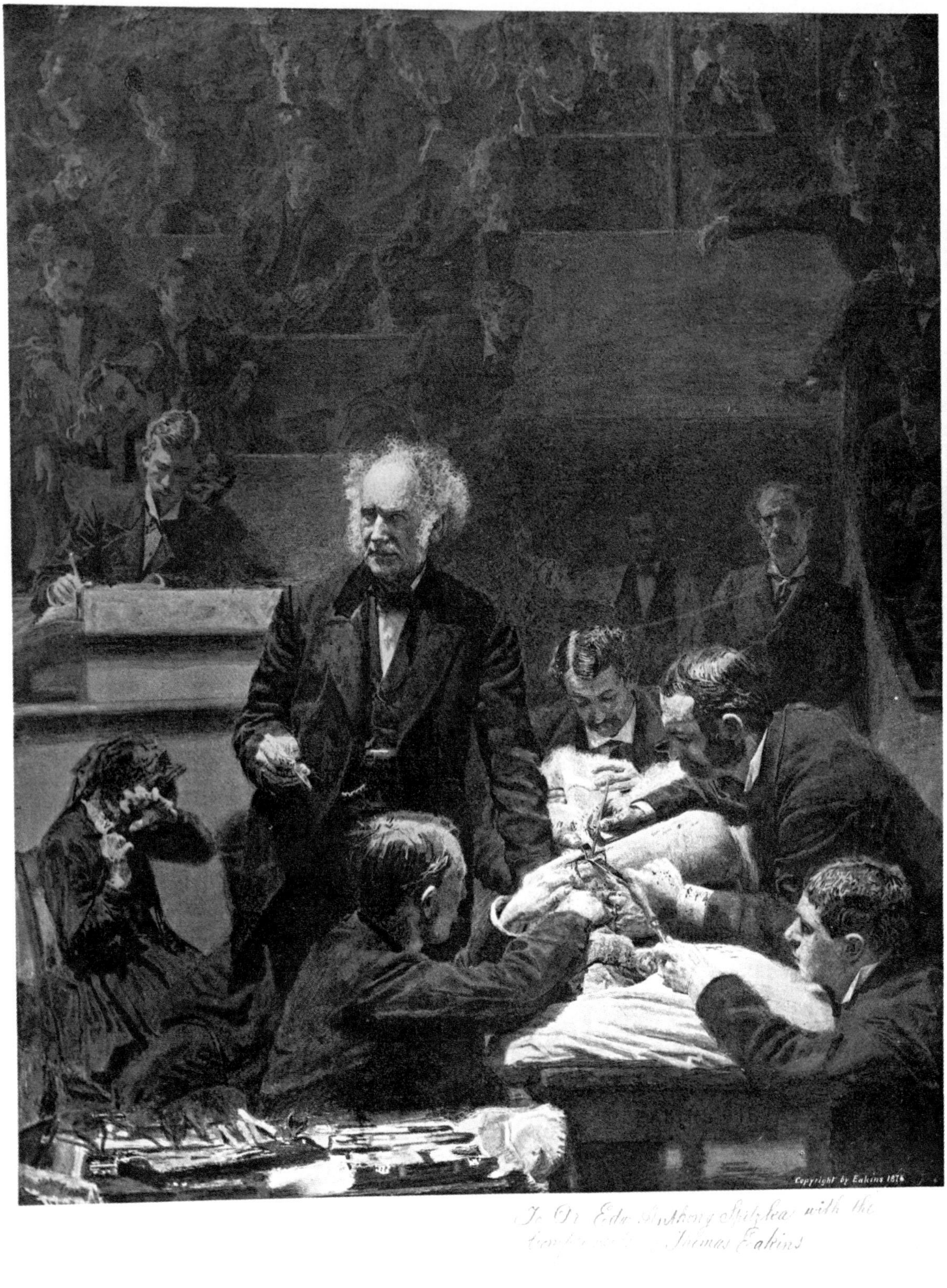

To Dr Edw Anthony Spitzka with the
[illegible] Thomas Eakins

Braun and Company was known for its fine reproductions of art works, both collotypes (a photomechanical process similar to lithography) and autotypes (a carbon print made from a negative). In the art history literature the terms collotype, autotype, photogravure, and photograph have all referred to Braun's reproduction of *The Gross Clinic.*[46]

It is not known how many reproductions were produced originally, but only a handful remain. Almost all known surviving collotypes were given by Eakins to friends and colleagues and inscribed by the artist. I discovered the Jefferson collotype serendipitously in the library of the department of anatomy where it was gathering dust on the unused top shelf of a bookcase. The framed print was inscribed with Thomas Eakins's "compliments" to Dr. Edward Anthony Spitzka (1876-1922), chairman of general anatomy from 1905 to 1914. A noted anatomist and criminologist specializing in the human brain, Dr. Spitzka was the subject of Eakins's last portrait which was begun in 1913.

Partly because the painting was being reproduced, Eakins applied for a copyright of *The Gross Clinic.* It is recorded on April 6, 1876 in the copyright office of the Library of Congress (Registration Number 4174).[47]

Forty years later Eakins still considered the painting one of his greatest achievements. He received a letter from the Library of Congress dated June 4, 1915 asking for photographic reproductions to add to the institution's collection of the "best modern work" of American artists. The library sent a receipt dated October 21, 1915 for photographs of *The Agnew Clinic, The Cello Player, The Gross Clinic,* and *Henry A. Rowland* (note titles of the clinic paintings).[48]

Eakins's expectation that the collotype would excite the public's anticipation of *The Gross Clinic* is shown by his exhibition of the print twice before the opening of the Centennial in May 1876. The first time was at a Penn Club art exhibition which opened March 7, 1876. This club had just been founded the year before to promote social intercourse among its members who included authors, artists, and men of science and the learned professions, and amateurs of music, letters, and the fine arts.[49] The founders hoped to make significant contributions to the city's plans for welcoming distinguished visitors to the Centennial. The original club members had belonged to a discussion group, the Penn Monthly Association, which published *The Penn Monthly Magazine.*

The clubhouse was located at Eighth and Locust Streets. Guests of honor at a reception on March 7, 1876 were foreign and American Centennial commissioners and judges of awards. The *Philadelphia Press* of March 8 reported that the reception's "new and very attractive feature was the display of paintings, drawings, and sculpture by American artists, the works being shown to advantage in the ample, well-lighted rooms." Thomas Eakins was listed among those artists who were invited, nearly all of whom were present that evening. Besides his "clever watercolor" (*Whistling for Plover*) there was also a "photograph of Mr. Eaken's *[sic]* remarkable portrait of Dr. S. D. Gross."

An article by Eakins's friend William J. Clark Jr. in the March 8, 1876 *Evening Telegraph* praised the "meritorious recent pictures by prominent Philadelphia artists." He explained that the works had been gathered in haste with no prior notice, and the exhibition was made up of works that were ready and could be conveniently loaned, yet it was a "good expression of the too little appreciated artistic talent of Philadelphia." He led off with a review of Eakins:

> The most striking works were the two contributed by Mr. Thomas Eakins, a young artist who is rapidly coming into notice as the possessor of unusual gifts. One of these was a photograph from his large portrait of Dr. Samuel D. Gross—representing that eminent surgeon holding a clinic. The original of this picture has never been out of the artist's studio, but reports of it have gone abroad and much curiosity has been excited with regard to it. It is a work of great learning and great dramatic power, and the exhibition of the photograph last night will certainly increase the general desire to have the picture itself placed on exhibition at an early day.

Eakins exhibited the collotype for a second time at the *Forty-seventh Annual Exhibition* at the Pennsylvania Academy of the Fine Arts, held from April 24 to June 5, 1876. The exhibition record listed Eakins's entry as "Photo from Painting of Dr. Gross, Surgical Clinic."

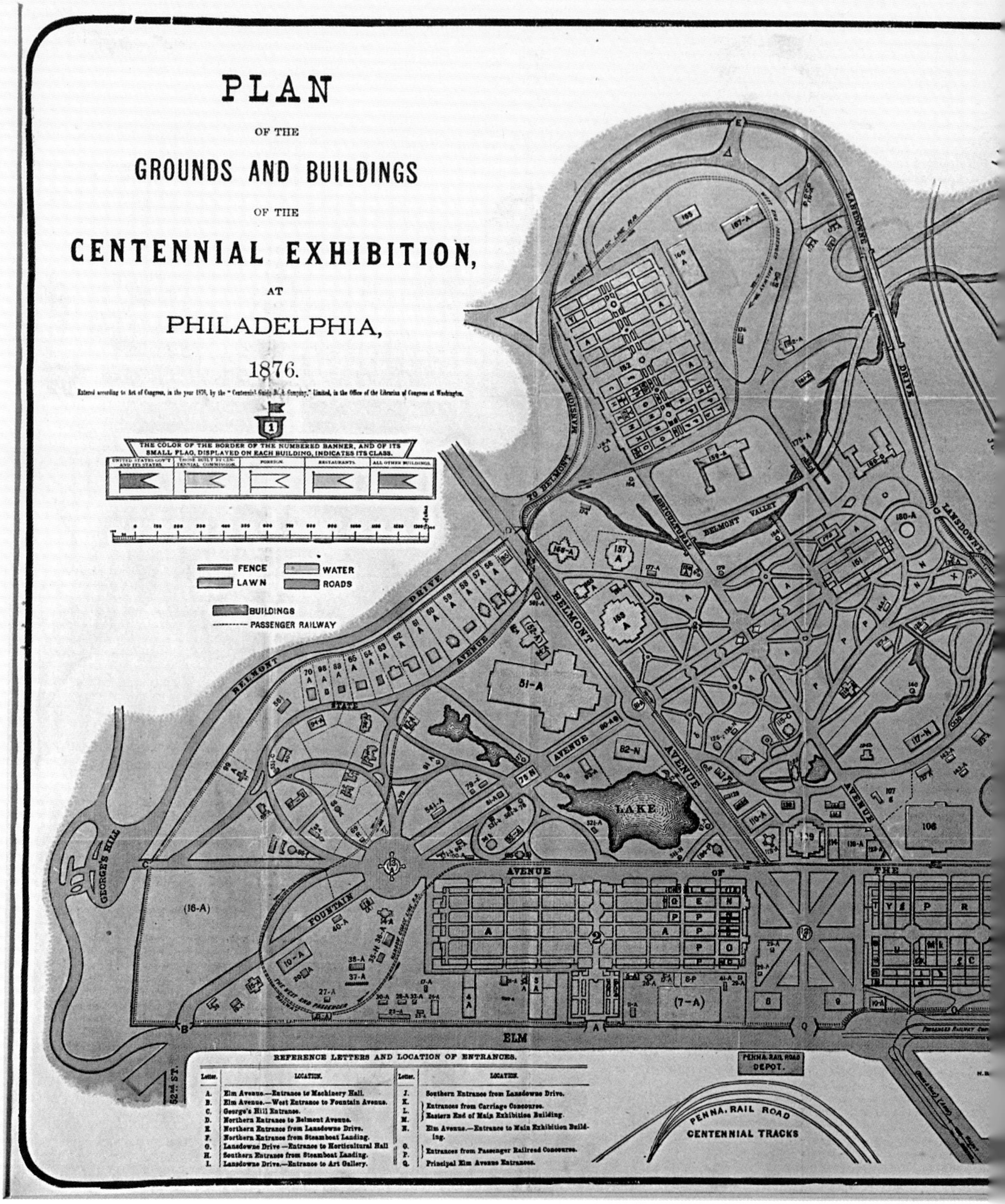
PLAN
OF THE
GROUNDS AND BUILDINGS
OF THE
CENTENNIAL EXHIBITION,
AT
PHILADELPHIA,
1876.
THE COLOR OF THE BORDER OF THE NUMBERED BANNER, AND OF ITS SMALL FLAG, DISPLAYED ON EACH BUILDING, INDICATES ITS CLASS.
FOREIGN.
RESTAURANTS.
ALL OTHER BUILDINGS.
FENCE
WATER
LAWN
ROADS
BUILDINGS
PASSENGER RAILWAY
BELMONT
DRIVE
AVENUE
STATE
FOUNTAIN
LAKE
ELM
52nd ST.
GEORGE'S HILL
TO BELMONT
BELMONT VALLEY
LANSDOWNE
DRIVE
PENNA. RAIL ROAD DEPOT.
PENNA. RAIL ROAD
CENTENNIAL TRACKS
REFERENCE LETTERS AND LOCATION OF ENTRANCES.
A. Elm Avenue.—Entrance to Machinery Hall.
B. Elm Avenue.—West Entrance to Fountain Avenue.
C. George's Hill Entrance.
D. Northern Entrance to Belmont Avenue.
E. Northern Entrance from Lansdowne Drive.
F. Northern Entrance from Steamboat Landing.
G. Lansdowne Drive —Entrance to Horticultural Hall
H. Southern Entrance from Steamboat Landing.
I. Lansdowne Drive.—Entrance to Art Gallery.
J. Southern Entrance from Lansdowne Drive.
K. L. Entrances from Carriage Concourse.
L. M. Eastern End of Main Exhibition Building.
N. Elm Avenue.—Entrance to Main Exhibition Building.
O. P. Entrances from Passenger Railroad Concourse.
Q. Principal Elm Avenue Entrances.

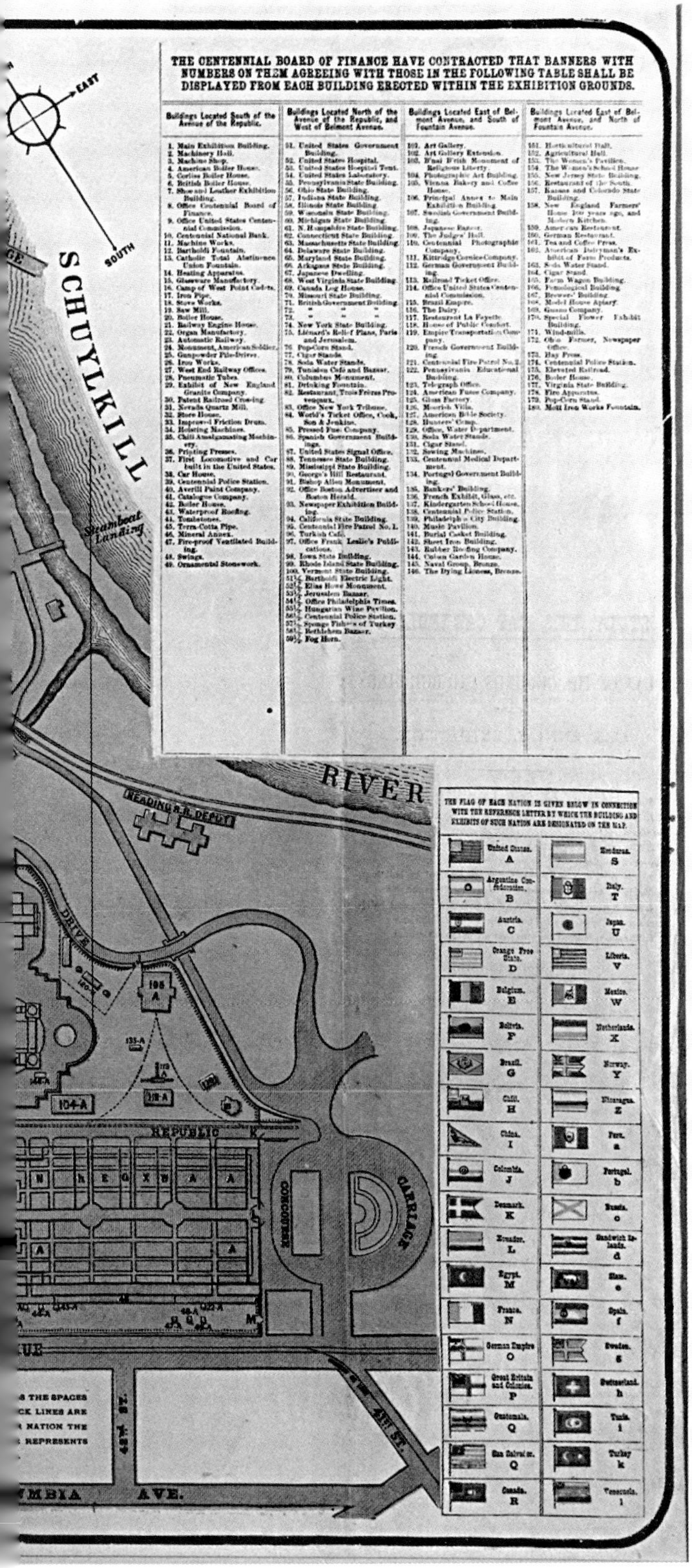

The Gross Clinic at the Philadelphia Centennial Exhibition

Plan of the Grounds and Buildings of the Centennial Exhibition

By unknown draftsman
Colored lithograph
1876
Image size: 16 3/4 x 23 1/4 in.
Sheet size: 17 1/4 x 23 1/2 in.

Folded page from *Authorized Visitors Guide to the Centennial Exhibition and Philadelphia 1876* (Philadelphia: J. B. Lippincott & Co., 1876)

Courtesy of Julie S. Berkowitz

John Sartain's "Report of the Chief of the Bureau of Art" explained the organization and management of the Centennial's art exhibit.[50] The American section was controlled by three committees, all of which were under the control of the director-general. Sartain superintended a six-member Advisory Committee (four administrators and two artists), a ten-member Committee on Selection (all artists), and a seven-member Committee on Arrangement (one administrator and six artists). The selection committee viewed submitted works in Boston, New York, and then Philadelphia.

When it was realized that Memorial Hall (Number 101 on the plan), the original art gallery planned to be a permanent structure, would be unable to accommodate all the chosen art works, an additional building just to the north, the Art Annex (Number 102), had to be erected at the last minute. Sartain admitted that the "unfinished condition of the Art buildings while the placing was going on was of course a serious embarrassment, and but one week before the opening little progress had been made." He added that a "respectable display" was possible by opening day on May 10 only by the "most energetic application to the business." Much to his consternation a ship bearing some American sculptures from Europe was delayed until after the opening.

A third building for art, Photographic Hall (Number 104), was located a short distance from Memorial Hall. According to Sartain, these art buildings were located on the "most commanding portion of the great Lansdowne Plateau," just north of one of the two largest buildings at the exposition, the Main Exhibition Building (Number One).

Sartain reported that 670 American artists contributed 2,621 objects. Thomas Eakins submitted four oils (*The Gross Clinic*, *Portrait of Dr. Benjamin H. Rand*, *The Chess Players*, and *Elizabeth at the Piano*) and two watercolors (*Base Ball* and *Whistling for Plover*) to the jury. All but *The Gross Clinic* were accepted. The portraits of Dr. Rand and the chess players were hung in Memorial Hall and the other pictures in the Annex.

Eakins exhibited his painting of *The Gross Clinic* at the Haseltine Galleries beginning in late April just before the Centennial opened, and about the same time that the collotype was on view at the Pennsylvania Academy. Though scholars have differed in the past, I agree with those who surmise that the impromptu decision to exhibit at Haseltine's in late April was made immediately *after* the painting's rejection for the Centennial art show.

Though he must have been terribly disappointed at the rebuff, Eakins made an effort to bring the painting before the public and to vindicate its worthiness. The tone of William Clark's lengthy and perceptive review in the April 28 *Daily Telegraph* bolsters this view. He explained that Eakins had exhibited very little in Philadelphia since returning from his artistic education in Europe, but had sent his "best things" to Paris where his sporting scenes especially had found a steady sale and were greatly admired. Clark continued,

> There is now on exhibition at Haseltine's galleries, No. 1125 Chestnut Street, Mr. Thomas Eakins' portrait of Dr. Samuel D. Gross, in which that eminent surgeon and teacher is represented as attending a clinic at the Jefferson Medical College. This picture until within a few days past has only been visible in the studio of the artist, but the reports of those who have seen it with regard to its many very striking qualities have stimulated the curiosity not only of art lovers but of people who do not under ordinary circumstances take much interest in art matters...The public of Philadelphia now have, for the first time, an opportunity to form something like an accurate judgment with regard to the qualities of an artist who in many important particulars is very far in advance of any of his American rivals. We know of no artist in this country who can at all compare with Mr. Eakins as a draughtsman, or who has the same thorough mastery of certain essential artistic principles. There are men who have a knack of choosing more popular and more pleasing subjects, who have a finer feeling for the quality that can best be described by the word picturesqueness, and who are more agreeable if not more correct in color. For these reasons it is not difficult to understand that the pictures of men who cannot pretend to rival Mr. Eakins as masters of technique should find more favor with the general American public than his have been able to do. With regard to Mr. Eakins' color, however, there is this to be said—and it is a point that must be considered by those who may be disposed to regard his color as odd, not because it does not represent nature, but because it does not look like what they have been accustomed to in other pictures—his aim in color, as in drawing, is to represent, as near as is possible with the pigments at command, the absolute facts of nature, and a misrepresentation of facts for the purpose of pleasing the eyes of those who do not know what nature looks like is something that his method does not contemplate. The genuineness of Mr. Eakins' method is abundantly exemplified in the picture under consideration, and on a sufficiently large scale for a just opinion with regard to it to be formed.

Clark continued with such a full and accurate description of Dr. Gross's clinic, one wonders if he had discussed his review with the artist in advance. He also countered some objections to the painting's subject matter and to its depiction of the patient, faults that must have been raised by the Centennial's selection committee. He concluded with probably the most ringing endorsement Eakins ever received in his lifetime:

> The principal figures are illuminated by a skylight immediately above their heads, which brings out the group in strong relief, while the students on the seats above and the persons in the background are in shadow. The picture being intended for a portrait of Dr. Gross, and not primarily as a representation of a clinic, the artist has taken a point of view sufficiently near to throw out of focus the accessories, and to necessitate the concentration of all his force on the most prominent figure...To say that this figure is a most admirable portrait of the distinguished surgeon would do it scant justice; we know of nothing in the line of portraiture that has ever been attempted in this city, or indeed in this country, that in any way approaches it. The members of the clinical staff who are grouped around the patient, the students and other lookers-on, are all portraits, and very striking ones, although from the peculiar treatment adopted they do not command the eye of the spectator as does that of the chief personage. The work, however, is something more than a collection of fine portraits; it is intensely dramatic, and is such a vivid representation of such a scene as must frequently be witnessed in the

amphitheatre of a medical school, as to be fairly open to the objection of being decidedly unpleasant to those who are not accustomed to such things. The only objection to the picture that can well be made on technical grounds is in the management of the figure of the patient. The idea of the artist has obviously been to obtrude this figure as little as possible, and in carrying out this idea he has foreshortened it to such an extent, and has so covered it up with the arms and hands of the assisting surgeons, that it is extremely difficult to make it out. It is a mistake to introduce a puzzle in a picture, and this figure is, at first glance, a decided puzzle.

Leaving out of consideration the subject, which will make this fine performance anything but pleasing to many people, the command of all the resources of a thoroughly trained artist, and the absolute knowledge of principles which lie at the base of all correct and profitable artistic practice, demand for it the cordial admiration of all lovers of art, and of all who desire to see the standard of American art raised far above its present level of respectable mediocrity. This portrait of Dr. Gross is a great work—we know of nothing greater that has ever been executed in America.

Post Hospital of the U.S. Army at the Centennial Exhibition

POST HOSPITAL OF THE U.S. ARMY AT THE CENTENNIAL EXHIBITION
By A. Zenone (active second half nineteenth century)

Wood engraving
1876
Image size: 6 3/4 x 4 1/4 in.
Page size: 8 1/2 x 5 3/4 in.

Signed lower left: "A. Zenone"
Caption: "POST HOSPITAL OF THE UNITED STATES ARMY"
From James D. McCabe, *The Illustrated History of the Centennial Exhibition* (Philadelphia: The National Publishing Co., 1876)

Courtesy of Julie S. Berkowitz

One wonders what behind-the-scenes negotiations were necessary for *The Gross Clinic* to be exhibited at the Centennial at all, after being rejected by the Committee on Selection. How was it decided to install the painting in the U.S. Government War Department's medical display? These circumstances have rarely been

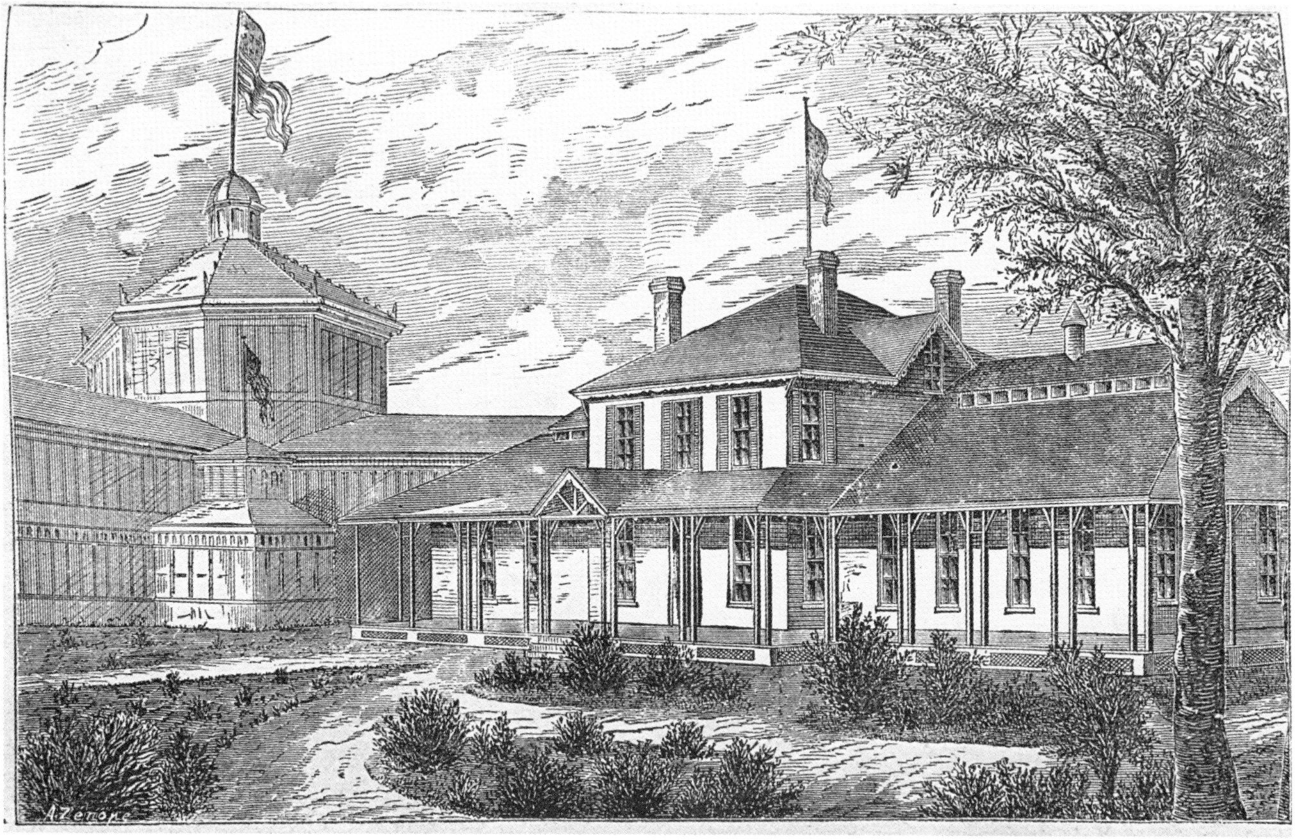

discussed, except in passing.

One can imagine that as a member of the Centennial's Committee on Selection Samuel B. Waugh would have agitated against the painting's inclusion, since it would overshadow his own depictions of surgeons, and it is likely that John Sartain's initial enthusiasm was tempered by concern over expected public aversion to the subject matter. But apparently arrangements were made quickly, for the painting was on view in the Post Hospital of the U.S. Army by late May.[51]

I agree with scholars who have presumed that Dr. Samuel D. Gross was a powerful advocate for displaying *The Gross Clinic* and choosing the Post Hospital as an alternative site. Since the painting includes several portraits of esteemed faculty members operating in the Jefferson Medical College amphitheater, Gross must have felt that Eakins's painting could further enhance his beloved alma mater's reputation in the history of American surgery.

This opinion is best justified by examining contemporary medical journals for information about medical activities in Philadelphia in 1876, so that one gets a better appreciation of Dr. Gross's participation in Centennial-related activities.[52] If he chose to exercise his power to influence the fate of Eakins's painting, this ability would be based not only on his international medical reputation, but also on his friendships with Centennial personnel, many of whom were Jefferson Medical College alumni and faculty, and his knowledge of forthcoming medical events in 1876.

As president of the Centennial Medical Commission Gross certainly would have approved social events already being planned in conjunction with the International Medical Congress in September. The secretary of the Committee on Entertainment was Gross's associate at Jefferson, Dr. J. Ewing Mears, who would make the reservations for the dinner on the first evening of the congress on September 4 when members of Philadelphia's medical profession would entertain delegates on the Centennial grounds in the Judges' Hall (Number 109 on the plan in the *Authorized Visitors' Guide*). Located midway between the two main exposition buildings, Judges' Hall reserved Room Four for the use of medical delegates to the Centennial. On the second evening receptions were being planned at the homes of Jefferson Medical College physicians: the ophthalmologist Dr. William Thomson, and alumnus and trustee Dr. Ellwood Wilson.

Gross would also have recognized that great numbers of physicians would be attending several other medical meetings in Philadelphia during the Centennial months: the American Medical Association, the Association of American Medical Editors, the Pennsylvania State Medical Society, the American Dermatological Association, and the Association of Medical Superintendents of American Institutions for the Insane, as well as dental and pharmaceutical associations. Another meeting was to be convened at Jefferson Medical College in June: the Association of the Representatives of American Medical Colleges, to which Drs. Samuel D. Gross and John B. Biddle were the Jefferson delegates.

Officers of the Medical Staff that would service the Bureau of Medical Services at the fair included Jeffersonians Dr. Samuel W. Gross and Dr. Hamilton Osgood, a lecturer in general symptomatology and microscopy. The Medical Department Building (Number 133) was centrally located not far from Judges' Hall. Several doctors with support staff would be constantly available in a hospital with six beds and a dispensary building to care for injured or ill visitors to the fair. By fair's end, Centennial physicians treated over six thousand patients among the almost ten million visitors. More than four hundred visiting physicians from all over the world recorded their names at the hospital.[53]

There were not only commercial medical exhibits, both American and foreign, throughout the fair, but others sponsored by the U.S. Army and the U.S. Department of the Interior's educational, Indian, and agricultural bureaus. Dr. Richard J. Dunglison contributed a regular column entitled "Medical Centennial Affairs" to *The Medical Record*, with detailed descriptions of various medical displays he outlined as tours for physicians attending meetings and visiting the fair in Philadelphia. Some of the objects to be viewed included advances in therapeutic apparatus, medicines, dietetic preparations, chemical and pharmaceutical products and apparatus, instruments of physical diagnosis, surgical and dental instruments and appliances, and vehicles and appliances for transportation of the sick and wounded.

Another active participant at the Centennial, Dr. Joseph J. Woodward (1833-84), was probably indispensable in helping Dr. Samuel D. Gross to place *The Gross Clinic* in a medical building after the painting was rejected for the art exhibition. A native Philadelphian and an assistant surgeon in the U.S. Army, Dr. Woodward was scheduled to lecture on typho-malarial fever at the first day's session of the International Medical Congress; and on the third evening of the congress he would deliver a special address in the lower lecture room at Jefferson Medical College on scientific work at the Surgeon General's office. Dr. Gross would honor Dr. Woodward by asking him to respond to a toast at the grand dinner on the final evening of the congress.[54]

Significantly, Dr. Woodward was "in charge of the representation of the Medical Department of the United States Army" at the Post Hospital display at the fair.[55] He had served as assistant surgeon with the Army of the Potomac and in 1862 was assigned to the Surgeon General's office in Washington, D.C. where he organized several military hospitals and then was put in charge of the Army Medical Museum. Woodward's pamphlets on Civil War hospitals and transport for field and medical supplies were distributed to visitors in the Post Hospital. He exhibited medical and surgical specimens and preparations from the Army Medical Museum as well as his own microphotographs at the fair.

A significant tie between Dr. Woodward and Dr. Gross was their mutual interest in military medicine. Woodward's work on the medical section of *The Medical and Surgical History of the War of the Rebellion (1861-65)* was published between 1875 and 1879. Surely he must have respected Dr. Gross's well known, pocket-sized *Manual of Military Surgery* of 1861 that encompassed the care of medical and surgical casualties. Gross's book was considered so valuable during the Civil War that the so-called "pirated edition" for the Confederate Army was republished in Richmond in 1862.[56]

Another Jeffersonian who was well known to Drs. Gross and Woodward and who might have played a role in securing the Post Hospital as a display place for *The Gross Clinic* was Dr. John H. Brinton, already mentioned as a Civil War surgeon, active participant in the U.S. Army Medical Museum, and contributor to the surgical section of *The Medical and Surgical History of the War of the Rebellion*. Although not appointed to Jefferson's permanent staff until the erection of the 1877 hospital, Brinton assisted Dr. Gross in establishing the alumni association and in raising alumni contributions for the hospital. He was also a "boon companion" to Dr. Samuel W. Gross in this period.[57] Eakins painted Dr. Brinton's portrait in 1876.

The U.S. Army Post Hospital (Number 52 on the plan) was an annex of the U.S. Government Building (Number 51) which was located at the intersection of two major thoroughfares, Belmont and Fountain Avenues. The Government Building was the largest structure at the Centennial after the five main buildings, and featured wide-ranging scientific and military exhibits from the Departments of War, Navy, Treasury, Interior, Post Office, and Agriculture, as well as the Smithsonian Institution and the Commission of American Food Fishes.[58]

Interestingly, all department displays of the U.S. government were "ornamented by oil portraits, many of them fine works of art representing distinguished personages connected with them."[59] This parallels the display of *The Gross Clinic* in the Post Hospital.

The U.S. Army's display of the twenty-four-bed hospital was intended to publicize the middle-sized, regulation hospital for use in military posts, adopted in 1867 and amended in 1871.[60] The frame building had a shingle roof and was surrounded by a veranda. The central administration area was two stories high, with a two-storied back building and two wings as wards, each containing twelve beds. Each ward was forty-five feet long, twenty-four feet wide, and fifteen feet high. Ridge ventilation with two boxed openings was provided for the summer months and a large stove for the winter months.

Ward Two displayed models of barrack hospitals, hospital steam vessels and railway cars, ambulances, and so forth, and specimens and photographs from the Army Medical Museum. The various administration rooms had exhibitions of medicines, medical stores, and chemicals; surgical instruments and dressings; photographed title pages of rare books on military medicine and surgery; mess furniture and utensils; prosthetic appliances; litters and stretchers; and medical panniers and knapsacks.

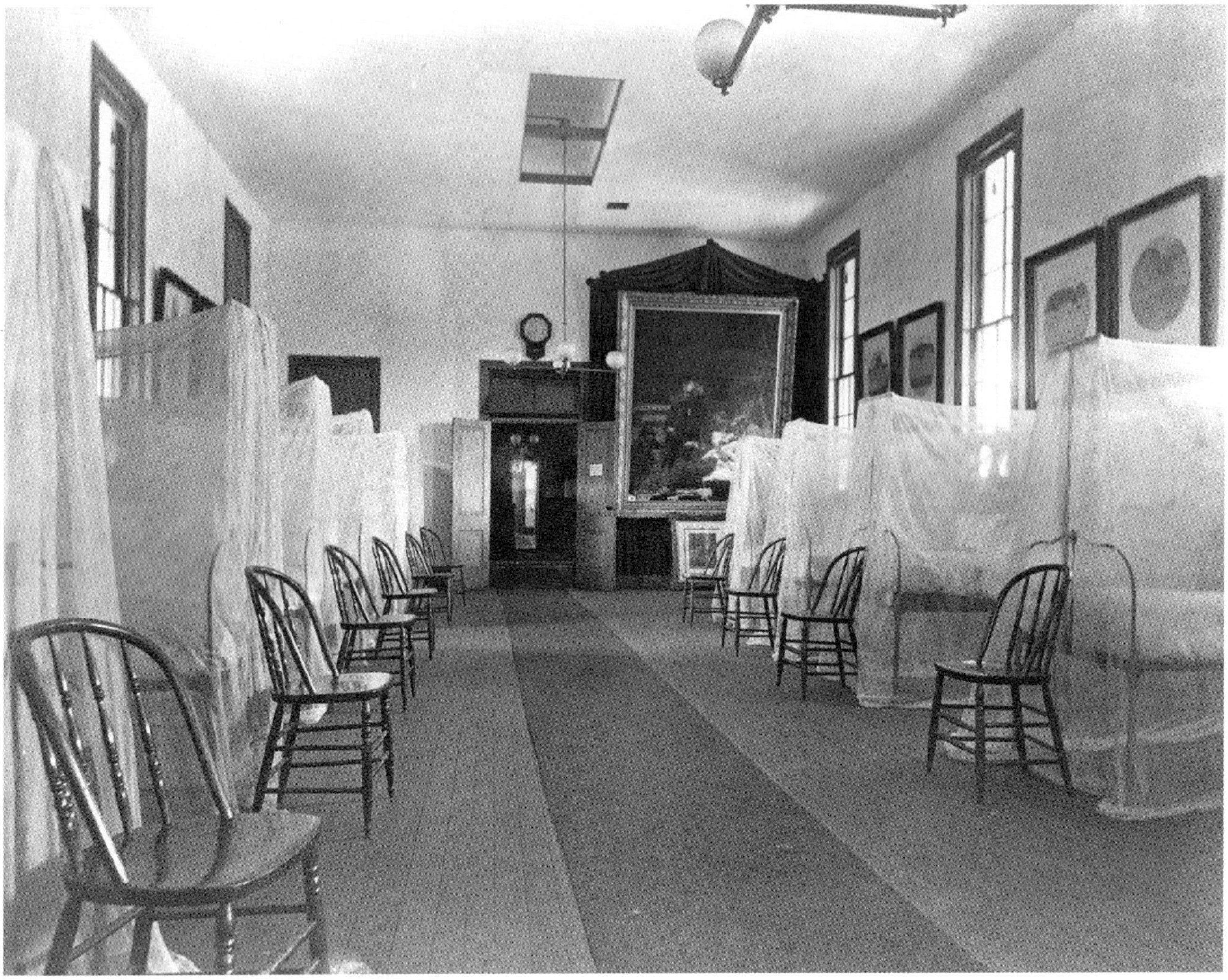

Ward One of the U.S. Army Post Hospital, Philadelphia Centennial

WARD ONE OF THE U.S. ARMY POST HOSPITAL
By unknown photographer

Vintage photograph
1876
8 x 10 in.

Courtesy of the Library of Congress

Ward One of the U.S. Army Post Hospital was fitted up to display hospital bedding, furniture, and clothing. The photograph from the Library of Congress shows two rows of beds covered with mosquito netting. *The Gross Clinic* can be seen hanging against a black cloth on the far wall. The edge of the frame is flush with the open door of a double doorway. A framed collotype of the painting rests on the floor below.

One illustrated, contemporary history of the Centennial Exhibition is unusual for even mentioning *The Gross Clinic* in the context of a description of the hospital. Its author, James D. McCabe, editorialized on the painting's installation:[61]

> The principal room on the lower floor showed the arrangement of the beds, and the conveniences provided in the army hospitals for attending to the wants of the sick and wounded. The treatment of wounds and other hurts was illustrated by papier-maché figures placed in the beds in the positions necessary to the proper treatment of such injuries. Upon the walls of the room and the halls adjoining it were photographs of difficult and successful amputations.
>
> In this room was Mr. Thomas Eakins' fine picture of Dr. Gross delivering a clinical lecture to a class of

> students. It was one of the most powerful and life-like pictures to be seen in the Exhibition, and should have had a place in the Art Gallery, where it would have been but for an incomprehensible decision of the Selecting Committee.

Although *The Gross Clinic* was virtually ignored by the lay press while on view at the Centennial except by the critic William J. Clark, the monumental painting *was* mentioned in several medical journals in the context of medical displays at the fair. Some authors remarked on the reasons for its rejection for display in the art building or its unbecoming installation in the Post Hospital, but none suggested that the building itself was an inappropriate or ignoble location. While the critical commentary was mixed, it was somewhat more positive than in the lay press.

The Medical and Surgical Reporter instituted a regular series of letters to the editor on medical features of the Centennial written by "various gentlemen, each a competent judge of the department he will undertake." On June 3, 1876, "A," the author of the first letter, urged the readers not to overlook the U.S. government building which "to the medical man has greater attractions than many of the larger and more crowded buildings." While praising the beautiful photomicrographs on the walls over the camp bedsteads with their "dummy" patients in Ward Two of the Post Hospital, he mentioned almost in passing a "large oil painting representing a clinic by Professor Gross" at the end of the room opposite the door. He criticized its installation saying, "Unfortunately, it is so hung that the figures are obscure, and I found much difficulty in recognizing the familiar faces which surround the operator."

The June 10 issue of *The Medical Record* referred to Eakins by name but described the surgical procedure inaccurately: a "large portrait of Prof. Gross in the act of performing an amputation in the presence of his class, painted by Mr. Thos. Eakins, of this city." The author was Dr. Richard Dunglison, a special correspondent to the New York journal. One suspects that the rejection of *The Gross Clinic* was a topic of gossip and rumors among artists and physicians, for Dunglison wrote,

> The picture has much merit, and the likeness is excellent; but the coloring is not pleasant, and the subject is so repulsive, the Professor's unnecessarily bloody hand being the conspicuous feature of the scene, that we are not surprised that, for this latter cause alone, it was refused a place in the Art Gallery by the Committee of Selection, to find a more appropriate niche in the Army Hospital.

A surprising analysis of Eakins's motives is found in a "Letter from Philadelphia" to the editor of the *Boston Medical and Surgical Journal* of August 3. The anonymous physician penned a full-page description of the "large oil painting by Eakens" [*sic*], "the most striking and attractive object" in the hospital structure.

His description of the scene echoes many of the comments in William J. Clark's lengthy and very complimentary article of April 28. The medical writer added a few colorful details such as that the clinical assistant was "mopping out" the wound while others "separate the lips of the cut," and that "about slipping to the floor from the operating table is a gouge-chisel, which suggests that the operation is for necrosis."

This author then said that Eakins was deliberately ambiguous about the patient's position because of his own apprehension about the subject, analogous to Clark's comment about Eakins's idea to "obtrude this figure as little as possible." In noting the faintheartedness of the art committee he made an ironic reference to unnamed "far more gory" paintings that were included in the art exhibition:

> It was originally offered to the art committee, but the details of the picture proved so shocking that two or three members of the committee actually became faint, and it was deemed wiser to reject it; so that although there are in memorial hall pictures which are far more gory, this fine work of art at last found its way to the government hospital building. Let me advise those of your readers who visit the Exhibition not to miss a view of it.

For the August 26 *Medical and Surgical Reporter*, physician/art critic "A" wrote another letter entitled "The Anatomist in the Art Gallery," claiming that physicians as anatomists have a "just title to be heard in reference to the proportion and hues of the human form" depicted in art works. He concurred essentially with Thomas Eakins in declaring that the painter needs "practical dissection as much as the surgeon," and "constant observation of the life model to catch the reflex of light from quivering flesh, the infinitely varied outlines of muscle in motion, and the harmonious action of living limbs.

"Painfully apparent to the anatomist" is his conclusion that "the works of nearly all the American artists show a deficient study of the life model," for to excel in portraiture they must "pass a much longer novitiate at the dissecting table, and give more attention to the living body." While never making an exception of the anatomically convincing and palpably energetic figures in Eakins's *Gross Clinic* or any of his other paintings at the Centennial, "A" made a wholesale denunciation of American artists as having "learned to draw from flat surfaces, from nerveless mannikins and plaster casts."

With unintended irony he singled out for praise only two works of art: dissection scenes by foreign painters. One was *The Anatomist* by the German artist Gabriel Max (1840-1915), "a masterly delineation, full of noble thought" of a "woman, young and fair," whose "wealth of golden hair lies in disorder around the pallid features" and whose "slight covering reveals the rounded outlines of/'The treasure/Of limbs too delicious for death.'" The other was *The Lesson in Anatomy* by the Frenchman F.-N.-A. Feyen-Perrin, in which Dr. Velpeau, who is surrounded by assistants and students, is "about to commence a demonstration on a male subject in the pathological rooms of La Charité." He said that "the faces are portraits and well painted," although the artist "failed to catch the peculiarly vivid and energetic light which marked Velpeau's countenance in lecturing." This is an intriguing comment, because in Eakins's painting Dr. Gross's forehead is bathed in such a light.

In a review of the Centennial's American art section in *The Evening Telegraph* of June 16, William J. Clark castigated blunders "beyond correction" of the art committee and the continuing confusion in the galleries as far as numbering and cataloguing the works. In commending Eakins's three portraits at the fair, he excoriated the selection committee's timidity and probable envy in rejecting *The Gross Clinic*:

> In commenting upon Mr. Thomas Eakins' portrait of Dr. Gross when it was on exhibition at Haseltine's galleries...we said that nothing finer had been done in this city. There is nothing so fine in the American section of the Art Department of the Exhibition, and it is a great pity that the squeamishness of the Selecting Committee compelled the artist to find a place for it in the United States Hospital building. It is rumored that the blood on Dr. Gross' fingers made some of the members of the committee sick, but, judging from the quality of the works exhibited by them we fear that it was not the blood alone that made them sick. Artists have before now been known to sicken at the sight of pictures by younger men which they in their souls were compelled to acknowledge were beyond their emulation. The figure of Dr. Gross in this picture is the representation of a man and not of a shadow.

Ironically, while the reputations of many painters on the selection committee and on the roster of chosen artists have not withstood the test of time, Eakins later became acknowledged as one of America's preeminent artists.

However, the indignation expressed by generations of art historians over the insult to Eakins has ignored some ameliorating evidence. My conclusion in no way justifies the art committee's decision to reject the painting, but instead makes a case for its alternative placement in the hospital building.

An analysis of displays of medicine at the fair demonstrates a serious effort to present to the public advances in American medical and surgical diagnosis and treatment. The advantageously situated Post Hospital was a major component of a relatively important complex of U.S. government buildings. The hospital was attractively constructed, and the displays were intellectually and visually stimulating. Though a majority of visitors to the hospital probably were individuals interested in medicine, science, and the military rather than just casual passersby, reports indicate steady attendance at this display. It was neither the uncouth place indignantly described by some early scholars nor the fair visitors' dispensary mistakenly identified by a few others.

The Centennial followed on the heels of the Civil War in which Drs. Gross and Woodward and so many other American physicians contributed their services to the wounded. The displays in the Post Hospital, especially the manikins of casualties in Ward One, were a sympathetic environment for the portrait of Dr. Gross operating on the diseased leg of a young man.

Controversy over *The Gross Clinic's* exhibition location at the Centennial and critical disapproval did not sway Jefferson Medical College from purchasing the painting in 1878, and these factors never lessened the institution's enthusiasm for displaying it. Jeffersonians wrote with pride about the picture's inclusion at the Centennial, never with shame over its exclusion from the art building.

Thomas Eakins was almost certainly bitterly disappointed and angered by the jury's rejection of *The Gross Clinic* for the art building, but he likely concurred with the decision for an alternative placement in the Post Hospital. Both of his exhibition record books list this location at the Centennial. No matter how great the artist's humiliation, pride did not keep him away from the Centennial site. His exhibitor's card in the collection of the Hirshhorn Museum and Sculpture Garden shows that he visited the fair grounds sixteen times in the months of September, October, and November alone.

Jefferson Medical College did not commission a painting from Thomas Eakins until the 1905 portrait of Dr. William S. Forbes, but this does not imply dissatisfaction with *The Gross Clinic*. The majority of art works acquired in the interim since 1878 were either sculptures or *gifts* of paintings. The only other painters commissioned in that twenty-seven-year period were Samuel B. Waugh, Bernard Uhle, Robert W. Vonnoh, and William Merritt Chase (one each), and George W. Pettit (three).

Later Exhibition of The Gross Clinic in the 1870s

Eakins's record books indicate that he exhibited *The Gross Clinic* at Haseltine's again "after the close of the Centennial" in November. In February 1879 Eakins borrowed the work from Jefferson Medical College to submit it to the *Second Annual Exhibition* of the Society of American Artists in New York.

Although Eakins had been represented for the first time at the National Academy of Design's annual exhibition in New York in 1877, he joined a group of independent and younger New Movement artists revolting from the conservative academy to form the Society of American Artists. He showed two paintings at the society's first exhibition in 1878, and although he was not made a member until 1880, the exhibition jury accepted *The Gross Clinic* for exhibition in 1879.

The show ran from March 10 to March 29, 1879 at the Kurtz Gallery and was extensively reviewed by New York newspaper critics. While many of them acknowledged Eakins's talent and the painting's power and authority, most critics found fault with the artist's composition and color, and agreed emphatically that the subject was objectionable. However, judging from its prominence in the reviews, the magnetic painting could not be ignored.

Several newspapers previewed the show on March 8, "varnishing day," just before the public opening. The critic for the *New York Daily Tribune* commented on Eakins's "large and important" work whose subject he confused with a dissection and whose bloodiness he compared with famous French scenes of death. He referred to *The Gross Clinic* as

> "The Anatomist," one of the most powerful, horrible and yet fascinating pictures that has been painted anywhere in this century—a match, or more than a match, for David's "Death of Marat," or for Géricault's "Wreck of the Medusa." But the more one praises it, the more one must condemn its admission to a gallery where men and women of weak nerves must be compelled to look at it. For not to look at it is impossible.

This comment in fact was high praise, for these paintings by Jacques-Louis David (1748-1825) and J.-L.-A.-Théodore Géricault (1791-1824) are among the finest works by these French masters.

On March 8 the *New York Times* reviewer wrote with only partial accuracy that Eakins was "an artist whose strength lies in anatomy, and whose life was begun in a surgeon's office," and that he had been *asked* to paint a great surgeon of Philadelphia. At least the reviewer got the subject right: "a portrait of a surgeon at a class lecture, surrounded by his students, and engaged in an operation on a man's thigh." The critic agreed with the previous reviewer that "the story told is in itself so dreadful that the public may be well excused if it turn away in horror." In addition to the offensive pincers, lancets, spurting blood, and blood on the surgeons' hands, the author listed a new object of moralizing scorn, the "ugly, naked unreal thigh."

He concluded, "The violent and bloody scene shows that at the time it was painted, if not now, the artist had no conception of where to stop in art, or how to hint a horrible thing if it must be said, or what the limits are between the beauty of the nude and the indecency of the naked. Power it has, but very little art."

The *New York Herald* of March 8 called *The Clinic* "decidedly unpleasant and sickeningly real in all its gory details," but a "startlingly lifelike and strong work."

By March 22 the *Tribune's* reviewer lamented the absence of poetry and the ideal in the exhibition as a whole. He launched immediately into a detailed and probing analysis of the "sickening scene" depicted in *The Gross Clinic*:

> The more we study Mr. Thomas Eakins's "Professor Gross," No. 7, the more our wonder grows that it was ever painted, in the first place, and that it was ever exhibited in the second. As for the power with which it is painted, the intensity of the expression, and the skill of the drawing, we suppose no one will deny that these qualities exist...
>
> This [painting] has occupied the time of an artist it has often been our pleasure warmly to praise, and that a society of young artists thinks it proper to hang in a room where ladies, young and old, young girls and boys and little children, are expected to be visitors. It is a picture that even strong men find it difficult to look at long, if they can look at it at all; and as for people with nerves and stomachs, the scene is so real that they might as well go to a dissecting-room and have done with it.

The critic, who assumed that the operation was of "great difficulty" because of the display of blood and the mother's agonized gesture, was ignorant of the fact that a certain amount of bleeding is unavoidable during such an operation as removal of a sequestrum. In the last paragraph the *Tribune* reviewer asked "what good can be accomplished for art or for anything else by painting or exhibiting such a picture." He opined that it would be a "very troublesome wall ornament" even for a medical college because the "amorphous member" (the patient's thigh) would create "doubts in the minds of neophytes" and "sarcasm in the minds of experts."

The reviewer asked, "Is it not unnecessary to introduce a melodramatic element—wholly hostile to the right purpose of art—into the scene, to show us this old woman writhing her body and twisting her hands as the Professor details the doings of the scalpel to the house of life of some one dear to her?"

He concluded that this "horrible story" is no fit subject for laymen and that "no purpose is gained by this morbid exhibition, no lesson taught—the painter shows his skill—and the spectator's gorge rises at it—that is all." As though to demonstrate a modicum of fairness he closed with the compliment: "No matter how slight the thing Mr. Eakins's people are doing, they always are doing it as effectually as if their painted bodies were real ones."

Although the artist left no written record of his reaction to the adverse reviews, among his papers were clippings of many notices.[62] The Bregler Collection of Thomas Eakins manuscripts at the Pennsylvania Academy of the Fine Arts includes several clippings dated between 1879 and 1899.

To balance the largely vituperative reviews were two others that praised both the execution and subject matter of *The Gross Clinic*. The *New York Daily Graphic* of March 8 even reproduced the work and its reviewer termed "The Clinic" a "large and important canvas which commands attention both from its subject and treatment." He thought the central figure of Dr. Gross was a "striking portrait" and he found no fault with the position of the patient or the gesture of the mother. In contrast to most other works in the exhibition, he said the picture is a "serious, thoughtful work, and we can readily understand what a fascination a subject like this must have for an artist who is himself a profound student of anatomy. There is thought and feeling of a high order in this painting."

The most knowledgeable review of this show was published in *The Nation* of March 20 and was probably written by Eakins's friend Earl Shinn.[63] He commented on the competition in style between those American exhibitors who had studied art in France and those who had studied in Germany, and pointed out that Eakins's "exact photographic realism" derived from his teacher Gérôme and his "robust realism" from Bonnat. Shinn emphasized Eakins's scientific teaching methods in perspective and anatomy. Then he asked whether "with all this patience in laying up facts" the artist has the "artistic faculty to apply them."

He astutely called *The Gross Clinic* a kind of challenge to Rembrandt's *Anatomy Lesson of Dr. Tulp*, with Dr. Gross "a contemporary Dr. Tulp, explaining the secrets discovered by his scalpel to an audience of respectful pupils," with the difference that Dr. Gross is treating a living patient, clearly evident from the chloroformed towel which conceals his head and from the anguish of his mother.

Shinn was one of the few to understand Eakins's complex composition of interconnected, life-scale figures and his dramatic use of light and shadow to differentiate groups, both techniques used by Rembrandt. He also praised the striking contrast between the "professional habitude" of "the aged and quiet professor, in a sharp perpendicular light, as he demonstrates very calmly with a gesture of his reddened fingers," and the "unaccustomed terror" of the mother clothed in the "decent and seedy dress of ceremony, overcome by a sudden horror which scatters ceremony to the winds." He added that "few professors have got themselves painted in so interesting a presentment for posterity."

In prescribing the appropriate place for the portrait's eventual display, Shinn repeated the inaccurate assumption that the painting had been *ordered for* Jefferson Medical College by a body of its alumni:

> The picture is no more amenable to questions of mere taste than Rembrandt's is. Rembrandt's has been removed from considerations of conventionality by the remoteness of its period and the interest of its art, and this *[The Gross Clinic]* may be held to be so removed by the remoteness of its destination in a college and the technical partiality of its future spectators.

After the close of the Society of American Artists show in New York, Eakins became embroiled in another controversy over *The Gross Clinic*. The society was invited to exhibit a selection of its members' work from the New York show at the Pennsylvania Academy of the Fine Arts' *Fiftieth Annual Exhibition* opening April 28, 1879. Eakins was teaching at the

Academy then and was asked to join the committee on exhibition.

It was agreed that the society's show should be hung together in a special gallery and treated as a unit in the catalogue. After initial disagreements between the society and the Academy and subsequent rearrangements, the society's paintings were finally installed together in a large gallery. However, *The Gross Clinic* was hung by itself near distant galleries of art works on paper and student works. Furthermore, the annual's place of honor was granted to a large painting by Philadelphia artist Thomas Moran, a work that had been rejected earlier for the New York show.

Eakins's and the society's protests caused such a public uproar that the society threatened to withdraw its entire exhibit. As a compromise, the Academy's exhibition committee decided to remove Moran's picture but adamantly refused to relocate *The Gross Clinic.*

The depth of Eakins's humiliation and confrontational indignation can be discerned in his letter of April 24, 1879 to the Academy's board of directors.[64] Eakins reminded the board that in the interval between the New York and Philadelphia shows the paintings had been redistributed to the artists and were to be recollected by agents of the Academy at the Academy's expense. He continued testily,

> In the redistribution my picture of Prof. Gross, a conspicuous and important part of the Society's exhibition was returned to Philadelphia and I then told Mr. Corliss [secretary of the Academy] that it was at Haseltine's where he could send for it at any time.
>
> I frequently asked about the arrival of the other New York pictures and on the arrival of the first of them I again reminded Mr. Corliss of my picture.
>
> He said nothing to me of his sly intention of sending for all the other pictures and neglecting mine and it was not until after the arrival of all the rest and on my again asking after mine that he informed me that he did not intend to send for mine without special orders from the committee on hanging.
>
> I am sure that he falsely accused me to the Committee of some neglect and misinformed them of the circumstances which he well knew for it was he who had finished all the business details of the arrangement with the Society having been sent by you to New York for that purpose.
>
> The committee acting on misinformation refused my picture.
>
> They reconsidered and decided to accept it if I assumed the trouble and expense of bringing my own picture which I did.
>
> I herewith enclose the receipted bill for that expense and ask your Board to refund me the amount.
>
> I ask in justice to myself and the Academy and in honest fulfillment of the compact between the Academy and the Society of American Artists that my picture be hung in the room with the other New York pictures and nowhere else and I suggest that the conduct of Mr. Corliss be investigated.
>
> I accuse him of acting the miserable and tricky partisan and not the honest servant of the Academy whose interest I have much at heart.

The Gross Clinic was not moved to another gallery. On the day after the opening the critic of the *Philadelphia North American* said that Eakins's "Portrait of Professor Gross" was a "large and pretentious production" that was "well but blackly painted, and is no doubt a good portrait." The professor and his assistant were "engaged in the thick of a serious surgical operation—the crimson evidences of which are more than obtrusively presented." He concluded:

> It may be seriously doubted whether the walls of Jefferson College have not been denuded without any sufficiently good reason. There is an especially objectionable finger and thumb, which will go far to cause the corner in which this grisly picture is hung to be severely left alone during the duration of the exhibition.

The critic who most ably described Eakins's aesthetic sensibility during this period was William C. Brownell in "The Younger Painters of America," an article in *Scribner's Monthly* of May 1880. In a discussion of contesting styles in American art in the late 1870s, Brownell praised Eakins's technical skills which he used to produce a powerful effect of actuality, or "intense realism":

> Mr. Eakins is another instance of a painter who knows how to paint. Whatever objection a sensitive fastidiousness may find to the subject of his picture, exhibited here a year ago, entitled "An Operation in Practical Surgery," none could be made to the skill with which the scene was rendered. It was a canvas ten feet high, and being an upright and the focus being in the middle distance, it presented many difficulties of a practical nature to the painter; the figures in the foreground were a little more, and those in the background a little less, than life size, but so ably was the whole depicted that probably the reason why nine out of ten of those who were startled or shocked by it were thus affected, was its intense realism; the sense of actuality about it was more than impressive, it was oppressive. It was impossible to doubt that such an operation had in every one of its details taken place, that the faces were portraits, and that a photograph would have fallen far short

of the intensity of reproduction which the picture possessed. What accuracy of drawing, what careful training in perspective and what skill in composition this implies, are obvious.

Listing Thomas Eakins among America's most able painters and also among a group criticized for being unpoetic, Brownell said that in Eakins's case his power "almost makes up for the lack of poetry":

> His "Surgical Operation" beforementioned as a masterpiece of realism in point of technique, is equally a masterpiece of dramatic realism, in point of art. The painter increased rather than diminished the intensity which it is evident he sought after, by taking for a theme a familiar and somewhat vulgar tragedy of everyday occurrence in American hospitals, instead of an historic incident of Rome or Egypt. The play of emotions which is going on is strong and vivid. The chloroformed patient is surrounded by surgeons and students whose interest is strictly scientific, his mother who is in an agony of fear and grief, and the operator who holds a life in his hand and is yet lecturing as quietly as if the patient were a blackboard. Very little in American painting has been done to surpass the power of this drama. But if the essence of fine-art be poetic, an operation in practical surgery can hardly be said to be related to fine-art at all. Many persons thought this canvas, we remember, both horrible and disgusting; the truth is that it was simply unpoetic. The tragedy was as vivid as that of a battle-field, but it was, after all, a tragedy from which every element of ideality had been eliminated. The same thing is true, with obvious differences of degree, of most of Mr. Eakins's work. He is distinctly not enamored of beauty, unless it be considered, as very likely he would contend, that whatever is is beautiful.

A discussion of aesthetics is beyond the range of this book, but from the late-nineteenth-century medical viewpoint, it was well known that the patient's life was never threatened, so the surgeons' efforts were considered valiant and uplifting because of the certain benefit to the patient and his family. A modern viewer finds it appropriate that Eakins gave heroic dimensions and drama to his powerful scene of healing. His objective transcended the mere scientific explication of "practical surgery."

Loans of The Gross Clinic Up to the Present

After the Pennsylvania Academy's show in 1879, *The Gross Clinic* was returned to Jefferson Medical College. Shortly before his trip to the Dakotas, Eakins wrote a letter dated June 23, 1887 to his former pupil and friend John Wallace in Chicago about exhibiting *The Gross Clinic* in that city, saying, "I am pretty sure the Faculty would not let the Gross Picture go, now that Gross is dead."[65] This might have been a reference to annual exhibitions at the Art Institute of Chicago that were to be inaugurated in 1888. Interestingly, the next important loan of the Gross painting was in Chicago, but at the World's Columbian Exposition in 1893. It was also shown at the Pennsylvania Academy with a group of paintings prior to their transport to the Chicago fair.

Today, many unfamiliar with Jefferson Medical College's loan policy presume that *The Gross Clinic* has seldom been seen away from the campus. In fact, a generous loan policy has long prevailed. Following the 1879 shows in New York and Philadelphia, *The Gross Clinic* was sent to world's fairs in Chicago (1893) where it was among a group of eleven paintings by Eakins that won a bronze medal collectively, and St. Louis (1904) where the painting received a gold medal.

This belated recognition was affirmed in 1904 in a book about contributions by Pennsylvanians to the St. Louis fair in which the painting was illustrated and called "especially noteworthy." The author praised Eakins's "seven powerful and realistic pictures, two of which, depicting the great Pennsylvania surgeons, Doctors Gross and Agnew, lecturing in their clinics, are among the finest achievements of American paintings."[66]

The Gross Clinic was loaned to memorial, retrospective, and centennial exhibitions on Eakins at the Metropolitan Museum of Art and the Pennsylvania Academy of the Fine Arts (1917-18); the Philadelphia Museum of Art (1930 and 1944); the National Gallery of Art, the Art Institute of Chicago, and the Philadelphia Museum of Art (1961-62); the Whitney Museum of American Art (1970); and the Philadelphia Museum of Art and the Museum of Fine Arts, Boston (1982).

Significantly, it was included in special mid-century anniversary shows of both major Philadelphia art institutions, the Museum of Art's *Diamond Jubilee Exhibition* (1950-51) and the Pennsylvania Academy's *150th Anniversary Exhibition* (1955). It was also on special loan to the Museum of Art five times in the 1960s during the summer months. Loans to numerous important medical art and other thematic shows have allowed the painting to be seen in Paris and major U.S. cities including New York, Boston, Baltimore, Washington, D.C., and Birmingham, Alabama.

Reaction to The Gross Clinic Then and Now

Although *The Gross Clinic* has long been acknowledged as a great work by one of America's preeminent artists, even today the monumental painting still has the power to shock, and many lay viewers react viscerally. At first some are unsettled by the pathetic terror of the mother, perplexed by the foreshortened view of the patient, disconcerted by the conspicuous display of blood, or dismayed by the lack of antisepsis.

In spite of any initial reservations, almost all viewers are immediately awed by the majesty of Eakins's conception and transfixed by the magnificent head of Dr. Gross. They are reassured by the surgeon's calm authority and dignity and impressed with the intense concentration and energy of the assisting surgeons.

The difference between then and now is that in the late nineteenth century many American viewers considered the subject repugnant, unfit, and brutal, and a century later it is considered boldly frank, immediate, and enlightening, an optimistic scene of healing. The artist's bravura paint style is no longer considered indelicate and uncouth, but rather powerful and dynamic. Most viewers sense the artist's respect for an older generation teaching a younger generation, and his underlying message about continuity in the practice of and progress of American surgery.

The reputation of Thomas Eakins and the importance of *The Gross Clinic* had been rehabilitated by the end of his life. The *Philadelphia Inquirer's* two column obituary on July 2, 1916 was headlined: "THOMAS EAKINS/DEAN OF ARTISTS/Lived Retired Life for Sev/eral Years Before His/Death/Masterpiece 'The Clinic of Dr./Samuel D. Gross' Hangs in/Jefferson Hospital."

The glowing summary of Eakins's career mentioned that he had studied anatomy at Jefferson Medical College. It referred to many of Eakins's public portraits including those of Drs. Forbes and Rand, the latter a "very important work by the painter, comparable with his best." It included a detailed description of *The Gross Clinic* which "may still be considered his masterpiece, certainly the masterpiece of his youth."

The obituary ended with an assessment of his importance,

> That his work will live when most of that produced by his contemporaries is forgotten has always been the firm conviction of those who know. Already he had begun to reap some of the fruits of his industrious and honorable life and work.
>
> The loss of such a figure in the history of American art cannot be reckoned. The effect upon the growing students is incalculable. Such an influence standing almost a solitary figure in the present state of commercialism, was greater than we knew.

1. Ellwood C. Parry III, "Thomas Eakins and *The Gross Clinic*," *Jefferson Medical College Alumni Bulletin* 16 (summer 1967): 3-6; and Parry, "*The Gross Clinic* as Anatomy Lesson and Memorial Portrait," *The Art Quarterly* 32 (1969): 373-75.
2. John Sartain, "Report of the Chief of the Bureau of Art," in United States Centennial Commission, *Report of the Director-General*, 2 vols. (1880), 1:148-49.
3. Lloyd Goodrich, *Thomas Eakins*, 2 vols. (Cambridge, Mass.: Harvard University Press for the National Gallery of Art, Washington, D.C., 1982), 1:130.
4. Elizabeth Johns, *Thomas Eakins: The Heroism of American Life* (Princeton: Princeton University Press, 1983), 55-63.
5. Samuel D. Gross, M.D., "A Century of American Medicine 1776-1876. II. Surgery," *American Journal of the Medical Sciences* 71 (Apr. 1876): 431-84.
6. *Philadelphia Medical Times* 5 (Apr. 24, 1875): 479.
7. Gross, *Autobiography of Samuel D. Gross, M.D.*, ed. Samuel W. Gross, M.D. and A. Haller Gross, 2 vols. (Philadelphia: George Barrie, 1887), 1:374-76.
8. Parry, "*The Gross Clinic* As Anatomy Lesson," 376-80; Johns, *Thomas Eakins*, 70-75; Neil Hyman, "Eakins' *Gross Clinic* Again," *Art Quarterly* 35 (1972): 159-64; Helen Osterman Borowitz, "The Scalpel and the Brush: Anatomy and Art from Leonardo da Vinci to Thomas Eakins," *Cleveland Clinic Quarterly* 53 (spring 1986): 61-73.
9. See Charles Frankenberger, "The Collection of Portraits Belonging to the College," *The Jeffersonian* 17 (Nov. 1915): 2. Frankenberger, Jefferson's librarian, identified the woman in *The Gross Clinic* as the patient's mother.
10. George M. Gould, M.D., *The Jefferson Medical College of Philadelphia: A History*, 2 vols. (New York: Lewis Publishing Co., 1904), 1:165.
11. See Kathleen A. Foster, *Thomas Eakins Rediscovered: Charles Bregler's Thomas Eakins Collection at the Pennsylvania Academy of the Fine Arts* (New Haven: Yale University Press and the Pennsylvania Academy of the Fine Arts, 1997), 108-09, 256 n. 12. Foster suggests that a photograph of Eakins in the Bregler Collection, with its eccentric pose and graphite rulings, hints at use in some planned composition, possibly *The Gross Clinic*: Eakins's leaning posture resembles that of Dr. Samuel W. Gross; and this photograph, cropped and reversed, appears on Eakins's exhibitor's pass to the Centennial. The angle of Eakins's head and the expression of his eyes in the photograph also resemble the self-portrait in the painting.
12. Gert H. Brieger, M.D., Ph.D., "A Portrait of Surgery: Surgery in America, 1875-1889," *The Surgical Clinics of North America* 67 (Dec. 1987): 1192-93.
13. Charles E. Rosenberg, *The Care of Strangers: The Rise of America's Hospital System* (New York: Basic Books, 1987), 116-28.
14. Reprinted as a condensed version of an 1880 address to the Jefferson Medical College alumni association by John H. Brinton, M.D., "Introductory Lecture: The Faculty of 1841," *The College and Clinical Record* 16 (Sept. 1895): 219-20.
15. Albert P. Brubaker, M.D., "Jefferson Medical College Then and Now—A Retrospect," *Jefferson Medical College Alumni Bulletin* 1 (May 1926): 5.
16. John Chalmers DaCosta, M.D., "Samuel David Gross," *The Jeffersonian* 13 (Apr. 1912): 9. Although DaCosta did not begin to study at Jefferson until 1882, he had attended didactic and clinical lectures by both his "surgical heroes," the elder and younger Gross, for many years during school holidays.
17. Richard J. Mullins, M.D. and Donald D. Trunkey, M.D., "Samuel D. Gross: Pioneer Academic Trauma Surgeon of 19th Century America," *The Journal of Trauma* 30 (May 1990): 536.
18. Gross, *A System of Surgery*, 6th ed., 2 vols. (Philadelphia: Henry C. Lea's Son & Co., 1882), 1:346.
19. Gross, *System of Surgery*, 5th ed., 2 vols. (Philadelphia: Henry C. Lea, 1872), 1:500.
20. Gross, "The Factors of Disease and Death after Injuries, Parturition, and Surgical Operations," in *Medical America in the Nineteenth Century: Readings from the Literature*, ed. Gert H. Brieger, M.D., Ph.D. (Baltimore: Johns Hopkins Press, 1972), 197.
21. "International Medical Congress: Surgical Section," *Philadelphia Medical Times* 6 (Sept. 30, 1876): 626-28.
22. "Letter from Philadelphia," *The Boston Medical and Surgical Journal* 95 (Sept. 21, 1876): 369.
23. Mullins and Trunkey, 537.
24. DaCosta, "Facts Concerning the Old Operating Table," *Jefferson Medical College Clinic* (1928), 86.
25. Gross, *System of Surgery*, 6th ed., 1:838.
26. Gross, *System of Surgery*, 5th ed., 1:868-70.
27. Gross, *System of Surgery*, 6th ed., 1:509.
28. DaCosta, "The Last Surgical Clinic in the Old Amphitheater of the Jefferson Medical College Hospital, Held before the Senior and Junior Classes, May 10, 1922, by Professor John Chalmers DaCosta," *Selections from the Papers and Speeches of John Chalmers DaCosta, M.D., LL.D.* (Philadelphia: W. B. Saunders Co., 1931), 338 (reprinted from the *Jefferson Medical College Alumni Bulletin* 1 (Feb. 1925): 8-19).
29. Gross, *Autobiography*, 2:111.
30. Gross, *System of Surgery*, 6th ed., 1:549-59.
31. W. Joseph Hearn, M.D., "The Administration of Anaesthetics," *The College and Clinical Record* (Jefferson Medical College) 7 (Feb. 1, 1886): 23-26.
32. "Sketch of W. Joseph Hearn, M.D.," *The Jeffersonian* 4 (April 1902): 11-14.

33. One notebook is in Charles Bregler's Thomas Eakins Collection, Archives, Pennsylvania Academy of the Fine Arts. On page 174, under "Pictures Sold Etc.," Eakins's second entry is "Gross 1878 200"; on page 25 in a section for exhibition records of individual paintings, Eakins wrote "Dr Gross Sold," with the latter word in larger size and heavier ink. A similar notebook is located at the Philadelphia Museum of Art.
34. See Goodrich, 1:323 n. 123:7; and Johns, 80 n. 71.
35. Frankenberger said the painting was exhibited in expositions in Chicago, Buffalo, and St. Louis. Perhaps Jefferson Medical College had considered sending the painting to the Pan-American Exposition of 1901, but no records at Jefferson attest to this, and the work is not listed in the catalogue of the fine arts exhibition in Buffalo.
36. "Art and Artists," *The Press*, Mar. 9, 1878, 4.
37. Goodrich, 1:123.
38. Goodrich, 1:128.
39. Letter in Charles Bregler's Thomas Eakins Collection, Archives, Pennsylvania Academy of the Fine Arts.
40. Goodrich, 1:128.
41. William Innes Homer, *Thomas Eakins: His Life and Art* (New York: Abbeville Press Publishers, 1992), 256 n. 32. Homer cites a perspective drawing mentioned in a letter from Charles Bregler to George Barker, June 18, 1939.
42. Letter from Susan Eakins in response to a request from Mrs. Lewis R. Dick, New Century Club, Philadelphia. In Charles Bregler's Thomas Eakins Collection, Archives, Pennsylvania Academy of the Fine Arts.
43. Seymour Adelman, "Thomas Eakins: Mount Vernon Street Memories," *The Moving Pageant* (Lititz, Pa: Sutter House, 1977), 160. This essay was first delivered in 1962 as a talk at the Philadelphia Museum of Art.
44. Charles Bregler, "Thomas Eakins as I Knew Him," manuscript in Charles Bregler's Thomas Eakins Collection, Archives, Pennsylvania Academy of the Fine Arts.
45. Foster, 109, 256 n. 16. Also see Theodor Siegl, *The Thomas Eakins Collection: Philadelphia Museum of Art* (Philadelphia: Philadelphia Museum of Art, 1978), 65. The Philadelphia Museum owns a collotype inscribed to Florence Einstein, an Eakins portrait subject.
46. A short notice in the *American Art Review* (Boston), 1880, 47, mentioned that Braun's collection of reproductions of art works numbered over 42,000, and that their agent for the United States was Mr. J. O. Stornay, at 1516 Chestnut Street in Philadelphia.
47. Phyllis D. Rosenzweig, *The Thomas Eakins Collection of the Hirshhorn Museum and Sculpture Garden* (Washington, D.C.: Smithsonian Institution Press, 1977), 59. The museum owns a collotype inscribed to Dr. Thomas H. Fenton, an Eakins portrait subject.
48. In Charles Bregler's Thomas Eakins Collection, Archives, Pennsylvania Academy of the Fine Arts.
49. Cortlandt van Dyke Hubbard, *History of The Penn Club* (Philadelphia: Winchell Co., 1976), 7, 35.
50. Sartain, 1:134-44.
51. *The Gross Clinic* was mentioned in a letter to the editor dated May 1876 in the June 3, 1876 issue of *The Medical and Surgical Reporter*, a weekly journal.
52. In addition to the *Transactions of the International Medical Congress of Philadelphia* (Philadelphia, 1877), the following journals reported on the Centennial's medical activities: *The Philadelphia Medical Times*, *The New York Medical Journal*, *The Boston Medical and Surgical Journal*, *The Medical and Surgical Reporter*, *The Medical News and Library*, and *The Medical Record*.

For a bibliography on other aspects of the Centennial Exhibition consult Robert W. Rydell, *The Books of the Fairs* (Chicago: American Library Association, 1992), 93-114.
53. *The Boston Medical and Surgical Journal* 95 (Dec. 7, 1876): 687.
54. *The Boston Medical and Surgical Journal* 95 (Sept. 21, 1876): 369.
55. "The U.S. Army Medical Department, Centennial Exhibition, May, 1876," *The Medical and Surgical Reporter* 34 (June 3, 1876): 457. See also *The Daily Evening Telegraph* of April 28, 1876 which reported that the medical department's model army hospital and "sets of all instruments and appliances used in military surgery and medicine" were "under charge of Assistant Surgeon J. J. Woodward."
56. Frederick B. Wagner Jr., M.D., *Thomas Jefferson University: Tradition and Heritage* (Philadelphia: Lea & Febiger, 1989), 66.
57. Wagner, 537.
58. United States Centennial Commission, *International Exhibition, 1876 Official Catalogue* (Philadelphia: John R. Nagle & Co., 1876), 65-75.
59. *Frank Leslie's Illustrated Historical Register of the Centennial Exposition 1876*, facsimile ed. (New York: Paddington Press Ltd., 1974), 102.
60. Joseph J. Woodward, M.D., *International Exhibition of 1876: Hospital of Medical Department, United States Army* (Philadelphia, 1876), 3-8; *International Exhibition, 1876 Official Catalogue*, 67.
61. James D. McCabe, *The Illustrated History of the Centennial Exhibition* (Philadelphia: National Publishing Co., 1876), 649-51.
62. Goodrich, 1:136.
63. Goodrich, 1:135.
64. Letter in Charles Bregler's Thomas Eakins Collection, Archives, Pennsylvania Academy of the Fine Arts.
65. Letter in Charles Bregler's Thomas Eakins Collection, Archives, Pennsylvania Academy of the Fine Arts.
66. James H. Lambert, *The Story of Pennsylvania at the World's Fair St. Louis, 1904* (Philadelphia: The Pennsylvania Commission, 1905), 2:52.

CHAPTER 5

Late Nineteenth Century: Growth of Clinical and Laboratory Facilities

In the late 1870s the quality of medical instruction and patient care was changed dramatically by the erection of the first detached Jefferson Medical College Hospital in 1877 and of a new laboratory facility attached to Medical Hall in 1879. College professors of medicine, surgery, and obstetrics each presided over a clinical teaching ward for medical students and could have assistants for whom they were responsible. The first select group of hospital staff appointees was well qualified for the challenges of the new hospital. The new laboratory building included facilities for operative and minor surgery, practical chemistry, microscopy, and physiology.

In 1895 Jefferson Medical College was reorganized from a proprietary school to a nonprofit organization of combined college and hospital under the absolute control of the board of trustees. Before then professors had collected fees directly from students for admittance to lectures, and the professors in turn had paid a rental fee to the board for use of the college and hospital. Now professors would no longer share profits but would serve on fixed salaries. Trustees now assumed responsibility for managing the property and the policy of the institution.

In 1891 a three-year course became mandatory and in 1895 the curriculum was upgraded to a four-year course including three years of preceptorship. The admission requirement was still only a high school diploma; by 1914 one year of college was required, in 1929 three years of college, and finally by 1940 an undergraduate bachelor's degree was required.

The art collection continued to expand. In addition to new portraits of many famous professors, the collection acquired portraits of two board members who served during the crucial decision-making years of 1894 and 1895: Joseph B. Townsend and Michael Arnold.

Portrait of Joseph B. Townsend

JOSEPH BARTON TOWNSEND (1822-96)
By Emma F. Leavitt Randall (active late nineteenth and early twentieth centuries)

Oil on canvas
1898
31 x 26 in.

Signed and dated lower left: "E. Randall/'98"

Given before 1915 by unknown donor
Accession number: 1898-1915.P.01

Joseph B. Townsend was a paradigmatic Philadelphia lawyer for more than fifty years. He was elected a trustee at Jefferson Medical College in 1878 and served as chairman of the board from 1894 until his death in 1896.

Joseph Townsend was born in 1822 in Philadelphia, and was admitted as an attorney of the Philadelphia courts in 1842. He served as vice chancellor (1891) and then chancellor (1894) of the Law Association of Philadelphia, and was a respected authority on trusts, estates, and real estate. In addition to Jefferson Medical

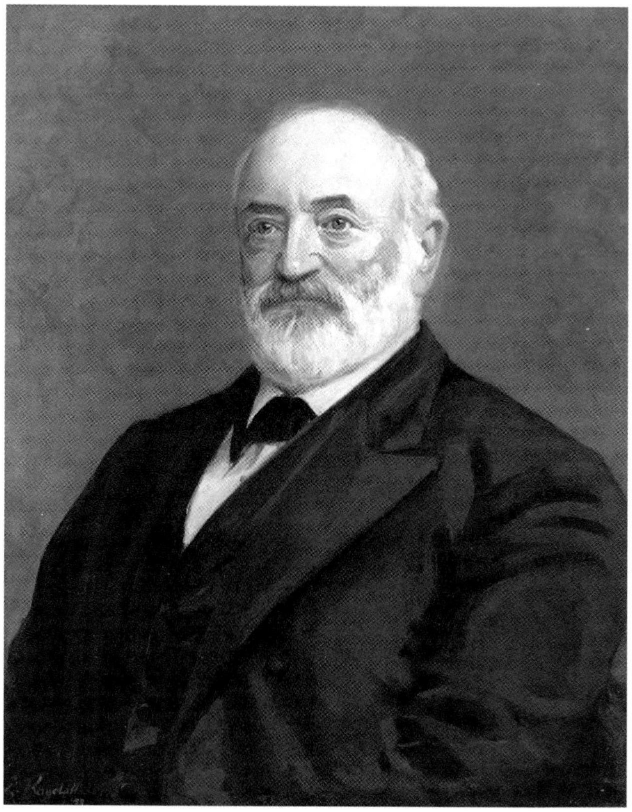

College he was active in the management of Pennsylvania Hospital, and received an honorary LL.D. degree from the University of Pennsylvania. He was also a manager of the Western Savings Fund Society. He was succeeded on Jefferson's board by his attorney sons, James P. Townsend and Charles C. Townsend.

Joseph B. Townsend's posthumous portrait was painted two years after his death by Emma F. Leavitt Randall. Although the artist was dependent on photographs, the attorney's bust-length portrait is surprisingly lifelike. His ample girth, ruddy complexion, and amiable expression correspond to descriptions of the attorney as kindly, lively, affectionate, and a lover of the outdoors.[1] The fluidly brushed strokes give an animation and energy to his face, white hair and beard, and costume.

Emma Leavitt Randall was a Philadelphian who studied at the Pennsylvania Academy of the Fine Arts and exhibited portraits there steadily between 1885 and 1897. In 1893 she married Dr. Burton Alexander Randall, an eminent clinical professor of diseases of the ear at the University of Pennsylvania.

Portrait of Michael Arnold

MICHAEL ARNOLD (1840-1903)
By Mary Van der Veer (b. 1865)

Oil on canvas
Before 1915
30 x 21 1/2 in.

Signed upper right: "M. Van der Veer"

Given before 1915 by unknown donor
Accession number: 1915+b.P.01

Judge Michael Arnold served as a Jefferson Medical College trustee from 1887 until his death in 1903. He was commended by the board for "thoughtful and careful attention to everything appertaining to the condition of the hospital and the welfare of its patients."

Michael Arnold was born in 1849 in Philadelphia and graduated from Central High School in 1857. He worked in business for a few years, then studied law with Edward Hopper, a son-in-law of the noted reformer Lucretia Mott. He was admitted to the bar in 1863. During the Civil War he served with the chief inspector of paymasters in the United States Army at Fortress Monroe and in New Orleans. After resuming his law practice in Philadelphia he was elected in 1882 to the first of three terms as a Democratic judge of the Common Pleas Court.

Besides serving as a trustee at Jefferson from 1887 until his death in 1903, Judge Arnold was a manager of the Edwin Forrest Home. An active Mason, he was a high priest of the Rising Star Lodge, and a grand master of the Ancient and Honorable Fraternity in Pennsylvania.

In his bust-length portrait by Mary Van der Veer, Judge Arnold is turned to the left and his eyes gaze off to the side. His bushy, light brown mustache offsets his thinning hair and calls attention to his long, aquiline nose, pointy chin, and angular jaw. His expression is serious, almost somber. It is not known if this was a posthumous portrait.

Mary Van der Veer was born in Amsterdam, New York in 1865. She studied at the National Academy of Design and with William Merritt Chase in New York, and at the Philadelphia Art School and the Pennsylvania Academy of the Fine Arts. She continued her studies abroad with James McNeill Whistler in Paris, and also in Holland.

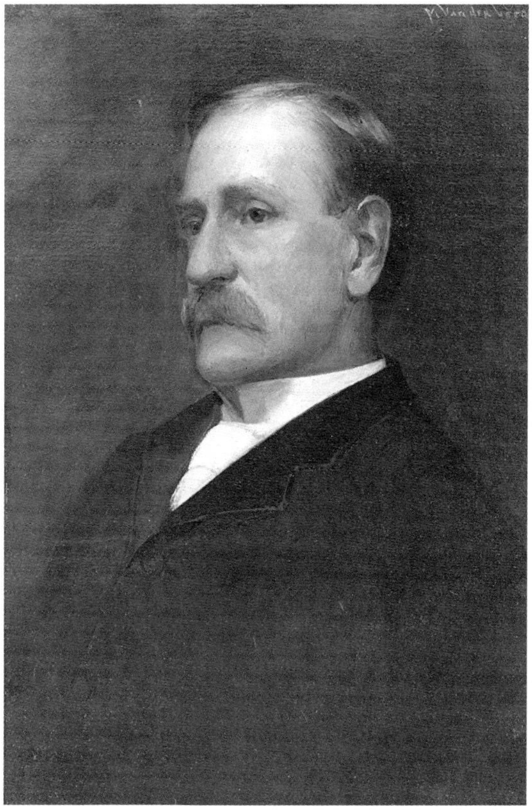

Best known for portraits, flower studies, and genre scenes set in Holland, Van der Veer exhibited at the National Academy of Design and the Water Color Club in New York and at the Pennsylvania Academy. She won a bronze medal at the Louisiana Purchase Exposition in St. Louis in 1904, and the Julia A. Shaw Memorial Prize (for painting or sculpture by an American woman) at the National Academy in 1911 for *The Geography Lesson*.

Jefferson Medical College Hospital Training School for Nurses, Class of 1893-94

TRAINING SCHOOL FOR NURSES, CLASS OF 1893-94
By unknown photographer

Vintage photograph
1894
8 x 9 3/4 in.

Given after 1894 by unknown donor
Accession number: 1894+f.Ph.03

This formal group photograph commemorated the graduation of members of the 1893-94 class from the Jefferson Medical College Hospital Training School for Nurses, the second class to graduate. The six stiffly posed young graduates symmetrically flank Susan C. Hearle, the "directress" of nursing who is enthroned in an ornately carved armchair. The rigid poses and somber faces of the newly minted nurses seem incongruous in the studio setting featuring soft floral draperies and a fur rug.

The nurses' pink, starched uniforms were floor-length, with buttons down the front, a bishop's collar, balloon sleeves, and long, tight cuffs. The costume's bib and apron were of one piece. The original peaked white cap was made of lawn, a delicate material used to make handkerchiefs, and

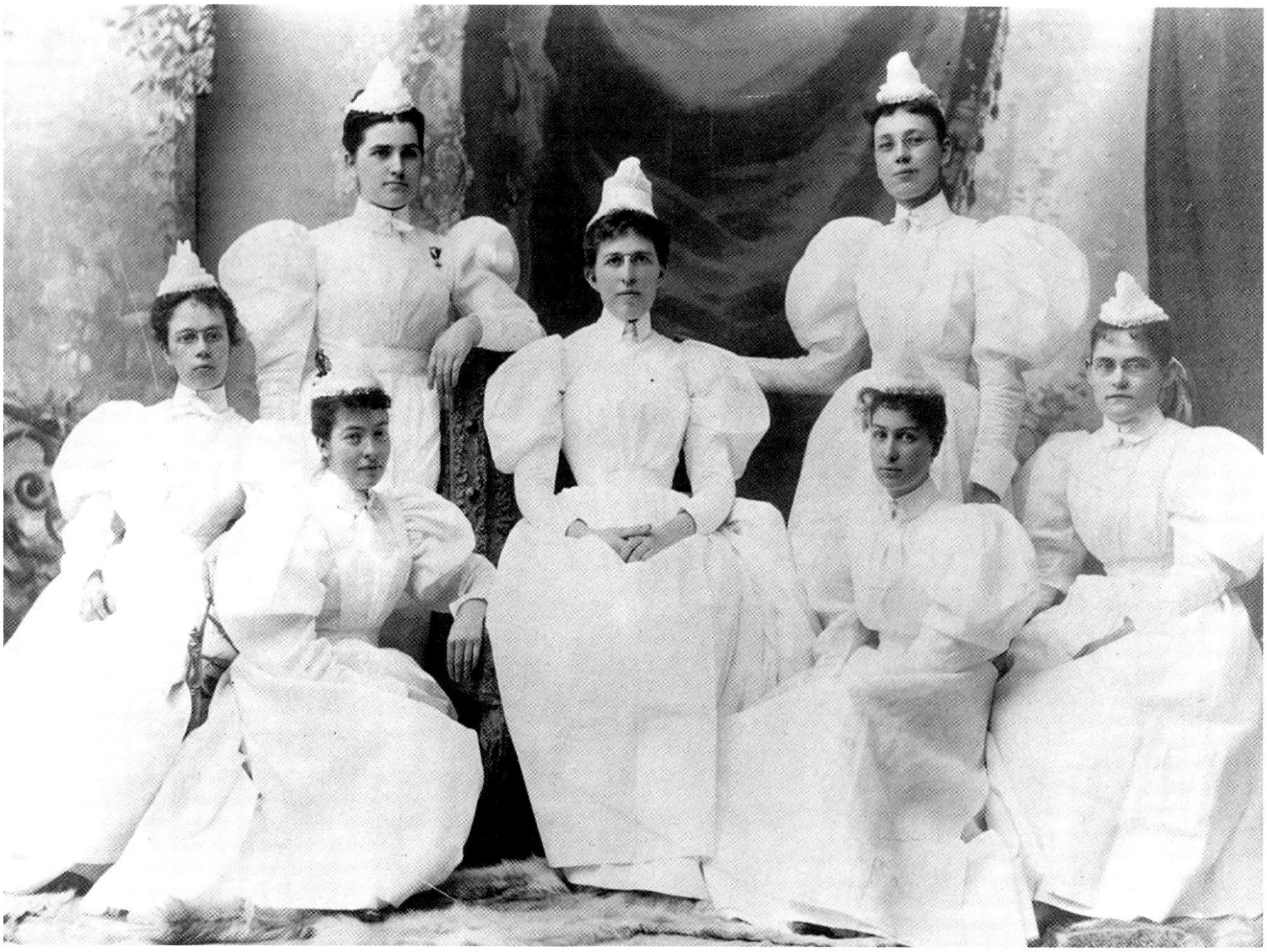

featured a high crown and a wide brim with ruffles around it.

After a resemblance to the Philadelphia General Hospital caps was noticed, the Jefferson cap became more distinctive. Starting in 1894-95 the material was changed to a stiffer organdy, the crown was lowered, the ruffle removed, and the brim narrowed, flattened, and spread like wing tips across the front of the cap.[2]

The School of Nursing of the Jefferson Medical College Hospital was founded in 1891. The earliest graduates survived rigorous entrance requirements and a two-year training program. By 1894 the course was expanded to three years.[3] Applicants for admission had to be between the ages of twenty-one and thirty-five, of "superior education, culture and refinement," and able to produce certificates of good health and testimonials of high moral character. Final acceptance was conditional upon completion of a thirty-day probation period.[4]

The students endured fourteen-hour work days beginning with reveille at dawn and classes from 7 A.M., as well as tours of duty in the hospital and visits to patients' homes. The curriculum covered general, medical, surgical, gynecological, and obstetrical nursing, and also dietetics. Students received board, lodging in the hospital, and laundry free of charge in addition to tuition. They received an allowance of six dollars per month the first year, seven dollars the second year, and eight dollars the third year. This stipend was not intended to compensate for services provided, but to cover expenses for uniforms, books, and other necessities.

Student nurses had little time for socializing, but were permitted to attend cultural events in chaperoned groups, and their "carefully screened" gentlemen friends could call one evening a week at the residence parlor. Starting in 1893 the board of trustees rented quarters at 518 Spruce Street for a special nursing residence, and soon after relocated to more spacious accommodations at 226 South Seventh Street, conveniently located next to the hospital's maternity section.

The imposing but kindly directress, Susan C. Hearle, had received her training first with Florence Nightingale in Great Britain and then at the nursing school of the Philadelphia General Hospital. Under her guidance as the Jefferson nursing school's third directress until her retirement in 1908, student enrollment rose rapidly. Though dignified and refined, Miss Hearle is said to have wielded a dry sense of humor to her advantage, and was popular with students as well as faculty. She was very proud of Jefferson graduate nurses who cared for American troops suffering from typhoid fever during the Spanish-American War of 1898, and for injured and sick civilians during the Galveston flood of 1900.

Portrait of Robert E. Rogers

ROBERT EMPIE ROGERS, M.D. (1813-84)
By Frederick Gutekunst (1831-1917)

Vintage photograph
1870-80
Image size: 5 3/4 x 4 1/4 in.
Board size: 6 1/2 x 4 1/4 in.

Signed lower right: "F. Gutekunst"

Given after 1880 by unknown donor
Accession number: 1880+f.Ph.02

Dr. Robert E. Rogers succeeded Dr. Benjamin H. Rand as chair of chemistry at Jefferson Medical College in 1877. He held the position until 1884 when he became emeritus professor.

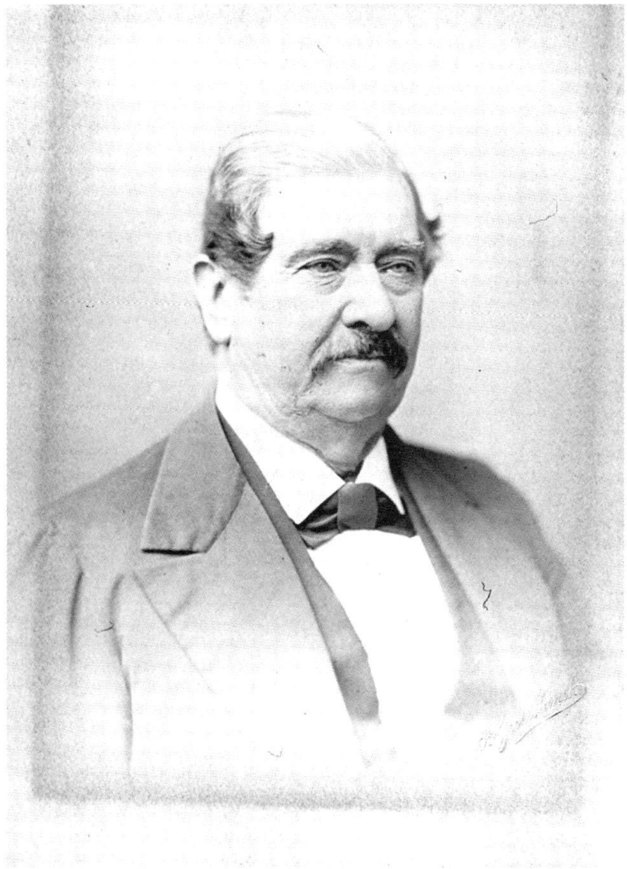

Robert E. Rogers was born in Baltimore in 1813, and studied at Dickinson College and William and Mary College before receiving a medical degree from the University of Pennsylvania in 1836. For the rest of his career he worked in the field of chemistry, initially as chemist to the first Geological Survey of Pennsylvania. His academic career began as professor of general and applied chemistry and materia medica at the University of Virginia (1842-52).

He succeeded his brother James as professor of chemistry at the University of Pennsylvania in 1852. In 1855 he published the American edition of *C. G. Lehman's Physiological Chemistry*. During the Civil War he served as acting assistant surgeon at the Satterlee Military Hospital in Philadelphia where in 1863 he lost his right hand while demonstrating the dangers in feeding a steam mangle. In 1877 he resigned the chair at the University of Pennsylvania to assume the post at Jefferson Medical College.

Dr. Rogers was the inventor of the Rogers and Black steam boiler, among other devices. He was active in many Philadelphia learned societies, including the Academy of Natural Sciences, the American Philosophical Society, and the Franklin Institute of which he was president (1875-79). He was an original member of the National Academy of Sciences and an organizer of the Association of American Geologists and Naturalists.

Rogers's affable nature is apparent in the photograph. It is said that his lecture room was always crowded and that he was beloved by his students for his gifts as a lecturer and experimenter, for his physical courage (in emergencies he had saved three strangers from certain death), and for his consideration and personal interest in all his students.

Portrait of Jacob M. DaCosta

(See color plate)

JACOB MENDEZ DaCOSTA, M.D. (1833-1900)
By Robert William Vonnoh (1858-1933)

Oil on canvas
1892
53 1/4 x 36 1/4 in.

Signed and dated lower right: "Vonnoh/1892"
Exhibition: Chicago, World's Columbian Exposition, 1893

Given in 1892 by friends and colleagues
Accession number: 1892+e.P.01

A sorrowful obituary in the October 1900 *Jeffersonian* said, "Death has robbed Jefferson of one of its most distinguished alumni, the late Professor Jacob M. DaCosta, a name which will live forever in medical literature as one of the brightest lights of the profession." The Jefferson board of trustees issued a resolution noting that the professor of the practice of medicine "was loved as few men are," and that "in his death the world loses one of those most rare men who have made it better by their character and attainments."

Jacob Mendez DaCosta was born in 1833 in St. Thomas, the West Indies where his father was a wealthy man of leisure whose ancestors were bankers

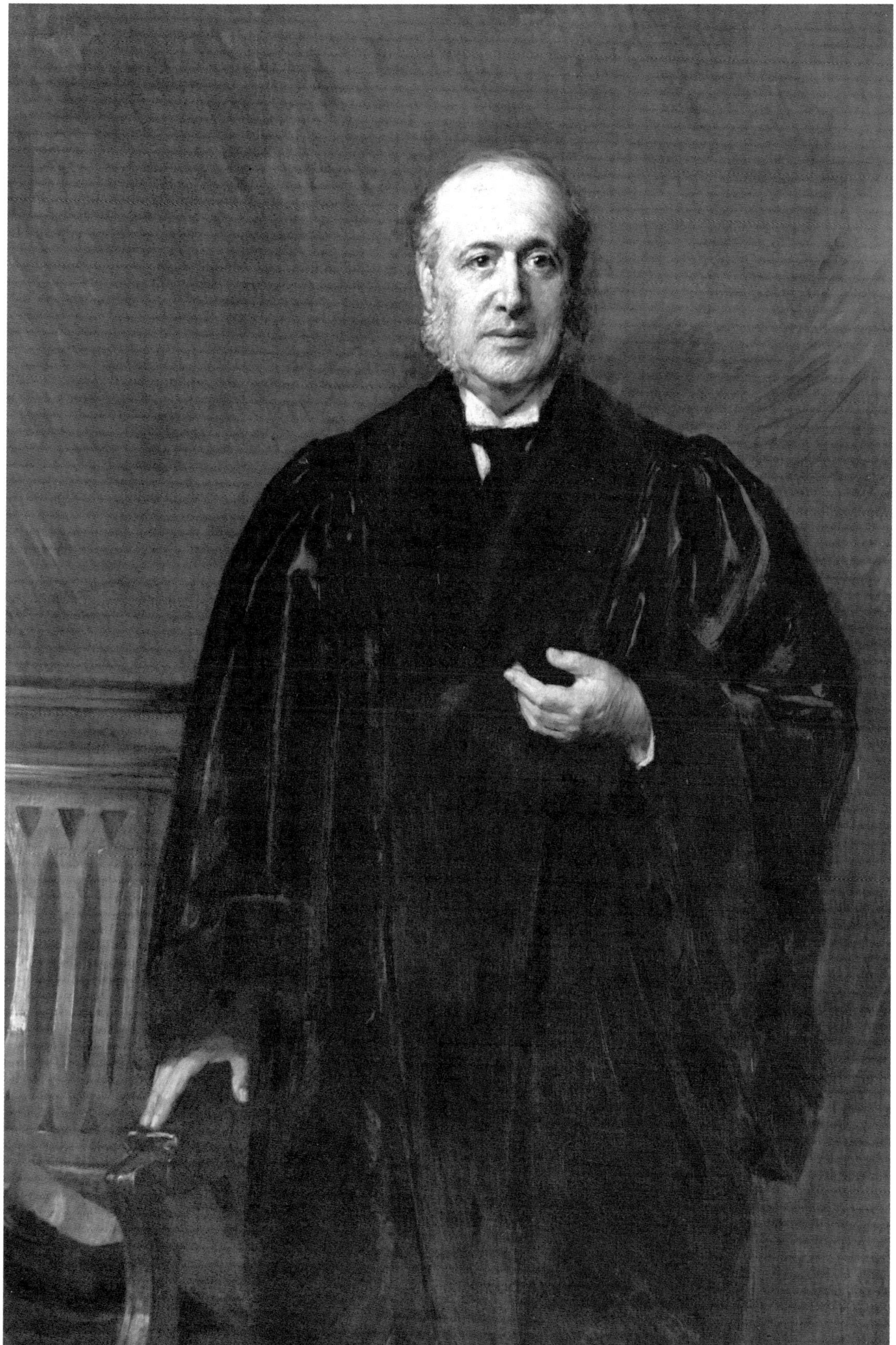

and planters. DaCosta was of Portuguese extraction, and was descended from a line which had emigrated to London in the sixteenth century. DaCosta was educated abroad, largely in Dresden.

He journeyed to Philadelphia in 1849 to become a pupil of Dr. Thomas Mütter and graduated from Jefferson Medical College in 1852. During this period he began a lifelong friendship with Dr. John H. Brinton whose sister, Sarah Frederica, he married in 1860.

After receiving his degree he spent eighteen months studying and attending clinics in Paris, Prague, and Vienna. Returning to Philadelphia, he taught physical diagnosis and clinical medicine privately and at the extramural Summer Association for Medical Instruction. His formal association with Jefferson Medical College began in 1858 as instructor, then as clinical lecturer in 1866. In 1872 he succeeded Dr. Samuel H. Dickson as the professor of the practice of medicine, a post he filled until 1891 when he was named emeritus professor. In addition to appointments at the Episcopal, Philadelphia, and Children's Hospitals, he was associated with Pennsylvania Hospital for thirty-five years.

Dr. J. M. DaCosta was a beloved teacher whose clinics were models of information and clarity, and he was widely admired as a skilled diagnostician and bedside teacher. His textbook *Medical Diagnosis, with Special Reference to Practical Medicine* (1864) was an immediate success; it went through nine editions during his lifetime and was translated into several foreign languages. While an acting assistant surgeon during the Civil War he gathered material for his 1871 article, "On Irritable Heart: A Clinical Study of a Form of Functional Cardiac Disorder and Its Consequences," a landmark study in the history of cardiovascular disease.

An active participant in medical and scientific societies, Dr. Jacob M. DaCosta was an organizer and president of the Pathological Society of Philadelphia, an original member and president of the Association of American Physicians, a fellow and two-term president of the College of Physicians of Philadelphia, and a fellow of the American Philosophical Society and of the Academy of Natural Sciences. He received honorary LL.D. degrees from Jefferson Medical College, the University of Pennsylvania, and Harvard University.

Jefferson Medical College's esteem and affection for DaCosta were reciprocated by the professor. Board of trustees minutes of October 4, 1900 recorded that DaCosta left his "entire teaching appliances" to the college. In November 1900 the trustees resolved to commemorate DaCosta's contributions by establishing the J. M. DaCosta Memorial Laboratory of Clinical Medicine, and a special fund to which friends and colleagues could subscribe.

Eight years earlier another subscription fund had been organized to honor Dr. Jacob M. DaCosta. On January 20, 1892, shortly after DaCosta's retirement, a group of his friends met at the home of Dr. S. Weir Mitchell. The invitation to the gathering stated that in recognition of DaCosta's

> distinguished labors in medical science, of his beneficent services to the community, and of the high personal esteem in which he is held, it has been proposed by a number of his friends to have two portraits painted—one to be presented to the College of Physicians of Philadelphia, of which he is an ex-President, and the other to the Jefferson Medical College, which for more than a quarter of a century has been the chief arena of his medical teaching.

Within a few days of the meeting the fund was oversubscribed and some contributions had to be returned![5] Philadelphia's *Evening Bulletin* of April 27, 1892 reported that "a magnificent portrait" of Dr. Jacob M. DaCosta was presented at the Jefferson Medical College commencement exercises by a representative of the alumni association.

In the painting by Robert W. Vonnoh the physician is shown life-sized and three-quarters length, in a standing frontal pose with one hand leaning against a chair arm. He is dressed in a black academic gown and his cap rests on the adjacent seat of the plain wooden chair. His large brown eyes look slightly to the right and his left hand is raised as though gesturing to an unseen visitor or group. He fills the picture space in a commanding manner and his expression is attentive and thoughtful. His face and left hand are beautifully articulated by a strong light coming from the left. The warm reds and maroons of the atmospheric background create luminous middle tones in this refined depiction.

On May 1, 1892 *The Philadelphia Press* reported on a presentation at the College of Physicians at which portraits of Drs. Alfred Stillé and Oliver Wendell Holmes were received at a festive banquet. The lengthy article mentioned that the portrait of Holmes was received by Dr. DaCosta, the college vice president, and that

> side by side with the two portraits was a splendid portrait of Dr. J. M. DaCosta. It is the property of the Jefferson Medical College, an exact duplicate of which is being painted by the artist shortly to be presented by the Jefferson Medical College Alumni and some of the patients of Dr. DaCosta to the College of Physicians with appropriate ceremonies.

Both of Vonnoh's portraits of Dr. J. M. DaCosta were painted while the artist was in Philadelphia teaching at the Pennsylvania Academy of the Fine Arts, the Jefferson portrait in 1892 and the College of Physicians portrait in 1893. During this same period, two other portraits of DaCosta were painted by Thomas Eakins.

Lloyd Goodrich wrote that Eakins was commissioned to paint one of the portraits proposed at the meeting in Dr. Mitchell's home, pointing out links between DaCosta and Eakins through Jefferson professors Samuel D. Gross, John H. Brinton, and William Pancoast.[6] Goodrich said that Eakins's completed portrait of DaCosta was exhibited in November 1892 at the Art Club of Philadelphia where it received unfavorable newspaper reviews and displeased the doctor's colleagues.

DaCosta wrote to Eakins asking him to continue working on it or paint another portrait using photographs. Offended by DaCosta's suggestion, Eakins destroyed the first canvas by cutting it into pieces, but out of respect for the eminent physician painted a second picture in 1893 which must have been approved. The archivist at Pennsylvania Hospital kindly provided me with board of managers minutes from January 1899 stating that Eakins's portrait was presented to the hospital by Charles L. DaCosta, the professor's son.

These events suggest the following sequence for the four DaCosta portraits. The first was the original Robert Vonnoh painting for Jefferson Medical College completed and presented in April 1892. The second was the original Thomas Eakins portrait painted in 1892, shown in late November, and destroyed. Because of the Eakins portrait's negative reception, Vonnoh must have received the second commission for the College of Physicians portrait, which he painted in 1893 and which was presented in 1894. The fourth portrait was Eakins's second attempt of 1893, presented to Pennsylvania Hospital in 1899. If Goodrich is correct that Eakins was commissioned to paint *one* of the original two portraits, then the *Philadelphia Press* article was either incorrect about the same artist painting an "exact duplicate," or else plans changed along the way.

Jefferson Medical College loaned the Vonnoh portrait of Dr. J. M. DaCosta to the Chicago World's Columbian Exposition in 1893. Photographs show the painting hanging in the library of the 1898 Medical College Building and then outside the dean's office in the 1929 College Building. Today it hangs near other historic portraits in the New Conference Center in the 1931 Curtis Building.

Most art scholars would disagree with Jefferson librarian Charles Frankenberger's assessment of Robert W. Vonnoh's style as "rather stiff and cold." The artist had established his reputation with "society" portraits and figure paintings, and was also a well known painter of impressionist landscapes.

The son of a German-born cabinetmaker, Vonnoh was born in Hartford, Connecticut in 1858, and spent his youth in Boston. He worked for a lithographic firm and studied at an evening art class, and then enrolled at the Massachusetts Normal Art School. During his formative years he made two trips to France, first studying at the Académie Julian under Gustave Boulanger and Jules J. Lefebvre, and later producing plein-air landscapes in the French countryside from 1887 to 1891.

In the middle 1880s he had been a popular teacher of figure and portrait painting in Boston at the Cowles Art School and at the School of the Museum of Fine Arts. In 1891 he became an instructor of figure and portrait painting at the Pennsylvania Academy of the Fine Arts where he stayed until 1896.

At the turn of the century he maintained studios in New York and Chicago where he had many portrait commissions, and starting around 1910 he divided his time between New York and Grez-sur-Loing, France. He returned to teach at the Academy in 1918, but by 1925 his eyesight started to fail, and he spent most of his remaining years in France with his second wife, the well known sculptor Bessie Potter Vonnoh (1872-1954) whom he had married in 1899.

Robert Vonnoh was made an academician of the National Academy of Design in 1906. His work was shown widely in European and American exhibitions, and retrospectives of his work were held in New York at the Ainslie Galleries in 1923 and the Durand-Ruel Galleries in 1926. He served on many local and international art juries, and he won awards and medals including the Paris Salon of 1889 (honorable mention), Paris Expositions of 1889 and 1900 (bronze medals), the National Academy of Design in 1904 (Thomas R. Proctor Prize for portraits), and international expositions in Buffalo in 1901, Charleston in 1902 (gold medal), and San Francisco in 1915 (gold medal).

Vonnoh's portraits and landscapes are represented in the collections of museums and institutions throughout the country, including the White House. In addition to the Philadelphia locations already mentioned, his works can be found at the Union League, the American Philosophical Society, and the Pennsylvania Academy of the Fine Arts.

Portrait of S. Weir Mitchell

SILAS WEIR MITCHELL, M.D.
(1829-1914)
By William Ordway Partridge
(1861-1930)

Plaster
1910-20
30 3/4 x 22 3/4 x 16 in.

Given after 1920 by unknown donor
Accession number: 1920+f.S.01

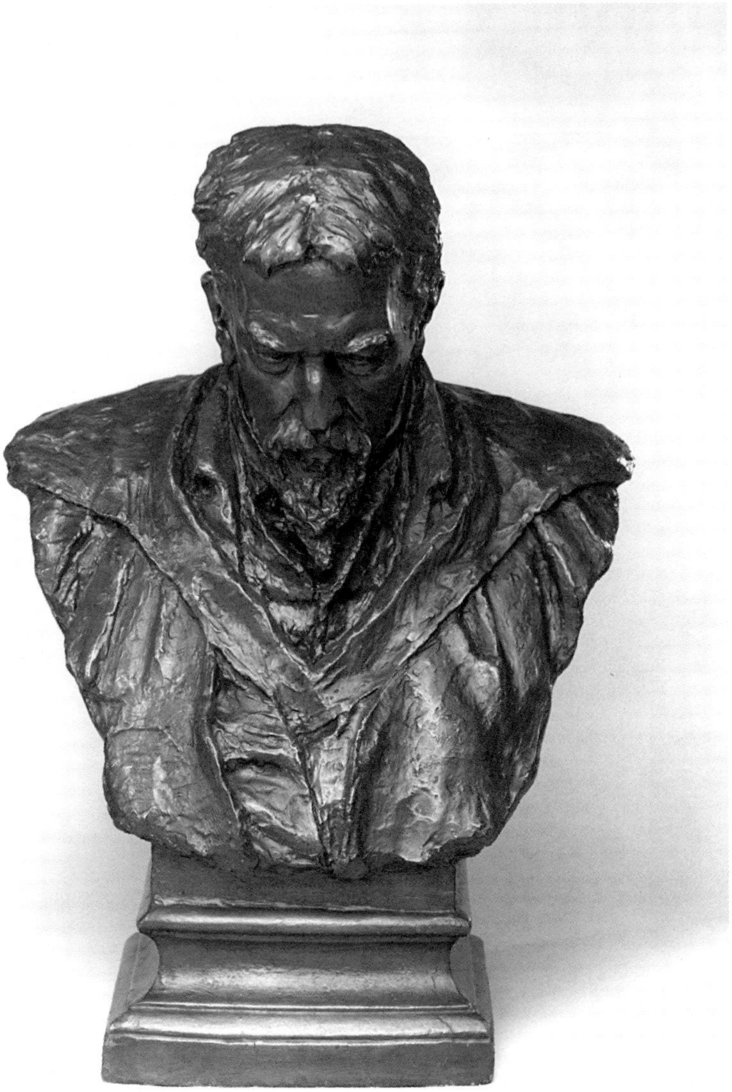

Dr. Jacob M. DaCosta's friend, the celebrated neurologist and therapist Dr. Silas Weir Mitchell, was a prolific poet and novelist, as internationally known in the world of literature as in the world of medicine where he helped to establish neurology as a specialty. Though an eminent practicing physician and renowned author, he was never a department chair at a major medical college.

S. Weir Mitchell was born in 1829 in Philadelphia, the son of Dr. John K. Mitchell, the Jefferson professor of the theory and practice of medicine, and he was also the grandson and great-grandson of physicians. After attending the University of Pennsylvania Mitchell graduated from Jefferson Medical College in 1850, then spent a year studying in Paris.

Upon returning to Philadelphia he entered general practice and published research in comparative physiology. He was a professor at the Philadelphia Polyclinic and College for Graduates in Medicine, and for more than forty years was associated with the Philadelphia Orthopaedic Hospital and Infirmary for Nervous Diseases.

When Mitchell was an acting assistant surgeon during the Civil War, wards were set aside for him in two large military hospitals in Philadelphia for the study and treatment of injuries of the peripheral nerves and central nervous system. In 1863 he had the opportunity to study several hundred patients at Turner's Lane Hospital in suburban Philadelphia, along with Drs. William W. Keen and George R. Morehouse. The trio published an important work, *Gunshot Wounds and Other Injuries of Nerves* (1864); giving most of the credit to Mitchell, Keen said in his *Memoirs* that the book "laid the foundation for all our modern neurological surgery."[7]

Dr. S. Weir Mitchell did pioneering research and writing in the description and treatment of various nervous disorders including red neuralgia, the physiology of the cerebellum, sleeping disorders, weather conditions and nerve injury and disease, erythromelalgia, causalgia, the psychological effects of amputations, reflex paralysis, and snake venoms. He made close observations on the effects of certain drugs and also introduced many nonmedical measures of treatment.

Mitchell gained international attention for the "rest cure," expounded in *Wear and Tear: or Hints for the Overworked* (1871), *Rest in the Treatment of Nervous Disease* (1875), and *Fat and Blood: and How to Make Them* (1877), in which he prescribed rest in bed, massages, a rich and full diet, isolation, and avoidance of disturbing events. Initially greeted with skepticism, his system was gradually accepted by many physicians worldwide. Later books expounding on his personal observations and skill in psychotherapy and psychoanalysis were *Lectures on the Diseases of the Nervous System, Especially in Women* (1881) and *Clinical Lessons on Nervous Diseases* (1897).

At age twenty S. Weir Mitchell submitted a book of poems to a Boston publisher, and was advised by physician/author Oliver Wendell Holmes to refrain from literary work until he was secure in the medical calling. Therefore, he published anonymously until about 1880 when he began to write under his own name, and continued through his middle eighties. Works include seven volumes of poetry and fifteen novels, among which are *Hugh Wynne, Free Quaker* (1897), *Constance Trescot* (1905), *The Red City* (1908), *John Sherwood, Iron Master* (1911), and *Westaways: A Village Chronicle* (1913).

Mitchell was the first president of the American Physiological Society, a president of the College of Physicians of Philadelphia, and a member of the National Academy of Science. He was honored with fellowship or honorary membership in several European societies including the Royal Society of Literature of the United Kingdom, the French Academy of Medicine, the Academy of Sciences of Bologna, the Royal Medical Society of Norway, the Academy of Sciences of Sweden, the Royal Academy of Medicine of Rome, and the Gesellschaft Deutscher Nervenärzte. He won honorary degrees from the Universities of Bologna, Edinburgh, Toronto, Princeton, and Harvard, and from Jefferson Medical College.

An obituary in the January 1914 *Jeffersonian* described Dr. Mitchell's appearance and vigorous lifestyle: "He is a tall man with a colossal head and a most impressive face, a lover of nature, addicted all his life to field sports, fishing, and camping in the wilderness, a believer in muscle and out-of-doors as a cure for disease and a stay for moral faculties, he is the embodiment of the wholesome and vigorous side of life."

In William Ordway Partridge's sculpture the physician is shown bust length, with wide shoulders and a massive head turned downwards. Under heavy, knitted brows his deepset eyes gaze somberly down as though lost in thought. The elongated triangular shape of his head is accentuated by his hair with its center part, his narrow face with high cheekbones, his long aquiline nose, and a full mustache that meets his long, pointed beard. All of these elements are echoed by the deep V-shaped mantle of his academic robe whose lively, irregular surface features deep folds. The powerful depiction accords with the description in the *Jeffersonian.*

The undated Jefferson bust is made of plaster painted brownish-umber to resemble bronze. It was located first in the reading room of the library in the 1898 College Building, then in the library of the 1929 building. Today it has pride of place in the department of psychiatry offices.

The sculpture is almost identical to a marble bust at the College of Physicians of Philadelphia, signed "Ordway Partridge" and presented to the college in 1910 by the physician's wife. Dr. Mitchell not only devotedly served the college for two terms as president (1886-88 and 1892-94), he was a generous benefactor to its museum, library, and various funds. The annual S. Weir Mitchell Oration was established in his honor.

Sculptor William Ordway Partridge shared a literary interest with his subject and was almost as versatile. He, too, was the author of several books of poetry and also of books and articles on the aesthetics and techniques of sculpture. Like Mitchell he came from a worldly background.

Partridge was born in 1861 of American parents in Paris where his father was a wealthy agent for a New York merchant. He studied at Columbia University and in Paris, Florence, Rome, and Stuttgart. He also attended the American Academy of Dramatic Arts in 1884 and gave public readings of poetry.

Partridge is best known for outdoor monuments to such notable figures as William Shakespeare (Chicago); Thomas Jefferson, Alexander Hamilton, and General Ulysses S. Grant (New York); Nathan Hale (St. Paul, Minnesota); and Pocahantas (Jamestown, Virginia). He also created a *Pietà* for New York's St. Patrick's Cathedral and a baptismal font for Washington's Cathedral of Sts. Peter and Paul, and numerous smaller sculptures. He exhibited widely in the United States and in Paris, London, and Berlin.

Partridge lectured on fine arts at George Washington University, the Concord School of Philosophy, Stanford University, and the Brooklyn Institute. In 1904 he was a founder of the Society of American Sculptors. He was ill the last few years of his life and Partridge's family was scandalized by unwelcome newspaper publicity about his being committed to a mental institution in Islip, New York in 1926. One wonders whether Partridge ever discussed his personal troubles with Dr. Mitchell when the latter posed for his marble bust.

The class of 1932 presented a pastel sketch of Dr. S. Weir Mitchell by Helen Warren Sears to the Jefferson collection in 1985.

Portrait of William W. Keen Jr.

(See color plate)

WILLIAM WILLIAMS KEEN Jr., M.D. (1837-1932)
By William Merritt Chase (1849-1916)

Oil on canvas
Ca. 1901
67 x 52 1/2 in.

Signed lower left: "Wm M Chase"

Given by JMC class of 1901
Accession number: 1901+e.P.01

Dr. William Williams Keen Jr. was another of Jefferson Medical College's internationally famous and talented surgeons. During his productive life of ninety-five years he participated in many of the new advances in surgery, and was personally acquainted with most of the great men in the field.

W. W. Keen's *Memoirs* describe his formative years. He was born in Philadelphia in 1837, the son of a prominent leather merchant. At Brown University he graduated as class valedictorian in 1859, then stayed an extra year to study the sciences and general culture. He entered Jefferson Medical College and became a private pupil of Dr. John H. Brinton and Dr. Jacob M. DaCosta, and graduated in 1862. Through Brinton he met Dr. S. Weir Mitchell with whom he formed a collegial friendship that lasted for over fifty-two years "without a cloud even as big as a man's hand coming between us."

Keen's military contributions will be described below. Following service in the Civil War, he studied abroad for two years in Paris, Vienna, and Berlin. Upon his return to Philadelphia in 1866 he opened an office for private practice. As already mentioned in connection with Thomas Eakins, Keen taught pathological anatomy at the summer school at Jefferson Medical College, and served as head of the Philadelphia School of Anatomy where he remained for nine years until it closed in 1875.

Keen's *Memoirs* stated that he suffered his "greatest disappointment" when defeated in a "very warm contest" for Jefferson's chair of anatomy after Dr. Joseph Pancoast's resignation in 1873; the post was awarded to his son, Dr. William H. Pancoast. Fearing that there were no prospects for having a successful teaching career in medicine, in 1876 he enthusiastically accepted the position as professor of artistic anatomy at the newly reopened Pennsylvania Academy of the Fine Arts where he remained until 1890. Keen later declined to consider the Jefferson chair of therapeutics even though Dr. Jacob M. DaCosta urged him to accept the position.

Keen's first academic appointment in surgery was as lecturer on surgical anatomy and then chair of surgery at Women's Medical College of Pennsylvania, the latter post from 1885 to 1889. During this period he edited a new American edition of Henry Gray's *Anatomy: Descriptive and Surgical* (1887), revising and largely rewriting the chapters on the physiological, pathological, and surgical anatomy of the nervous system. In his *Memoirs* Keen expressed pride that the appearance of his name on the title page made him known to the entire medical profession.

Before his appointment at Jefferson Medical College in 1889 he had been approached by Harvard University for the chair of anatomy, and by Rush Medical College and the University of California in San Francisco for their respective chairs of surgery, but for various reasons never seriously considered these offers. When he was approached by the University of Pennsylvania for the demonstratorship of anatomy and eventually the chair, his election was opposed by Drs. Joseph Leidy and D. Hayes Agnew. In his *Memoirs* Keen labelled his rejection of these and other offers as "fortunate escapes."

Finally in 1889 at age fifty-two Keen succeeded Dr. Samuel W. Gross in the "un-dreamed-of distinction of the Professorship of Surgery in the Jefferson Medical College, a position of such eminence and influence that in my early professional life, I had never considered it as a possibility; nor even up to 1889 did I ever seriously aspire to it."

Finding no current textbook on surgery satisfactory with regard to the importance of pathology, he coedited with Dr. J. William White of the University of Pennsylvania *An American Text-Book of Surgery for Practitioners and Students* (1892). This text was the forerunner to the comprehensive, eight-volume *Surgery, its Principles and Practice* (1906-21), edited by Dr. Keen.

Keen published almost continuously on a wide variety of medical, historical, and religious subjects including, among others, *The Surgical Complications and Sequels of Typhoid Fever* (1898), *The Bi-centennial Celebration of the Founding of the First Baptist Church of the City of Philadelphia* (1899), *Addresses and Other Papers: W. W. Keen, M.D.* (1905), *Animal Experimentation and Medical Progress*

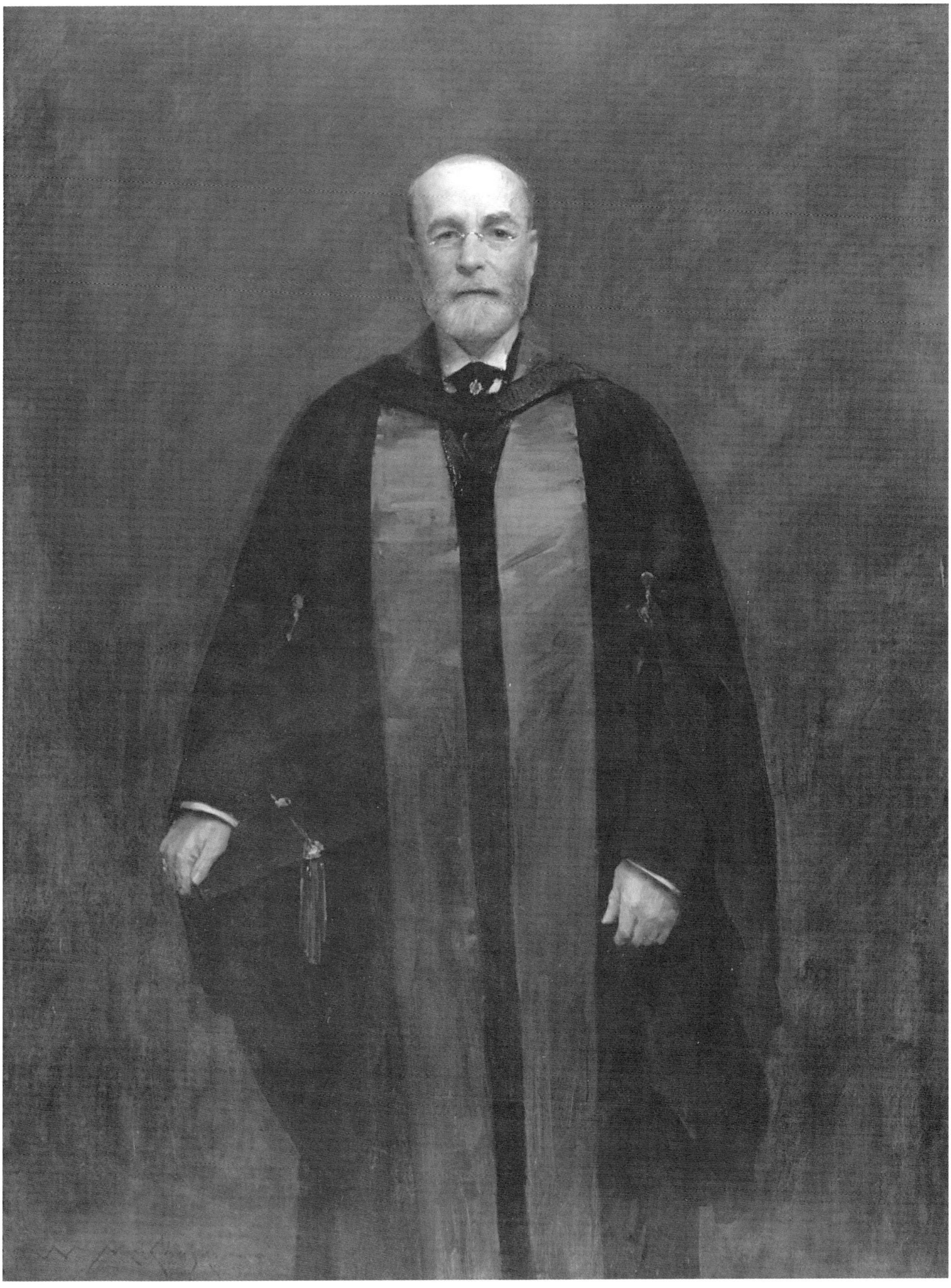

(1914), *The Treatment of War Wounds* (1917), *Medical Research and Human Welfare* (1917), *I Believe in God and Evolution* (1922), *Selected Papers and Addresses by William Williams Keen* (1923), and *Everlasting Life; A Creed and a Speculation* (1924).

A fascinating chapter in Keen's *Memoirs* is entitled "Presidents I Have Known." These included President McKinley on whose wife he performed a "minor operation," and with whom he had a social relationship, often lunching at the White House *en famille*; President Taft whom he convinced to state opposition to the antivivisectionists, and for whose daughter he arranged orthopaedic treatment while she was attending Bryn Mawr College; President Cleveland on whom he operated twice, secretly, for carcinoma of the maxilla with a team of surgeons on the yacht *Oneida* off Long Island Sound; and President Wilson on whose wife and two daughters he operated. After publicity about Grover Cleveland's operation was leaked, Keen set the record straight in an account published in 1917, *The Surgical Operations on President Cleveland in 1893*.

Dr. W. W. Keen served as president of the American Surgical Association, the American Medical Association, the College of Physicians of Philadelphia, the Philadelphia Academy of Surgery, the Philadelphia County Medical Society, the American Philosophical Society, the American Baptist Missionary Union, an American Congress of Physicians and Surgeons in 1903, and an International Congress of Surgery in 1917.

Few surgeons have been so universally admired and honored. Dr. Keen was awarded the Henry Jacob Bigelow Gold Medal from the Boston Surgical Society and the Colver-Rosenberger Medal from Brown University. He was elected an honorary fellow or member in the Royal Colleges of Surgeons of England, Edinburgh, and Ireland; the Italian, Belgian, and German surgical societies; and the Berlin, Paris, and Palermo surgical societies. He was named an Officer of the Order of the Crown of Belgium and Officer of the Legion of Honor of France.

He received honorary LL.D. degrees from Brown, Northwestern, Yale, Toronto, Edinburgh, and St. Andrews Universities, and the University of Pennsylvania. He was awarded Sc.D. degrees from Jefferson Medical College and Harvard University. He received an honorary Ph.D. from the University of Uppsala, and an honorary M.D. from the University of Greifswald.

To paint the portrait of this extraordinary man, the Jefferson Medical College class of 1901 commissioned the internationally lionized artist William Merritt Chase. He was one of the foremost figures in American art, a tastemaker who was an uncommonly successful teacher, painter, and activist for his profession.

Over 750 students, faculty, and friends crowded into Jefferson's amphitheater for the portrait presentation in 1901. Afterward the painting was installed in the library of the 1898 College Building. Its next installation was beside *The Gross Clinic* on the second floor landing of the 1929 College Building, and the Keen portrait still hangs there.

The rather formal depiction emphasizes the subject's august reputation and noble character. Professor Keen is shown full length in an absolutely frontal stance, with hands down at his side and confidently looking directly toward the viewer. The figure's face and hands are rendered solidly and convincingly in three dimensions. Dr. Keen wears a black academic robe with red panels, and holds his academic cap in his right hand. This costume signifies his honorary membership in the Royal College of Surgeons of England, awarded in 1900 the year before the portrait was painted.

Although Keen was short in stature and slight of build, he appears tall and robust in the portrait. The long, twin red panels elongate his height, and the brilliant red color lends energy and excitement to the depiction. The warmth is repeated in his ruddy skin tones. In fact, it was reported that Dr. Keen "needed a rest" and asked for and was granted a "long vacation" at the end of the term in 1901.[8]

This portrait is a relatively reticent depiction by the usually more dazzling artist, but Chase makes the most of opportunities for sparkle in the red satin panels, the gold tassel of the cap, the brilliant white shirt collar and jeweled tie pin, and the gleam on the physician's spectacles.

In a 1905 address to the W. W. Keen Surgical Society of Jefferson Medical College, Keen described the ceremony at which he was awarded his honorary degree from the Royal College of Surgeons of England.[9] The elaborate public ceremony in Burlington House, London inducted more than thirty surgeons from throughout the world, no more than four from any one country. The distinguished American contingent also included Drs. J. Collins Warren from Harvard, Robert F. Weir from Columbia, and William S. Halsted from Johns Hopkins, and Keen was honored to deliver a short address in their behalf. Attendees wore either academic gowns and hoods of every color, military uniforms, or full evening dress. The College of Surgeons robe, which was not worn during the ceremony, could be purchased later by honorees, and Keen proudly described his robe of black alpaca faced with crimson which he wears in Chase's painting.

Although William Merritt Chase and Thomas Eakins were contemporaries and friends who exchanged portraits of each other, they were opposites in temperament and style. Chase painted more varied scenes of American life. His portraits were rendered with virtuoso brush work in impressionistic or avant-garde styles, and in a wider range of media, including tempera, pastels, and prints. Unlike Eakins who dressed strictly for comfort and often looked unkempt, Chase dressed like a dandy. A gentleman artist with Vandyke beard, he was often attired in cutaway, spats, boutonnière, gold-rimmed pince-nez, top hat, and cane. In contrasting their places of work Eakins said meaningfully, "Chase's studio is an atelier; this is a workshop."[10]

William M. Chase began this dazzling career inauspiciously as a clerk in the family shoe store in Indianapolis at age sixteen. Reportedly he lost this job for wasting too much wrapping paper by painting on it, so his father sent him to study with a local painter and then to the National Academy of Design in New York. The young artist was able to sell enough pictures in New York to finance a move to St. Louis where his family had relocated.

There he produced paintings for local art patrons who financed further study at the Royal Academy in Munich in 1872, where he learned to emulate the dark palette and bravura brush work of his teachers. Chase's portraits in Munich brought enough recognition that he was asked in 1878 to join the academy's faculty, but he declined in favor of returning to America to teach at the newly formed Art Students League in New York.

Chase had legions of admiring students during a long teaching career, first at the Art Students League and later at the Brooklyn Art School, the Chicago Art Institute, the Pennsylvania Academy of the Fine Arts, and his own schools in New York and Shinnecock, Long Island. He even took groups of students on tours of Europe and conducted summer classes abroad. Many of his pupils became leading American modernists. His famous New York studio which was magnificently appointed with his collection of fine and decorative arts, costumes, and props became a chic meeting place for artists and collectors.

Like his eminent portrait subject Dr. Keen, William Merritt Chase was a dynamic leader in his profession. He participated in the first exhibition of the Society of American Artists and later served the society as president for ten years. He was a founding member of the Society of Painters in Pastel in 1884. He was named an academician of the National Academy of Design in 1890. The artist joined the progressive Ten American Painters in 1902.

Chase had his first one-man show at the Boston Art Club in 1886. He was a consistent prizewinner in exhibitions in the U.S. and abroad, including four gold medals in three years (1900-02) at the Paris Exposition, the Pennsylvania Academy of the Fine Arts, the Pan-American Exposition in Buffalo, and the Charleston Exposition. He showed more pictures than any other American at the Paris Exposition of 1889, was assigned a whole gallery to himself at the Panama-Pacific Exposition in San Francisco in 1915, and won silver medals in both shows. William Merritt Chase was one of the few Americans honored with a commission of a self-portrait for the famed collection at the Uffizi Gallery in Florence.

Professor William W. Keen's Clinic at Jefferson Medical College

PROFESSOR WILLIAM W. KEEN'S CLINIC
By Edgar Newton Fought, M.D. (d. 1944)

Vintage photograph
1902
7 1/2 x 9 1/2 in.

Handwritten inscription at bottom of image: "Professor William W. Keen's Clinic/Jefferson Medical College hospital/December 10th. 1902." Handwritten inscription on left side of image: "COPYRIGHTED '02/BY E. N. FOUGHT"

Given in 1961 by George F. Doyle, M.D. (JMC 1905)
Accession number: 1961+e.Ph.01

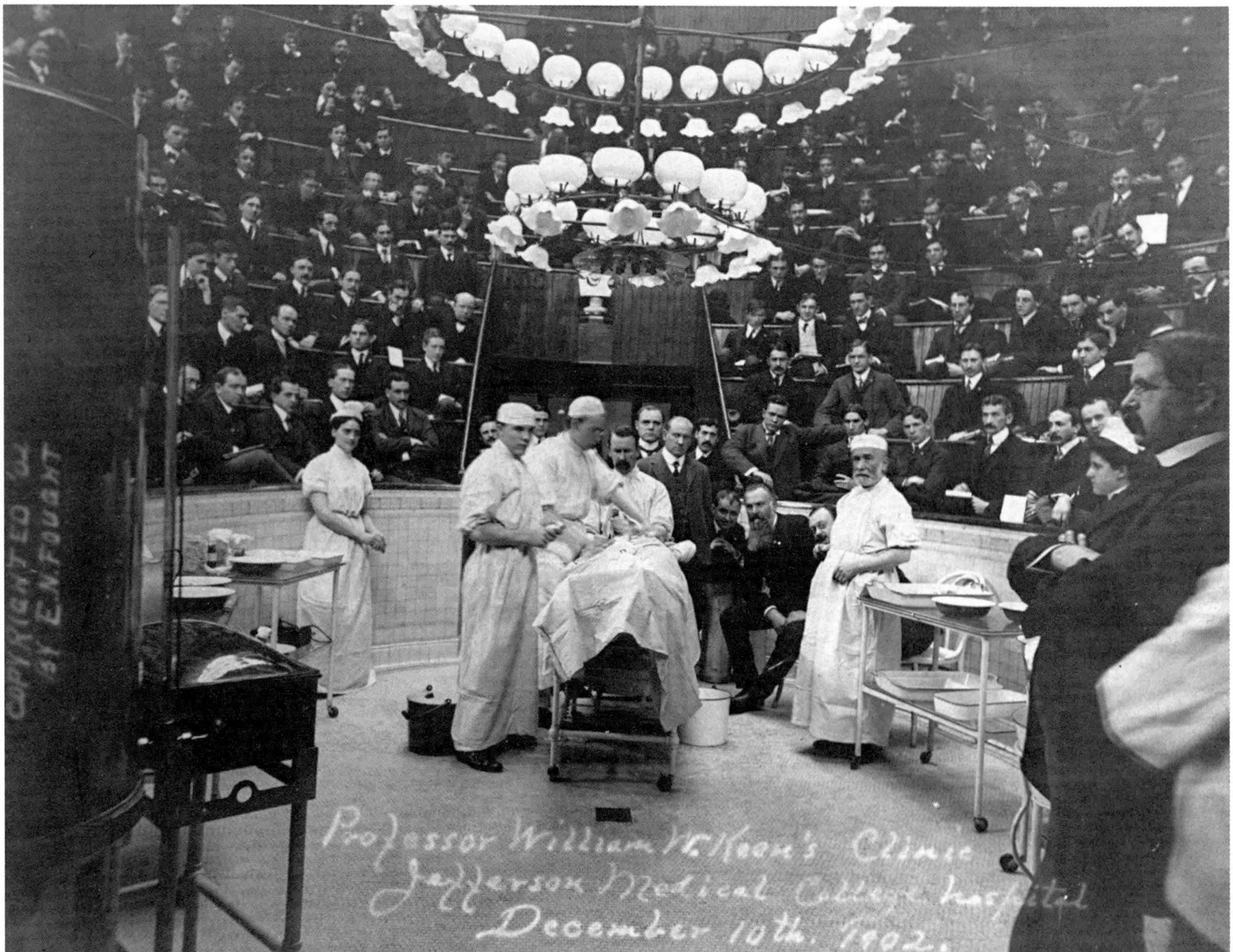

When Dr. W. W. Keen heard Dr. Joseph Lister's lecture at the International Medical Congress in September 1876 in Philadelphia, he became fully convinced at once of the value of antiseptic surgery. Keen was the first surgeon in Philadelphia and one of the first in America to adopt Lister's principles, employing them in a case at St. Mary's Hospital on October 1, 1876. In 1887 at this same hospital he successfully localized and removed a large brain tumor, the first case of modern cerebral surgery in America. Over sixty of Keen's four hundred published case reports concerned neurological surgery of the brain, spinal cord, and peripheral nerves. Antiseptic surgical technique and progress in neurological localization made advancements possible.[11]

Best known as America's pioneer neurosurgeon, Dr. Keen's contributions also included the development of his own faradic battery and flexible bipolar electrode for brain stimulation. He was an early proponent of an operation for hydrocephaly and described three approaches for puncture and drainage of the lateral ventricles. He contributed to linear craniotomy for microcephalus in 1890. He performed his first successful gasserian ganglionectomy by a temporal method in 1893. He attempted to treat cerebral hemorrhage by carotid ligation. Other areas of cranial surgery in which he published included cerebral abscess, scalp and bone reconstruction, and diagnostic radiology. He devised his own chisel, osteotome, and rongeur forceps for bone work.[12]

This vintage photograph of 1902 taken by Dr. Edgar Newton Fought (JMC 1905) shows Dr. William Williams Keen's surgical clinic in the amphitheater of the 1877 Jefferson Medical College Hospital. In contrast to the earlier *Gross Clinic,* Keen is following some antiseptic principles. Keen (standing on the right next to an instrument table) and the assisting surgeons and a nurse are wearing caps and gowns, and all have their sleeves rolled up. Equipment includes buckets near the operating table and a number of small tables with instruments and materials around the walls. The scene looks posed rather than candid, judging by the number of participants facing the camera. The amphitheater seats are filled with students, and there are several visitors inside the operating arena. Keen's clinics were often crowded with extra students, faculty, and visiting American and foreign surgeons. The Jefferson archives possesses several sets of instruments used by Keen.

Dr. John Chalmers DaCosta first encountered Dr. Keen when DaCosta was an assistant in the surgical outpatient department of the hospital. DaCosta wrote in the April 1907 *Jeffersonian* upon the occasion of the surgeon's resignation:

> He always knew his subject most thoroughly, and was always perfectly prepared in every thing that related to its literature and its history...He clearly differentiated the essential and fundamental from the nonessential and extraneous...
>
> As an operator, he...is absolutely fearless, and his judgment seems at its very best when the surgical situation appears at its very worst. I have helped him in operations in which there have been presented the very greatest difficulties and dangers; but, to drop into the vernacular, in all these years I have never seen him turn a hair...Over and over again, in an operation, I have seen him calmly and thoughtfully originate a valuable new step as he went along. These new steps have in many instances become part of the literature of surgery.

Portrait of William W. Keen Jr.

WILLIAM WILLIAMS KEEN Jr., M.D.
By Gilbert Bacon (?)

Vintage photograph
1917
Image size: 7 x 4 1/2 in.
Card size: 10 7/8 x 6 3/8 in.

Signed on card below image: "Gilbert & Bacon"
Inscriptions below photograph written by two different people: "W. W. Keen Major, Medical/Reserve Corps U.S. Army July 1917."/"First commission dated July 1, 1861/First Lt and Asst Surgeon 5th Mass. Vol./Professor of Surgery/1890-1907"

Given after 1917 by unknown donor
Accession number: 1917+f.Ph.01

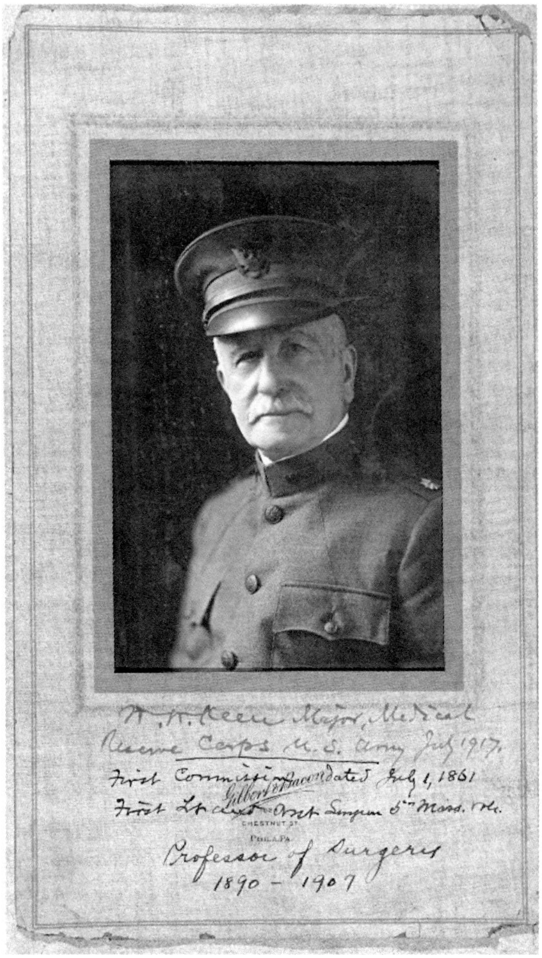

Dr. W. W. Keen's sense of patriotism was extraordinary and his service in the military spanned more than fifty years. In 1917 at the age of eighty he was named a major in the U.S. Army as a consultant in the Reserve Corps during World War I, as depicted in this photograph.

When he was a student at Jefferson Medical College, his preceptor Dr. John H. Brinton recommended Keen as a replacement for a vacated position as assistant surgeon in the Fifth Massachusetts Regiment. He saw action at the first Battle of Bull Run in his brief service between July and September 1861, then resumed his studies and graduated in March 1862. The following May he was commissioned an acting assistant surgeon in the U.S. Army.

He was ordered to report to the office of Dr. Jonathan Letterman (JMC 1849), the medical director of the Army of the Potomac in Washington. Keen was sent out from Washington to the encamped army with a large supply train, and tended wounded at the second Battle of Bull Run.

In September 1862 he was sent to Frederick, Maryland after the Battle of Antietam and was assigned to the First Hospital. He later wrote in detail about the "dreadful mortality" in military surgery in those years before antisepsis and first aid packages.[13] While in Frederick as Dr. John H. Brinton's agent for the Army Medical Museum in Washington, he forwarded his notes and specimens from military hospitals, many of which were published in *The Medical and Surgical History of the War of the Rebellion*.

In the winter of 1862 Dr. Keen was sent to the Satterlee Hospital in Philadelphia where secondary hemorrhage cases occurred with "dreadful frequency" after the Battle of Gettysburg. With no hemostatic forceps the physicians' "only resource" was to pass a tenaculum through the vessel and tie it with silk, a procedure which usually took several attempts. His work on nervous diseases and injuries in Civil War soldiers has already been discussed.

Keen volunteered for the Spanish-American War but his services were not required. In the Jefferson archives is Keen's certificate of commission as a first lieutenant in the Medical Reserve Corps, dated December 28, 1909 and signed by President William H. Taft.

Portrait of Emma Borden (Mrs. William W.) Keen

EMMA BORDEN (MRS. WILLIAM W.) KEEN (d. 1886)
By unknown photographer

Old copy of vintage photograph
1870-80
Image size: 9 1/4 x 6 1/2 in.
Card size: 16 x 12 3/4 in.

Given after 1932 by unknown donor
Accession number: 1932+f.Ph.02

In 1867 Dr. Keen married Emma Corinna Borden of Fall River, Massachusetts, and the devoted couple had four daughters: Corinne, Florence, Dora, and Margaret.

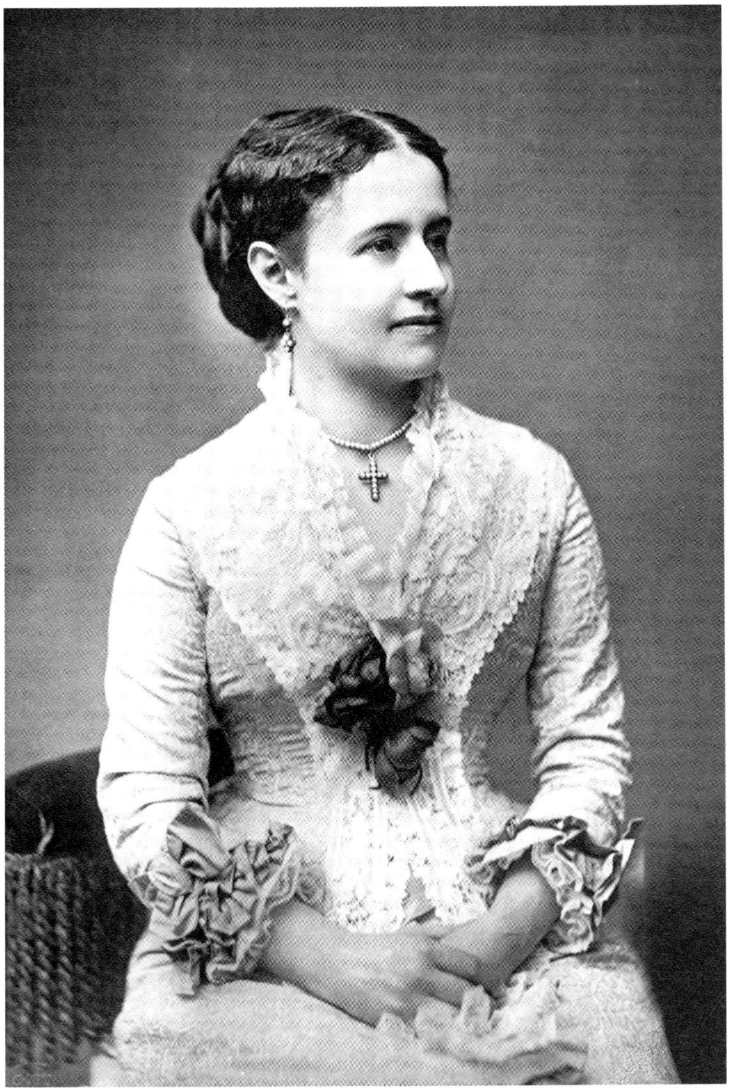

Dr. and Mrs. Keen shared an interest in singing. In his *Memoirs* Keen expressed pride that both were members of the Centennial Choir which performed at the opening day of the Centennial Exposition in Philadelphia in 1876. The performance was held in the open in front of an audience of one hundred thousand visitors, and President Grant initiated the program which was a "glorious triumph."

In the undated photograph Mrs. Keen sits demurely with hands in her lap, turned slightly to the right. Her dark hair has a center part and is pulled back to display her youthful and attractive features arranged in a welcoming smile. Her ornate dress is adorned with lace, ribbons, and ruffles. She wears pearl drop earrings and a necklace with a pendant cross. One wonders if this choice of ornament signifies that Mrs. Keen was as devoutly religious as her husband.

Although glued to heavy board impressed with the name "F. Gutekunst" and placed in a presentation folder marked with the name "The Gutekunst Studio," this photograph is marked "copy" in the lower left corner, and so one cannot be absolutely certain that the original photograph was taken by Frederick Gutekunst.

The couple's happy marriage came to an untimely end when Mrs. Keen died suddenly on July 12, 1886. Keen wrote frankly about the "one appalling disaster of my life" in his *Memoirs*,

> In the autumn of that year, I found that my grief was threatening to impair both my health and my ability to care for my dear girls...
>
> One day, while I was in this condition, Mr. Henry C. Lea proposed that I edit a new edition of Gray's *Anatomy*...and I accepted the offer. I would have done it for nothing at all, for I was in such a mental condition that I felt that such congenial and absorbing work was just what I needed to take me out of myself.

Portrait of Roberts Bartholow

ROBERTS BARTHOLOW, M.D.
(1831-1904)
By George W. Pettit
(d. 1910)

Oil on canvas mounted on wood
1892
30 x 25 in.

Signed lower left: "G. W. Pettit"

Given by JMC class of 1892
Accession number: 1892+e.P.02

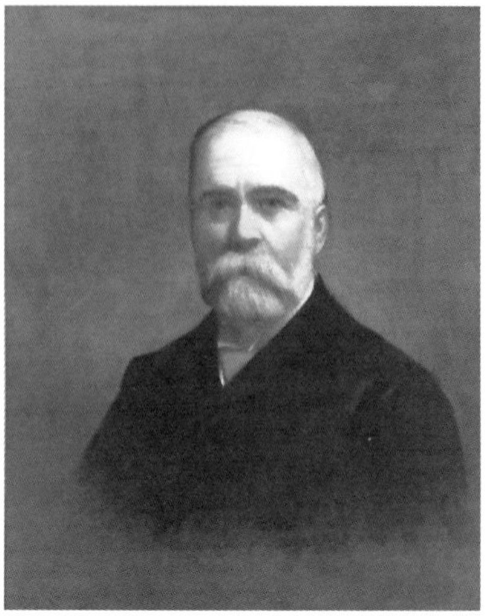

Like many of his contemporaries at Jefferson Medical College Dr. Roberts Bartholow had a varied career. He was a physician, chemist, sanitary reformer, army surgeon, and author.

The most informative biography of Dr. Bartholow is an affectionate memoir by Dr. James W. Holland read before the College of Physicians in 1905, the year after his death.[14] Roberts Bartholow was born in 1831 in New Windsor, Maryland. He graduated from Calvert College (later New Windsor College) in 1848 where he received a master of arts degree in 1854, after having earned his medical degree from the Medical Department of the University of Maryland in 1852.

He joined the regular army as an assistant surgeon in 1857, and his unit was sent to Utah to preserve order among the pioneer population and government officials from the "fanaticism" of the Mormons and from frequent disputes with Native Americans. After the outbreak of the Civil War Dr. Bartholow served in military hospitals in Maryland, New York, Washington, D.C., and Tennessee. During this period he wrote *A Manual of Instruction for Enlisting and Discharging Soldiers* (1863), and a series of papers for the instruction of the United States Sanitary Commission.

He left the army in 1864 and established a busy private practice in Cincinnati, where he accepted the chair of medical chemistry at the Medical College of Ohio. He was transferred to the chair of materia medica in 1867. He published on varied subjects such as spermatorrhea, bromides, and hypodermic medication. His textbook *Practical Treatise on Materia Medica and Therapeutics* (1877) was immensely popular and went through twelve editions.

In a famous case, Bartholow received immediate censure in 1874 (and later, sanction) after he published in *The American Journal of the Medical Sciences* the results of a daring experiment. A patient with rapidly spreading epithelioma of the scalp with exposure of the dura mater consented to a procedure in which Bartholow applied electrical stimulation to the posterior lobes of the cerebrum. This was a pioneer attempt to localize brain activity. Many felt that the patient's death soon after was due to injury from this rather than extension of the cancer itself. Despite the controversy he was elected professor of the practice of medicine at the Medical College of Ohio.

Dr. Bartholow came to Philadelphia to succeed Dr. John Biddle as chair of materia medica and therapeutics at Jefferson Medical College in 1879. Like his predecessor, Bartholow served as dean for a few years starting in 1883. Dr. Holland wrote that Bartholow resigned the deanship in 1887 because his "growing business made the official duties irksome." His consultation practice, teaching responsibilities, and attendance at the Jefferson and Philadelphia hospitals were handled with distinction until his abrupt resignation in 1890.

A year after he arrived in Philadelphia Bartholow published *A Treatise on the Practice of Medicine, for the Use of Students and Practitioners* which incorporated his course of lectures on that subject and eventually went through eight editions, and in 1881 he published *Medical Electricity: a Practical Treatise on the Applications of Electricity to Medicine and Surgery*. In 1882 the talented Dr. Bartholow became an original member of the editorial staff of the reorganized *Medical News*, a Philadelphia weekly.

Among Bartholow's honors was an LL.D. degree from Mount St. Mary's College. He was a member of the American Philosophical Society and the College of Physicians, and an honorary member of the Royal Medical Society of Edinburgh and the Society of Practical Medicine of Paris.

In spite of Dr. Bartholow's prominence in Philadelphia medicine, the end of his career was tragically fraught with bitterness and conflict over his fragile mental state. Jefferson board of trustees minutes of October

14, 1890 indicate that his struggle had already begun. The board regretted that "it is now requisite that Dr. Bartholow should be relieved from further duty and have an opportunity given him to take needed rest...[and] lay aside the arduous duties of his chair."

Authorities at the school were chagrined that news of the board's action was made public. A headline in the October 16 *Record* was: "WORN OUT IN HARNESS/Dr. Bartholow's Professorship/Soon to End./A VERY PAINFUL AFFLICTION./The Famous Physician's Mind Has suffered from the Wear and Tear of Too Active Work."

Bartholow's indignant refusal to resign was supported by students. *The Times* of October 18 reported on a "tumultuous" student meeting with the headline: "A STUDENTS' UPRISING/JEFFERSON COLLEGE MEN STANDING/BY PROFESSOR BARTHOLOW/THEY WANT HIM TO STAY." The board granted Bartholow a six-month leave of absence in the hope that rest from his labors would better prepare him to perform the duties of his chair. He refused this offer in a painful letter.

Dr. Holland's memoir stated succinctly that Bartholow had suffered a mental breakdown, and had explained the "attack" as diabetes, and for a cure had been put upon a course of opiates which were seconded with other drugs, enabling him to continue his work until he "reached the limit of his endurance."

The board resolved unanimously to vacate the chair of therapeutics. It was decided to postpone the election for the rest of the 1890-91 session and to appoint a temporary lecturer. In April 1891 Dr. Hobart A. Hare was elected successor to the chair of therapeutics. After a period of rest, Dr. Bartholow made a partial recovery and resumed his office practice and literary career. He was appointed emeritus professor in 1893.

Still admiring their professor of therapeutics, the Jefferson Medical College class of 1892 presented Bartholow's portrait at the spring commencement ceremonies, and the painting was installed in a reading room of the library in the 1898 College Building.

George W. Pettit's portrait of Bartholow is bust length with the subject's body turned slightly to the left. The most distinguishing feature is his luxurious white mustache and short beard. His deepset eyes look straight ahead and are almost hidden in a dark shadow, perhaps symbolic of his inner troubles and the somber recent events. His expression is unusually neutral and bland. Holland's memoir had noted that Bartholow's bearing was reserved and lacking in geniality: "While his professional expertness was of undoubted value to society, as an unremitting student, with the habit of seclusion, the social life had few charms for him."

Another possible reason for the almost inanimate expression is that the portrait was not done from life. The blurred lower contour of his torso suggests that it was copied after a photograph or print. The timing of the presentation suggests that perhaps Dr. Bartholow was not in good enough health to sit for a portrait and that the artist used another source for his image.

Portrait of Jacob da S. Solis-Cohen

JACOB da SILVA SOLIS-COHEN, M.D. (1838-1927)
By Agnes Allen (b. 1897), after William T. Thomson

Oil on canvas
1966-67
30 x 24 in.

Inscription and signature lower right: "AGNES ALLEN/after/W.T. Thomson"

Given in 1967 by JMC trustees
Accession number: 1967+e.P.03

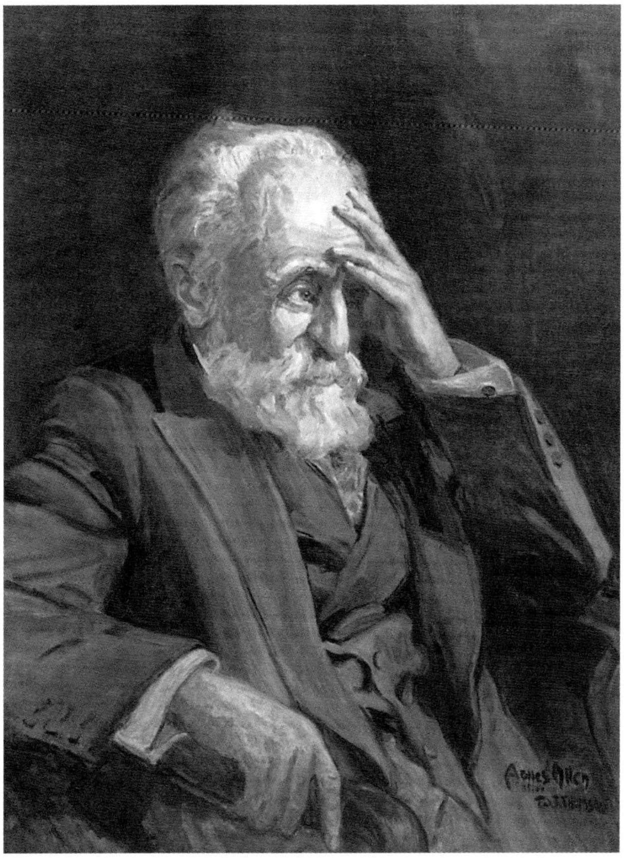

A pioneer laryngologist at Jefferson Medical College, Dr. Jacob da Silva Solis-Cohen was descended from some of the earliest Sephardic Jewish settlers who arrived in America in 1654, a group who traced their history back to medieval Spain and Portugal.

A few members of the Hays branch of the family who came to America in the early 1700s made their way to Philadelphia just before the Revolution. The marriage of Jacob D. Solis-Cohen's mother, Judith da Silva Solis, to his father, Myer David Cohen, added the Ashkenazic Eastern European tradition to the family. This family is unusual for the number of distinguished members who have made important contributions to Philadelphia medicine, law, business, the arts, education, civic reform, and philanthropy.[15]

Jacob da Silva Solis-Cohen was born in 1838 in New York and moved with his family to Philadelphia when he was aged two. After his graduation from Central High School he earned a medical degree from the University of Pennsylvania in 1860.

His residency training at Old Blockley (Philadelphia General Hospital) was interrupted by the Civil War in which he first served as assistant surgeon in the Twenty-sixth Regiment, Pennsylvania Volunteers. He resigned to accept an appointment in the U.S. Navy. From 1864 to 1865 he was visiting surgeon to the two military hospitals in Philadelphia.

He resumed practice in Philadelphia in 1866, soon specializing in the diagnosis and treatment of diseases of the throat and air passages, and he gave lectures on this topic at the Philadelphia School of Anatomy. In 1867 he was appointed lecturer on electro-therapeutics at Jefferson Medical College, and in 1869 lecturer on laryngoscopy and diseases of the throat and chest. In 1883 he was named honorary professor of laryngology and lectured regularly until 1888.

He was the first visiting physician on the staff of the Jefferson Hospital and supervised the throat clinic until the late 1890s. He also served on the staffs of German Hospital (now Lankenau) and the Jewish Hospital. In 1883 he became professor of diseases of the throat and chest in the Philadelphia Polyclinic and College for Graduates in Medicine.

Solis-Cohen's reputation was established early in his career with the publication of *Inhalation, its Therapeutics and Practice: A Treatise on the Inhalation of Gases, Vapors, Nebulized Fluids, and Powders* (1867) and his classic *Diseases of the Throat and Nasal Passages: A Guide to the Diagnosis and Treatment of Affections of the Pharynx, Esophagus, Trachea, Larynx, and Nares* (1872).

Dr. Solis-Cohen was president of the Northern Medical Association, and twice president of the Philadelphia County Medical Society. He was a founder and two-term president of the American Laryngological Association, and a founder of the *Archives of Laryngology*. He was an honorary member of the American Philosophical Society, the Neurological Association of New York, the Société Française de Laryngologie, and the British Association of Laryngology and Rhinology.

The portrait of Dr. Solis-Cohen by Agnes Allen was ordered by Jefferson Medical College trustees and presented in 1967. It is a copy after an original portrait made in 1927 when the subject was close to ninety years old. According to records at the College of Physicians of Philadelphia where the original portrait is located, it was painted by William T. Thomson in the last year of the doctor's life "simply because of the interest of the artist in the subject." It was found in the artist's studio by his physician, a fellow of the College of Physicians, and presented to that institution by the section on otolaryngology in 1939.[16]

Dr. Solis-Cohen is depicted half length, seated, and turned halfway to the right. He rests his arms on the chair arms, and the long fingers of his left hand support his head. His most distinguishing features are his thick white hair, eyebrows, mustache, side whiskers, and beard. His high domed forehead, deepset eyes, and long and bumpy nose are emphasized by highlights. Although the traditional head-on-hand pose usually denotes meditation or even brooding, the subject's fair complexion, ruddy cheeks, and bright eyes seem to radiate energy, and this liveliness is emphasized by the artist's rapid, calligraphic brush strokes.

Jacob da S. Solis-Cohen Examining a Patient

JACOB da SILVA SOLIS-COHEN, M.D. EXAMINING A PATIENT
By unknown photographer

Ferrotype
1869
6 1/8 x 4 1/8 in.

Given after 1929 by family of Dr. Solis-Cohen
Accession number: 1929+f.Ph.13

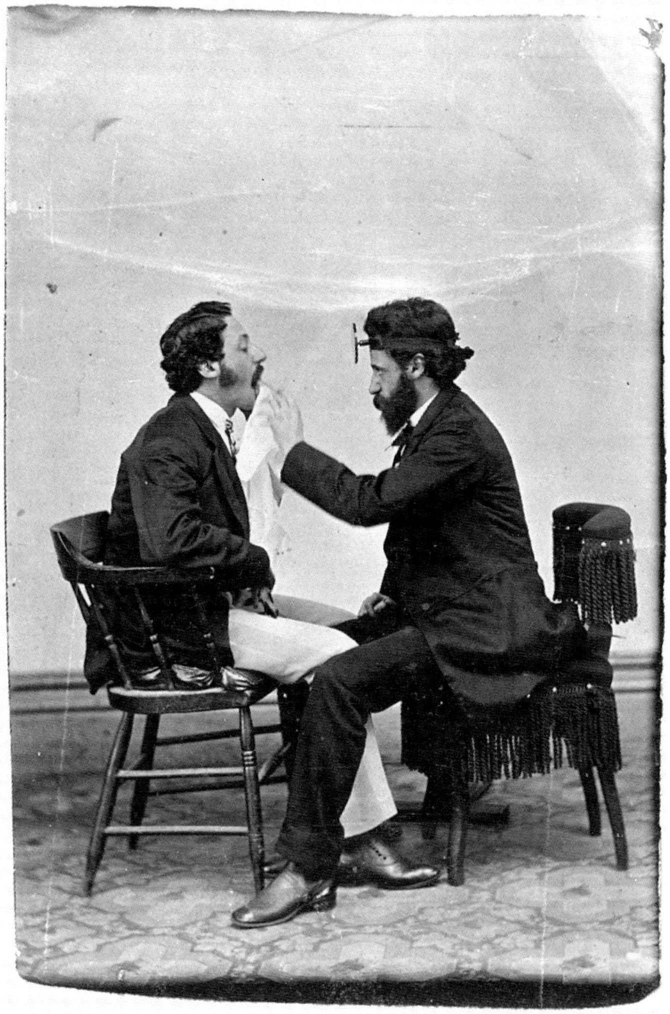

An unusual photograph of a physician at work features Dr. Jacob da Silva Solis-Cohen. The ferrotype (photograph on an iron support, often called "tintype") is dated 1869 on the back. A letter in the Jefferson archives states that it was probably made for an illustration of Solis-Cohen's early paper on laryngoscopy.

The young physician is shown leaning forward to examine his patient's larynx. He wears a head mirror and performs the laryngoscopy by holding the patient's tongue with a cloth and inserting a laryngeal mirror. In the profile double portrait, the two men sit facing each other with their legs in alternating positions. In contrast to the patient's plain wooden chair, the upholstered back and seat of the physician's chair are decorated with a long fringe and studded with brass nails.

Dr. Jacob D. Solis-Cohen was unusual for specializing, and at first was derided by many eminent generalists of the day including Dr. Samuel D. Gross, but through his teachings and publications he helped establish laryngology as a distinct specialty. He was one of the first Americans to study the use of the laryngoscope. In 1868 Solis-Cohen performed the first successful laryngotomy in the world for cancer of a vocal cord. In 1884 he performed the first complete laryngectomy in this country, and his patient survived eleven years and without recurrence.

Portrait of James W. Holland

JAMES WILLIAM HOLLAND, M.D.
(1849-1922)
By Adolphe Borie (1877-1934)

Oil on canvas
1909
43 x 35 in.

Signed and dated upper left: "Adolphe Borie 1909"
Exhibitions: Philadelphia, *Annual Exhibition*, Pennsylvania Academy of the Fine Arts (incorrectly listed as "Portrait of Dr. T. W. Holland"), 1910; Philadelphia, McClees Art Gallery, 1910

Given in 1910 by JMC alumni association
Accession number: 1910+e.P.01

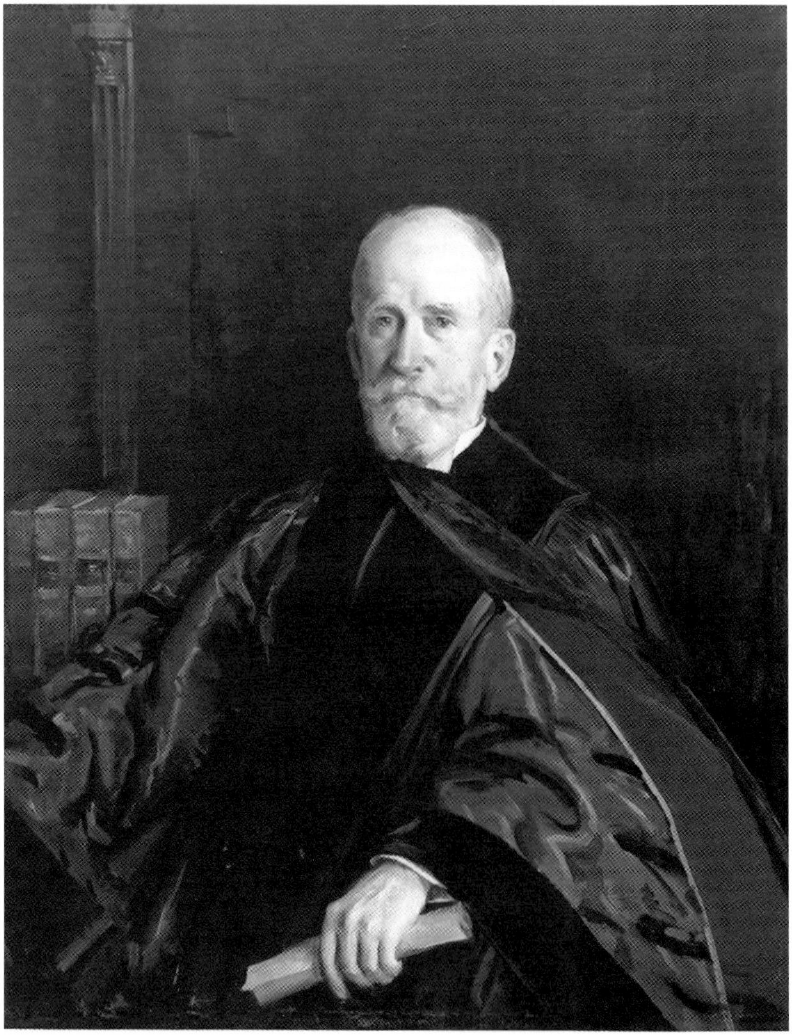

Dr. James W. Holland was more suited temperamentally to fill the Jefferson deanship than was Dr. Roberts Bartholow, and he served admirably in that post from 1887 until 1916. Noted for his professional longevity, he was also professor of medical chemistry and toxicology for twenty-seven years.

James Holland was born in Nashville, Tennessee in 1849. His physician father moved the family to Louisville, Kentucky during the 1852 cholera epidemic. Holland earned a bachelor's degree from the University of Louisville in 1865, and then a master's degree there in 1868, the same year he graduated from Jefferson Medical College.

He returned to Kentucky to enter practice with his father and immediately received a teaching post as assistant demonstrator of anatomy at the University of Louisville. In 1872 he became professor of medical chemistry and clinical neurology, and then successively occupied the chairs of materia medica, clinical medicine, and the practice of medicine and clinical medicine. He served as president of the Kentucky State Medical Association and editor of the *Louisville Medical News*.

Dr. James W. Holland was called to Jefferson in 1885 to become professor of medical chemistry and toxicology. During his long tenure he expanded the curriculum to include a full year of lectures and laboratories in both inorganic and organic chemistry. He emphasized the applications of chemistry in its toxicological, therapeutic, and diagnostic uses, rather than its physiological functions.

Just two years after joining the faculty, Holland began serving as dean. He could look with pride on the favorable rating of Jefferson in the 1911 Flexner Report which evaluated all U.S. and Canadian medical schools, and the A+ rating given Jefferson by the American Medical Association in 1914.

The May 1912 *Jeffersonian* announced Dr. Holland's resignation from teaching "with a thousand regrets" felt by all the graduates who were so fortunate to have attended his lectures and laboratory, who would "always remember him as a faithful, loyal teacher, ever ready to help each man out of any difficulty." He was named professor emeritus in 1912 and received an honorary Sc.D. degree the following year.

Dr. Holland was the author of several books on medical chemistry and toxicology including: *Diet for the Sick* (1880), *The Urine and the Clinical Chemistry of the Gastric Contents, the Common Poisons, and the Milk* (1895), and *Textbook on Medical Chemistry and Toxicology* (1905). He was also an editor of *Medical News*. Holland served as president of the Association of American Medical Colleges and was a member of the Council of Medical Education of the American Medical Association.

In 1909 Jefferson trustee Simon Gratz chaired a committee to raise voluntary contributions for a portrait of Dr. James W. Holland. Circulars were sent around the country hoping that every alumnus "will be loyal to his Alma Mater and contribute to this portrait of the Veteran Teacher and Dean of Old Jeff." The May 1909 *Jeffersonian* reported that support was very gratifying.

The following January's *Jeffersonian* reported that the portrait was completed and accepted by the committee in charge, and was on view at McClees Art Gallery at 1411 Walnut Street. Alumni and students were urged to visit the gallery and "see the admirable portrait of our beloved Dean and Teacher" made by "noted" artist "Adolph [*sic*] Borie."

Philadelphia's *Evening Bulletin* gave a full report of the Jefferson commencement at the Academy of Music on June 6, 1910. Highlights of the occasion included an honorary LL.D. degree awarded to Dr. S. Weir Mitchell on the sixtieth anniversary of his graduation, Dr. W. W. Keen's address memorializing Dr. Samuel D. Gross, and the presentation of Dr. Holland's portrait. The newspaper reproduced the painting and complimented Borie's "masterly technique," calling the work an "excellent likeness."

Dr. Holland is shown half length, seated in an interior space featuring a paneled wall and Corinthian pilaster above a table with four books. The subject's large blue eyes look directly toward the observer, but his expression is somewhat reticent. The narrowness of his oval-shaped face is emphasized by his high domed forehead and gray-blond mustache, beard, and side whiskers. He holds a rolled paper in his left hand, possibly a diploma.

The most striking feature of the portrait is the dean's costume: a loosely brushed, black academic gown with green velvet trim and voluminous sleeves that seem to engulf the figure. One can sense that he was rather small-boned and short in stature.

Adolphe Borie was as well educated and prominent in his own field as his subject. Born in Philadelphia in 1877, he graduated from the Lawrenceville School in 1895. He spent the following year at the University of Pennsylvania after which he studied for three years at the Pennsylvania Academy of the Fine Arts. Following the path of many art and medical students, Borie decided to continue his studies in Europe and chose the Royal Academy in Munich, like his teacher at the Pennsylvania Academy, William Merritt Chase.

Borie revisited Europe frequently but forged his career in Philadelphia except for the years 1915 to 1919 in New York. When the United States entered World War I he worked for a year at camouflaging ships, and contributed portraits in exchange for subscriptions to the last Liberty Loan. While his landscapes, still lifes, and nudes show the influence of European impressionism and modernism, the artist supported himself mainly from traditional portrait commissions.

Borie's father was a prosperous banker (until his bank failed in 1905) and was initially displeased with his son's choice of profession. The artist's biographer and friend George Biddle described Borie as "in every sense...an aristocrat—in looks, manners, grooming, and social background—and that manner he carried with the same ease and detachment with which he painted."[17] Biddle said that as a professional portrait painter Borie was "subjected to the petty family criticisms and sartorial strictures of his clients." Biddle quoted Borie wittily describing himself as

> "a fashionable tailor at the final fitting. Today there was a post-mortem and the family were delighted with the face. But the coat had to be re-cut. I took it in at the waist, put some padding in the shoulders, and finally achieved the right note by substituting a pearl gray Charvet cravat for a Christmas-sale necktie from Wanamaker's. And as I chalked the alterations on the canvas, I could feel my mouth bristling with pins."

While Borie deprecated his reliance upon portraiture and the traditional dilemma it imposed upon artists of squaring their vision with the client's self-image, he felt that photography had liberated the art of portraiture from merely rendering an exact, mechanical likeness. Many of his portraits are suffused with an air of gentle sympathy and geniality.

Adolphe Borie was well recognized by the art establishment and was made a full academician at the National Academy of Design in 1934. A one-man show of his work was held at the Folsom Gallery in New York in 1915, and memorial exhibitions were held at the Philadelphia Museum of Art in 1935 and the Corcoran Gallery of Art in Washington in 1942.

Among his many awards were: the Pennsylvania Academy's Carol Beck Gold Medal for portraiture; the Maynard Portrait Prize at the National Academy of Design; silver medals at the San Francisco Panama-Pacific International Exposition and the Philadelphia Sesquicentennial; the Third Clark Prize and bronze medal at the Corcoran Gallery, Washington, D.C.; a gold medal at the Philadelphia Art Club; and the Norman Wait Harris Bronze Medal at the Art Institute of Chicago.

As in the cases of Drs. Samuel D. Gross and Jacob M. DaCosta, rival artists including Thomas Eakins painted images of the same subject. In 1899, ten years before Adolphe Borie's commission from Jefferson Medical College, Eakins had asked Dr. Holland to pose for a portrait, expecting that the college would purchase it. His full-length depiction of Dr. Holland calling the roll of new graduates at commencement is known as *The Dean's Roll Call.*

The dean's son, Leicester Holland, recalled that the sittings lasted for at least five months starting in January 1899:

> My Father was never physically very strong and by that season of the year was always pretty well fagged out. What made it worse was that Eakins always insisted that he take the full standing pose, with the light from the skylight full in his face. He would not let him sit down even when working on the head alone. It was quite an ordeal and the result was a tense, almost haggard expression...Alas, when it was all done, the college and the alumni who knew father in more genial moods...didn't like it at all and wouldn't buy it. So Eakins, having no general market at the time had the painting on his hands,...and as a friendly gesture gave the picture to my mother.[18]

A reproduction of Eakins's painting of Dr. Holland was chosen for the title page of the Jefferson Medical College yearbook of 1900, showing at least partial institutional regard for the portrait. Clearly, Dr. Holland approved of the depiction and did not rule out a potential Jefferson purchase, as noted in an undated (ca. 1900) letter from Dr. and Mrs. Holland to Eakins:

> Your very kind letter of the 29th inst. has been received. Mrs. Holland has been informed of your intention to present her the portrait of myself "with the understanding that if at any time the trustees of the Jefferson Medical College may wish to purchase the picture the ownership of it will not be a bar to selling it on your account."
>
> She wishes me to say that she is grateful to you for your kindness and accepts the present as a trust under the conditions I have quoted above.
>
> She joins me in repeating the expressions of admiration you have already heard from us for the fidelity of the likeness and the artistic merit of the work.[19]

There are no extant Jefferson Medical College archival documents relating to Eakins's portrait of Holland. The painting was on long-term loan at the Philadelphia Museum of Art until it was purchased from Dr. Holland's children in 1943 by the Museum of Fine Arts, Boston. In 1983 the latter museum borrowed *The Gross Clinic* for the exhibition *A New World: Masterpieces of American Painting, 1760-1910*, and lent the Holland portrait to Jefferson where it was enthusiastically, if ruefully, admired.

Portrait of William S. Forbes

(See color plate)

WILLIAM SMITH FORBES, M.D. (1831-1905)
By Thomas Eakins (1844-1916)

Oil on canvas
1905
84 x 48 in.

Signed and dated lower right: "Eakins/1905"
Inscription carved in the amphitheater wall, right center: "GVLIELMVS S. FORBES, M.D./QVI LEGEM NOVAM DE RE ANATOMICA/GVBERNIO STATVS PENNSYLVANIAE/PROPOSVIT COMMENDAVIT DEFENSIONE STVDIOSA/EX SENATVS CONSVLTV/FERENDEM CVRAVIT"[20]
Exhibitions: Philadelphia, *Annual Exhibition*, Pennsylvania Academy of the Fine Arts, Jan. 22-Mar. 3, 1906; Philadelphia, *Memorial Exhibition of the Works of the Late Thomas Eakins*, Pennsylvania Academy of the Fine Arts, Dec. 23, 1917-Jan. 13, 1918; Philadelphia, *Thomas Eakins 1844-1916*, Pennsylvania Museum of Art, ca. Mar. 5-ca. Apr. 15, 1930; Philadelphia, *150th Anniversary Exhibition*, Pennsylvania Academy of the Fine Arts, Jan. 15-Mar. 13, 1955; Philadelphia, *The Art of Philadelphia Medicine*, Philadelphia Museum of Art, Sept. 15-Dec. 7, 1965; Philadelphia, summer loan, Philadelphia Museum of Art, June 15-Aug. 30, 1969; New York, *Thomas Eakins Retrospective Exhibition*, Whitney Museum of American Art, Sept. 22-Nov. 21, 1970; Birmingham, Ala., *The Art of Healing: Medicine and Science in American Art*, Birmingham Museum of Art, Feb. 7-Mar. 29, 1981

Given in 1905 by JMC classes of 1905-08 and junior alumni
Accession number: 1905+e.P.01

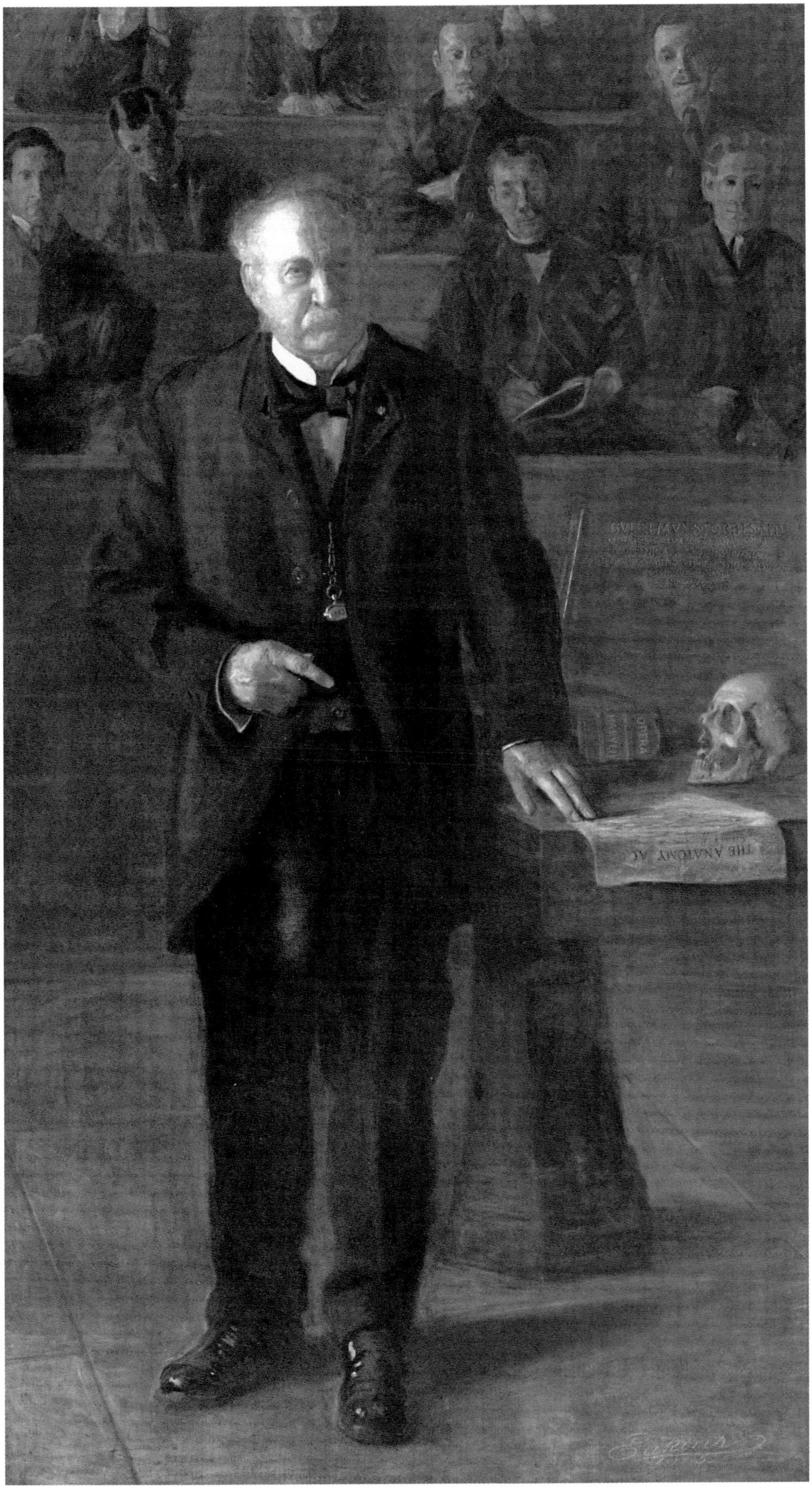

Dr. William Smith Forbes was a professor of anatomy and clinical surgery at Jefferson Medical College from 1886 until his death in 1905. He is most renowned for pioneering the legislation known as the Anatomy Act of Pennsylvania.

William S. Forbes was born in 1831 in Falmouth, Virginia, descended from a family who arrived in America in 1657. After a classical education at the Fredericksburg and Concord Academies, he began his medical education in 1850 at the University of Virginia. While completing his medical degree at Jefferson Medical College in 1852, he worked in the office of Dr. Joseph Pancoast. During a residency at the Pennsylvania Hospital he also took courses in anatomy and medicine at the University of Pennsylvania.

He left the country in March 1855 to study military surgery abroad, and visited England, France, Switzerland, Austria, and Germany before sailing for Constantinople. His steamer, *The Africa*, ran aground, but the adventurous young man made his way unscathed to Scutari, where he was assigned to the surgical staff of the barrack hospital of the British army. Although the Treaty of Paris was signed just five months later, Forbes was commended for his work in the Crimea and offered a commission with the rank of major in the British medical services, but he declined the honor. The famous English nurse, Florence Nightingale (1820-1910), gave Forbes her instrument kit in memory of their close professional association at the end of the Crimean War. Following the war he audited courses in surgery and anatomy in Paris and then traveled to Belgium.[21]

Upon his return to Philadelphia in 1857 Dr. William Forbes opened a private school of anatomy which primarily served dental students from the southern states. The school closed during the Civil War but reopened later and continued until about 1872. Although Forbes was a native Virginian and his family was naturally loyal to the Confederacy, the young physician had married a woman from Philadelphia and was determined to forge his career there, so with some anguish he sided with the North during the Civil War.

He was commissioned as a surgeon of volunteers with the rank of major in the port of Philadelphia, then served as medical director of the Thirteenth Army Corps under General Grant during the siege at Vicksburg. He handed in his commission abruptly in 1863, possibly in reaction to the death of his brother who was killed at the Battle of Chancellorsville.

Dr. Forbes returned to Philadelphia and in 1866 received a second medical degree from the University of Pennsylvania. For a time he was professor of anatomy at the Pennsylvania Dental College. Starting in 1862 he was surgeon to the Episcopal Hospital, a post he held for twenty-five years. Although Forbes became one of several aspirants who failed in their quest to succeed Dr. Joseph Pancoast as chair of anatomy at Jefferson Medical College, in 1879 he was appointed demonstrator of anatomy there. He secured the chair of anatomy and clinical surgery in 1886, and introduced formal courses in histology in 1896 and embryology in 1900.

Among Dr. Forbes's best-known papers are "The Removal of Stone in the Bladder" (1894) in which he described the invention of a new lithotrite (designed with his engineer son, John S. Forbes), an instrument for the breaking and measuring of vesical calculi into small pieces; and "Liberation of the Ring-finger in Musicians by Dividing the Accessory Tendons of the Extensor Communis Digitorum Muscle" (1898), a continuation of a paper of 1884.[22] He was the first to perform this procedure.[23]

Dr. Forbes was admired and beloved by his students, and in 1893 they sought his assistance in establishing a society devoted to the propagation of anatomical knowledge. The W. S. Forbes Anatomical League was the first such officially sanctioned student anatomical organization in American medicine. Although Forbes had been ill with heart trouble since late November 1905, he thought himself sufficiently well two weeks later to deliver a lecture, but his condition worsened and he died on December 17.

Dr. Forbes's greatest legacy to medical education is the Anatomy Act. In 1866 he had attempted unsuccessfully to guide passage of such an act through the Pennsylvania legislature, to solve the problem of insufficient bodies available for the great number of students studying anatomy in Philadelphia. Forbes described the unfortunate circumstances necessary for obtaining unclaimed dead bodies in his *History of the Anatomy-Act of Pennsylvania*:[24]

> [The bodies] are therefore buried, and are afterward obtained surreptitiously by a third party, the so-called "resurrectionists," who engage in a degrading traffic, and sell them to the highest bidder...and the practical teachers here and elsewhere find themselves in unworthy competition with each other. Consequently the price demanded, and often obtained, is such as to tempt the resurrectionist to enter private cemeteries and graves, and even to commit murder...all tending to bring obloquy on anatomical teaching.

In February 1867 Forbes proposed that the College of Physicians of Philadelphia appoint a committee of three for the purpose of urging passage of a law sanctioning the dissection of human bodies. With the untiring efforts of Forbes as committee chairman, along with Drs. Samuel D. Gross and D. Hayes Agnew, the Anatomy Act was passed later that year. It provided that:

> the Inspectors and Superintendent of any county prison, the Board of Guardians of any City or County Almshouse, the Coroner of any County, or any other public officer having charge thereof or control over the same, shall give permission to any physician or surgeon of the same county, upon his request made therefor, to take the bodies of such persons dying in such prison, almshouse, or county, as are required to be buried at the public expense, to be by him used within the State for the advancement of medical science, preference being given to medical schools, public and private; and said bodies to be distributed to and among the same, equitably, the number assigned to each being proportioned to that of its students; provided, however, that if the deceased person, during his or her last sickness...shall request to be buried; or if any person...satisfying the proper authorities that he is of kindred to the deceased, shall ask to have the body for burial, it shall be surrendered for interment.

After the Anatomy Act's passage a voluntary association of anatomy demonstrators in chartered and private schools was formed in Philadelphia to agree upon an equitable distribution of bodies. This association continued until it was superseded by the Anatomy Act passed in June 1883. The revision was necessary because the original phrase "shall give permission" to take the unclaimed bodies did not actually bind certain officials who had control over the bodies.

At Forbes's insistence the 1883 law removed this ineffectual phrase and substituted "shall deliver." It specifically provided an anatomy board for the distribution and delivery of material from all sixty-seven counties in the state to all medical and dental schools in the commonwealth. The board was to be composed of no less than five scholars, and its first president was Dr. Joseph Leidy from the University of Pennsylvania.

All officers and agents of almshouses, prisons, morgues, and hospitals having charge of unclaimed bodies were required to notify the anatomy board and *deliver* the bodies without fee, and the schools or physicians had to give bond to the state before receiving the bodies. The 1883 Anatomy Act was a model soon adopted by many other states, and Dr. Forbes served on the Pennsylvania board for more than twenty years.

The triumph of pioneering this legislation which proved so important for medical education came at great personal cost to Dr. Forbes. By his account, the amended, second version of the Anatomy Act came as a direct result of a conflict between him and the city coroner who owned and conducted the Philadelphia School of Anatomy in competition with Jefferson Medical College. The coroner said that it was his duty to bury the bodies not to deliver them. He supplied enough bodies for his own school but would not deliver an equitable number to Jefferson.

In December 1882 detectives arrested three men who were hauling bodies from a common grave of "colored persons" in deep pits in the Lebanon Cemetery in Philadelphia. Dr. Forbes was soon arrested as an accomplice and accused of receiving stolen bodies from the ring of grave robbers. Of the several men accused, Dr. Forbes was the only one acquitted of charges, but the trial cost him many erstwhile friends who were alienated by the humiliating public proceedings.

A thoroughly researched account by University of Georgia historian Horace Montgomery, Ph.D. implicates Dr. Forbes and Jefferson Medical College in this particular case and other anatomists and schools in general in the necessity of collaborating with grave robbers.[25]

Montgomery says that several Philadelphia journalists and a "few Negro leaders" suspected that resurrectionists were continuing to rob graves at the Lebanon Cemetery for years after the 1867 legislation. This group was joined by a Pinkerton detective for months of surveillance which was rewarded by discovering an organized gang of dealers in dead bodies including doctors, graveyard superintendents, and undertakers.

Local newspapers reported that on the night of the arrest, the grave robbers said that the six bodies disinterred were destined for Jefferson Medical College. When these bodies were identified by horrified and anguished friends and families at the morgue, and other graves at Lebanon Cemetery were subsequently opened and empty coffins were revealed, the ghoulish disclosures so disturbed the Philadelphia community that widespread public protests were held.

Some Jefferson professors and administrators thought that the attendant notoriety could ruin the college, and Dean Ellerslie Wallace, M.D. succeeded in convincing local authorities to guard college property against possible assault by angry citizens. Dr. William H. Pancoast and a few others took the lead in persuading influential physicians in Philadelphia to exhort the Philadelphia Anatomical Association to frame an amended anatomy act to prevent future such crises.

Their petition was signed by members of the various

Philadelphia anatomy and medical schools. With the assistance of Dr. William J. McKnight, a state senator (ironically a confessed grave robber as a young physician in western Pennsylvania), the suspicions of rural Pennsylvania legislators were appeased, and the revised Anatomy Act was signed into law on June 13, 1883.

Sensational press treatment and the resulting public clamor were an ordeal for the gentlemanly and dignified Professor Forbes, but letters in the Jefferson archives indicate loyal support from many colleagues, friends, and family, including one from Dr. Samuel D. Gross who congratulated Forbes on his acquittal. In January 1884 a letter on Forbes's behalf was circulated by Drs. D. Hayes Agnew, Richard J. Levis, and J. William White to Jefferson faculty and alumni and to medical societies throughout the state. It appealed for funds totalling four thousand dollars to reimburse Forbes for his "unjust and expensive" lawsuit and to emphasize his "complete vindication," noting that he had acted not as a private teacher, but for the good of a public institution and medical science.

With the money collected and his reputation intact, honors and promotions were accorded him at Jefferson Medical College after the notorious case. According to Dr. William I. Forbes, when his great-grandfather was made professor of anatomy in 1886, Jefferson students presented him with a gold watch and chain as a token of their esteem. In 1887 the trustees elected him to conduct the general surgical clinic in addition to his work in anatomy, and Forbes resigned as surgeon to Episcopal Hospital to devote his full time to Jefferson.

The class of 1889 presented Dr. Forbes with a cane that expressed their admiration in an unusually personalized form: the signatures of students carefully carved in parallel rows down the length of the wooden shaft. Students from the Forbes Anatomical League presented their sponsor with a gold-headed cane during the session of 1900-01, and both canes were later donated to the Jefferson archives by family members.

In 1905 Dr. William S. Forbes was doubly honored for almost fifty years of contributions to medical education at a unique ceremony which brought together alumni from two rival medical schools at the eightieth annual Jefferson Medical College commencement. Dr. Addinell Hewson, assistant professor and demonstrator of anatomy and representative of the classes of 1905-08 and "junior alumni," presented Thomas Eakins's portrait of Forbes to the trustees of the college. He said that the portrait had been painted in less than four months, and that subscriptions achieved a surplus which was turned over to the Jefferson library.

Next, Dr. George A. Piersol, professor of anatomy and a representative of the medical alumni association of the University of Pennsylvania, presented a silver loving cup to Dr. Forbes. He explained that the cup symbolized their recognition of Forbes's initiative in securing the "adoption of wise laws protecting and promoting anatomy" for the benefit of the "entire medical profession throughout the length and breadth of this great land."

Dr. Forbes responded to the presentation of portrait and cup:

> Your hearty applause and these memorials...go far beyond my deserts. I did but do my duty...at a critical moment in the history of medical education in this country...
>
> I rejoice that I was thought worthy to bear a part of the obloquy and even peril which once surrounded this important study, and which, thanks to the legislation of 1883, has now, I trust, passed away forever.
>
> It is most gratifying to me that my services in this behalf have been the occasion of such a fraternization of our two great medical schools as we witness here today. Let us hope this co-operation will continue...
>
> To you, Professor Piersol...convey to our fellow-alumni of the University of Pennsylvania the loving regards of one who has never ceased to be grateful for what he learned at the feet of Professor Joseph Leidy... Professor Hewson, I would express to the students and alumni of our own college my sense of the great honor they have done me in placing my portrait on her walls along with those of men whose names are imperishable in the history of medical science.

As depicted by Thomas Eakins, Dr. William S. Forbes is shown lecturing to students in the clinical amphitheater of the 1877 Hospital Building. On a nearby table are three significant objects relating to Forbes's accomplishments: a book, *Opera Harveii*, the collected works of William Harvey (1578-1657), the English anatomist he admired[26]; a parchment document hanging over the edge of the venerable operating table and whose inverted title, "The Anatomy Act," is legible; and a skull that bears silent witness to Forbes's tribulations in achieving this legislation. The skull is not only an appropriate attribute for the teacher of anatomy, it is also a *memento mori*. Both subject and artist were of advanced age, and both were nearing the end of their careers. A Latin inscription carved into the amphitheater wall in front of the attentive students credits Forbes for implementing the Anatomy Act.

At first glance Forbes is an imposing figure, tall and stocky, occupying center stage of the amphitheater, with all eyes on him. Then one notices signs of frailty and vulnerability. His posture is stooped and he seems to be leaning on the table for support and appears unsteady on his feet. Though he is fashionably dressed in black frock coat and shirt with winged collar, his rumpled and baggy trousers pool around his ankles. Even the heavy pedestal of the operating table leg echoes Forbes's ponderous figure. His graying hair and whiskers are thin and wispy, and the skin on his neck is slack and wrinkled. Deep lines are etched into his forehead and face. There are dark circles under his eyes. The stolid, almost halting figure seems to lack the energy or strength for action. Indeed, the seventy-four-year-old professor died six months after the portrait was presented.

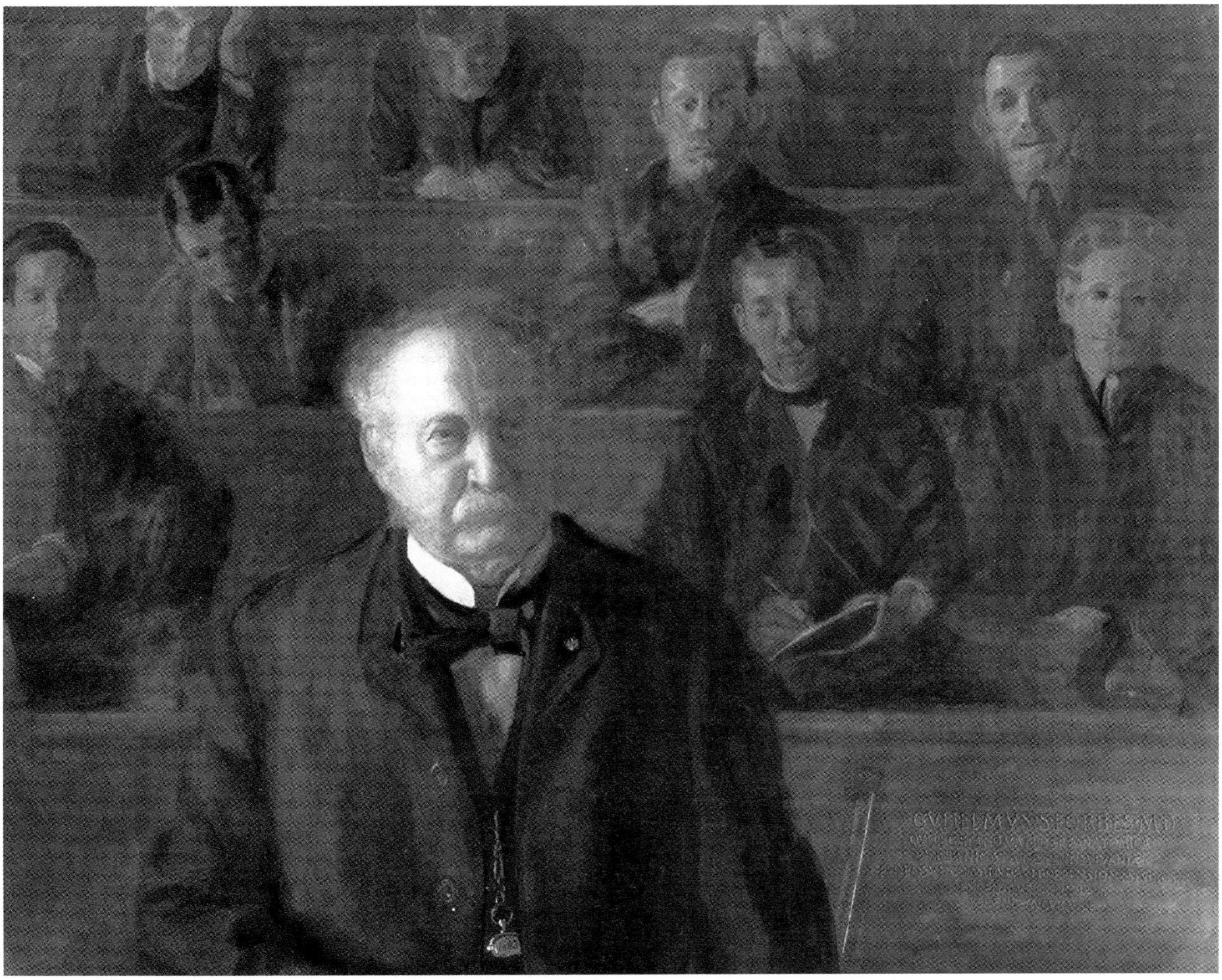

Detail: Head of Dr. Forbes

Yet his still-strong hands interact with the objects and allude to a once vigorous career. The index finger of his right hand points to the Anatomy Act proclamation, and the fingertips of his left hand rest on this parchment. Above the pointing finger hangs a glistening gold chain and watch seal, probably the gift from admiring students mentioned above. It is inscribed with the date 1883, the year of the revised Anatomy Act. A pointer used in anatomy lectures leans against the wall and aims diagonally toward the tiers of attentive students. Dr. Forbes wears another ornament that relates to his military career, the lapel pin of the Military Order of the Loyal Legion of the United States.

The amphitheater in the 1877 hospital was of similar proportions to that of the Ely Building depicted in *The Gross Clinic*. But in contrast to the earlier, more active and dramatic scene, crowded with physicians performing multiple tasks and crowned with the imperious figure of Dr. Samuel D. Gross, here time and motion have slowed down and the mood has become more reflective. This expresses both the portrait subject and the artist's outlook: Eakins had painted *The Gross Clinic* in the energetic ambition of youth, but created the Forbes portrait near the close of a long and difficult career. The space depicted in the amphitheater is shallower. The full-length, life-sized figure of Professor Forbes stands alone in the foreground, and only three rows of attentive students can be seen in the background.

A warm glow emanating from the skylight above highlights the side of the professor's head and his hand, shirt collar, and watch. The students, too, are suffused in golden tones. The slow movement of lines and forms, and the somber, almost monochromatic, brown and tan, autumnal tones allude to the doctor's stately dignity and meditative mood, and the waning of his life. There is an all-pervasive stillness in the room. By these metaphorical means Eakins's empathetic portrayal becomes a quiet celebration of a once heroic physician's past triumph. It is a fitting tribute to an outstanding figure in the history of American medical education.

Jefferson students requested that the Forbes portrait be hung "in a prominent place in the college." It was installed in the upper amphitheater of the 1877 hospital, and later near *The Gross Clinic* in the 1929 College Building.

As it is situated today in the Eakins Gallery across the room from the painting of Dr. Benjamin H. Rand, there is a curious dialogue between the late public portrait of 1905 and the private portrait made thirty-one years earlier. Both professors, surrounded by objects relating to their specialty, appear introspective and lost in their thoughts. Each portrait features a white paper suspended over the edge of a desk or table. The thin tissue paper in the Rand portrait is

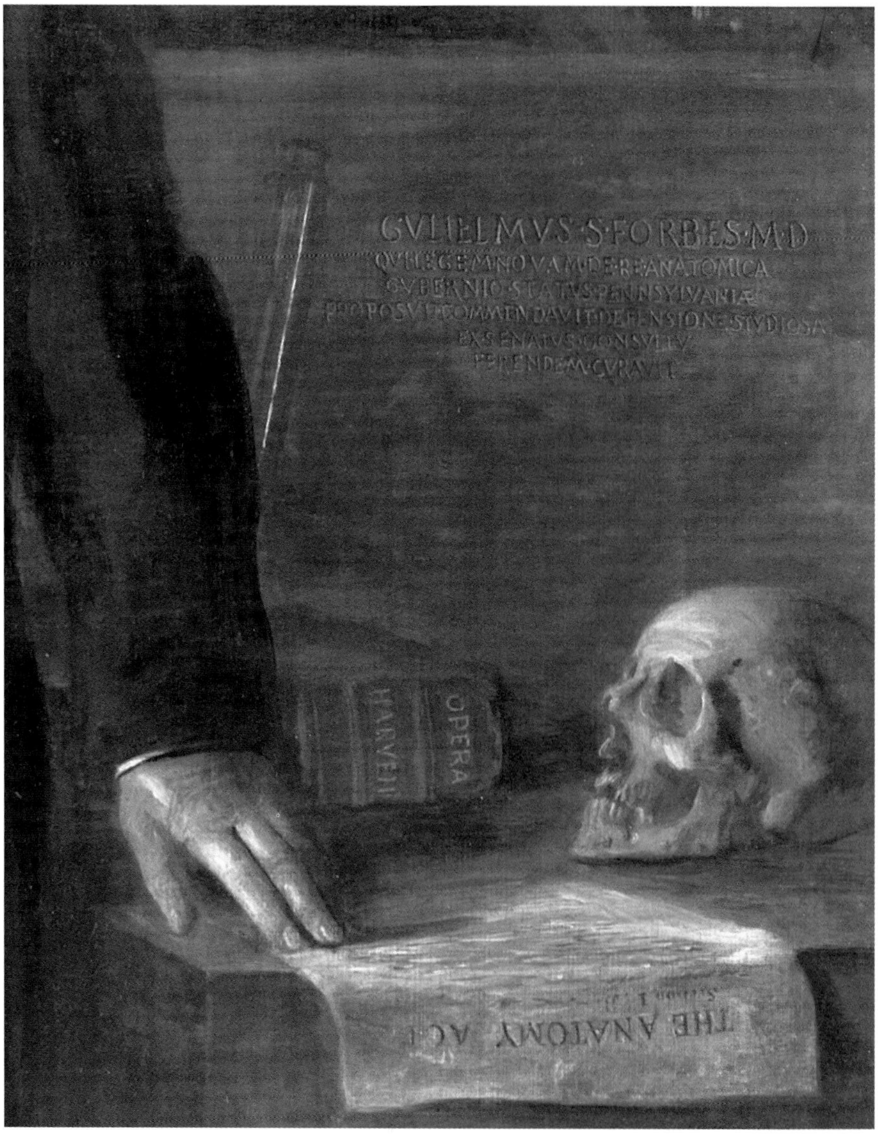

Detail: Hand of Dr. Forbes and Objects on Table

not really relevant to an understanding of the subject's profession, but is merely an eye-catching vehicle for displaying Eakins's ability to render a difficult material. In contrast, the stiffer parchment proclaiming the Anatomy Act in the Forbes portrait is vital to understanding the subject's important professional contribution.

Jefferson Medical College administrators must have admired Eakins's portrait of Dr. Forbes, for copies were given to all subscribers of the portrait fund in 1905. The *Jeffersonian* of December 1908 offered reproductions of the painting and copies of Forbes's *History of the Anatomy Act* to its readers for ten cents. The Jefferson collection also possesses a photomechanical reproduction of the portrait made by the Electro-tint Company of Philadelphia, donated in 1943 by Dr. Charles W. Bonney (JMC 1904).

Loving Cup Presented to William S. Forbes

LOVING CUP PRESENTED TO WILLIAM SMITH FORBES, M.D.
J. E. Caldwell & Co.

Silver
1905
14 1/8 x 14 x 8 1/4 in.

Inscription on the front: "PRESENTED TO/WILLIAM S. FORBES, M.D./BY THE/MEDICAL ALUMNI ASSOCIATION/OF THE/UNIVERSITY OF PENNSYLVANIA/IN RECOGNITION OF HIS EMINENT SERVICES TO THE CAUSE OF/MEDICAL SCIENCE"
Stamped on bottom of base: "J.E. CALDWELL & CO/925/STERLING/1000/PHILADELPHIA"

Given in 1989 by descendants of Dr. William S. Forbes: William I. Forbes Jr., Francis C. Forbes, and Charles B. W. Forbes
Accession number: 1989+e.DA.01
Photograph by Robert Neroni

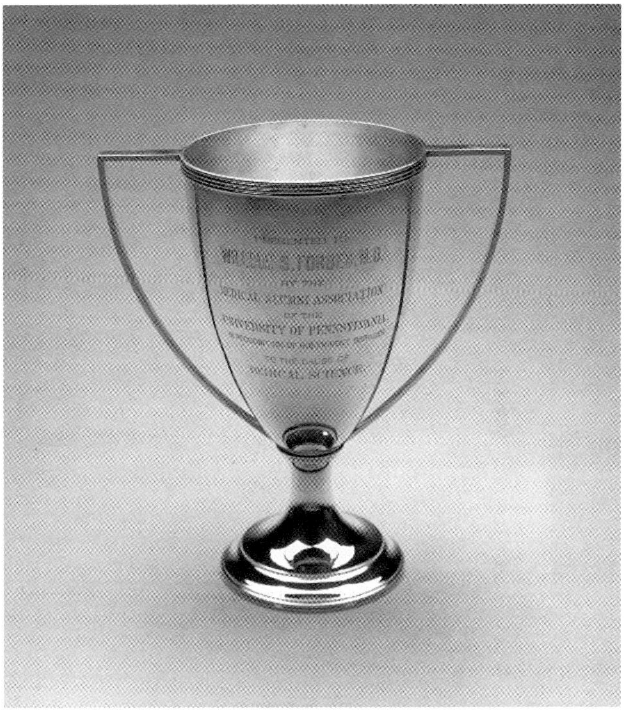

The medical alumni association of the University of Pennsylvania circulated a flyer soliciting two-dollar subscriptions from alumni for the "notable occasion" of presenting a silver loving cup and an "engrossed set of resolutions" to Dr. William S. Forbes at the Jefferson commencement exercises in 1905.

When researching the portrait of Dr. Forbes, I was surprised to read about the silver cup, because it was not present on the Jefferson campus, and no one queried even knew of its existence. Then I discovered that Jefferson alumnus Dr. William I. Forbes III of Watertown, New York, had already donated to the archives manuscript material and artifacts relating to his illustrious great-grandfather. When contacted, Dr. Forbes vaguely remembered such a cup and kindly put me in touch with his father and uncle who resided in the Philadelphia suburbs. They recalled that in the distant past the family had transformed the loving cup into a lamp, and, in turn, they directed me to Dr. Forbes's cousin in whose garage the lamp could probably be found.

I arrived at Mr. Forbes's home just in time, as he was relocating permanently to Sydney, Australia later that week. In the garage was a blackened and battered silver presentation piece with frayed wires extending from its chipped wooden base. After consulting his family he allowed us to borrow the cup/lamp and to entrust the original maker, J. E. Caldwell and Company, with restoration. Soon thereafter, the Forbes family graciously donated the beautifully refurbished cup, so that it could be reunited with the portrait in the Eakins Gallery at Thomas Jefferson University.

The sterling silver cup is of a standard presentation type. The shape is an inverted helmet, with a steeply tapered round bowl standing on a splayed pedestal. It is fitted with a pair of C-shaped, angular strapwork handles joining the reeded rim of the bowl. On the front is a presentation inscription, and on the back an applied silver seal of the University of Pennsylvania.

Portrait of William S. Forbes

WILLIAM SMITH FORBES, M.D.
By unknown photographer

Vintage photograph mounted on card
Ca. 1905
Image size: 7 1/4 x 4 1/4 in.
Card size: 10 1/2 x 8 1/4 in.

Given after 1905 by unknown donor
Accession number: 1905+f.Ph.04

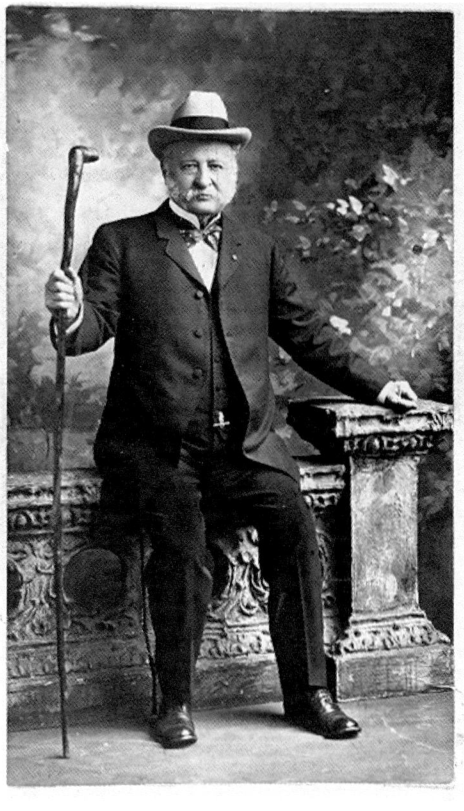

A photograph in the Jefferson collection shows Dr. William S. Forbes looking more robust than in the contemporary oil painting by Thomas Eakins. Though on first impression the aging physician's posture seems erect and stable, one realizes that he is actually buttressing his position by leaning on the wall with his left hand and holding an unusually long cane with his right hand.

Though one cannot always accept handwritten dates on art works (the photograph is marked "ca. 1905" on the back of the card), the professor's white side whiskers and mustache and wrinkled neck lend credibility to the date.

In the photograph his hair is fuller and his face more angular than in the Eakins portrait where he looks drawn and fatigued, yet there is evidence of studio retouching on the vintage photograph, so comparisons of physical characteristics are difficult. Yet certainly the posture, mood, and setting of painting and photograph are very different.

Depicted in a photographer's studio rather than his place of work, the subject is placed in a stage setting with an ornately carved, low wall in front of a painted backdrop of dappled foliage. His costume includes a hat, cane, and a jaunty polka-dotted tie, suggesting that he has just sat down while out for a stroll. Yet his expression is incongruously severe as he stares directly towards the camera as though impatient with posing for the photograph. He does not appear meditative or introspective as depicted by Eakins.

Osler at Old Blockley

(See color plate)

OSLER AT OLD BLOCKLEY
By Dean Cornwell (1892-1960)

Oil on canvas backed with masonite
1939-40
48 x 66 in.

Signed lower left: "DEAN/CORN/WELL"
One in a series of six paintings, *Pioneers of American Medicine,* commissioned by Wyeth Laboratories; presented in 1952 to Philadelphia General Hospital where it hung until 1977 when it was turned over to TJU on long-term loan

Accession number: 1977+e.P.03L

Osler at Old Blockley is an important chronicle of Philadelphia medical history for its portrayal of an eminent American doctor when he was attending physician at an old public hospital that was the foundation of training for so many physicians. Blockley supplied a wealth of clinical material for professors from Jefferson Medical College and the University of Pennsylvania. By 1870 competitive examinations were held for residencies, and in 1884 training for nurses was added.

Blockley had been established originally as an almshouse in 1732, the first place in Philadelphia that not only served the poor, but also the insane, and, in addition, provided a lying-in hospital and a foundling hospital for infants. By 1828 it had outgrown its quarters and moved west across the Schuylkill River to the village of Blockley. The name was changed to Philadelphia Hospital in 1835, but "Blockley" or "Old Blockley" remained its popular designation. In 1902 the name was changed again to Philadelphia General Hospital. In 1920 the almshouse component was eliminated when the oc-

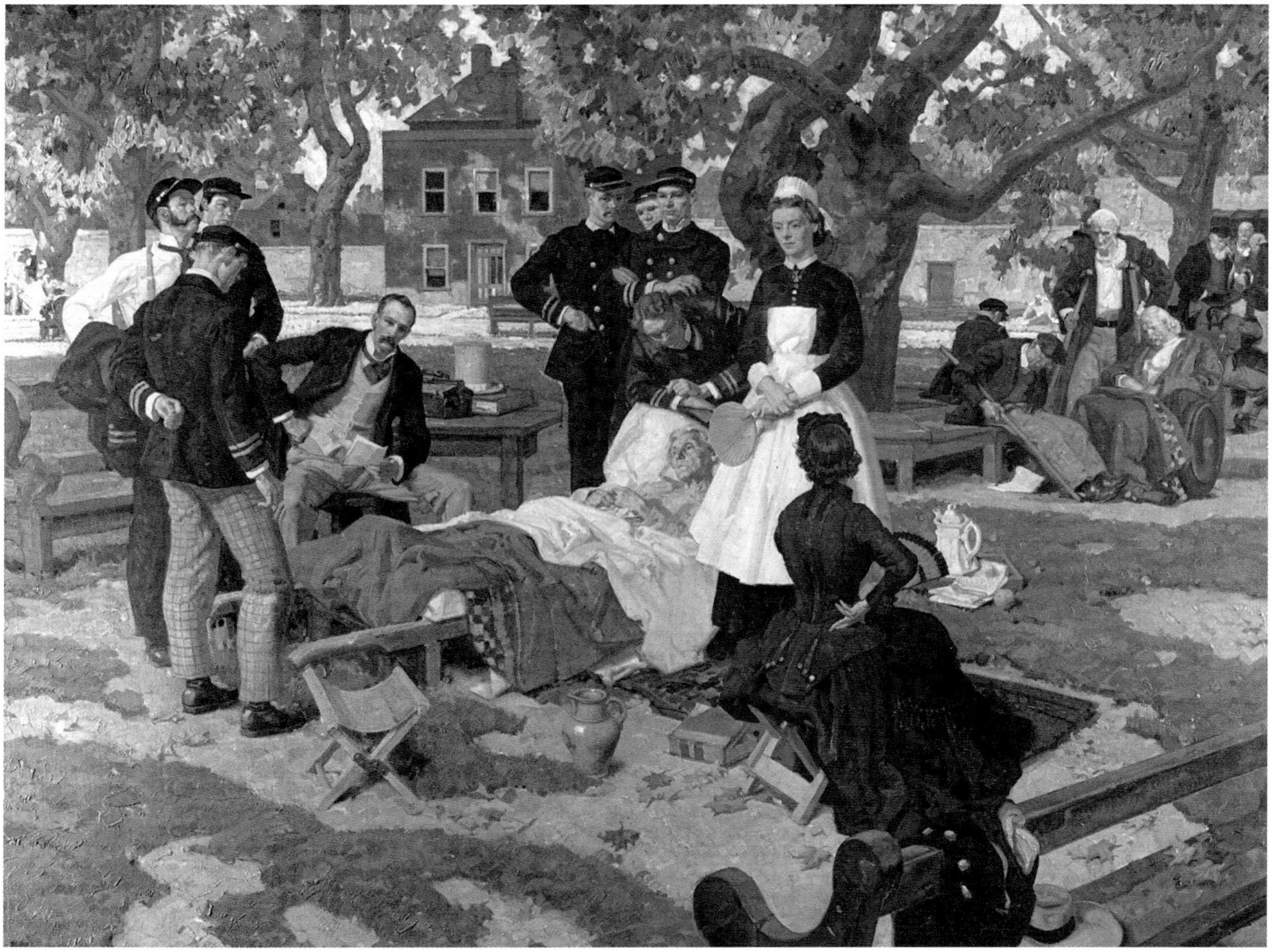

cupants were transferred to the Home for the Indigent, and in 1926 the mentally disturbed patients were transferred to the Philadelphia State Hospital at Byberry.

When Dr. William Osler left McGill University to become professor of clinical medicine at the University of Pennsylvania in 1884 he declared that "not the least of the reasons for his coming was the promise of a position on the Blockley staff."[27]

Born in 1849 in Bond Head, Ontario, Canada, Dr. William Osler was a renowned clinician, scientist, teacher, medical historian, and bibliophile. He graduated from Trinity College, Toronto (1868) and received his M.D. degree from McGill University, Montreal (1872) where his lifelong interest in pathological anatomy was born. After two years abroad studying in London, Berlin, and Vienna, he returned to McGill as lecturer and then professor of the institutes of medicine. While at McGill Osler began to perfect his teaching methods: having students perform autopsies and keep records in great detail, followed by the systematic demonstration of lesions in the clinic.

At age twenty-five Osler described the blood platelets and their relation to coagulation. Among other contributions, Osler was the first to emphasize the relationship between mycotic aneurism and mycotic endocarditis, and to describe the ball-valve thrombus at the mitral orifice, and was among the first to describe amoebae as the cause of dysentery.

In 1884 he accepted a professorship at the University of Pennsylvania, and he remained in Philadelphia for five years. He continued his bedside teaching methods in the university hospital wards in the mornings, followed by afternoons at Blockley where he demonstrated the results of postmortem examinations.[28] In 1887 Osler was appointed attending physician at the new Philadelphia Orthopaedic Hospital and Infirmary for Nervous Diseases.

In 1889 Osler left Philadelphia to undertake the organization of the medical service at the Johns Hopkins Hospital in Baltimore, and he occupied the chair of medicine in the new medical school when it opened in 1893. Osler's insistence on clinical instruction, particularly bedside teaching, was to have lasting influence, as was his insistence on precise laboratory methods and exact science in clinical medicine.

He moved to England in 1905 when he was called to Christ Church at Oxford University for the Regius Professorship of Medicine, and in 1911 he was created baronet by King Edward VII. Sir William Osler became a fellow of the Royal College of Physicians, and served as president of the Classical Association at Oxford and of the Bibliographical Society of London. Not only was Osler a prolific writer on medicine, but his monograph *Incunabula Medica: A Study of the Earliest Printed Medical Books, 1467-1480* was published posthumously (1923), as was an annotated catalogue of his own rich library of books illustrating the history of medicine and science, *Bibliotheca Osleriana* (1969).

While in Philadelphia Osler became the social and professional friend of many Jefferson faculty members, and some of these friendships continued throughout his life. An address that Osler was unable to deliver in September 1914 was published in the October *Jeffersonian*, and in it he warmly praised "old Jeff men" he had known: Drs. Robley Dunglison, Samuel D. Gross, Samuel H. Dickson, and John K. Mitchell. He credited his appointment at the University of Pennsylvania to the "good offices" of the editorial committee of the *Medical News*, especially Dr. Samuel W. Gross, as well as Drs. I. Minis Hays and Theophilus Parvin.

Osler's letter continued,

> No small measure of the happiness of the five happy years I spent in this city came from my association with Jefferson men. Among the surgeons, Keen and Samuel W. Gross became intimate friends. They, with Brinton, Mears and Hearn, maintained the splendid surgical traditions of the school. With the seniors in medicine, Bartholow and DaCosta, I never got on quite so intimate terms, but they were always encouraging and friendly. The younger Jefferson set became my fast friends, particularly Wilson and Hare.

Dr. Hobart A. Hare was on the committee that offered Osler the position of chairman of the practice of medicine at Jefferson Medical College. Although Osler declined the offer in favor of Johns Hopkins Hospital, he recommended his friend Dr. James C. Wilson who promptly accepted in 1891. It was Osler who recommended Dr. Thomas McCrae to succeed Wilson in 1911.[29]

Osler had also been a frequent guest at the home of Dr. and Mrs. Samuel W. Gross. He was one of four physicians who attended Gross during his last illness in 1889, and who promised Gross on his deathbed to take care of his wife, the former Grace Linzee Revere of Boston. Three years later she married Dr. Osler.

Osler's achievements were so well recognized that when Wyeth Laboratories commissioned illustrator Dean Cornwell to paint a series of six oil paintings on the subject "Pioneers of American Medicine," *Osler at Old Blockley* was the second picture to be completed. The series was executed between 1939 and 1945, and pictures of other medical heroes included: *The Dawn of Abdominal Surgery* (Dr. Ephraim McDowell), *The Father of American Pharmacy* (William Proctor Jr.), *That Mothers Might Live* (Dr. Oliver Wendell Holmes), *Conquerors of Yellow Fever* (Dr. Carlos Finlay), and *Beaumont and St. Martin* (Dr. William Beaumont). Reproductions of the entire series were widely circulated by Wyeth Laboratories.

Osler at Old Blockley shows the physician sitting on the hospital grounds and discussing the condition of a patient with a group of interns or residents who, along with a nurse holding a fan and a fashionably dressed woman visitor, surround the patient. The unresponsive, elderly, female patient lies on a cot covered with a red blanket. To the right of the main characters are other patient groups resting in the sun-dappled, park-like setting.

The old brick Post House where Osler led students through autopsies can be seen between the foliage of buttonwood trees in the background. For authentic period touches, Cornwell has included wooden park benches, canvas folding chairs, ceramic pitchers, and a table behind Dr. Osler with a medical bag, a book, and his hat. The interns' blue uniforms with brass buttons and braid and their caps with stiff visors were patterned after those of a surgeon in the U.S. Navy.[30]

In 1931 the old Post House was saved and designated the Osler Memorial Building in tribute to the celebrated physician, when the autopsy and pathological departments were installed elsewhere.[31] The dedication of the restored building and the installation of Cornwell's painting in Osler's old autopsy room took place on June 8, 1940.

One former resident who spoke at the dedication recalled that Osler was worshipped for his "great personal charm...wide learning and deep scholarship, a most persuasive teacher and a most convincing leader." Another said that students wanting to attend his autopsies were "so numerous that the overflow had to look down through the open ceiling from the room above."

Dean Cornwell spoke about his preparatory research for the painting. After reading numerous biographies and essays and studying photographs of Dr. Osler, he visited Old Blockley on a late summer day. There he composed the picture in his mind's eye and soon devised means to create the proper ambiance:

> Osler, leaving his ward rounds, accompanied by his uniformed students—stopping at the bedside of an old lady for a chat, and characteristically he reads a letter from the old patient's son, handed him by a charitable woman visitor. He offers words of hope to the patient followed by some philosophical observations for the benefit of his students, and then they are off to the "Post House" for an afternoon's work...
>
> I purchased costumes of the period from a variety of sources and a "want ad" in the New York Times brought an authoritative physician's bag of Osler's time. The internes were modeled by Cornell Medical School students, but the other figures were professional models...I built the patient's bed with my own hands, which, along with the canvas stool was authenticated by photographs taken by Brady during the Civil War. In gathering technical material an artist must always use objects which date well before the time of his picture. The grey pitcher in the foreground is the property of "Old Blockley."

Cornwell also responded to a group of ex-residents who questioned the picture's historical correctness by describing his artistic prerogatives (and perhaps those of his corporate sponsor):

> An artist does not pretend to make an exact photographic presentation of a scene, but rather to suggest the topic...[It is] better to depict a pleasant setting than...to show Osler working over a cadaver. The warm red blanket afforded contrast of color...as did the light and shade under the trees, and the well dressed lady visitor helped relieve the drab monotony of the hospital garb, and added a touch of what one might have hoped for, rather than what one actually saw at the old institution.

It is interesting to contrast this artist's view with the hard-hitting realism of Eakins in *The Gross Clinic*.

Osler at Old Blockley was moved at a later date to the main lobby of Philadelphia General Hospital. When "PGH" was closed and cleared away for urban renewal in 1976, Wyeth Laboratories agreed to place the painting on long-term loan at Thomas Jefferson University the following year.

Key factors in the decision to relocate the painting at Jefferson were the warm relationships between Osler and Jefferson faculty members; the fact that Lady Osler had established the Grace Revere Osler Professorship of Surgery at Jefferson Medical College in memory of her first husband, Dr. Samuel W. Gross; and that the impressive painting would be a welcome addition to Jefferson's already significant art collection.

Noted mural painter and illustrator, Dean Cornwell, was born in 1892 in Louisville, Kentucky. He studied at the Art Institute of Chicago and began his career with *The Chicago Tribune* drawing maps of World War I battlefields. Soon after he was making illustrations for books and leading magazines. Typically he made assiduous preparations for depicting geographical locales and historical periods. While at the height of his career as an illustrator in the mid-1920s he apprenticed himself to the English muralist Frank Brangwyn (q.v.), and soon thereafter looked upon mural painting as his true vocation.

Among Cornwell's best-known murals are those for the General Motors Building at the New York World's Fair of 1939, a forty-foot-square history of California for the Los Angeles Public Library, a history of transportation for the Eastern Airlines office at Rockefeller Center, and the history of Tennessee for the new State Building in Nashville. Abroad he executed murals for the International Labor Office in Geneva, and for the Battle Monument at the American Cemetery in Neuville-en-Condroz, Belgium. He assisted Brangwyn in a series of murals in the King's Robing Room at the House of Lords in London.

Dean Cornwell was awarded prizes by the Wilmington Society of Fine Arts, the Art Institute of Chicago, the Allied Artists of America, and the Architectural League of New York. He was a president of the National Society of Mural Painters and the Society of Illustrators, and a trustee of the American Academy in Rome. He was a fellow of the Royal Society of Arts, and an academician of the National Academy of Design.

Portrait of Ephraim McDowell

EPHRAIM McDOWELL, M.D. (1771-1830)
By F. Ziegler
(active mid-nineteenth century)

Bronze medal
1909
2 7/8 in. diameter

Signed lower left, obverse and reverse: "F. ZIEGLER"
Inscription obverse: "TO COMMEMORATE THE FIRST OVARIOTOMY/EPHRAIM M^c^DOWELL/1809-1909"
Inscription reverse: "THE AMERICAN GYNECOLOGICAL SOCIETY/1876"

Given after 1909 by Anna E. Biswanger
Accession number: 1909+f.M.01

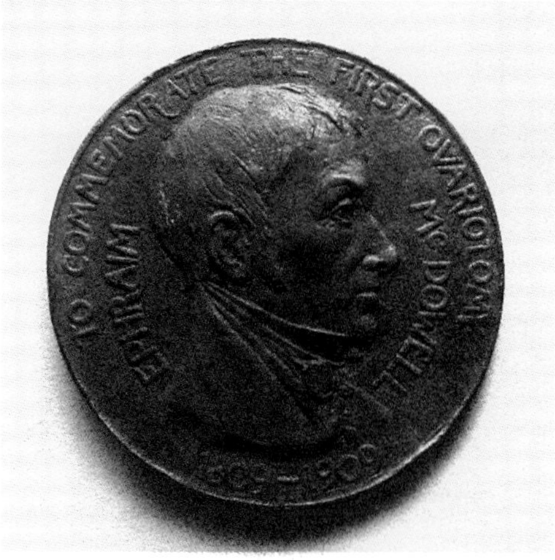

The Jefferson archives contain a bronze medal of Dr. Ephraim McDowell, known as the "Father of Ovariotomy."

Ephraim McDowell was born in Rockbridge County, Virginia in 1771, and moved with his family to Danville, Kentucky. He studied medicine with a physician in Staunton, Virginia and went abroad to attend lectures at the University of Edinburgh in 1793-94 and to study privately with John Bell, the famous Scottish surgeon. McDowell did not receive a medical degree until an honorary M.D. was conferred upon him by the University of Maryland.

McDowell returned to practice surgery in Danville, a small village on the western outpost. Within a few years he became known as the best surgeon throughout the southern and western states, and performed virtually every operation then practiced.

In 1809 he was called to see a patient afflicted with a rapidly growing ovarian tumor. When he decided that the only hope for relief was the excision of the diseased mass and explained the nature and hazards of the experimental operation, the courageous patient opted for the procedure. The operation was successful and the patient lived thirty-one more years. McDowell did not publish the case until October 1816 in the *Eclectic Repertory and Analytical Review*, after he had repeated the operation twice more. His feat of performing an untried procedure without anesthesia is all the more remarkable considering his isolated circumstances: he had no colleagues to consult and was nearly one thousand miles from the nearest hospital or dissecting room.

The bronze medal by F. Ziegler was issued on the centenary of McDowell's first ovariotomy by the American Gynecological Society. The obverse shows a head-and-neck profile of Ephraim McDowell facing to the right. The reverse has a design based on the seal of the society: a circle formed by a serpent with its tail in its mouth surrounding a seated figure of Juno Lucina (protectress of birth) with a baby in the crook of her arm.

1. "Bar Meeting," *The Legal Intelligencer*, Oct. 23, 1896, 423-24.
2. "The History of the Jefferson Cap," *Nurses Alumni Association Bulletin* (Thomas Jefferson University), Fall 1991, 52.
3. Clara Melville, R.N., *History of the School of Nursing of the Jefferson Medical College Hospital* (booklet printed for the college, 1937), 3-4.
4. Andrew W. Shearer, *A Commitment to Excellence: A History of the School of Nursing, College of Allied Health Sciences, Thomas Jefferson University, 1891-1982* (Wynnewood, Pa.: Heden-Livingston, 1982), 6-13.
5. James C. Wilson, M.D., "Memoir of J. M. DaCosta, M.D., LL.D.," read before the College of Physicians of Philadelphia, Nov. 5, 1902, and reprinted in *The Jeffersonian* 8 (Dec. 1906): 40.
6. Lloyd Goodrich, *Thomas Eakins*, 2 vols. (Cambridge, Mass.: Harvard University Press for the National Gallery of Art, Washington, D.C., 1982), 2:81-82.
7. William Williams Keen, M.D., *Memoirs*, ed. W. W. Keen James (Doylestown, Pa.: privately printed, 1990), 34.
8. From an unidentified newspaper clipping about the portrait presentation in the Jefferson archives.
9. Keen, "The Graduation Ceremony," *Selected Papers and Addresses* (Philadelphia: George W. Jacobs & Co., 1923), 13-17; and Keen, *Memoirs*, 228-29.
10. Goodrich, 2:8, 220-22.
11. James L. Stone, M.D., "W. W. Keen: America's Pioneer Neurological Surgeon," *Neurosurgery* 17 (1985): 1001.
12. Stone, 1003-05.
13. For Keen's military experiences, see *Memoirs* and Keen, "Surgical Reminiscences of the Civil War," *Addresses and Other Papers* (Philadelphia: W. B. Saunders & Co., 1905), 420-41.
14. James W. Holland, M.D., "Memoir of Roberts Bartholow, M.D.," *The Jeffersonian* 6 (Jan. 1905): 96-103.
15. See Eric C. Levin, "The Solis-Cohens: Philadelphia's Grandees," *Philadelphia Inquirer*, Sept. 12, 1976, *Today* magazine section, 18-20.
16. Julie S. Berkowitz, *The College of Physicians Portrait Catalogue* (Philadelphia: The College of Physicians, 1984), 198.
17. George Biddle, *Adolphe Borie* (Washington: American Federation of Arts, 1937), 4.
18. Barbara N. Parker, "The Dean's Roll-call by Eakins," *Bulletin of the Museum of Fine Arts Boston* 41 (Dec. 1943): 60.
19. Letter in Charles Bregler's Thomas Eakins Collection, Archives, Pennsylvania Academy of the Fine Arts.
20. I am grateful to Maryanne Quinn, chair of the language department at The Haverford School (Haverford, Pa.) for the following translation: "William S. Forbes, M.D., who proposed to the legislature of the state of Pennsylvania the new law concerning anatomy, by his studious defense initiated [it] and saw to [its] enactment by decree of the senate."
21. Many of the personal details of Forbes's life were recounted by his great-grandson, William Innes Forbes III, M.D., Ph.D., in "William Smith Forbes, M.D. 1831-1905," an unpublished paper written in 1969. Dr. William I. Forbes III received his Ph.D. from Jefferson in 1972 and his M.D. in 1973.
22. Frederick P. Henry, M.D., "Memoir of Dr. William S. Forbes," read before the College of Physicians of Philadelphia, Jan. 2, 1907, and printed in *Transactions of the College of Physicians of Philadelphia*, 1907, 9.
23. "William Smith Forbes, M.D.," an obituary in *The Jeffersonian* 7 (Jan. 1906): 88.
24. William S. Forbes, M.D., *History of the Anatomy-Act of Pennsylvania* (Philadelphia: The Philadelphia Medical Publishing Co., 1898), 8-9.
25. Horace Montgomery, Ph.D., "A Body Snatcher Sponsors Pennsylvania's Anatomy Act," *Journal of the History of Medicine* 21 (Oct. 1966): 374-93.
26. In 1878 Forbes read a paper to the College of Physicians of Philadelphia on the tricentennial of the birth of William Harvey: "Harvey and the Transit of the Blood from the Arteries to the Veins 'per Porositates.'"
27. John Francis Marion, *Philadelphia Medica: Being a Guide to the City's Historical Places of Health Interest* (Philadelphia: SmithKline Corp., 1975), 85.
28. Address by W. G. MacCallum, M.D., "Osler at Blockley," at ceremonies, "Dedication of the Osler Memorial Building of the Philadelphia General Hospital, 'Old Blockley,' June 8, 1940," *Bulletin of the History of Medicine* 10 (June 1941): 78.
29. Details about Sir William Osler's connections with Jefferson Medical College faculty come from Frederick B. Wagner Jr., M.D., "Department of Retrospection: The Jefferson Medical College Connection: A Letter from Sir William Osler," *Transactions & Studies of the College of Physicians of Philadelphia* 8 (1986): 277-82; and Wagner, *Thomas Jefferson University*, 243-46.
30. Marion, 85.
31. Descriptions of Osler and the Post House are found throughout the addresses in "Dedication of the Osler Memorial Building of the Philadelphia General Hospital," 57-104.

CHAPTER 6

The Turn of the Century: Expansion of the Medical School and Hospital

The Jefferson Medical College reforms of 1895, including the change from a proprietary to a nonprofit-sharing corporation and an expansion of the curriculum to a four-year course, contributed to the need for new buildings. Up-to-date college and laboratory structures were required to provide an increased number of students with facilities in keeping with the advancements in science.

The college assembled a large property on the northwest corner of Tenth and Walnut Streets after a decision not to relocate at Broad and Christian Streets in South Philadelphia. The new Medical Hall was opened in 1898. Also, by the turn of the century the 1877 hospital was too antiquated to meet the escalating demand for patient beds and dispensary facilities. A new hospital that opened in 1907 at Tenth and Sansom Streets later became known as "Old Main." Still in use today, "Main" is an integral part of Jefferson's hospital facilities.

New Medical Hall and Laboratory Building of Jefferson Medical College

NEW MEDICAL HALL AND LABORATORY BUILDING
By James Hamilton Windrim (1840-1919)

Ink over graphite pencil on artist's board
Ca. 1896
Image size: 15 x 22 3/8 in.
Sheet size: 18 1/4 x 25 1/4 in.

Signed lower left: "Jas. H. Windrim/Architect/1107 Walnut St. Phila."
Inscription on the cornice: "1825 JEFFERSON MEDICAL COLLEGE 1898"

Drawing prepared for Jefferson Medical College
Accession number: 1896+c.D.01

James H. Windrim, who had completed the Ely Building renovations in 1881, was selected to design Jefferson's new Medical Hall and Laboratory. Preserved in the Jefferson archives are architectural renderings in ink and another in graphite and crayon by the James H. Windrim firm.

Medical Hall fronted on Walnut Street, and its side joined the Laboratory Building on Tenth Street. A large light well was placed between the two fireproof buildings. Medical Hall was built in Baroque Revival style, with a gray granite basement and a superstructure of gray brick with terra cotta trim. Interestingly, an inscription on the top cornice of the facade, "1825 JEFFERSON MEDICAL COLLEGE 1898," reflected an inaccurate view of the founding date which was later determined to be 1824.

The Walnut Street facade was divided horizontally into three sections by a molded string course between the second and third floors, and an ornamental main cornice between the fifth story and the attic sixth story. It was also divided into three parts vertically corresponding to the arrangement of rooms within. The lateral sections flank a classic portico with its entrance surrounded by columns and topped with a split, arched pediment. The porch is surmounted by five tiers of triple windows and balconies. Each floor of the lateral zones is defined by diverse styles of windows, balconies, and trims including quoins and keystones.

The basement of Medical Hall was occupied by rooms that serviced the recess hours of students, including a gymnasium with lockers and showers, and rooms for billiards, reading, and smoking, and for storage of bicycles. The first floor contained a reception room for visitors and a ladies' waiting room, a clerk's room with the telephone communication center, the dean's office and trustees room, the library, and a kitchen and pantry. It also held the first story of the lower semi-amphitheater, recitation rooms, professors' offices, and a laboratory for pharmacy, materia medica, and experimental therapeutics.

On the second floor were the second story of the amphitheater, laboratories for the study of morbid anatomy and of medical chemistry and toxicology, professors' rooms, and a museum. The museum housed the collections of Professors Samuel D. Gross, M.D. and Jacob M. DaCosta, M.D., in addition to other assorted models, preparations, and specimens.

The third floor was occupied by a large lecture hall connecting with a chemical apparatus room, a smaller lecture hall, and the physiology apparatus room and laboratory. The fourth floor contained the upper part of the two lecture halls on the floor below, a laboratory for normal histology, and a laboratory for obstetrics and bandaging. The fifth floor contained the first story of the upper semi-amphitheater, dissecting rooms, laboratories for surgery and morbid histology, and professors' offices. On the sixth floor were the second story of the upper amphitheater and dissecting rooms, a chart room, and a bacteriology laboratory.

There was a commodious stairway in the center of the building and an inside fire escape and smoke-proof tower extending from the sixth floor to the entrance.

There was a large light well between Medical Hall and the Laboratory Building. The latter contained rooms for recitation, offices, student societies, private and experimental research, and storage; and laboratories devoted to pharmacy, toxicology, histology, and bacteriology. Student laboratories were well lighted by windows on three sides and incandescent electric light; equipment included 150 microscopes and a complete outfit for electric lantern projection and photography.

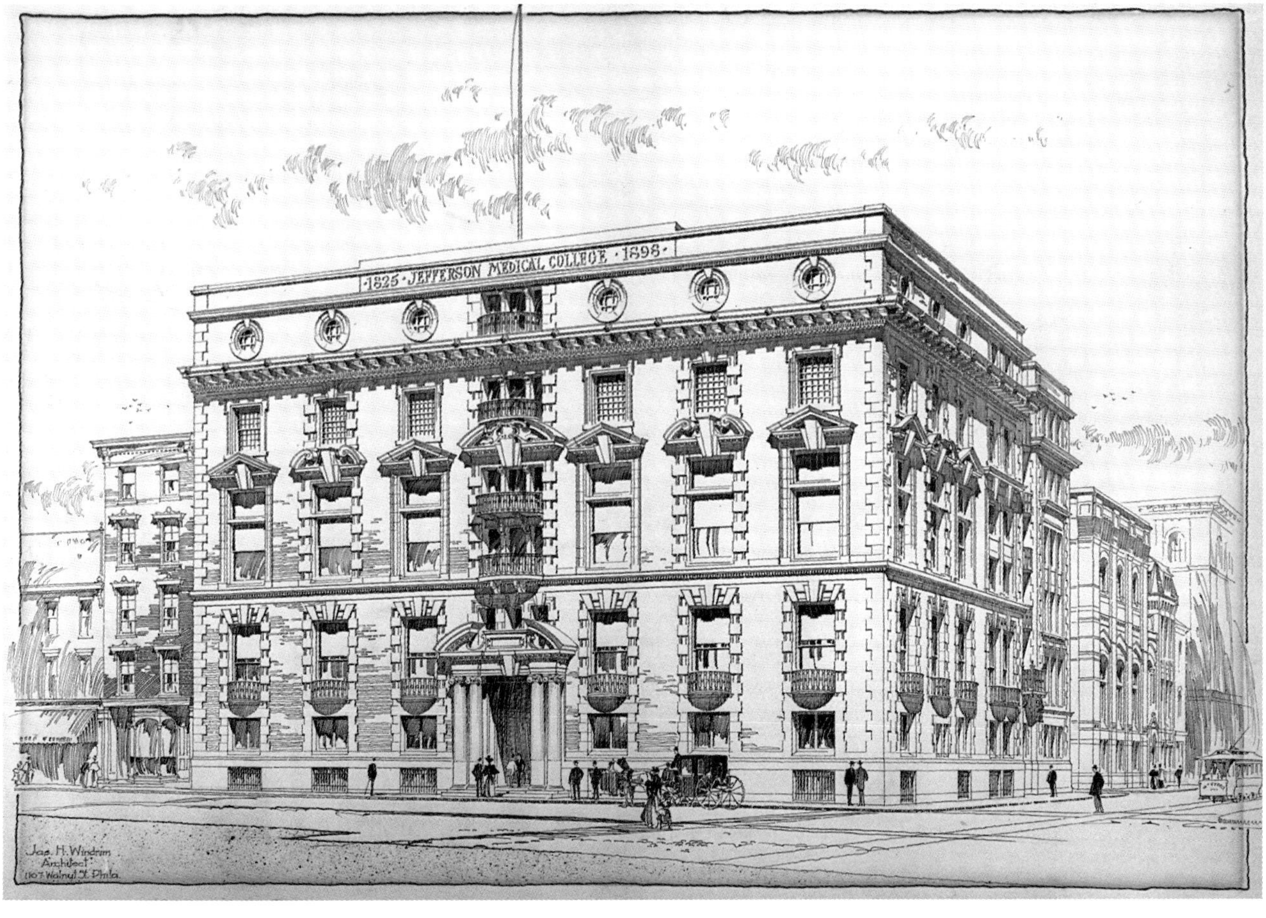

Portrait of Thomas Jefferson

THOMAS JEFFERSON (1743-1826)
By unknown artist

Cast stone
Ca. 1898
23 1/4 x 19 x 5 in.

Made for facade of Medical Hall
Accession number: 1898+c.S.01

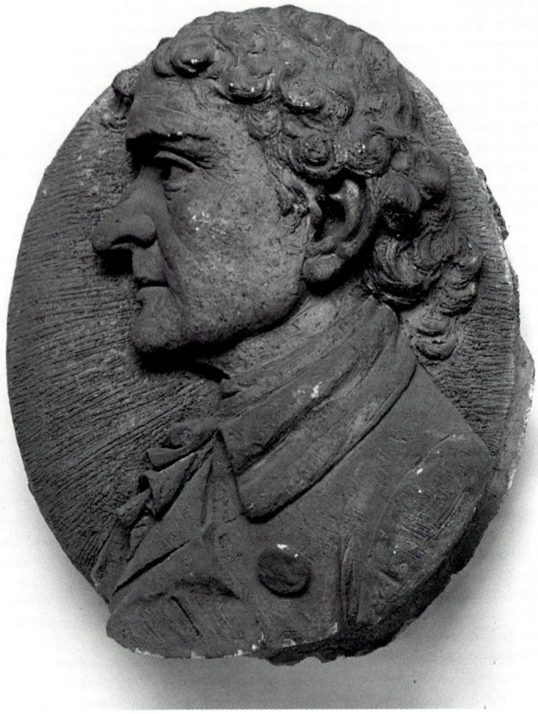

When the 1898 Medical Hall was demolished and replaced in 1931 by the current Curtis Building, a large, cast stone bust of Thomas Jefferson from the building's facade was salvaged, but then long forgotten. Recently it was discovered serendipitously in a wooden crate in a deep storage area on the Jefferson campus, while I was searching for another artifact.

The image of Thomas Jefferson is not included in the early architectural rendering of Medical Hall above, but is visible in a contemporary photograph of the building taken by Edgar N. Fought, M.D., an alumnus of 1905. The larger than life-sized profile bust of Jefferson was placed in the curved pediment of the fourth-floor window in the central bay of the facade. The photograph shows other minor changes after the rendering was made.

Because the oval plaque containing the roughly carved bust was so high off the ground, the subject's features are exaggerated for visibility to passersby from the pavement below: deepset eyes and overhanging brow, long and bulbous nose, jutting chin, and extra large ears. Equally overstated is the thick, flowing, curly hair nestling into the collars of his coat and jabot.

Vestibule of Medical Hall

VESTIBULE OF MEDICAL HALL
By Bond Brothers (active early twentieth century)

Vintage photograph
1920-28
8 x 10 in.

Made for Jefferson Medical College
Accession number: 1920+f.Ph.02

The focal point of the ornate vestibule entrance of the new Medical Hall was a cast stone rondel with a profile bust of Thomas Jefferson, another sculptural work that was salvaged when the building was razed. An inscription around the bust reads "JEFFERSON MEDICAL COLLEGE OF PHILADELPHIA FOUNDED 1826" (another incorrect date).

This round Jefferson bust and the oval bust on the Medical Hall facade are both loosely based on the well known "medallion profile" of Thomas Jefferson painted from life in 1805 by Gilbert Stuart (Fogg Museum, Harvard University), which the sculptor could have known from numerous copies. Compared with the exterior bust, the surface of the interior portrait medallion is comparatively smoother, the carving shallower, and the subject's features less exaggerated. These differences exist because the interior bust was to be seen at closer range.

The vestibule bust is placed in the center of a large group of plaques over the doorway which has an inscription on the left, "ESTABLISHED 1825/THE COLLEGE SEAL/ADOPTED 1826," and on the right, "INDEPENDENT CHAR/TER WITH VNIVERSITY/POWERS

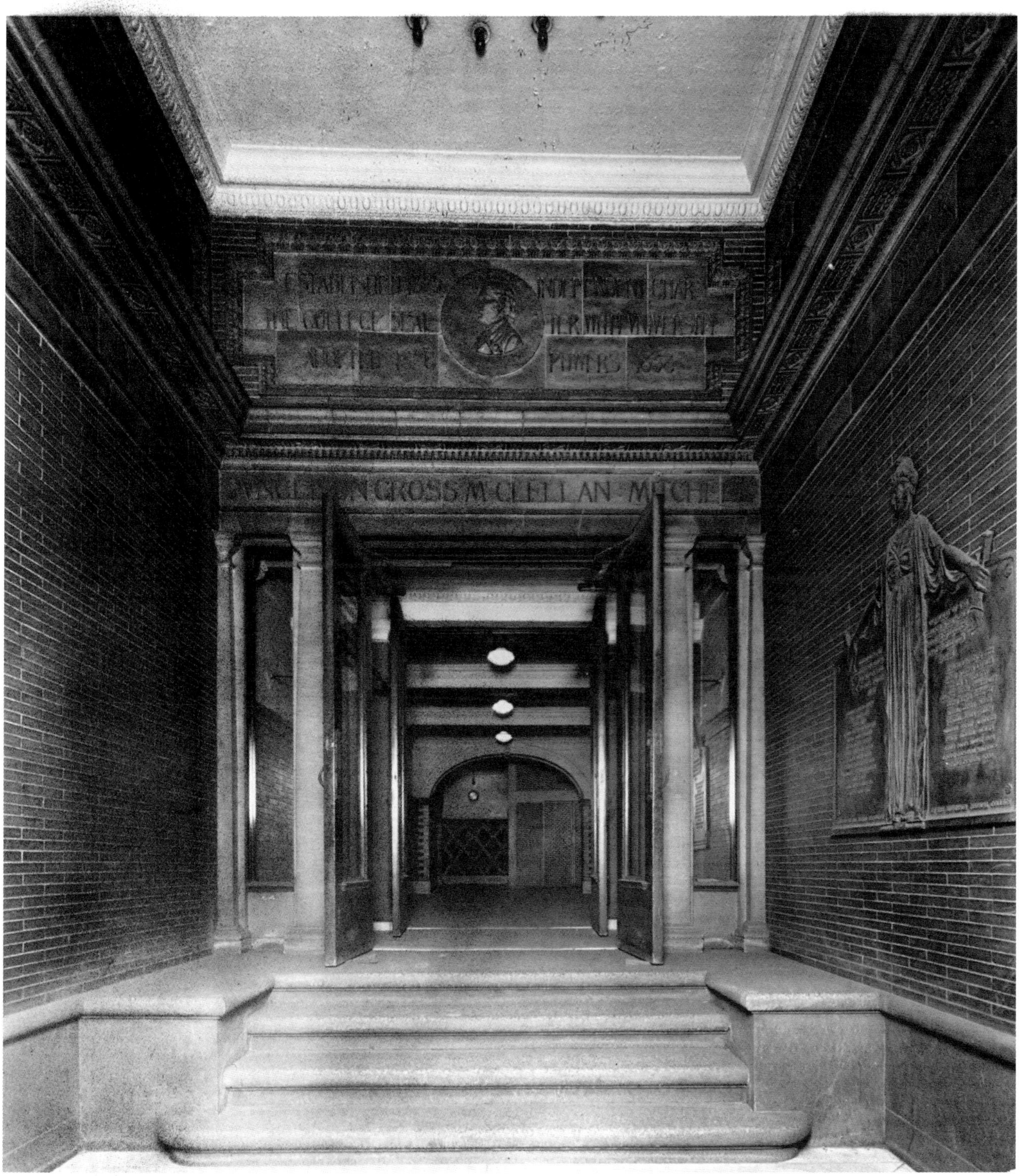

1838." Names of celebrated Jefferson faculty, "DVNGLISON GROSS McCLELLAN MITCHELL," are carved on the doorway lintel under the bust.

Names of other Jefferson luminaries continue on the right hand wall: "MEIGS SIMS DRAKE DICKSON." Above the professors' names is another large panel inscribed, "FIRST SVRGICAL CLINIC 1825/FIRST ANESTHETIC CLINIC IN PHILADELPHIA 1846/JEFFERSON COLLEGE HOSPITAL OPENED 1877."

Below is a large bronze plaque erected in memory of twenty-six college physicians who died during World War I. Seven were killed in ground action, two were lost at sea, and seventeen died in military camps or hospitals. More than one in four living Jefferson graduates served during World War I, and sixty-five percent of the graduates of the five years preceding 1918 served in the armed forces.[1]

The plaque is signed "DOYLE-PHILA" and dated 1920, and measures six feet high and wide. It features an allegorical female figure clad in classical garb rising above a rectangular panel. Her outstretched arms hold inverted torches. Flanking the standing figure are the names of the deceased. An inscription above the names reads, "DEDICATED TO THE GRADUATES OF THE/JEFFERSON MEDICAL COLLEGE IN THE WORLD/WAR WHO GAVE FULL MEASURE OF DEVOTION/TO THEIR COUNTRY THAT CIVILIZATION/MIGHT ENDURE." An inscription below reads, "ERECTED BY THE ALUMNI ASSOCIATION OF THE JEFFERSON MEDICAL COLLEGE."

Jefferson Medical College Student Navy Training Corps Unit

STUDENT NAVY TRAINING CORPS UNIT
By Bell & Fischer (active early twentieth century)

Vintage photograph mounted on board
1919
Image size: 6 3/4 x 16 in.
Board size: 9 1/2 x 19 1/4 in.

Signed lower left: "BELL & FISCHER/PHILA"
Inscription lower right: "JEFFERSON/MEDICAL COLLEGE/NAVAL UNIT/-1918-1919"

Made for Jefferson Medical College
Accession number: 1919+f.Ph.02

The Student Training Corps at Jefferson Medical College trained thirty-three men sworn into the navy and 398 inducted into the army. In addition, the college provided graduate refresher courses and board for army and navy medical officers.[2]

The photograph shows three rows of men in the Jefferson Student Navy Training Corps whose unit was mobilized in September 1918. Standing at attention on the steps of a building, the young men wear white caps, pea jackets, knickers, and spats. Their officer, dressed in a long coat, gloves, and a peaked hat, stands in the middle of the bottom row. The unit was demobilized in 1919 when the war came to a close.

In 1918 Jefferson was one of four Philadelphia hospitals that volunteered to staff base hospitals in France for the Armed Forces Medical Corps. The effort was orga-

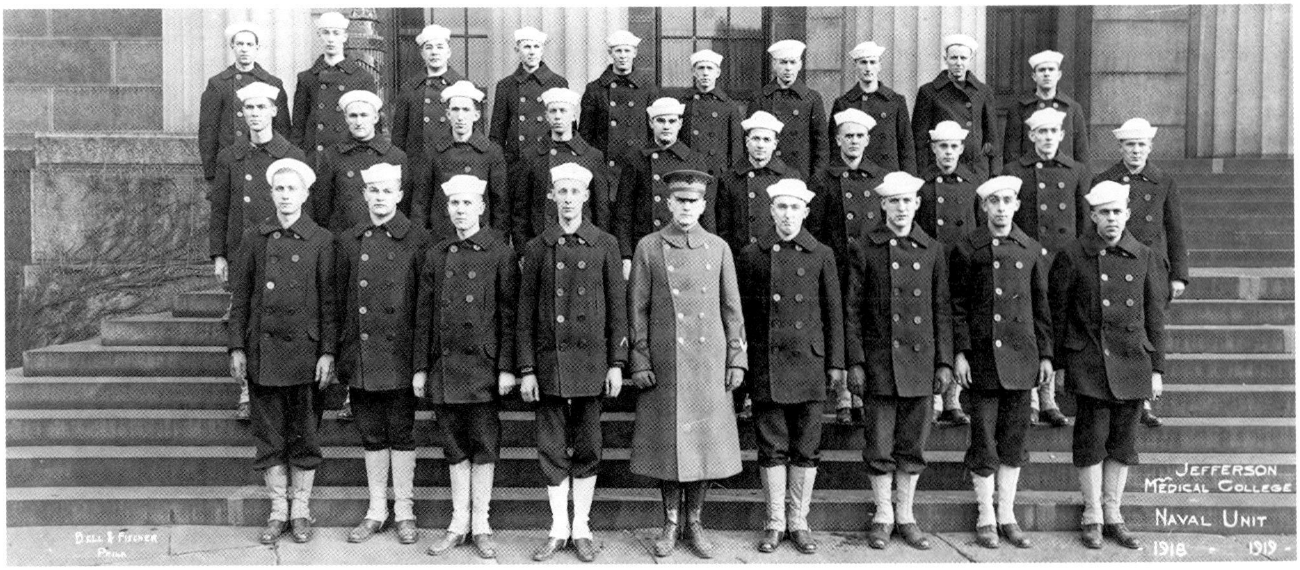

nized by the Red Cross to support the American Expeditionary Forces, and the objective was to assemble a cohesive staff that could function quickly and efficiently before mobilization abroad. Eight months of preliminary didactic and practical training for the volunteer personnel took place at Philadelphia's Second Army Regiment and at several area hospitals.

Jefferson Base Hospital Thirty-eight in Nantes, France had twenty-one wards for casualties, and was staffed by thirty-five officers, one hundred registered nurses, two hundred enlisted men, and several civilians. Hastily erected facilities also included kitchens, barracks, and mess halls for officers and nurses. Enlisted men lived in incomplete tarpaper buildings, and their equipment was in short supply. Nearly nine thousand patients were treated for infections, effects of gassing, fractures, gunshot wounds, gangrene, and communicable diseases.

Portrait of William M. L. Coplin

WILLIAM MICHAEL LATE COPLIN, M.D. (1864-1928)
By F. Davidson (active early twentieth century)

Pastel on paper
1906
23 1/2 x 19 1/2 in.

Signed and dated lower right: "F. Davidson 1906"

Given in 1967 by John K. Leister
Accession number: 1967+e.P.01

In 1896 Dr. William M. L. Coplin was named professor of pathology and bacteriology at Jefferson Medical College, and gave the first systematic courses in morbid histology, hygiene, bacteriology, and clinical microscopy. In May 1917 he was selected to be director and chief of the laboratory division of the U.S. Army Base Hospital Thirty-eight in Nantes.

Dr. Coplin proved to be an energetic organizer of the hospital and served until September 1918 when he was appointed director of the laboratory division of the Third Army with headquarters in Coblenz, Germany. At the time of his discharge in April 1919 he had risen to the rank of colonel and was cited for meritorious service.

A native of Clarksburg, West Virginia, Coplin was born in 1864 and graduated from Jefferson Medical College in 1886. During his senior year he did much of the pathological work on specimens from the practice of Dr. Samuel W. Gross. The next year he was appointed assistant pathologist to the Jefferson Hospital and became a member of the surgical and gynecological staffs. In 1892 he was made demonstrator of pathology at Jefferson and curator of the pathology museum, and was also appointed pathologist to the Philadelphia Hospital. Coplin's best-known literary works were produced in this period: *Textbook of Practical Hygiene* (1893) and *Lectures on Pathology* (1894-95).

In 1895 Coplin was called to Vanderbilt University as professor of pathology, and then returned to Jefferson as chair of pathology and bacteriology the following year to succeed Morris Longstreth, M.D. He was president of the hospital's medical staff from 1908 until 1912. He remained as pathology chair until his retirement in 1922. The following year he published a book about his military experiences in France.[3]

While he was director of the Department of Public Health and Charities for the City of Philadelphia, Coplin's committee exposed corruption and graft among administrators and wretched conditions endured by the city's poor and insane, and was responsible for instituting

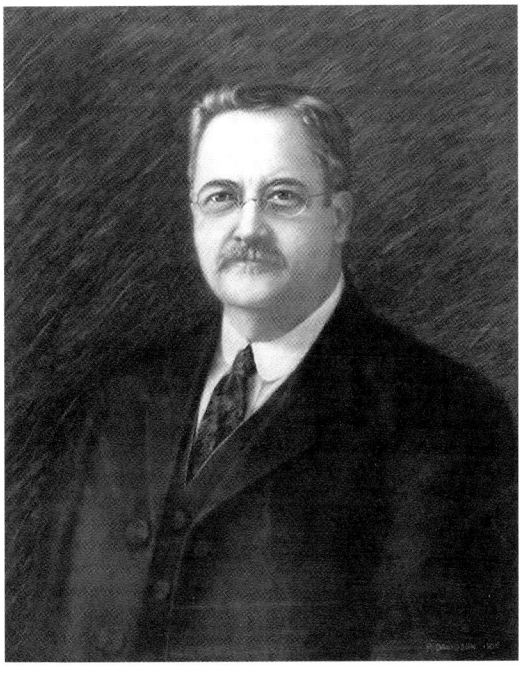

beneficial changes. He was also bacteriologist to the Pennsylvania State Board of Health and the Friends Asylum for the Insane.

In 1901 Jefferson students formed the Coplin Pathological Society in his honor. One of Coplin's chief interests was the organization and equipping of the pathology museum which was enlarged and relocated in 1914 to the top floor of the 1898 College Building. A type of grooved glass jar which allows slides to stand separated in a staining solution is named the "Coplin jar," and is still used today in histology and bacteriology laboratories.

A bust-length, pastel portrait shows Dr. Coplin at age forty-two. His amiable expression belies his reputation as a prodigiously talented and dedicated, but hard-driving and demanding teacher and researcher. The picture has the appearance of being copied from a photograph. There are no records about the artist, F. Davidson, who signed and dated the painting in 1906, or the donor, John K. Leister, who presented the portrait in 1967.

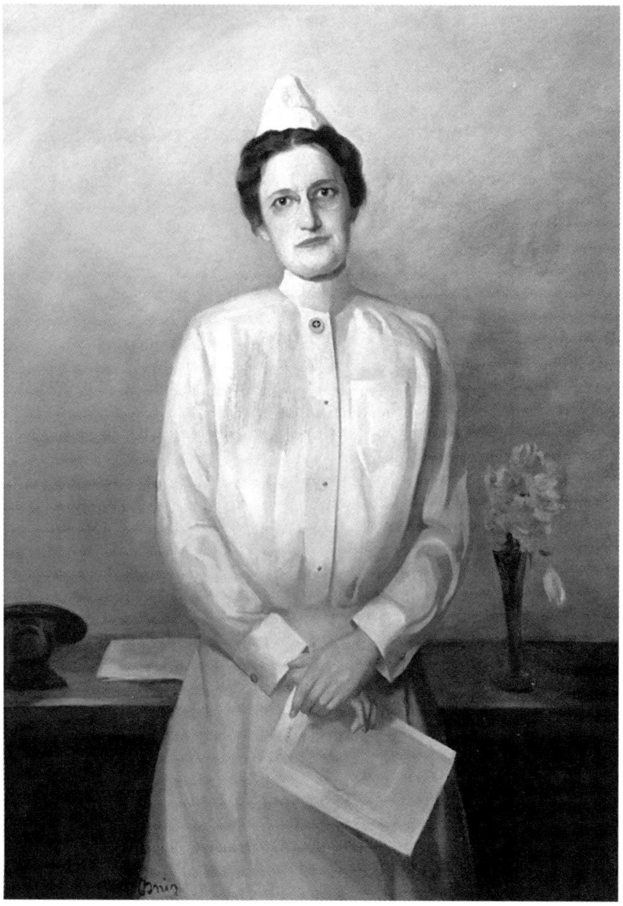

Portrait of Clara Melville

CLARA MELVILLE, R.N. (d. 1937)
By Benedict Anton Osnis (1872-1941)

Oil on canvas
1935
51 x 37 in.

Signed and dated lower left: "B. A. Osnis/1935"

Given in 1935 by the Jefferson nurses alumnae association
Accession number: 1935+e.P.01

Clara Melville, R.N. was directress of nurses at Jefferson Medical College Hospital Training School for Nurses from 1915 until her death in 1937. Dr. W. M. L. Coplin chose her as chief nurse for the Jefferson Base Hospital Thirty-eight in France.

Following her graduation from Jefferson's nursing school in 1910 Clara Melville was appointed supervisor of operating rooms of the Jefferson Hospital. She left briefly to become supervisor of the Trouro Infirmary in New Orleans, and returned in 1914 to become assistant directress of nurses and was appointed directress the following year. During her twenty-two-year term she was known for unselfish devotion and wise guidance, and was unsurpassed in meeting emergencies and responsibilities.

In 1917 Miss Melville volunteered to obtain one hundred trained nurses to supply Jefferson's base hospital, and Dr. Coplin's memoir recounted their heroic contributions.[4] The requisite number of nurses was mustered into service in March 1918 and sailed for France. The majority were detailed to advanced stations where more urgent needs existed, and some were even placed in mobile units which followed the troops on the front lines.

As the chief nurse Clara Melville was left with just seven assistants to organize nursing activities in a hospital which had begun with five hundred beds and later reached a daily census of more than twenty-four hundred. Their hospital was the first in the open field to receive patients and was woefully handicapped by inadequate supplies.

The temporary buildings were cold, dark, and surrounded by mud. There were between forty and one hundred patients under one nurse. Miss Melville's group coped with operations, epidemics, the arrival of hospital trains, the departure of convalescents, and the bringing of comfort to despondent patients. Finally, they were joined by a nursing unit from Chicago. Nurse Melville and her group returned home in March 1919 after the Armistice was signed.

Upon her return to Jefferson as directress of the Training School for Nurses, Clara Melville found that in the aftermath of the war the hospital required more beds, necessitating an increased number of staff nurses and nursing students. The indefatigable directress supervised the implementation of several initiatives including: new laboratories, demonstration areas, classroom space, and a library; new appointments of a full-time instructor of nurses, a nursing supervisor for the Samuel Gustine Thompson Annex (opened 1924), and a nurse superintendent for Ivycroft (a convalescent center for men); nurses-in-charge at the maternity department and the medical and surgical clinics; and a new residence for staff nurses.[5]

After Clara Melville's death from pneumonia in 1937 the nurses alumnae association established a scholarship in her memory. Two years earlier the association had commissioned her portrait in recognition of her devotion and contributions during her long tenure as directress. Her portrait hung in various nursing residences until its relocation to McClellan Hall in 1981.

In the three-quarters-length, life-sized depiction by Benedict Osnis, Melville stands in a frontal pose gazing sternly and directly toward the viewer. Her hands are crossed primly in front of her body and she holds a sheaf of papers. Placed on a table behind her are a telephone and papers, and as a softening element, a vase of pink roses. The portrait embodies the following description of her steely personality:

> Perhaps the most fabled figure in the lore of the School, she made an indelible impression on all who knew her. Stern of visage and brusque in manner, she ruled with an iron hand rarely veiled in velvet. Not one to mince words, she informed one hapless student that she didn't like redheads. Another was admonished to comb out her spit curls. Her charges soon learned to toe the line of piety because a fall from Miss Melville's grace could be disastrous. Nonetheless, Clara Melville's loyalty and devotion to the School were beyond question.[6]

Benedict A. Osnis was a Russian immigrant who arrived in Philadelphia as a teenager, and studied at the Pennsylvania Academy of the Fine Arts. His wife, Daisy, was also an Academy graduate, and they exhibited jointly at the Art Club of Philadelphia in 1936.

Benedict Osnis was noted for oil and charcoal portraits of society, military, religious, and political figures, such as Dennis Cardinal Dougherty, General Charles P. Summerall, and members of the prominent duPont, Montgomery, and Clothier families. Other notable portrait subjects included President Calvin Coolidge who granted him thirty sittings for a series of charcoal sketches, and General John J. Pershing for whom Osnis painted an oil portrait and several charcoal sketches.

Reading Room in Library of Medical Hall

READING ROOM IN LIBRARY OF MEDICAL HALL
By James Hamilton Windrim (1840-1919)

Vintage photograph
By unknown photographer
1929
8 x 10 in.

Given after 1929 by unknown donor
Accession number: 1929+f.Ph.11

The Jefferson archives is fortunate to have amassed many vintage photographs of the interior of the 1898 Medical Hall. Many rooms were decorated with oil portraits, sculpted portrait busts and other figures, and prints, drawings, and photographs. These pictures not only demonstrate how the art was displayed, but provide a *terminus ante quem* for undocumented works entering the collection.

A typical photograph is a 1929 view of the library's large reading room which served as an unofficial gallery, just as Dr. Samuel D. Gross had envisioned in his speech to the alumni association in 1871. The 1929 Jefferson Medical College yearbook described the room as "a corner of the old library. On all sides were busts and pictures of men famous in Jefferson and medical lore."

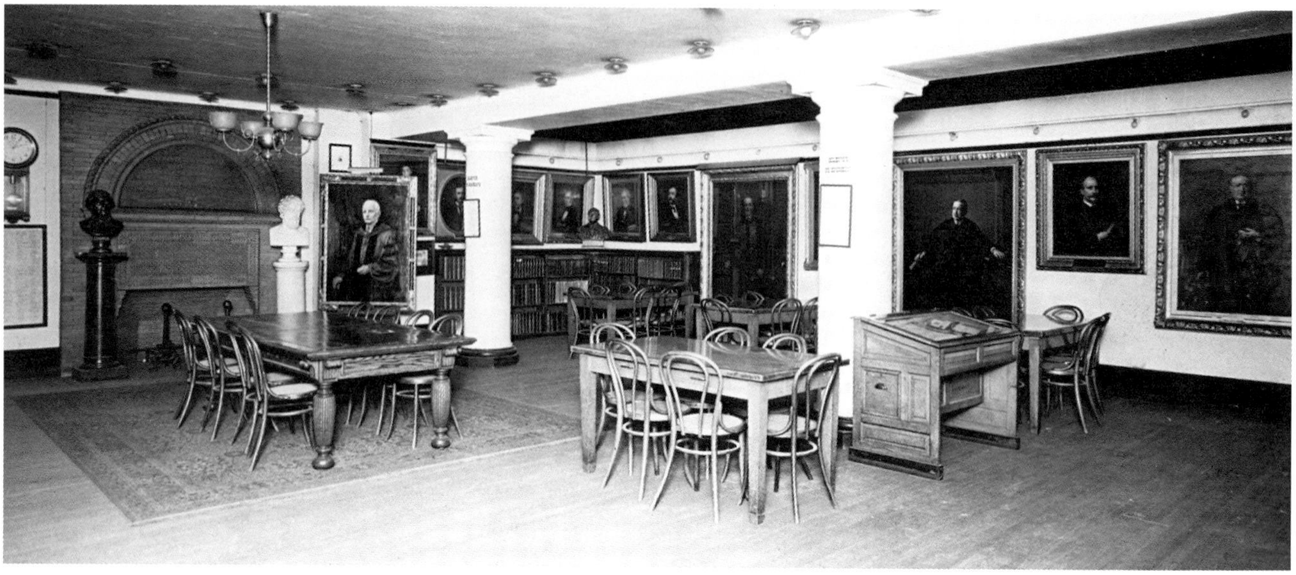

The two sculptures on pedestals flanking the fireplace are busts of Thomas Jefferson and William Harvey. On an easel in front of the fireplace is the most recent acquisition, a portrait of Dr. Hiram R. Loux, and immediately behind him is a painting of Dr. John Chalmers DaCosta.

Continuing from left to right on the back wall are portraits of Drs. Francis F. Maury, James A. Meigs, and Robert M. Huston. In the corner is a bust of Dr. James C. Wilson. On the side wall are oil portraits of Drs. Robley Dunglison, Joseph Pancoast, and William W. Keen. Partially hidden behind the pole is a painting of Dr. James W. Holland. The remaining portraits are of trustee William Potter, and Drs. William H. Pancoast and Jacob M. DaCosta.

Another vintage photograph shows a continuation of the portrait wall with depictions of Drs. Roberts Bartholow and Samuel D. Gross, and sculpted busts of Drs. J. Marion Sims, S. Weir Mitchell, and George McClellan. Additional objects are numerous framed works on paper which are too small to decipher, but presumably many are portraits.

Spinario (The Thorn Extractor)

SPINARIO
Replica of ancient Roman sculpture

Bronze
Second half of nineteenth century
27 5/8 x 19 1/4 x 24 1/2 in.

Inscriptions at bottom of stump and on rear of integral base: "TIFFANY & CO."
Inscription on rear of integral base: "NELLI [or NELLO] ROMA"

Given in 1899 by Jonathan Ackerman Coles, M.D. in memory of his father, Abraham Coles, M.D. (JMC 1835)
Accession number: 1899+e.S.02

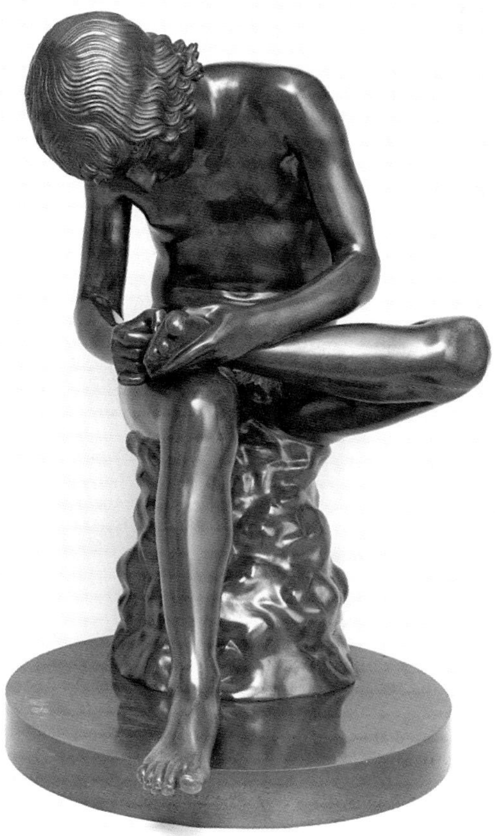

Photographic records show that another bronze sculpture, *Spinario (The Thorn Extractor)*, has always been placed in the library reading room in the 1898 Medical Hall, the 1929 College Building, and the Scott Memorial Library where it is regarded affectionately by students today.

The bronze statue of a nude young boy extracting a thorn from his foot is a replica of one of the most famous antique sculptures, *Spinario*. The original bronze work was first recorded in the mid-twelfth century in Rome where it stood outside the Lateran Palace. It was transferred to the Palazzo dei Conservatori (now the Capitoline Museum) by Pope Sixtus IV in 1471 where it has remained except for the years 1797 to 1816 when it was ceded to the French.

Spinario was one of the first antique sculptures to be copied in bronze and marble during the Renaissance period, and replicas of the popular work continued to be made in later centuries. Although it is disputed, many scholars think that the original is a pastiche dating from the late Republican or early Imperial Roman period, taken from an early Greek head and a later Greek body.[7]

The nude figure is seated on a tree stump, with his head tilted down. While he holds his foot with one hand, the other hand extracts a thorn from his sole. The carving is smooth and polished, except for the wavy, thick strands of shoulder-length hair.

Scholars' interpretations of the boy's identity have included: Absalom, the Old Testament male beauty; Priapus, the ancient fertility god; a victorious athlete in the Greek games; and Martius, a shepherd boy who bore a message to the Roman Senate with such conscientious dispatch that he stopped to remove a thorn from his foot only after his arrival.

Renaissance and Baroque copies of the popular antique statue proliferated in museums throughout Europe and the United States. One was displayed at the Philadelphia Centennial Exposition of 1876 in the Art Annex, among a group of archeological marbles owned by the Italian collector Alessandro Castellani.

It is likely that the Tiffany Company was responsible for the base of the Jefferson version and for manufacturing the sculpture, which was signed by Nello, or Nelli, of Rome.

Jefferson Medical College Dean James W. Holland, M.D. was very grateful for Dr. Jonathan Ackerman Coles's donation of *Spinario*, seeing in it a "striking fidelity to nature shown in the pose and clean form of the body."

Dr. Coles (1843-1925) was a native of Scotch Plains, New Jersey and earned his medical degree from Columbia University. After studying abroad he established a medical practice in New York, and then became a partner of his father in Newark.

The younger Dr. Coles was a noted collector of paintings, sculptures, rare books, manuscripts, letters, and autographs of famous authors. In addition to the *Spinario* his generous donations to Jefferson Medical College included a portrait relief sculpture of his father, sculpted busts of William Harvey and Thomas Jefferson, and an oil portrait once believed to be of William Harvey.

Dr. Coles also gave art works to other institutions including the New Jersey State House in Trenton; the Metropolitan Museum of Art; Columbia, Yale, Harvard, Oxford, and Cambridge Universities; and the American Embassy in London.

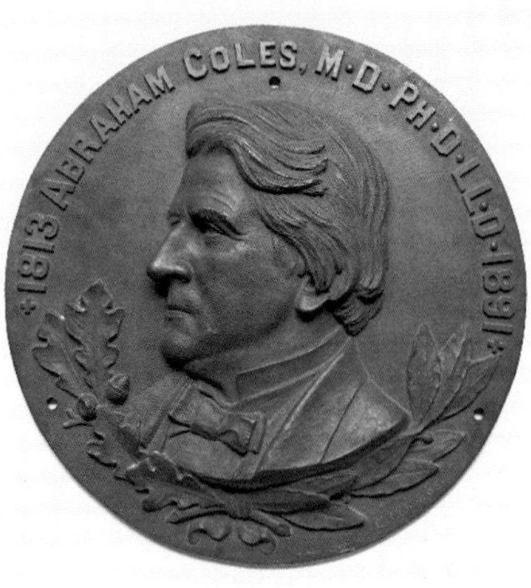

Portrait of Abraham Coles

ABRAHAM COLES, M.D. (1813-91)
By Carl H. Conrads (b. 1839)

Bronze
1891-98
19 3/4 x 19 3/4 x 2 1/4 in.

Inscription: "1813 ABRAHAM COLES, M.D. PH.D. LL.D. 1891"
Signed lower right: "C. Conrads."

Given in 1899 by J. Ackerman Coles, M.D., son of the subject
Accession number: 1899+e.S.03

When Dr. J. Ackerman Coles donated the *Spinario* in 1899 in memory of his father, Abraham Coles, M.D., he also gave a bronze relief portrait sculpture of the elder Dr. Coles. A contemporary photograph shows the medallion hanging on the wall above *Spinario* in the reading room of the 1898 Medical Hall.

Abraham Coles was born in Scotch Plains, New Jersey in 1813, a descendent of James Coles who landed at Plymouth, Massachusetts in 1630.[8] After a classical education at the Bond Academy in Plainfield, he began to study law but soon switched to medicine. He studied first at the College of Physicians and Surgeons of Columbia University and then took his degree at Jefferson Medical College in 1835. His medical and surgical practice in Newark was interrupted by two study trips to Paris in 1848 and 1854.

When elected president of the Medical Society of New Jersey, Dr. Coles wrote a long poem as his inaugural address: "The Microcosm," a compendium of science concerning the human body in verse. Coles was widely admired for the publication of eighteen different versions of the Latin hymn "Dies Irae," his translations of medieval Christian hymns and Hebrew psalms, and "The Evangel," a life of Christ in verse.

In addition to medical and literary work Coles was involved with educational, historical, and religious organizations in Newark. His diverse activities earned him honorary degrees: a Ph.D. from Lewisburg University (later Bucknell) and an LL.D. from Princeton University.

Dr. Coles possessed an exceptional library and collection of art works. The most outstanding were replicas of antique sculptures and works by eighteenth- and nineteenth-century European sculptors and American sculptors who studied in Rome. Coles hired an English landscape gardener to design seventeen acres of his ancestral farm at Scotch Plains, Deerhurst.

The bas-relief, bronze medallion of Dr. Abraham Coles was sculpted by Carl H. Conrads. The profile, head-and-shoulders figure is surrounded by a curved inscription above and oak and laurel leaves tied with a ribbon below. The subject's strong, angular features are crowned by thick, wavy hair.

Carl H. Conrads was born in 1839 and emigrated from his native Germany to New York in 1860. He served in the Union Army during the Civil War and resided in Hartford, Connecticut after 1866. He returned to Munich in 1871 to further his studies. His public sculptures include figures of Alexander Hamilton in New York, Daniel Webster in the Capitol at Washington, D.C., and a huge, granite figure of an American soldier created for the Philadelphia Centennial Exposition and placed in front of Memorial Hall.

Jefferson Medical College Hospital ("Old Main")

JEFFERSON MEDICAL COLLEGE HOSPITAL
By James Hamilton Windrim (1840-1919)
Completed 1907

Vintage photograph
By unknown photographer
1931-40
13 3/8 x 10 1/2 in.

Made for Jefferson Medical College
Accession number: 1940+f.Ph.02

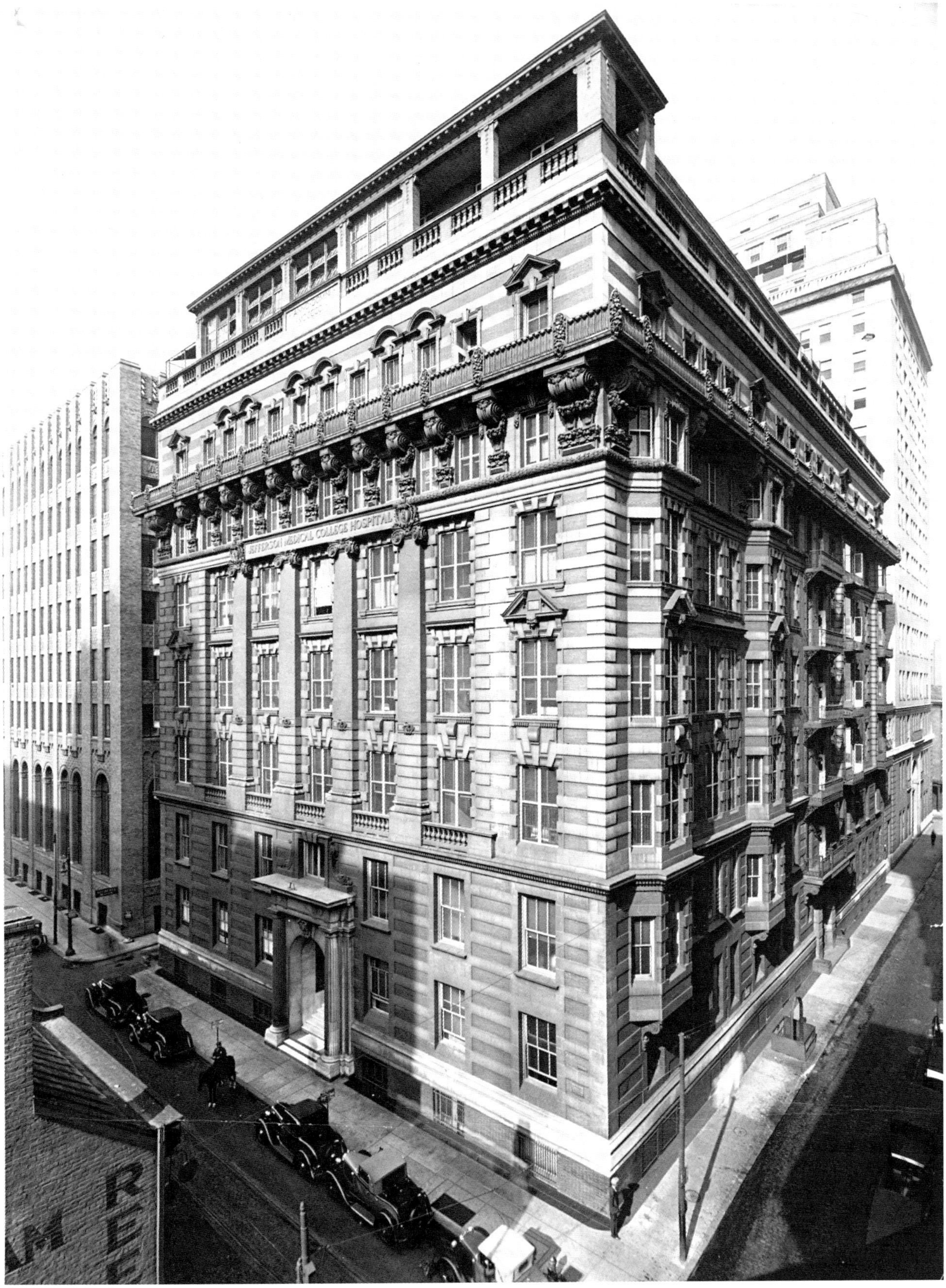
JEFFERSON MEDICAL COLLEGE HOSPITAL

The architectural firm of James H. Windrim designed a new hospital for Jefferson Medical College to replace the antiquated 1877 hospital. The modern eight-story, steel-framed, fireproof building opened in 1907, at Tenth and Sansom Streets where the Ely Building had stood.

The hospital's exterior was pale brick with stone dressing. The variation in tone produced a horizontal striped effect, contrasting with the three-story Ionic pilasters. The small, arched entrance portico was marked by engaged columns. The sixth story featured huge brackets surmounted by balconies, and the eighth story had a balustrade.

The interior contained more than three hundred beds in fourteen wards each with adjoining balconies. On the top floor was a roof garden for heliotherapy. Modern facilities included electric lighting, steam heating from an outside plant, a vacuum cleaning system, and a noiseless exhaust system.

The photograph shows the side of the Curtis Clinic Building (opened 1931) to the left of the hospital, and the Samuel Gustine Thompson Annex (opened 1924) rising up on the right. With the opening of "Old Main," the 1877 hospital had been converted to a nurses' residence and school. The amphitheater at the earlier hospital remained in use for surgical cases until it was superseded by the third and last "pit" in the Thompson Annex.

When the new hospital was dedicated on June 8, 1907, Dr. John Chalmers DaCosta gave a stirring speech on the venerated history of the old Jefferson hospital and its celebrated physicians.[9] But it was DaCosta's opinion that the progress of the machine age resulted in the decline of urban life, necessitating expanded hospital facilities:

> The need of hospital accommodation is every year becoming more and more pressing. This is an age when dangerous occupations multiply. The streets are filled with rapidly moving and death-dealing vehicles; every few stories of a great modern building mean one man dead and many injured...great machine shops and factories crush and mutilate...Closely adjacent to the hospital are the slums, the inhabitants of which, when injured or diseased, know no resource but the hospital...The very situation of the building means a wealth of clinical material, because it is placed where it is most needed. In the slums... plagues are ever lurking.

Ambulance of the Jefferson Medical College Hospital

AMBULANCE
By unknown photographer

Vintage photograph mounted on card
Ca. 1911
Image size: 7 3/8 x 9 3/8 in.
Card size: 7 3/8 x 9 3/8 in.

Made for Jefferson Medical College Hospital
Accession number: 1911+f.Ph.04

The 1907 Jefferson Hospital was the first in Philadelphia to utilize an electric ambulance to supplement the service of horse-drawn ambulances. The electric vehicle was a gift from Jefferson trustee and benefactor, Daniel Baugh.

The ambulance had a speed of fifteen miles per hour, and could run forty miles without recharging its battery. The chauffeur had a room near the accident ward so that he could respond quickly. In 1913 the trustees purchased a new Packard ambulance, so that the use of horse-drawn, electric, and gasoline vehicles overlapped briefly.[10]

The posed photograph shows attendants loading a patient onto the ambulance with a crowd of curious onlookers, including children on the street and two women watching from the window of a nearby building. The photograph might have been taken by the company whose sign hangs from the second story, "C. H. GRAVES, LANTERN SLIDES."

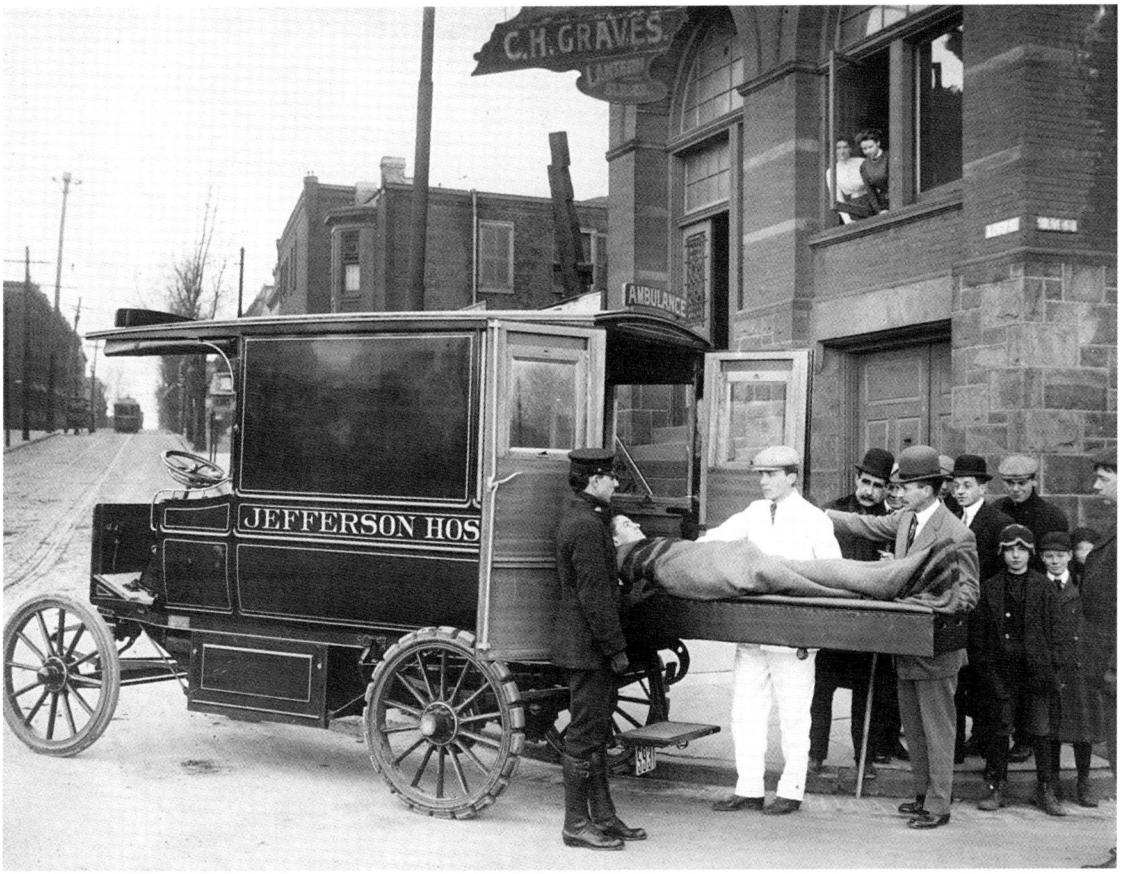

Outpatient Clinic Waiting Room at Jefferson Hospital

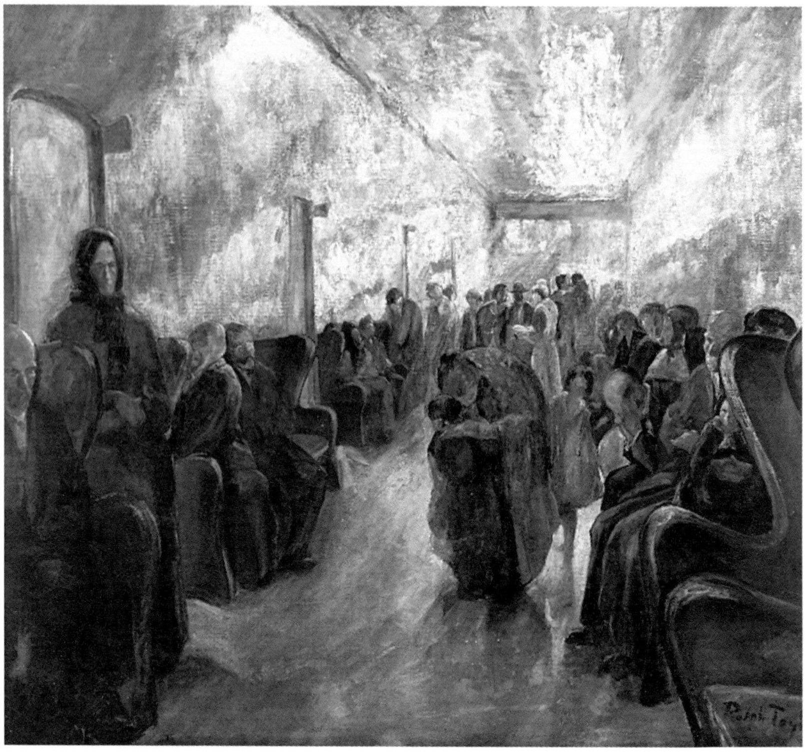

OUTPATIENT CLINIC WAITING ROOM
By Ralph Taylor (1896/97-1978)

Oil on canvas
Ca. 1924
47 1/2 x 52 in.

Signed lower right: "Ralph Taylor"

Purchased in 1979 from Mrs. Ralph Taylor, wife of the artist
Accession number: 1979+e.P.04

The Jefferson Medical College Hospital outpatient clinic, or dispensary, was depicted about 1924 by Philadelphia artist Ralph Taylor. The clinics were located on the ground floor of the Main Hospital Building of 1907, and remained there until the Curtis Clinic Building opened in 1931.

The waiting area is shown teeming with patients of all ages, some standing and others sitting on wooden benches which line the corridor. In this genre scene of an urban hospital the patients have not removed their coats and hats and babushkas. A mother comforts a child while a second child looks on, another group surrounds a student nurse, some huddle together for solace, some stare absently into space, some lean their heads on their hands. All are waiting to be ushered into the various treatment rooms lining the left wall.

Ralph Taylor's rendition may accord with Dr. John C. DaCosta's description of patients thronging the outpatient departments. Or it may be exaggerated and unduly somber, for it differs from a contemporary photograph showing an orderly group of patients seated calmly on the benches lining the corridor. Although crowded and probably overheated, the dispensary was a humane and vital service which provided treatment for all who entered. The downcast emotion expressed by the postures of the anonymous character types seems at odds with the animated, freely brushed, and colorful surface of the painting itself.

This picture was not commissioned by Jefferson Medical College, and it is not known what motivated Taylor to paint the scene or whether it was done from life.

Ralph Taylor was a Philadelphia painter, printmaker, and art teacher. When he was a child, his family emigrated from Russia to Philadelphia. At an early age he studied art at the Graphic Sketch Club and music at the Settlement Music School. After receiving a scholarship to the Pennsylvania Academy of the Fine Arts he decided on art as a career. A Cresson traveling scholarship allowed him to continue his studies abroad in Paris, Florence, and Rome.

Later awards from the Pennsylvania Academy's Fellowship were the Harrison S. Morris Watercolor Prize (1952) and the Mary Butler Memorial Prize (1954). He also won awards from the DaVinci Alliance, the Philadelphia Art Alliance, and the Graphic Sketch Club. Taylor exhibited nationally and had one-man shows at the Bower Gallery in New York, Philadelphia's Little Gallery, the University of Pennsylvania, and the Philadelphia Art Alliance.

Taylor also designed and carved frames, was an art dealer, and served on art committees and juries. He once painted a self-portrait with a violin, and many other pictures reflect his lifelong interest in music. Another of his paintings in the Jefferson collection depicts the surgical clinic in the 1877 hospital.

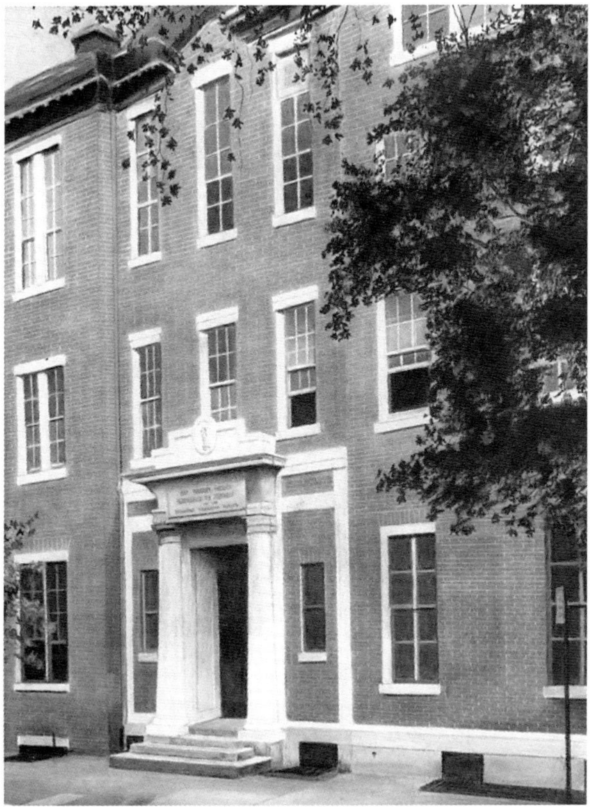

Daniel Baugh Institute of Anatomy

DANIEL BAUGH INSTITUTE OF ANATOMY
By John Torrey Windrim (1866-1934)
Adaptation 1910-11 of two earlier structures

Painting by Hobart A. Reimann, M.D. (1897-1986)
Pastel, pencil on paper
1978
27 1/2 x 21 1/2 in.

Signed and dated lower right: "H. A. REIMANN/1978"

Commissioned and given in 1981 by Joe Henry Coley, M.D. (JMC 1934) and Mrs. Coley
Accession number: 1981+e.P.01

The Daniel Baugh Institute of Anatomy was another important building added to the Jefferson facilities in the early twentieth century. In order to relieve overcrowded conditions in the anatomical rooms in the 1898 College Building, in 1910 Jefferson trustee Daniel Baugh purchased and pledged renovations for a building and adjoining residence at the northeast corner of Eleventh and Clinton Streets, a site formerly occupied by the Pennsylvania Dental College.

Daniel Baugh hired the firm of John T. Windrim to refurbish and enlarge the structures, aiming to place the facility in the forefront of anatomical instruction and research. When completed in 1911, the first floor of the four-story, brick building included offices, library, study hall, museum, and lower amphitheater. On the second floor were the histology and embryology laboratories, a professors' laboratory and research room, and a fireproof incubating and imbedding chamber. The third floor was occupied by eight dissecting rooms and four demonstration rooms, and the upper amphitheater. Operative surgery was conducted on the fourth floor.

The institute was named in honor of Daniel Baugh, and many distinguished American and European anatomists were among the guests at the dedication in September 1911. "DBI" served Jefferson Medical College for fifty-seven years until the anatomy department moved to Jefferson Alumni Hall in 1968.

The pastel painting of the Daniel Baugh Institute of Anatomy was executed in 1978 by Hobart A. Reimann, M.D., the Magee Professor of Medicine and chair of the department (1936-51).

The picture shows the building largely as it still exists. Though the original fire escapes are gone and the window trim has been somewhat augmented, the columned entrance with marble plaque and caduceus identifying the building is still in place today, though the building is no longer owned by the university.

John T. Windrim began the study of architecture with his father, James H. Windrim, in 1882. While the elder Windrim was director of public works for the City of Philadelphia in 1892, the younger Windrim assumed operation of their firm, and after that it is difficult to allocate responsibility for various projects. Among other buildings John T. Windrim did design, at least partially, are the John Wanamaker department store, the Franklin Institute, and the Family Court Building in Philadelphia.

Portrait of Daniel Baugh

DANIEL BAUGH (1836-1921)
By Lazar Raditz (1887-1958)

Oil on canvas
1911
38 1/2 x 30 1/2 in.

Signed and dated upper right: "Lazar Raditz/1911"
Exhibition: Philadelphia, *Lazar Raditz*, Art Club of Philadelphia, 1913

Given in 1911 by JMC alumni and friends
Accession number: 1911+e.P.01

Industrialist, philanthropist, and art patron, Daniel Baugh was a noted figure in Philadelphia business and society. He was an active board member and generous donor to numerous local, nonprofit institutions.

Born in 1836 near Downingtown, Pennsylvania, Baugh studied at the Fremont Seminary in Norristown. He entered the family tanning business at an early age because his assistance was needed, thus deviating from plans to attend college. In 1855 Baugh and his brother joined with their father to inaugurate a new enterprise, Baugh and Sons, a manufacturer of superphosphates for crop fertilization.

Within a few years the business grew to include other chemicals, and was known as the Delaware River Chemical Works, one of the leading companies of its kind in the world. By 1888 Daniel Baugh became head of Baugh and Sons, and its subsidiaries, the Baugh Chemical Company in Baltimore and the Chemical Works in Norfolk, Virginia.

Baugh achieved exceptional success in the business world, but was equally known as a philanthropist and tireless worker for numerous medical and cultural institutions. He joined the Jefferson board of trustees in 1896 and became one of its moving spirits. As chairman of the hospital committee he raised a great deal of the funds for the 1907 building, superintended its construction with trustee Alba Johnson, and personally donated the electric ambulance and X-ray equipment.

By the time of his death his benefaction to the Daniel Baugh Institute of Anatomy amounted to two hundred thousand dollars, and he left an additional sum in trust for the salary of the professor of anatomy. In 1915 he had pledged one hundred thousand dollars of unrestricted funds to start a general endowment if that sum would be matched within one year, a successful strategy. President William Potter called Daniel Baugh the "most valuable man" ever to serve on the board, not only for his generosity but for his time and intelligence as well. The Jefferson Medical College yearbook of 1914 was dedicated to Baugh and referred to him as "The Benefactor."

Baugh was also a trustee or manager of the Rush and Howard Hospitals. He was a member of the Permanent Relief Committee of Philadelphia and president of the Sanitarium Association. As president of the Philadelphia Medical Publishing Company he published the *Philadelphia Medical Journal* until it merged with the *New York Medical Journal*. He was a director of Girard National Bank, the Delaware Insurance Company, and the Philadelphia Bourse.

He served as president of the School of Design for Women (later Moore College of Art and Design), as trustee of the Philadelphia Museum of Art, and as founder and long-term president of the Philadelphia Art Club. He was a founder and first president of the Art Federation whose original purpose was to secure a grand boulevard running diagonally from City Hall to Fairmount Park (where the Philadelphia Museum of Art stands). The federation was later superseded by the Parkway Association.

Daniel Baugh traveled abroad for five or six months each year. His lavishly appointed home at Sixteenth and Locust Streets contained a notable collection of art works and antiquities acquired during his extended journeys. He was a donor of funds and objects to the University of Pennsylvania Museum of Archaeology and Palaeontology.

When Jefferson's alumni association and his many friends initiated the Daniel Baugh portrait fund in 1910, it was so heavily subscribed that excess monies were donated to the hospital's endowed room fund. The following year the painting was installed in the library of the Daniel Baugh Institute of Anatomy, and it still hangs today in the department's offices in Jefferson Alumni Hall. Portraitist Lazar Raditz included the work in his one-man show at the Art Club of Philadelphia in 1913.

In the half-length, life-sized portrait, Daniel Baugh is shown seated with his head turned slightly to gaze directly at the observer and with his arms resting on the chair arms. Though seventy-five years of age, he sits very erectly and emanates physical and intellectual strength. His expression is serious and confident, punctuated by his firmly pressed lips and square jaw. His fashionable costume includes gold cuff links and watch

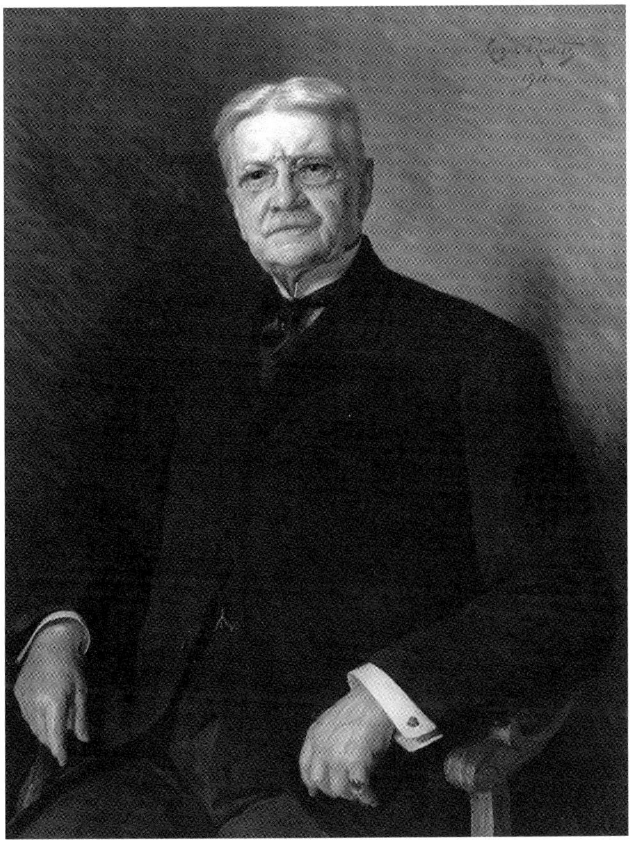

chain, as well as a jewelled tie pin and ring.

Baugh's complexion is ruddy and his silver hair is accented with strokes of blue. Flesh tones on face and hands are painted with thick, impasto strokes, as are highlights on the white shirt collar and cuffs. Diagonal brush strokes are also visible in the light and shadow areas of the atmospheric background, enlivening the whole surface. The shadow behind the figure gives a sense of depth to the surrounding space.

The personal backgrounds of subject and artist could not have been more divergent. Daniel Baugh's great-great-grandfather had emigrated from Germany shortly before the Revolutionary War, and he and his descendants had acquired substantial estates in Chester County.

Lazar Raditz was born in 1887 in the small town of Dvinsk in Russia, one of only three survivors in a family of eleven children. His family was disappointed that he adamantly refused rabbinical study in favor of becoming an artist. The penniless youth was ineligible for admission to the art academy in Riga and the only work he could find was assisting a German decorator.

His older brother had fled to America to avoid arrest after protesting the massacre of two siblings in a pogrom. He brought Lazar to his home in Philadelphia in 1903 to help the young man realize his artistic ambitions. Lazar's luck turned almost immediately, for some of his Russian sketches were detained in customs, and an agent showed the drawings to Philadelphia Judge Mayer Sulzberger (interestingly, a Jefferson trustee). The judge was favorably impressed and arranged for the sixteen-year-old to study at the Pennsylvania Academy of the Fine Arts.

Though the Raditz brothers were constantly on the edge of poverty, Lazar spent four years at the Academy where officials considered him one of the most promising students, and his instructor, William Merritt Chase, even arranged for a portrait commission. This led to other commissions and he was awarded two Cresson traveling scholarships to Europe in 1907 and 1908. At the Academy he also won the Second Charles Toppan Prize for Portraits in 1906 and the First Charles Toppan Prize in 1909. After graduation he sought further study in portrait painting in Boston under Edmund C. Tarbell, and made one final study trip to Europe before opening a studio in his adopted home of Philadelphia.

Success followed quickly and his portrait commissions included prominent business, political, and professional people in Philadelphia, Boston, Providence, and Lancaster, including two paintings of Daniel Baugh and one of Mrs. Baugh. Public portraits can be found at the following Philadelphia institutions: the American Philosophical Society, the University of Pennsylvania, Temple University, the Academy of Natural Sciences, the Franklin Institute, the College of Physicians of Philadelphia, the Free Library, and the Pennsylvania Academy. Other portraits hang at the State Capitol in Harrisburg, and at Brown and Yale Universities.

As early as 1913 he had a one-man show of forty-two portraits at the Art Club of Philadelphia. Raditz was widely admired for his ability to render the figure and to delineate the character of the subject. He had another show at McClees Galleries in Philadelphia in 1935. His work won a bronze medal at the Panama-Pacific Exposition in 1915 and the Julius Hallgarten Prize at the National Academy of Design in 1918.

Lazar Raditz was an instructor of drawing and painting at the Graphic Sketch Club. He was married to Henrietta Herman, a professional pianist. She and her family had been among the first to befriend and encourage Raditz upon his arrival in Philadelphia.

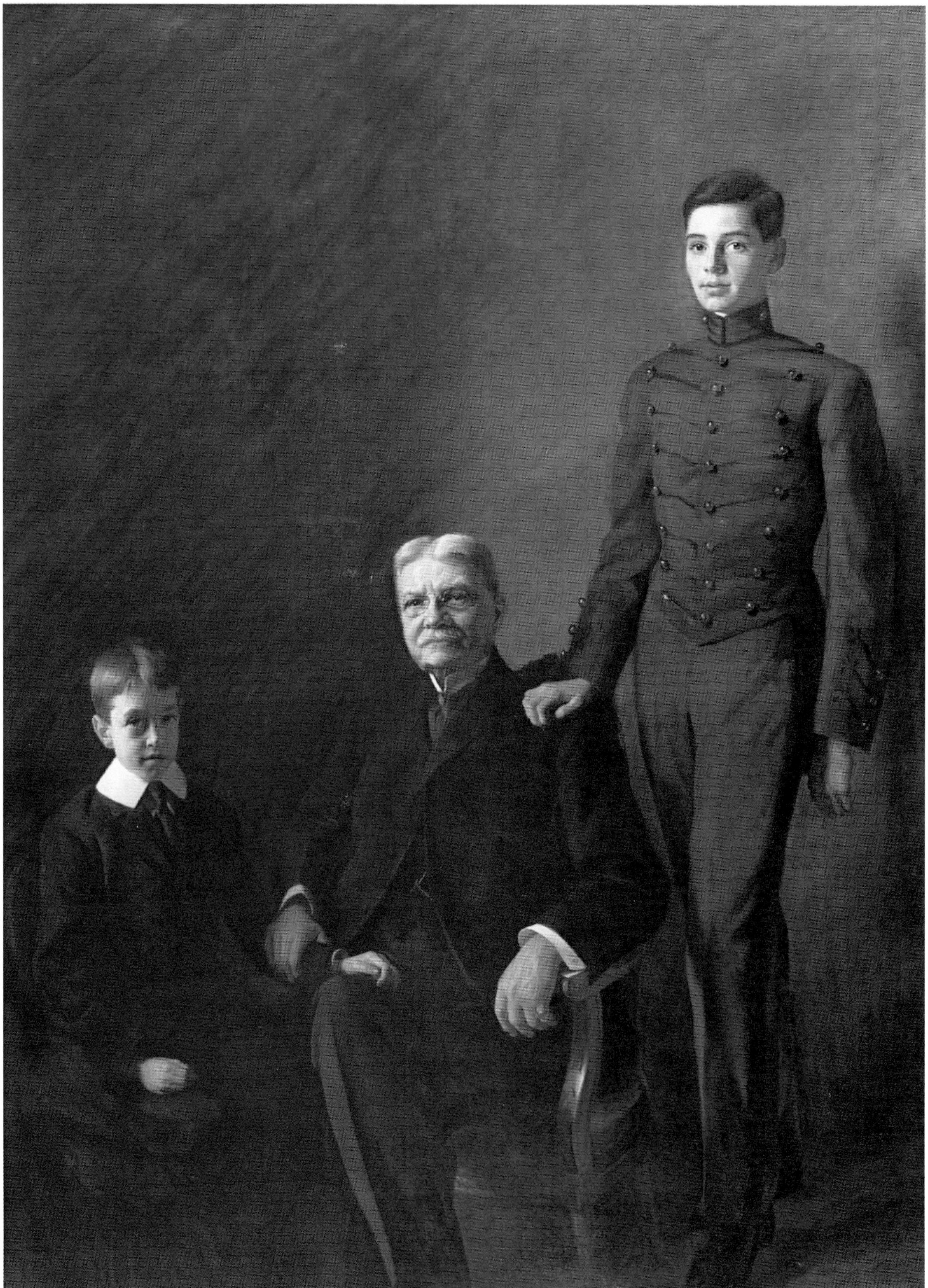

The Three Daniels (Portrait of Daniel Baugh and His Grandsons)

THE THREE DANIELS (DANIEL BAUGH AND HIS GRANDSONS)
By Lazar Raditz

Oil on canvas
1911
84 x 62 1/2 in.

Signed and dated lower right: "Lazar Raditz/Feb. 1911"
Exhibition: Philadelphia, *Lazar Raditz*, Art Club of Philadelphia, 1913

Given between 1915 and 1931 by the Baugh family
Accession number: 1915-1931.P.01

It is a testament to Raditz's artistic ability and fortunate social connections that Daniel Baugh, a wealthy businessman and patron of the arts, commissioned two portraits from the twenty-four-year-old artist so early in his career. Both Baugh portraits were painted in 1911, soon after Raditz had completed his studies and foreign travels and returned to Philadelphia to open his studio.

The full-length group portrait shows Daniel Baugh seated between his two grandsons, Daniel Baugh Brewster standing on the right, and Daniel Baugh III seated on the left. The torso and face of the grandfather is virtually identical with his other portrait by Raditz in pose, costume, and facial expression. The only variation is his right hand which grasps the forearm of his younger grandson.

As in the other portrait by Raditz, Daniel Baugh is seated in the same high-style armchair of the 1860s, a Second Empire type adapted from the Louis XVI style. The larger group portrait also includes an oriental rug on the floor. Another elegant note is the younger grandson's fashionably wide Eton collar. The older grandson wears a gray cadet's uniform.

The prevailing mood of this formal portrait is a quiet stateliness and dignity. One senses family pride and the importance of tradition, further emphasized by the painting's title, *The Three Daniels*. Though the figures are reserved and austere in expression and pose, there is a hint of tenderness in the intertwining of gestures that connect them. While the standing figure of the older grandson rises far above the other figures, the contrast of light and shadow in the loosely painted, atmospheric background helps to unite the group. Another unifying factor is the strong raking light from the left which spotlights the faces of all three figures.

The imposing group portrait was originally installed in the upper amphitheater of the Daniel Baugh Institute of Anatomy, but there are no records pertaining to its exact date of donation. In 1981 Daniel Baugh III said that he remembered sitting for the portrait when he was about eight years old and recalled seeing the work at his grandfather's house. Documents show that the painting arrived at Jefferson sometime between 1915 and 1931.

When the institute was relocated to Jefferson Alumni Hall in 1968, the monumental painting could not be accommodated in the department offices, so it was put in storage, and as often happens, forgotten. Years later it was "rediscovered" and found to be suffering from water damage. Following splendid restoration, *The Three Daniels* was rededicated in a special ceremony in 1981 and installed in the second floor landing of the College Building (after *The Gross Clinic* was moved to Jefferson Alumni Hall).

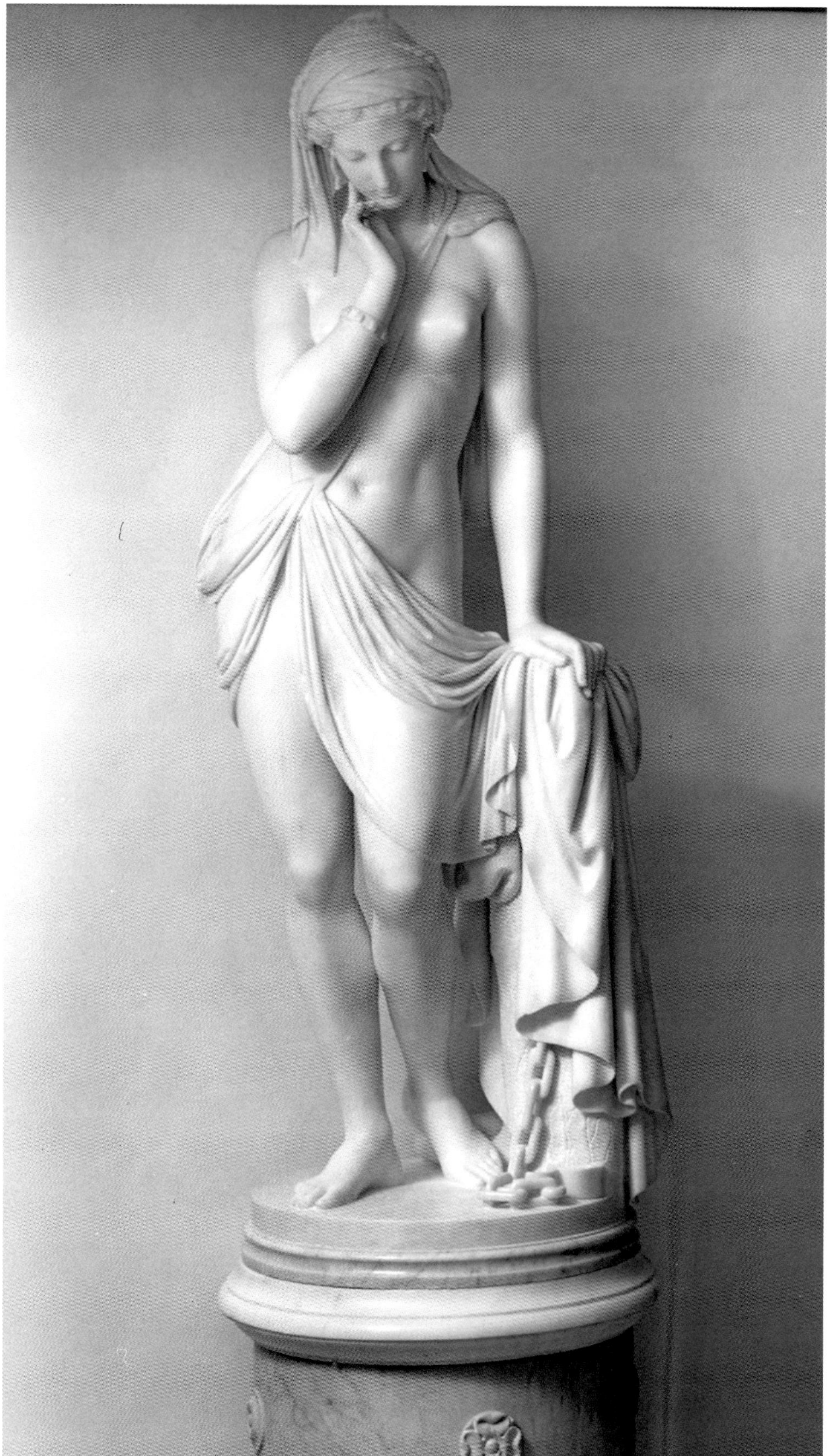

The Greek Slave

THE GREEK SLAVE
By Scipione Tadolini (1822-92)

Marble
Ca. 1875
57 1/4 x 23 3/8 x 20 1/4 in.

Signed on rear edge of integral base:
"EQ^{s}.SCIPIO.TADOLINI.ROMAE"

Given ca. 1921 by estate of Daniel Baugh[11]
Accession number: 1921+c.S.01

The Daniel Baugh Institute of Anatomy not only had its own library stocked with rare medical books, but also a large group of associated art objects, presumably donated by Daniel Baugh and perhaps gathered on his foreign travels.

Beside the two oil portraits of the founder, art works included oil copies of two famous paintings depicting anatomists Andreas Vesalius and Nicolaas Tulp, a marble sculpture of *The Greek Slave*, a large engraving of William Harvey, a collotype of Thomas Eakins's *Gross Clinic*, large engravings after paintings of notable European surgeons Ambroise Paré, Theodor Billroth, and Jules Péan, vintage photographs of numerous professors connected with the institute, and two antique clocks.

The Greek Slave is a fifty-seven-inch, marble sculpture of a nude female standing in a *contrapposto* pose with her weight on her right foot, and her left hand leaning upon the top of a tree stump. The chin of her downcast head rests upon her right hand. A narrow, curving drapery which begins at her elaborate turban cascades over her back, falls diagonally across her hips, and ends in deep folds over the tree stump. At her left foot is an opened anklet attached to the end of a chain secured to the tree stump.

A leather strap forming an opposing diagonal on her torso holds the various sections of drapery in place. Her jewelry includes a bracelet on her right arm, key-shaped earrings, and a spiral necklace inscribed with a combination of Greek and Latin letters. The long, flowing headdress complements her elaborate hair arrangement of waves, braid, and ponytail.

Though the style and proportions of the figure recall the classical canons of beauty seen in ancient figures of Venus, the subject is really one of modern history relating to the Greek War of Independence (1821-30). A virtuous, Christian, Greek maiden has been captured in the conflict and is about to be sold in the Muslim Turkish slave markets in Constantinople.

This subject was favored by mid-nineteenth-century artists and writers, because they looked to Greece as the ancient center of art and literature. A celebrated example of the subject was created about 1844 by the expatriate American sculptor, Hiram Powers (1805-73). A number of artistic figures, notably Lord Byron, actually went to Greece to fight on the side of the beleaguered nation.

Contemporary society understood that Tadolini's sculpture is a personification of oppressed Greece. The opened link of her chain symbolizes the possibility of liberation. The idealized figure expresses pensiveness and serenity, in the style of ancient Greek sculptures, rather than despair or humiliation at her plight. The downward tilt of her head suggests modesty and chasteness in the midst of the unsavory slave traders.

Scipione Tadolini was born in Rome in 1822 and trained in the sculpture studio of his celebrated father, Adamo Tadolini (1788-1868). Among the younger sculptor's best-known works are a Santa Lucia (Gonfalone Church, Rome), a St. Michael (now in Boston), an equestrian portrait of Simon Bólivar (Lima), and a bust of King Vittorio Emanuele I (Senate, Rome). Museums in Glasgow, Madrid, and Sydney also have versions of Tadolini's *Greek Slave*.

Number Two Regulator Wall Clock

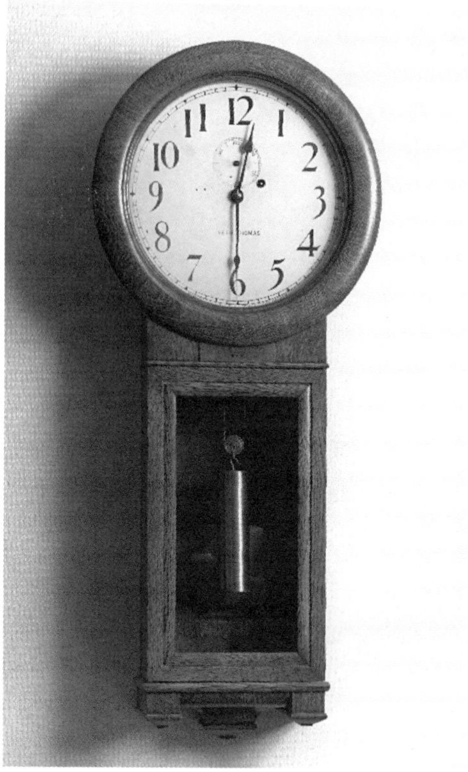

NUMBER TWO REGULATOR WALL CLOCK
By Seth Thomas Clock Co.

Oak, glass, brass, tin
1890-1920
36 3/4 x 15 1/2 x 5 1/2 in.

Stamped inscription on clock face: "SETH THOMAS"
Inscription on brass plaque under dial: "DANIEL BAUGH INSTITUTE OF ANATOMY/JEFFERSON MEDICAL COLLEGE/1911-1968"

Purchased before 1931 by the Daniel Baugh Institute of Anatomy
Accession number: 1931+b.DA.01

Bracket Clock

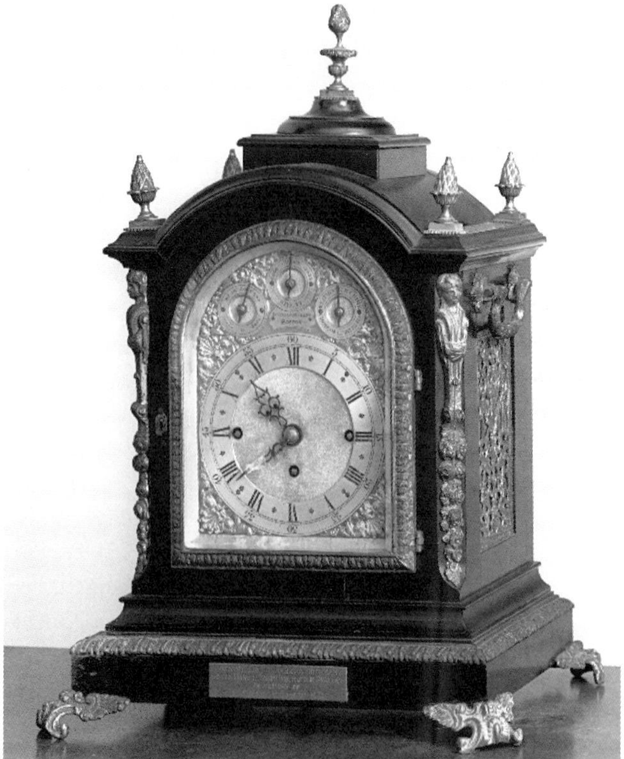

BRACKET CLOCK
Works by Elliott of London (?)

Ebonized wood, gold plated brass, glass
1880s-1890s
23 1/2 x 16 7/8 x 11 3/4 in.

Plaque on block face with inscription: "SHREVE CRUMP & LOW/BOSTON"
Plaque on clock base with inscription: "PRESENTED BY FREDERICKA HOFFMAN/TO THE DANIEL BAUGH INSTITUTE OF ANATOMY/IN MEMORY OF/CLARENCE HOFFMAN, M.D."

Given in 1927 by Fredericka Hoffman, widow of Clarence Hoffman, M.D. (JMC 1906), demonstrator of anatomy
Accession number: 1927+e.DA.01

Two antique clocks that had decorated the Baugh Institute of Anatomy are of contrasting types and styles, reflecting the output of their makers: the Seth Thomas Clock Company of Thomaston, Connecticut and Elliott of London.

The Number Two oak regulator clock made by Seth Thomas is a wall clock of a very common type, used in public places such as offices, train stations, and banks or other businesses. Very popular from 1870 to 1920, it was sometimes called a "railroad clock." Characteristic features are a protruding drum case above a vertical, rectangular trunk above pilaster pendants. A hinged, glazed door reveals a brass pendulum with cylinder weights.

Today this clock hangs in the reception room of the Thomas Jefferson University president.

In contrast to the regulator clock, the late Victorian bracket or mantle clock, still located in the anatomy department, is a very high-style piece with works probably by Elliott of London. Its case is probably of English origin, too, and is made of ebonized wood and mounted with brass to look like gilt bronze. Its design recalls English clocks of about 1730 from the George II period.

The clock's domical cornice is surmounted with a recessed rectangular plinth holding a flaming urn finial, flanked by brass corner finials of pine cone design. The chamfered corners of the cornice are mounted with brass floral strips suspended from female herm figures draped with swags. The domical glazed door with a waterleaf repeat border encloses a brass dial with a silvered chapter ring of black enamel Roman and Arabic numerals.

The very fine clock works include a slow-fast adjustment dial, a chime silent dial, and a dial for choosing either Westminster chimes or chimes on eight bells, both accompanied by a large coil gong.

The sides are decorated with pierced brass grille work of Renaissance style enclosing a cloth protective dust cover. Below the grille work are quarter round brass moldings of husk (resembling triple bellflowers) and gadroon repeats. The feet are elaborate rococo scroll work of Regency style, and the sides are mounted with brass carrying handles.

Portrait of George McClellan

(See color plate)

GEORGE McCLELLAN, M.D. (1849-1913)
By Julian Russel Story (1857-1919)

Oil on canvas
1894
45 x 36 in.

Signed and dated upper right: "Julian Story 1894"
Exhibition: Philadelphia, *Annual Exhibition*, Pennsylvania Academy of the Fine Arts, 1894

Given in 1982 by Mrs. Mary Fleeming Penn-Gaskell Hall White, grand-niece of the subject
Accession number: 1982+e.P.04

Dr. George McClellan was a noted anatomist who was appointed chair of applied anatomy at Jefferson Medical College in 1906. He was the son of Dr. John Hill Brinton McClellan and was the namesake of his grandfather, the founder of the college.

Born in 1849 and reared in Philadelphia, the younger McClellan initially studied for three years in the arts department at the University of Pennsylvania. He graduated from Jefferson Medical College in 1870 and practiced surgery immediately afterwards. A turning point in his career occurred in 1872 when he studied under the famous Viennese anatomist, Josef Hyrtl, one of the first comparative anatomists of his day. This stimulating learning experience caused McClellan to concentrate on

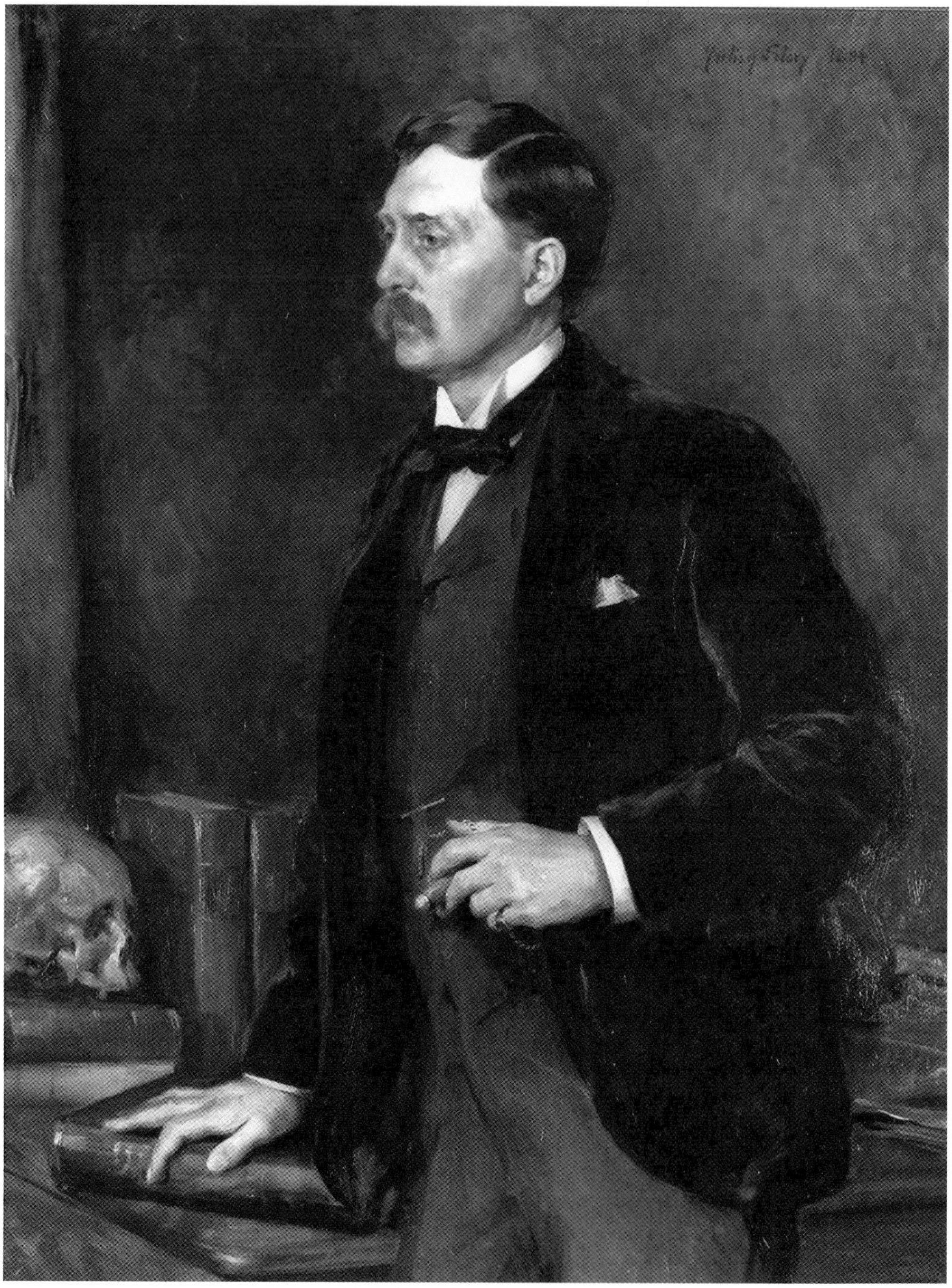

the teaching of anatomy as a career.

Upon his return to Philadelphia he continued surgical practice at the Philadelphia, St. Joseph's, and Howard Hospitals. In 1881 he founded the Pennsylvania School of Anatomy and Surgery where he taught until 1893. Dr. John C. DaCosta, one of many Jefferson students who attended McClellan's nearby school, wrote a colorful description in the April 1914 *Jeffersonian*:

It was an axiom when I was a student that if you would really like and understand anatomy you must go to McClellan's demonstrations. I was charmed with his teaching. His perfect familiarity with his subject, the beauty of his dissections, the clearness of his demonstrations, the pictures which he drew on the board with such marvellous speed, accuracy and dexterity, excited the warmest admiration of his class. His anatomy was art. He dissected a body as a great sculptor would carve a statue...I thought then, and I think now, that nobody ever gave more useful anatomical lectures.

In the autumn of 1890 McClellan succeeded Dr. W. W. Keen as professor of artistic anatomy at the Pennsylvania Academy of the Fine Arts and taught there until his death in 1913. According to the Academy's *Circular of the Committee on Instruction 1891-1892,* his lectures were illustrated by preparations, live models, photographs, and extempore drawings on the blackboard. Dissection of the muscles were shown and demonstrations of the cadaver appropriate to art students were made. Special attention was given to the mechanism and action of the joints; the prominences of the skeleton and the interaction of the muscles affecting the contour of the body; and the fine surface markings due to fatty tissue and the relative elasticity of the skin. The anatomy of human expression included comparative anatomy.

Following the death of Dr. William S. Forbes in 1905, Jefferson's department of anatomy was divided. Dr. McClellan was named chair of applied anatomy and Dr. Edward A. Spitzka was named chair of general anatomy. McClellan had aspired to the chair of general anatomy and was greatly disappointed that at age fifty-six he was appointed to teach practical anatomy and had to share the chair with the twenty-nine-year-old Spitzka. Apparently the experiment of a divided chair was unsuccessful because after McClellan's death the chairs were reunited under Dr. Spitzka.

A kind, loyal, and refined gentleman of the old school, Dr. George McClellan could also be acerbic when standing up for his convictions. Yet he was admired and beloved by the students, and "his boys" in the class of 1913 dedicated their yearbook to him, shortly before his death that year.

Dr. George McClellan's best-known literary work is the two-volume *Regional Anatomy in Its Relation to Medicine and Surgery* (1890-92) which went through four American and two French editions. For this work McClellan made his own dissections, took the photographs, and colored the illustrations. An important publication on artistic anatomy is his *Anatomy in Its Relation to Art: an Exposition of the Bones and Muscles of the Human Body with Especial Reference to Their Influence upon Its Actions and External Form* (1900).

In Julian R. Story's portrait of 1894 the physician is shown two-thirds length facing the left, standing next to a desk with his hand resting on a book. The warm, reddish-brown, atmospheric background includes a gray drapery on the left edge, suggesting an interior domestic location such as a study. McClellan's dashingly handsome profile is accentuated by wavy hair and a thick, curling mustache. He holds a cigar in his left hand and wears a maroon velvet smoking jacket over his gray trousers and vest. Accessories include a gold watch chain and jeweled pinky ring. In spite of his urbane attire, the subject glances downward as though lost in thought during a private moment, and his reticent expression has a tinge of sadness.

Other objects on the table include a variety of papers and books, and most importantly a conspicuous skull propped up on books. An article of great significance to McClellan, it is the actual skull of George Frederick Cooke, a flamboyant, early-nineteenth-century, Shakespearean actor, idolized by English and American theatergoers. McClellan acquired the skull from a physician patient who had inherited it from his father, a young doctor who in 1812 assisted at Cooke's autopsy and could not resist the temptation to add it to his collection of skulls.

McClellan prized the skull and was greatly relieved when his office was ransacked but the burglars missed finding this artifact. In 1922 Mrs. George McClellan willed the relic to her personal physician, Jefferson's Dean Ross V. Patterson, who, in turn, bequeathed it to Jefferson Medical College in 1937.

According to an obituary in the Philadelphia *Evening Bulletin,* Julian Story was related to the McClellan family. Another article in the same newspaper mentioned specifically that he was a cousin of Dr. George McClellan. Story's portraits of the physician and of Mrs. McClellan were exhibited at the Pennsylvania Academy of the Fine Arts in 1894.

Julian R. Story, the social counterpart of his portrait subject, was born in 1857 at Walton-on-Thames, England. He was the son of William Wetmore Story, a famous poet and sculptor who lived most of his life abroad. The painter's grandfather, Joseph Story, was a noted legal authority and justice on the United States Supreme Court. Julian Story received the classical education of an English gentleman at Eton and Oxford where he received an A.M. degree in 1879. On the continent he studied art with Frank Duveneck in Florence and with Jules-Joseph Lefebvre and Gustave Boulanger in Paris.

He exhibited portraits and other figurative works throughout Europe and the United States. Among other awards he received a third class medal and honorable mention at the Paris Salon of 1889; a gold medal at Berlin in 1891; a bronze medal at the Paris Exposition of

1899, and a silver medal at the Paris Exposition of 1900; and medals at the Pan-American Exposition in Buffalo in 1901 and the Panama-Pacific Exposition in San Francisco in 1915. He was made a chevalier of the French Legion of Honor and an associate of the National Academy of Design. Story was a member of the Society of American Painters in Paris, the Society of American Artists in New York, and the London Society of Portrait Painters.

He often spent winters in the United States and kept a studio in the St. James Hotel in Philadelphia. His portrait sitters included the cream of Philadelphia society as well as civic and business leaders here and elsewhere. He also had studios in Paris and at a four-hundred-acre estate at Vallombrosa, near Florence. One of his most famous subjects was King Edward VII painted when he was still the Prince of Wales. Numerous other portraits can be found in museums and private and institutional collections throughout America.

Mr. Story led a colorful life as attested by the number of newspaper stories about him. While a struggling painter in Paris in 1891 he married a famous opera singer, Emma Eames. Soon after they were divorced in 1907 the soprano was named a "psychic" co-respondent in another divorce of baritone Emilio De Gogorza with whom she had performed, and to whose wife Eames was rumored to have paid one hundred thousand dollars to secure the singer's freedom to marry her. While in London in 1909 Julian Story quietly married a Philadelphia woman just recently divorced, Mrs. Elaine Sartori Bohlen.

Portrait of William Potter

(See color plate)

WILLIAM POTTER (1852-1926)
By Hugh Henry Breckenridge (1870-1937)

Oil on canvas
1910
62 1/2 x 52 1/2 in.

Signed lower right: "Hugh H. Breckenridge/1910"
Exhibition: Philadelphia, *Annual Exhibition*, Pennsylvania Academy of the Fine Arts, 1911

Given in 1910 by JMC alumni and trustees
Accession number: 1910+e.P.02

In 1896 William Potter succeeded Joseph B. Townsend as president of the Jefferson Medical College board of trustees. He steered the college's expansion and development very effectively during an event-filled, thirty-year term.

The value of Jefferson's buildings rose dramatically with the new Medical Hall, "Old Main" Hospital, and the Daniel Baugh Institute of Anatomy, already mentioned. In 1924 the Samuel Gustine Thompson Annex was opened on Sansom Street between Tenth and Eleventh Streets on the site of the original 1877 hospital. Another notable event during Potter's tenure was Jefferson's first endowed professorship, the Samuel D. Gross Professorship of Surgery.

Potter's board considered mergers with Medico-chirurgical College, the Temple University School of Medicine, and the University of Pennsylvania School of Medicine. All such potential alliances were rejected, as was an overture for coeducation from Women's Medical College.

William Potter was born in 1852 in Philadelphia, and was descended from a general who served under George Washington in the Revolutionary War. He entered the University of Pennsylvania in 1874, but because of his father's illness Potter had to take over direction of the family's oilcloth manufacturing company, Thomas Potter, Sons, and Company. While engaged in business he received a law degree from the University of Pennsylvania and was admitted to the bar in 1896.

An unusually public-spirited citizen, he was appointed to several important international positions by President Benjamin Harrison. In 1890 his work as special commissioner to London, Paris, and Berlin in behalf of the Post Office Department resulted in modernizing transatlantic mail delivery. In recognition of his work as American ambassador to Italy, in 1897 he received from King Umberto the decoration of Commander of the Order of Sts. Maurizio and Lazzaro, and in 1908 from Victor Emanuel III the decoration of Grand Officer of the Order of the Crown of Italy.

Upon his return to Philadelphia he subsequently declined President William McKinley's offer of the ambassadorships to Germany and Russia. During the Spanish-American War he was sent by the National Relief Commission to distribute medical and hospital supplies in Puerto Rico.

William Potter was a member of Philadelphia's Board

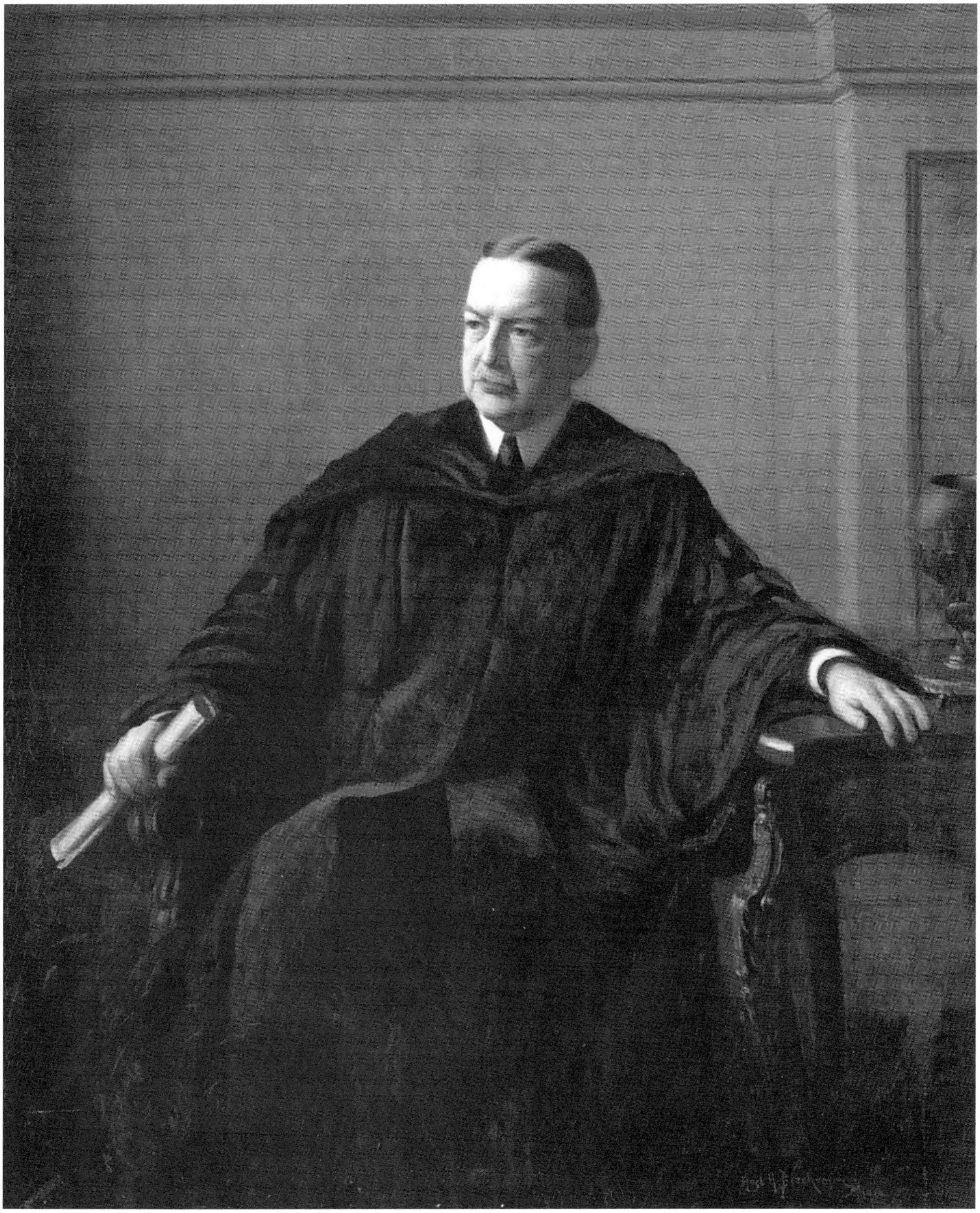

of City Trusts and involved in the management of Girard College. He was also a manager of the Pennsylvania Institute for the Deaf and Dumb, and a member of the Citizens' Permanent Relief Committee. Active in reform politics, he was a member of the Committee of One Hundred and chairman of the Advisory Board to the Mayor. Potter ran as the Fusion candidate for mayor of Philadelphia in 1907 but was defeated. President Woodrow Wilson appointed him Fuel Administrator for Pennsylvania to conserve coal and other fuels during World War I.

He received an honorary B.A. degree from the University of Pennsylvania in 1919, and an honorary LL.D. degree from Washington and Jefferson College in 1921.

William Potter's son-in-law, Joseph W. Wear, and his grandson, William Potter Wear, also served on the Jefferson board of trustees. William Potter Wear endowed the annual William Potter lectureship in honor of his grandfather. The Jefferson Medical College class of 1904 dedicated its yearbook to this energetic leader.

Potter's expansive, full-length, life-sized portrait by Hugh H. Breckenridge shows the subject wearing an academic gown and seated in a panelled room. He gazes to the left with a confident expression. His voluminous black robe is trimmed with a purple hood, stripes on the sleeves, and front panels. His right hand holds a rolled object, possibly a diploma or blueprint. He is seated in an American Victorian armchair, and his left hand rests on a Louis XVI-style table featuring a cabriole leg with ormolu decoration. An ornate, silver bowl and stand is a centerpiece on the table. A framed tapestry or painting hangs on the wall behind the table.

Though the sitter's erect pose and neutral facial expression are straightforward and conventional, the artist's shimmering dashes of color and loose brush strokes radiate a sense of energy. Visible brush strokes of pinks, purples, and blues animate the sitter's flesh tones and the light and shaded portions of the background wall. The large dimensions of the canvas, the confident spread of the sitter's arms, and the inclusion of high-style decorative objects all suggest a man of means and position.

The impressive painting has always hung in favorable locations, initially in the library of the 1898 College Building. In 1930 it was installed across from *The Gross Clinic* on the second floor landing of the 1929 College Building where it remained until its relocation in 1973 to the boardroom in the Scott Building.

Hugh H. Breckenridge, a well established and influential Philadelphia painter, was commissioned to paint William Potter's portrait in 1910. Almost a match for his illustrious subject in prestige, Breckenridge was actively engaged in teaching, exhibiting, and judging art at the local and national level throughout his career.

He was born in 1870 in Leesburg, Virginia, the son of a cabinetmaker. He entered the Pennsylvania Academy of the Fine Arts in 1887, merited the First Charles Toppan Prize in 1890, and spent a year in Paris studying on a Cresson traveling scholarship.

Breckenridge became a painting instructor at the Pennsylvania Academy where he served for more than four decades from 1894 until 1937. In 1900 he opened a summer school in a barn with painter Thomas Anshutz in Darby, Pennsylvania, then moved the school to larger quarters in Fort Washington where it remained from 1902 until 1918. In 1919 he directed the Department of Fine Arts at the Maryland Institute in Baltimore. He also conducted the Breckenridge Summer School of Art in East Gloucester, Massachusetts from 1920 until his death in 1937.

Breckenridge was widely admired for a variety of subjects: academic portraits, loosely handled, impressionistic landscapes, more solidly handled still lifes, and later in his career, intensely colored abstractions. He exhibited regularly at the large annual exhibitions in Chicago, St. Louis, and Philadelphia and at most of the world's fairs. He served on more than fifteen juries of selection, and was appointed the painter member of the Municipal Art Jury for Philadelphia from 1911 until 1922.

One-man shows of his work were held at the Pennsylvania Academy in 1904 and 1934, and he exhibited fourteen works at the Academy's annual exhibition in 1917. Memorial shows were held at the Philadelphia Art Alliance in 1938, and the Valley House Gallery in Dallas in 1967. His work is found in numerous public and private collections throughout the United States. Before his death in 1937 he had almost completed a book on the theory of color.

Among Hugh Breckenridge's awards were a medal at the Atlanta Exposition (1895), an honorable mention at the Paris Exposition (1900), the Corcoran Prize at the Society of Washington Artists (1903), a silver medal at the International Exposition in Buenos Aires (1910), a gold medal at the Panama-Pacific Exposition in San Francisco (1915), and the Edward T. Stotesbury Prize and Jennie Sesnan Gold Medal at the Pennsylvania Academy of the Fine Arts.

Portrait of James C. Wilson

JAMES CORNELIUS WILSON, M.D. (1847-1938)
By Samuel Aloysius Murray (1869-1941)

Bronze
1917
19 x 22 1/2 x 10 7/8 in.

Inscription on rear of non-integral base: "SAMUEL MURRAY ©1917"
Foundry mark on bottom edge of non-integral base: "Roman Bronze Works, NY"
Inscription on front of non-integral base: "JAMES CORNELIVS WILSON/MEDICAM ARTEM ET CLINICEN PROFESSVS/AB MDCCCXCI AD MCMXI A.D."

Given in 1917 by William H. Greene, M.D. (JMC 1873)
Accession number: 1917+e.S.01

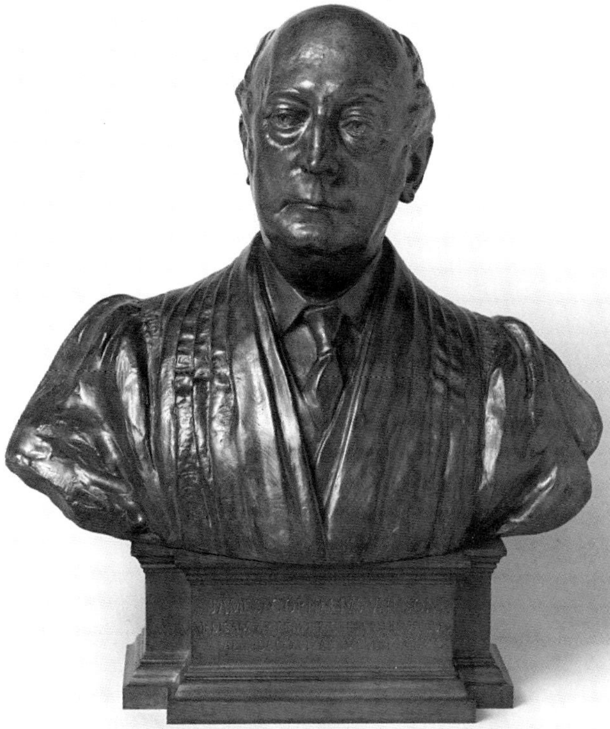

Dr. James C. Wilson succeeded Jacob M. DaCosta, M.D. as chair of the practice of medicine at Jefferson Medical College in 1891 and served until his resignation in 1911. In addition to teaching and administrative duties he maintained a large private practice.

James C. Wilson was born in Philadelphia in 1847, the son of Ellwood Wilson, M.D. (JMC 1845), a teacher, an assistant to Professor Charles D. Meigs, M.D., and for many years a Jefferson trustee.

The younger Wilson graduated from Phillips Exeter Academy and Princeton University (1867), and took his medical degree at Jefferson (1869) where he was a private pupil of Dr. W. W. Keen. He also received a master's degree at Princeton in 1869. He further enhanced his strong academic credentials by studying in Vienna and Dresden, after completing a term as resident physician at the Wills Eye and Pennsylvania Hospitals.

After his return to Philadelphia Wilson was made chief of the medical dispensary at the Jefferson Hospital, chief clinical assistant to Professor Jacob M. DaCosta, M.D., and lecturer on physical diagnosis. In 1876 he was appointed a physician at the Philadelphia Hospital where he served until 1889, and the German (now Lankenau) Hospital where he was physician-in-chief from 1897 to 1924.

In 1891 Dr. Wilson succeeded DaCosta as chair of the practice of medicine and practical medicine at Jefferson, and in 1895 was appointed physician at Pennsylvania Hospital. He resigned the Jefferson chair in 1911 because of chronic ill health, but continued in his private practice for many years afterward.

Wilson was renowned as a diagnostician and also as a gifted teacher. The J. C. Wilson Medical Society was founded by Jefferson students in 1892. He was further honored by the class of 1905 which dedicated its yearbook to him.

Wilson was editor of *An American Text-book of Applied Therapeutics* (1896) and the author of *A Manual of Fever Nursing* (1887) and *A Handbook of Medical Diagnosis* (1909). He served as president of the Philadelphia County Medical Society, the College of Physicians of Philadelphia, the American Academy of Medicine, the American Climatological Society, and the Association of American Physicians.

In 1973 Dr. Wilson's daughter, Beatrice Wilson, bequeathed one and one-half million dollars for the establishment of the James C. Wilson Professorship of Medicine, to be filled by the director of the division of cardiology in the department of medicine.

William H. Greene, M.D., donor of the bust, was also a donor to Jefferson's new library in the 1898 College Building. A vintage photograph of art works in the library's reading room shows the Wilson sculpture on top of a bookcase.

It is not known who originally commissioned this bronze bust by Samuel A. Murray. There is an almost identical plaster copy at the College of Physicians of Philadelphia. The latter bust is dated 1924 and was donated by Mrs. Samuel A. Murray that year.

Murray's bust-length, bronze portrait shows Dr. J. C. Wilson garbed in an academic robe over his suit, with his necktie slightly askew. His balding head is turned slightly to the left, and he has the characteristic, deeply grooved features and fleshy face and neck of a seventy-year-old man. His expression is tight-lipped and rather austere as he glances to the side. Yet he has broad shoulders and seems to exude physical power and strength. His robe has deep, curving, vertical folds which echo the predominant oval shape of his head. The sculptor's skill at modeling a solid, three-dimensional, realistic likeness gives the figure a nearly palpable presence in the room.

Samuel A. Murray is best known today as a student, assistant, and younger companion of Thomas Eakins, and their lives and careers were intertwined. However, he also forged an independent career as a noted sculptor and teacher in Philadelphia.

Murray was born in Philadelphia, the eleventh of twelve children of an Irish immigrant who worked as a stonemason. In 1886 he entered the Art Students League which had just been organized. He studied with Eakins who considered him his favorite pupil, encouraged him to be a sculptor, and in 1892 chose him as his studio assistant at the school. In 1890 Eakins also helped Murray obtain a position as instructor in modeling and lecturer on artistic anatomy at the Philadelphia School of Design for Women (now Moore College of Art and Design), a position he retained for fifty years.

Murray even shared Eakins's studio at 1330 Chestnut Street from 1892 until 1900. He was on close personal terms with the members of Eakins's household and their extended families. The two artists took bicycling, swimming, hunting, and fishing trips together, and accompanied each other to the theater, boxing matches, and museums in Philadelphia and New York.

The painter and sculptor made portraits of each other and their respective families. Murray was almost exclusively a portraitist and many of his subjects were also depicted by Eakins. Murray assisted Eakins with some sculptural commissions and Eakins offered criticism and collaborated with Murray on several of the latter's projects.[12]

After an engagement of almost twenty years, in 1916 Murray married Jennie Dean Kershaw, a graduate of the Pennsylvania Academy of the Fine Arts, and teacher of perspective at the Philadelphia School of Design for Women.[13]

Murray's reputation was mainly local and his style remained resolutely naturalistic, eschewing contemporary expressionist and modernist aesthetics. But he received numerous commissions and exhibited his works widely to an appreciative public. His full-length, bronze statues of Commodore John Barry, Dr. Joseph Leidy, Monsignor William Corby, Admiral George Wallace Melville, and Senator Boies Penrose were well received and displayed prominently. Other large-scale works include ten terra cotta *Prophets* for the Witherspoon Building in Philadelphia, reliefs and a monumental *Winged Victory* for the Pennsylvania State Memorial at Gettysburg National Military Park, and a *Crucifixion* for the Bishop Shanahan Memorial at St. Patrick's Cathedral in Harrisburg.

Samuel Murray exhibited regularly for almost four decades at the Pennsylvania Academy, twice at the National Academy of Design, and at the world's fairs in Chicago in 1893 (honorable mention), Buffalo in 1901 (honorable mention), St. Louis in 1904 where he exhibited thirteen works (silver medal), and Philadelphia in 1926. He won a gold medal in 1894 at the Art Club of Philadelphia and an honorable mention there in 1897.

The only one-man show during his lifetime was held in 1896 at the Academy, under the auspices of the Fairmount Park Commission. A two-person show in 1931 at the Fifty-sixth Street Galleries in New York was entitled *Paintings by Thomas Eakins, Sculpture by Samuel Murray*. A posthumous show devoted to Murray was held in 1982 at the Hirshhorn Museum and Sculpture Garden in Washington, D.C.

Portrait of William H. Greene

WILLIAM HOUSTON GREENE, M.D. (1853-1918)
By Samuel Aloysius Murray

Plaster
1916
25 1/4 x 20 5/8 x 11 5/8 in.

Signed and dated on rear below collar: "SAMUEL MURRAY/1916"
Exhibition: Philadelphia, *Annual Exhibition*, Pennsylvania Academy of the Fine Arts, 1917

Given in 1919 by the artist
Accession number: 1919+e.S.01

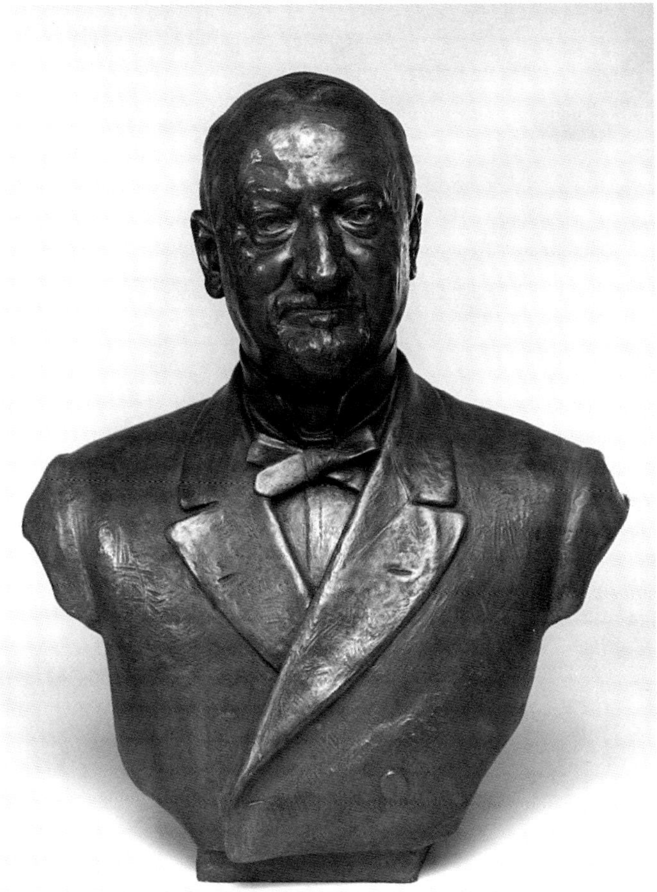

Dr. William H. Greene,[14] who gave the bust of Dr. James C. Wilson, was also the subject of a bust by Samuel Murray. Greene was a faculty member at Jefferson Medical College only briefly, but he was associated with Dr. Benjamin H. Rand and there are parallels between their careers.

William H. Greene was born in Columbia, Pennsylvania but his family soon moved to Philadelphia. He graduated from Jefferson Medical College in 1873, became an assistant to Professor Benjamin H. Rand, M.D., and in 1875 was made a demonstrator of chemistry. After pursuing research in Paris with Adolph Wurtz he returned to Philadelphia and was made demonstrator of chemistry at the University of Pennsylvania. In 1881 he was elected professor of chemistry at Central High School, a post once held by Dr. Rand. He resigned the chair in 1892 to pursue the printing business with his father.

Greene's literary productions include a translation and editing of Wurtz's *Elements of Modern Chemistry* (1879) and his own textbook, *A Practical Handbook of Medical Chemistry Applied to Clinical Research and the Detection of Poisons* (1880). He was a member of the American Philosophical Society, the American Association for the Advancement of Science, the Société Chimique of Paris, and the Chemical Society of London.

As in the naturalistic bust of Wilson, Samuel Murray's depiction of Greene suggests the robust physicality of the subject. However, Dr. Greene seems less somber and more animated, his expression suggesting a sense of curiosity or interest in the observer. There is a certain jauntiness and informality in the asymmetrical points of his shirt collar and bow tie, and in his suitcoat which is unbuttoned and has one lapel hanging open. This bust is made of plaster and painted dark greenish-brown to resemble bronze. A bronze version is in the collection of the Hirshhorn Museum and Sculpture Garden.

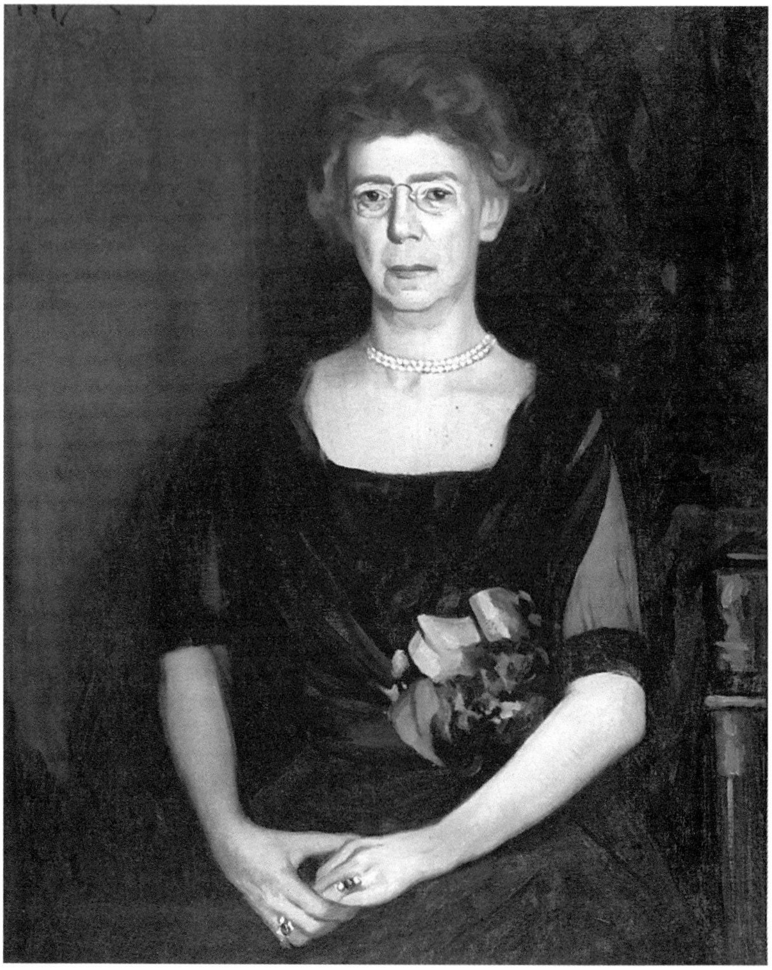

Portrait of Anna J. Magee

(See color plate)

ANNA JUSTINA MAGEE (1843-1923)
By Hugh Henry Breckenridge (1870-1937)

Oil on canvas
1917
37 x 30 in.

Signed upper left: "Hugh H. Breckenridge"

Commissioned in 1917 by JMC board of trustees
Accession number: 1917+e.P.01

Anna J. Magee was a grateful patient of Dr. James C. Wilson. A noted Philadelphia philanthropist, she was a generous benefactor to Jefferson Medical College, among many institutions.

Miss Magee was descended from Dutch immigrants who arrived in Philadelphia in 1753.[15] Her ancestors were very successful manufacturers and merchants of saddlery hardware. Her father expanded the business to New Orleans where he also invested in real estate. He was an incorporator and director of the Pennsylvania Railroad and a director of the Harrisburg Railroad. He was also the founder and first president of the Westmoreland Coal Company.

Little is known of Anna's childhood except that she was one of seven children. As an adult she was interested in many civic and religious organizations, including the Philadelphia Society of the Colonial Dames of America, the Philadelphia Chapter of the Daughters of the American Revolution, and the Pennsylvania School of Industrial Art. She was particularly generous to St. Stephen's Episcopal Church where her father was a vestryman, and donated a huge Venetian mosaic of *The Last Supper*, a choir screen, and furniture.

Anna J. Magee died in 1923 and left a bequest of over $1,250,000 to establish the Magee Memorial Hospital for Convalescents. She stipulated that her institution would receive patients regardless of sex, color, ethnic origin, or religion, excluding only children under fourteen years. Dr. Wilson was named a director of the hospital's first board.

During the intervening years before the institution opened in 1958 as Magee Rehabilitation Hospital, medical advances had made significant improvements in convalescent care, and so the original emphasis changed from convalescence to rehabilitation and "new hope for the disabled." Almost from its beginning the hospital has maintained an important affiliation with Jefferson.

Anna Magee also gave a gift of sixty thousand dollars to Jefferson Medical College in memory of her parents. The board of trustees resolved that the professorship of medicine should be designated the Magee Professorship of the Practice of Medicine and Clinical Medicine. The trustees also resolved that Miss Magee be requested to sit for a portrait.

It is said that Anna J. Magee was very aware of modern business trends but that socially she clung to the nineteenth century, preferring to use a horse-drawn carriage rather than an automobile. She was retiring and revealed little about herself even to acquaintances.

In the two-thirds-length, life-sized portrait by Hugh Breckenridge, Anna Magee is shown sitting erectly with hands clasped stiffly on her lap next to a French-style console table. Her black silk evening gown has gauzy, short sleeves and a large corsage with a pink, silk bow at the waist. Her conspicuous jewelry consists of a double strand, diamond necklace and two rings, one of diamonds and rubies, the other of diamonds and emeralds. Her choice of costume and accessories are in stark contrast to her prim posture and sober expression, emphasized by her fixed look behind a pince-nez, aquiline nose, pursed lips, and strong, angular jaw.

Hugh Breckenridge has captured Anna Magee's more confident and resolute demeanor rather than her mysterious and retiring side. Yet this confidence and resolution are not paralleled by the painting's loosely brushed surface and its prevailing brown and pink colors which are harmoniously and delicately balanced.

In 1958 Jefferson Medical College placed the portrait on long-term loan to Magee Rehabilitation Hospital. Today the painting is installed in the hospital's solarium, next to bust-length portraits of her parents, James and Caroline Magee, depicted by Samuel B. Waugh in 1878 and 1884, respectively.

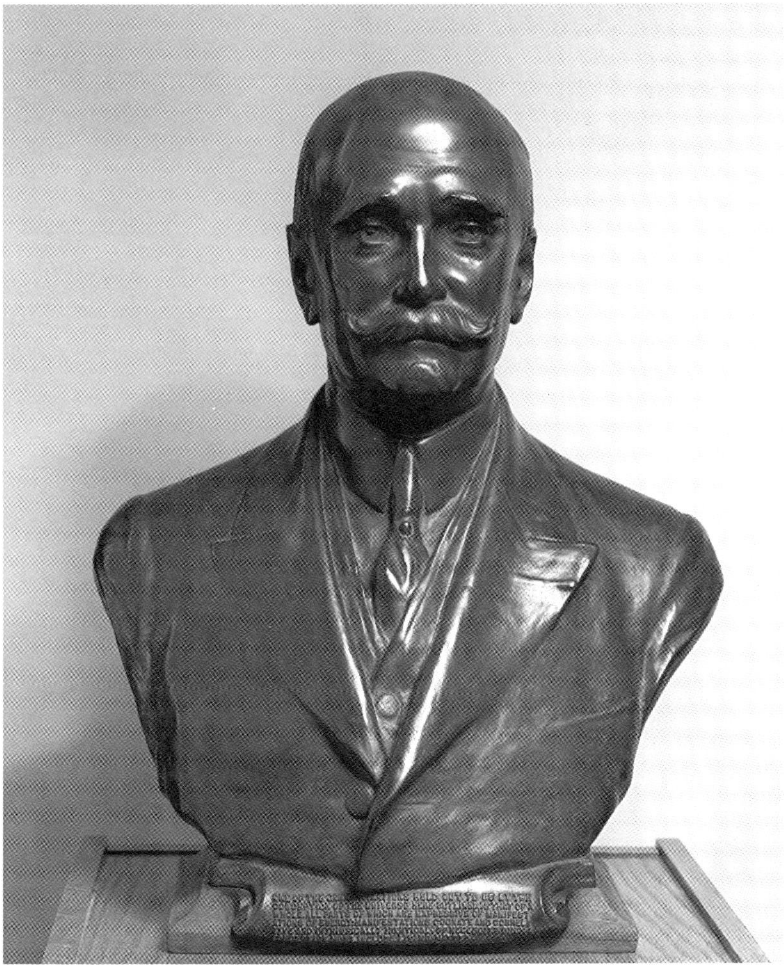

Portrait of Francis X. Dercum

FRANCIS X. DERCUM, M.D., Ph.D. (1856-1931)
By Carl Augustus Heber (1875-1956)

Bronze
1925
23 3/4 x 18 3/4 x 13 in.

Signed and dated right side of base: "C.A. HEBER/1925"
Inscription on rear of integral base: "Francis X. Dercum."
Inscription on front of integral base: "ONE OF THE GENERALIZATIONS HELD OUT TO US BY THE/ CONCEPTION OF THE UNIVERSE HERE OUTLINED, IS THAT OF A/WHOLE, ALL PARTS OF WHICH ARE EXPRESSIVE OF MANIFEST/ATIONS OF ENERGY: MANIFESTATIONS COGNATE AND CORRELA/TIVE AND INTRINSICALLY IDENTICAL, OF NECESSITY SUCH A/ CONCEPTION MUST INCLUDE LIVING MATTER/FRANCIS X. DERCUM, M.D."
Exhibition: Philadelphia, *Annual Exhibition,* Pennsylvania Academy of the Fine Arts, 1926; replica exhibited at the Academy, 1939

Given 1925-26 by Mrs. Francis X. Dercum, wife of the subject
Accession number: 1925-1926.S.01

With the appointment of Dr. Francis X. Dercum as clinical professor of nervous and mental diseases in 1892, the field of neurology was first established as a specialty at Jefferson. Through his writings and lectures, his reputation was worldwide.

A native Philadelphian, Dercum was born in 1856. He graduated from Central High School in 1873, received a master's degree the following year from the school, and earned doctorates in medicine and philosophy from the University of Pennsylvania in 1877. He was appointed chief of clinic and instructor of diseases of the nervous system at the university. Dr. Dercum was also made pathologist to the State Hospital for the Insane at Norristown, Pennsylvania, and consulting neurologist to the Philadelphia Hospital, among many other institutions.

In 1892 Dr. Francis X. Dercum was called to Jefferson Medical College, and by 1900 his chair was expanded to a full professorship of nervous and mental diseases. He headed this department until his retirement in 1925 when he was named emeritus professor. He was honorary president of the Francis X. Dercum Neurological Society, founded by Jefferson students in 1900. The class of 1911 dedicated its yearbook to him.

In 1884 Dr. Dercum had been a founder of the Philadelphia Neurological Society and he served twice as its president in 1892 and 1898. He also was president of the American Neurological Association and the American Philosophical Society. He was elected to several eminent European societies including the Society of Physicians of Vienna, the Royal Society of Medicine of London, the Psychiatric and Neurological Society of Vienna, and the Royal Medical Society of Budapest. He was one of only fifty members worldwide of the Société de Neurologie de Paris. In 1923 he was made a chevalier of the French Legion of Honor. In addition he received an honorary doctor of science degree from Jefferson Medical College in 1928.

He described a new disease, adiposis dolorosa, known abroad as Dercum's disease. He was editor of *A Text-book on Nervous Diseases by American Authors* (1895), and author of the following texts: *Rest, Mental Therapeutics, Suggestion* (1903), *A Clinical Manual of Mental Disorders* (1913), *Hysteria and Accident Compensation: Nature of Hysteria and the Lesson of the Post-litigation Results* (1916), *An Essay on the Physiology of Mind: An Interpretation Based on Biological, Morphological, Physical and Chemical Considerations* (1922), and *The Biology of the Internal Secretions: the Endocrine Factor in Development, in Subnormalities, in Neoplasms and Malignancy, in Nervous and Mental Diseases and in Heredity* (1924).

Dercum was admired by students and colleagues for his ability to develop the signs and symptoms of his cases with descriptive clarity and precision. He enjoyed a special reputation as an expert witness in medicolegal cases concerning questions of nervous diseases and insanity. Dercum was called to the bedside of President Woodrow Wilson and headed the team of consulting neurologists attending the president during his stroke.

While an instructor at the University of Pennsylvania Dercum participated in Eadweard Muybridge's experiments with serial motion photography there. The neurologist contributed an essay on the clinical aspects of certain nervous afflictions, "A Study of Some Normal and Abnormal Movements," to the publication *Animal Locomotion: The Muybridge Work at the University of Pennsylvania: The Method and the Result* (1888).[16]

The bronze sculpture of Dr. Francis X. Dercum by Carl A. Heber is a straightforward, bust-length depiction. Dressed in business attire, the physician gazes directly at the viewer with deepset eyes and a neutral expression. The subject's almost totally bald head is contrasted with his luxuriant, upswept mustache. The sculpture's smooth surface reflects and absorbs light and shadow dramatically. An unusual addition is the volute-shaped, integral base bearing a philosophical quotation from Dercum.

The bust was presented by Mrs. Francis X. Dercum and was displayed in the library. It was exhibited at the Pennsylvania Academy of the Fine Arts in 1926 at the *Annual Exhibition.* A replica owned by Mrs. Dercum was exhibited at the Academy in 1939.

Sculptor Carl A. Heber was born in Stuttgart, Germany in 1875. He studied art at the Art Institute of Chicago, and at the Académie Julian and École des Beaux-Arts in Paris. In addition to portrait busts he sculpted many public monuments including the *Schiller Monument* in Rochester, New York, *Benjamin Franklin* at Princeton University, the *Soldiers and Sailors Monument* in Geneva, Illinois, *Roman Epic Poetry* at the Brooklyn Museum, and *Pastoral* at the St. Louis Museum of Fine Arts. Other works in Philadelphia can be found at the U.S. Post Office, the University of Pennsylvania Museum, and St. Ann's Church.

Heber's awards include bronze medals at the St. Louis Exposition (1904) and the Panama-Pacific Exposition in San Francisco (1915), and a prize at the American Institute of Architects and T-square Club joint exhibition in Philadelphia. He exhibited works at the National Sculpture Society in 1923.

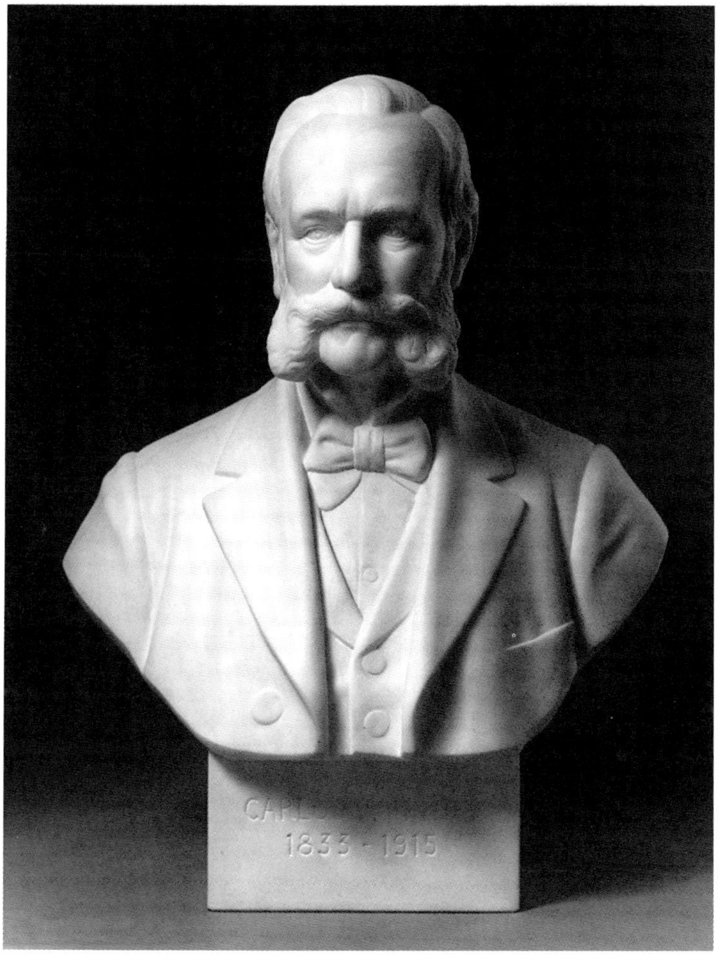

Portrait of Carlos J. Finlay

CARLOS JUAN FINLAY, M.D. (1833-1915)
By Tony Lopez (b. 1918), after Auguste Maillard

Marble
1955
30 3/8 x 23 3/4 x 14 1/4 in.

Signed and dated on beveled edge of left shoulder: "Tony Lopez HAbANA/CUBA 1955"
Inscription on front of integral base: "CARLOS J. FINLAY/1833-1915"

Given in 1955 by the Republic of Cuba
Accession number: 1955+e.S.01

One of Jefferson Medical College's most celebrated alumni was Dr. Carlos J. Finlay, a native of Cuba. He was the discoverer of the transmitting agent of yellow fever, a scourge that was soon eradicated from the tropics.

Carlos J. Finlay was born in 1833 in Camagüey, the son of a Scottish-born physician and a Frenchwoman from Trinidad. After a secondary education in France and Germany, Finlay graduated from Jefferson Medical College in 1855.

During this period the city had another virulent epidemic of yellow fever. Finlay was impressed with the views about experimental corroboration of scientific theories of his professor, Dr. John K. Mitchell, and his preceptor, Mitchell's son Dr. S. Weir Mitchell. When Finlay returned to Cuba he maintained a busy practice while developing a reputation in epidemiology.

In 1879 he was appointed the representative to the American Yellow Fever Commission in Havana. In 1881 Finlay presented the results of his experiments first to the International Sanitary Commission in Washington, D.C., and then to the Royal Academy of Medical Sciences of Havana with a paper, "The Mosquito Hypothetically Considered as the Agent of Transmission of Yellow Fever." Even though initial reactions to his work ranged from indifference to ridicule, he continued to publish his results that the disease was not transmitted by contact or through the air, but by the bite of a mosquito. He identified the female mosquito, *Culex fasciatus*, today known as *Aedes aegypti*, as the vector, but he was unable to provide indisputable proof.

The control of yellow fever became an urgent challenge to the United States during the Spanish-American War and the occupation of Cuba. When the United States Army Commission headed by Dr. Walter Reed arrived in Cuba in 1900, the skeptical major at first rejected Finlay's theories. But after eliminating other causes, Reed set up an isolated, controlled experimentation camp with civilian and army volunteers, even commission members. They discovered why Finlay had been unable to prove his theory that yellow fever was not contagious.

Although some participants felt that certain commission members deflected too much credit from Finlay at first, he later became an international hero. He became Cuba's first Director of Health in 1902. His many honors included the Mary Kingsley Medal of the Liverpool School of Tropical Medicine, the Insignia of the French Legion of Honor, and membership in the French Academy of Medicine. He received an honorary Sc.D. degree from Jefferson Medical College in 1902 and honorary fellowship in the College of Physicians of Philadelphia.

Finlay's work made practicable the building of the Panama Canal, and the cleaning up of Havana and other cities. Finlay institutes and laboratories were established in Havana and in Panama. The Pan-American Medical Congress celebrated Finlay's birthday as the official Day of American Medicine. The centenary of his birth was also celebrated by the Academy of Medicine of Paris, and the city named a street after him.

In 1955 Jefferson Medical College celebrated the centenary of Finlay's graduation from the school with a two-day international symposium on yellow fever, in cooperation with officials of the Cuban government and the Pan American Sanitary Bureau. Cuba conferred upon Jefferson Medical College the Great Cross of the National Order of Merit Carlos J. Finlay.

Cuba had erected a bust of Finlay in the great hall of its Academy of Medical, Physical, and Natural Sciences in Havana. This work was sculpted by Auguste Maillard. A replica signed by Cuban artist Tony Lopez was presented by the Republic of Cuba to Jefferson Medical College at the Finlay Day celebration.

It can be seen that the marble bust of Finlay is an idealized, neoclassical depiction, when compared with contemporary photographs of the physician. His serious expression is emphasized by knitted eyebrows. His upper lip is totally obscured by the thick, wavy mustache and mutton chop whiskers which look more solid and dense than natural hair. The carving is utterly smooth with no visible tool marks.

It is unknown when the original bust of Finlay was sculpted, and no biographical information about Auguste Maillard has yet been found. The copyist Tony Lopez was born in Havana in 1918, the son and grandson of sculptors originally from Spain. Lopez studied at the Escuela Tecnica where his father was a professor, and where he was appointed an assistant professor in 1936. After joining revolutionary protests against Fulgencio Batista, in 1958 Lopez was ordered to leave the country on two days' notice, and relocated to Miami where he maintained his studio ever since.

Lopez's portrait busts and monuments can be found in public buildings, parks, and museums in Latin America and the United States. In Miami there are busts of Booker T. Washington, presidents Washington, Jefferson, and Andrew Jackson, a monument entitled *Torch of Friendship*, and an altar at St. Bernardino Church. Lopez sculptures are also located in Washington, D.C., Chicago, and Baltimore.

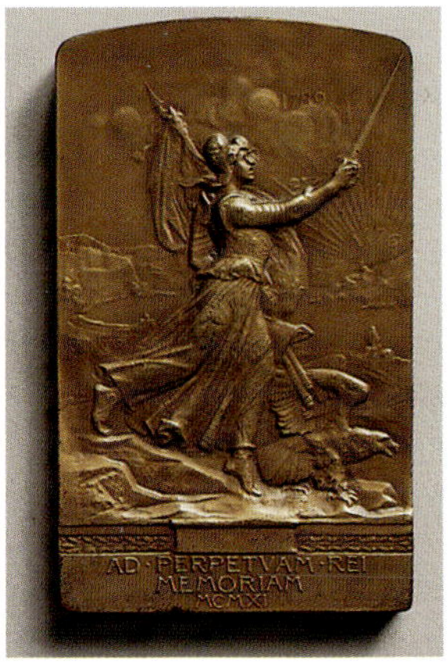

Medal of the Marquis de Lafayette (reverse) (see page 613)

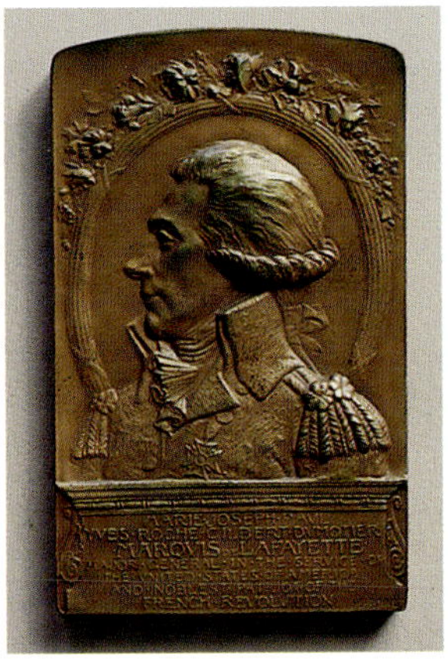

Medal of the Marquis de Lafayette by Jules Edouard Roine (obverse) (see page 613)

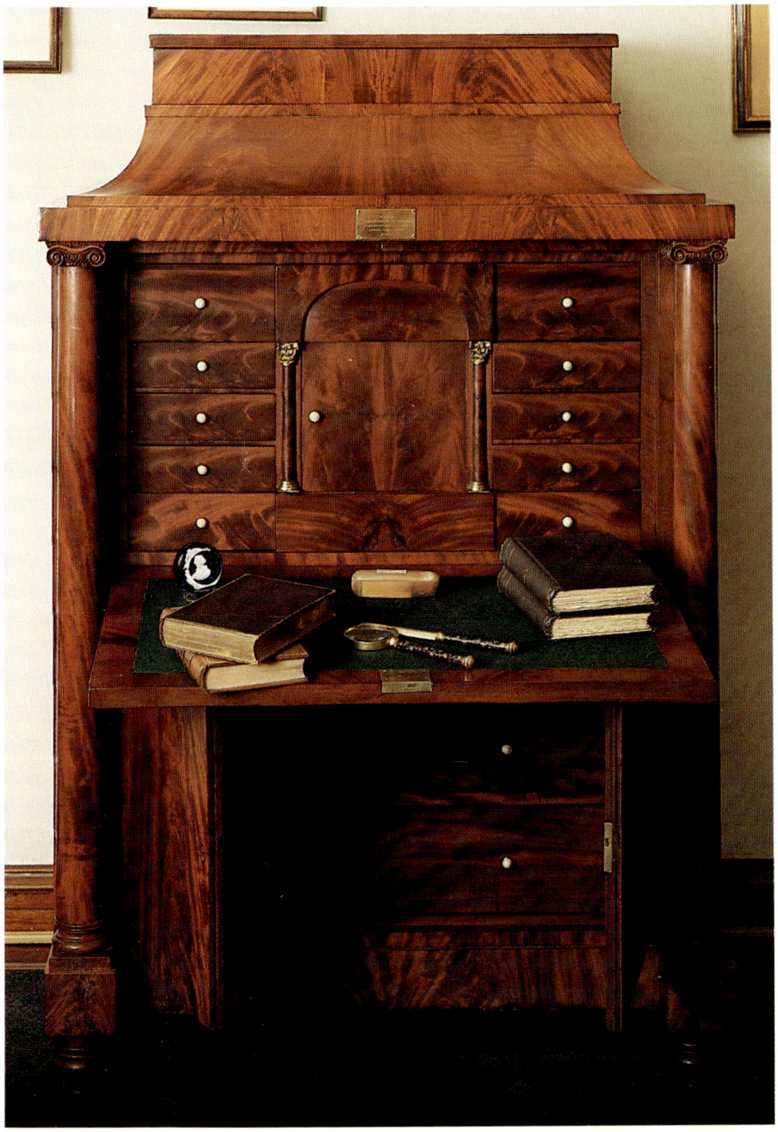

Desk of George McClellan (the founder) (see page 43)

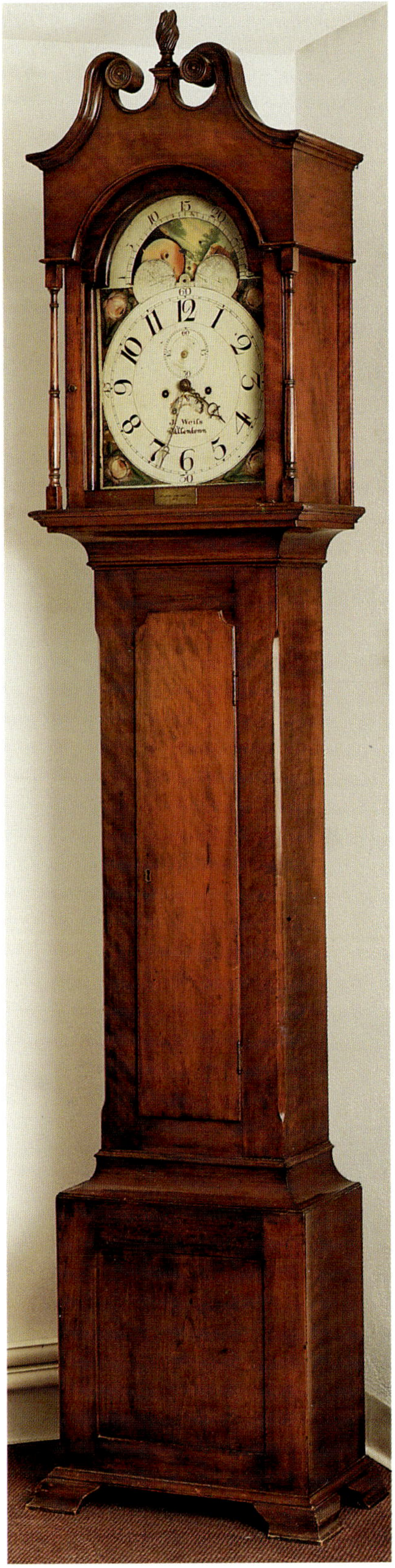

Tall Case Clock by Joseph Weiss (see page 474)

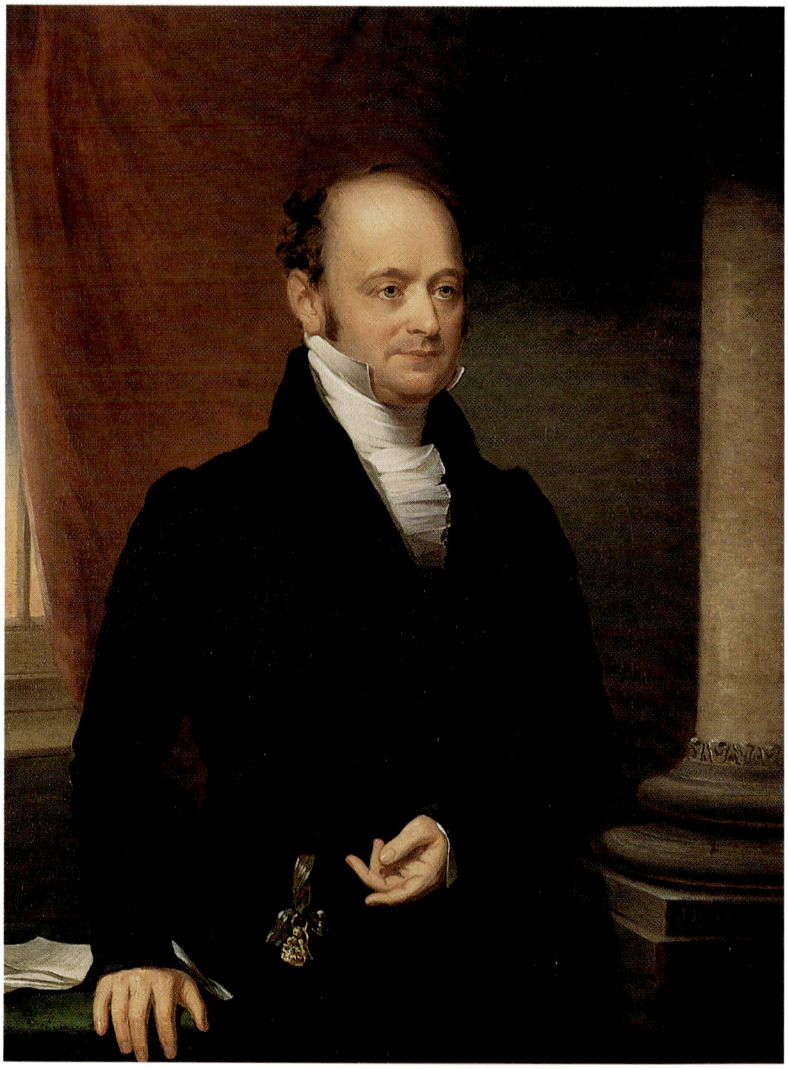

Portrait of John Eberle
by Jacob Eichholtz
(see page 47)

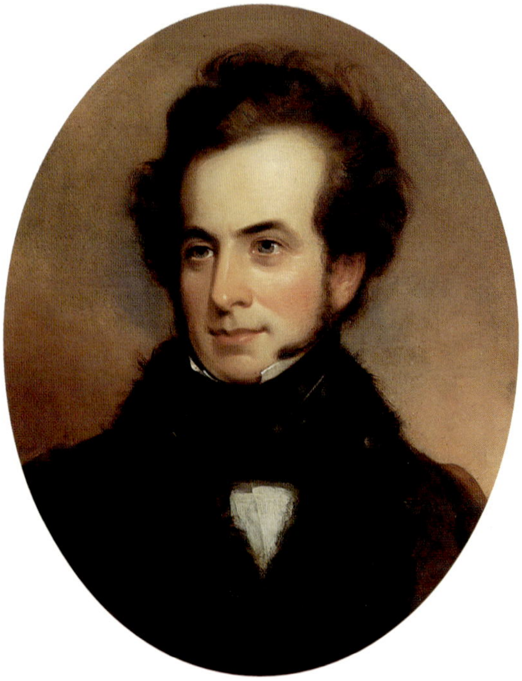

Portrait of Thomas D. Mütter
by Thomas Sully
(see page 72)

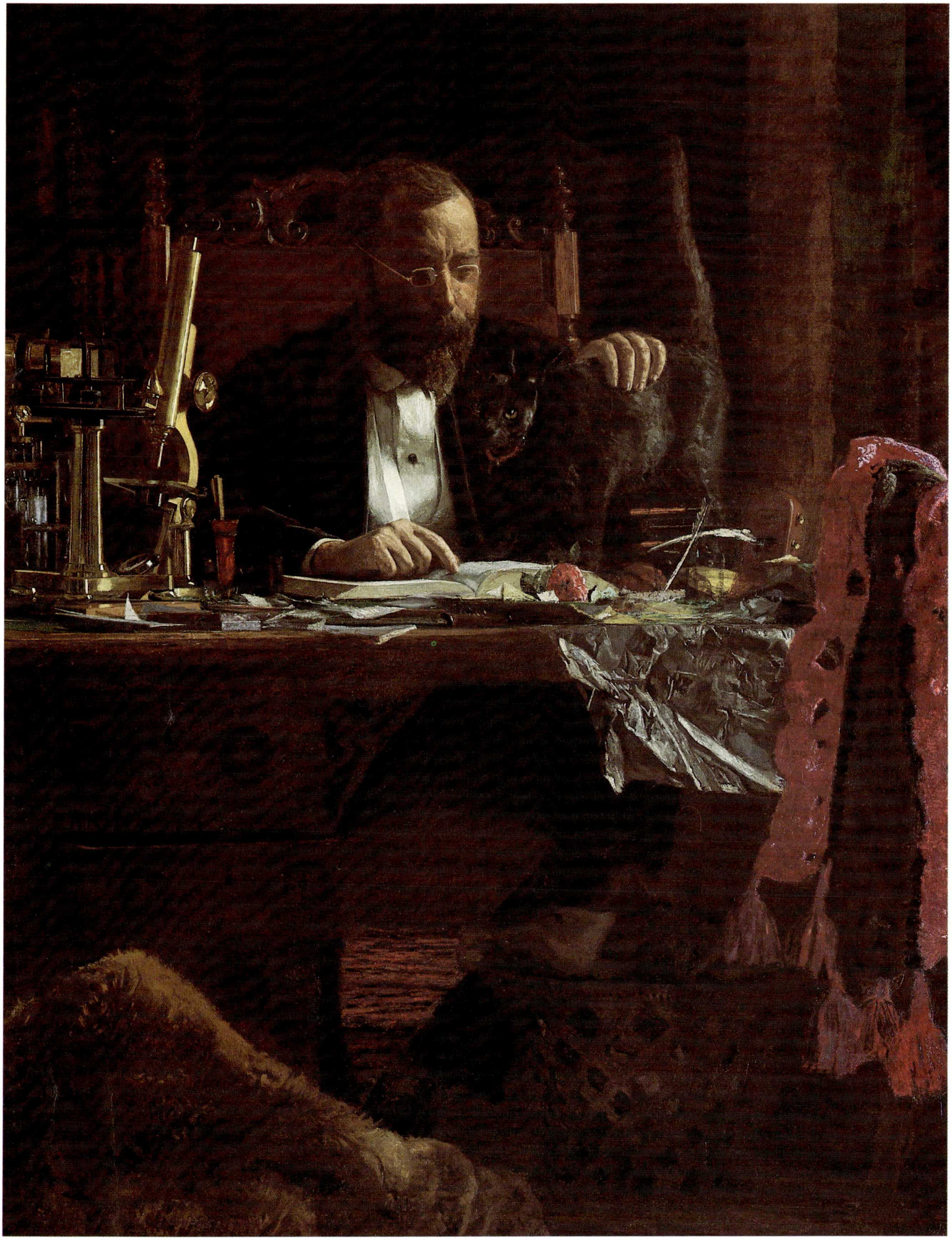

Portrait of Benjamin H. Rand by Thomas Eakins (see page 135)

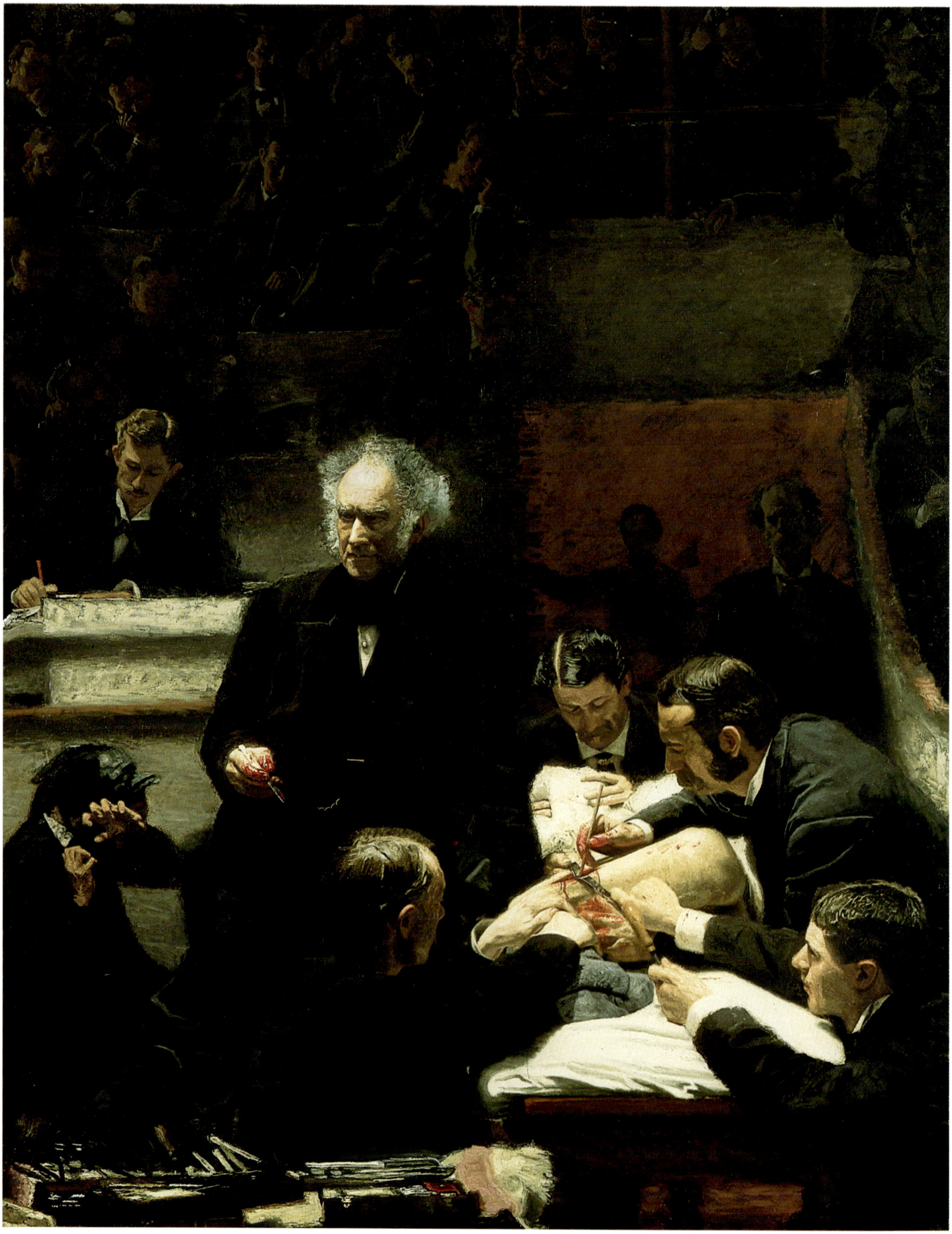

The Gross Clinic by Thomas Eakins (see page 162)

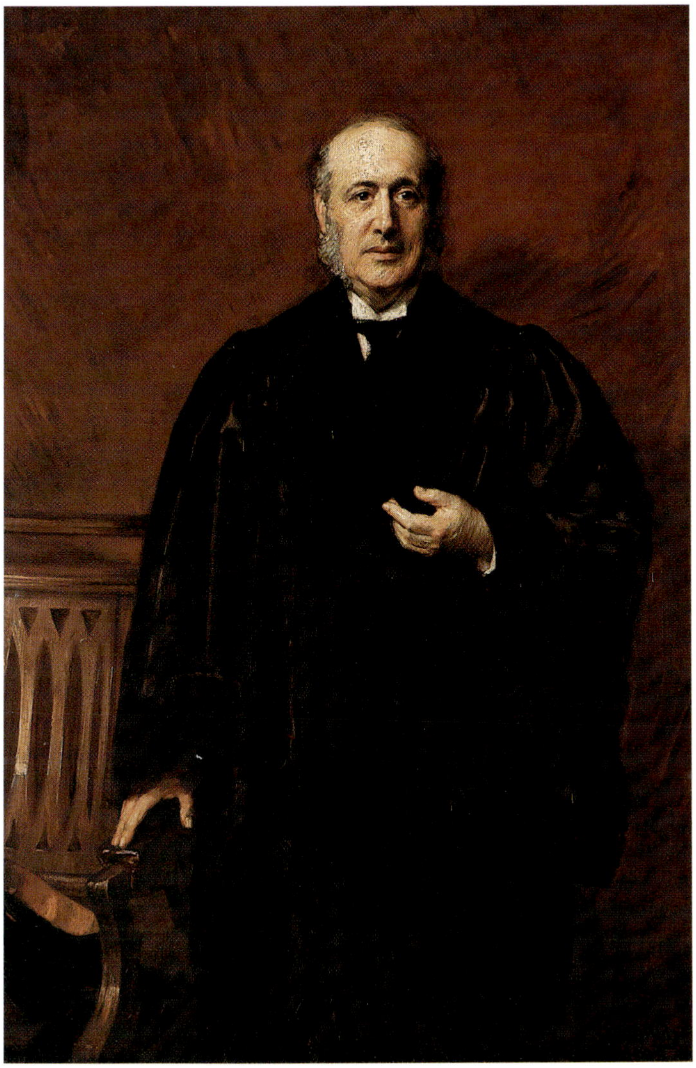

Portrait of Jacob M. DaCosta
by Robert W. Vonnoh
(see page 218)

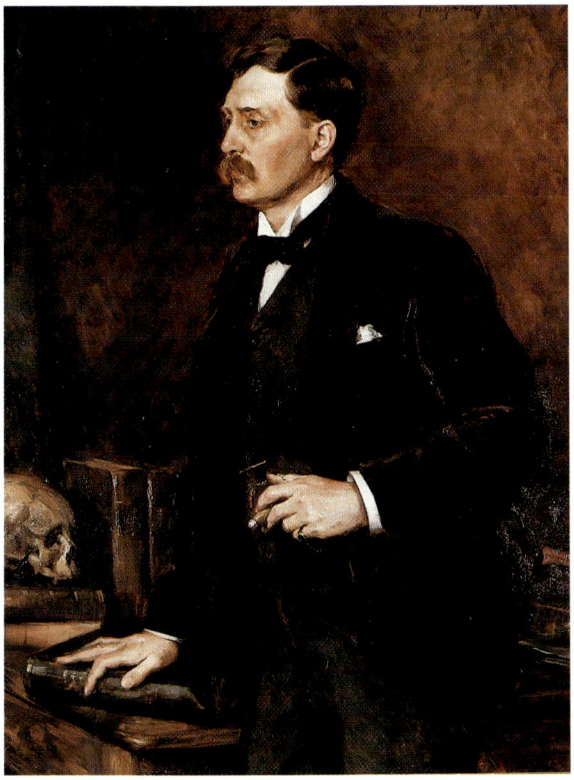

Portrait of George McClellan
(grandson of founder)
by Julian R. Story
(see page 275)

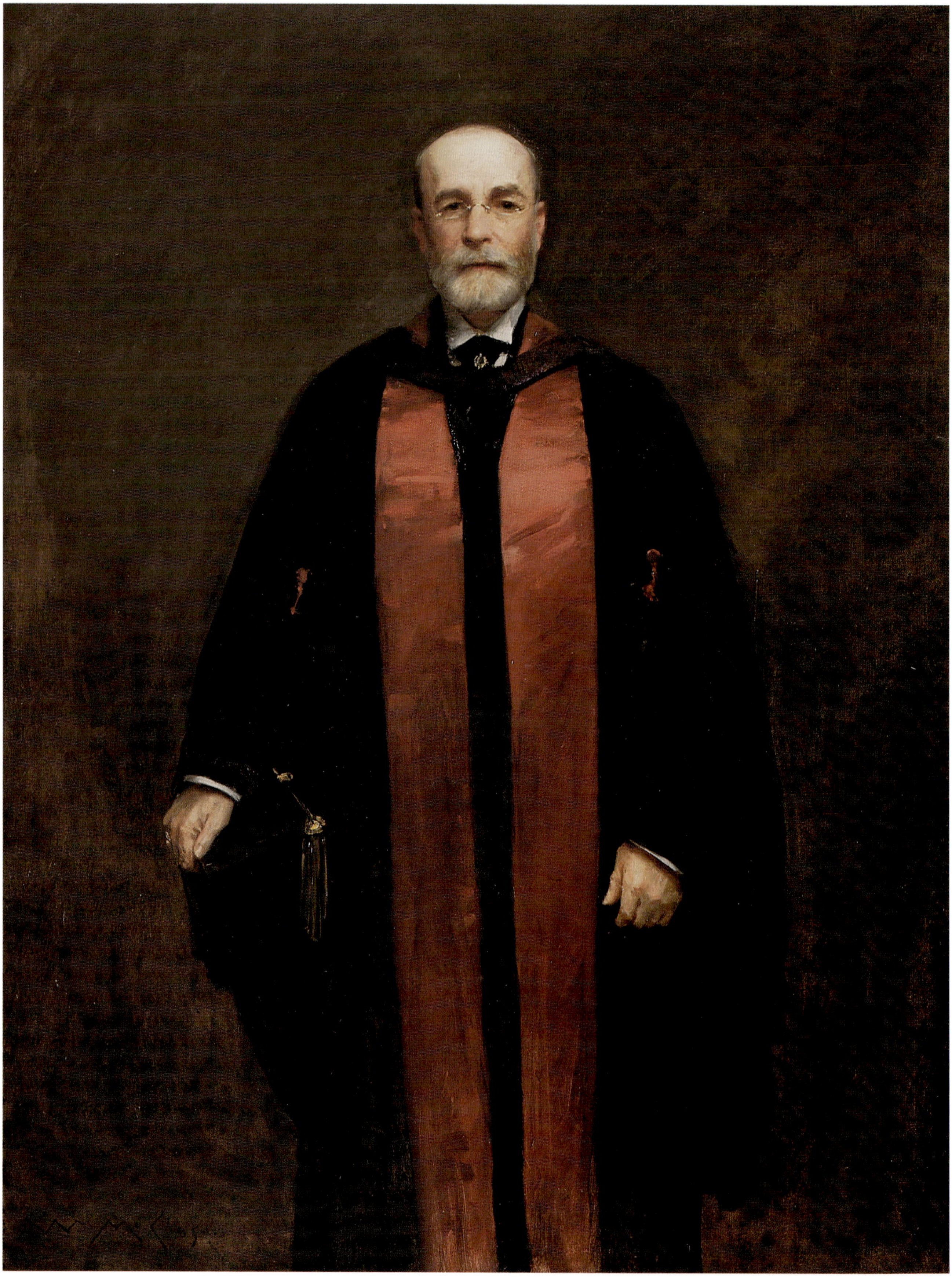

Portrait of William W. Keen Jr. by William Merritt Chase (see page 224)

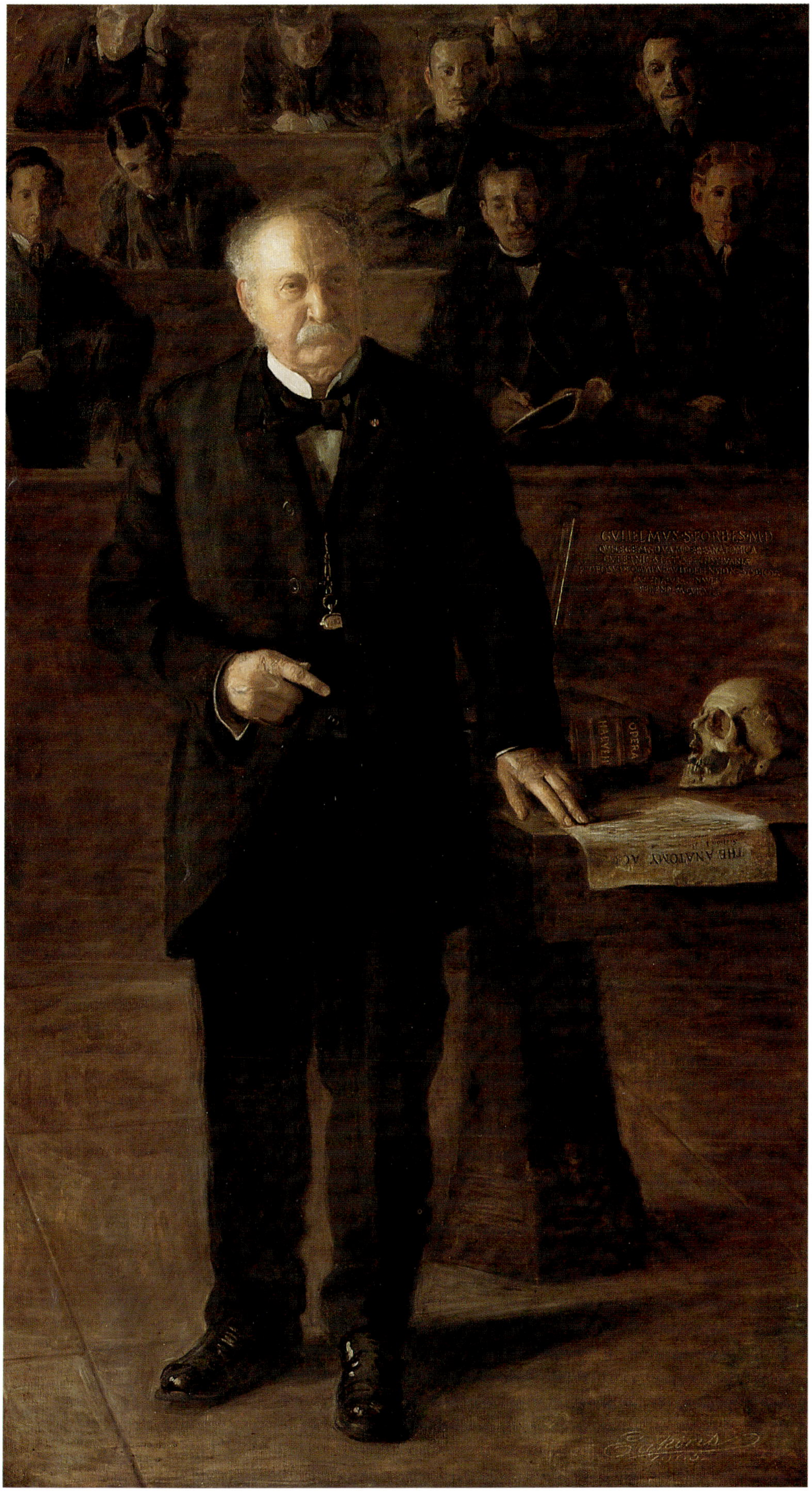

Portrait of William S. Forbes
by Thomas Eakins
(see page 238)

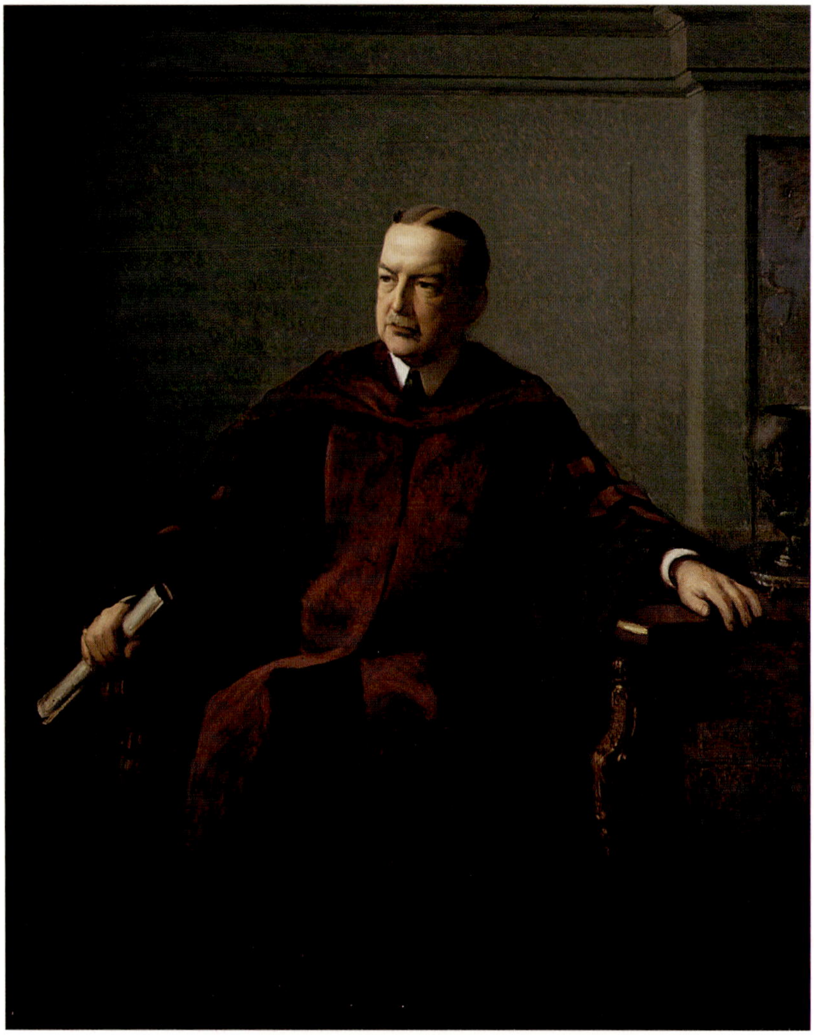

Portrait of William Potter
by Hugh H. Breckenridge
(see page 278)

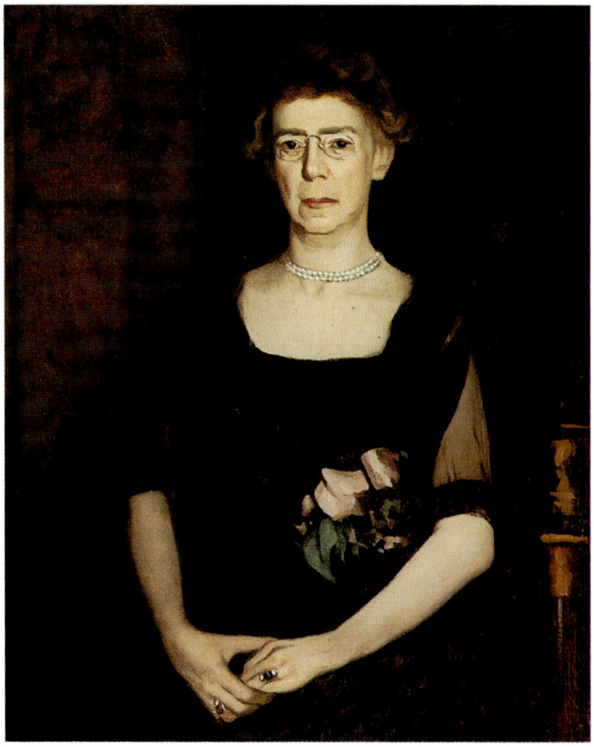

Portrait of Anna J. Magee
by Hugh H. Breckenridge
(see page 284)

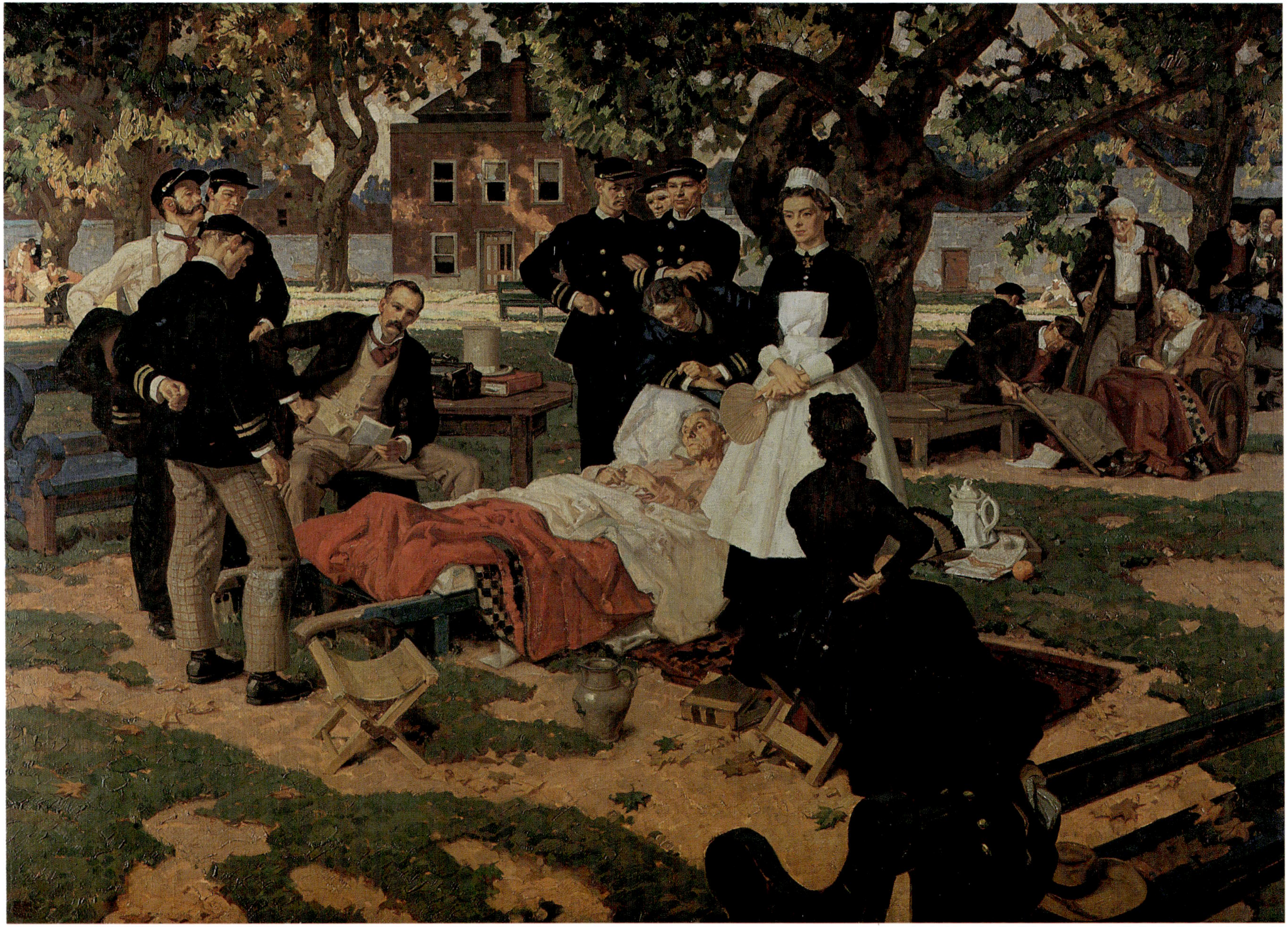

Osler at Old Blockley by Dean Cornwell (see page 247)

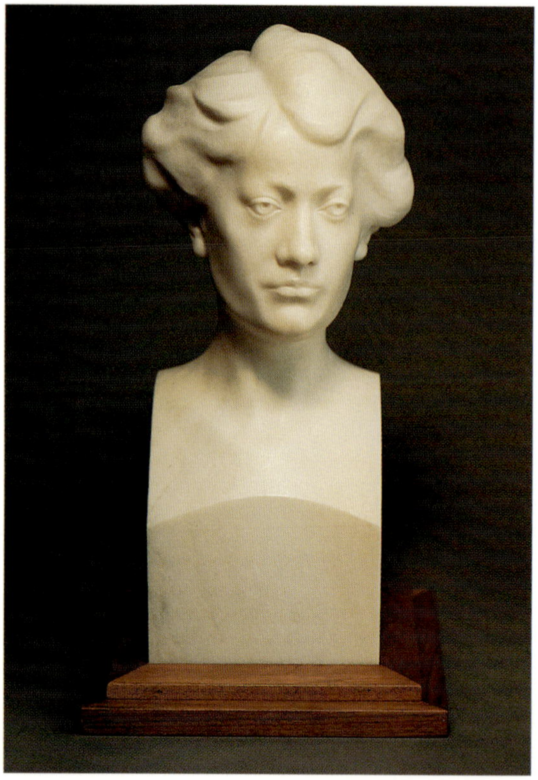

Portrait of Mary R. Cardeza
by Liamji (?) Kolomeier
(see page 348)

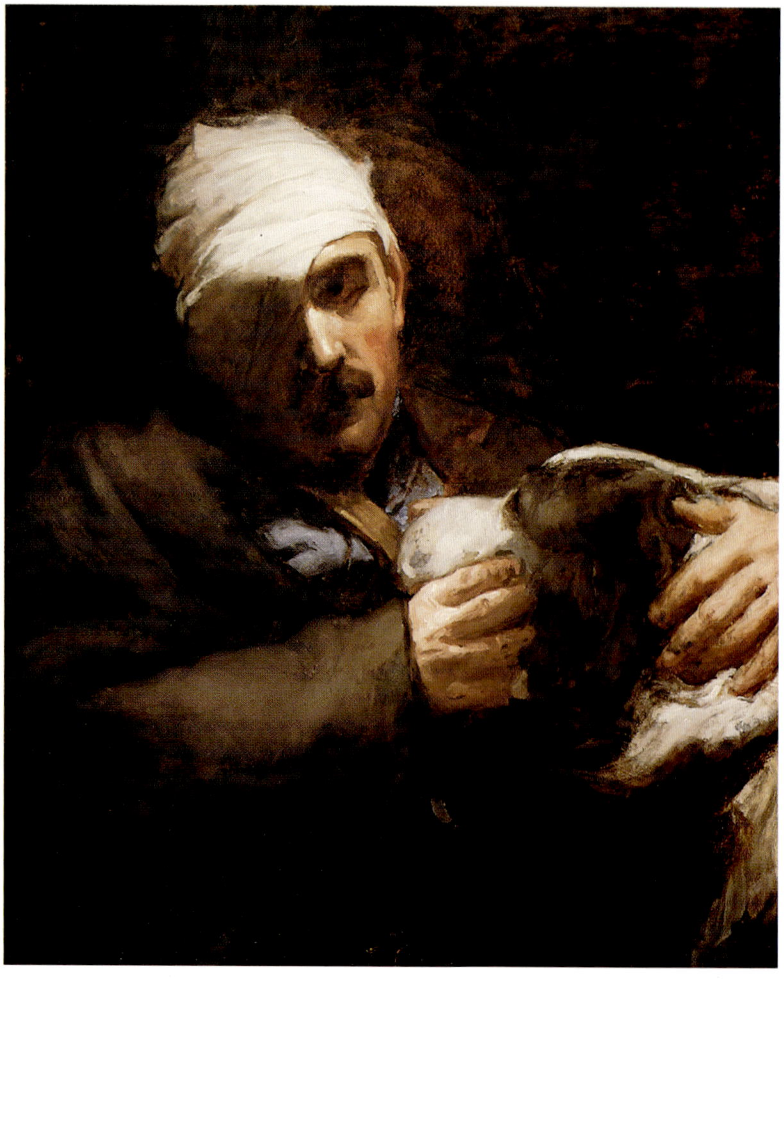

Portrait of a Soldier
by Susan M. Eakins
(see page 614)

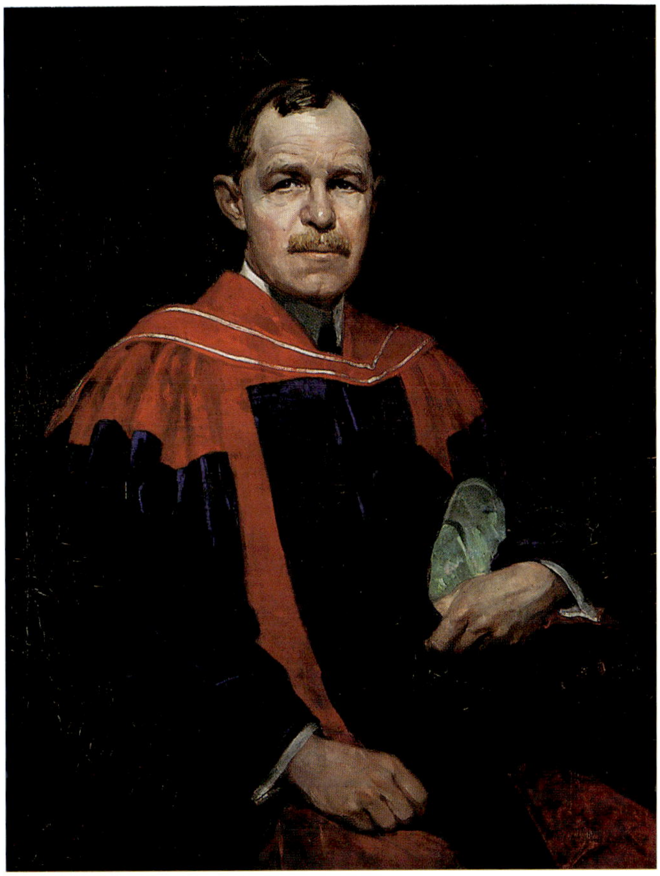

Portrait of Thomas McCrae
by William T. Thomson
(see page 334)

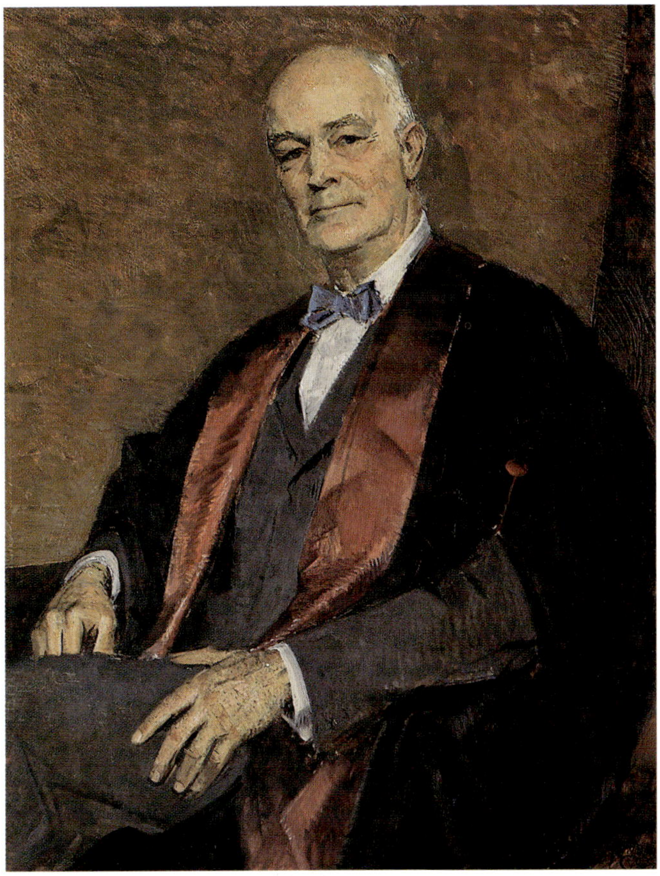

Portrait of John H. Gibbon Jr.
by Gardner Cox
(see page 429)

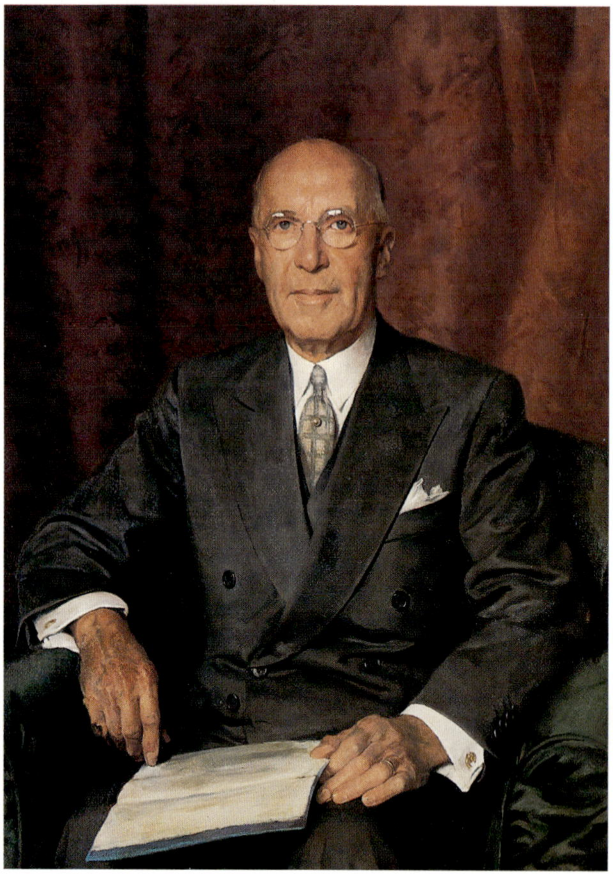

Portrait of Percival E. Foerderer
by Sir Gerald F. Kelly
(see page 398)

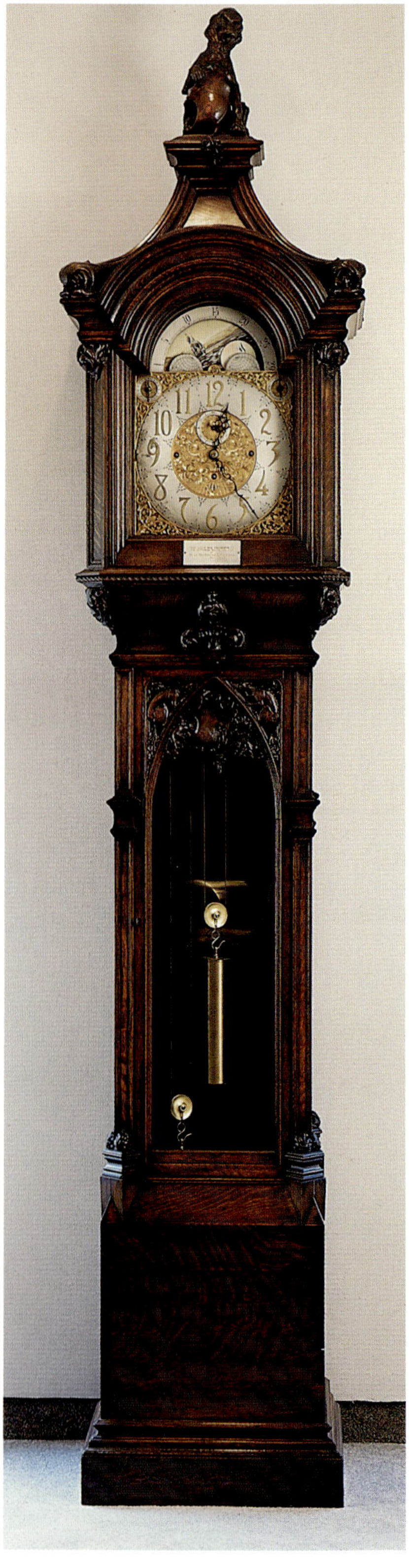

Tall Case Clock donated by Percival E. Foerderer (see page 403)

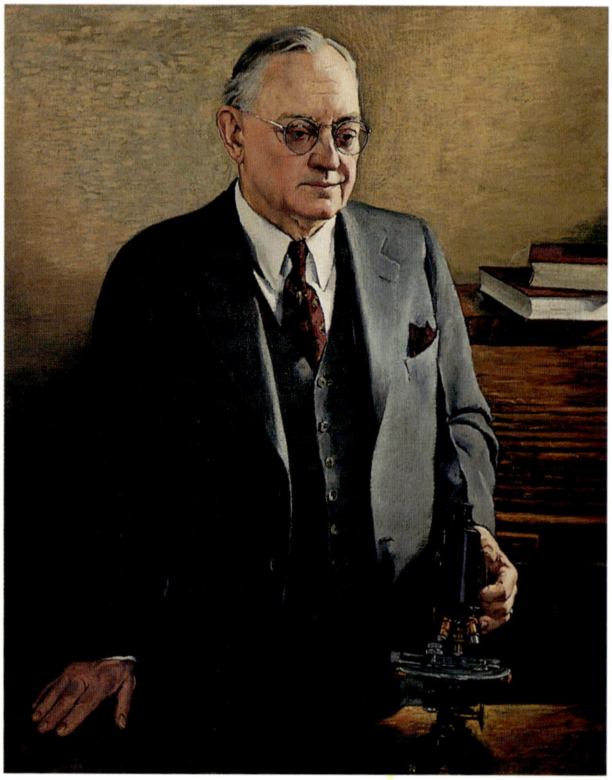

Portrait of Henry E. Radasch
by Roy C. Nuse
(see page 376)

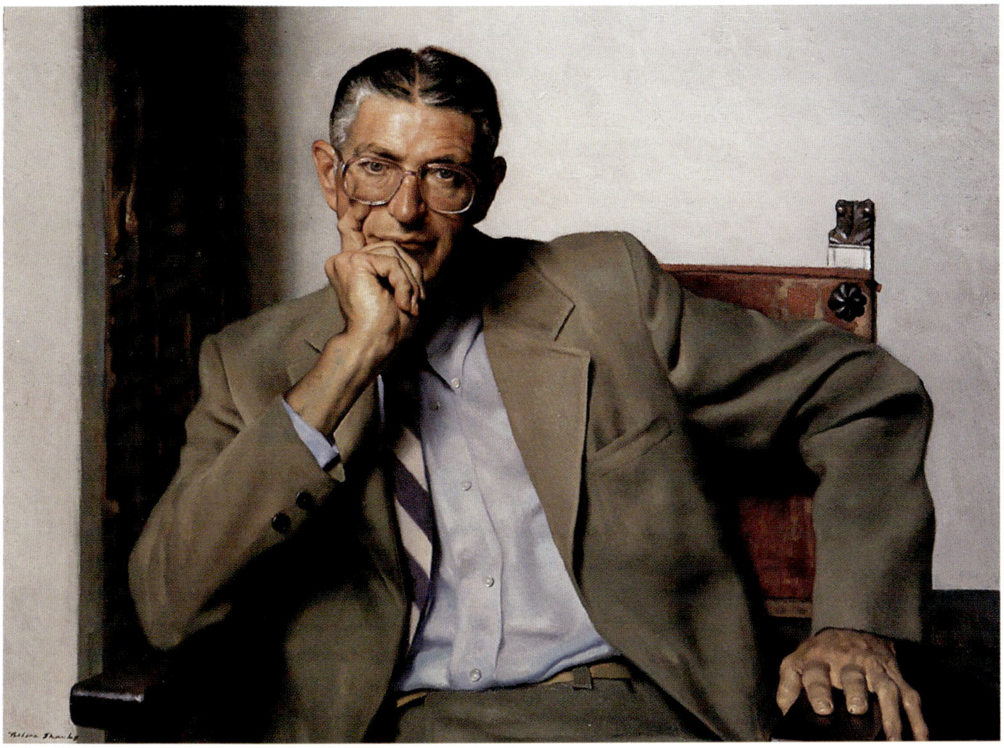

Portrait of Thomas D. Duane
by Nelson Shanks
(see page 513)

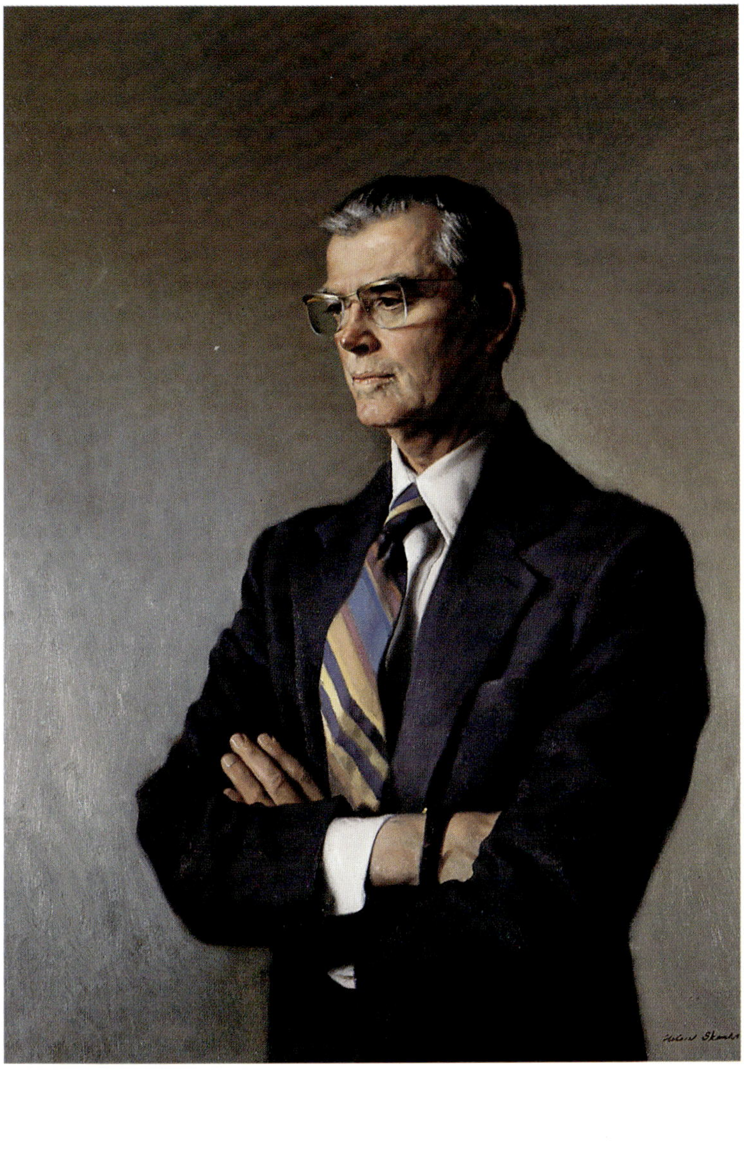

Portrait of John Y. Templeton III
by Nelson Shanks
(see page 500)

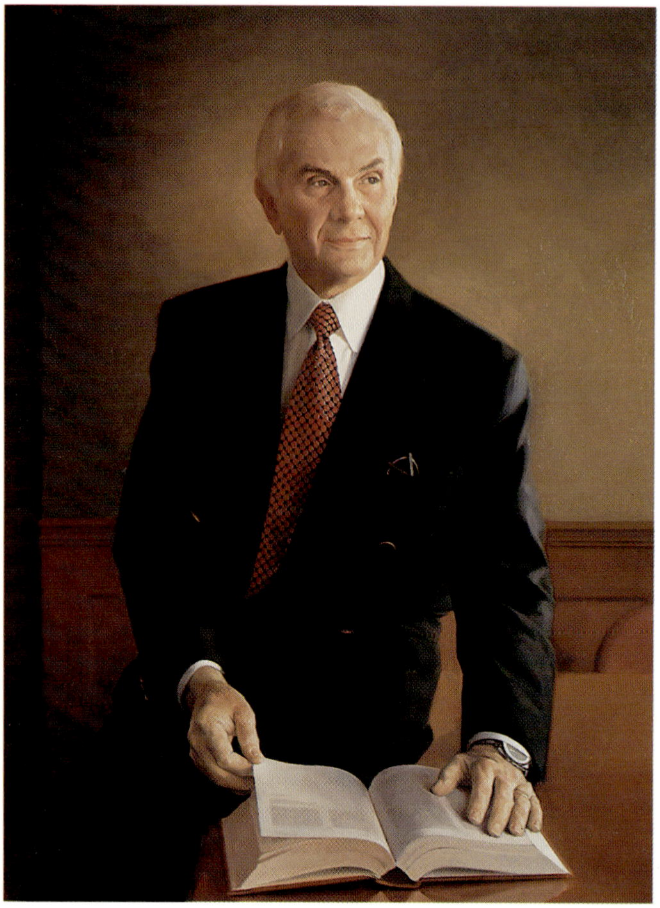

Portrait of Jewell L. Osterholm
by Mark E. Skolsky
(see page 575)

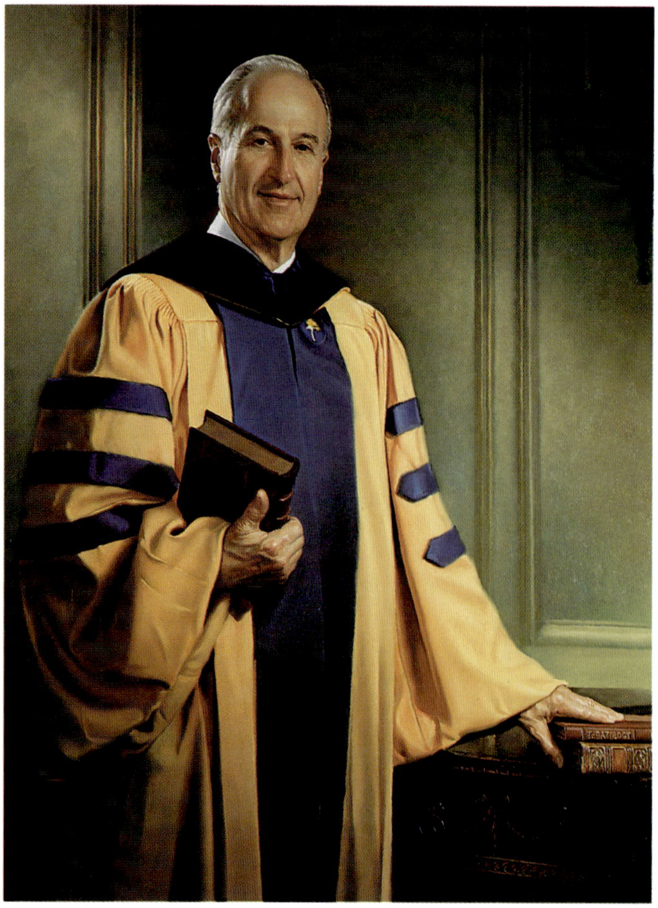

Portrait of Robert L. Brent
by Dean L. Paules
(see page 559)

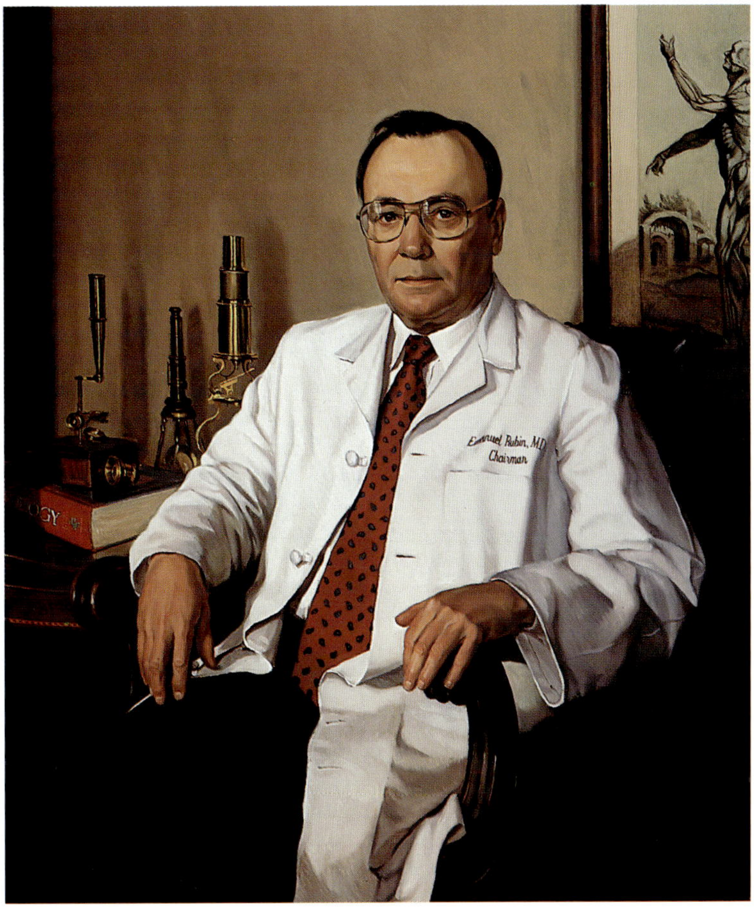

Portrait of Emanuel Rubin
by Russell W. Recchion
(see page 583)

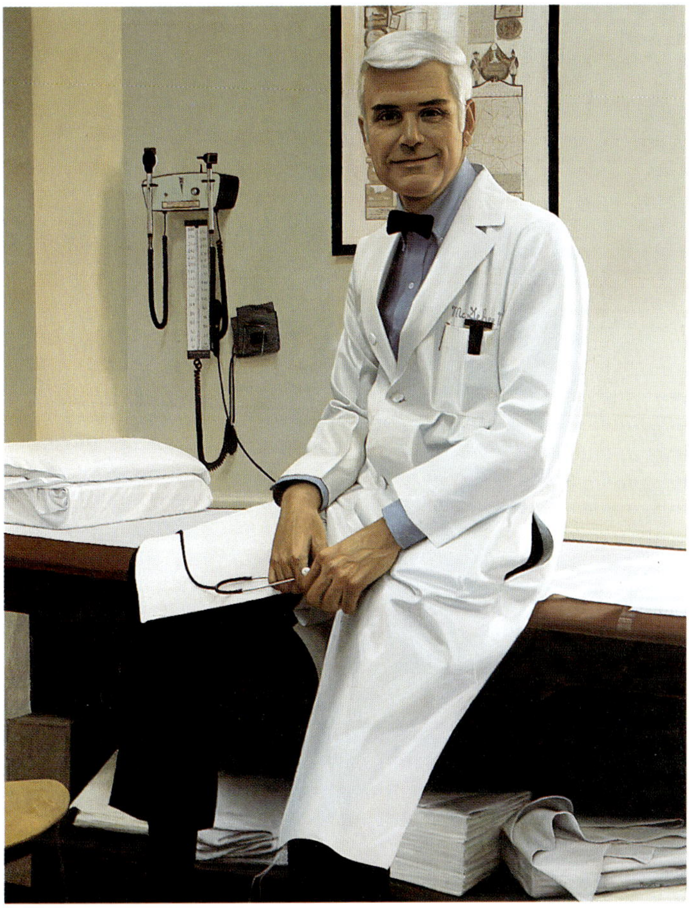

Portrait of Edward H. McGehee
by José F. Marcote
(see page 554)

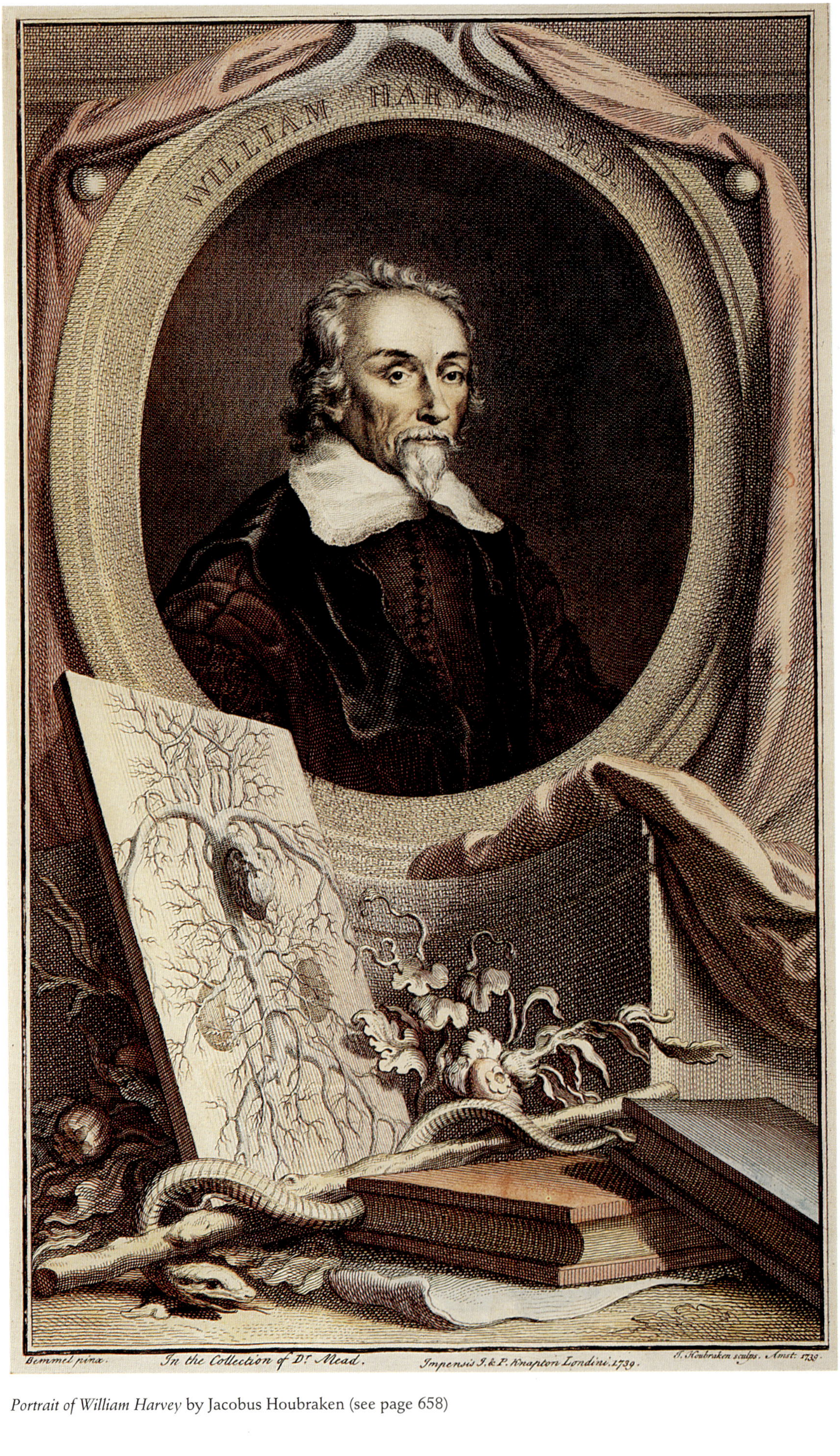

Portrait of William Harvey by Jacobus Houbraken (see page 658)

Department for Diseases of the Chest

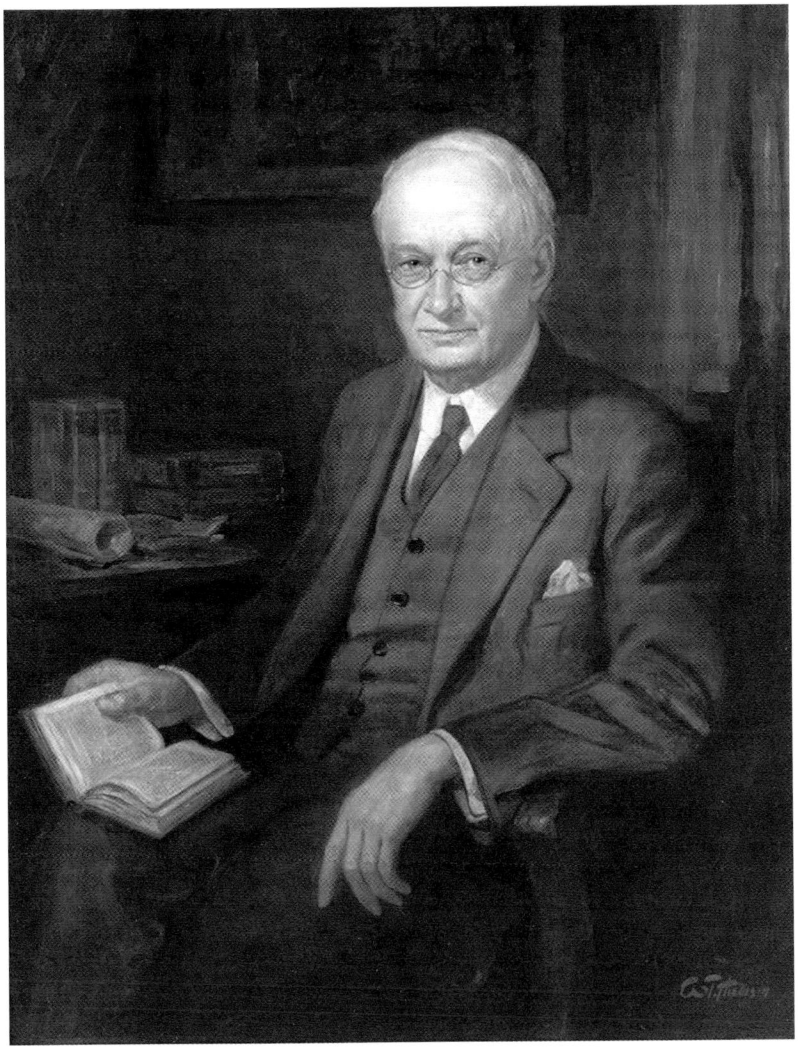

Portrait of Lawrence F. Flick

LAWRENCE FRANCIS FLICK, M.D. (1856-1938)
By William Taylor Thomson (1858-1941)

Oil on canvas
Before 1934
50 x 40 in.

Signed lower right: "W. T. Thomson"
Exhibition: Philadelphia, Bellevue-Stratford Hotel, at a meeting of the Pennsylvania Tuberculosis Society in conjunction with the Fiftieth Annual Meeting of the National Tuberculosis Association, May 6-9, 1942

Given in 1934 by unknown donor
Accession number: 1934+e.P.01

Dr. Lawrence F. Flick was a pioneering physician and crusader for the understanding and treatment of tuberculosis. He was responsible for the establishment of a department for diseases of the chest at Jefferson Medical College.

Lawrence F. Flick was born in 1856 in Cambria County, Pennsylvania.[17] He had to leave St. Vincent's College just before graduation because of a bout with tuberculosis from which he recovered without treatment. After graduating from Jefferson Medical College in 1879 he interned at Blockley and opened an office for the practice of medicine in Philadelphia.

After becoming ill with tuberculosis again he first attempted to recuperate by resting and walking in the countryside, then agreed to "go west" for a cure. He finally returned to his father's farm where he concentrated on a regime of rest, fresh air, milk, and eggs, and gradually improved so that he could resume his medical practice in Philadelphia by 1882.

He had early accepted the principle of communicability and began a crusade to promote medical and lay understanding of the contagiousness of tuberculosis. A scholarly paper he delivered in 1890 contributed to the organization of the Rush Hospital for Consumption and Allied Diseases and to the Society for the Prevention of Tuberculosis. This society evolved into the Pennsylvania Tuberculosis Society which laid the groundwork for the National Tuberculosis Association.

The society's programs for public education convinced local legislatures to pass laws against public spitting and against the sale of milk and meat from tuberculous cows, and for the compulsory disinfection of houses which had been occupied by consumptives, and for appropriations for hospitals and sanitariums.

Dr. Flick was a leader in fund-raising to pay for hospital care for tuberculosis patients. Since few hospitals would accept these patients, he established the Free Hospital for Poor Consumptives and the White Haven Sanatorium in the Pocono Mountains near Hazelton, Pennsylvania in 1901. The sanatorium promulgated Flick's principles of rest, nutritious food, fresh air, and limited exercise, and he was its president and medical director until 1935. The sanatorium was turned over to Jefferson in 1946 and was sold to the Commonwealth of Pennsylvania in 1956.

In 1903 Dr. Flick was also responsible for establishing the Henry Phipps Institute for the Study, Treatment, and Prevention of Tuberculosis in Philadelphia where he introduced the clinical and pathological conference which discussed patients at regular meetings and placed emphasis on autopsy findings. When the institute was taken over by the University of Pennsylvania in 1910 Flick was replaced as director.

Dr. Flick and the Phipps Institute were in the forefront of establishing the National Association for the Study and Prevention of Tuberculosis in 1904, and convening international conferences on tuberculosis in Paris in 1905 and in Washington in 1908. Flick was instrumental in organizing the department for diseases of the chest at Jefferson. It occupied the brick row houses at 236-38 Pine Street which had been vacated by the Phipps Institute in 1913.

Among Flick's contributions to the literature are: *Contagion: Its Meaning and Its Limitations* (1899), *Consumption, a Curable and Preventable Disease: What a Layman Should Know about It* (1903), *The Crusade against Tuberculosis in Pennsylvania* (1908), and *Tuberculosis, a Book of Practical Knowledge to Guide the General Practitioner of Medicine* (1937).

Curiously, Flick's last contribution to medicine was not in the field of tuberculosis, but was his position as the first president of the Philadelphia Institute for the Study and Prevention of Nervous and Mental Diseases.

In William T. Thomson's three-quarters-length, life-sized portrait of Dr. Lawrence F. Flick, the physician is seated at a desk in his study or office, surrounded by books, papers, and a framed picture on the wall. He looks up from a book resting in his lap and turns away from his desk as though to acknowledge a visitor. His gaze is direct and cordial, and there is a faint trace of a smile on his face. Though the elderly physician has thinning hair and a jowly jaw line, his complexion is ruddy and he still exudes energy and great intelligence.

William T. Thomson was a Philadelphia portrait painter, landscapist, and illustrator. Born in 1858, he studied at the Pennsylvania Academy of the Fine Arts and at the Drexel Institute, and pursued his career in Philadelphia. Thomson exhibited at the Pennsylvania Academy, the Philadelphia Art Club, the Philadelphia Sketch Club, the American Art Society, and the Newspaper and Illustrators' Club. He also exhibited in Cincinnati and Chicago, and at the Omaha Trans-Mississippi and International Exposition of 1898.

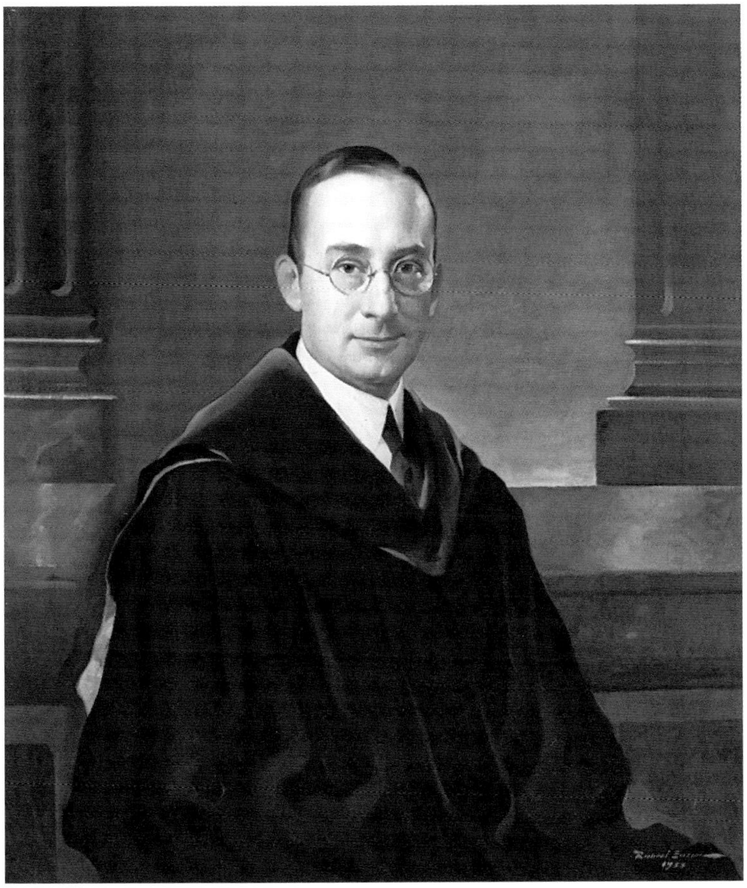

Portrait of Elmer H. Funk

ELMER HENDRICKS FUNK, M.D. (1886-1932)
By Robert S. Susan (1888-1957)

Oil on canvas
1933
40 x 35 in.

Signed and dated lower right: "Robert Susan/1933"

Given by JMC class of 1933
Accession number: 1933+e.P.01

Dr. Elmer H. Funk was a widely admired clinician, teacher, investigator, and administrator. He was the first director of the pulmonary department of Jefferson Medical College.

A native Philadelphian, Dr. Funk was born in 1886 and graduated from Jefferson Medical College in 1908. He served as resident physician at the Philadelphia Hospital for Contagious Diseases and at Jefferson Medical College. After the resignation of Dr. James C. Wilson as chair of medicine at Jefferson in June 1911, Dr. Funk was appointed to a committee to administer the department until the arrival of Dr. Thomas McCrae in September 1912.

By 1913 Funk was acting medical director of the Jefferson Hospital and acting secretary of the board of trustees. He joined the Jefferson faculty as instructor in medicine in 1913 and rose in the ranks to clinical professor of medicine and therapeutics. In 1931 he succeeded Dr. Hobart A. Hare as the Sutherland M. Prevost Professor of Therapeutics, unfortunately serving only one year until his untimely death in 1932.

At McCrae's request Funk had resigned his position as acting medical director of the hospital in 1913 to take charge of Jefferson's new department for diseases of the chest. As medical director and physician-in-charge until 1926, Funk was an energetic leader much acclaimed by the students who also learned to emulate his compassionate bedside manner. "Pine Street" was remembered as fostering an unusually close relationships between physicians, social workers, students, and patients most of whom were there for prolonged periods.

Students noted the emphasis on the "sociologic features" of tuberculosis, and they visited patients' homes under the supervision of social service workers. Social services included assistance to families of patients who had to cope with both the financial and medical aspects of the disease. Some patients were sent to sanatoria for more aggressive treatment. Nursing care and instruction were also priorities of the department.

Dr. Funk himself developed tuberculosis and spent a period at White Haven in 1915-16. He was a visiting physician there during most of his career.

He was an active clinical investigator and the author of *The Diagnosis and Treatment of Chronic Diseases of the Respiratory Tract: with Especial Reference to the Lesions of the Trachea, Bronchi, Lungs, Pleura, and Diaphragm* (1929). He was coeditor with Dr. McCrae of the third edition of Dr. William Osler's *Modern Medicine: Its Theory and Practice in Original Contributions by American and Foreign Authors* (1925-28). Dr. Elmer Funk also served as president of Jefferson's alumni association.

A posthumous portrait by Robert S. Susan was given by the class of 1933. At the ceremony Dr. Thomas McCrae said about Dr. Funk, "I have known very few men who planned for the future as systematically and with as broad a vision as he did."

The half-length figure is shown seated in front of a stone wall flanked by fluted columns. He wears a black academic gown with a green mantle. In spite of the imposing and imaginary setting, he turns to look directly at the observer with a pleasant and amiable expression. The fluidly painted portrait is naturalistic in both modeling and color, but the background is dominated by the eccentric, glowing hues favored by the artist. The wall and columns are painted rust, copper, bronze, and pink, and the space behind the figure varies from rust and green to acidic yellow.

At the presentation Dr. McCrae also endorsed the college's growing portrait tradition as a vehicle for teaching Jefferson history: "While the written word does something in this regard, it would seem that the portraits of the men who worked here do much more. As the years go by the number of portraits will increase and will be more and more representative of those who have labored in our halls."

Born in 1888, society portraitist Robert S. Susan was a native of Amsterdam, Holland. He studied art in Philadelphia at the Pennsylvania Museum School of Art, the Graphic Sketch Club, and the Pennsylvania Academy of the Fine Arts where he won two Cresson scholarships allowing him to travel and study abroad from 1911 to 1913. He exhibited consistently in *Annual Exhibitions* at the Academy from 1915 until 1943, and his portrait *June* was voted the most popular painting in the 1932 show by visitors.

Susan was especially noted for his portraits of prominent lawyers, judges, and high elected officials, including Pennsylvania Governor Gifford Pinchot and Pennsylvania Supreme Court Chief Justice Horace Stern. His portraits are represented in the collections at Philadelphia's City Hall, the Capitol at Harrisburg, Pennsylvania, and the United States Supreme Court in Washington.

Robert Susan was the first president of the Graphic Sketch Club when that school became incorporated. The painter's personality could be alternatively modest or flamboyant. When he was honored in 1934 by the Big Brothers Association for conducting art classes for inmates at Philadelphia's Eastern State Penitentiary, he refused to discuss his work there except to say that "an act of kindness is not a matter for publication."

On the other hand, he declared provocatively in a newspaper interview that "lips are the real windows of the soul," attributing the personalities of pretty, young, Philadelphia society women to an analysis of their mouths.[18] The artist was the father of actress and novelist Jacqueline Susann, and is said to have depicted her face on a reclining nude he painted.

Tall Case Clock

TALL CASE CLOCK
Works by Waltham Clock Co.

Mahogany
1900-25
87 x 29 x 18 in.

Signed in dial: "WALTHAM CLOCK CO."

Given in 1980 by Elmer H. Funk Jr., M.D. (JMC 1947) and Rachel W. Funk Jenkins in memory of their parents, Dr. and Mrs. Elmer H. Funk
Accession number: 1980+e.DA.01

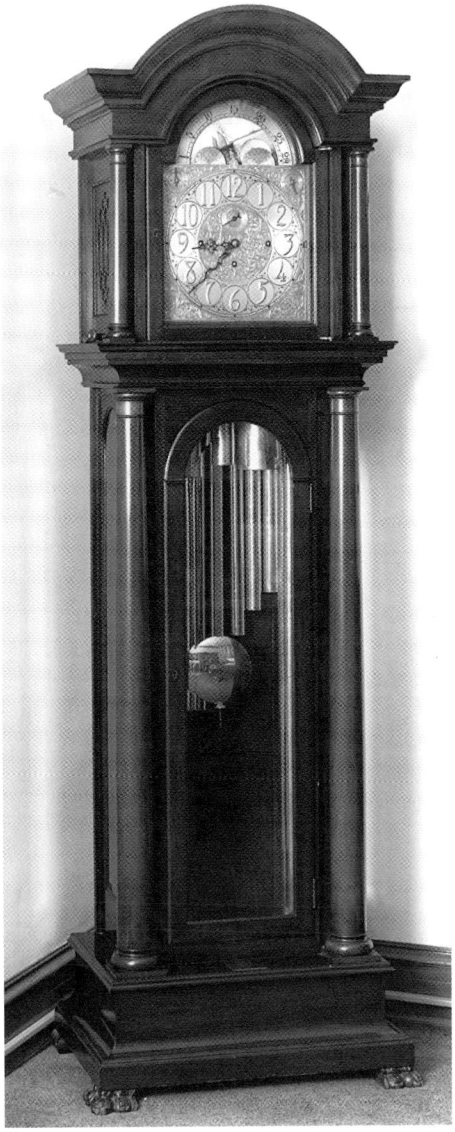

An American, tall case clock originally owned by Dr. and Mrs. Elmer H. Funk was given in their memory by their children, Dr. Elmer H. Funk Jr. and Rachel W. Funk Jenkins, in 1980.

The younger Dr. Funk graduated from Jefferson Medical College in 1947. He joined the Jefferson faculty in 1953 as coordinator of clinical research under Dr. Leandro Tocantins, and worked on collaborative clinical trials with Wyeth Laboratories.

Soon after, Funk became medical director of the Ives-Cameron Company of Wyeth Laboratories. After transferring to the Merck Sharp and Dohme Research Laboratories in 1959, he rose through the ranks to become director of advanced clinical research and director of cardiovascular/renal clinical research. In 1982 Dr. Funk received the Henry W. Elliott Award for Distinguished Service to the American Society for Clinical Pharmacology and Therapeutics.

After joining the pharmaceutical industry Dr. Funk continued to see patients at the Jefferson Hospital and to teach. He was clinical assistant professor of medicine from 1968 to 1990. He served as president of the alumni association in 1968-69.

The works of the Funk family clock were made by the Waltham Clock Company. The heavy, mahogany, Chippendale-style case has a hood with a domical cornice raised on a pair of freestanding ringed and tapered Tuscan columns. The broad trunk has a domical pendulum door with bevelled glass panel, exposing the chromed tubular chimes and brass cylinder weights and brass pendulum, flanked by ringed Tuscan columns. The entire case is raised on a tall, molded base supported by paw feet. The tubular chimes has a graduated set of full octave of eight chimes plus a gong on the side, and a choice of typical English chime sounds: Westminster, Whittington, and Oxford. The dial is brass mounted with a steel chapter ring with arabic numerals. The painted lunette moon phase operates on the same mechanism as the clock and rotates with the seasons.

Landscape, Bucks County

LANDSCAPE, BUCKS COUNTY
By Walter Emerson Baum (1884-1956)

Oil on canvas
1920-40
30 x 36 in.

Signed lower right: "W.E. BAUM"

Purchased in 1949 by Barton Memorial Committee of the women's board of JMC Hospital, in honor of Mrs. Natalie Hubschman
Accession number: 1949+e.P.02

Jefferson Medical College's department for diseases of the chest remained at its Pine Street address from 1913 until 1946 when it moved to the old Broad Street Hospital at Broad and Fitzwater Streets. Here it was known as the Barton Memorial Division, honoring a generous bequest from Emily Barton Pendleton and named in memory of her mother, Mrs. Betty Chase Barton. Patients at Barton received active treatment and surgery, while White Haven provided chronic sanatorium rest care. The chest department moved to newly renovated quarters in the Main Hospital around 1961.

Pine Street and Barton employed many methods to boost the morale of their chronically ill patients within the limitations of their close confinement. In addition to handwork for women and woodworking for men, the offerings included sketching and oil painting lessons by an instructor from Moore Institute of Art (later Moore College of Art and Design). In the late 1930s the Philadelphia Art Alliance provided a rotating selection of paintings to decorate the hospital.

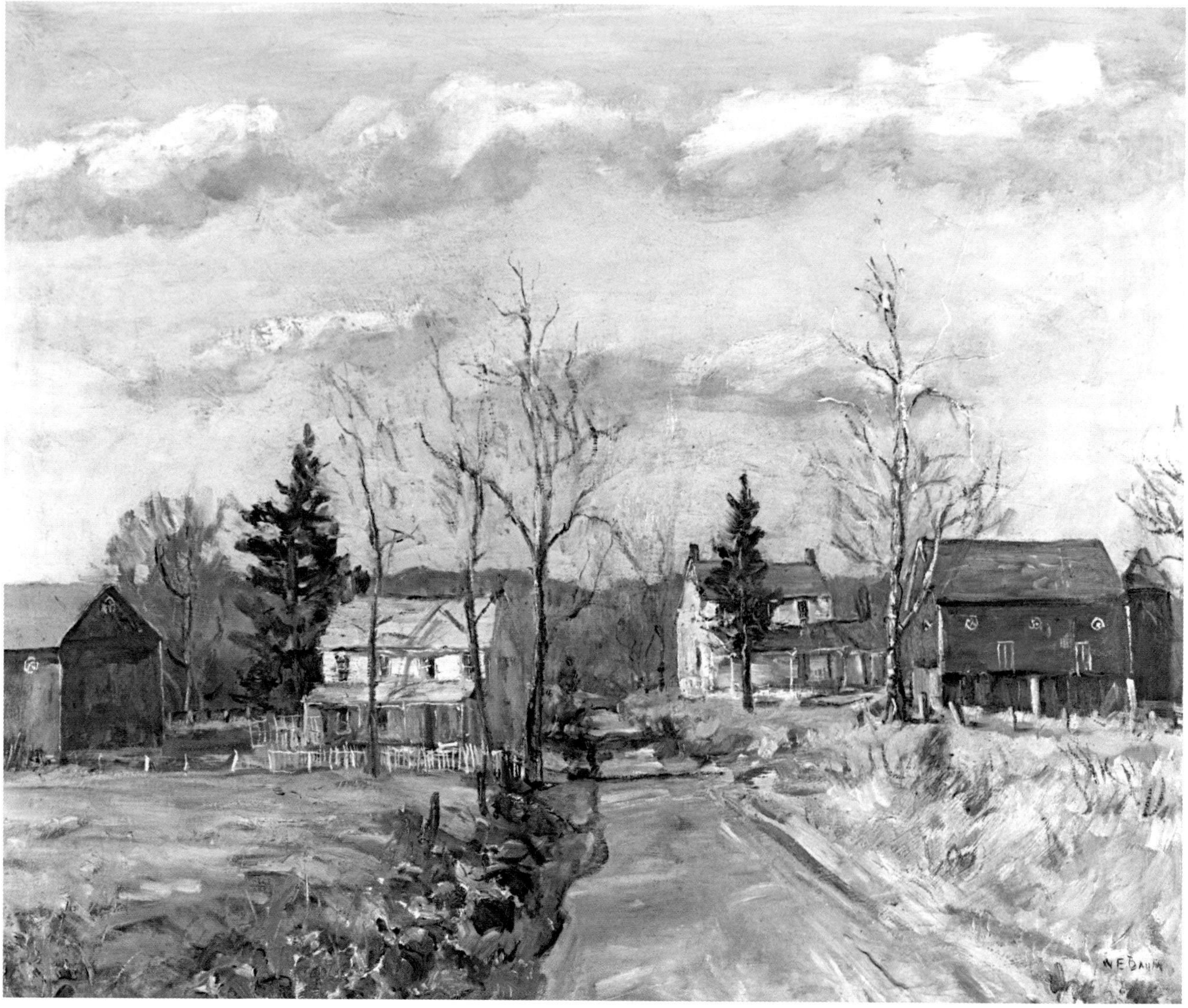

A letter dated April 3, 1947 from Mrs. Melrose E. Weed, executive secretary of the Jefferson Medical College alumni association, to Dr. Burgess L. Gordon, physician-in-charge, recounted a thriving loan program of paintings by fourteen artists used to beautify public areas and patients' rooms. The whereabouts of the works are unknown, with the exception of four landscapes by Walter E. Baum. Many of the artists are also represented by portraits in the Jefferson collection.

In 1949 the Barton Memorial Committee of the women's board of Jefferson Hospital purchased two oil paintings by Walter E. Baum. They were dedicated to the memories of two active and beloved members, Natalie Hubschman and Paula Weiss. Bronze plaques bearing the women's names are attached to the paintings: *Landscape, Bucks County* and *Road to Trumbauersville*, respectively.

Even today these are displayed in the pulmonary department of the department of medicine in the College Building, along with two additional paintings by Baum: *Autumn, Pennsylvania Dutch Country*, given in honor of Mrs. J. Parsons Schaeffer, and *Autumn, Edge of Allentown*, given in honor of Mrs. J. Horace Williams. Presumably these were also purchased by the Barton Memorial Committee before the move in 1961.

Landscape, Bucks County is a characteristic work by Walter E. Baum, a modest-sized, oil landscape depicting the eastern Pennsylvania countryside in late autumn. The artist was a well known painter, teacher, arts activist, and author, born in 1884 in Sellersville, a village about fifty miles from Philadelphia. He said, "I have spent my life painting scenes from my backyard."

Baum is best known for brightly colored, impressionistic landscapes, thickly painted and filled with an almost somber light and cool blue shadows. The scenes are infused with stillness and quiet, even when occasional figures appear. The red barns, white frame houses, curving road, stone wall, and trees in *Landscape, Bucks County* are typical of the artist's stock subject matter. He also exhibited large-scale watercolors and urban street scenes.

Baum's artistic education began with six years of study with a local artist near Sellersville, and then a brief period at the Pennsylvania Academy of the Fine Arts in 1905-06. A turning point in his career occurred when his painting *Sunlight and Shadow* won the Jennie Sesnan Gold Medal for landscape at the Academy in 1925. He later won the Academy's Fellowship prize, and other awards from the American Water Color Society, the National Arts Club, and the Pennsylvania Society of Miniature Painters, among others. Baum exhibited in many national exhibitions and his works are owned by numerous public and private collections. A one-man show in 1933 at the McClees Gallery in Philadelphia featured his recent landscapes. Another one-man exhibition of large landscapes was held at the Allentown Art Museum in 1996.

For many years Baum was an art reviewer for the *Philadelphia Evening Bulletin*. For supplementary income he began a Saturday art school first in his home in Sellersville, then relocated to nearby Allentown in 1926. By 1930 four of his students were accepted in the Circulating Picture Club of the Philadelphia Art Alliance and other exhibitions.

He orchestrated a grassroots effort to establish the Circulating Picture Club in Allentown and the Allentown Art Gallery, both of which were housed in public school facilities. By 1934 the Allentown Art Museum opened formally and two years later it moved into its own building with galleries devoted to the work of artists from the Lehigh Valley, Philadelphia, and the Midwest. Baum continued to direct both his art school and the museum until his death in 1956. He received an honorary doctorate from Lehigh University in 1946 for his contributions to the artistic community.[19]

Portrait of John C. DaCosta

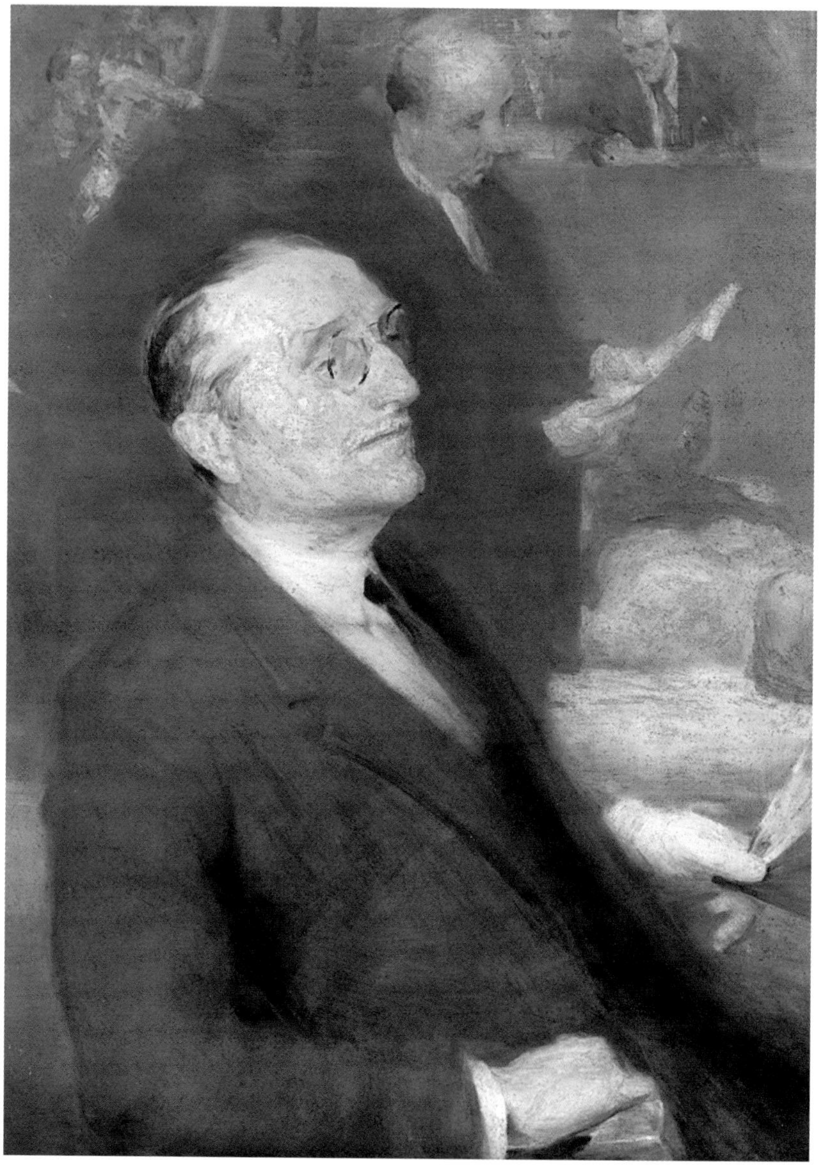

JOHN CHALMERS DaCOSTA, M.D.
(1863-1933)
By Richard Blossom Farley (1875-1954)

Oil on canvas
1924
38 x 28 in.

Signed and dated lower left: "RB Farley 1924"

Given by JMC class of 1924
Accession number: 1924+e.P.01

It is gratifying that the Jefferson collection has acquired so many art works and artifacts pertaining to one of its favorite sons, Dr. John Chalmers DaCosta, successor to Dr. William W. Keen as chair of surgery and the first Samuel D. Gross Professor of Surgery. These comprise four oil portraits, numerous photographic and printed portraits, a set of surgical instruments, a gold-headed cane, two silver presentation cups, a jeweled badge, and five embellished certificates.

DaCosta was often called a "Renaissance man" because of his many talents: a brilliant surgeon, a beloved and respected teacher, an inspiring orator, a noted author, and a student of history and literature. Contemporary colleagues often spoke admiringly of his unusual devotion to medical students and of his dogged determination to overcome the effects of progressive rheumatoid arthritis which struck him in 1922. Like Dr. Thomas McCrae, DaCosta continued to deliver lectures, conduct clinics, and give speeches from a wheelchair and he never referred publicly to his affliction.

Originally of Spanish descent, DaCosta's first ancestor to arrive in this country emigrated from London to Boston in 1697. The family settled in Philadelphia about a century later. His grandfather was engaged in the East India shipping trade and was a cofounder and first president of the Camden and Atlantic Railroad. His father also became president of the railroad.

The DaCosta family maintained an important presence at Jefferson Medical College in the late nineteenth and early twentieth centuries. His uncle, also named John Chalmers DaCosta, was a Jefferson alumnus (1878) and a gynecologist at the Jefferson Hospital from 1884 to 1901. His cousin, Dr. John Chalmers DaCosta Jr., known as "Black Jack," graduated from Jefferson in 1893 and taught internal medicine at the college. The surgeon and subject of this biography was affectionately known as "Jack" DaCosta. His family was not related to that of Dr. Jacob Mendez DaCosta.

John Chalmers DaCosta was born in 1863 in Washington, D.C. when his father was serving in the infantry of the Army of the Potomac during the Civil War. DaCosta's otherwise happy childhood in Philadelphia was marred by an accident at age nine resulting in the loss of vision in his right eye. Many biographers date the beginning of his interest in medicine from this event and the ensuing kindness accorded him by his physician.

He attended the University of Pennsylvania from 1880 to 1882, but could not complete his college course in chemistry because of his father's death and the family's subsequent financial reverses. During his college career he attended surgical clinics at the University and Blockley Hospitals. DaCosta chose Jefferson Medical College for medical studies and graduated in 1885 as class valedictorian. After a residency at Old Blockley he became assistant physician to the Insane Department there. In 1887 he became assistant physician to the Pennsylvania Hospital for the Insane and began a private practice.

That same year he received his first appointment at Jefferson Medical College as assistant demonstrator of anatomy and a clinical assistant at the surgical outpatient department under Dr. Samuel W. Gross. After Gross's untimely death in 1889, Dr. W. W. Keen acceded to the professorship and took on DaCosta as an office assistant. DaCosta later credited Keen's instruction, friendship, and support as crucial to his development.

His spare time was spent editing a medical dictionary and preparing a classic textbook, *A Manual of Modern Surgery: General and Operative*, which went through ten editions between 1894 and 1931. By 1895 this book and numerous articles helped him achieve the rank of clinical professor of surgery at Jefferson, and in 1900 he was appointed full professor at the age of thirty-seven. In 1907 he succeeded Keen as the cochair of surgery with Dr. John H. Gibbon. DaCosta was named the first Samuel D. Gross Professor of Surgery in 1910, Jefferson's first endowed chair, and held this until his retirement in 1931. DaCosta also served as surgeon to the Philadelphia General Hospital and consultant to St. Joseph's and Misericordia Hospitals.

In 1926 he received the Strittmatter Award of the Philadelphia County Medical Society. Jefferson Medical College classes of 1906 and 1923 dedicated their yearbooks to their beloved professor. In May 1927 the Jefferson alumni association erected a plaque that recorded a gift of a hundred thousand dollars in his honor for the establishment of a department of experimental medicine and an alumni endowment fund. As a token of its admiration the Jefferson Medical School class of 1926 presented him with a gold-headed cane of the Samuel D. Gross Professorship, inscribed with his name on a gold plaque. At their fiftieth reunion this class endowed a fund to add the names of succeeding Gross professors, so the artifact has been a continuous symbol of Jefferson distinction in surgery from 1926 to the present.

Dr. J. C. DaCosta served as president of the Jefferson Medical College alumni association in 1908. On the national level he belonged to the Society of Clinical Surgery, the American Surgical Association, the American College of Surgeons, and the American Philosophical Society. Internationally, he was a member of the International Surgical Society and an honorary fellow of the Society of Surgery of Bucharest, Rumania.

Richard Blossom Farley's 1924 portrait shows Professor DaCosta presiding over a surgical clinic. Aged sixty-one and already suffering from crippling arthritis, DaCosta is shown half-length and seated in a wheelchair in the foreground, turned almost in profile. Standing to the right is his assistant, Dr. Henry Seelaus, reading the history of the patient lying on a litter. An unidentified figure leans on a railing, and a few students in the audience are seen behind the wall. The artist has chosen not to include other spectators in DaCosta's clinics such as colleagues, alumni, and visiting physicians who often attended.

Compared with Benedict Osnis's portrait of Dr. Thomas McCrae in a similar clinic setting in which the more reticent McCrae seems squeezed between the patient's bed and the nearby table, the larger figure of Dr. DaCosta is alone in the foreground and extends almost the entire width of the canvas. His authority is established with greater impact, in spite of the seated position dictated by his disease.

Unlike McCrae, DaCosta was in his glory in front of a large audience, as his assistants Drs. Henry Seelaus and Thomas A. Shallow wrote in a memoir in the student yearbook of 1934:

> Dr. DaCosta's didactic lectures and surgical clinics were tremendously popular as his wit, brilliance of style and philosophical discourses made the hearers of his speeches and the readers of his writings treasure them...It is not an exaggeration to say that he was a master of the art of teaching; he presented every day surgical problems in such a manner as to arouse and hold the interest, not only of the students but graduates as well because many of the latter attended the famous Wednesday clinics...[which] were models of preparation, clearness and emphasis in statement...he will be remembered as one of the greatest clinical surgical teachers that this country has ever produced.

The commissioning of a portrait of a beloved professor by the Jefferson Medical School class of 1924 began a unique annual portrait tradition that continues to this day. An article in the *Jefferson Medical College Alumni Bulletin* of summer 1967 described the circumstances of this first senior class portrait in an interview of a 1924 graduate, Dr. Robert K. Y. Dusinberre. He remembered that a classmate, Dr. Albert Feinberg, "talked it up and found a lot of sentiment for it." Feinberg contacted artist Richard B. Farley who agreed to paint the portrait for six hundred dollars, far less than his usual fee, and the committee assessed each class member five dollars. Farley's preparations included sketching Dr. DaCosta at his home and occasionally attending his surgery clinics.

In order to earn additional money for portrait and frame expenses, the enterprising Feinberg organized and trained a team of Jefferson basketball players to challenge students from the University of Pennsylvania School of Medicine. Although Jefferson suffered an ignominious defeat at Penn in front of medical students and nurses, they made their expenses.

Born in 1875, Richard Blossom Farley was a native of Poultney, Vermont and studied at the Pennsylvania Academy of the Fine Arts from 1893 to 1898. He won a Cresson traveling scholarship and was one of the first pupils at the Whistler School in Paris. Best known as a marine and portrait painter, Farley was awarded the Academy's Fellowship Prize in 1912, the Philadelphia Art Club's gold medal in 1912 and a prize in 1913, a prize from the Corcoran Gallery of Art in 1914, and a medal at the Panama-Pacific Exposition in San Francisco in 1915.

He was acclaimed for a huge, four-panel historical mural, *The Unity of Life*, installed in the national headquarters of the American Theosophical Society in Wheaton, Illinois in 1933. Other works by Richard B. Farley are in the collections of the Pennsylvania Academy, the Corcoran Gallery, and the Reading, Pennsylvania Museum.

In 1914 Farley married the former Abigail Rosenthal, daughter of Max Rosenthal and sister of Albert Rosenthal, both of whom are represented in the Jefferson art collection.

A group of four oil portraits of Dr. John Chalmers DaCosta is unprecedented in the Jefferson art collection. In addition to the painting by Farley, there are three others by William T. Thomson. Further depictions of DaCosta include numerous vintage photographs and an etching by Erwin F. Faber.

The largest of the Thomson portraits was given jointly in 1929 by the Jefferson Medical College class of 1902 and the artist. It depicts DaCosta seated in front of a maroon drapery. A second portrait shows DaCosta standing informally with one hand in his trouser pocket. It was given between 1929 and 1936 by an unknown donor. The setting of the third Thomson work is particularly appropriate because it shows Dr. DaCosta seated at an open desk in his office or study. He holds a book in his left hand, and other books are on the desktop and on a shelf above the desk. It was given before 1929 by an unknown donor.

The surgeon was an articulate and well-read scholar with a broad knowledge of medicine, history, and literature; a graceful and dynamic orator; and a prolific author and editor of diverse medical and historical works. His speeches, lectures, and writings utilized historical and philosophical underpinnings to appeal to the imagination of his audience.

In 1905 DaCosta published a new, American, revised edition of Henry Gray's *Anatomy, Descriptive and Surgical*. DaCosta coedited volumes four and five of Keen's monumental eight-volume *Surgery, Its Principles and Practice, by Various Authors* (1906-21). Other books sampling DaCosta's extensive writings include: *Selections from the Papers and Speeches of John Chalmers DaCosta* (1931), *Poems of John Chalmers DaCosta* (1942), and *The Trials and Triumphs of the Surgeon and Other Literary Gems* (1944).

DaCosta's Set of Surgical Instruments

SURGICAL INSTRUMENTS
Manufactured by J. H. Gemrig & Son

Steel and ivory instruments, walnut box lined in velvet
Late nineteenth century
Box: 1 1/8 x 17 x 11 1/4 in.

Each stamped "Gemrig/Phila."

Accession number: 1933+f.DA.03-31

Dr. John Chalmers DaCosta was as effective a teacher at the operating table as at the lectern. A memoir in the 1934 *Clinic* said, "To the operating room he brought a profound knowledge of practical anatomy, an uncanny surgical judgment, a broad grasp of surgical literature and a diagnostic acumen which amounted to positive genius."

Despite his handicap of blindness in one eye, he was respected by his peers as a practicing surgeon, although the cases he performed would be considered elementary by today's standards, and he often depended upon

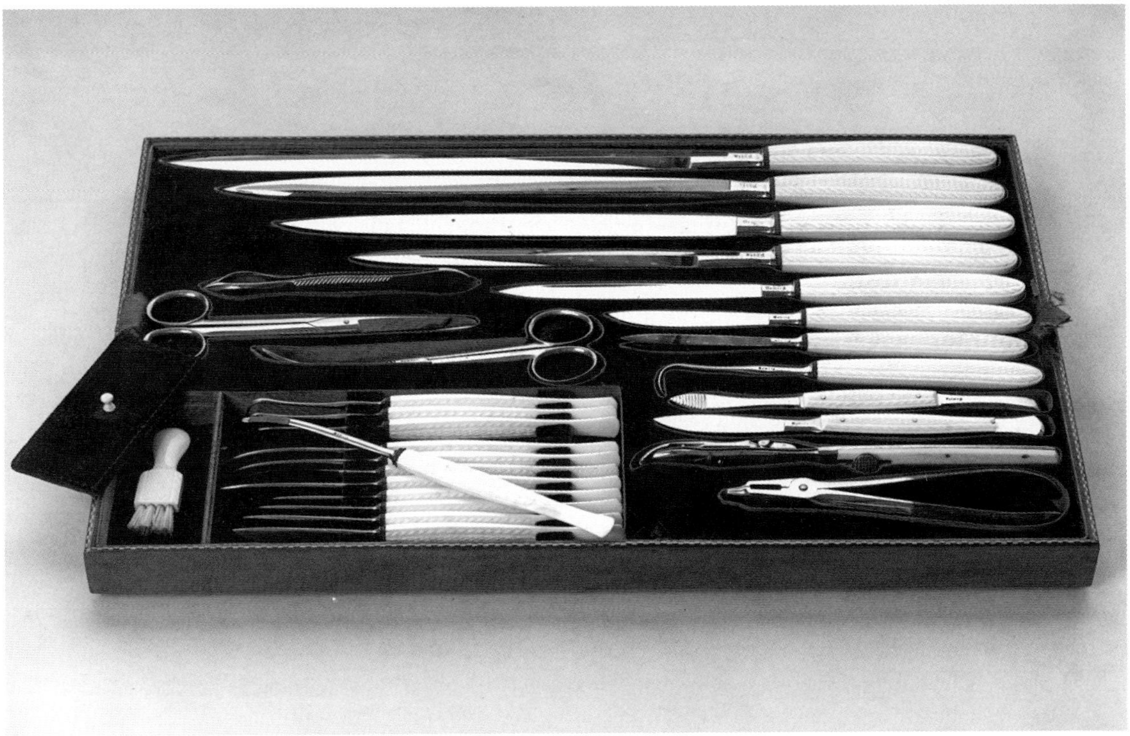

assistants when his handling of tissues was somewhat rough and when there was excessive bleeding.[20]

A prized artifact in the Jefferson archives is a set of DaCosta's surgical instruments with steel blades and ivory handles, made by the Philadelphia firm of J. H. Gemrig and Son. The instruments are placed in a walnut box lined in red velvet. All are still in very good condition. Included are seven amputation knives in graduated lengths ranging from eleven to three inches, as well as a rasp, scalpel, bone shears, two small hooks, ten other scalpels, forceps, a tenaculum, curved and straight scissors, and a brush.

DaCosta's Deputy Fire Chief's Badge

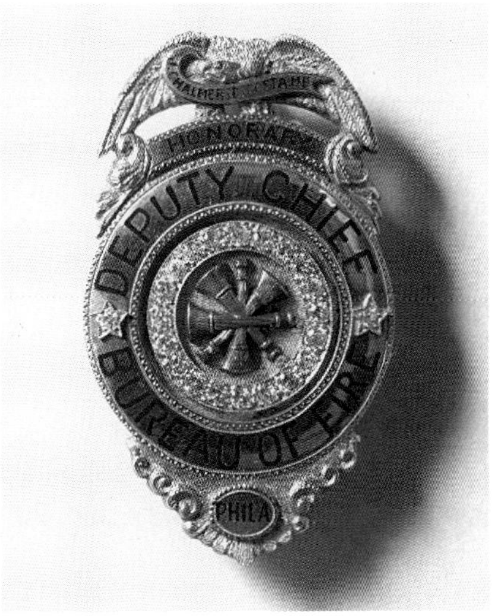

DEPUTY FIRE CHIEF'S BADGE
By unknown craftsman

Gold plate, enamel, diamonds, ruby
1910-30
2 1/8 x 1 1/4 x 1/8 in.

Inscription on front of badge: "J. CHALMERS DA COSTA, M.D./HONORARY/DEPUTY CHIEF BUREAU OF FIRE/PHILA"
Inscription on back of badge: "PRESENTED TO/J. CHALMERS DACOSTA, M.D./BY THE OFFICERS BUREAU OF FIRE/FOR FAITHFULL *[sic]* SERVICE/TO ALL MEMBERS OF THE BUREAU/1891-1931"

Given in 1951 by Mrs. Thomas B. K. Ringe, niece of Mrs. J. C. DaCosta and president, women's board of Jefferson Medical College Hospital
Accession number: 1951+e.DA.01

Friends recalled that in private life Dr. John Chalmers DaCosta avoided occasions like dinner parties and other social gatherings, but he pursued two hobbies ardently throughout his life: fire fighting and locomotives.

He shared his grandfather's and father's participation in the Volunteer Fire Department. For about thirty-five years Dr. DaCosta was a surgeon without salary to the Firemen's Pension Fund and maintained an extension of the city's fire alarm system in his home. He often accompanied the chief to fires on horse-drawn fire wagons and rendered immediate care to injured firemen. The physician was not only acquainted with fire fighters in Philadelphia, but also in New York, Atlantic City, and Baltimore.

He was so admired and respected by the fire association that during his last illness two firemen were assigned to tend him at his home, and many fire department officials visited the homebound physician to reminisce with him. In 1931 his contributions were recognized in a unique way: city and fire department officials came to his surgical clinic and presented DaCosta with a jeweled badge signifying his new rank as honorary battalion chief.

The gold plated badge has a central trophy panel of four crossed water hoses surrounded by a circle of small faceted diamonds, enclosed within a dark blue enamel perimeter with an inscription whose are separated by two star-shaped diamonds. Above is a crest featuring a spread eagle with an inscribed banner in its beak and an inscribed plaque in its claws. Below the circular inscription is a scrolled apron enclosing an inscribed cartouche.

The Jefferson archives was also given an embellished certificate awarded to Dr. DaCosta in 1901, installing him as a member in good standing of the Firemen's Association of the State of Pennsylvania. The elaborate pictorial document features various kinds of fire apparatus and heroic fire fighting scenes.

Another of Dr. DaCosta's hobbies was railroads, probably because of his father's and grandfather's railroad business. He collected large-scale photographs of famous locomotives. He was concerned about safety procedures and offered free first aid training to employees of railroads with trains entering Philadelphia. Colleagues recalled his unique routine for correcting student examinations: he purchased enough tickets for a one-thousand-mile trip, boarded a train, and continued to ride until all the papers were corrected.

DaCosta's Naval Medical Reserve Corps Certificate

NAVAL MEDICAL RESERVE CORPS CERTIFICATE
By unknown designer

Photolithograph of engraving
1913
19 x 15 1/2 in.

Given after 1933 by unknown donor
Accession number: 1933+f.Pr.05

Dr. John C. DaCosta served for eight years in the Medical Reserve Corps of the U.S. Navy, reaching the rank of commander in 1921. In 1919 DaCosta was sent on a special mission to care for the ailing President Woodrow Wilson while negotiations for the peace treaty ending World War I and the League of Nations were being conducted.

The Jefferson archives contains several certificates related to DaCosta's military career in the army and the navy. The earliest commissioned him a first lieutenant in the Medical Reserve Corps of the Army in 1908, and was signed by President Theodore Roosevelt.

The second, shown here, commissioned him an assistant surgeon in the Medical Reserve Corps of the Navy with the rank of lieutenant, junior grade in 1913, and was signed by President William H. Taft. This design includes a spread eagle above and an arrangement below with trophies, banners, and weapons.

Under the text is a complex and fanciful sea scene with sailing ships on the horizon. Riding the high waves in the foreground are classical deities: Neptune, ruler of the sea, holding a trident and gesturing toward the distance; his sea-nymph wife, Amphitrite, holding a banner and sitting on a scallop shell being pulled by straining sea horses; their son, Triton, a merman blowing a conch horn; and a Nereid, a mermaid who leans on Amphitrite's shell.

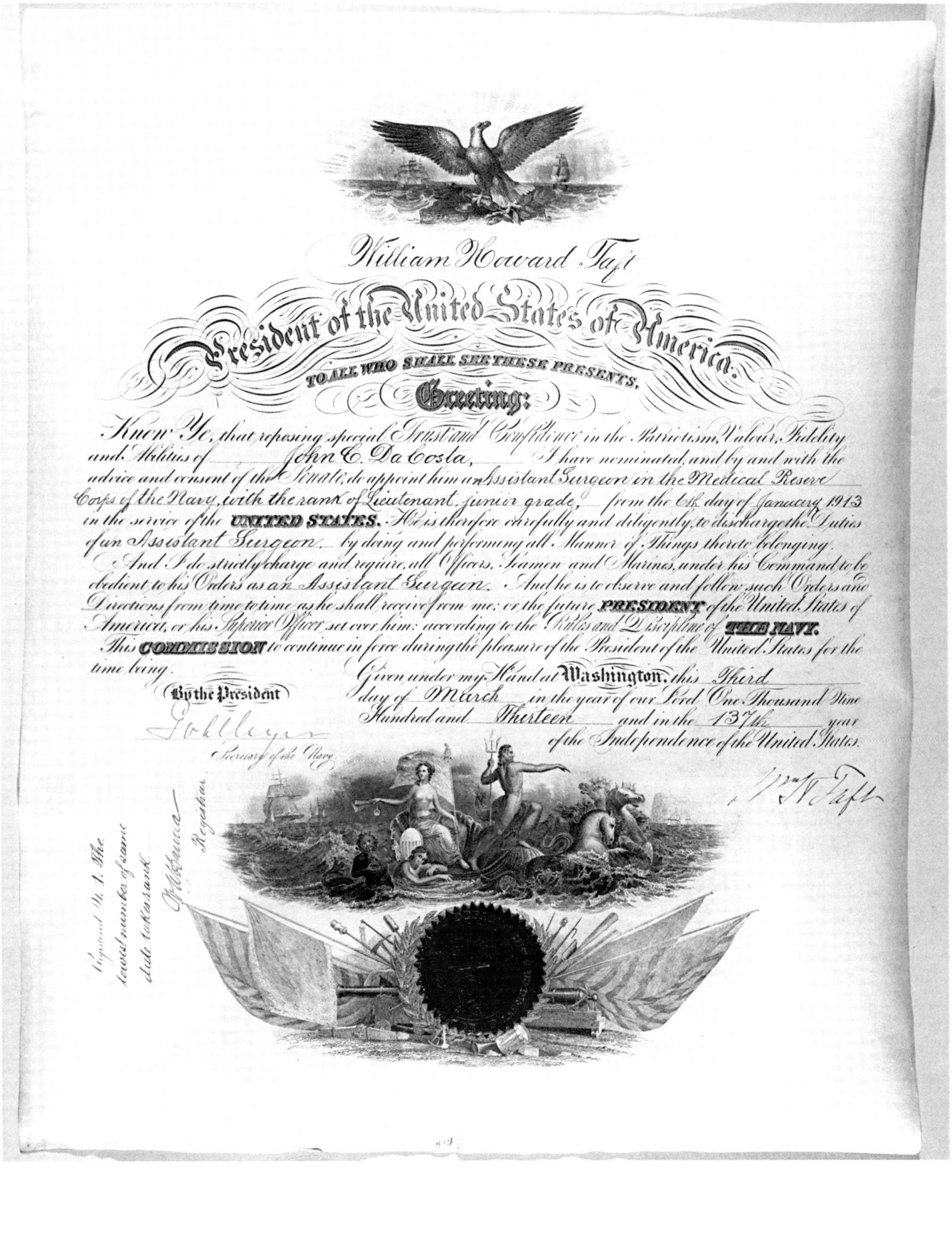

William Howard Taft

President of the United States of America.

TO ALL WHO SHALL SEE THESE PRESENTS,

Greeting:

Know Ye, that reposing special Trust and Confidence in the Patriotism, Valour, Fidelity and Abilities of John E. Da Costa, I have nominated, and by and with the advice and consent of the Senate, do appoint him an Assistant Surgeon in the Medical Reserve Corps of the Navy, with the rank of Lieutenant, junior grade, from the 6th day of January 1913 in the service of the UNITED STATES. He is therefore carefully and diligently, to discharge the Duties of an Assistant Surgeon by doing and performing all Manner of Things thereto belonging.

And I do strictly charge and require, all Officers, Seamen and Marines, under his Command to be obedient to his Orders as an Assistant Surgeon. And he is to observe and follow such Orders and Directions from time to time as he shall receive from me, or the future PRESIDENT of the United States of America, or his Superior Officer set over him, according to the Rules and Discipline of THE NAVY.

This COMMISSION to continue in force during the pleasure of the President of the United States for the time being.

Given under my Hand at Washington, this Third day of March in the year of our Lord One Thousand Nine Hundred and Thirteen and in the 137th year of the Independence of the United States.

By the President

Secretary of the Navy

Register

Wm H Taft

Portrait of John H. Gibbon

JOHN HEYSHAM GIBBON, M.D. (1871-1956)
By Alice Kent Stoddard (ca. 1884-1976)

Oil on canvas
1931
44 x 36 in.

Signed lower left: "A. STODDARD"
Exhibition: Philadelphia, *Annual Exhibition*, Pennsylvania Academy of the Fine Arts, 1932

Given by JMC class of 1931
Accession number: 1931+e.P.03

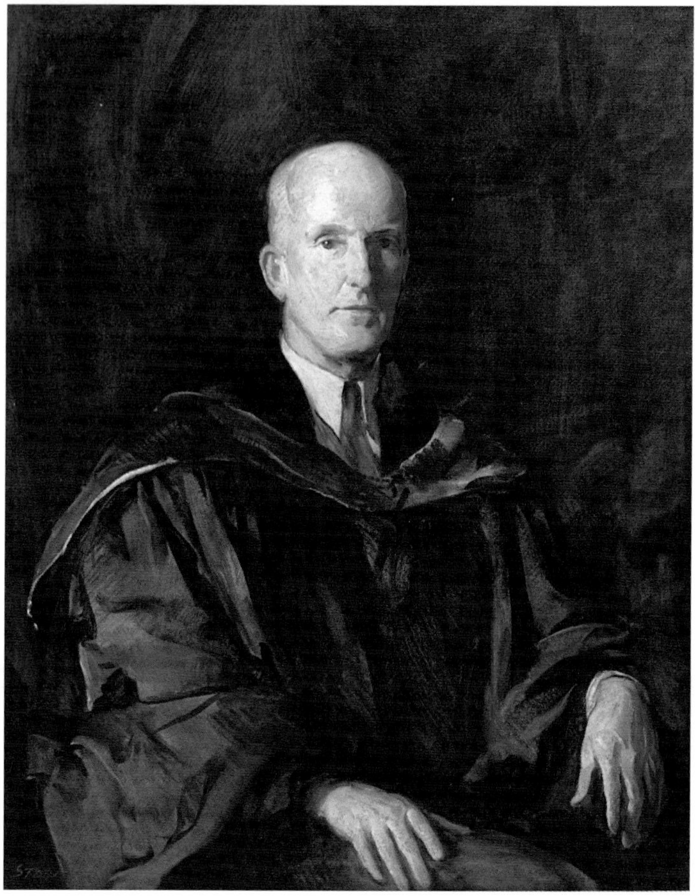

In 1907 Dr. John H. Gibbon succeeded Dr. John H. Brinton as professor of the practice of surgery and clinical surgery. He served as cochair of the department with Dr. John C. DaCosta until they both retired in 1931. They worked as a harmonious team and even coedited the Saunders *Year Book of Surgery* for many years.

John Heysham Gibbon was born in Charlotte, North Carolina in 1871 and came from a distinguished medical lineage: his great-grandfather, grandfather, father (JMC 1847), and brother (JMC 1888) were physicians. After graduating from Jefferson Medical College in 1891 Dr. Gibbon interned at the Polyclinic Hospital and spent three years as resident physician at the Pennsylvania Hospital. In 1895 he was appointed assistant demonstrator of anatomy at Jefferson. In 1899 he was made chief of the surgical clinic under Dr. W. W. Keen, a position he held until 1901 when he was made professor of surgery at the Philadelphia Polyclinic.

He returned to Jefferson as associate professor of surgery, and in 1907 became full professor. Almost from the beginning he also performed surgery at Pennsylvania Hospital. Appointments at other institutions included the Philadelphia Hospital, Children's Hospital, and Bryn Mawr Hospital.

During the Spanish-American War Gibbon served as first lieutenant and assistant surgeon in the Third U.S. Volunteer Engineers. In April 1917 he was commissioned major in the Medical Reserve Corps of the U.S. Army, and was attached to Pennsylvania Base Hospital Ten in Le Treport, France as chief of surgical services, followed by assignments in Belgium and England. He had achieved the rank of colonel by the time of his discharge in January 1919.

Dr. Gibbon was an original member of the Society of Clinical Surgery, and served as president of the American Surgical Association, the College of Physicians of Philadelphia, and the Philadelphia Academy of Surgery. Upon his retirement he was made emeritus professor and in 1948 Jefferson awarded him an honorary D.Sc. degree.

In addition to his clinics at Jefferson Hospital Gibbon conducted a weekly clinic at the Pennsylvania Hospital. This drew medical students from throughout Philadelphia to observe his technical prowess and superior judgment.

The graduating class of 1931 commissioned Alice Kent Stoddard to paint Professor Gibbon's portrait. In the lifesized, half-length portrait, Gibbon wears an academic gown and he looks directly out at the observer. He is seated against a neutral, atmospheric background. A dramatic contrast of light and shade calls attention to the angularity of his long, narrow face and high domed forehead. The paint application of the academic robe and background is thin and vivacious, in contrast to the more impasto and stolid handling of the subject's face and hands.

Gibbon was regarded with esteem and affection by his students, but his amiable nature is not even suggested by his somber, rather bland facial expression in the portrait. Yet there is strength in his hands, and a confident expansiveness in the way his robed figure fills the width of the canvas. The portrait must have been considered a success, because the artist showed it at the *Annual Exhibition* of the Pennsylvania Academy of the Fine Arts in 1932.

Students reminisced about their teacher in the 1925 yearbook:

> John Gibbon never called the roll. It was not necessary. We were always there...Will we ever forget "Hyperextension, Traction and Flexion"? He made hernias simple, the understanding of which we had previously considered an intellectual feat well nigh impossible. He gave us the inside practical dope on Surgery as he splashed soap suds around in the pit at the Pennsylvania Hospital...
>
> We like him...because he has a smiling, friend-winning and lovable, humorous yet professional personality; and because we appreciate his simple, accurate, forever-to-be-remembered teachings.

Alice Kent Stoddard was a colorful personality who forged an unusually successful and versatile career for a woman artist of her generation. She was born around 1884 in Watertown, Connecticut and was a cousin of the famed painter and illustrator Rockwell Kent.

She studied at the Philadelphia School of Design for Women and at the Pennsylvania Academy of the Fine Arts. An outstanding student at the Academy, she twice won the Cresson traveling scholarship, but in 1907 publicly rejected a third Cresson award because of her "well-bred rage" at not having received the top prize of two thousand dollars which she thought she deserved.

Alice Kent Stoddard was a practicing artist for seventy years, and painted portraits of numerous prominent Philadelphians. She was equally famous for depicting children and animals. Summers were spent at a family home in Monhegan Island, Maine where she delighted in painting seascapes and sailing vessels. She was not only a successful artist but helped many aspiring young artists to secure an art education.

Stoddard contributed to the war effort during both world wars. During World War I she served with the Y.M.C.A. in France and made drawings and paintings on the battlefield. During World War II she worked as a technical instructor for the Edward G. Budd Manufacturing Company. Her charcoal sketches of enlisted men at the Stage Door Canteen were shown at the Philadelphia Art Alliance in 1943.

Stoddard exhibited regularly at the Pennsylvania Academy of the Fine Arts from 1908 through 1964, and won the Academy's Mary Smith Prize, Fellowship Prize, and Carol Beck Gold Medal. She received two prizes at the Philadelphia Art Club. She won the Isidor Medal in 1917 and the Thomas P. Clark Prize in 1928 at the National Academy of Design where she was elected an associate in 1938. There was a solo exhibition of her work at the Woodmere Art Gallery in Philadelphia in 1951. Retrospective exhibitions were held at Philadelphia's David David Galleries in 1978 and the Monhegan Museum in 1984.

Alice Kent Stoddard did not marry until 1948 when she wedded a lifelong friend, Joseph T. Pearson Jr. The couple had known each other since their student days at the Pennsylvania Academy. Pearson enjoyed a national reputation for his landscape paintings and had won numerous awards. He was an instructor at the Academy for twenty-five years before resigning in a tiff over his failure to accept modernism. The Academy accorded him a memorial exhibition.

Portrait of Francis T. Stewart

FRANCIS TORRENS STEWART, M.D.
(1874-1920)
By Leopold Gould Seyffert (1887-1956)

Oil on canvas
1930
30 1/4 x 25 1/4 in.

Signed and dated lower right: "Leopold Seyffert/1930"

Given 1930-47 by Mrs. Francis T. Stewart, wife of the subject
Accession number: 1930-1947.P.01

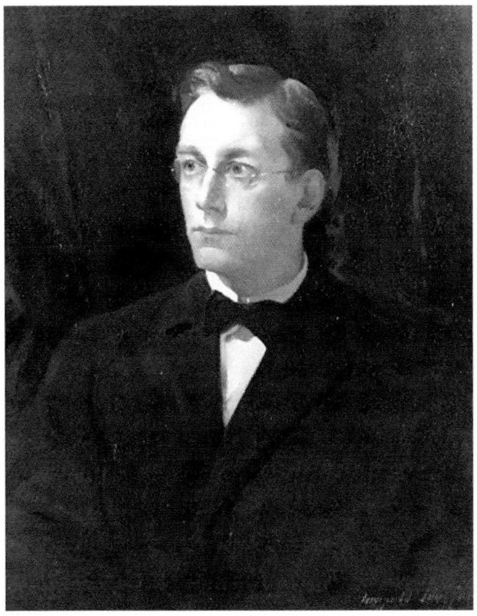

Dr. Francis Torrens Stewart was professor of clinical surgery at Jefferson Medical College from 1910 to 1920.

Had it not been for his untimely death at age forty-six, most colleagues expected that the brilliant surgeon would succeed Dr. John C. DaCosta as chair of surgery.

A native of Philadelphia, Francis T. Stewart was born in 1874 and graduated from Central High School and Jefferson Medical College (1896). He interned at the Philadelphia Polyclinic and served a residency at the Pennsylvania Hospital.

His first appointment at Jefferson Medical College occurred in 1902 when he was named assistant to Dr. W. W. Keen. He was also surgeon to Germantown Hospital from 1903 to 1918 and professor of surgery at the Philadelphia Polyclinic from 1903 to 1910. That year Stewart succeeded Dr. W. Joseph Hearn as professor of clinical surgery at Jefferson. He was also surgeon to the Pennsylvania Hospital.

Dr. Stewart was a frequent contributor to the medical literature, most notably papers on surgery of the heart and blood vessels. In the faculty minutes of March 29, 1920, Dr. John H. Gibbon called Stewart's *Manual of Surgery* (1907) "one of the best text-books for students ever written." His transverse incision for mastectomy was known as the "Stewart Incision."

The obituary by Dr. John C. DaCosta in the class yearbook of 1920 called Dr. Stewart one of Jefferson's most able men, saying, "had he lived the ordinary span of life his name would have belonged with our two or three greatest celebrities." Admirers of the original and skillful surgeon's "wizard hands" commended Stewart's calmness and deliberate speed in the operating room.

The portrait of Dr. Francis T. Stewart by Leopold Seyffert was painted in 1930, ten years after his death. Today the painting's surface shows signs of heavy restoration, but the subject's face is still in good condition. The level gaze of his pale blue eyes through wire-rimmed glasses and the force of his tightly pressed lips accord with descriptions of the surgeon as modest, but frank to the point of bluntness.

Presumably Stewart's portrait was commissioned by his family. It was given to Jefferson Medical College by Mrs. Stewart sometime before 1947 when it is mentioned in documents. His widow also endowed the Francis Torrens Stewart Prize for excellence in clinical surgery.

Portraitist Leopold Seyffert was born in the small town of California, Missouri in 1887 and his family relocated to a log cabin on a farm in Colorado Springs, Colorado. After moving to Pittsburgh in 1904 he first studied art at night at the Stevenson Art School while he worked by day as a stock boy for a senior geologist at the Standard Oil Company. His boss was so impressed with the young man's talent that he underwrote his studies at the Pennsylvania Academy of the Fine Arts. Seyffert won Cresson traveling scholarships in 1910 and 1912 and studied in Italy, Spain, and Holland.

In 1912 he was befriended by Philadelphia Orchestra conductor Leopold Stokowski who sat for a portrait that won both the Fellowship Prize and the Popular Prize at the Academy's *Annual Exhibition* in 1913. This was the first in a series of more than four hundred portraits of notable figures in industry and the arts.

Leopold Seyffert began teaching early in his career, starting in 1909 at Philadelphia's Graphic Sketch Club. From 1914 to 1921 he was instructor in portrait painting at the School of Design for Women, and then head instructor at the Art Institute of Chicago from 1921 to 1927. Thereafter he moved to New York. Seyffert was a public-spirited citizen, and during World War I he presented his portraits of a sailor and soldier to groups that subscribed one hundred thousand dollars for Victory Bonds.

Seyffert exhibited nationally and was a consistent prizewinner for his portraits and figure paintings. He won four awards at the Pennsylvania Academy, a silver medal at the Panama-Pacific Exposition in San Francisco, a gold medal at the Sesqui-centennial Exposition in Philadelphia, and the Popular Prize at the *Carnegie International Exhibition* in Pittsburgh in 1930.

Seyffert was made an academician of the National Academy of Design where he won four prizes over the years. The Art Institute of Chicago gave him three awards. His last prize was the Gold Medal of Honor at the *Allied Artists Exhibition* in New York in 1946.

During his lifetime Seyffert was featured in solo exhibitions in Boston, Detroit, New York, Pittsburgh, Chicago, Washington, D.C., and Columbus, Ohio. A retrospective exhibition was held in 1985 at the Berry-Hill Galleries in New York.

Portrait of D. Braden Kyle

DAVID BRADEN KYLE, M.D.
(1863-1916)
Attributed to Henry R. Rittenberg
(1879-1969)

Oil on canvas
Ca. 1900
50 x 36 in.

Given in 1938 by Mrs. D. Braden Kyle, wife of the subject
Accession number: 1938+e.P.02

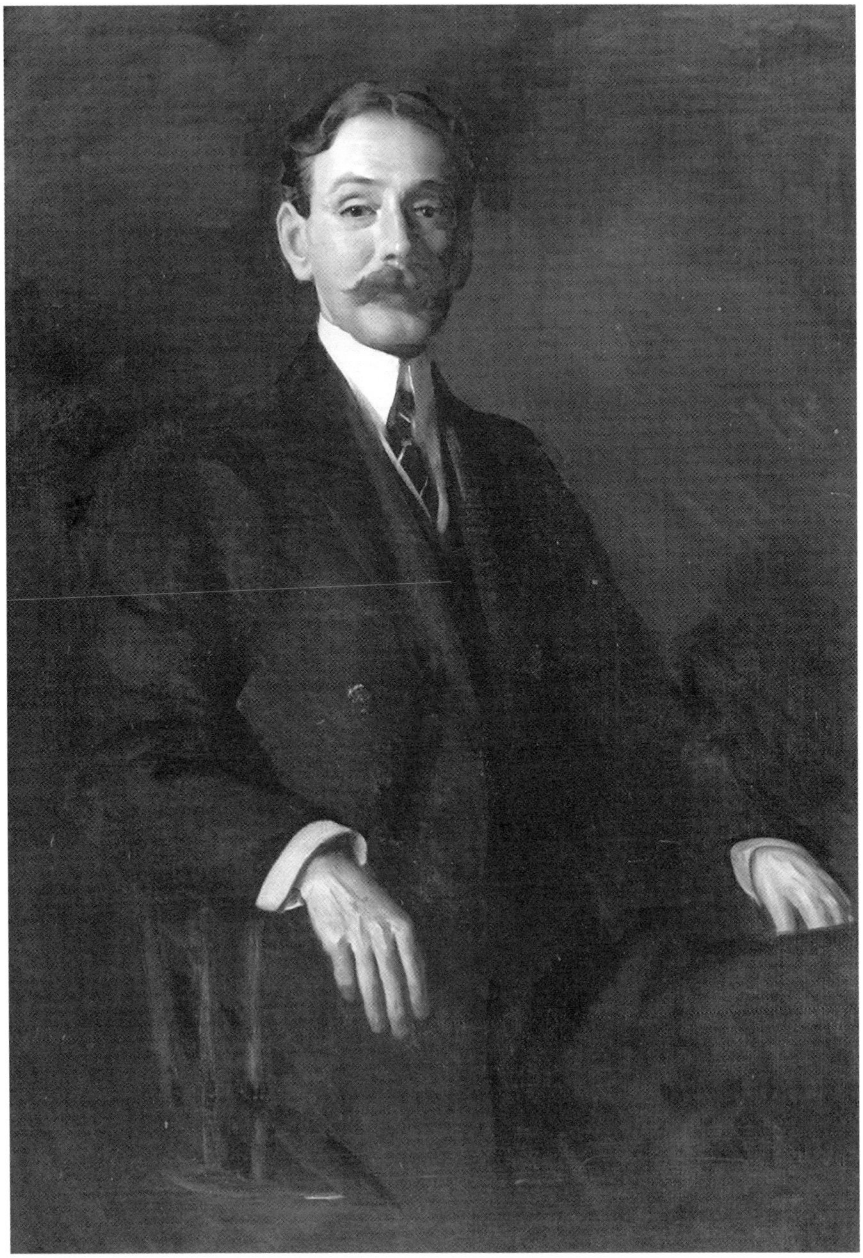

Dr. David Braden Kyle was an early and noted specialist in otolaryngology. He was the first chairman of laryngology at Jefferson Medical College, serving from 1904 until his death in 1916.

D. Braden Kyle was born in 1863 in Cadiz, Ohio, and after studying at Muskingum College in Ohio he graduated from Jefferson Medical College in 1891. He took private instruction from Drs. William Coplin and John C. DaCosta and was an office student of Dr. W. Joseph Hearn. In the year of his graduation he was appointed assistant demonstrator of pathology at Jefferson and established a private laboratory for instruction in clinical microscopy, bacteriology, and pathology. He also served as laryngologist, rhinologist, and otologist at St. Mary's and St. Agnes Hospitals.

By 1896 he was elected clinical professor of laryngology at Jefferson Medical College while maintaining a busy practice devoted to diseases of the ear, nose, throat, and chest. He was admired for personally overseeing the convalescence of his patients. He invented several instruments used by throat and nose specialists. He was made a full professor in 1904, a post he held until his sudden death from pleuropneumonia in 1916.

Kyle was president of the American Laryngological, Rhinological, and Otological Society in 1900, and president of the American Laryngological Association in 1911. His chief literary contribution was *A Text-book of Diseases of the Nose and Throat* (1899) which went through five editions.

In 1938 Jefferson's board of trustees accepted the gift of Dr. Kyle's portrait from his widow, and directed that the painting be installed in the library of the College Building. The portrait has no visible signature and board minutes do not record the artist's name. Subsequent records associate the portrait with artist Henry Rittenberg and the work bears a strong resemblance stylistically to two other Rittenberg portraits in the Jefferson collection.

Judging from Kyle's relatively youthful appearance

and direct, lively gaze, the work was painted from life around the turn of the century. Seated erectly in a wooden armchair, his legs are crossed and he turns slightly to the right. His handsome features are accented by a luxuriant, dark brown mustache and wavy hair with a center part. His complexion is florid, and his face and hands are broadly painted and well described. His business attire and the atmospheric background are so dark that his white shirt collar and cuffs stand out markedly in contrast.

Henry R. Rittenberg was another talented, early-twentieth-century artist who emigrated from Russia to the United States. Born in Libau, Russia in 1879, he arrived with his family in this country in 1885. Rittenberg attended Philadelphia's Northeast Manual Training High School, then studied art at the Pennsylvania Academy of the Fine Arts from 1897 to 1900, and at the Bavarian Academy in Munich.

Rittenberg maintained his home and studio in New York where he taught at the Beaux-Arts Institute of Design and the Art Students' League. He also held special portrait classes at the National Academy of Design where he was made an associate in 1921 and an academician in 1927. He exhibited widely throughout the country and was awarded the First Cresson traveling scholarship at the Pennsylvania Academy, honorable mention at the Art Club of Philadelphia, the Norman Waite Harris Medal at the Art Institute of Chicago, and the Isaac N. Maynard Portrait Prize and Thomas R. Proctor Portrait Prize at the National Academy of Design.

He was secretary of the Allied Artists of America, treasurer of the National Commission to Advance American Art, and a council member of the National Academy of Design. During World War I Rittenberg was active in Liberty Loan drives and in the Division of Publicity.

His works are represented in many private collections as well as museums, universities, libraries, hospitals, and civic buildings in New York, Philadelphia, and Harrisburg. One of his best-known portraits depicts a group of dignitaries including President Harry S. Truman at the Potsdam Conference in 1945.

Portrait of Edward P. Davis

EDWARD PARKER DAVIS, M.D. (1856-1937)
By Henry R. Rittenberg (1879-1969)

Oil on canvas
1905-15
48 1/2 x 38 1/2 in.

Given 1937-39 by unknown donor
Accession number: 1937-1939.P.01

Dr. Edward Parker Davis succeeded Dr. Theophilus Parvin as chair of obstetrics at Jefferson Medical College in 1898. He served with distinction until his retirement in December 1924 when he was elected emeritus professor.

Edward P. Davis was born in 1856, a native of Baldwinville, New York. He obtained bachelor's and master's degrees from Princeton University in 1879 and 1882, and graduated from Rush Medical College in 1882. He was a resident physician to the Cook County Hospital in Chicago. He continued obstetric and gynecologic studies abroad in Vienna, Berlin, and Prague.

In 1887 Dr. Davis joined the faculty at Jefferson Medical College as assistant demonstrator of obstetrics and became assistant to Dr. Theophilus Parvin, while earning a Jefferson medical degree the same year. Davis was named clinical professor of obstetrics in 1895 and professor in 1898. One of his most important contributions was directing the expansion of obstetrical patient facilities and clinical teaching.

Jefferson's first real maternity unit was established at 327 Pine Street in 1892. Because this facility soon proved inadequate to the increasing numbers of patients, a new maternity home opened in 1894 at 224 South Washington Square.

Around the turn of the century when Pennsylvania regulations required medical students to attend twelve deliveries, arrangements were made for each student to witness six deliveries in the maternity unit and six home deliveries. In 1910 another obstetric clinic was established at 2545 Wharton Street in South Philadelphia. This facility continued until 1946. Before his abrupt retirement Dr. Davis supervised the planning and construction of the maternity ward in the new Thompson Annex.

He was also professor of obstetrics and diseases of infancy at the Philadelphia Polyclinic, and visiting obstetrician and gynecologist to the Philadelphia Hospital.

He was one of the first to use X-rays for pelvimetry and the diagnosis of pregnancy. In 1910 Davis was a special American representative to the International Obstetrical and Gynecological Society meeting in St. Petersburg, Russia. That same year he was president of the American Gynecological Society and the Obstetrical Society of Philadelphia.

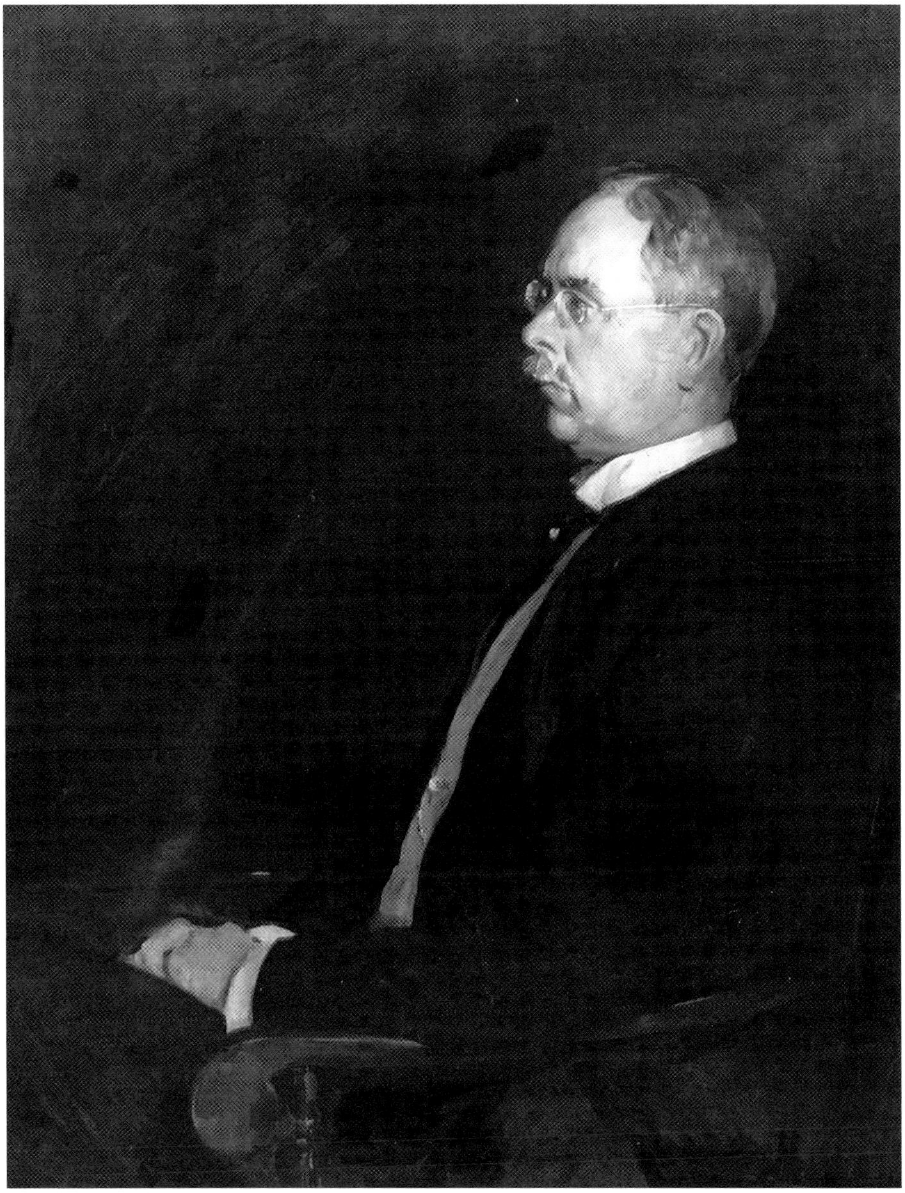

Dr. Davis had been a Princeton classmate and longtime friend of President Woodrow Wilson, and was attending obstetrician at the birth of the president's grandson at Jefferson Hospital in 1919. That same year he even published a small volume of poetry about President Wilson entitled *The Man and the Hour*.

Dr. Edward P. Davis was editor of the *American Journal of Medical Sciences* from 1890 to 1898. He was a prolific author of the following widely used obstetric texts: *A Manual of Practical Obstetrics* (1891), *Mother and Child* (coauthor with John Keating, 1892), *A Treatise on Obstetrics for Students and Practitioners* (1896), *Obstetric and Gynecologic Nursing* (1901), *Operative Obstetrics; Including the Surgery of the New Born* (1911), *Manual of Obstetrics* (1914), and *Complications of Pregnancy* (1923).

The physician was depicted in a most unusual profile portrait by Henry R. Rittenberg. Shown life-sized and two-thirds length, he is seated in an armchair with hands clasped in his lap. He gazes through rimless spectacles into the distance with a meditative expression. He is attired in the customary black street clothes of the day. The mood of the subject is quiet and reserved.

One can just barely differentiate the outline of the chair from the sitter's dark attire and the black, atmospheric background. The curving lines of the chair's back and arms subtly echo the physicians's spherical head, vest watch, tie pin, shirt collar, and spectacles.

The prevailing dark tones of this beautifully designed and executed composition are subtly enlivened by the golden tones of the subject's watch chain, tie pin, and spectacle temples, and a fragmentary view of his mustard-colored vest. The physician's sculptural head and hands are freely brushed with particular attention to his wavy gray hair and thick mustache. Reflections and highlights on his face, spectacles, and white shirt collar contrast with the prevailing smooth and dark tones.

This unsigned and undated portrait is almost certainly by Henry R. Rittenberg, because of a statement by Dr. Davis and because of the portrait's close resemblance to others by the artist. However, there are problems with its provenance.

Dr. Davis wrote a letter on May 7, 1932 to Dr. William P. Bradley (a collector of data on portraits of Philadelphia physicians) stating that "the artist of his portrait was Henry R. Rittenberg." There is no reason to doubt this. But Davis continued, "A few years after painting this portrait he moved to New York where he is successful as a portrait painter. I cannot give the exact date, I think 1900."[21] Neither the signature nor the date is visible today because of heavy restoration. It is ambiguous whether the "1900" in Davis's letter refers to the creation of the portrait or Rittenberg's move to New York.

If 1900 refers to the date of the painting, it seems unlikely that Professor Davis would have selected Rittenberg, then a twenty-one-year-old artist just finishing his studies at the Pennsylvania Academy of the Fine Arts in 1900, before he went to Europe. The work's dark palette and bravura brush work accord with an influence by the Bavarian Academy in Munich where he studied in 1902. If 1900 refers to the date he moved to New York, that is certainly incorrect. Rittenberg's address in exhibition listings at the Pennsylvania Academy (1906-34) and the National Academy of Design (1907-49) show that he moved from Philadelphia to New York in 1917 or 1918.

Therefore, the painting probably dates from about 1905 to 1915. This period better accords with the subject's appearance and with the artist's reputation, style, and whereabouts.

Dr. Davis's portrait was first mentioned in Jefferson documents in 1939, but the work could have arrived immediately after his death in 1937. Jefferson inventories of the 1950s and 1960s assert that the portrait's donor was Cyrus H. McCormick of Chicago, but no documents survive to prove this. The inventor of the reaping machine died in 1884, and it is possible that a family member might have contributed the portrait. Dr. Davis had spent a few years in Chicago in the early 1880s, but it would take further research to establish a relationship between him and the McCormicks.

Portrait of Edward E. Montgomery

EDWARD EMMET MONTGOMERY, M.D. (1848-1927)
By Robert S. Susan (1888-1957)

Oil on canvas
1921
40 1/4 x 30 1/4 in.

Given in 1941 by Mrs. Pascal Brooke Bland, daughter of the subject and widow of Dr. Bland, former chair of obstetrics
Accession number: 1941+e.P.01

Dr. Edward E. Montgomery was the chair of gynecology at Jefferson Medical College from 1892 to 1920. A leader in his field, he was also an outstanding clinician and teacher.

Edward E. Montgomery was born in Newark, Ohio in 1848. He graduated from Denison University in 1871 and received his medical degree from Jefferson Medical College with the class of 1874, and served as class president at both institutions. During the next few years he was a resident physician at the Blockley Hospital; taught private classes at Jefferson in physiology and anatomy; taught classes at Women's Medical College in operative surgery; and was clinical surgeon to the Women's Hospital.

In 1878 Montgomery joined the obstetric staff of Blockley where he performed the first successful ovariotomy at that hospital (although not the first in Philadelphia). He was the first in Philadelphia to intubate the larynx through the mouth for diphtheria.

From 1886 until 1892 Dr. E. E. Montgomery was professor of gynecology at the Medico-chirurgical College. He was gynecologist at St. Joseph's Hospital for thirty-five years and served as president of the medical staff there.

Until 1891 there had been a single department of obstetrics and diseases of women and children at Jefferson Medical College. The following year when three separate departments were created—gynecology, obstetrics, and diseases of children—Dr. Montgomery was named the first chair and professor of clinical gynecolo-

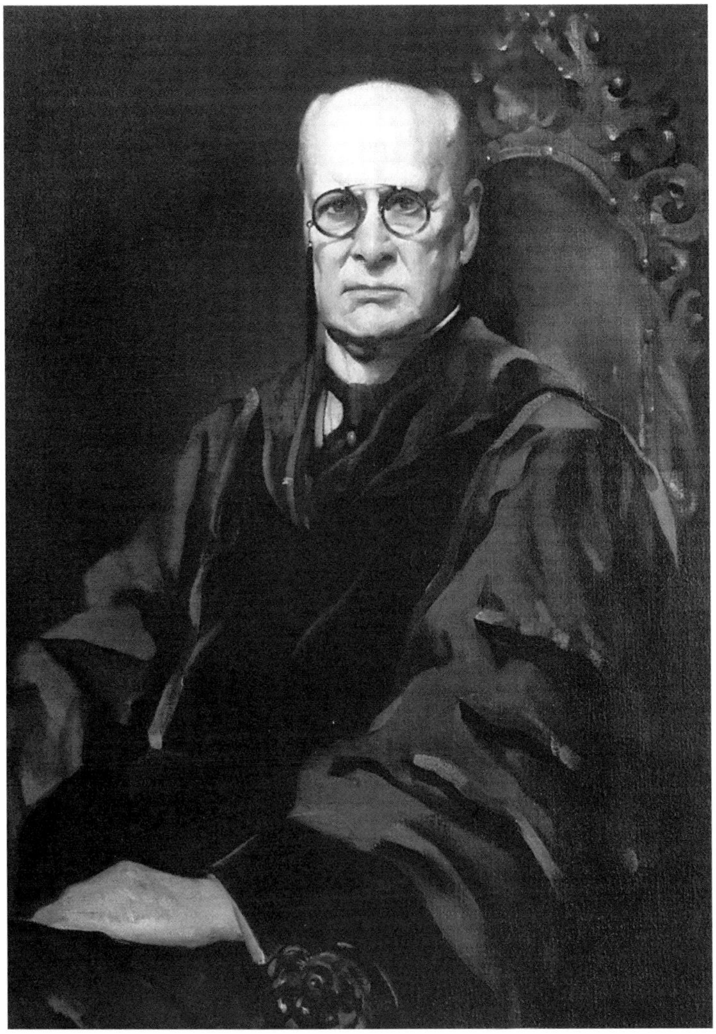

Robert Susan's half-length portrait of Dr. Edward Emmet Montgomery shows the physician seated with his body turned partly to the left and his head facing front to look directly at the observer. The coloration and setting for the Montgomery portrait are as idiosyncratic as in Susan's portrait of Dr. Elmer Funk.

Dr. Montgomery wears an academic robe with a purple hood lined in pinkish red, and brilliant green stripes on the sleeves. The atmospheric background is dark with slashes of purple. The sitter's thronelike chair, of Baroque Revival style, has a curved, high back which is upholstered in brilliant, orange-pink velvet. The cresting rail is elaborately carved and the chair arms terminate in lion heads resting on paws.

Equally arresting is the physician's face. His demeanor is so stern and grim as to be almost Mephistophelean, especially with his steely gaze behind the heavy, dark-framed pince-nez, his brooding mouth, and his wispy fringes of hair that resemble rudimentary horns framing his high-domed forehead. The subject's face is depicted with loosely brushed pink, purple, green, and blue highlights and shadows. The total coloristic effect gives the portrait an almost iridescent glow.

The author of an obituary in the *Jefferson Medical College Alumni Bulletin* of May 1927 confirmed the physician's rather austere manner. Dr. Montgomery had confided his great desire to be friendly, but said it was difficult for him "to come out of his shell among strangers." Yet in contrast to the forbidding, imperial image depicted in the portrait, Dr. Montgomery was admired by his students for his integrity and staunch principles. He was compassionate and generous to his patients.

On successive Saturday evenings senior students were invited to his home for a program of student papers followed by refreshments and musicales. His devotion to his students was reciprocated. The E. E. Montgomery Gynecological Society was established by Jefferson students in 1901 and the 1917 Jefferson yearbook was dedicated to him.

Mrs. Pascal Brooke Bland, the daughter of Dr. Montgomery, gave the portrait with the understanding that it and the portrait of her husband would be placed "above the alcove set aside for the Bland Collection of Books." Today, the two portraits are adjacent to the library's archives where the Bland donation is housed.

gy. On the death of Dr. Theophilus Parvin in 1898 Montgomery was named professor of gynecology.

Dr. Montgomery established history-taking and clinical instruction as priorities in the curriculum, section demonstrations in the operating room and the wards, and for the first time, permission for students to examine patients in the clinic under staff supervision. Upon his retirement in 1920 Dr. E. E. Montgomery was named emeritus professor.

His best-known book was *Practical Gynecology: a Comprehensive Text-book for Students and Physicians* (1900). Active in national and local medical societies, Montgomery was a founding member and president of the American Association of Obstetricians and Gynecologists and a trustee and first vice president of the American Medical Association. He was president of the Philadelphia Obstetrical Society, the Philadelphia County Medical Society, the Pennsylvania State Medical Society, and the alumni association of Jefferson Medical College.

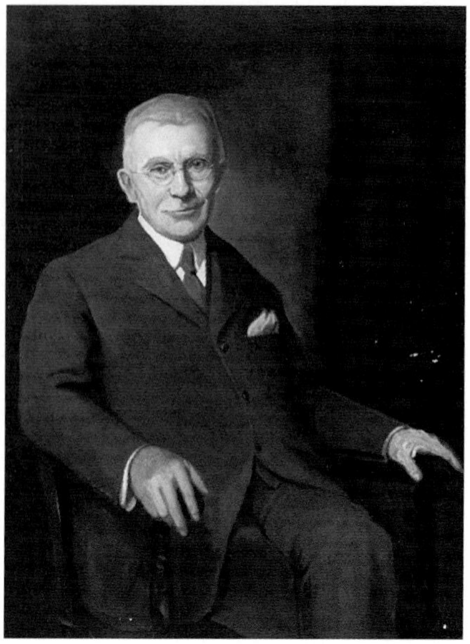

Portrait of John M. Fisher

JOHN MONROE FISHER, M.D. (1858-1937)
By Benedict Anton Osnis (1872-1941)

Oil on canvas mounted on board
1931
45 x 34 1/2 in.

Signed and dated lower right: "B. A. OSNIS/1931"

Given in 1931 by JMC alumni, friends, and colleagues
Accession number: 1931+e.P.02

Jefferson Medical College gynecologist John Monroe Fisher, M.D. was associated with the college for his entire career.

A native of Hanover in Lebanon County, Pennsylvania, John M. Fisher was born in 1858. After graduating from Jefferson in 1884 he became a resident at the Jefferson Hospital and was named a private assistant to Dr. Samuel W. Gross. In 1890 he was appointed assistant attending gynecologist to the Jefferson Hospital. Shortly after Dr. Edward E. Montgomery was appointed professor in 1893, Dr. Fisher was made chief of the clinic and demonstrator of gynecology.

He was made assistant attending surgeon at the Jefferson Hospital in 1900, and rose to associate professor of gynecology in 1910. In 1933 he was made clinical professor. He was also associated with the St. Agnes, Philadelphia, and Phoenixville Hospitals. He served as president of the Jefferson Medical College alumni association, the Philadelphia Medical Club, and the Philadelphia Obstetrical Society.

Dr. John M. Fisher's portrait by Benedict A. Osnis was presented by alumni friends immediately after the Ex-interne Day program in 1931. The subject is shown three-quarters length and life-sized, seated in a wooden armchair. Although the portrait has suffered considerable damage, the observer can still sense Dr. Fisher's warm and kindly personality. He is said to have been a faithful alumnus, a conscientious teacher, and a compassionate physician with a large following.

Portrait of George E. de Schweinitz

GEORGE EDMUND de SCHWEINITZ (1858-1938)
By Erwin F. Faber (1866-1939)

Etching
1915-25
Image size: 11 1/4 x 8 1/4 in.
Plate size: 13 1/4 x 9 3/4 in.
Sheet size: 17 1/2 x 12 in.

Signed in plate lower left: "E. F. Faber"
Inscribed in ink on plate lower right: "To Dr. P. Brooke Bland/from his former teacher/G. E. de Schweinitz"
Signed in pencil in border, lower right: "Erwin F. Faber"

Given in 1940 by bequest of Pascal Brooke Bland, M.D., chair of obstetrics
Accession number: 1940+e.Pr.33

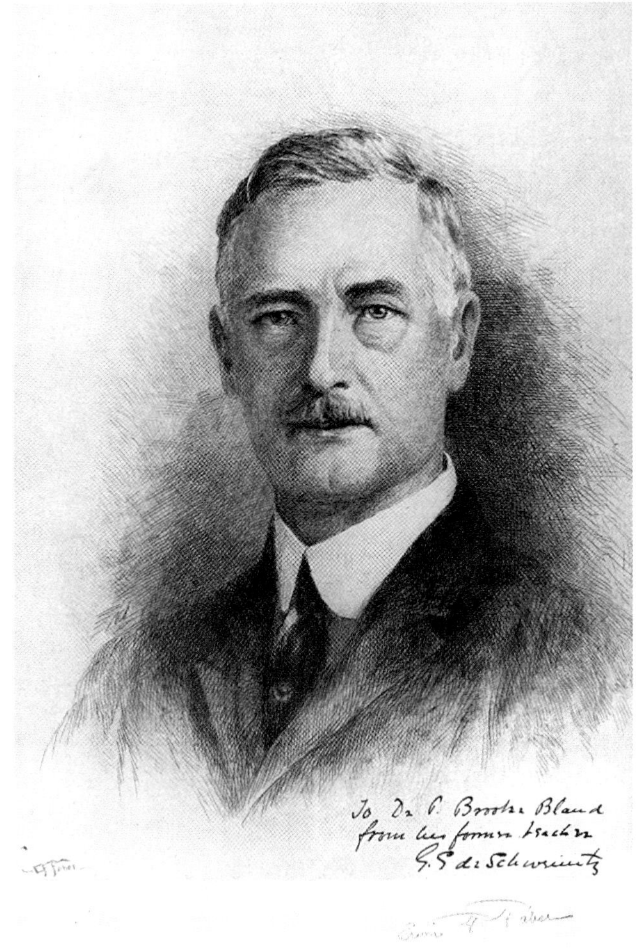

Dr. George Edmund de Schweinitz was a nationally known ophthalmologist and a leader in his field. His career at Jefferson Medical College spanned the decade 1892 to 1902.

Descended from distinguished Huguenot and Silesian ancestors, George E. de Schweinitz was born in 1858 and reared in Bethlehem, Pennsylvania. He graduated in 1876 from Moravian College where his father was president. After receiving his medical degree from the University of Pennsylvania in 1881 he spent two years as prosector of anatomy for Dr. Joseph Leidy there.

After serving as assistant to Dr. William F. Norris, professor of ophthalmology at the university, de Schweinitz was appointed ophthalmic surgeon to the Children's Hospital, Philadelphia Hospital, and the Orthopaedic Hospital and Infirmary for Nervous Diseases. He was also lecturer in medical ophthalmology at the University of Pennsylvania and professor of ophthalmology at the Philadelphia Polyclinic and College for Graduates in Medicine.

Dr. George E. de Schweinitz was appointed clinical professor of ophthalmology at Jefferson Medical College in 1892 and then chair of ophthalmology in 1897, succeeding Dr. William Thomson. He resigned his post in 1902 to follow his mentor, Dr. Norris, as chair of ophthalmology at the University of Pennsylvania where he remained for the rest of his career.

As a clinician de Schweinitz was known for his attention to the effects of systemic diseases upon the eyes. He was one of the first to list the symptoms common to glaucoma and one of the first to use the tonometer for detection of that disease. His best-known literary contribution was *Diseases of the Eye; a Hand-book of Ophthalmic Practice, for Students and Practitioners* (1892), which went through ten editions. The first American to deliver the Bowman Lecture in London, de Schweinitz chose as his topic the ocular aspects of pituitary disorders.

Dr. de Schweinitz guided many professional societies as president of the College of Physicians of Philadelphia, the American Ophthalmological Society, the American Medical Association, and the International Congress of Ophthalmology. He received honorary degrees from the Universities of Pennsylvania and Michigan, Harvard University, and Moravian College. He was a member of the American Philosophical Society, and a trustee of the University of Pennsylvania and the Library Company of Philadelphia.

In Erwin F. Faber's meticulously rendered portrait etching, Dr. George E. Schweinitz is shown bust length and wearing business attire. The regularity of his features is emphasized by subtle tonal contrasts of light and shade. The delicacy of line achieved in the etching process continues in the background shading behind the figure. The subject's piercing gaze and confident bearing make him appear a bit austere. The portrait was inscribed by Dr. de Schweinitz to Dr. Pascal Brooke Bland "from his former teacher."

In addition to his fame as a portraitist, Erwin F. Faber was a well known anatomical artist who taught pathological drawing at the University of Pennsylvania School of Medicine for more than twenty years. He was born in Philadelphia in 1866 to an artistic family. He collaborated with his father, Hermann, and brother, Ludwig, to illustrate George A. Piersol's *Human Anatomy* (1907), on which they labored for twelve years to produce over fifteen hundred illustrations. The brothers also illustrated Gwilym G. Davis's *Applied Anatomy* (1910).

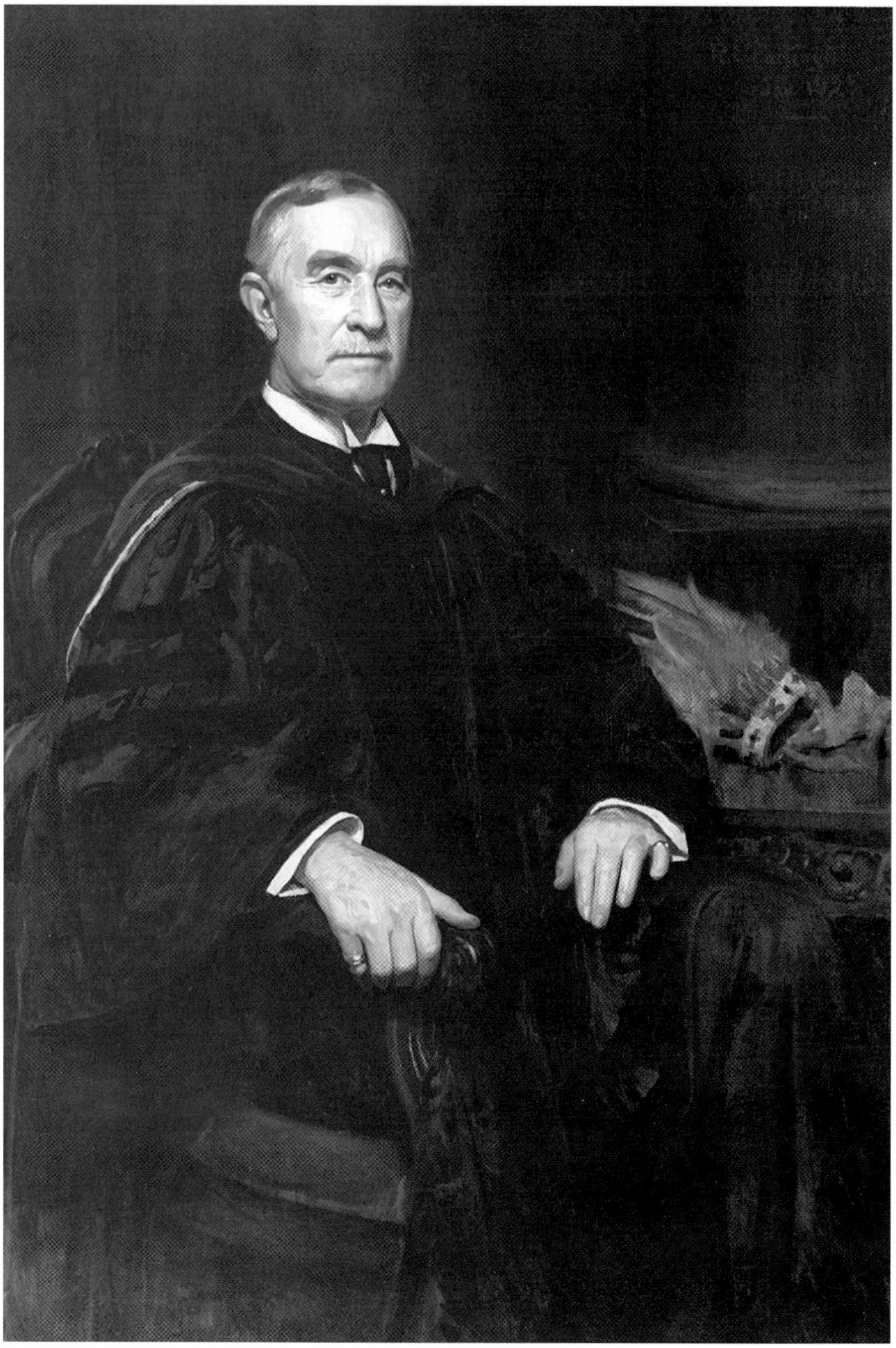

Portrait of L. Webster Fox

LAWRANCE WEBSTER FOX, M.D.
(1853-1931)
By Richard Langtry Partington
(1868-1929)

Oil on canvas
1925
54 1/2 x 38 1/2 in.

Signed and dated upper right: "R. L. Partington/Jan. 1925"

Given after 1931 by C. Beatrice Fox Griffith, daughter of the subject
Accession number: 1931+f.P.01

Another noted eye surgeon with connections to Jefferson Medical College was Dr. Lawrance Webster Fox. He was the son of Dr. Thomas G. Fox (JMC 1852).

L. Webster Fox was born in 1853 in Hummelstown, Dauphin County, Pennsylvania, the descendant of James Fox who had bought five thousand acres of land from William Penn in 1685. He was educated at the Millersville State Normal School (1872) and Jefferson Medical College (1878) where he was class president. He spent the next four years studying and working in Paris, Berlin, Vienna, and London where he was the first American to become house surgeon and clinical assistant at the Royal London Ophthalmic Hospital, Moorsfields.

Upon his return to Philadelphia in 1881 Dr. Fox was appointed assistant ophthalmologist and clinical assistant to Dr. William Thomson at Jefferson Medical College where he remained until 1883 when he became ophthalmic surgeon at Germantown Hospital, a post he held for ten years.

In 1893 he was appointed professor of ophthalmology at Medico-chirurgical College and retained that post when that institution became the Graduate School of Medicine of the University of Pennsylvania.

He also served as expert ophthalmologist for the U.S. Board of Pensions, the Baptist Orphanage, and the U.S. Indian schools in Carlisle, Pennsylvania, and was appointed a manager of the Orthopaedic Hospital.

Dr. L. Webster Fox was coauthor with George M. Gould, M.D. of *A Compend of the Diseases of the Eye: Including Refraction and Surgical Operations* (1886), and author of *A Practical Treatise on Ophthalmology* (1910). In 1924 Dr. Fox served as president of the board of trustees of the Pennsylvania Military College and in 1925 was appointed a member of the newly created State Council for the Blind. He received an honorary LL.D. from Dickinson College in 1908.

Dr. Fox's wife, the former C. Beatrice Bickerton of London, served as national president of the Daughters of the British Empire. Dr. and Mrs. Fox traveled to the southwestern United States during the summers in the 1920s, and were particularly interested in the schools and medical care of Native Americans.

Working through the Indian Medical Service of the Indian Bureau, Dr. Fox volunteered to establish trachoma clinics in Gallup and Albuquerque, New Mexico. He was especially noted for his work at the Blackfoot Reservation adjoining Glacier National Park in Browning, Montana where he conducted demonstration clinics especially for Indian Service physicians. In gratitude for his work in helping to eradicate trachoma, the Blackfoot Tribe made Dr. Fox a formal member in a 1925 ceremony before several hundred men robed in brilliant leather and fur garments decorated with beaded ornaments. During the ceremony Dr. Fox was given the name of Chief Eagle, after the bird prized for its keen sight. Members of more than three hundred families of the tribe had been saved from certain blindness.

In 1925 Mrs. L. Webster Fox arranged for her husband to be portrayed in his academic gown. But the physician resolved that the depiction must also include the eagle-feathered headdress awarded by the Blackfoot Tribe, his favorite gift among all the honors he had ever received.[22]

The artist chosen was Mrs. Fox's fellow Briton, Richard Langtry Partington, who was born in 1868 in Stockport, England. He studied art under his father, J. H. Partington, and with Sir Hubert von Herkomer in England, as well as at the Beaux-Arts Institute in Antwerp, Belgium. A nationally known portrait painter in America, he lived at various times in Philadelphia, San Francisco, and Detroit. Among his notable Philadelphia portrait subjects were Mr. and Mrs. Cyrus H. K. Curtis, Governor William C. Sproul, Edward T. Stotesbury, and Dr. John B. Deaver.

In the full-length portrait Dr. Fox is shown life-sized, seated erectly in a carved armchair and facing partly to the right. His deepset and hooded blue eyes look into the distance, and his narrow mouth topped by a neat mustache is set in a sober expression. Bright lights catch the winged collar of his shirt visible under his black academic robe with its colorful purple and green hood lined in yellow and red. Details of his costume include a pearl stick pin and two gold pinky rings.

The elaborate Indian headdress with its red and white feathers, ornamental beading, fur, and leather rests on a Rococo Revival carved table in the lower right corner. The atmospheric black background contains the base and shaft of a symbolic column. The predominant darkness and restraint of the artist's paint application and the somber facial expression and elegance of costume and furniture create a mood expressing the sitter's refinement, confidence, and dignity. The presence of the Indian headdress in an otherwise traditional setting hints at the sitter's dedication to an uncommon cause and his sense of adventure.

1. John Chalmers DaCosta, M.D., "Address Presenting Memorial Tablet to Jefferson Medical College, October 7, 1920," *The Trials and Triumphs of the Surgeon and Other Literary Gems* (Philadelphia: Dorrance & Co., 1944), 335-36.

2. Frederick B. Wagner Jr., M.D., *Thomas Jefferson University: Tradition and Heritage* (Philadelphia: Lea & Febiger, 1989), 1027-32.

3. W. M. L. Coplin, M.D., *American Red Cross Base Hospital No. 38 in the World War: United States Army Base Hospital No. 38 Organized under the Auspices of the Jefferson Medical College and Hospital* (Philadelphia: E. A. Wright Co., 1923).

4. Coplin, 87-99.

5. For a first-person account of the period, see Clara Melville, R.N., *History of the School of Nursing of the Jefferson Medical College Hospital* (booklet printed for the college, 1937).

6. Andrew W. Shearer, *A Commitment to Excellence: A History of the School of Nursing, College of Allied Health Sciences, Thomas Jefferson University, 1891-1982* (Wynnewood, Pa.: Heden-Livingston, 1982), 18.

7. Francis Haskell and Nicholas Penny, *Taste and the Antique* (New Haven: Yale University Press, 1981), 308.

8. For biographies of Dr. Abraham Coles see: Fred B. Rogers, M.D., "Abraham Coles, Poet-physician of New Jersey," *Journal of the Medical Society of New Jersey* 51 (Feb. 1954): 61-65; and Jonathan A. Coles, M.D. and Emilie S. Coles, ed., *Abraham Coles: Biographical Sketch, Memorial Tributes, Selections from His Works* (New York: D. Appleton & Co., 1893).

9. John Chalmers DaCosta, M.D., *Selections from the Papers and Speeches* (Philadelphia: W. B. Saunders Co., 1931), 205.

10. Wagner, and J. Woodrow Savacool, M.D., ed., *Jefferson Medical College of Thomas Jefferson University: Legend and Lore* (Devon, Pa.: William T. Cooke, 1996), 560.

11. Donation information courtesy of Theresa Powers, former director of the Audiovisual Center, originally established in 1970 by the Baugh Institute of Anatomy. Dr. Andrew J. Ramsay told me he remembered the statue on the first floor outside the library of the old anatomy building.

12. For biographical information see Michael W. Panhorst, *Samuel Murray: The Hirshhorn Museum and Sculpture Garden Collection* (Washington, D.C.: Smithsonian Institution Press, 1982).

13. Lloyd Goodrich, *Thomas Eakins,* 2 vols. (Cambridge, Mass.: Harvard University Press for the National Gallery of Art, 1982), 2:109.

14. Early Jefferson documents and other publications spell his name as listed. Some later publications spell the name "Green."

15. For information about Anna Magee and the hospital, see Thomas L. Ashcom Jr. and Edith W. Schmidt, *A History of Magee Rehabilitation Hospital 1923-1983* (Philadelphia: Magee Rehabilitation Hospital, 1983).
16. Gordon Hendricks, *Eadweard Muybridge: The Father of the Motion Picture* (New York: Grossman Publishers, 1975), 162-63.
17. For biographical details see J. Woodrow Savacool, M.D., "Philadelphia's Doctor Flick—Medical Crusader," *Philadelphia Medicine* 78 (Apr. 1982): 148-51.

J. Woodrow Savacool, M.D. (JMC 1938), honorary clinical associate professor of medicine, has been a distinguished Jefferson faculty member in the department of medicine and community health and preventive medicine, and was a pulmonary consultant to the Philadelphia Department of Public Health.

In 1984 Dr. Savacool's colleagues established the J. Woodrow Savacool Prize in Medical Ethics in his honor.

In addition to many other contributions to the literature, Dr. Savacool is author of the chapter "Division of Pulmonary and Critical Care Medicine" in Wagner, *Thomas Jefferson University: Tradition and Heritage*. He is also coeditor with Dr. Wagner of *Thomas Jefferson University: A Chronological History and Alumni Directory 1824-1990* (Philadelphia: Thomas Jefferson University, 1992), and *Jefferson Medical College of Thomas Jefferson University: Legend and Lore*.
18. *The Record* (Philadelphia), Apr. 8, 1934.
19. Martha Hutson-Saxton, Ph.D., "Walter Emerson Baum: Pennsylvania Artist, 1884-1956," *American Art Review* 6 (Dec. 1994-Jan. 1995): 150-57. Dr. Hutson-Saxton was the curator of the exhibition *Sunlight and Shadow: The Art of Walter Emerson Baum* at the Allentown Art Museum, and author of a monograph on the artist.
20. Wagner, *Thomas Jefferson University: Tradition and Heritage*, 545.
21. William N. Bradley, M.D., Collection of Letters, Historical Collections, College of Physicians of Philadelphia, 1:74.
22. For L. Webster Fox's experiences with Indian medicine, see the biography by his daughter: Beatrice Fox Griffith, *Pennsylvania Doctor* (Harrisburg, Pa.: The Stackpole Co., 1957), 203-21. The author also mentions that the face of L. Webster Fox appears among the students in *The Gross Clinic*, but since she misspells the name of Thomas Eakins and says that his painting was hung in Memorial Hall at the 1876 Centennial Exhibition, one should put little credence in the assertion.

CHAPTER 7

The Nineteen-twenties through World War II

Jefferson Medical College celebrated the centennial of its founding in 1924. The college launched a construction campaign around this time leading to three major buildings, the College and Curtis Buildings and the Samuel Gustine Thompson Annex, all still in active use today. The Depression necessitated a period of austerity during which some programs were canceled or deferred, but the number of graduates continued at a high level. When the United States entered into World War II in 1941 Jefferson Medical College met the emergency by accelerating the curriculum from four years to three, and shortening the hospital internship from one year to ten months.

Samuel Gustine Thompson Annex

SAMUEL GUSTINE THOMPSON ANNEX
By John Torrey Windrim (1866/67-1934)
Erected 1924
Reproduction of original etching
By Earl Horter (1883-1940)
Ca. 1925-30

Image size: 6 1/4 x 4 1/4 in.
Sheet size: 12 x 9 1/4 in.

Signed on plate lower right: "E. Horter"
Inscription below image: "Jefferson Hospital, Philadelphia/The New Samuel Gustine Thompson Annex"

Given in 1996 by Julie S. Berkowitz, the university art historian
Accession number: 1996+e.Ph.01

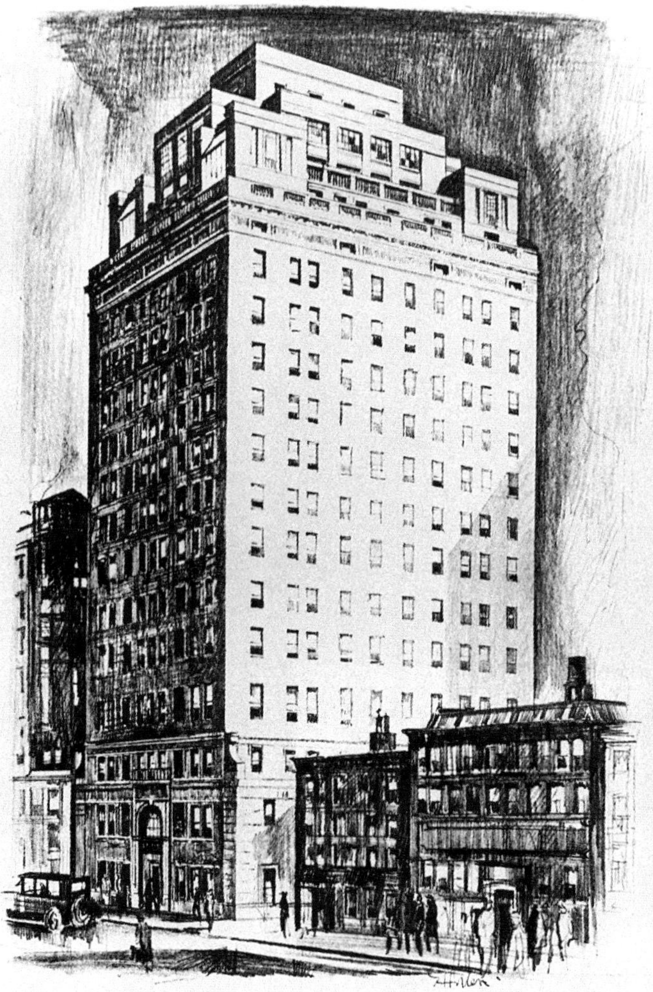

Jefferson Hospital, Philadelphia
The New Samuel Gustine Thompson Annex

According to Henry K. Mohler, M.D., medical director of the Jefferson Hospital, it was thought that planning for the Main Hospital of 1907 had allowed for ample growth and extension for many years into the future.[1] But within a decade many patients had to be turned away for lack of adequate accommodations, and so it was decided to build a major new addition on the site of the first hospital of 1877. Initial funds were provided by a legacy from William Thompson who stipulated that the building be named in memory of his brother, Samuel Gustine Thompson, a Jefferson trustee (1895-1909) and chief justice of Pennsylvania's Supreme Court.

By July 1922 demolition began of the old hospital located on Sansom Street between Tenth and Eleventh

Streets. The centennial of Jefferson's founding was celebrated on October 13, 1924 with the dedication of the Samuel Gustine Thompson Annex.

The annex connected with the first seven floors of the Main Hospital of 1907 at Tenth and Sansom Streets. The new brick building had sixteen floors devoted to clinical facilities, and was then the tallest hospital in the world. The clinical amphitheater occupied the basement, first, and second floors and had a seating capacity of five hundred. It replaced the 1877 hospital's pit. The outpatient neurological, orthopaedic, medical, and gastrointestinal departments were also located in the basement. The first floor contained administrative offices and the social service and occupational therapy departments. On the second floor were X-ray rooms and the dental and bronchoscopic clinics. Nurses' quarters were located on the third to the sixth floors. Patients' private rooms were on the eighth to the thirteenth floors. The fourteenth floor was occupied by the operating and delivery rooms. The two setback upper floors contained laboratories and a roof garden.

The architect for the Thompson Annex was John Torrey Windrim, best known for designing the John Wanamaker store, the Franklin Institute, and the Family Court building, as well as many office, college, and other hospital buildings in Philadelphia. He was the son and partner of architect James H. Windrim.

Earl Horter's etching of Thompson Annex is one in a series of American hospitals created in the late 1920s. A native Philadelphian born in 1883, Horter was a gifted draftsman who evidently never had formal fine arts training. After working in advertising for N. W. Ayer and Son from 1917 to 1923, he turned to freelance illustration, especially of urban architectural subjects. A group of his etchings won a silver medal at San Francisco's Panama-Pacific Exposition in 1915.

During the 1920s and 1930s he began to paint in watercolor and oils. After traveling abroad he assembled a notable private collection of avant-garde French Post-impressionist and Cubist paintings. He exhibited his own works at the Wildenstein Gallery in New York and at a number of Philadelphia galleries. The Philadelphia Art Alliance gave him a one-man show in 1936, and memorial exhibitions in 1940 and 1954.

In addition to instructing private pupils, Earl Horter taught for two decades at the Graphic Sketch Club, the Philadelphia Museum School of Art, and the Tyler School of Art at Temple University. By means of teaching, collecting, and his own painting, Earl Horter was instrumental in introducing modern art to Philadelphia.

Athena/Minerva

ATHENA/MINERVA
By unknown artist(s)

Marble
Ca. second century, with eighteenth- or nineteenth-century additions
47 1/4 x 23 5/8 x 13 1/2 in.

Given before 1939 by unknown donor
Accession number: 1939+b.S.01

In 1989 I "re"-discovered a rare antiquity located in a niche in the ground floor elevator lobby of the Thompson Building. Although the full-length marble statue of Athena/Minerva had probably been in that location for decades, it had been overlooked as "art" in contemporary times. The statue was mentioned in only two of more than twenty art inventories, and it was curiously called a "bust" and not described as antique.

With the assistance of several scholars of ancient art and archeology, it was established that Athena's torso was created in the early Roman Imperial period around the second century and that the head and arms were added to the damaged work in the eighteenth or nineteenth century.[2] Clues about dating stemmed from the style and carving of the costume, the attachment of an exterior metal pin, the stance and anatomy of the figure, the Roman-type moldings of the attached base, and the condition of the marble surface.

The slightly smaller than life-sized figure stands on a four-inch plinth integral to the statue. Her classical costume includes a chiton (the thin, linen, tubular undergarment buttoned along the upper arm to form sleeves) and a peplos (the heavy wool overgarment belted over the overfold). The softly draped folds of the drapery are inexactly rendered, but do reveal the figure's underlying forms.

She is identified as Athena/Minerva by her customary attributes of a helmet decorated with rams' horns and an aegis (breastplate), the goatskin of her father, Zeus. Used as an amulet for magical protection, the aegis is carved with writhing snakes on the border and the central head of Medusa, the fearful Gorgon.

Her *contrapposto* stance is a traditional posture with body weight carried on one leg and the other leg bent at the knee. The figure has elongated proportions with narrow shoulders and a high waist. The surface of the marble is a tawny color with pockmarks and irregularly scattered, dark accretions. The accretions are the result

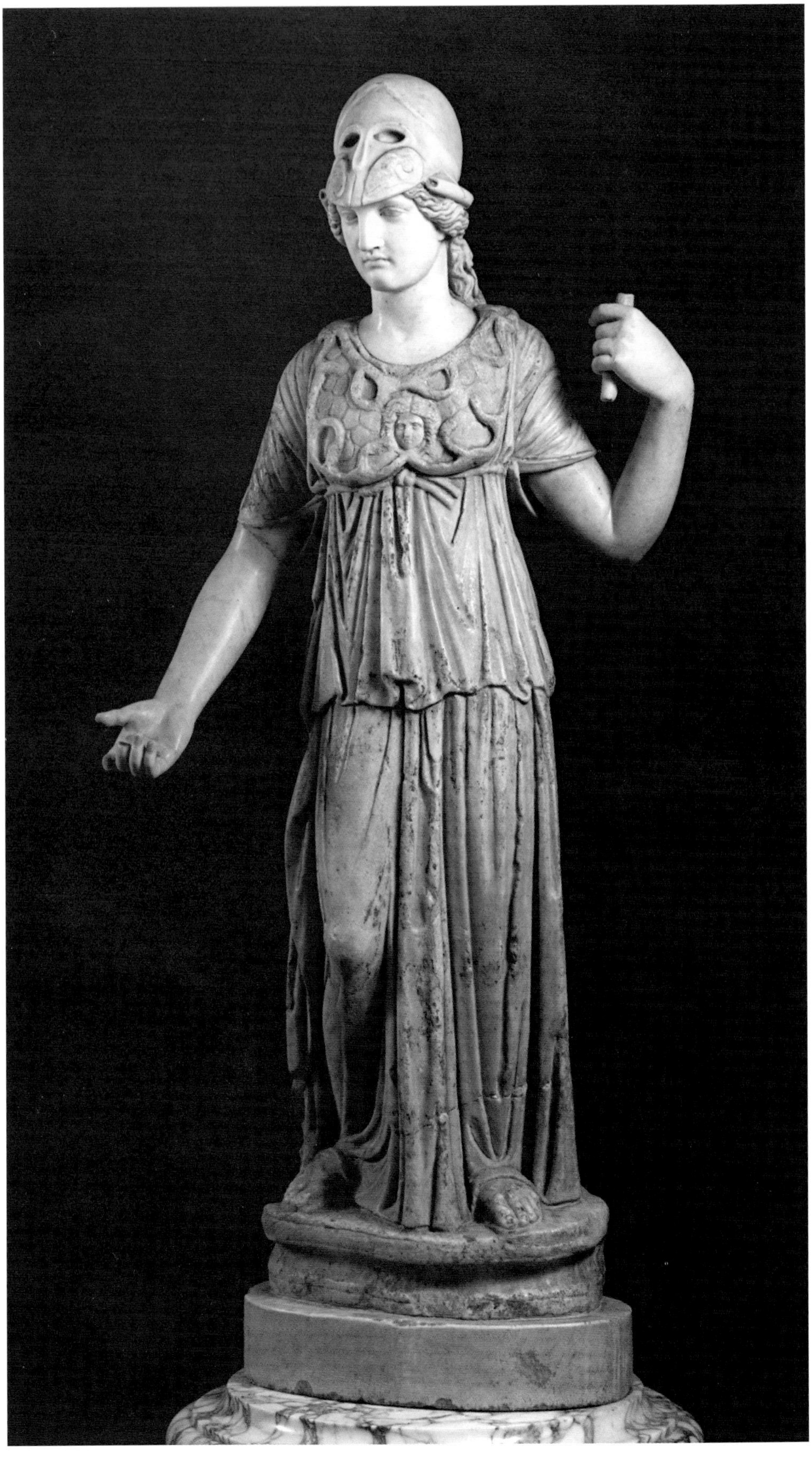

of chemical reactions between marble crystals and minerals in the soil, suggesting probable burial in antiquity and long exposure to the elements.

Although best known as the deity of war and wisdom and as the patron goddess of Athens, she was also worshipped as the protectress of the skilled arts and crafts including medicine. In Greece there are references to the deity in art and literature as Athena Hygeia, a healer, especially before the popularity of Asklepios in Greece. In Rome the cult of Athena blended with that of Minerva and she was the special deity of physicians. Temples were dedicated to Minerva Medica and her connections with medicine are attested to in the literature.

The statue's torso is a free, inventive, and eclectic interpretation of prototypes, rather than a direct copy of a specific earlier Athena/Minerva. The scholars who consulted on Athena's research felt that the overly thick and awkwardly restored arms probably did not recall the gestures of the original Roman statue before it was damaged, and that originally the statue's right arm had held a spear and the left arm a shield. However, the especially fine carving of the helmeted head suggests that the neoclassical restorer in the eighteenth or nineteenth century was aware of a specific fourth-century source, most likely the *Athena Giustiniani* (now in the Vatican Museum), itself a Roman marble copy of an original Greek bronze of about 400 B.C.

When sculpture conservators declared that the statue was safe to move, Athena was relocated to the Eakins Gallery in 1989. In spite of excitement caused by the find, no records about the work's provenance, donor, or date of donation have emerged.

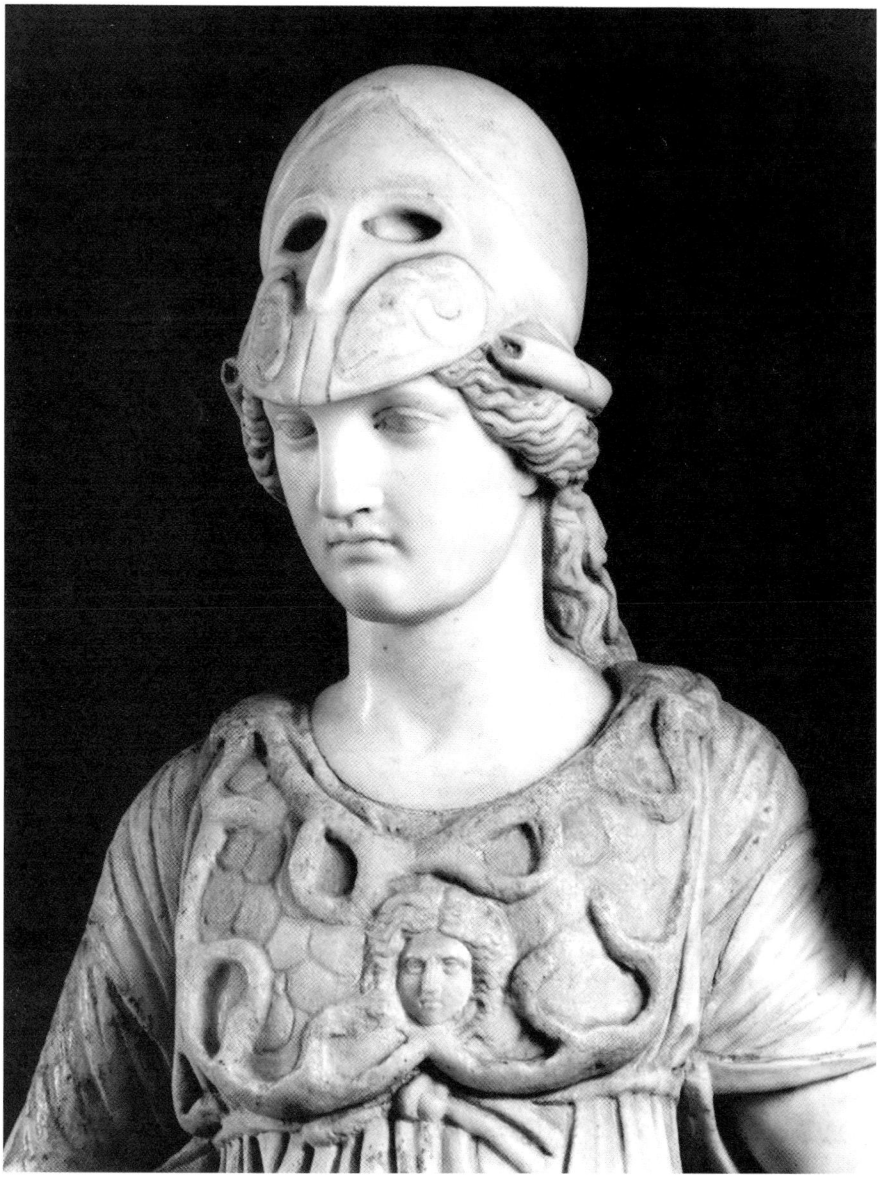

Because the Thompson lobby niche is depicted in the architect's original drawings, and because the Jefferson art collection included no other object appropriate for such a space, it is my guess that the statue was already owned or was a promised gift in 1924. A former Jefferson nurse who was a student at the time of the annex's dedication thought she recalled the statue being in its niche then. The first published photograph of Athena appeared in a Jefferson nursing school yearbook of 1939.

One can speculate that the statue was the gift of an alumnus or faculty member who had traveled to Rome. More likely it was a gift from a generous contemporary trustee such as Daniel Baugh or William Potter. Baugh's antiquarian interests were discussed in the previous chapter. Potter not only served as the American minister to Italy, but was also a vice president of the American and British Archeological Society of Rome and a member of the Committee of the American Schools at Rome for the Study of Archeology.

Portrait of Alba B. Johnson

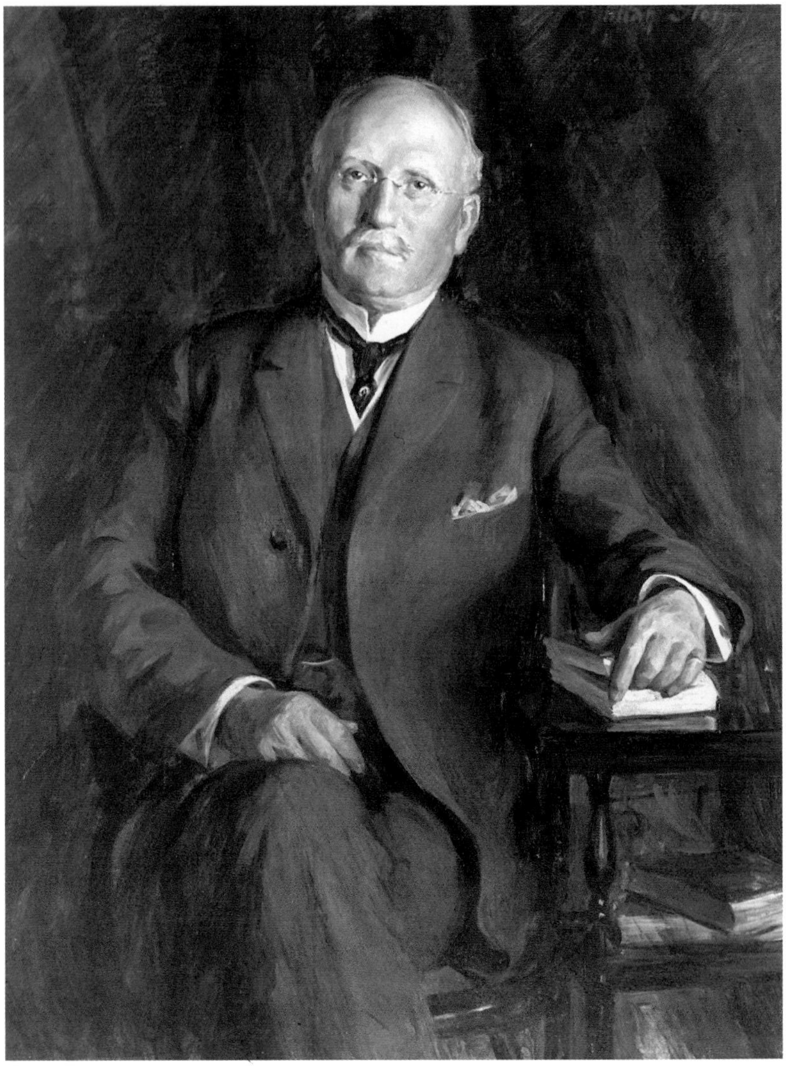

ALBA BOARDMAN JOHNSON (1858-1935)
By Julian Russel Story (1857-1919)

Oil on canvas
Ca. 1913
45 x 35 in.

Signed and dated upper right: "Julian Story"
Exhibition: Philadelphia, *Annual Exhibition*, Pennsylvania Academy of the Fine Arts, 1913

Given 1935-48 by unknown donor
Accession number: 1935-1948.P.01

The Thompson Annex was planned and constructed when Alba B. Johnson was president of the board of trustees. The distinguished industrialist and civic leader was a Jefferson trustee for more than thirty years.

Born in 1858 in Pittsburgh, Alba B. Johnson was descended from an English forbear who arrived in Massachusetts in 1677. After graduating from Philadelphia's Central High School in 1876, Johnson entered the Baldwin Locomotive Works as a junior clerk. He made that industry his life's work and rose progressively in the firm until he became partner in 1896 and president in 1911, a position he held until 1919.

This public-spirited Philadelphian also found time to serve as president of the Philadelphia and the Pennsylvania Chambers of Commerce, the Railway Business Association, and the American Manufacturers Export Association; chairman of the Southwark Foundry and Machine Company, the Standard Steel Works Company, and the National Foreign Trade Council; and a director of the Federal Reserve Bank of Philadelphia and the New York Life Insurance Company. He was an originator and prime mover in the early efforts of Philadelphia's Sesqui-centennial Exposition. He served as president of the Presbyterian Social Union and the YMCA of Philadelphia, and was chairman of the China Famine Relief Committee. He was awarded honorary LL.D. degrees from Ursinus College in 1909 and the University of Vermont in 1928.

A cultivated and scholarly gentleman, Johnson possessed an outstanding private library including many rare volumes on early mechanical discoveries and inventions. He was a member of the Art Jury of Philadelphia and the Fairmount Park Art Association. He was also a prizewinning horticulturalist.

Alba Johnson chaired the hospital committee of the 1924 Centennial Fund. The Ivycroft Farm and Convalescent Home for Men in Wayne, Pennsylvania was a gift to Jefferson Hospital from Mr. and Mrs. Johnson in 1917. In addition to numerous contributions during his lifetime, he left the college a bequest of $250,000.

Alba B. Johnson merited three portraits at Jefferson Medical College, the most of impressive of which was painted by Julian R. Story. The donor and year of donation of the portrait are undocumented, but the portrait probably arrived shortly after Johnson's tenure on the board of trustees ended with his death in 1935. In 1913 Story exhibited a portrait of Alba Johnson at the *Annual*

Exhibition of the Pennsylvania Academy of the Fine Arts (presumably this one).

The three-quarters-length depiction shows the subject seated in an armchair with his legs crossed and facing the viewer. His left hand marks the place in his book, and he looks up as if just interrupted in his reading. His fastidious attire includes a jeweled tie pin and gold cuff links, watch chain, and "pinky" ring. Johnson's expression is serious and his posture rather stiff, but Story's paint style is free in its fluid and expressive handling of the flesh tones, costume, and background drapery.

A second portrait of Alba B. Johnson is a half-length depiction by Henry R. Rittenberg, purchased from Philadelphia art dealer Robert Carlen by Jefferson's board of trustees in 1961. Carlen stated that the previous unidentified owner had acquired it from the American Railroad Association which had commissioned it in 1928 on the occasion of Johnson's seventieth birthday and his tenth anniversary as president of the association.

Jefferson documents refer to another half-length portrait of Alba Johnson painted in 1929 by Benedict A. Osnis, and presented by the alumni association in 1930. By 1961 the Osnis work was in "ruinous" condition, and it was decided to "substitute" the Rittenberg portrait for the Osnis, and the latter disappeared.

Jefferson Medical College Building

JEFFERSON MEDICAL COLLEGE BUILDING
By firm of Horace Trumbauer (1868-1938)

Graphite, crayon, ink on artist's board
Ca. 1927
Image size: 23 x 18 1/4 in.
Sheet size: 29 1/2 x 22 1/4 in.

Signature lower right: "Horace Trumbauer Architect"
Inscription below image: "JEFFERSON MEDICAL COLLEGE/WALNUT AT CLIFTON STREETS/PHILADELPHIA"

Prepared for Jefferson Medical College
Accession number: 1927+c.D.01

This graphite and crayon rendering of the new Jefferson Medical College Building was probably presented by architect Horace Trumbauer for the board's approval about 1927. Not intended to be a precise working drawing of the architectural elevation, instead it situates the building in its urban environment. Thus it includes neighboring buildings, pedestrians, automobiles, and a trolley. The drawing's shading of sky and street is quite dramatic.

The new College Building accommodated all college activities except for anatomy classes which continued at the Baugh Institute on Clinton Street. The building was planned in tandem with an adjoining outpatient clinic building which would soon replace the 1898 College Building on Walnut Street between Tenth and Eleventh Streets.

The College Building had a frontage of 158 feet on Walnut Street. A large auditorium (later named the Herbut Auditorium) occupied the central portion of the ground and first floors. Student rooms, meeting rooms, and storage and locker facilities completed the ground floor. A library on the first floor extended the depth of the building, 108 feet. Adjacent to the library were the board room and offices of the president, dean, and registrar. On the second floor were lecture rooms and an auditorium (later named McClellan Hall) large enough to seat the entire student body and faculty. The third floor housed all the facilities for the teaching of chemistry and clinical medicine. The departments of physiology and pharmacology occupied the fourth floor, and the pathology department and its museum were on the fifth floor. The bacteriology department and facilities

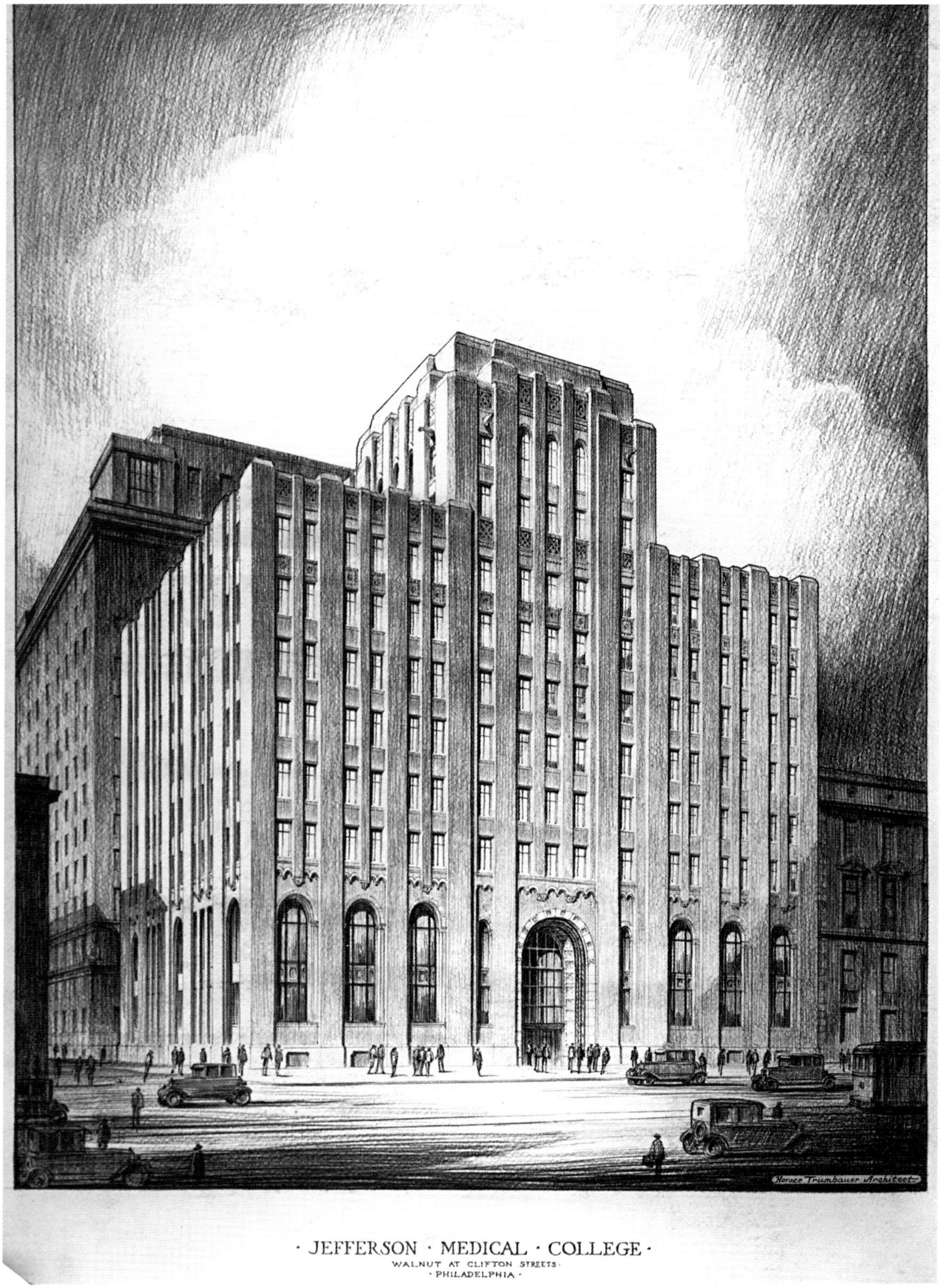
Horace Trumbauer Architect
· JEFFERSON · MEDICAL · COLLEGE ·
WALNUT AT CLIFTON STREETS ·
· PHILADELPHIA ·

for research and experimental animals occupied the sixth floor. The upper floors were not yet allocated.

The facade of the College Building of 1929 was constructed of orange brick with terra cotta ornamentation. It is ten stories high with an attic under the eaves. The dominant features of the facade are its Romanesque arched windows alternating with strong vertical elements in the Moderne style. A central tower is stepped back in masses resembling Mexican or Mayan design. Lively terra cotta ornament consists of reliefs of animals and stylized plant forms below; griffins, squirrels, and rams above; rows of lions' heads; and griffin and eagle gargoyles.

A native Philadelphian, Horace Trumbauer was born in 1868. He entered the architectural firm of G. W. and W. D. Hewitt in 1884 as an office boy, and after eight years of training he established his own practice. He defied tradition by hiring an African American associate, Julian Abele. The first black architecture student to graduate from the University of Pennsylvania, Abele was put in charge of most of the architectural drawing in Trumbauer's office.

Trumbauer launched his reputation soon thereafter with Grey Towers, a spectacular Gothic mansion for sugar tycoon William H. Harrison. Grey Towers is now a landmark on the Beaver College campus in Jenkintown, Pennsylvania. Trumbauer also designed imposing residences for other industrialists: Peter A. B. Widener, Edward B. Stotesbury, and William L. Elkins.

Horace Trumbauer was awarded commissions for important commercial buildings in Philadelphia including the Ritz-Carlton, Adelphia, St. James, and Benjamin Franklin Hotels; the Stock Exchange and the Beneficial Savings Fund Society Building; the Philadelphia Museum of Art and the Free Library; the Racquet Club and the Union League addition; the Public Ledger, Widener, and Bankers Security Buildings; and the Hahnemann Medical College.

In New York he designed the Evening Post, Wildenstein, and Duveen Buildings; and homes for Cornelius Vanderbilt and James B. Duke. His university buildings also included the Widener Memorial Library at Harvard and the Gothic buildings at Duke.

Entrance of the Jefferson Medical College Building

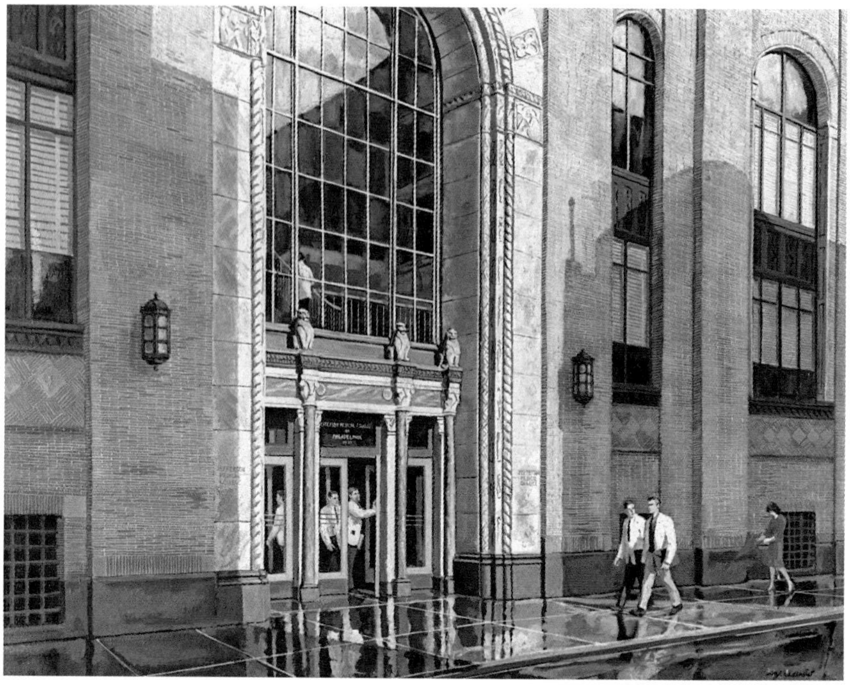

ENTRANCE OF THE 1929 COLLEGE BUILDING
By Benjamin Eisenstat (b. 1915)

Oil on canvas
1965
28 1/4 x 36 1/4 in.

Signed lower right: "Benj Eisenstat"

Given in 1965 by E. R. Squibb & Sons
Accession number: 1965+e.P.01

In 1965 E. R. Squibb and Sons, the New York pharmaceutical manufacturer, sponsored a project known as "Collegia Medica Squibb" in connection with the bicentennial of medical education in America. It aimed at creating a collection of original oil paintings of significant buildings located at the eighty-three accredited, four-year American medical schools.

Jefferson Medical College was honored with being the first subject of the Squibb project because it had graduated more physicians than any other American medical college, over twenty thousand by that date. It was also a natural choice because the great-grandfather of the current vice president for marketing at Squibb was the firm's founder, Edward R. Squibb, M.D. (JMC 1845). Reproductions of the series appeared in numerous medical journals, and copies were mailed to alumni of each school.

The 1929 College Building was chosen as best typifying Jefferson architecture, and specifically its Walnut Street entrance as the aspect best remembered by every graduate. The colorful painting by Ben Eisenstat shows the building on a rainy day, focusing on the two-story entrance with its windowed archway above the tripartite portal and all its diverse architectural ornamentation. Medical students in white jackets are entering and leaving the building and mounting the steps inside. The wet sidewalk and street contain reflections from the building. Apparently the rain has just stopped, because a blue sky is reflected in the upper windows and the building bears patterns of light and shade. An eye-catching figure on the sidewalk is the shapely young woman dressed in red who is lowering her matching umbrella.

Ben Eisenstat is best known for his paintings of landmark buildings in historic sections of Philadelphia, including murals commissioned by several banks, churches, libraries, and insurance companies. Eisenstat's illustrations appeared so often in the *Philadelphia Inquirer*'s Sunday magazine section that he was virtually the paper's "official artist." His work also appeared in the *New York Times* and the *Saturday Review*, among others.

Eisenstat was born in Philadelphia in 1915. After studying at the Fleisher Art Memorial and the Barnes Foundation, he won a scholarship to the Pennsylvania Academy of the Fine Arts. For thirty-eight years he taught painting, watercolor, drawing, and illustration at the Philadelphia College of Art and was chair of the illustration department. He also taught at the Philadelphia Museum of Art, Fleisher, the Cambridge (England) College of Art, Syracuse University, the Parsons School of Design in New York, and the Academy of Art in San Francisco.

Eisenstat exhibited his works nationally and was honored with more than thirty solo shows. His works are owned by numerous museums, businesses, and educational institutions. He won three Harrison Morris Prizes at *Annual Exhibitions* of the Fellowship of the Pennsylvania Academy of the Fine Arts, the Thornton Oakley Prize and the Medal of Achievement at the Philadelphia Water Color Club, and first awards at the Philadelphia Art Directors Annual and the Watercolor U.S.A. show at the Springfield Museum.

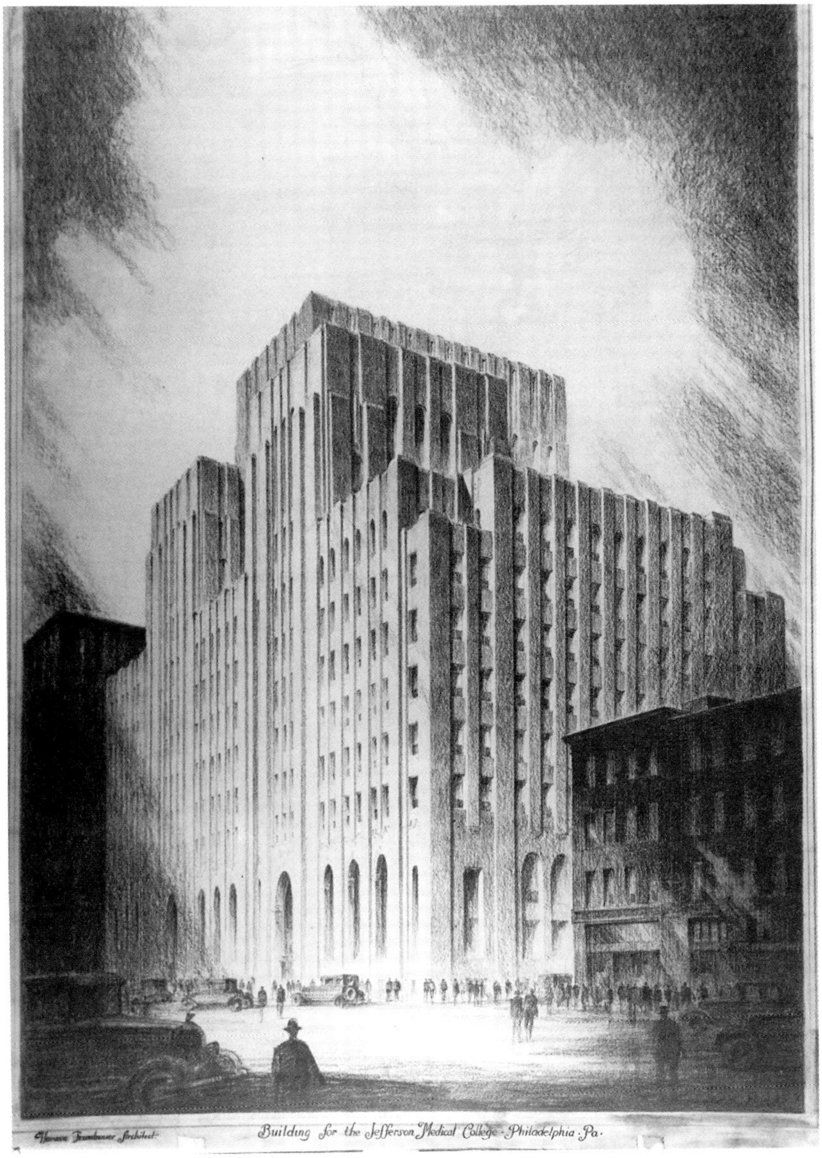

Jefferson Medical College and Curtis Clinic Buildings

COLLEGE AND CURTIS CLINIC BUILDINGS
By firm of Horace Trumbauer

Graphite, crayon, ink on artist's board
Ca. 1929
Image size: 29 1/2 x 21 1/4 in.
Sheet size: 31 1/4 x 23 in.

Signed under image lower left: "Horace Trumbauer Architect"
Inscription below image: "Building for the Jefferson Medical College Philadelphia Pa."

Prepared for Jefferson Medical College
Accession number: 1929+c.D.01

An architectural rendering of Jefferson's College and Curtis Buildings was produced by the Horace Trumbauer firm around 1929. The demolition of the 1898 College Building and its replacement with the Curtis Building for clinical activities were deferred until the new College Building was completed in 1929 and opened in February 1930. The twin structures occupied a total frontage of 268 feet on Walnut Street between Tenth and Eleventh.

According to the *Jefferson Medical College Alumni Bulletin* of January 1932 the eight-story building with four tower floors was "one of the most modern and completely equipped outpatient clinics in existence." By grouping together the various medical, surgical, and specialty divisions, the Curtis Building showed Jefferson's special regard for utilizing the clinic for teaching purposes as well as convenience for patients and physicians. Each department had its own patient waiting room, history-taking booths, examining rooms, student classrooms, and offices for physicians and a social service worker.

On the ground floor was the department of physical therapy. The first floor accommodated admission desks, the drug store, waiting and examining rooms, and the emergency ward with a special entrance on Tenth Street for receiving patients from the ambulance or police patrol. Accident and emergency cases could be transferred directly to the hospital if necessary. The second floor was occupied by the social service and X-ray departments, and had a passageway connecting it with the Main Hospital.

The third floor contained the maternity and children's departments; the fourth floor housed the nose and throat and the ophthalmological clinics; on the fifth floor were the general surgery and gynecological departments, and the tumor clinic; the sixth floor contained the orthopaedic and neurological clinics; on the seventh floor were the genito-urinary, dermatology, and syphilitic clinics. The department of medicine and the clinical laboratory occupied the whole eighth floor. The ninth-floor tower was occupied by the dental department. The three upper floors contained the training school for nurses.

This drawing is even more romantic in style than the drawing of the College Building above. The massive buildings look almost ghost-like and weightless, and the draftsman has emphasized their verticality. He has included dramatic shadows on the buildings, the street, and the stormy sky. The buildings are shown at an angle and set back into the middle ground, while the denizens of the city on foot and in their automobiles occupy the foreground.

Portrait of Cyrus H. K. Curtis

CYRUS HERMANN KOTZSCHMAR CURTIS
(1850-1933)
By William Taylor Thomson (1858-1941)

Oil on canvas
1931
58 1/4 x 42 1/4 in.

Signed lower right: " W. T. Thomson/after R. L. Partington"

Given in 1931 by JMC Hospital medical staff
Accession number: 1931+e.P.01

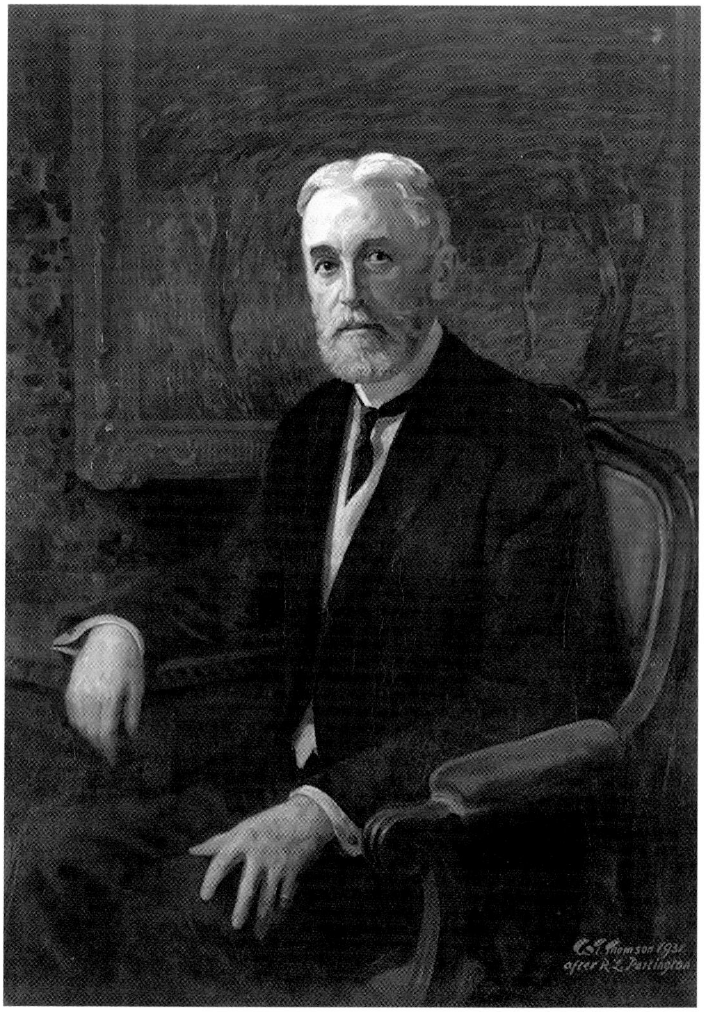

The Curtis Clinic Building was named in honor of Cyrus H. K. Curtis, the Philadelphia publishing magnate who had contributed an initial gift of five hundred thousand dollars to the building fund.

Cyrus H. K. Curtis was born in 1850 and reared in Portland, Maine. He was a ninth-generation member of the American line of the Curtis family who had emigrated from Great Britain to America in 1632. By the age of fifteen Curtis began publishing a weekly paper while still attending school. After relocating to Boston he became associated with several newspapers before founding the *People's Ledger* in 1872.

He moved to Philadelphia in 1876 and was connected with the *Philadelphia Press* before he established the *Tribune and Farmer* in 1879 and the *Ladies' Home Journal* in 1883. He organized the Curtis Publishing Company in 1890 and in 1893 erected the Curtis Building at Fourth and Arch Streets. Curtis purchased the *Saturday Evening Post* in 1897 and the *Country Gentleman* in 1911.

He bought the *Public Ledger* in 1913 and the following year started the *Evening Public Ledger*. In 1918 he added the *Evening Telegraph* to gain an Associated Press franchise. In 1920 he purchased the *Philadelphia Press* and merged it with the morning *Public Ledger*, and in 1925 purchased and merged the *Philadelphia North American* with it as well. He acquired the *New York Evening Post* in 1923. Curtis Publishing also owned the *Philadelphia Inquirer* briefly in the 1930s.

In addition to Jefferson Medical College, Curtis's philanthropies extended to several other educational institutions in the city. He was a director of several banks, insurance companies, and the Academy of Music Corporation. A lasting legacy of the Curtis family is the world-renowned Curtis Institute of Music, founded by Cyrus H. K. Curtis's daughter, Mary Louise Curtis Bok. In 1913 Cyrus Curtis received an honorary M.A. degree from Bowdoin College and an LL.D. degree from Ursinus College.

A portrait of Cyrus H. K. Curtis was presented during the dedication ceremonies of the Curtis Clinic Building on December 17, 1931. On behalf of the medical staff, Dr. Pascal Brooke Bland noted that the portrait and accompanying bronze plaque would be installed at the entrance to the building where "countless thousands of sick and maimed...will look with grateful hearts into the kindly eyes of their benefactor."

The portrait by William T. Thomson is a copy of an original work by Richard L. Partington of 1926, still hanging at the Curtis Institute of Music. In the two-thirds-length depiction Curtis is seated in an elegant Louis XV-style armchair facing the left, but with his head turned to gaze upward and to the right, as though expecting a reply from an unseen visitor. His posture is erect and somewhat stiff. Thomson's animated paint style is especially conspicuous in the sitter's whitish hair and beard with their flecks of green, his skin tones rendered in deep pinks and greens, and the background elements: a beautifully framed, impressionistic landscape painting and flocked, floral wallpaper.

Portrait of Wilfred W. Fry

WILFRED WASHINGTON FRY (1875-1936)
By Leopold Gould Seyffert (1887-1956)

Oil on canvas
1937
45 x 35 in.

Signed and dated lower left: "Leopold Seyffert 1937"

Given 1937-48 by family of the subject
Accession number: 1937-1948.P.01

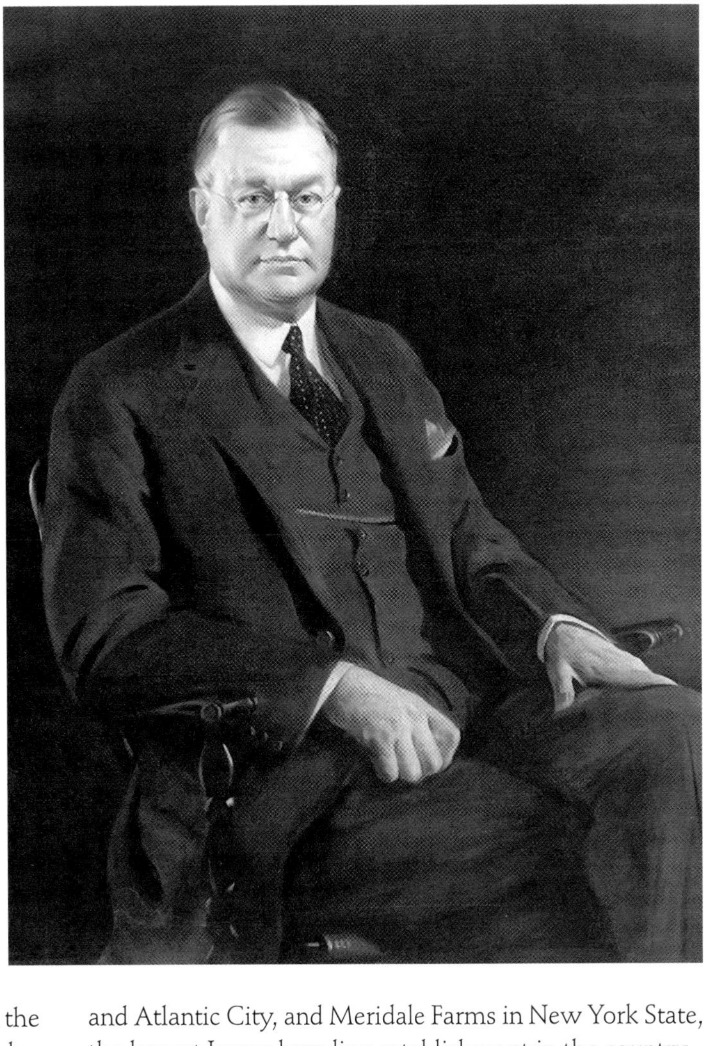

Prominent businessman Wilfred W. Fry succeeded Alba B. Johnson as Jefferson's president of the board of trustees in March 1935, but unfortunately his death occurred only a year later. He had been elected a member of the board in 1931.

Wilfred Fry was born in 1875 in Mount Vision, New York, the son of a Protestant minister. While attending the Mount Hermon School in East Northfield, Massachusetts he had to leave in order to care for his widowed mother. His interest in community service led to a series of positions with the YMCA in several different cities. A few years after his marriage to Anna G. Ayer, he moved to Philadelphia and joined the advertising firm of his father-in-law, N. W. Ayer and Son.

He was made managing partner in 1916, head of the company in 1923, and president in 1929 when the advertising company was incorporated. He was also president of Meridale Dairies of New York, Philadelphia, and Atlantic City, and Meridale Farms in New York State, the largest Jersey breeding establishment in the country.

Fry was actively engaged in philanthropic and civic affairs. A resident of Camden, New Jersey, he served as president of the Camden and Suburban Railway Company and the Camden Horse Railroad Company. Church activities also claimed his attention in Camden, where he was president of the YMCA from 1923 to 1935 and president of the board of trustees of the North Baptist Church. In 1932 he was made chairman of the International Committee of YMCAs of the U.S. and Canada.

Fry was an accomplished organist and president of the Musical Art Society of Camden. He was a trustee at Colgate and Brown Universities, and a board member at the Crozer Theological Seminary and the Franklin Institute. He was awarded an honorary LL.D. degree from Colgate University in 1927.

The posthumous portrait of Wilfred W. Fry was painted in 1937 by Leopold G. Seyffert and donated by the sitter's family before 1948, when it was first mentioned in a Jefferson insurance appraisal. In the three-quarters-length portrait the subject sits in a plain, wooden armchair with his legs crossed. Although his body faces partly right, his head is turned to gaze directly toward the viewer with a pleasant and confident expression. The figure is rendered in solid, three-dimensional forms. The atmospheric background is quite dark and the painting's surface is very smooth.

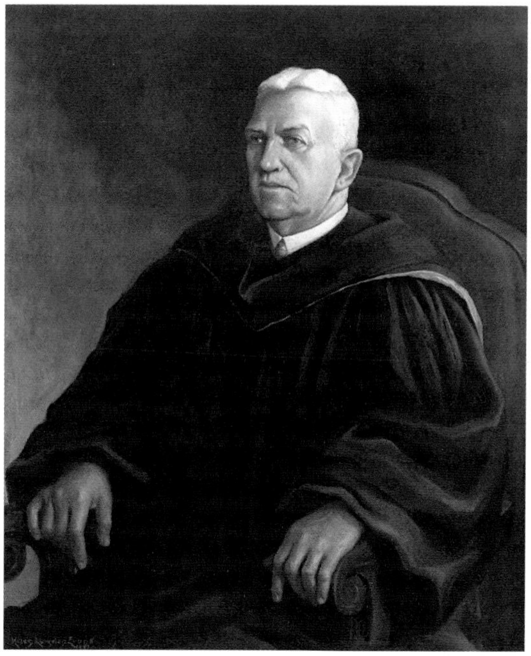

Portrait of Robert P. Hooper

ROBERT POOLE HOOPER (1872-1958)
By Helen Lowden Evans (1898-1993)

Oil on canvas
1947
40 x 34 in.

Signed and dated lower left: "Helen Lowden Evans/1947"

Given in 1947 by JMC alumni association
Accession number: 1947+e.P.01

Robert P. Hooper was elected to Jefferson Medical College's board of trustees in 1920, and he succeeded Wilfred W. Fry as president in 1936. In 1949 it was decided that Jefferson operations and administration had become so complex that it required a full-time president, and Mr. Hooper was elevated to chairman of the board, a post he held until 1950.

During his tenure the Charlotte Drake Cardeza Foundation was organized in 1938 as the division of hematology, and the Barton Memorial Division was organized in 1946 as the department of diseases of the chest at the former Broad Street Hospital.

Robert P. Hooper was born in Baltimore in 1872 to a prominent Maryland family and was educated at the Hill School. After serving as a draftsman for the Poole and Hunt Engineering Company he acted as agent in New York for various southern manufacturers of cotton products. He moved to Philadelphia in 1896 where he formed a commission house to handle this southern output. In 1902 he became president of the Hooper Sons' Manufacturing Company which later merged with another family company, the William E. Hooper and Sons Company, founded in 1800 as a manufacturer of cotton duck for the sails of clipper ships. The company's research laboratories developed and patented a fire-, water-, and mildew-resistant finish for textiles, a product used extensively by the armed forces during the war.

An early owner and advocate of the automobile, Robert P. Hooper was an organizer and president of the American Automobile Association and its Good Roads Board, of the Pennsylvania Motor Federation, and of the

Automobile Club of Philadelphia. He was a director of several insurance companies and banks, and also an enthusiastic yachtsman. Hooper received an honorary LL.D. degree from Jefferson Medical College in 1940.

The portrait of Robert P. Hooper by Helen L. Evans was presented by Jefferson's alumni association in 1940. The subject is depicted wearing a black academic gown with a blue-violet hood lined in pale blue. He is seated in a red upholstered armchair and his head and body are turned to the left. His expression is somber and he seems to stare stonily into space. His hands and facial features are rendered solidly with an emphasis on linear detail.

Helen Lowden Evans was a Philadelphia-area portraitist born in 1898. She studied at the School of Industrial Art (now University of the Arts) and privately with Robert Susan. During World War I she was a draftsman working on airplane designs at the Philadelphia Navy Yard. During the Depression she conducted adult and children's art classes.

Evans produced a series of thirty portraits of historical and contemporary political and military figures for the Valley Forge Military Academy in Wayne, Pennsylvania, in exchange for free tuition at the academy for her son, Samuel Evans III. Other portraits by Helen Evans can be found at the Pentagon in Washington, D.C., the Capitol in Harrisburg, Pennsylvania, the Pennsylvania State University, and the University of Pennsylvania.

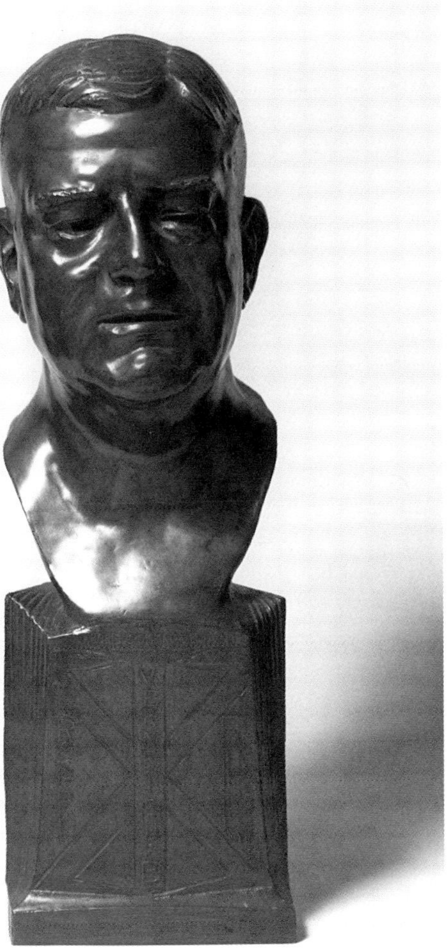

Portrait of Ross V. Patterson

ROSS VERNET PATTERSON, M.D. (1877-1938)
By Giuseppe Donato (1881-1965)

Bronze
1934
23 5/8 x 8 1/8 x 9 3/8 in.

Signed and dated on back lower right: "G. DONATO/34"
Inscriptions on integral base: front, "DN/LABORIBUS.OMMNIA [*sic*].VENDUNT" and name in three columns "ROSS VERNET MD.SD/PATTERSON," right side, "PRESENTED/4.31.35," and left side, "BY ALUMNI AND OTHER FRIENDS"
Exhibition: Philadelphia, *Annual Exhibition*, Pennsylvania Academy of the Fine Arts, 1937

Given in 1935 by JMC alumni and friends
Accession number: 1935+e.S.01

Dr. Ross V. Patterson was dean of Jefferson Medical College from 1916 until his death in 1938. A confirmed bachelor and dedicated Jeffersonian, he left his estate to establish the Ross V. Patterson fellowships in research.

Ross Patterson was descended from Scottish and French forbears who had arrived in America before the Revolution. He was born in New Orleans in 1877. After studying at Washington University in St. Louis, he graduated from Jefferson Medical College in 1904.

Following two years as intern and resident at Philadelphia Hospital, he established a private medical practice and was appointed sub-dean at Jefferson Medical College and also a teaching assistant in the department of medicine. In steady succession he was appointed dean in 1916, physician in charge of electrocardiography in the hospital in 1918, associate professor of medicine in 1927, and the Sutherland M. Prevost Professor of Therapeutics in 1934.

Patterson was noted for his strong executive ability, and was appointed the fifteenth dean of Jefferson Medical College, succeeding Dr. James W. Holland. He was dean during a period of architectural expansion at Jefferson, a period of change in medical education, research, and practice, and during the protracted negotiations and ultimate rejection of a proposed merger with the University of Pennsylvania School of Medicine.

Patterson was among the first group commissioned in the Medical Reserve Corps by President William H. Taft in 1911. In 1917 he served on active duty as cardiovascular examiner at Camp Dix, New Jersey until ordered to resume his academic duties by the surgeon-general. He was directly instrumental in securing funds to establish the Jefferson Base Hospital Thirty-eight, and in organizing the Students' Army Training Corps.

In addition, Patterson is credited with conceiving, planning, and establishing the Bureau of Professional Education in Pennsylvania. He was president of the Medical Society of the State of Pennsylvania and the Association of American Medical Colleges. He served three terms as president of Jefferson's alumni association. He was awarded D.Sc. degrees from LaSalle College and Colgate University, and LL.D. degrees from Ursinus College and Wake Forest College.

In spite of his heavy working schedule, Patterson retained a lifelong interest in sports including football, tennis, and baseball. Ever since his boyhood days on the western plains he remained an avid fisherman, deer hunter and trap-shooter.

Dean Patterson's physical prowess and forceful personality inspired equally strong reactions among his colleagues and students. In a particularly revealing obituary drawn up as a faculty resolution and printed in the *Alumni Bulletin* of May 1938, Dr. Thomas A. Shallow noted the "loss of his magnetism," adding,

> No more colorful figure ever graced the halls of our institution. We have had Masters in Medicine, Surgery and Science, but never such a character in whom pride, egotism, arrogance and intelligence were so finely blended to make the super-man...
>
> His tenure as Dean was filled with trials, tribulations and triumphs. A man of courage, he feared no one. He entered into combat willingly against strong foes who frequently outnumbered him, sometimes outmanoeuvered him, but never out-generaled him...
>
> Doctor Patterson was not without personal ambition. What red-blooded man is? His enemies unjustly accused him of being ambitious as though this were a crime and on this ground they pilloried him unmercifully, while he, apparently unaffected by their animosity, suffered quietly and at times reached a state almost of depression. On these occasions he was quite morose and seclusive, retiring to a hunting lodge for trap-shooting or fishing from which he would return in a few days his courtly, genial self...
>
> To his intimate friends—the few he permitted himself to have—Doctor Patterson was a man of sterling character. They enjoyed his genteel influence, his comradeship and his hospitality and they were devoted to him.

An oil portrait of Dean Patterson by Benedict A. Osnis depicts him as a formidable icon with a dour expression and stiffly erect posture. The painting was commissioned by the alumni association and presented in 1930, along with the Osnis portrait of Alba B. Johnson.

In contrast to the painting, the sculpted head of Dr. Ross V. Patterson by Giuseppe Donato is more successful in emphasizing the physical presence of the man and his underlying ruggedness. Though limited to head and neck, the image alludes to the subject's athleticism by means of the powerful, thick neck and the slight asymmetry of his features. His lips are parted with a trace of a smile as though engaging in friendly dialogue with a student or colleague, and the dark surface of the smoothly carved bronze head sparkles with reflected light.

The unusual base represents an open book which narrows to a spine in the back where a scroll and flames are carved. On the front of the book Patterson's name is inscribed vertically and flanked by an abstracted caduceus below the Latin inscription "DN/LABORIBUS. OMMNIA[*sic*].VENDUNT." This defies easy translation, but "laboribus" (by means of hard work) probably refers to Patterson's ethic.

The 1919 Jefferson yearbook was dedicated to Dean Ross V. Patterson with "affection, admiration and gratitude" for his sympathetic understanding of students and for being their "friend in court." The 1925 yearbook "unmasked" his alleged austerity:

> The real Ross V. isn't the stern and unapproachable "Dean" who makes opening addresses and sits in judgment in the "College Offices." It's when he is in intimate contact with the classes in his Junior lectures and Senior quizzes that the mask is off, and the real Ross V. Patterson with his kindliness of manner and inexhaustible store of real humor is disclosed. Ever true to his convictions, unbendable, four-square, he has been a source of real inspiration to all of us.

The artist himself was a widely known, sometimes controversial figure in the art world, a good match with his portrait subject. In 1908 Donato was involved in a controversy with the city of Baltimore which refused two of his nude allegorical figures. In Philadelphia he successfully forced painters who were gilding bronze stairways in City Hall to cease covering the ornamental originals with "gold dust and banana oil."

Born in Maida, Calabria, Italy in 1881 Donato came to Philadelphia with his family in 1892. He studied at the Pennsylvania Academy of the Fine Arts and the Philadelphia Industrial Art School. He won the Academy's Stewardson Sculpture Prize and the Cresson traveling scholarship. He continued his studies in Paris at the École des Beaux-Arts, the Académie Julian, and the Académie Colarossi, and also under Auguste Rodin.

Donato belonged to the New York Architectural League, the National Sculpture Society, the Society of Medallists, the American Arts Association of Paris, and the International Society of Arts and Letters. He exhibited portraits and allegorical figures throughout the United States. Commissioned portraits and monuments were located at Philadelphia's City Hall, Municipal Court Building, and Logan Circle, and in Harrisburg and Easton, Pennsylvania.

Portrait of Henry K. Mohler

HENRY KELLER MOHLER, M.D. (1887-1941)
By Maurice Molarsky (1885-1950)

Oil on canvas
1940
45 x 35 in.

Signed and dated lower right: "Maurice Molarsky 1940"

Given by JMC class of 1940
Accession number: 1940+e.P.01

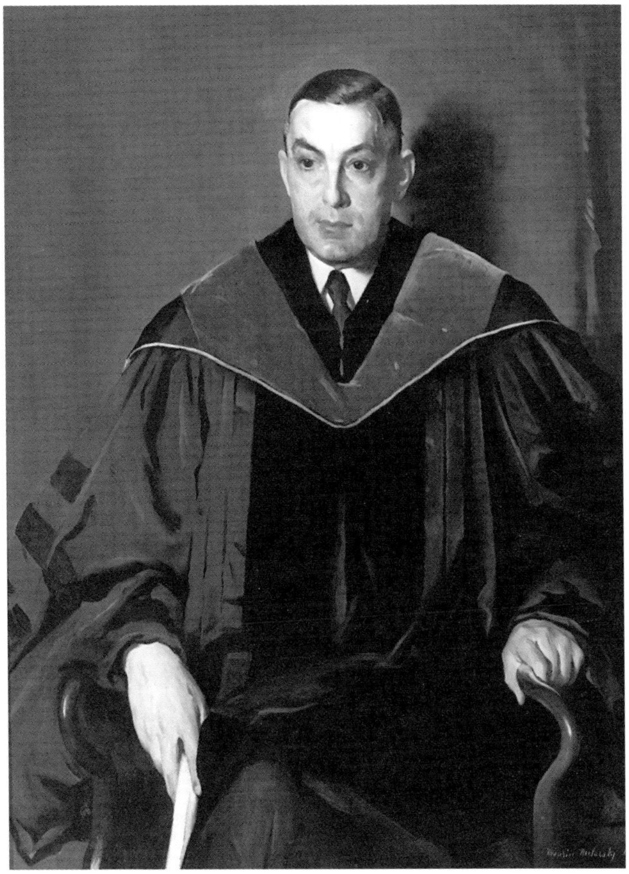

In 1938 Dr. Henry K. Mohler succeeded Dr. Ross V. Patterson as dean and served until his death in 1941. Although his tenure was brief, he was admired and respected for his executive ability and his untiring devotion to Jefferson Medical College and Hospital.

Henry Mohler was born in 1887 and reared in Ephrata, Pennsylvania near "Mohler's Corner" where his forbears had settled in 1732. Postponing a medical education for lack of funds, in 1907 he earned a degree at the Philadelphia College of Pharmacy where he was first in his class in spite of working long night hours in a drugstore. He graduated from Jefferson Medical College in 1912 with highest honors, as class president and its "most popular man."

After interning at Jefferson he was placed in charge of the laboratory of clinical medicine and appointed instructor in medicine in 1914. He rose through the ranks to become clinical professor of medicine in 1936. Two years later he was named the Sutherland Prevost Professor of Therapeutics.

Mohler was in charge of the cardiology department and was the medical director of the hospital until 1938 when he was named dean of the college. As dean he guided the growth of the department of clinical investigation and the completion of its laboratories. Medical students showed their esteem by inaugurating the Mohler Therapeutics Society and dedicating the yearbook to him in 1939. That same year he was elected president of the alumni association.

Dr. Mohler was commissioned a captain in World

War I, and served at the U.S. Army Base Hospital Thirty-eight where he was chief of the medical service. After the Armistice he rose to the rank of lieutenant colonel in the Medical Reserve Corps, serving until 1938. He served as president of the Philadelphia Heart Association and of the Pennsylvania Hospital Association. He received honorary D.Sc. degrees from LaSalle and Juniata Colleges.

A 1940 yearbook article praised his modesty, determination, clear thinking, and ability to judge human nature. It is questionable whether these personal qualities are evident in Maurice Molarsky's portrait presented by the class of 1940. The subject is shown in a frontal pose seated in an armchair in front of a maroon curtain and holding a rolled document. He is garbed in a full-flowing academic gown. Yet his averted eyes, heavy "five o'clock shadow," crooked mouth, and yellowish complexion create an unintentionally lugubrious effect. Coupled with his iconic pose, voluminous robe, and his tight grip on the chair arm, he appears tense and withdrawn rather than kind and judicious. Nevertheless, the canvas is freely painted and the subject appears solidly three-dimensional.

Maurice Molarsky is another well known, Russian emigré artist represented in the Jefferson collection. Born in Kiev in 1885, he studied at the Pennsylvania Museum School of Industrial Art and the Pennsylvania Academy of the Fine Arts where he won the Henry Thouron Prize for Composition and the Cresson traveling scholarship which allowed him to study in France and England.

Molarsky was a consistent exhibitor at the Academy's annuals, and in 1950 its museum presented a memorial exhibition of his portraits, figure studies, still lifes, and landscapes. His awards include the Art Club of Philadelphia gold medal, the Pennsylvania Academy Fellowship Prize, silver medals at the Panama-Pacific Exposition and the Sesqui-centennial Exposition, and a gold medal at the Philadelphia Sketch Club.

Molarsky was best known for his commissioned portraits of distinguished Philadelphians. Such portraits can be found in Philadelphia's City Hall, and in numerous colleges and cultural institutions, banks, social clubs, and hospitals, as well as in private collections. He also created several murals for the Elks Home and other public buildings.

Clinicians in the Medical Specialties

Portrait of Thomas McCrae

THOMAS McCRAE, M.D. (1870-1935)
By Benedict Anton Osnis (1872-1941)

Oil on canvas
1936
72 x 44 in.

Signed and dated lower left: "B. A. OSNIS/1936"

Given in 1937 by JMC alumni association, colleagues, and students
Accession number: 1937+e.P.02

Dr. Thomas McCrae succeeded Dr. James C. Wilson in the chair of medicine in 1912, and was named the first Magee Professor of Medicine and Clinical Medicine in 1917. An outstanding clinician, teacher, and author, he was loved and admired by faculty and students alike.

Prior to his arrival at Jefferson McCrae underwent unusually rigorous academic training. A native of Guelph, Ontario, Canada, McCrae was born in 1870. Early in his training he received three degrees from the University of Toronto: the bachelor of arts (1891), bachelor of medicine (1895), and doctor of medicine (1903), and later an honorary doctor of science degree (1927).

In 1895 he was a resident at Toronto General Hospital, and then went to the Garrett Hospital for Children in Baltimore and the Johns Hopkins Hospital in the fall of 1896. He was an assistant resident for five years at Hopkins, and then resident physician in the medical clinic under Sir William Osler for an additional three years. In 1899 he went abroad to study medicine and pathology at the University of Göttingen, and during the next few years spent summers studying in London and Paris. In 1901 he was made a member, and in 1907 a fellow, of the Royal College of Physicians in London, one of the highest honors in English medicine.

By 1906 he was made an associate professor of medicine at Johns Hopkins. He had become a close friend and colleague of Dr. Osler and in 1908 married Osler's niece, Amy Gwyn. McCrae collaborated with Osler on *Cancer of the Stomach: A Clinical Study* in 1900.

Osler was the editor and McCrae his assistant in the monumental, seven-volume work, *Modern Medicine: Its Theory and Practice, in Original Contributions by American and Foreign Authors* (1907-10). McCrae also helped Osler revise later editions of his *Principles and Practice of Medicine; Designed for the Use of Practitioners and Students of Medicine.*

Dr. McCrae accepted the offer to become professor of medicine at Jefferson Medical College in 1912, for which post Osler had recommended him. The following year he was made attending physician to the Pennsylvania Hospital. His abilities as a teacher and clinician soon endeared him to his students, colleagues, and the medical community in Philadelphia. He occupied the chair of medicine for twenty-four years, longer than any predecessor.

During his subsequent literary career McCrae published more than one hundred articles on a variety of clinical subjects and was an associate editor of the *Annals of Medical History*. In 1924 he was honored to deliver the Lumleian lectures at the Royal College of Physicians of London on the topic, *Foreign Bodies in the Bronchi*. In 1934 he was made an honorary foreign member of the Association of Physicians of Great Britain and Ireland. McCrae also served a term as president of the Association of American Physicians and was a member of the American Philosophical Society.

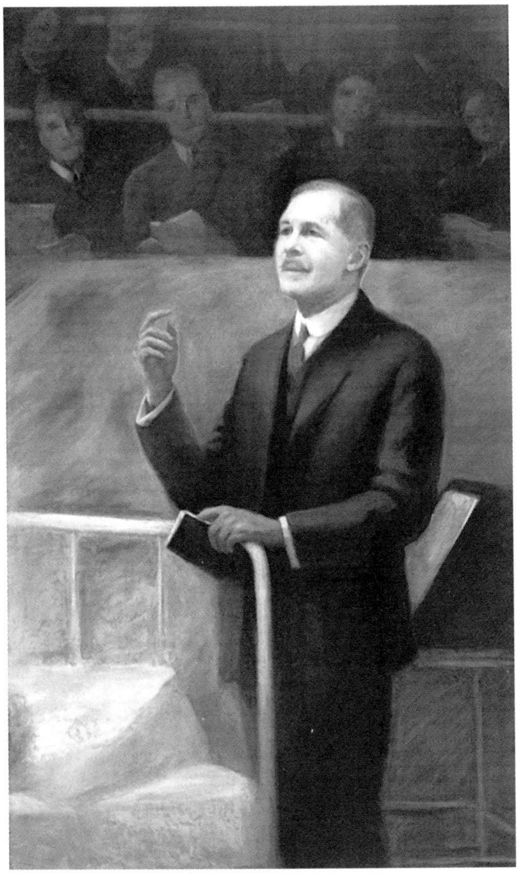

For the last two years of his life Dr. Thomas McCrae suffered from an increasing loss of power and dulling of tactile senses in his legs, symptoms whose origins baffled his consulting physicians. He never surrendered to his condition, but near the end of his life had to deliver his lectures from a wheelchair.[3]

In 1936 Benedict Osnis was commissioned by Jefferson Medical College to paint a posthumous portrait of McCrae, and it was presented the following year by the alumni association, colleagues, and students. The large scale work shows McCrae conducting a medical clinic in the amphitheater of the Thompson Annex, Jefferson's third pit. With a characteristic gesture of his right hand the professor is explaining a clinical point to the students seated in the surrounding benches of the arena. His left hand, holding his place in a small roll book, is resting on the rail of a hospital bed. An X-ray light box is on a nearby table.

Dr. Thomas McCrae made use of a wealth of clinical material for teaching small groups in clinics and the wards, preferring this more intimate method to didactic, formal lecturing. Though kindly and considerate to students, he expected precision and conscientiousness from them and would "wax irate" if met with laziness or ignorance.

The Jefferson Medical College yearbook of 1925 summarized the students' respect and admiration for their professor,

> We shall never forget the fear, the apprehension and the feeling of abject mental blankness we experienced when first we saw Dr. McCrae draw from his pocket a certain little black book, open it to a certain page, and after due deliberation heard him say, "Will Mr. Blank please come down?" All our carefully learned methods of examination departed from us completely and we were as unfamiliar with the manner in which the spleen should be palpated as the most verdant of Freshmen. But the kindliness with which he treated us, the patience he displayed and the gentlemanly manner in which he dealt with us endeared him to us for all times.

Portrait of Thomas McCrae

(See color plate)

THOMAS McCRAE, M.D.
By William Taylor Thomson (1858-1941)

Oil on canvas
1925
40 1/4 x 32 1/4 in.

Signed and dated lower left: "W. T. Thomson/1925"

Given by JMC class of 1925
Accession number: 1925+e.P.01

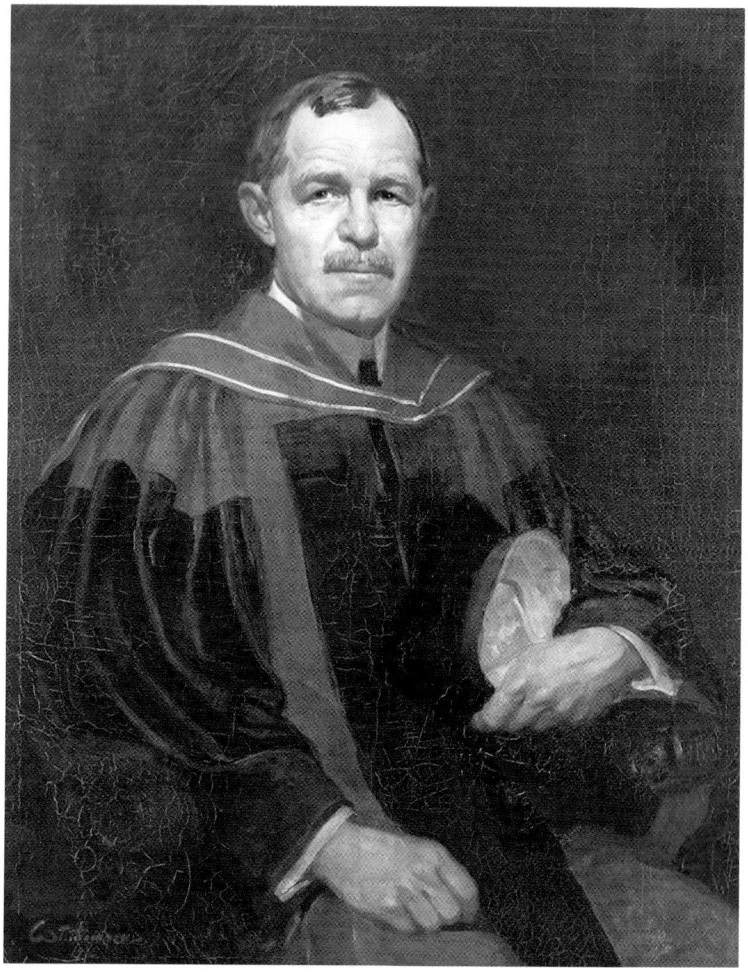

An earlier portrait of Dr. Thomas McCrae by William Thomson had been the special centennial gift of the Jefferson Medical College class of 1925. The imposing portrait shows the subject two-thirds length and life-sized, seated and facing slightly right. He gazes toward the observer with a forthright and serious expression. His right hand is placed in his lap and his left hand rests on the chair arm and holds an academic cap lined in green. The face and hands are solidly rendered in smooth brush strokes. The most striking element is the color of Dr. McCrae's Royal College of Physicians academic gown: royal blue with a brilliant red yoke and front panels, and a red mantle with white stripes.

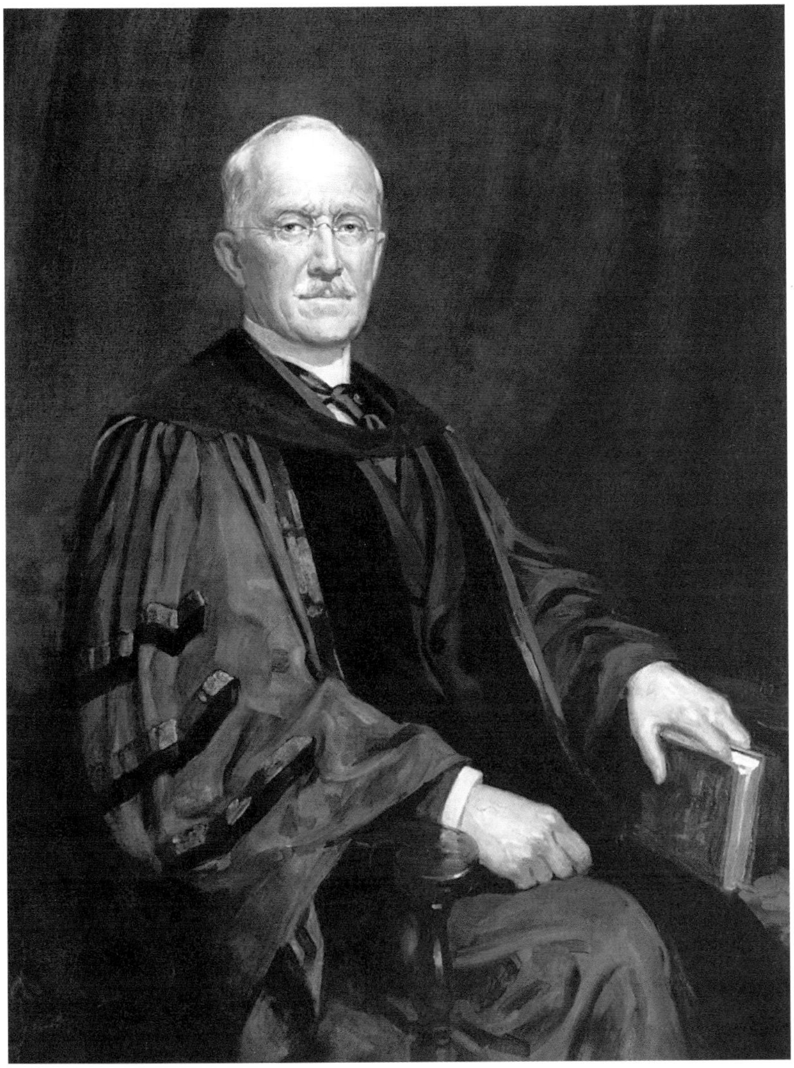

Portrait of Hobart A. Hare

HOBART AMORY HARE, M.D. (1862-1931)
By William Taylor Thomson (1858-1941)

Oil on canvas
1927
50 1/2 x 40 1/2 in.

Signed lower left: "W. T. Thomson"

Given by JMC class of 1927
Accession number: 1927+e.P.01

In 1891 Dr. Hobart Amory Hare became professor of therapeutics and materia medica at Jefferson Medical College. He served with distinction for forty years, and died "while in harness."

A native Philadelphian born in 1862, Hobart A. Hare earned a medical degree in 1884 from the University of Pennsylvania, and then studied physiology abroad in Leipzig, Berne, and London. Upon his return to Philadelphia, the University of Pennsylvania appointed him an instructor in physical diagnosis and a demonstrator of medicine. In 1890 he was made a clinical professor of the diseases of children.

Between 1885 and 1890 Dr. Hobart A. Hare won awards for research on such diverse topics as the physiological effects of tobacco, new and altered form of diseases, antipyretics, respiration, intestinal obstruction, and epilepsy. These prizes were awarded by the Rhode Island Medical Society, Harvard University, Massachusetts General Hospital, the College of Physicians and Surgeons of New York, and the Royal Academy of Medicine of Belgium. He was the only American to receive the Fothergillian Gold Medal of the Medical Society of London for his work on mediastinal diseases.

In 1891 Dr. Hare succeeded Dr. Roberts Bartholow at Jefferson, and in 1916 he was named the first Sutherland M. Prevost Professor of Therapeutics, Materia Medica, and Diagnosis.

His most enduring literary contribution was his *Textbook of Practical Therapeutics* (1890) which went through twenty-one editions in his lifetime. He was also the author of *Practical Diagnosis: the Use of Symptoms in the Diagnosis of Disease* (1896), and *A Textbook of the Practice of Medicine: for Students and Practitioners* (1907), and the editor of *A System of Practical Therapeutics* (1891-97) and *Modern Treatment: the Management of Disease with Medicinal and Non-medicinal Remedies* (1910-11). He served as editor of the journals *Medical News*, *Progressive Medicine*, and *Therapeutic Gazette*.

Hare served on the Philadelphia Board of City Trusts, and was president of the Jefferson Medical College alumni association and the College of Physicians of Philadelphia. In 1921 he was awarded an honorary LL.D. degree from the University of Pennsylvania.

Dr. Hare was equally respected and beloved by his colleagues on the Jefferson faculty and his students as an outstanding clinician, educator, and author. He was awarded a Jefferson diploma in 1893 and named honorary president of the class. He died just one month after the Jefferson Medical College class of 1932 had dedicated a bronze plaque expressing the affection and admiration of forty graduating classes.

Students had already honored him repeatedly in organizing the Hobart Amory Hare Medical Society in 1899, giving the bronze statue of Mercury in 1916, dedicating the student yearbooks to him in 1908 and 1925, and naming him the class portrait honoree in 1927.

In William T. Thomson's depiction Dr. Hare is seated in front of a purplish-maroon drapery. He wears a black academic gown embellished by green front panels, green stripes on the sleeves, and a maroon mantle. He has marked his place in a book with his index finger, and paused in his reading to glance directly toward the viewer with a serious and inquiring expression. The large and imposing portrait is painted fluidly with loose and lively brush strokes. The prevailing dark colors are punctuated with violets, pinks, blues, and greens in the shadows of his face and hands.

Mercury

MERCURY
Cast of original by Jean-Baptiste Pigalle (1714-85)

Bronze
Before 1916
22 7/8 x 13 1/4 x 12 5/8 in.

Signed on bottom of rear: "PIGALLE"
Founder's mark on left bottom of integral base: "MUSÉES NATIONAUX/MOULAGE"

Given in 1916 to Hobart A. Hare, M.D. by JMC students; donated after 1931 by his family
Accession number: 1931+f.S.01

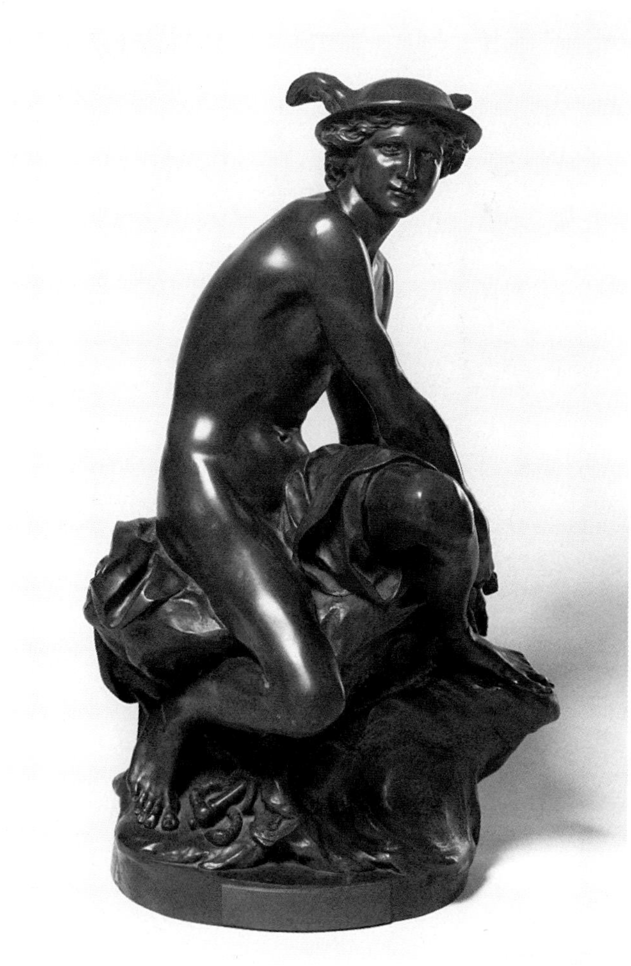

It was standing room only in the clinical amphitheater on April 11, 1916 when six hundred students, faculty, and friends gathered to commemorate Dr. Hobart Amory Hare's twenty-fifth anniversary as the professor of therapeutics, materia medica, and diagnosis. A bronze state of Mercury was presented to the professor by the entire student body as a token of their love and esteem.

It was reported in the May 1916 *Jeffersonian* that for several minutes after the guest of honor arrived, "a storm of applause spoke the sentiment of the crowd who had assembled to do honor to one of the most beloved members of the Faculty." The master of ceremonies was Francis X. Dercum, M.D., professor of nervous and mental disorders, who remarked, "We come today not to celebrate the termination of his career, but to mark an epoch of a great career."

Mercury is best known as one of the twelve gods of Mount Olympus who acted as a messenger of the gods or as a guide. He is easily recognizable by his winged sandals and winged hat, for swift travel, and for his winged caduceus with entwined snakes, an attribute which evolved into a symbol of physicians and of the medical profession. In allegorical terms Mercury also personifies eloquence or reason, the hallmarks of an effective teacher and a fitting tribute to Professor Hare.

The statue of Mercury was cast from a famous marble statuette at the Louvre Museum in Paris, made in 1744 by the French sculptor Jean-Baptiste Pigalle. Pigalle was celebrated for his many statues of Mercury tying on his sandals, made in various sizes and of various media such as terra cotta, stone, and plaster. Although Pigalle studied antique statuary in Rome and his style recalls ancient statues in a general way, this work does not copy a specific Greek or Roman sculpture of the god.

The smoothly carved, gleaming, nude bronze figure is full of motion as he twists his upper body to bend over and fasten his sandals. He sits on a tree stump covered with flowing drapery which also decorously covers his left thigh and groin. His caduceus lies on the ground under his right foot. The athletic figure exudes energy and appears poised to spring into action. Mercury's unlined face and thick, wavy hair, his *contrapposto* posture, and his lean and muscular body personify an idealized youth.

The Jefferson collection also contains a Hamilton gold watch presented to Dr. Hare on December 4, 1914 by house staff of the hospital. The exterior of the outer lid is engraved with a rabbit and an amusing inscription: "I wold my master were an Hare." The watch was left by bequest of Dr. Thomas A. Shallow in 1956.

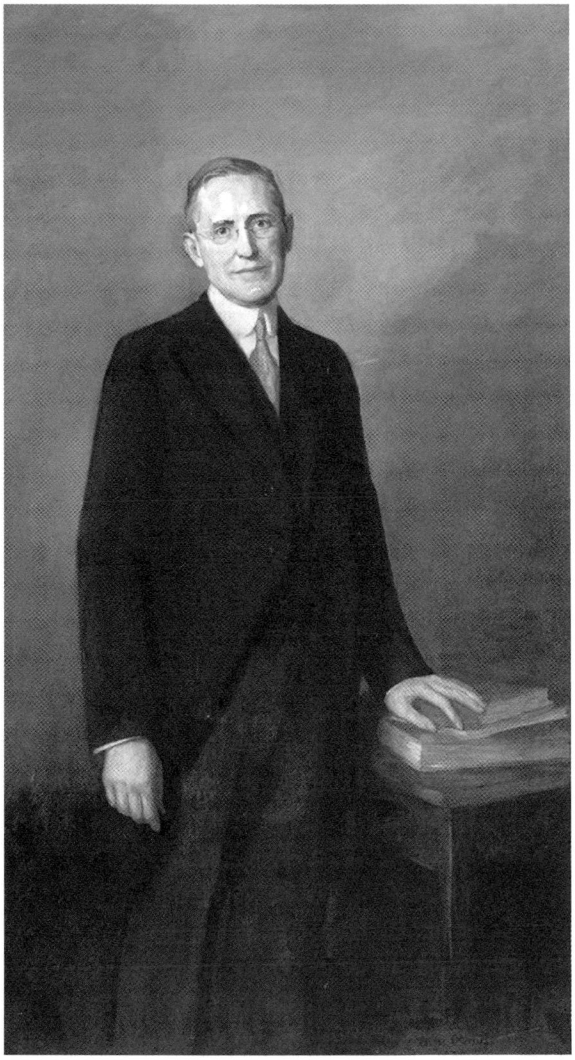

Portrait of E. Quin Thornton

EDWARD QUIN THORNTON, M.D. (1866-1945)
By Benedict Anton Osnis (1872-1941)

Oil on canvas
1930
70 1/2 x 40 1/2 in.

Signed and dated lower right: "B. A. OSNIS/1930"

Given by JMC class of 1930
Accession number: 1930+e.P.02

After the death of Dr. Hobart A. Hare in 1931, the Sutherland M. Prevost Professorship of Therapeutics, Materia Medica, and Diagnosis passed in rapid succession from Dr. Elmer H. Funk who died in 1932 during his first year, to Dr. E. Quin Thornton.

E. Quin Thornton was born in 1866 in Marion, Alabama where he attended Howard College. He came to Philadelphia in 1886 and earned degrees at the Philadelphia College of Pharmacy in 1889 and Jefferson Medical College in 1890. He served as demonstrator of materia medica at Jefferson from 1890 to 1900, and rose through the ranks to become associate professor in 1900. In 1932 he was named the Sutherland M. Provost Professor, a post he held until 1934 when he retired from teaching and was made emeritus professor. The class of 1934, which referred to itself as "Poppy Thornton's Class," dedicated a bronze tablet in his honor expressing their gratitude and esteem for his four decades of teaching.

Dr. Thornton's best-known literary works were *Dose-book and Manual of Prescription Writing* (1895), *The Medical News Pocket Formulary* (1899), and *A Manual of Materia Medica for Medical Students* (1911).

The portrait of Dr. E. Quin Thornton by Benedict A. Osnis was commissioned by the class of 1930. Shown almost full length, the physician stands next to a table with his left hand resting on a pile of books and his right arm hanging down at his side. He is dressed formally in a cutaway coat. His head is tilted in a friendly way and his expression is amiable, as he looks directly toward the observer.

Dr. Thaddeus L. Montgomery, an alumnus of 1920, reminisced about Thornton's lectures in the winter 1993 *Jefferson Medical College Alumni Bulletin*. The former student recalled Thornton's customarily elegant appearance and tall, youthful-looking figure. He and his classmates appreciated Thornton's lucid lecture style in which he presented instances from his own practice in discussing every disease, thus combining the study of drugs and their place in the treatment of disease with instruction in physical diagnosis.

Tray of E. Quin Thornton

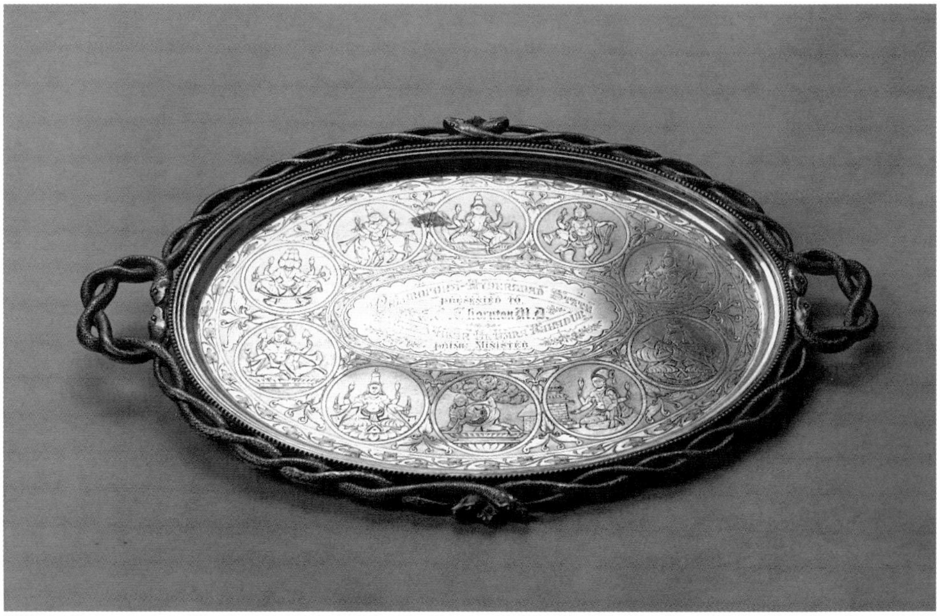

TRAY OF E. QUIN THORNTON, M.D.
By P. Orr & Sons

Silver
Ca. 1890
16 x 11 x 1/2 in.

Inscription: "CHLOROFORM-HYDERABAD STATE/NAWAB VIKAR UL UMRA BAHADUR/PRIME MINISTER," enclosing "PRESENTED TO E. Q. THORNTON M.D."
Stamped on back: "P. ORR & SONS/MADRAS"

Given in 1941 by Dr. and Mrs. E. Quin Thornton
Accession number: 1941+e.DA.01

In 1889 His Highness, the Nizam of Hyderabad in India, honored Drs. E. Quin Thornton and Hobart A. Hare by inviting them to join an Anglo-American commission to investigate the cause of death in chloroform anesthesia. The Nizams were rulers of fabled wealth whose authority once extended over much of southern India. The controversial subject of death following the administration of chloroform had come to the attention of the current Nizam, a philanthropist with an interest in science.

When the results of the first commission had failed to satisfy the medical profession, the Nizam financed a second commission in 1889. The results, *A Study of the Influence of Chloroform upon the Respiration and Circulation*, showed conclusively that the cause of death was chiefly respiratory, and were published by Thornton and Hare in 1893.

As a mark of appreciation for the difficult investigation the government awarded each commission participant a ceremonial silver tray. The tray's decoration is atypical of Indian domestic pieces, but probably was made for English export by English or Indian craftsmen. The manufacturer was P. Orr and Sons of Madras, jewelers and silversmiths.

The oval, silver tray has bead borders surrounded by an open work perimeter of intertwined snakes ending in intertwined handles at both ends. The interior field features ten rondels depicting various multiarmed deities. The rondels surround an oval reserve with its engraved inscription dedicated to Dr. Thornton.

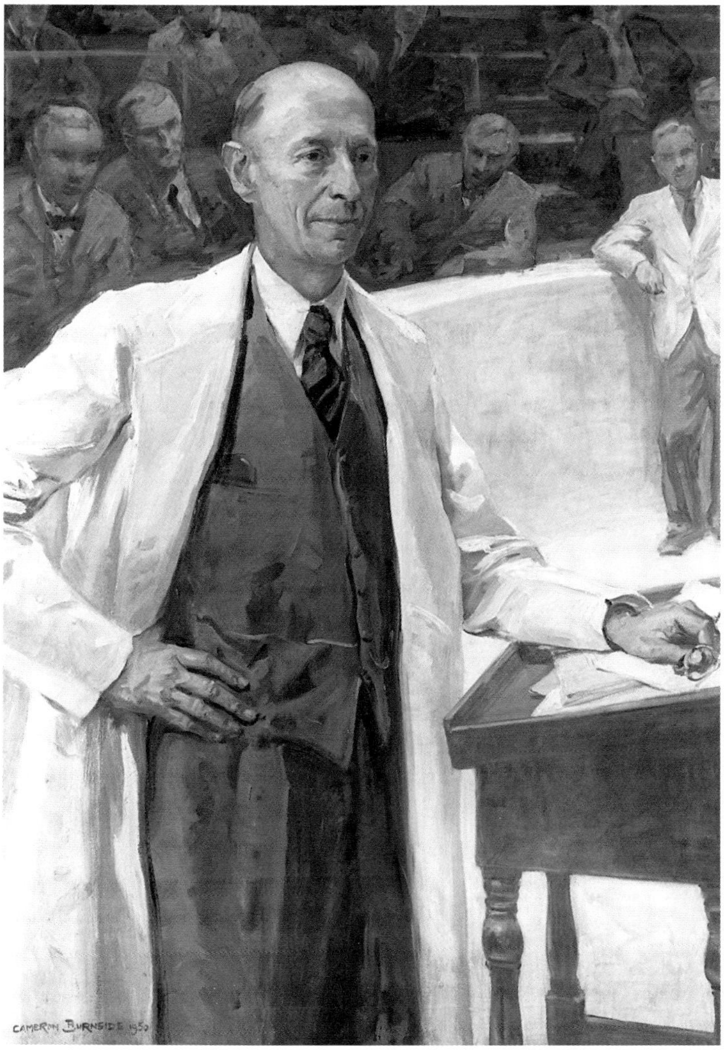

Portrait of Hobart A. Reimann

HOBART ANSTETH REIMANN, M.D. (1897-1986)
By Cameron Burnside (1887-1952)

Oil on canvas
1950
50 x 36 in.

Signed and dated lower left: "CAMERON BURNSIDE 1950"
Exhibition: Philadelphia, *Cameron Burnside Memorial Exhibition*, Woodmere Art Gallery, 1953

Given by JMC class of 1951
Accession number: 1951+e.P.02

With the death of the beloved Dr. Thomas McCrae in 1935 it was wondered with some anxiety who would succeed him as the Magee Professor and chairman of the department of medicine. After a year the appointment was given to Dr. Hobart A. Reimann who proved to be a creative and forceful administrator, and an indefatigable worker. His career was unusual for its breadth of pursuits and travels.

Reimann was born in 1897 in Buffalo, New York and received his medical degree from the University of Buffalo in 1921. After an internship at the Buffalo General Hospital he was sent to the Hospital of the Rockefeller Institute for investigative clinical research. In 1926 he was a fellow in pathology at the Anton Ghon Institute in Prague. From 1927 to 1930 he was elected an associate professor of medicine at Peking Union Medical College in China under the auspices of the Rockefeller Institute.

Upon his return to the United States in 1930 the University of Minnesota appointed him an associate professor of medicine. He was made professor there in 1936 at the age of thirty-nine, but later the same year he accepted an appointment as Magee Professor and chair of medicine at Jefferson Medical College. In 1945 he took a two-month leave of absence to join a cholera team in Chungking, China which issued a report advocating prompt fluid replacement to lower the mortality rate.

During Dr. Reimann's tenure as chairman at Jefferson, he merged the department of therapeutics with the department of medicine, began the development of divisions within the department, established the first residency program in medicine, and initiated a program in clinical investigation. He inaugurated the clinical clerkships in the teaching of medicine and placed third-year students in the medical wards instead of the outpatient departments. He also founded the student health service.

Chafing under departmental administrative problems Dr. Hobart A. Reimann resigned in 1951, and he spent the next nine years abroad as a visiting professor at the American University of Beirut in Lebanon, the University of Indonesia in Djakarta, and the University of Shiraz in Iran. In 1960 he returned to Philadelphia as professor of medicine at Hahnemann Medical College and associate medical director of its hospital. During this period he also continued his work abroad with educational and consulting projects in Vietnam, Afghanistan, Honduras, and Colombia. He was made visiting professor of medicine at Jefferson in 1979 and retained his connections there until his death in 1986.

Professor Reimann's outstanding literary contributions were chiefly on infectious diseases including the first description of viral pneumonia, the viral diseases of the intestinal tract, and periodic disease. He also contributed to the knowledge of pneumonia and the pneumococcus, typhus and Rocky Mountain spotted fever, plasma proteins in amyloid disease, prolonged fevers, focal infection, typhoid fever, trichinosis, and histoplasmosis.

Among Reimann's best-known books are *The Pneumonias* (1938), *Treatment in General Medicine* (edited by Reimann and published in 1939), and *Periodic Diseases* (1963). He was also editor of *Acute Respiratory Tract Diseases: Prevention and Treatment* (1975) and coauthor of *Infectious and Parasitic Diseases of the Intestine* (1977). Dr. Reimann wrote over forty consecutive annual reviews of infectious diseases for *Archives of Internal Medicine* and the *British Postgraduate Medical Journal*.

His honors and awards included the Charles V. Chapin Medal from the Rhode Island State Medical Society, the Citation for Distinguished Service in Medical Education from the University of Buffalo, the Order of Cedars, Lebanon, the Hahnemann Corporation Medal for Distinguished Service, the Clarence E. Shaffrey, S.J. Award from St. Joseph's College, and an honorary doctor of science degree from Jefferson Medical College.

Dr. Hobart A. Reimann was chosen as subject for the senior class portrait in 1951. Cameron Burnside was commissioned as portraitist. Professor Reimann is depicted in a characteristic pose lecturing in the Thompson pit. Gazing across the amphitheater to students on the opposite side, he stands with his right hand on his hip, and his left hand holding his glasses and resting on papers and pamphlets covering the lectern. He wears his long, white laboratory coat. A student leans against the wall, and three rows of physicians and students are visible in the tiers of seats.

The printed program for the presentation proceedings is unusual for commenting on the content of the painting:

> The portrait...depicts Dr. Reimann in the pose that all of his students at Jefferson will best remember—in the Pit, black roll book close at hand, calling upon students to "come down and examine this patient."...During these rigorous sessions or on his "grand rounds" students, house officers, and faculty were frequently subjected to intense quizzing which moved one to commit the clinical facts on 20 or 30 patients to memory so as not to be embarrassed by the *Professor*. How many times has one looked back on these sessions with continued fear and trembling only to give eternal thanks for the excellent training and habits that were instilled.

At the portrait ceremony Professor Reimann humorously revealed that Cameron Burnside's sometimes off-color stories kept him occupied while holding his pose for hours. He also commented on the decision-making process for the portrait's composition. Since no one could picture him in academic cap and gown, "those relics of the middle ages," working clothes seemed more fitting, but he did not want to resemble the fraternity house caricature of him with a chart under his arm and white coattails flying.

Reimann said that the posture caused an argument because at first he was to lean over the lectern, but then he and Mrs. Burnside insisted that he straighten up to "look more authoritative." He also mentioned that students would miss a few characteristic objects not present: the stethoscope in his left pocket, and his "little black book" which causes "so much apprehension, sweaty palms and tachycardia." One wonders if the black roll book was painted out, since it was mentioned in the written program.

A confident and sophisticated artist like Cameron Burnside must have been aware of numerous portraits in the Jefferson collection showing doctors lecturing or operating in the amphitheater, starting with Thomas Eakins's portraits of Drs. Gross and Forbes. Almost assuredly Burnside studied Benedict A. Osnis's portrait of Dr. Thomas McCrae, because the setting and pose are similar. However, the Burnside depiction is more insightful due to his clarity of drawing and liveliness of brush strokes.

Cameron Burnside was born in 1887 to American parents in London where his father was a foreign correspondent for a New York newspaper. He was the great-grandson of Simon Cameron, secretary of war in the Lincoln administration and a United States Senator from Pennsylvania, and of Judge Thomas Burnside, a Pennsylvania Supreme Court justice.

Burnside studied art first in London and then in Paris at the Grand Chaumière and privately. He lived in France for most of his career and was closely associated with the European art scene. He exhibited at the Royal Academy and Royal Institute in London, and in Paris with the Artistes Français, the Société Nationale des Beaux-Arts, the Salon d'Automne, the Salon des Independents, the Salon des Tuileries, and the Société Internationale des Aquarellistes. His works are owned by the French government and by collectors in England, France, and Japan. At the close of World War I Burnside worked as an official artist to the American Red Cross in France.

The artist and his wife left Paris abruptly in 1940 when the German army occupied the city, and they lost all of their belongings in their haste to catch the last train. They resettled in Philadelphia, and occasionally also lived in Washington, D.C. Burnside exhibited oil paintings, watercolors, pastels, and drawings of figurative subjects, landscapes, and cityscapes at the National Academy of Design, the Pennsylvania Academy of the Fine Arts, the Corcoran Gallery in Washington, and solo and group shows at numerous galleries.

He received commissions for portraits of judges, lawyers, political leaders, and business leaders, for such institutions as City Hall, the University of Pennsylvania, the Hahnemann Medical College, the American Philosophical Society, the Philadelphia Bar Association, the Union League, and the Curtis Institute. Although the poses and settings of his sitters are often traditional, his painting style favors freely brushed and sometimes sparkling surfaces, hinting at his French training.

His awards include a silver medal at the Panama-Pacific Exposition in San Francisco and a gold medal at the Exposition Coloniale de Marseilles in 1922.

Portrait of Irene (Mrs. Cameron) Burnside

IRENE (MRS. CAMERON) BURNSIDE
By Cameron Burnside

Oil on canvas
1943
30 x 25

Signed and dated upper left: "CAMERON BURNSIDE 1943"

Given in 1972 by Dwight R. Ashby, M.D. (JMC 1946)
Accession number: 1972+e.P.01

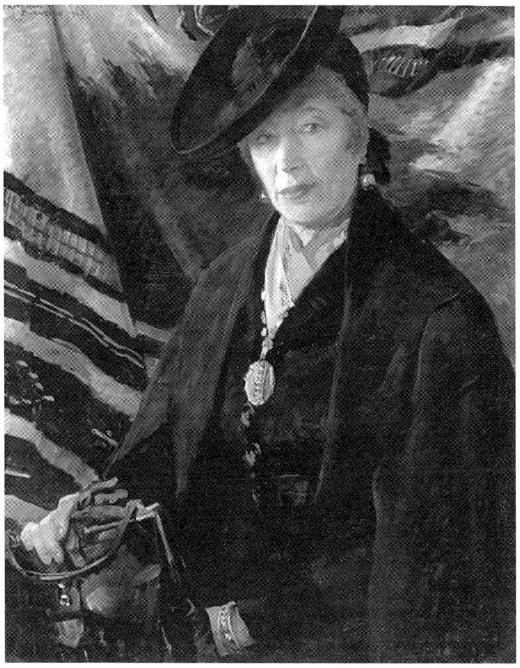

Apparently Cameron Burnside enjoyed a close relationship with Jefferson Medical College in the 1940s and early 1950s. In addition to the portrait of Dr. Hobart A. Reimann, he received four other commissions for distinguished Jeffersonians: Drs. Edward L. Bauer, Frederick H. Mills, William H. Perkins, and Martin E. Rehfuss.

Further, board of trustees minutes of March 17, 1952 record that Burnside generously offered to give "certain drawings and paintings" for resale by the college as his contribution to the hospital building fund. The matter was never settled because the artist died on March 26, 1952. In addition, Jefferson received two other Burnside paintings from alumni: a portrait of the artist's wife, Irene, and a picture of Dr. Thomas A. Shallow operating.

Burnside's first wife, the former Lucile Hitt, was an artist who died in 1927. His second wife, Irene, was also an artist who exhibited flower and landscape paintings in Paris. It has been seen that she took an active role in her husband's career. A year after the artist's death she organized his memorial exhibition at the Woodmere Art Gallery in Philadelphia, for which she borrowed the Jefferson portraits of Drs. Reimann and Perkins. The widow helped support herself by giving painting classes privately.[4]

As depicted by her husband in 1943, Irene Burnside is posed in front of an artfully gathered fabric of green, yellow, and blue diagonal stripes. Her colorful attire consists of a royal blue hat perched at a rakish angle, a dark blue dress and cape accompanied by a bright green scarf, blue gloves, and a purse. Her jewelry includes gold pendant earrings, a large gold locket, and a bracelet. Purplish lipstick and vivid, red nail polish add to her theatrical appearance, as does her somewhat coquettish, almost haughty expression. The portrait's surface sparkles with bright colors and brilliant contrasts of lights and darks in the skin tones and jewelry.

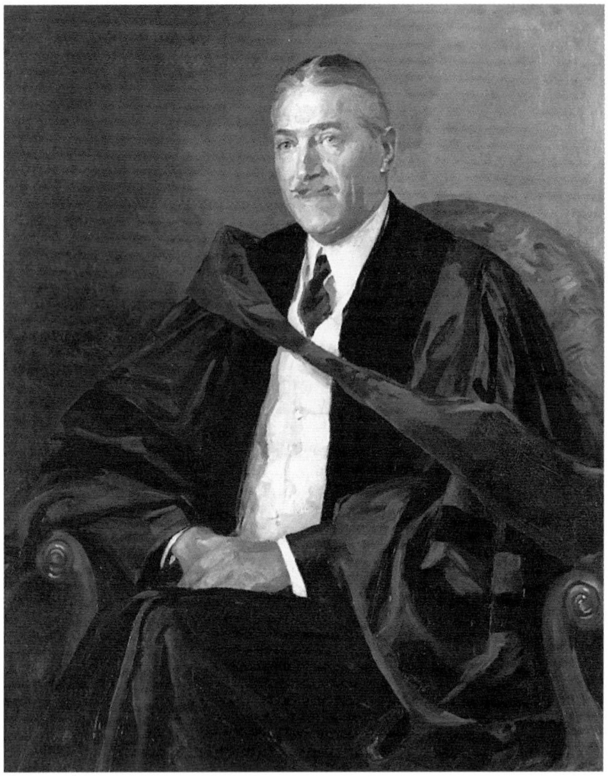

Portrait of Martin E. Rehfuss

MARTIN EMIL REHFUSS, M.D. (1887-1964)
By Cameron Burnside

Oil on canvas
1943
44 1/2 x 36 1/2 in.

Signed and dated lower left: "CAMERON BURNSIDE 1943"

Given in 1943 by JMC class of January 1944
Accession number: 1943+e.P.02

Dr. Martin E. Rehfuss was named the Sutherland M. Prevost Professor of Therapeutics in 1941. The renowned gastroenterologist was a member of the Jefferson faculty for thirty-eight years.

Born in 1887, Martin Rehfuss was a native Philadelphian and educated at Central High School and the University of Pennsylvania where he earned a medical degree in 1909. After an internship at the Hospital of the University of Pennsylvania he continued his education abroad. He was a resident physician at the American Hospital in Paris and a student at the Pasteur Institute, then studied for a year in Berlin, Munich, and Vienna.

He developed an interest in diseases of the gastrointestinal tract. During this period he invented a new kind of gastric tube, later known as the "Rehfuss tube," which permitted removal of multiple specimens of gastric secretions over a period of hours. This technique led to the development of the test known as fractional gastric analysis.

Upon his return to Philadelphia in 1914 Rehfuss was appointed to the medical staff of the Jefferson Hospital as an instructor in medicine. His eight years of research on normal and pathological gastric digestion with Dr. Philip Hawk, professor of biochemistry, resulted in many publications recognized worldwide.

Rising through the academic ranks, Rehfuss's appointments progressed from an associate in medicine in 1918 to professor of clinical medicine in 1936. He was named the Sutherland Prevost Professor of Therapeutics in 1941 succeeding Dr. Henry K. Mohler. When trustees discontinued this professorship in 1949 Rehfuss continued the course of therapeutics as a lectureship in the department of medicine. He was made emeritus professor in 1952, and received an honorary doctor of laws degree from Jefferson in 1954.

Among Rehfuss's major literary contributions were: *Diagnosis and Treatment of Diseases of the Stomach, with an Introduction to Practical Gastro-enterology* (1927), *The Medical Treatment of Gall Bladder Disease* (with Dr. Guy M. Nelson, 1935), *Indigestion: Its Diagnosis and Management, with Special Reference to Diet* (1943), and *A Course in Practical Therapeutics* (with Drs. F. Kenneth Albrecht and Alison Howe Price, 1948).

In addition to his reputation as a researcher, teacher, and author, Dr. Rehfuss was admired for being an astute, meticulous, and compassionate clinician. Notable among his patients were Mr. and Mrs. Percival E. Foerderer. A Philadelphia industrialist, Foerderer was chairman of Jefferson's board of trustees, and the couple endowed the Martin E. Rehfuss lectureship in internal medicine to honor their physician.

Dr. Rehfuss was also respected by Jefferson students. The class of 1936 dedicated their yearbook to this "scientist, scholar, excellent teacher, brilliant clinician, gastroenterologist of international reputation, widely recognized writer of medical literature, students' friend, and above all, a gentleman."

The wartime class of January 1944 selected Dr. Rehfuss as portrait honoree and presented the painting to the college on November 29, 1943. He was depicted by Cameron Burnside two-thirds length and seated in an upholstered armchair with clasped hands. Rehfuss chose to be depicted wearing an academic gown, unlike his contemporary, Dr. Hobart A. Reimann. The debonair physician looks out toward the viewer with a pleasant and confident expression.

Contemporary accounts note that he was a handsome man with ruddy coloring and a neat waxed mustache, impeccably attired, almost always in a white vest, as can be seen under his open robe in this portrait. Burnside used the robe's green mantle as a compositional device to create a strong diagonal across the subject's chest and connect the flowing material in the gown's voluminous sleeves.

Correspondence indicates that in August 1943 Jefferson offered Burnside the modest fee of six hundred dollars for the Rehfuss portrait, saying, "This...in no way compensates for your work but in the past most artists have appreciated the fact that the students do not have a large amount to expend...They have been willing to contribute their services for this small amount." Burnside agreed that while the sum "represents about half of my present wartime fee, I should feel it an honor to be of service to...the Jefferson Medical College."

Portrait of Martin E. Rehfuss

MARTIN EMIL REHFUSS, M.D.
By Agnes Yarnall (d. 1989)

Bronze
1963-66
20 3/4 x 9 7/8 x 9 7/8 in.

Signed on rear of right shoulder: "A. Yarnall"

Given 1963-66 by unknown donor
Accession number: 1963-1966.S.01

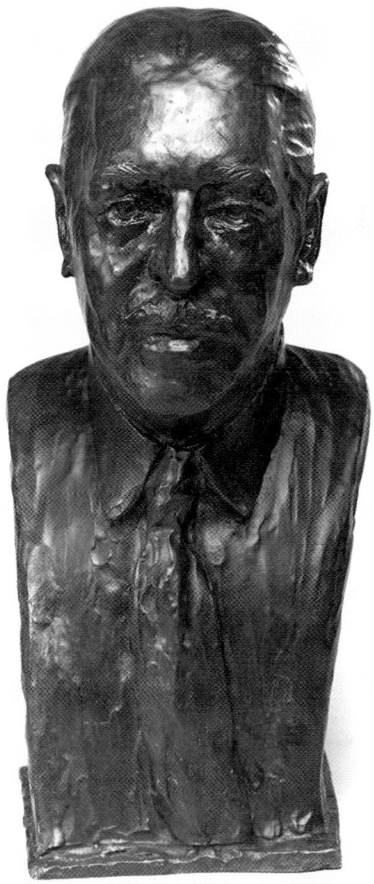

In contrast to Cameron Burnside's expansive depiction of Dr. Martin E. Rehfuss, Agnes Yarnall's bronze portrait bust of Rehfuss is rather stark and attenuated, with little indication of the sitter's shoulders or chest. Uncharacteristically, his costume consists of shirt and tie only, with no suit coat or vest.

However, the portrayal is penetratingly naturalistic in the subject's narrow, oval face; deepset, penetrating eyes; long, aquiline nose; high cheekbones; and pursed lips and jutting jaw. The unevenly modelled surface picks up shadows and highlights which add a sense of animation to the bronze figure.

Although no documents have yet been found about the provenance of Yarnall's work, the sculpture appeared in a 1966 photograph of the auditorium where the honorary Rehfuss Lecture took place. Today the bust is still relocated to the auditorium stage for the annual Rehfuss Lecture to remind the audience of the physician's visage.

Sculptor and poet Agnes Yarnall was born in Drifton, Pennsylvania and her mother, a painter, sent Agnes as a child to study sculpture at the Liberty Tadd School of Modeling in West Philadelphia.[5] Later she studied at the Pennsylvania Academy of the Fine Arts with Charles Grafly and Boris Blai. She furthered her studies in New York with Paul Manship and Alexander Archipenko.

Sometimes her work has an edge of biting sarcasm or social comment, for example her 1962 series of thirty-nine small, bronze figures commemorating the centennial of the Civil War. She captured the grief and pathos of the event by showing its effect on ordinary soldiers, planters, drummer boys, and slaves. This work was first unveiled at Philadelphia's Union League where it was seen by former President Eisenhower. The year before Yarnall had created another series, *World of the Circus*, which revealed the bittersweet life of its performers. Both series were shown around the country.

She was also well known for dynamic, naturalistic, bronze portrait busts of famous figures in the arts such as Dame Judith Anderson, Edna St. Vincent Millay, John Keats, Maurice Evans, John Gielgud, and Carl Sandburg. Agnes Yarnall's life-sized statue of Benjamin Franklin with a kite is located at Philadelphia's Franklin Institute Laboratories. Her head of the Marquis de Lafayette was commissioned by the Chicago Historical Society. Her work was featured in solo exhibitions from Maine to Florida.

Agnes Yarnall's own books of poems include *Hesperides*, illustrated with photographs of her bas-reliefs, and *Pandora and Other Poems*. She attributed her interest in Greek art and literature to her mother reading the Greek myths to her as a child. She accepted with good humor newspaper articles early in her career that described her attractive appearance and referred to her as a "society woman," at the expense of critiquing her work.

Portrait of Solomon Solis-Cohen

SOLOMON SOLIS-COHEN, M.D.
(1857-1948)
By Maurice Molarsky (1885-1950)

Oil on canvas
1929
40 x 36 in.

Signed and dated upper right: "M. Molarsky 1929"

Given in 1929 by friends and colleagues
Accession number: 1929+e.P.03

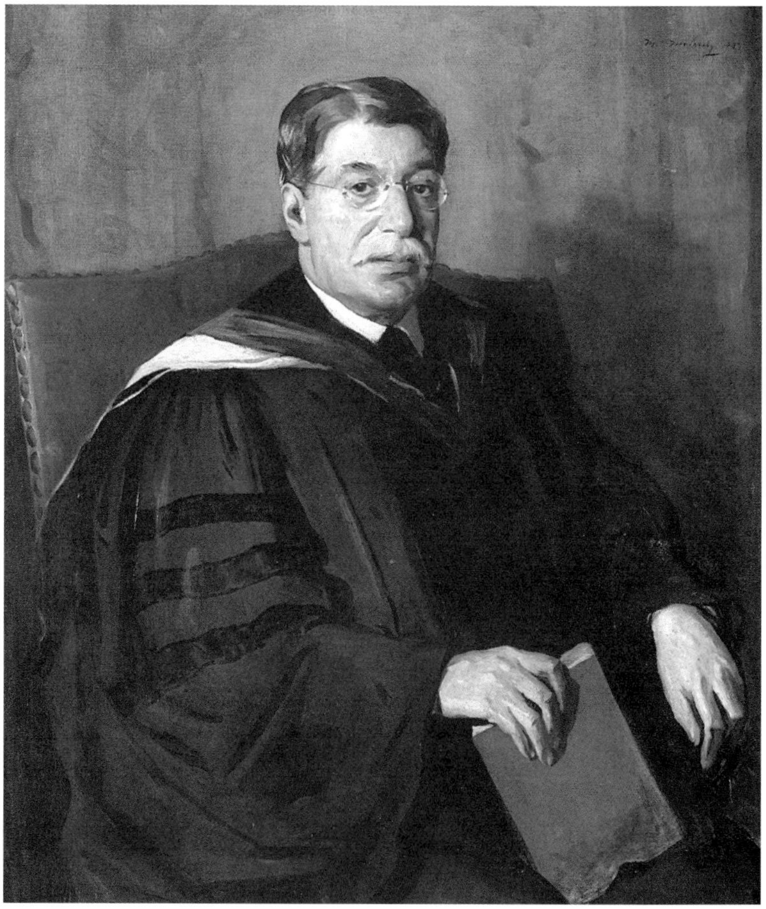

Dr. Solomon Solis-Cohen was a member of the Jefferson Medical College faculty for four decades, including twenty-three years as professor of clinical medicine. He was widely known for developing standard diagnostic and therapeutic techniques.

A native Philadelphian, Solomon Solis-Cohen was born in 1857, twenty years after his brother Jacob da Silva Solis-Cohen. After receiving a bachelor's degree (1872) and master's degree (1877) from Central High School, he graduated from Jefferson Medical College (1883). Dr. Solomon Solis-Cohen's first position at Jefferson was as chief clinical assistant to Drs. Jacob Mendez DaCosta and Roberts Bartholow in the outpatient medical department.

After serving as lecturer on therapeutics, he rose through the ranks to become assistant professor of clinical medicine in 1902, and then was named the first professor of clinical medicine in 1904. He was attending physician at the Jefferson Hospital from 1887 until 1927 when he was named emeritus professor.

Dr. Solis-Cohen was also physician to the Philadelphia General Hospital, the Jewish Hospital, and the Rush Hospital for Consumptives, and consulting physician to the Pennsylvania State Hospital for the Insane. He was professor of clinical medicine and therapeutics and physician to the Philadelphia Polyclinic.

Solis-Cohen was one of the first physicians to recommend hydrotherapy in the treatment of typhoid fever and among the first to use adrenal therapy for hay fever, asthma, and hives. He was the first to name and describe vasomotor ataxia. He was a trustee of the U.S. Pharmacopoeial Convention from 1920 to 1940. He received honorary D.Sc. degrees from Jefferson Medical College in 1933 and the Philadelphia College of Pharmacy and Science in 1939.

Among his contributions to the medical literature were *Essentials of Diagnosis: Arranged in the Form of Questions and Answers Prepared Especially for Students of Medicine* (1892) and *Pharmacotherapeutics, Materia Medica and Drug Action* (with Thomas S. Githens, M.D., 1928). He was editor of the eleven-volume *A System of Physiologic Therapeutics: a Practical Exposition of the Methods, Other than Drug-Giving, Useful in the Treatment of the Sick* (1901-05).

During his lifespan of ninety years Dr. Solis-Cohen also participated in wide-ranging medical, literary, religious, and philanthropic activities. As president of the Philadelphia County Medical Society and chairman of its committee on water supply, he was instrumental in introducing effective filtration to the system. As a long-term member of the Philadelphia Board of Education he was influential in introducing diphtheria immunization. His memory is perpetuated in the Solomon Solis-Cohen Elementary School in North Philadelphia. He was also a director of the School of Design for Women (later Moore College of Art and Design) and of Gratz College.

Dr. Solomon Solis-Cohen was also a published poet. His best-known poem, "When Love Passed By," appeared in 1887 in *Scribner's Magazine* and was translated into more than twenty languages. Another poem was included in an anthology of poetry edited by John Greenleaf Whittier in 1890. He was acclaimed for his translations of medieval Hebrew poets. A commemorative book of his writings and addresses, *Judaism and Science* (1940), was published by several bibliophile friends. He received an honorary doctorate of Hebrew literature from the Jewish Theological Seminary of America in 1928.

A group of friends and colleagues presented a portrait of Dr. Solomon Solis-Cohen by Maurice Molarsky in 1929. In the life-sized, two-thirds-length depiction, the professor sits in an armchair facing partially to the right. The voluminous sleeves of his black academic gown fill the lower left section of the composition. He holds a closed book and looks toward the viewer through rimless spectacles with a serious expression. The colors are neutral except for the greenish background and the red upholstered chair. Molarsky's loosely brushed style creates an allover fluidity to the surface. Though a good likeness of the subject, the portrait falls somewhat short of capturing the professor's towering intellectual attainments and forceful personality.

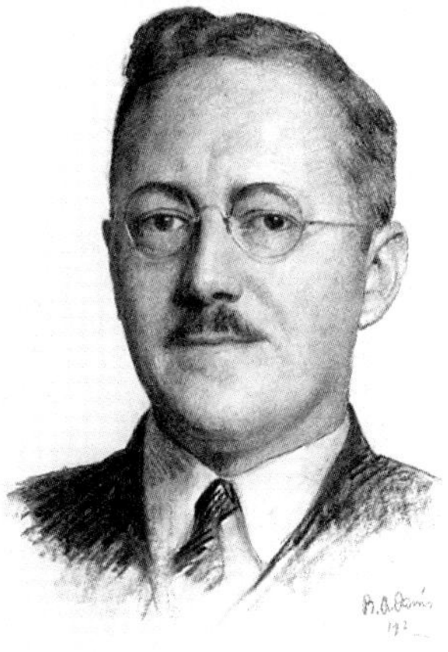

Portrait of Harold W. Jones

HAROLD WELLINGTON JONES, M.D. (1891-1959)
By Benedict Anton Osnis (1872-1941)

Charcoal on paper
1929
21 1/2 x 15 in.

Signed and dated lower right: "B. A. Osnis/1929"

Given after 1929 by unknown donor
Accession number: 1929+f.D.01

Dr. Harold W. Jones was a pioneer investigator in blood disorders at Jefferson Medical College. It was under his leadership that the Division of Hematology was established.

Dr. Jones graduated from Jefferson Medical College in 1917, and became chief resident after his return from World War I. He practiced as a general internist and then was named director of Jefferson's laboratory of clinical medicine, during which period he developed an interest in blood disorders.

Distressed by the lack of medical research at Jefferson, Jones proposed three areas in urgent need of organization to Dr. Thomas McCrae, the chair of medicine: facilities for the accurate study of patients with blood disorders by trained personnel; adequate laboratories and equipment for a long-term study of the fundamental aspects of blood diseases; and a service to provide transfusions of carefully matched blood.

Until funds were collected, Jones conducted independent studies of blood diseases and blood transfusions and wrote several textbook chapters dealing with blood disorders. He was also the author of *Application of Laboratory Methods to Clinical Medicine* (1924) and an editor of *Blakiston's New Gould Medical Dictionary* (1949). He was a founder of the Jefferson Society for Clinical Investigation.

With the encouragement of the new Magee Professor of Medicine, Dr. Hobart A. Reimann, substantial backing for the extensive project in hematology was achieved in the late 1930s with the largesse of a Philadelphia society woman, Mary (Mrs. Thomas) Cardeza. She was acutely aware of the importance of blood transfusions from her experiences as a Red Cross nurse during World War I. She herself had been referred by New York physicians to Dr. Harold W. Jones for treatment of a chronic blood disorder, and had spent almost two years as a patient at Jefferson Hospital and at home. She was an admirer of Dr. Jones's research efforts.

Mary Cardeza and her husband, Thomas Drake Cardeza, formally incorporated the Charlotte Drake Cardeza Foundation For Hematologic Research in 1941 in memory of Mr. Cardeza's mother who had died in 1939. Thomas Cardeza's generous gift included annual grants of fifty thousand dollars for not less than ten years, and after his death in 1952 he left more than three million dollars to establish a trust for the Cardeza Foundation.

Dr. Jones was the foundation's first director and the first Thomas Drake Martinez Cardeza Professor of Clinical Medicine and Hematology. Upon his retirement in 1954 Jones was named emeritus professor.

Although the Jefferson collection has no formal portrait of Dr. Harold W. Jones it is fortunate to have a charcoal sketch by Benedict A. Osnis made in 1929. The head-and-shoulders depiction is a straightforward study of a youthful but confident-looking man. No documents about the circumstances of the drawing's creation and donation have been found.

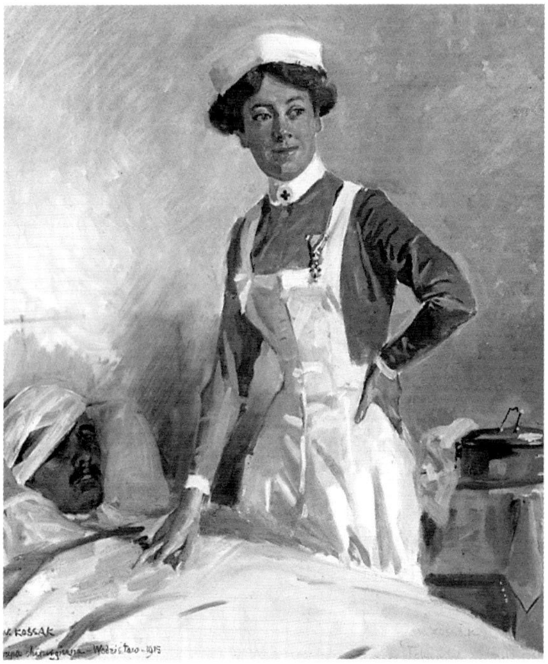

Mary Cardeza as a Nurse

MARY RACINE (MRS. THOMAS) CARDEZA (1880-1943)
By Woiciech von Kossak (1857-1942)

Oil on artist's board mounted on wood
1915
21 1/4 x 18 1/4 in.

Signed lower left and right: "W. KOSSAK," and dated lower left: "1915"
Inscriptions below image: left, "Grupa chirurgiuna/Wodzistaw-1915" (surgical ward), and right, "Feldspital [*sic*] Wodzistaw" (field hospital)

Given 1941-52 by unknown donor
Accession number: 1941-1952.P.01

A headline referring to Mary Cardeza in the April 23, 1917 *New York Evening Telegram* read, "Wealthiest Woman Ever to Hold Office Aims to Teach Aliens Patriotism." Of all Jefferson benefactors Mary Racine Cardeza undoubtedly led the most colorful life, as both a pampered society woman and a heroic Red Cross nurse.

Mary Racine was born in 1880 in Besançon, France, and her earliest years were spent in France and Switzerland. Her parents emigrated to Philadelphia where her father kept a small bakery and confectionery shop in South Philadelphia. At age seventeen she worked first in a department store and then opened a little manicure parlor where, *The Philadelphia Evening Bulletin* reported, "nearly all the men-about-town were her steady customers."

About 1900 after moving to New York the so-called former "shop girl" announced to the newspapers that she had been secretly married for a year to Thomas Drake Martinez Cardeza, much to the chagrin of his formidable mother, Charlotte Drake Cardeza. Thomas Cardeza was a wealthy Philadelphia club man, big-game hunter, and explorer whose maternal grandfather had been an industrialist and a founder of the Fidelity Trust Company. Mary Racine Cardeza became famous for lavishing her new-found wealth on designer gowns and then being photographed wearing them.

The senior Mrs. Cardeza was one of the few female big-game hunters of her day and owned hunting lodges in Maine and Austria and a shooting ranch in Montana. She twice skippered her oceangoing yacht around the world. Her stone mansion, Montebello, was filled with art works collected on her travels. According to one account, after being ordered over the side of the sinking *Titanic*, she refused to enter the lifeboat until places were found for her son and their two servants.[6] Newspapers reported that their accommodations had cost several thousand dollars and that Mrs. Cardeza had brought aboard fourteen trunks of gowns, furs, and jewelry.

In 1901 Mary and Thomas Cardeza went to Vienna and established one of their several homes and hunting estates in Central Europe. When not lavishly entertaining guests they went on diverse hunting expeditions to Asia and Africa, some of which were directed by former president Theodore Roosevelt. Underneath her flamboyant exterior was a woman of great intelligence who could speak five languages fluently, and who was always cognizant of the poor during her travels around the world.

The outbreak of World War I caught the Cardezas on their estate near the Russian-Austrian border. While guests of the ambassador at the U.S. Embassy in Vienna they were asked to volunteer their services in the war effort. Thomas Cardeza became an under-secretary and Mary Cardeza gave her services to the Red Cross. She led a surgical group of eight doctors, fifteen nurses, and two hundred orderlies carrying medical supplies for wounded soldiers behind the firing lines in Galicia, Poland. Her unit was one of the most successful due to her leadership and resourcefulness, including billing her husband for necessary medical supplies. She was publicly commended by the Red Cross in 1916 for her courage and efficiency, and was awarded the War Order of Franz Joseph by the Austrian emperor.

In 1915 Polish artist Woiciech von Kossak depicted Mary Cardeza as a nurse standing at the bedside of a wounded soldier. Garbed in her Red Cross uniform, she stands with her left arm akimbo and rests her right hand on the blanket-covered chest of a patient. Behind is a table holding towels and a metal pot or kettle. The patient's head and right eye are bandaged and he appears barely conscious. Cardeza's uniform bears two pins: the Red Cross insignia on her round starched collar and a colorful gold cross with striped ribbon on her apron strap.

Mary Cardeza's expression registers unexplained surprise as she looks away from the patient. The artist's illustrative style incongruously emphasizes her shapely body rather than suggest her heroism under the primitive and frightening conditions behind the front lines. The location is identified as a field hospital in Wodzistaw, in southernmost Poland near the Czech border.

Woiciech von Kossak was born in 1857 in Paris of Polish parents and studied with his father, a painter. He won medals at several European expositions around the turn of the century, was made a chevalier of the French Legion of Honor in 1904, and was named painter to the court of Prussia. He was best known for portraits and military subjects.

After Mary Cardeza recovered from exhaustion following her two and one-half years of service abroad she returned to New York. In 1917 she organized a society to undertake the rebuilding of the farms and villages of Galicia which had been wasted by the war. Her immediate concern was to alleviate the suffering of eighty thousand orphaned children who remained starving and disease-ridden in concentration camps in Russia and Austria.

That same year she was appointed assistant secretary of the New York State Bureau of Industries and Immigration. Although some newspaper articles relentlessly fixated on descriptions of her luxurious suite at New York's Ritz Carlton Hotel, Mrs. Cardeza toiled indefatigably to inspect immigrant labor camps and to educate, i.e. "Americanize" and teach patriotism to three million Central European "enemy aliens," immigrants working for the war effort in New York. She assured them of President Wilson's proclamation that no one who obeyed the law would be ill-treated.

After the war Thomas Cardeza expanded his interests from business and hunting to inventing numerous devices for deep-sea fishing and furnishing specimens for museums and zoos. He was a member of the Royal Geographic Society of London and a director of the Philadelphia Zoo and the Morris Arboretum. In 1939 he joined Jefferson's board of trustees. Mary Cardeza died in 1943 and her husband in 1952. The couple had no children.

Portrait of Mary R. (Mrs. Thomas) Cardeza

(See color plate)

MARY RACINE (MRS. THOMAS) CARDEZA
By Liamji (?) Kolomeier (active early twentieth century)

Marble
1915
19 5/8 x 8 3/4 x 10 in.

Signed and dated lower right side of integral base: "Liamji [?] Kolomeier 1915"

Given 1941-52 by unknown donor
Accession number: 1941-1952.S.01

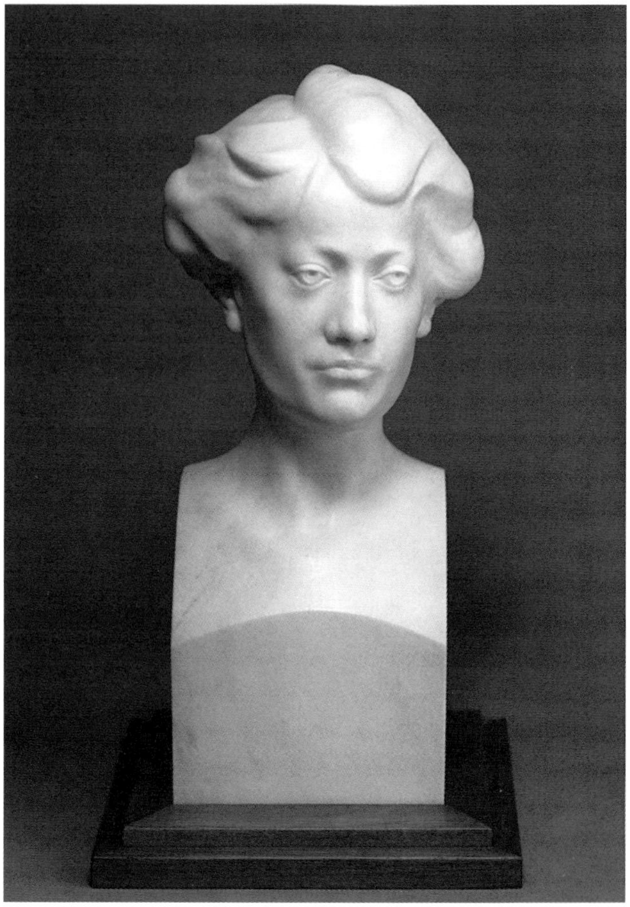

Mary Racine Cardeza was about thirty-five years old when a marble portrait head was created. The sculpture is dated 1915, so presumably it was commissioned in Central Europe during the early days of World War I.

At first an observer is struck by the delicate carving of the pinkish marble streaked with gray, the sitter's regular features, and her fashionable hairdo. Then one notices the pursed lips, clenched jaw, and knitted brows, features that give the young woman a look of steely determination and formidable character.

There is no record at Jefferson of the donation of either the painting or sculpture of Mary Cardeza, and nothing is known about the sculptor Kolomeier. Presumably the works were given between 1941 when the Cardeza Foundation was established and 1952 when Thomas Cardeza died.

Portrait of Frank C. Knowles

FRANK CROZER KNOWLES, M.D. (1881-1957)
By Frederick James Gill (1906-74)

Oil on canvas
40 1/2 x 30 in.

Signed and dated: "Frederick Gill/1939"

Given by JMC class of 1939
Accession number: 1939+e.P.01

Dr. Frank C. Knowles was professor of dermatology at Jefferson Medical College. He chaired the department from 1920 until his retirement in 1946 when he was made emeritus professor.[7]

A native Philadelphian, Frank Crozer Knowles was

born in 1881 and was a graduate of the William Penn Charter School (1898) and the University of Pennsylvania School of Medicine (1902). He interned at Presbyterian Hospital and subsequently studied with Drs. Henry Stelwagon, Louis A. Duhring, and Arthur Van Harlingen, all distinguished clinical dermatologists.

Knowles's principal outpatient dispensaries were at the Philadelphia General, University of Pennsylvania, Howard, Pennsylvania, and Children's Hospitals. He was assistant professor of dermatology at the University of Pennsylvania. For ten years he was clinical professor of dermatology at Women's Medical College.

Dr. Knowles spent twenty-three months overseas during World War I. At first he was dermatologist to the Pennsylvania Hospital unit, U.S. Base Hospital Ten in Le Treport, France. Later he became dermatologic consultant to the American Expeditionary Forces. In 1919 he was sent to Washington, D.C. to write the section on dermatology in the permanent medical war records. He was later commissioned a colonel in the Medical Officers Reserve Corps.

Dr. Knowles became assistant professor of dermatology at Jefferson Medical College and then succeeded Dr. Henry Stelwagon as professor of dermatology. Knowles was one of the original members of the American Academy of Dermatology and Syphilology, and in 1939 was elected president of the American Dermatological Association. His widely used textbook, *Diseases of the Skin* (1914), went through four editions.

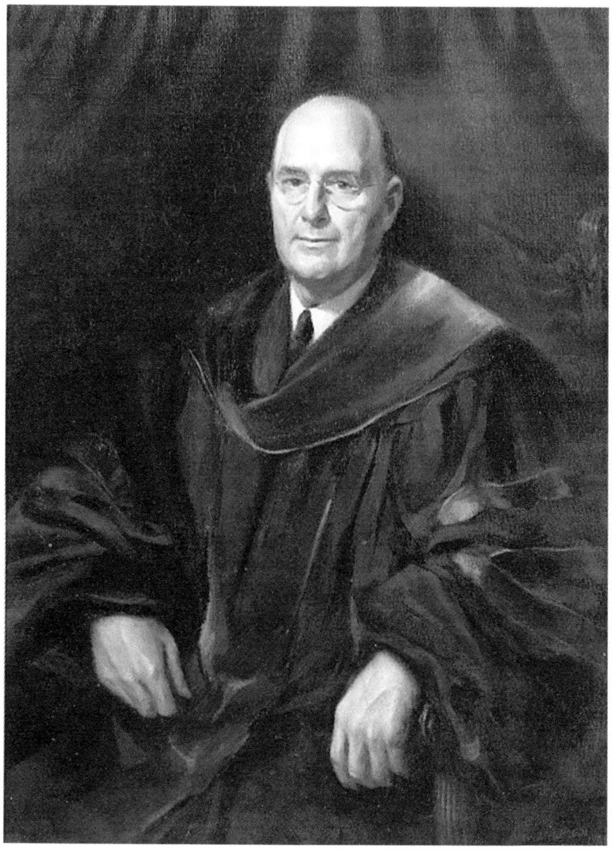

Jefferson students in the class of 1937 dedicated their yearbook to him. The Frank Crozer Knowles Dermatological Society was named in his honor by students, and his portrait was presented by the class of 1939. In 1951 Jefferson Medical College awarded him an honorary doctor of science degree.

In Frederick Gill's three-quarters-length, life-sized portrait Dr. Knowles is seated in an armchair facing slightly to the left, with his hands hanging over the chair arms. His richly painted black academic robe is trimmed in green velvet in the front panels, mantle, and sleeves. The subject has a high domed forehead and looks straight ahead through rimless spectacles. His wide mouth has the trace of a smile. Though the figure is convincingly three-dimensional, in comparison with contemporary photographs his eyes appear blank and his smile looks artificial as though forced. The bland portrait barely suggests the sitter's warm personality and a man with diverse interests in sports and the arts.

Artist Frederick J. Gill was a well known Philadelphia painter, educator, and musician. A native of the city, he received a bachelor of fine arts degree in education from the University of Pennsylvania and a master's degree from the Tyler School of Art of Temple University. He headed the art department at Central High School for many years, and also taught at the Philadelphia Museum School of Art, the Philadelphia College of Art, Lehigh University, and privately.

Gill worked his way through college by playing the saxophone and continued to perform professionally in jazz combos throughout his life. His art career began in earnest about 1936 with portraits and other representational subjects. However, he gradually found his real métier with abstract paintings and collages that often depicted instrumentalists or expressionist subjects focusing on the rhythms and textures of music.

Frederick Gill exhibited in group shows nationally and in many one- or two-person shows at local galleries. He was a consistent prizewinner for oils and watercolors at annual shows of the Art Teachers Association of Philadelphia. During the late 1940s and 1950s he won the Zabriskie Prize of the American Water Color Society in New York, the Grumbacher Prize of the Audubon Artists, the Woodmere Prize and Harrison Morris Prize of the Woodmere Art Gallery in Philadelphia, and the Dana Water Color Medal of the Philadelphia Water Color Club, among others.

Portrait of Edward L. Bauer

EDWARD LOUIS BAUER, M.D. (1891-1976)
By Cameron Burnside (1887-1952)

Oil on canvas
1945
40 x 32 in.

Signed and dated: "CAMERON BURNSIDE 1945"

Given by JMC class of 1945
Accession number: 1945+e.P.01

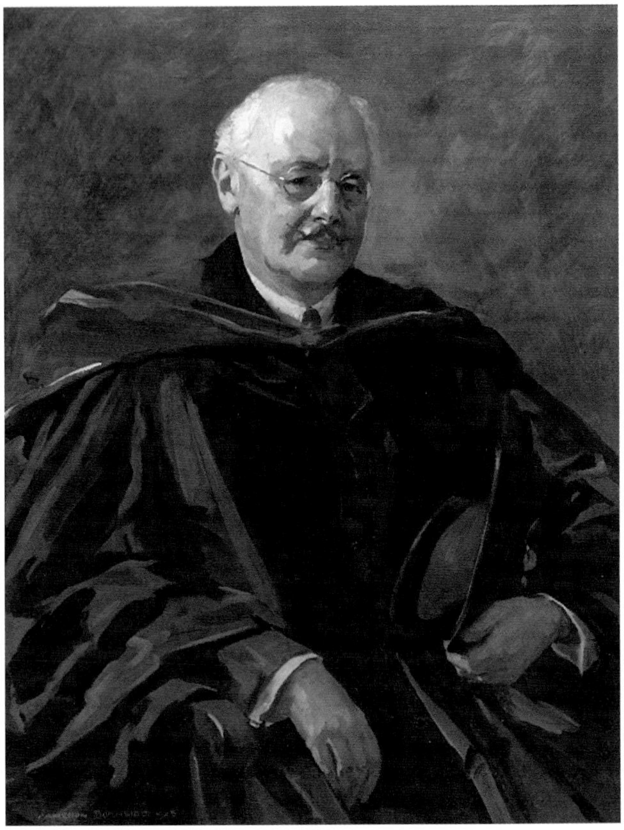

Dr. Edward L. Bauer headed the department of pediatrics at Jefferson Medical College from 1926 until his retirement in 1961. He was a leading advocate of pediatric public health measures.

A native Philadelphian, Edward L. Bauer was born in 1891. He was a graduate of Central High School and Jefferson Medical College (1914). He was the seventh generation of physicians in his family and the third Jefferson alumnus, and his son Richard was a member of the class of 1945 that presented his portrait. Dr. Richard Bauer presented a portrait of his mother in 1982 to the Jefferson School of Nursing, one of her interests as a member of the women's board.

Dr. Edward Bauer interned at Germantown Hospital and was a resident physician at the Children's Seashore House in Atlantic City, the Philadelphia Hospital for Contagious Diseases, and the Children's Hospital of the Mary J. Drexel Home. During World War I he was a first lieutenant assigned to tuberculosis examining boards in several army camps.

In 1918 Dr. Bauer was a leader in an uphill battle to introduce modern methods of immunizing children against diphtheria, and during his fourteen years as the chief immunologist in Philadelphia, outbreaks of this dreaded disease were virtually eliminated. He also helped revise the Health Code of Philadelphia and was a member of the state's Certified Milk Commission and the Advisory Committee in Maternal and Child Care.

He served on the staff of the Philadelphia Hospital for Contagious Diseases from 1921 until its closure in 1953. He also served for twenty-four years as medical director of health services for Girard College. Many of his original ideas on immunization, scarlet fever prevention, celiac diseases, rheumatic diseases, and warnings against contamination in commercial baby food were acrimoniously criticized at first and then later confirmed.

Dr. Bauer taught at the University of Pennsylvania School of Medicine before joining the faculty of Jefferson Medical College. During his tenure as chair of pediatrics Bauer enlarged the department and redesigned the pediatric outpatient clinic and the infant hospitalization unit. He developed new programs including neuropsychiatric services for children and a rotation for medical students at the Philadelphia Hospital for Contagious Diseases.

Dr. Bauer served as president of the Philadelphia Pediatric Society and of the pediatric section of the Pennsylvania Medical Society. He was cited for his contributions in the advancement of pediatrics at the seventy-fifth anniversary of the Philadelphia Pediatric Society.

Bauer was named emeritus professor of pediatrics in 1952. Among his most significant contributions to Jefferson Medical College is a history of the institution, *Doctors Made in America* (1963). He served as president of the alumni association and received an honorary degree from Jefferson Medical College in 1970.

The class of 1945 presented a portrait of Dr. Edward L. Bauer by Cameron Burnside. The professor is shown two-thirds length and life-sized, sitting in a wooden armchair. He wears a flowing, black academic gown with abundant sleeves and a green mantle, and holds his ceremonial cap in his left hand. His brows are knitted as he gazes slightly down and to the right through steel-rimmed glasses. His serious, tight-lipped expression is heightened by a trim, waxed mustache. Burnside's characteristic lively and fluid paint style features bright pinks and reds in the flesh tones and striking highlights on the physician's high domed forehead.

Clinicians in the Surgical Specialties and Radiology

Portrait of Thomas A. Shallow

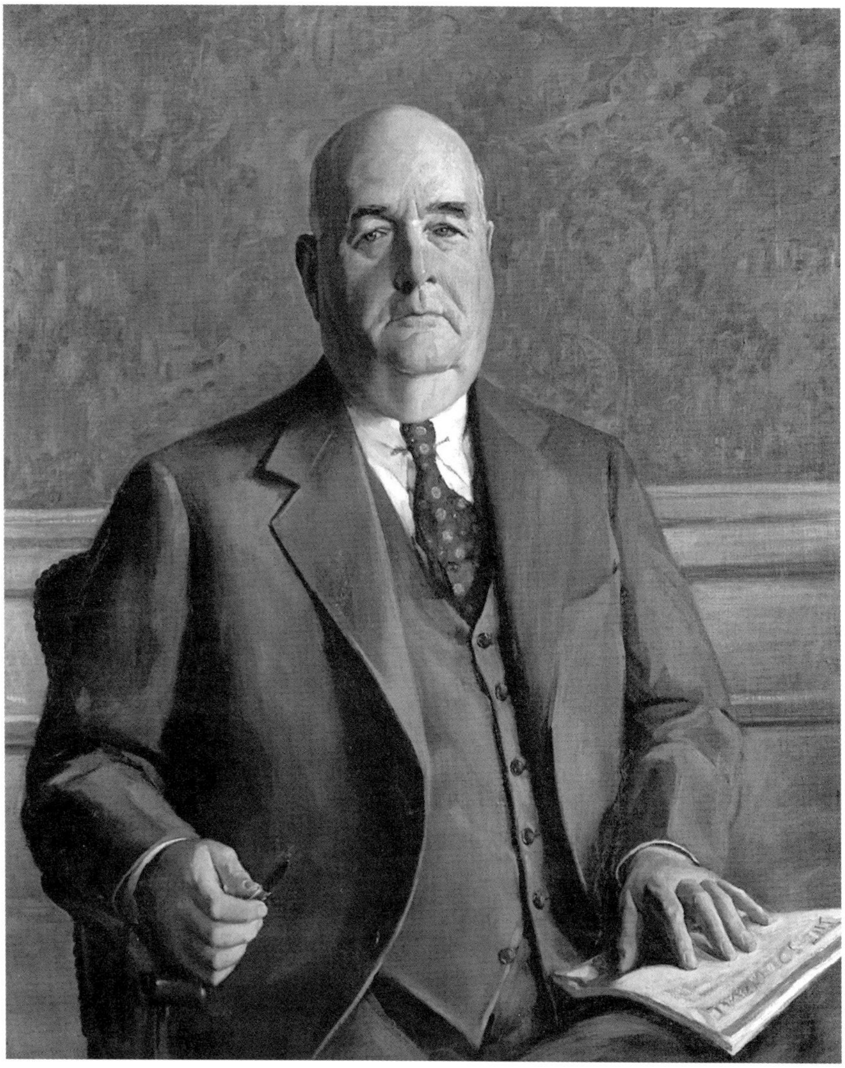

THOMAS ALOYSIUS SHALLOW, M.D. (1886-1955)
By Roy Cleveland Nuse (1885-1975)

Oil on canvas
1950
40 x 34 in.

Signed and dated lower left: "RN./'50"

Given by JMC class of 1950
Accession number: 1950+e.P.02

Dr. Thomas A. Shallow served as cochair of surgery from 1931 to 1955. As a member of the executive faculty his advice was sought for solving complex administrative problems of both college and hospital.

Thomas Shallow was a native Philadelphian born in 1886. He was motivated to attend clinics and postmortem examinations at Medico-chirurgical College Hospital while still attending Central High School. He became an outstanding student at Jefferson Medical College where he graduated in 1911 with the highest grade average.

While taking his internship and residency at Jefferson Hospital Dr. Shallow worked with Drs. Hobart A. Hare and Albert Brubaker, but was most proud of serving as personal assistant to Dr. John C. DaCosta from 1914 to 1925. It was DaCosta who later championed him for the post of surgery department chair. Shallow was a captain in the Medical Corps during World War I, and served as surgeon to the Evacuation Hospital Center Twenty-five in France.

When the cochairs of surgery, Drs. John C. DaCosta and John H. Gibbon, both resigned in 1931, Jefferson trustees stipulated that DaCosta retain the Samuel D. Gross Professorship and temporarily oversee the surgery department which was then being run by two newly appointed professors of equal ability and reputation: Drs. Thomas A. Shallow and Edward J. Klopp. In 1939 Shallow was named the second Samuel D. Gross Professor, and kept this and the chairmanship until his death in 1955.

Admired by colleagues for his dexterity and sound judgment, Shallow pioneered the one-stage operation of pharyngeal diverticulectomy requiring a surgeon and an esophagoscopist, devised his own operation for gastrostomy, and invented an intestinal crushing clamp for the extraperitoneal closure of colostomy.

Dr. Shallow's formidable demeanor was well described by Dr. Frederick B. Wagner Jr., Jefferson surgeon and university historian, and long-term private assistant to Dr. Shallow:

> He was among the last in the era of "Geheimrat" and dictatorship in Surgery at Jefferson and other institutions. Known as "the boss," he welcomed being addressed as such.
>
> Dr. Shallow's rough edge made him controversial in academic circles, but in the operating room he was a superb technician with the soundest of judgment...His Wednesday afternoon clinics were models of preparation for case presentations in which he would call four students into the "pit" and quiz them as well as members of his staff...Immediately after the clinic he would perform major surgery before the assembled class, most of whom would remain. It was the last of the type of teaching immortalized in the *Gross Clinic.*[8]

In 1978 the Jefferson art collection acquired a small watercolor and gouache depiction of Dr. Shallow operating. Painted in 1945 by Cameron Burnside, the impressionistic work was a gift of Gerard S. Serino, M.D., an alumnus of the class of 1932.

Shallow's energy and talent also afforded him time for leadership roles in medical societies and civic affairs. He was a president of the Philadelphia Academy of Surgery and a founding member of the American Board of Surgery. At Jefferson he was president of the alumni association in 1938 and the recipient of an honorary LL.D. degree in 1953. He was a member of the Board of City Trusts of Philadelphia, and a board member of Wills Eye Hospital and the Philadelphia House of Detention.

Dr. Thomas A. Shallow's portrait by Roy C. Nuse was presented by the class of 1950. The physician is shown half length and life-sized, sitting in an armchair in front of a wall, and turned very slightly to the right. He wears a three-piece business suit. His left hand rests on a pamphlet entitled "THE JOURNAL," while his right hand holds a pen.

His arresting facial features include an almost bald head, thick black eyebrows, narrow and slanting blue eyes, asymmetrical nose, thin tight lips, deep facial creases, and fleshy cheeks and chin. The subject's facial expression is intense, severe, and unyielding. This must be his "official" look, because despite his sternness and high standards as a teacher and surgeon, he was also known for his sunny disposition and ready wit in social situations.

Though he is portly, Shallow's broad shoulders and thick chest under his gray suit exude physical strength. Nuse has created a sculptural and solid figure who fills the space in front of the wainscotted wall with its oriental-style wallpaper. Nuse's paint style is loose and free with deep shadows and a scattering of reds and maroons in the sitter's bright necktie and ruddy complexion, the wallpaper, and the pamphlet.

Born in 1885, Roy C. Nuse was a native of Springfield, Ohio. He studied at the Cincinnati Art Academy between 1905 and 1912, then briefly at the John Herron Art Institute in Indianapolis, Oberlin College, and the University of Chicago. He transferred to the Pennsylvania Academy of the Fine Arts where he won Cresson traveling scholarships in 1917 and 1918, and the First Thouron and the First Toppan Prize in 1918.

After brief teaching stints at the Cincinnati Art Academy and Oberlin College, Nuse capped his teaching career as director and professor at the Beechwood School of Fine Arts at Beaver College (1915-32) and as instructor of drawing and painting at the Pennsylvania Academy (1925-54) where he was also coordinator of courses held in conjunction with the University of Pennsylvania. He was president of the Academy's Fellowship in 1937, was awarded the Fellowship's gold medal in 1940, and was honored with a one-man exhibition at the Academy in 1947. Nuse was known for his portraits and landscapes, and was the author of *Treatise on Pastel Painting*.

Portrait of Edward J. Klopp

EDWARD JONATHAN KLOPP, M.D.
(1880-1936)
By Benedict Anton Osnis (1872-1941)

Oil on canvas
1937
36 1/2 x 26 in.

Signed and dated lower left: "B. A. Osnis/1937"

Given by JMC class of 1937
Accession number: 1937+e.P.01

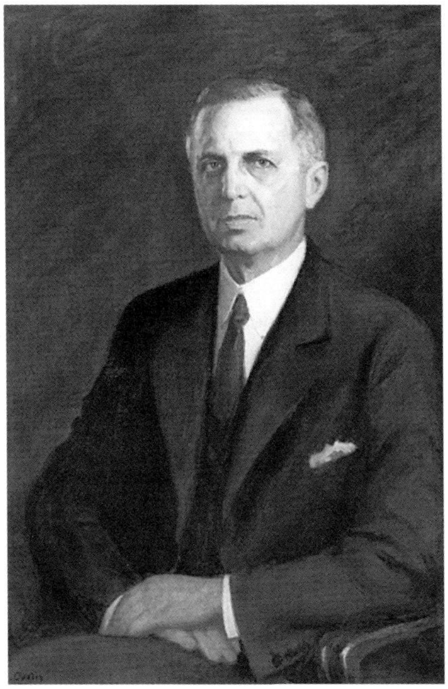

Dr. Edward J. Klopp was a professor of surgery at Jefferson. He died suddenly of infectious disease in 1936 during his fifth year as cochair of the department.

Edward Klopp was born in Sheridan, Pennsylvania in 1880. He graduated from the Philadelphia College of Pharmacy and Science in 1901 and from Jefferson Medical College in 1906. After serving as intern and chief resident at Jefferson he began a surgical career with Dr. Francis T. Stewart, assisting with revisions of the fourth edition of Stewart's *Manual of Surgery*.

After Stewart's death in 1920 Klopp was associated with Dr. John H. Gibbon at Jefferson and Pennsylvania Hospitals, and by 1931 he was elected professor of surgery upon the resignation of Dr. Gibbon. In 1936 he was elected a chief of service in the surgical department at Pennsylvania Hospital. He also was attending physician at Roxborough Memorial Hospital and Delaware County Hospital.

Dr. Klopp was a member of the Medical Advisory Board in Philadelphia during World War I, and a member of the United States Naval Reserve until 1930. He was president of the Philadelphia Medical Club and of Jefferson's alumni association in 1930. In 1931 he delivered the first Grace Revere Osler Lecture. Admired for his diagnostic acumen and for the delicacy and dexterity of his surgical technique, he was widely known for excellent results in a large number of colonic and rectal resections for cancer.

Benedict A. Osnis was commissioned by the class of 1937 to paint Dr. Klopp's portrait the year after he died. The surgeon is shown half length and life-sized, dressed modestly in business attire. He sits stiffly in an armchair, with his crossed hands resting in his lap. He looks directly out toward the viewer with a benign expression. The harsh lighting of the posthumous portrait appears to be copied from the tones of the original photograph.

Portrait of George P. Muller

GEORGE P. MULLER, M.D. (1877-1947)
By Alice Kent Stoddard (ca. 1884-1976)

Oil on canvas
1945
44 x 35 in.

Signed lower left: "A. K. Stoddard 45"

Given by JMC class of 1946
Accession number: 1946+e.P.01

Dr. George P. Muller succeeded Dr. Edward J. Klopp as professor of surgery and cochair of the department in 1936. He was a dynamic leader in American surgery and a pioneer thoracic surgeon.

Muller was a native Philadelphian who graduated from Central High School in 1895 and the University of Pennsylvania School of Medicine in 1899. After serving under Dr. John B. Deaver as an intern at the German Hospital (later Lankenau) for three years, his career was forged at the University of Pennsylvania.

Starting as an instructor in the university's department of anatomy, Muller took his initial surgical training as a junior assistant to the chair of surgery, Dr. Charles H. Frazier. From 1918 until 1933 he served as chair of surgery at the University of Pennsylvania's Graduate School of Medicine, and was also chair of the Postgraduate Clinics of Philadelphia for several years.

In 1933 Dr. Muller was appointed professor of clinical surgery at the University of Pennsylvania. He was named senior surgeon at Lankenau Hospital following the death of Dr. Deaver in 1931, and was surgeon to the Misericordia Hospital, Children's Hospital, and the Mary J. Drexel Home.

At age fifty-nine Dr. Muller was already a distinguished surgeon and activist when he came to Jefferson Medical College in 1936 as cochair of surgery. Muller had already served as president of the American College of Surgeons, the American Association for Thoracic Surgery, the College of Physicians of Philadelphia, the Philadelphia Academy of Surgery, and the Philadelphia County Medical Society.

An early practitioner of thoracic surgery, Dr. Muller performed many pulmonary resections in the late 1930s. He was innovative in his use of intravenous fluids and the new sulfonamide drugs. He was admired for his acumen in diagnosis and his skill in the treatment of the surgical patient. His lectures were meticulously prepared and dynamically delivered. He continued the Grace Revere Osler Lectures initiated by Dr. Klopp in 1931, and in 1939 was named the first Grace Revere Osler Professor. He was named emeritus professor of surgery after his retirement in 1946.

Dr. Muller was an editor of *Annals of Surgery* and he revised the sixth edition of Gwilym G. Davis's *Applied Anatomy* (1924). He was one of the earliest writers on diseases of the vascular system. He was awarded an honorary M.S. degree by Villanova University (1916) and an honorary D.Sc. degree by Muhlenberg College (1937). The Jefferson class of 1940 dedicated its yearbook to him, and the class of 1946 commissioned his portrait.

Alice Kent Stoddard's half-length portrait of Professor Muller shows him larger than life, appropriate for this surgical giant. He is seated in an armchair and turned slightly to the left, with his hands tightly clasped in front of his body. He gazes directly toward the observer through a pince-nez with an intense expression

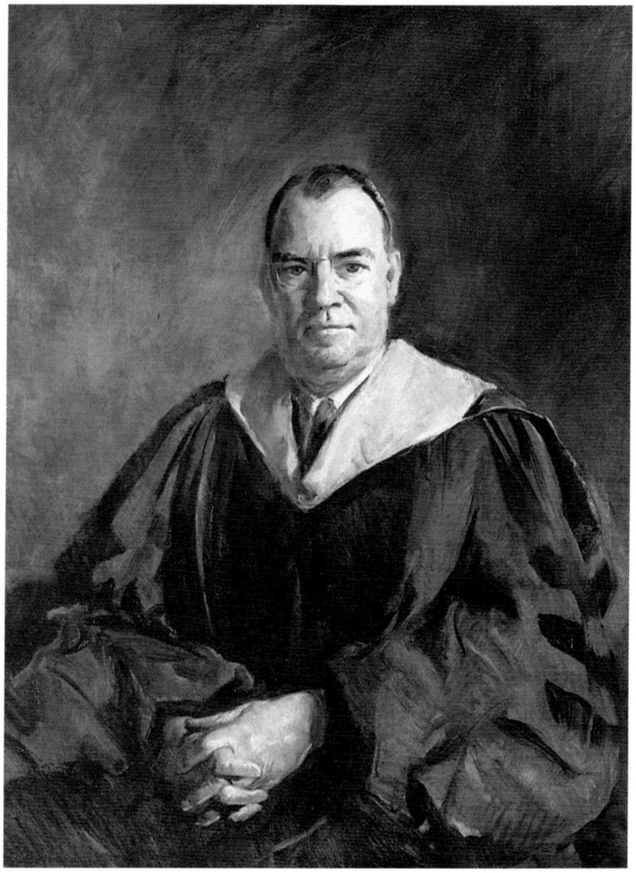

as though waiting for a reply. The voluminous sleeves of his black academic gown fill the entire bottom half of the painting. The robe has a brilliant yellow hood which shows a trace of its red lining.

As in several other portraits discussed in this chapter, the subject's posture in this depiction appears rigid and stiff, while the artist's paint style is animated and free. Stoddard's rapid and fluid feel is most evident in the sitter's richly painted face and hands whose forms are molded by flickering strokes of reds, oranges, yellows, pinks, greens, and blacks.

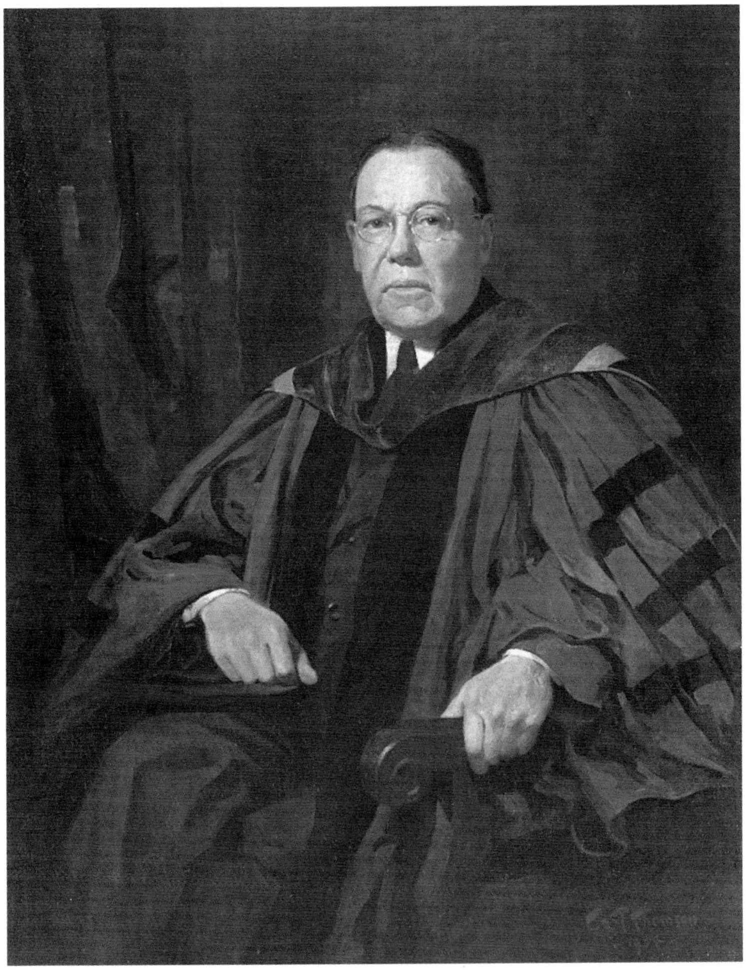

Portrait of James T. Rugh

JAMES TORRANCE RUGH, M.D. (1867-1942)
By William Taylor Thomson (1858-1941)

Oil on canvas
1934
50 x 40 1/4 in.

Signed and dated lower right: "W. T. Thomson/1934"

Given by JMC class of 1934
Accession number: 1934+e.P.02

Dr. James Torrance Rugh succeeded Dr. H. Augustus Wilson in 1918 to become the second chair of the department of orthopaedic surgery at Jefferson Medical College.

James T. Rugh was born in 1867 in New Alexandria, Westmoreland County, Pennsylvania. He was the son of Dr. Jacob W. Rugh (JMC 1851) and brother of Dr. Carroll B. Rugh (JMC 1885). Dr. James Rugh graduated from Michigan's Adrian College in 1889 and Jefferson Medical College in 1892. After serving as resident physician at the Jefferson Hospital, he practiced medicine with Drs. Jacob Solis-Cohen and H. Augustus Wilson.

Prior to his appointment at Jefferson as chair of orthopaedic surgery in 1918 he had acquired extensive teaching and clinical experience both in civilian and military practice. At Jefferson he had taught in the departments of pathology and laryngology, and after 1908 in orthopaedic surgery. In 1895 he was associated with the Philadelphia Polyclinic and was adjunct professor of orthopaedic surgery there from 1897 to 1899. In 1905 he was appointed the first orthopaedic surgeon at the Methodist Hospital. He was made orthopaedic surgeon to the Philadelphia General Hospital in 1912 and clinical professor of orthopaedics at the Women's Medical College in 1914.

In 1916 he was promoted from the Medical Reserve Corps to captain and orthopaedic surgeon to Base Hospital Thirty-eight, the Jefferson unit. In 1917 he advanced to supervising orthopaedic surgeon in charge of southern camps. In 1918 he was transferred to the Surgeon General's office and placed in charge of the precombat orthopaedic work in all United States camps. He was named senior consulting orthopaedic surgeon for all United States camps and base hospitals. His last post was as director of orthopaedic instruction in the Student Army Training Corps for all the medical colleges in Pennsylvania, Maryland, Virginia, and West Virginia. He was discharged in 1919 as a commissioned colonel in the Medical Reserve Corps.

Dr. James T. Rugh served as chair of orthopaedic surgery at Jefferson until his retirement in 1939 when he was made emeritus professor. In 1930 he was named the first James Edwards Professor. He was orthopaedic surgeon to Jefferson, Methodist, Philadelphia General, Women's, and Lying-in Hospitals, and was consulting surgeon to several others. Rugh is credited with gradually shifting the treatment of orthopaedic disabilities from the more old-fashioned mechanical methods to modern, open, surgical correction.

Dr. Rugh was well liked and admired by the students for his clear, simple, and forceful lectures and clinical demonstrations, and for his patient and optimistic demeanor. The class of 1921 dedicated their yearbook to him and the class of 1934 presented his portrait to the college.

In the painting by William T. Thomson, Dr. Rugh is shown two-thirds length and life-sized, facing slightly left. He is seated in front of a dark drapery which lightens to maroon behind his head. His narrow eyes look directly ahead toward the viewer through steel-rimmed glasses. He wears a black academic gown with a hood featuring purple, green, and yellow stripes. The ruddy complexion of his face and hands are painted with a lively touch. The sitter's conventional pose and serious, almost stern, expression give little hint of his outgoing personality. Contemporary biographies note that he was fond of good music and often entertained by accompanying his rich baritone voice on his guitar.

Portrait of James R. Martin

JAMES REID MARTIN, M.D. (1886-1956)
By John Christen Johansen (1876-1964)

Oil on canvas mounted on wood
1958
39 x 31 in.

Signed lower right: "J. C. JOHANSEN"

Given in 1959 by JMC faculty
Accession number: 1958+e.P.02

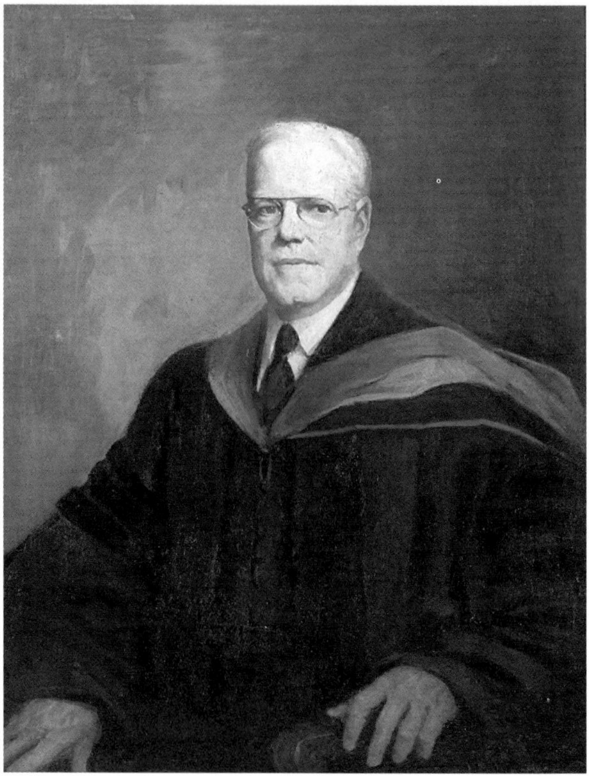

Dr. James Reid Martin joined the orthopaedic department at Jefferson Medical College in 1913 and served as assistant to Dr. James T. Rugh. In 1939 Dr. Martin succeeded Rugh as the third chairman of orthopaedics and James Edwards Professor.

James R. Martin was a native Philadelphian who graduated from Central High School in 1906 and from Jefferson Medical College in 1910. After serving as intern and chief resident at the Jefferson Hospital he rose in the department of orthopaedics to become assistant professor of orthopaedic surgery in 1930 and chief of the outpatient clinic in 1938. That year he resigned to become chief surgeon at the State Hospital for Crippled Children at Elizabethtown and director of the Social Security program for crippled children in the Commonwealth of Pennsylvania.

He returned to Jefferson in 1939 when appointed to the chair of orthopaedics. Under Martin's chairmanship many of the methods of surgical corrections introduced by Dr. Rugh were discarded in favor of the former mechanical treatments. In spite of this reversal of progress, Martin made a major contribution to the department by establishing the orthopaedic residency education program. Upon Martin's resignation in 1950 he was named emeritus professor and appointed associate dean. He served in that capacity until his death in 1956.

During World War I Dr. Martin served overseas from 1917 to 1919 as medical officer in the 109th Infantry of the Twenty-eighth Division. After the Armistice he served on the orthopaedic surgical staffs of various base hospitals of the American Expeditionary Forces. In addition to his long service at Jefferson he was also associated with Philadelphia General Hospital, Delaware County Hospital, Roxborough Memorial Hospital, and Pottsville Hospital.

Martin was president of Jefferson Medical College's alumni association in 1948 and received an honorary doctor of science degree from the college in 1951. His generous bequest made possible the James R. Martin Student Nurses' Residence which opened in 1959.

Unlike his predecessor, Dr. Martin is remembered as a quiet and modest person, retiring and unobtrusive. He was devoted to his church and served as an elder and Sunday school teacher. He was admired by his small circle of friends for his integrity, tolerance, wisdom, and sense of duty.

John C. Johansen's portrait suggests these personal qualities. The physician is shown half length and life-sized, seated with both arms resting on the chair arms. Turned slightly to the left, he looks out directly to the observer with a pleasant and kindly expression. The color scheme, including the greenish atmospheric background, is subdued throughout except for the bright yellow lining of the green hood of Martin's black academic gown. Today the painting is marred by heavy restoration.

The posthumous portrait was commissioned at the initiative of Dr. Anthony F. DePalma, Martin's successor as chair of orthopaedics. Minutes from meetings of the executive faculty portrait committee describe "difficulties" with the portrait. It had to be returned to the artist to remove "objectionable white specks" and to straighten the creased canvas. It was sent to a local framer to correct "other flaws" that resulted from inadequate framing and the fir-wood backing of the canvas.

Such complaints were highly unusual for an artist of John C. Johansen's stature. The Martin portrait was his sixth Jefferson commission since 1953. A reasonable explanation is that by 1958 the artist was eighty-two years of age and perhaps the flaws escaped his notice. Incredibly, Johansen continued his distinguished and lengthy career until a few months before his death in 1964.

Born in 1876 in Copenhagen, Denmark, Johansen was brought to America as a young child. After studying at the Art Institute of Chicago, he traveled abroad and attended the Académie Julian in Paris. Upon their return to New York Johansen and his painter wife, Jean, established separate studios there and also in Stockbridge, Massachusetts where they spent the summers. John C. Johansen taught briefly at the Art Institute of Chicago and then at the Art Students League in New York. He was made an academician of the National Academy of Design in 1915.

Johansen's most significant commission was to paint the signing of the peace treaty at Versailles after World War I. The huge group portrait hangs today in the National Portrait Gallery in Washington, D.C. He was also known for his portrait of President Herbert Hoover which hung in the White House, and a portrait of Abraham Lincoln delivering his famous Cooper Union address which belongs to the school in New York. His last completed portrait was that of Bishop Fulton J. Sheen.

Johansen won numerous awards in important national exhibitions including the Municipal League Purchase Prize, the Young Fortnightly Prize, the Norman Waite Harris Gold Medal, and the William M. R. French Gold Medal, all at the Art Institute of Chicago. He also won a gold medal at the Buenos Aires Exposition of 1910, the J. Sanford Saltus Gold Medal at the National Academy of Design, the H. S. Morris Prize at the Newport Art Association, a gold medal at the Panama-Pacific Exposition in San Francisco, and a silver medal at the Sesqui-centennial Exposition in Philadelphia.

John C. Johansen's portraits are represented in private and university collections throughout the country and in the following institutions: the Art Institute of Chicago, the National Gallery of Art, the Metropolitan Museum of Art, the National Academy of Design, the Carnegie Institute in Pittsburgh, the Wadsworth Atheneum in Hartford, Connecticut, the Pennsylvania Academy of the Fine Arts, and the National Gallery in Santiago, Chile.

Portrait of Charles E. G. Shannon

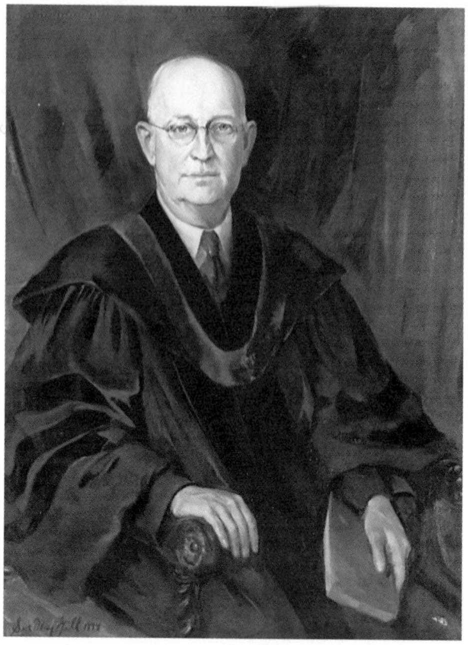

CHARLES EMORY GOULD SHANNON, M.D. (1875-1965)
By Sue May Wescott Gill (b. 1890)

Oil on canvas
42 x 32 in.
1944

Signed and dated lower left: "Sue May Gill 1944"

Given by JMC class of September 1944
Accession number: 1944+e.P.02

Dr. Charles E. G. Shannon succeeded Dr. William M. Sweet as chair of ophthalmology at Jefferson Medical College in 1927. He held the post until his retirement in 1948.

Charles E. G. Shannon was born in Saco, Maine in 1875, descended from a forbear who had settled in Massachusetts in 1623. He was encouraged to study medicine by his cousin, George M. Gould, M.D. (JMC 1888), a Philadelphia ophthalmologist who devised cemented bifocal lenses. Gould was the author of *The Jefferson Medical College of Philadelphia* (1904), a two-volume history, and editor of the widely used *Gould Medical Dictionary*.

Charles Shannon graduated from Colby College in Waterville, Maine in 1899 and from Jefferson Medical College in 1902. He interned at the Pottsville Hospital and then pursued postgraduate work in ophthalmology at the Massachusetts Eye and Ear Infirmary. In 1904 he returned to Jefferson as office and hospital assistant to Professor Howard F. Hansell, M.D., chair of ophthalmology. He became chief of the outpatient eye clinic and an associate in ophthalmology.

In 1911 Shannon was appointed assistant ophthalmologist to the Philadelphia General Hospital and with the resignation of Dr. Hansell he became attending ophthalmologist there. In 1917 he was commissioned a first lieutenant in the Medical Corps and was discharged with the rank of captain in 1919.

Dr. Shannon continued to rise through the ranks at Jefferson until he was named a full professor in 1927. He served as president of the Jefferson Medical College alumni association. He retired in 1948 and was named emeritus professor. He returned to Maine where he resumed a private practice. He was awarded an honorary D.Sc. degree from Colby College in 1954.

Dr. Shannon was regarded with esteem and affection by his students. His portrait by Sue May Wescott Gill was commissioned by the wartime class that graduated in September 1944. The class yearbook featured a candid photograph of the artist dressed in a floral smock, holding a palette and a long-handled brush, adding the finishing touches on Shannon's portrait.

The two-thirds-length, life-sized portrait shows the professor seated in an armchair with his body facing slightly right. His left hand holds a book bound in red. He wears a black academic robe with green velvet trim in the mantle. His wide blue eyes gaze straight ahead through rimless glasses and his expression is benign. The loosely painted background drapery of green, blue, rose, and umber relates to the colors in the upholstered chair, costume, and book.

At the portrait presentation a student speaker recalled the professor's earnestness and modesty in humorous situations:

> We shall all remember...the difficult time we had trying to tell him that our class wanted him to sit for a portrait. He was so engrossed in showing us some lantern slides that we just couldn't squeeze in a word; and the time he came all prepared to quiz us one Friday afternoon, only to discover after calling a few names that he had last year's roll book with him. Then there are all those A's in Ophthalmology that the bespectacled members of our class are pledged to make this year in payment for their visits to Dr. Shannon's office.

Sue May Wescott was born in 1890 in Sabinal, Texas. She followed an elder sister, Sarah, to study at the Pennsylvania Academy of the Fine Arts. She won the Academy's Cresson traveling scholarship and First Toppan Prize, and studied abroad at the Académie Julian in Paris. It was there that she first met Paul L. Gill, a fellow student whom she married in 1928.

Sue May Gill was first known for landscapes and then for portraits and flower paintings. She received solo exhibitions at the Philadelphia Art Club, the Philadelphia Art Alliance, the Syracuse Museum of Fine Arts, and the Oklahoma City Art Center. She won an honorable mention at the Ogunquit Art Center in 1931, the Penman Memorial Prize of the National Association of Women Painters and Sculptors in 1932, the Fellowship Prize of the Pennsylvania Academy in 1933, and awards at the Philadelphia Plastic Club and the Philadelphia Sketch Club in the 1940s.

Sue May Gill was awarded a sculpture commission from the Military Academy at West Point, and was commissioned for numerous fountain sculptures in private collections. Her portrait of Pennsylvania Academy of the Fine Arts president Alfred G. B. Steel was purchased by the institution in 1956.

Portrait of Pascal B. Bland

PASCAL BROOKE BLAND, M.D.
(1875-1940)
By Lazar Raditz (1887-1958)

Oil on canvas mounted on board
1935
42 x 36 in.

Signed and dated lower right: "Lazar Raditz/1935"
Exhibition: Philadelphia, *Annual Exhibition*, Pennsylvania Academy of the Fine Arts, 1936

Given by JMC class of 1936
Accession number: 1936+e.P.01

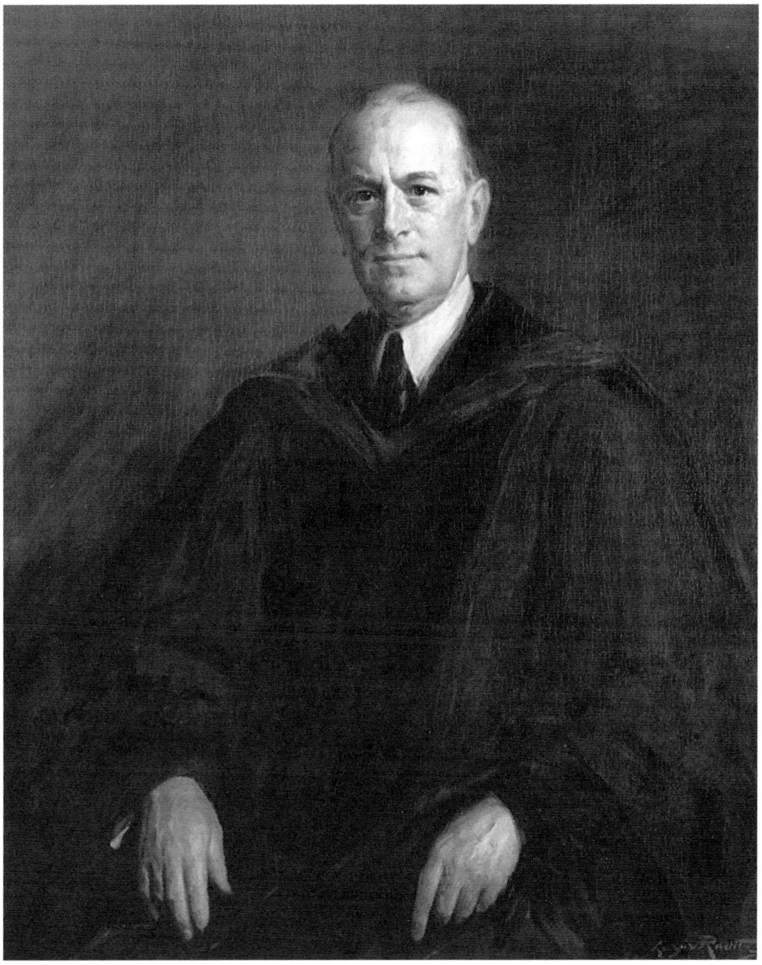

Dr. Pascal Brooke Bland became chair of obstetrics at Jefferson Medical College in 1925, succeeding Dr. Edward P. Davis. He was instrumental in strengthening the department academically and in improving its facilities.

Pascal B. Bland was born in 1875 in Monocacy, Berks County, Pennsylvania, to a family whose English forbear had emigrated to Virginia in 1654. Bland was president of his senior class and graduated with honors from Jefferson Medical College in 1901.

After his residency at the Jefferson Hospital he became an assistant to Dr. Edward E. Montgomery and a demonstrator in the department of gynecology, while establishing a private practice. During this early period of his career he also visited clinics abroad and did postgraduate work in Vienna and Berlin.

Upon his return to Jefferson he was made an assistant professor of gynecology in 1910. His rise in the faculty ranks culminated with his appointment as chair and professor of obstetrics in 1925. In the early 1930s he became aware that structured specialty training in obstetrics and gynecology in hospitals (rather than merely serving as an assistant to an established specialist) was becoming recognized across the country. Although his efforts to reorganize his department met with some resistance, he was successful in improving the didactic and clinical instruction in obstetrics. He established the first residency in obstetrics at Jefferson in 1937.

After Bland retired that same year and was named emeritus professor, he continued his busy, private practice in obstetrics until his sudden death in 1940. Tragically, he died from a self-inflicted gunshot wound to the head, as reported in local papers.

Dr. Pascal B. Bland had been an associate or consulting obstetrician or gynecologist to ten other hospitals in the Philadelphia area, and served as president of the Obstetrical Society of Philadelphia in 1928. His texts, *Gynecology: Medical and Surgical* (1924) and *Practical Obstetrics: for Students and Practitioners* (1932), became standard works in medical education.

In addition to numerous American medical societies, Bland was also a fellow of the Royal Society of Medicine of London, first vice president of the International College of Surgeons, corresponding member of the Society for Clinical Study of Havana, and foreign corresponding member of the Royal Medical Society of Budapest.

Dr. Bland was a noted bibliophile and passionate collector of rare books and incunabula on the subjects of anatomy, obstetrics, and gynecology. His considerable medical library was bequeathed to Jefferson and it formed the core of the college's historical collections. Bland's enthusiasm as chairman of the executive faculty's library committee also inspired other physicians to make donations.

In gratitude for his generous gift trustees resolved that a Bland Memorial Alcove be set aside in the library for the collection. Dr. Bland also bequeathed to the department of obstetrics and gynecology over one million dollars which was used to establish the Bland fellowships in obstetrics and gynecology.

The student yearbook of 1929 was dedicated to Dr. Pascal B. Bland. The professor was equally esteemed by Jefferson nursing students who dedicated their 1941 yearbook to his memory.

Dr. Bland was the class portrait honoree in 1936. In the half-length, life-sized portrait by Lazar Raditz, the physician is seated in an armchair facing slightly to the left. He turns his head to look directly toward the viewer with an inquiring expression. He is attired in a black academic robe. The atmospheric background deepens subtly from maroon to black. Raditz's ability to depict a sitter in a convincingly lifelike way is manifest here in the loosely brushed, solidly rendered face and hands. One senses the volume of the sitter's body underneath his gown.

The artist must have been pleased with the portrait because he submitted it to the 1936 *Annual Exhibition* at the Pennsylvania Academy of the Fine Arts. The show ended just before the portrait was presented to Jefferson. Mrs. Bland requested that her husband's portrait be placed in the Bland Alcove in the library near the portrait of her father, Dr. Edward E. Montgomery.

Portrait of Norris W. Vaux

NORRIS WISTAR VAUX, M.D. (1881-1958)
By Maurice Molarsky (1885-1950)

Oil on canvas
1947
35 x 35 in.

Signed and dated lower left and upper right: "Maurice Molarsky 1947"

Given by JMC class of 1947
Accession number: 1947+e.P.02

In 1937 Dr. Norris W. Vaux succeeded Dr. Pascal B. Bland as chair of obstetrics at Jefferson Medical College. He was an esteemed teacher and a national figure in his field.

Norris Wistar Vaux was born in 1881 in Rosemont, Pennsylvania, a descendant of four distinguished Philadelphia families: the Wistars, Peppers, Norrises, and Vauxes. His grandfather, Richard Vaux, had been mayor of Philadelphia. Norris Vaux received his medical degree from the University of Pennsylvania in 1905, interned at the Pennsylvania Hospital for two years, and did postgraduate work in obstetrics at the Rotunda Hospital, Dublin University.

While establishing a general practice in Philadelphia he began an academic career at Jefferson as instructor in obstetrics under Dr. Edward P. Davis. World War I intervened and he served with the American Expeditionary Forces at Base Hospital Ten, the Pennsylvania Hospital unit, and with the British General Hospital Sixteen. He was discharged in 1919 with the rank of major after twenty-three months of overseas duty.

In 1919 Dr. Vaux became chief obstetrician to the Bryn Mawr Hospital. In 1925 he was appointed clinical professor of obstetrics at Jefferson, and in 1937 he was made chairman, succeeding Dr. Bland. He held that post until 1946 when he was made emeritus professor, and continued as a consultant in obstetrics and gynecology until his death in 1958. In 1951 he received an honorary LL.D. degree from Jefferson Medical College.

Dr. Vaux held several other significant obstetrical positions. When Pennsylvania Hospital and the Philadelphia Lying-in Hospital merged in 1938 he became director of the department of obstetrics and gynecology and held that post until 1946. He was also president of the Philadelphia Obstetrical Society, member of the American Board of Obstetrics and Gynecology, and president of the American Gynecological Society. He was director of health of the Commonwealth of Pennsylvania from 1947 to 1951.

His best-known literary works were his revision of Dr. J. Clifton Edgar's *Practice of Obstetrics: for Students and Practitioners of Medicine* (sixth edition, 1926) and *The Mechanics of Obstetrics* (coauthor with Mario A. Castallo, M.D., 1943). He also published numerous papers on postpartum hemorrhage, prenatal care, eclampsia, and pyelitis.

Students greatly valued Dr. Vaux's pragmatic viewpoint in teaching a system of obstetrics with clear and well organized lectures that emphasized practical facts. The class of 1947 chose Vaux as its portrait honoree the year after his retirement.

In the two-thirds-length, life-sized portrait by Maurice Molarsky, Dr. Vaux is seated in an armchair turned slightly to the left, and his legs extend to the lower edge of the picture. He holds a book bound in red in his right hand. His piercing gaze and the sharp, downward slant of his thick, dark eyebrows create a slightly menacing expression. His black academic gown with its massive sleeves has a green mantle with red lining. The background consists of olive green drapery and the partial view of a framed picture on the left. The unusual square format, combined with the sitter's firmly modeled body, somber scowl, and forward placement in the pictorial space, create the imposing presence of a figure to be reckoned with.

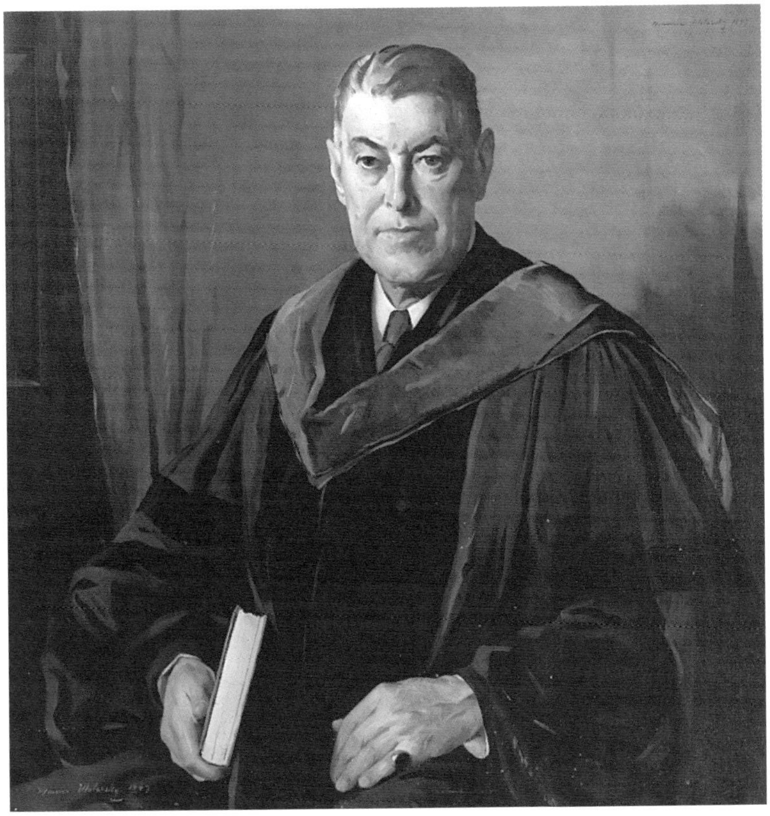

Portrait of George A. Ulrich

GEORGE ALVIN ULRICH, M.D. (1873-1944)
By Roy Cleveland Nuse (1885-1975)

Oil on canvas
1941
40 1/4 x 34 1/4 in.

Signed and dated lower right: "RN/1941"

Given by JMC class of 1941
Accession number: 1941+e.P.02

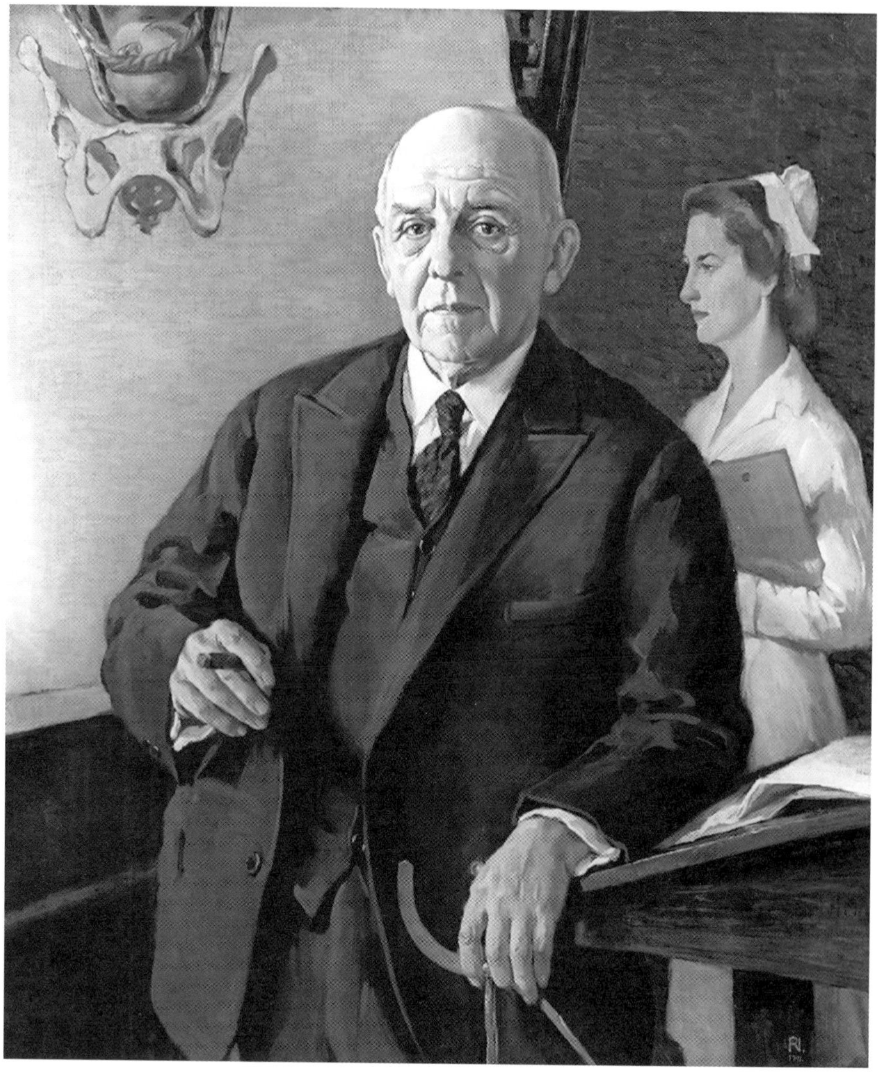

Dr. George A. Ulrich was a clinical professor of obstetrics at Jefferson Medical College. The gifted and beloved obstetrician spent almost his entire career at the institution.

George Ulrich was born in 1873 near Lebanon, Pennsylvania. He received bachelor of science (1897) and master of science (1899) degrees from Lebanon Valley College. He also taught at the local public schools before earning a medical degree at Jefferson Medical College in 1901. A winner of the gold medal for excellence in midwifery, he became associated with the maternity department at Jefferson Hospital immediately after graduation. Ulrich advanced steadily in the department of obstetrics and was appointed a clinical professor in 1931. He was an active staff member until his death in 1944. He also had a long association with the Polyclinic Hospital.

For twenty-five years Dr. Ulrich was responsible for the greater part of the clinical teaching of obstetrics at Jefferson, and was known for conveying information by anecdote and apt illustrations from his extensive practice. The Jefferson yearbook of 1941 described his advocacy of patience and condemnation of haste and intervention when dealing with obstetrical problems, by repeating his famous aphorism that "the best and most generally useful obstetrical instrument is a big black cigar." Supposedly he always had a pocketful of cigars in readiness to soothe his nerves as he awaited indications from Mother Nature as to the proper course.

Loved and esteemed by the students who affectionately referred to him as "Pop" or "Uncle George," Dr. Ulrich was the first clinical professor to be honored by a senior class portrait.

The physician as teacher is depicted two-thirds length and life-sized. He stands in front of his "coat of arms," an anatomical chart depicting the female pelvis with fetus. His left arm rests on lecture notes on the lectern and his hand holds a pelvimeter. His right hand holds his ever present cigar. Dr. Ulrich's features are very sharply delineated in strong contrasts of light and shade, and emphasized by the creases in his high-domed forehead, corners of his eyes, cheeks and mouth, the circles below his eyes, and the slack skin of his neck.

Although the physician's facial expression is stern, his posture is relaxed as he addresses the class. The students are not shown in this painting, unlike some other group portraits of clinical lectures already encountered. However, an unexpected character is a uniformed nurse clasping a chart who enters the scene immediately behind and to the right of Dr. Ulrich. Her profile figure is small in scale compared with the professor, and she inexplicably appears to be just "passing through."

The portrait's harmonious color scheme is prevalently cool, especially the professor's dark blue suit and blue and maroon dotted necktie, the bluish white of the nurse's uniform, and the pale gray background of the anatomical illustration. Nuse's loosely brushed paint style is very animated, enhancing the feeling of energy emanating from the subject.

Even today observers conjecture on the presence and identity of the nurse. The good-natured obstetrician set the record straight in remarks at his portrait presentation,

> I have taken a good deal of teasing about that [the nurse]. Some fellow would say, "Is that your favorite nurse?" One asked, "Is that your pet?" and Doctor Vaux said, "Why, Bill, you don't know George, he pets them all."
>
> And the artist and I had a little bit of an argument when he wanted to put a nurse on the picture. I wanted to know why he couldn't accommodate five or six. Some asked, "Where did you find her?" Roughly, about twenty years ago, I was on the reception committee, the head usher at her coming-out party. When she emerged she was fifty centimeters in length and weighed nine pounds, two ounces. Now here she is, popping up again. Which just proves the fact that chickens will come home to roost.

Jefferson documents state that the woman who posed for the figure of the nurse was actually Marie Riley, a technician at the Pennsylvania Hospital. The *Philadelphia Record* of March 7, 1941 reporting on the portrait ceremony said that the obstetrician was "always running into ex-babies he had 'sponsored.'" Dr. Ulrich was well respected by the nurses, and among the overflow crowd at the portrait ceremony was a large contingent of Jefferson Hospital nurses who presented the sitter with a bouquet of roses.

Portrait of Brooke M. Anspach

BROOKE MELANCTHON ANSPACH, M.D. (1876-1951)
By Benedict Anton Osnis (1872-1941)

Oil on canvas
1938
35 1/4 x 30 1/4 in.

Signed and dated upper left: "B. A. OSNIS/1938"

Given by JMC class of 1938
Accession number: 1938+e.P.01

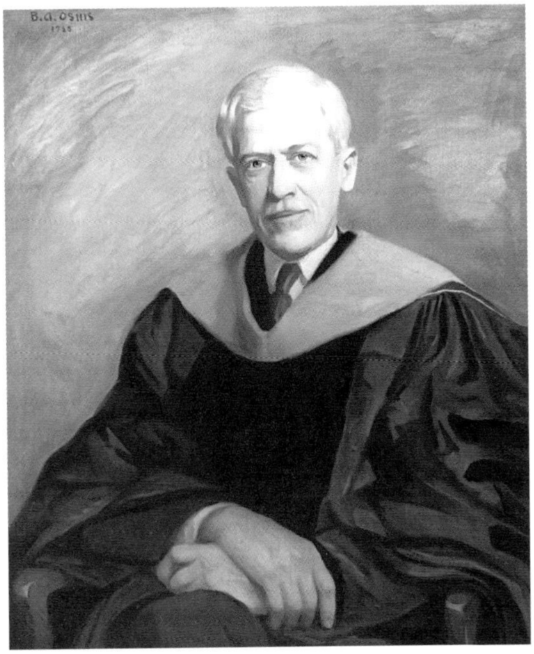

Dr. Brooke M. Anspach was named the chair of gynecology at Jefferson Medical College in 1921, succeeding Dr. Edward E. Montgomery. The second head of the department, Anspach retained the post until 1940 when he was named emeritus professor.

Brooke M. Anspach was born in 1876 in Reading, Pennsylvania. After one year at Lafayette College he entered the medical department of the University of Pennsylvania and graduated in 1897. After serving as a resident physician at the University Hospital he joined the staff of Dr. John G. Clark, professor of gynecology, and also trained briefly at the Johns Hopkins Hospital and in Berlin. He advanced to the post of associate in gynecology at the University of Pennsylvania. At this time he was also associated with the Philadelphia General, Kensington, and Bryn Mawr Hospitals.

Upon accepting the chair of gynecology at Jefferson in 1921 Dr. Anspach relinquished all of his prior associations except with Bryn Mawr Hospital. He continued the curriculum initiated by Dr. Montgomery: didactic lectures in the third year; section teaching including demonstrations in the operating room, clinical conferences, and examination and treatment of clinic patients in the fourth year. Laboratories for gynecologic endocrinology research were expanded in the new 1929 College Building, and clinical gynecologic facilities increased with the opening of the Curtis Building in 1931.

Anspach's best-known literary work was *Gynecology* (1921) which soon became a standard text and reached its fifth edition by 1934. He served as president of the Obstetrical Society of Philadelphia and of the American Gynecological Society. He was a member of the board of governors of the American College of Surgeons. During World War I Dr. Anspach was enrolled in the Reserve Corps of the University of Pennsylvania Base Hospital Twenty. He received honorary D.Sc. degrees from Lafayette College (1936) and from Jefferson Medical College (1946).

The class of 1938 chose Dr. Brooke M. Anspach as its portrait honoree. Benedict Osnis depicted the physician half length and life-sized, turned very slightly to the left in his armchair. He wears a black academic gown with a yellow mantle lined in red. These dark and bright colors contrast with the subject's fair complexion: silver hair and mustache, pale blue eyes, and pink skin tones. His expression is pleasant and the observer feels engaged by his direct but kindly gaze.

Portrait of Chevalier Jackson

CHEVALIER JACKSON, M.D. (1865-1958)
By Gilbert Bacon (?)

Old copy of photograph mounted on board
Original photograph 1930-40
Image size: 9 x 7 in.
Sheet size: 12 1/4 x 9 1/2 in.

Signatures below image: ink, "Chevalier Jackson" and pencil, "Gilbert Bacon" (?)

Given in 1953 by unknown donor
Accession number: 1953+e.Ph.01

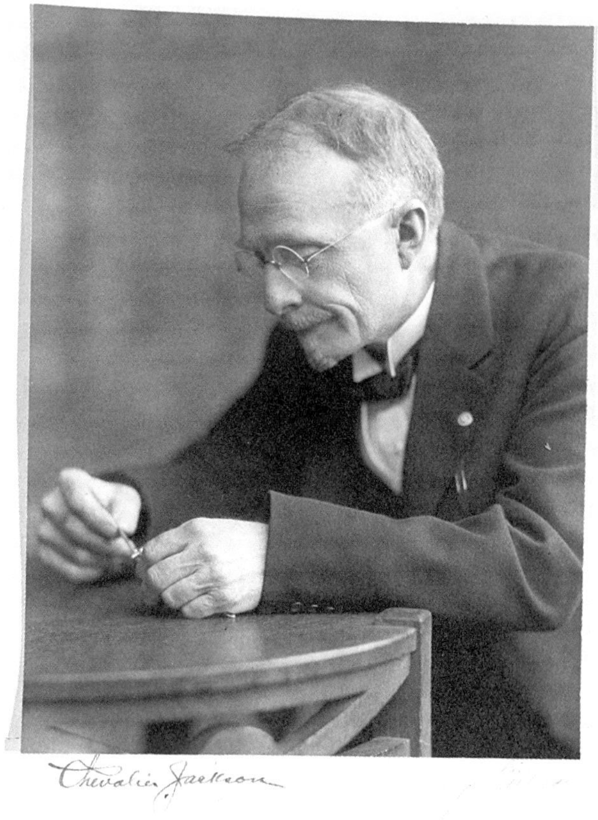

Dr. Chevalier Jackson became the second chairman of laryngology at Jefferson Medical College, and several years later a new chair of bronchoscopy and esophagoscopy was created especially for him. He was a world-famous, pioneering authority in his field, and one of Jefferson's most distinguished alumni.

Chevalier Jackson was born in Pittsburgh in 1865 and studied at the Western University of Pennsylvania (now the University of Pittsburgh). While attending Jefferson Medical College Jackson became impressed by the work of Dr. Jacob da Silva Solis-Cohen and other Philadelphia specialists in diseases of the nose and throat. After his graduation in 1886 he went abroad to study at the clinic of Dr. Morell Mackenzie, a leading laryngologist in London.

In his initial years of practice among the poor in Pittsburgh Dr. Chevalier Jackson became associated with the Western Pennsylvania Medical College. One of his earliest contributions was to advocate the control of tonsillar hemorrhage by the use of hemostatic forceps, torsion, and ligation. Around 1890 he developed the prototype for the esophagoscope. He also constructed a practical bronchoscope, developed a technique for its safe passage, and devised accessory instruments. He became widely acclaimed for removing foreign bodies inspirated into the lungs and other air passages, replacing the more dangerous methods of surgical intervention used at the time.

In his autobiography Jackson described how Dr. D. Braden Kyle invited him to Philadelphia during the session of the American Laryngological Association to remove a price-tag fastener from a child who had swallowed it while at work in a stocking factory.[9] He said, "The novelty of the procedure attracted many celebrated physicians of the day," and they initially doubted that the child's life would be saved. He recalled another case in which Dr. J. Chalmers DaCosta refused to treat a young patient who had swallowed a scarf pin, and instead referred him to Dr. Jackson out in Pittsburgh. The photograph shows Dr. Jackson about 1930 to 1940 intently examining a metallic, clip-like object apparently just removed from a patient's trachea or esophagus.

In 1911 Dr. Jackson was stricken twice with tuberculosis and his recovery period took almost a full year. In 1912 he was elected to the chair of laryngology at the Western Pennsylvania Medical College, and was also appointed to the staff of fourteen hospitals in Pittsburgh. Most of the local laryngologists there referred him patients who required bronchoscopy, esophagoscopy, gastroscopy, and endolaryngeal surgery. Then in 1915 he was elected professor of bronchoscopy at the New York Post-graduate Medical School and Hospital where he commuted regularly. He was forced to resign two years later to recuperate from a debilitating, third bout of tuberculosis.

In 1916 Dr. Chevalier Jackson accepted the chair of laryngology at Jefferson Medical College. He resigned that professorship in 1924 to assume Jefferson's first chair of bronchoscopy and esophagoscopy, a post he held until 1930. In addition to treating patients from a wide geographic area, he dedicated his career to teaching. As a testament to his reputation and stamina, he also held a chair or lectureship at the Graduate School of Medicine of the University of Pennsylvania, the School of Medicine of the University of Pennsylvania, the Temple University School of Medicine, and the Women's Medical College. He was president of the latter institution from 1935 until 1941.

Another of Jackson's great contributions was his work in the prevention of caustic lye burns of the pharynx and esophagus. As chairman of the Committee on Lye Legislation of the American Medical Association, his initiative in organizing physicians in every state resulted in the passage of a Federal Caustic Poison Law in 1927.

Dr. Jackson's prodigious literary output included twelve textbooks, six monographs, and chapters in thirteen "systems" of medicine and surgery. He was author or coauthor of more than seven hundred articles. His most notable texts are: *Tracheo-bronchoscopy, Esophagoscopy, and Gastroscopy* (1907), *Peroral Endoscopy and Laryngeal Surgery* (1915), *Bronchoscopy and Esophagoscopy: A Manual of Peroral Endoscopy and Laryngeal Surgery* (1922), *Diseases of the Air and Food Passages of Foreign-body Origin* (coauthor with his son, Chevalier L. Jackson, M.D., 1936), and *The Larynx and Its Diseases* (with Chevalier L. Jackson, M.D., 1937).

Dr. Chevalier Jackson served as president of the American Laryngological, Rhinological, and Otological Society, the American Bronchoscopic Society of which he was a founder, and the American Laryngological Association. He was also president of the Pan-American Medical Association and of the American Therapeutic Society. Jackson was a founder of the American College of Surgeons. He held honorary membership in ten American medical societies and twenty others in Europe and South America.

With five honorary degrees, Dr. Jackson was one of the most decorated physicians of his era. Among his most prestigious civic and medical awards were: the Philadelphia (Bok) Award and the John Scott Award of the City of Philadelphia, Officer of the Legion of Honor of France and Knight of the Order of Leopold of Belgium, the De Roaldes Award of the American Laryngological Association, the gold medal of the Radiological Society of North America, Commander of the Order of the Crown of Italy, Grand Master of the Southern Cross of Brazil, the Bellion Prize of the Academy of Sciences of Paris, and the Distinguished Service Medal of the American Medical Association.

Dr. Chevalier Jackson was also an accomplished painter and printmaker, and often illustrated his own medical articles. His interest in woodworking and machinery helped him devise many instruments to solve foreign body removal problems. His most oft-quoted aphorism is, "Being purely mechanical, the problem must be soluble." He aimed to share his discoveries freely, so refused to patent them. He continued to review articles and revise his own textbooks almost until his death at age ninety-three in 1958.

Portrait of Chevalier Jackson

CHEVALIER JACKSON, M.D. (1865-1958)
By Luigi Maraffi (b. 1891)

Plaster
1937
21 3/4 x 13 x 11 1/4 in.

Signed and dated rear center right: "Luigi Maraffi/1937"

Given in 1952 by Dr. Louis H. Clerf (JMC 1912)
Accession number: 1952+e.S.01

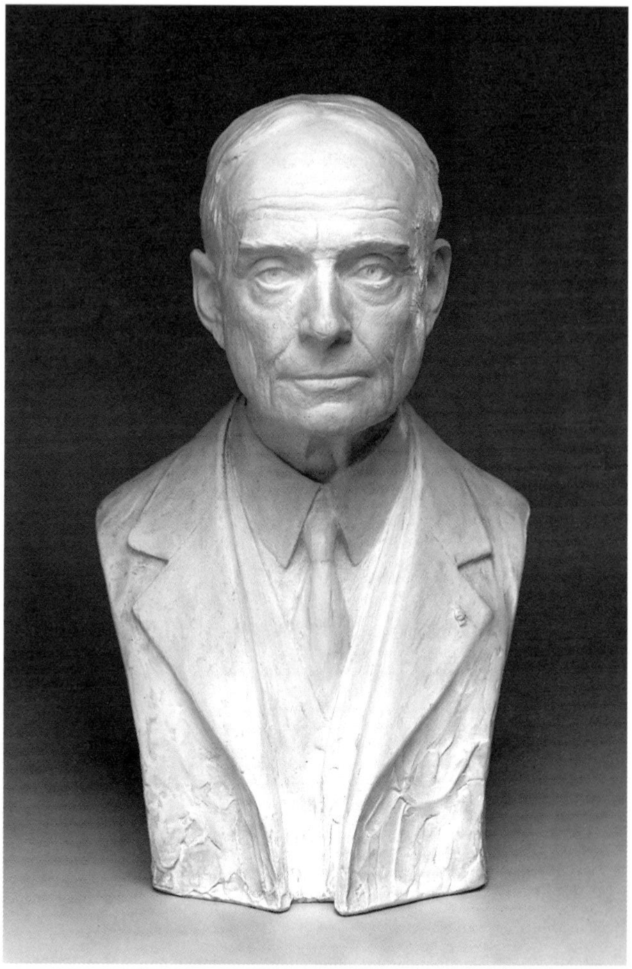

The Jefferson art collection includes one painted and two sculpted portraits of Dr. Chevalier Jackson. The oil painting was created in 1956 by Robert L. Lukens, M.D., a Jefferson alumnus of 1912; in it he faithfully copied the photograph shown above. A bronze bust was created by Maurine Ligon in 1941 showing Dr. Jackson wearing an operating cap and gown, with a surgical mask hanging from his neck. The bust was a centennial gift in 1970 to the Jefferson alumni association from Dr. Sterling A. Barrett, an alumnus of 1934, and Mrs. Barrett.

A white, plaster portrait bust modeled in 1937 by Luigi Maraffi was presented to Dr. Chevalier Jackson by a group of his pupils and colleagues that same year.[10] The sculpture is a naturalistic description of the physician at age seventy-two. The textured surface of the portrait bust emphasizes his sloping forehead and flattened hair, deepset eyes and protruding eyebrows, hooked nose, thin lips and wide mouth, and deep wrinkles in his forehead and cheeks. His determined gaze and tightly closed lips add to the forcefulness of Maraffi's characterization.

Luigi Maraffi was born in 1891 in Aversa, a small Italian town near Naples, and emigrated to Philadelphia with his family in 1903. He studied sculpture at the Fleisher Art Memorial and then at the Pennsylvania Academy of the Fine Arts (1913-17) where he won a Stewardson Prize and two Cresson traveling scholarships. Maraffi was best known for traditional portrait sculptures, but also contributed stone carvings to the Cathedral of the Church of the New Jerusalem in Bryn Athyn, Pennsylvania and to the main building of the Free Library of Philadelphia.

Portrait of Fielding O. Lewis

FIELDING O. LEWIS, M.D. (1878-1965)
By David H. Gettens (active 1960s)

Oil on canvas
1966
32 x 26 in.

Signed and dated upper right: "David H. Gettens/1966"

Given in 1966 by Mrs. Morris H. Dixon, daughter of the subject
Accession number: 1966+e.P.02

Dr. Fielding O. Lewis was the third chairman of laryngology at Jefferson Medical College. He was an acclaimed otolaryngologist whose career was tragically halted by a stroke at age fifty-six.

Fielding O. Lewis was born in 1878 in Hebbardsville, Kentucky, a descendant of the Revolutionary War hero, Fielding Lewis. After attending Georgetown College in Kentucky, in 1901 he graduated from the Philadelphia College of Pharmacy, and in 1906 from Jefferson Medical College where he was senior class president.

Following an internship at Jefferson Hospital he

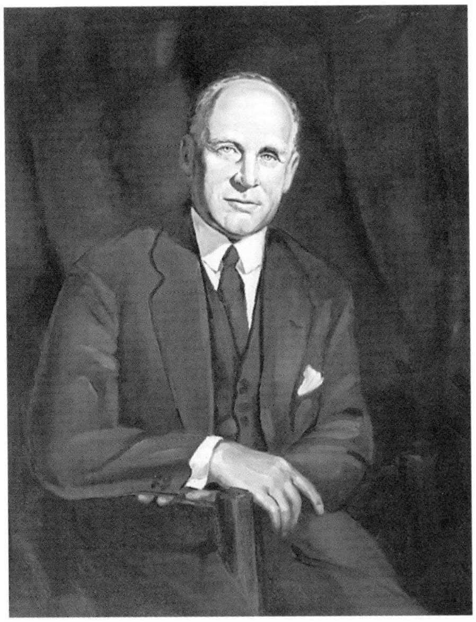

began private practice and was associated with Dr. D. Braden Kyle from 1907 to 1912. He rose through the academic ranks until his appointment as chair of laryngology in 1924. He was also associated with the Philadelphia General Hospital and the Hospital for Contagious Diseases in Philadelphia. During World War I he served as captain in the Medical Corps and was stationed at Base Hospital Nine at Camp Green.

When he returned from the war Dr. Fielding O. Lewis became interested in surgical treatment of cancer of the larynx, and soon became a pioneering authority on the operation of total laryngectomy in Philadelphia. He also was respected for his work in sinus surgery, rhinoplasty, tonsillectomy, mastoid surgery, and laryngeal surgery.

Dr. Lewis was at the height of his career when illness struck in 1934. He was compelled to retire from practice and teaching but maintained an active interest in Jefferson affairs until his death in 1965. He was elected emeritus professor. Dr. Lewis had served a term as president of the Jefferson alumni association.

The posthumous portrait of Dr. Fielding Lewis was painted in 1966 by David H. Gettens, and was donated that same year by Mrs. Morris H. Dixon, daughter of the subject. The smaller-than-life-sized portrait shows the physician two-thirds length and seated in an armchair. He looks out toward the viewer with an amiable expression. The portrait's disconcerting notes of overly bright skin tones and unconvincing anatomy suggest that David H. Gettens was an amateur artist.

Portrait of Louis H. Clerf

LOUIS H. CLERF, M.D. (1889-1989)
By Frederick Roscher (1890-1968)

Oil on masonite
1948
48 x 36 in.

Signed and dated lower left: "Roscher/1948"

Given by JMC class of 1949
Accession number: 1949+e.P.01

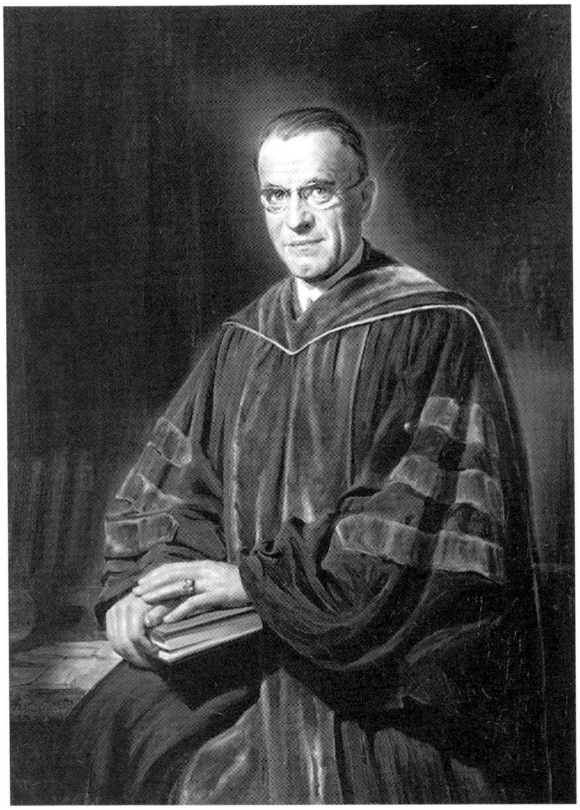

Dr. Louis H. Clerf was the successor to Dr. Chevalier Jackson in the development of bronchoesophagology at Jefferson Medical College. Dr. Clerf, too, was an outstanding American laryngologist, and his honors were legion.

Louis H. Clerf was born in 1889 in Ellensburg, Washington where his family ran a cattle ranch. After attending St. Martin's College in Olympia, Washington he began medical school at the University, but transferred to Jefferson Medical College and graduated with the class of 1912. After two years of internship he was chief resident at the Jefferson Hospital from 1914 to 1916.

Dr. Clerf served in the U.S. Navy medical department during World War I, and was an instructor in otolaryngology at the Naval Medical School. He was later commissioned a captain in the reserves. Before his appointment in 1922 as demonstrator in laryngology at Jefferson Medical College he continued his training at the New York Eye and Ear Infirmary.

Dr. Clerf became the personal assistant to Dr. Chevalier Jackson and under his tutelage became adept at handling the bronchoscope. In 1930 Dr. Clerf succeeded him as professor of bronchoscopy and esophagoscopy at the Jefferson Medical College, and continued to build upon the worldwide reputation of the bronchoscopic clinic founded by Jackson. Six years later he succeeded Dr. Fielding O. Lewis as chairman of laryngology, and held both posts until his retirement in 1954 when he was elected emeritus professor. Dr. Clerf was also bronchoscopist to the Philadelphia General, Jewish, Pennsylvania, and Germantown Hospitals. He lived until the age of one hundred at his Florida retirement home.

In a memoir William H. Baltzell, M.D., an alumnus of 1946, described Dr. Clerf's meticulous operating room procedures:

> There were painted dots on the floor for the position of every piece of equipment. There was no talking at the table except the business at hand, the patient, the anatomy, or the surgery. There was never a wasted motion. To drop an instrument on the floor was a sin. Dr. Clerf would never hurry, but when one looked at the clock at the end of an operation it was always a surprise how little time had passed.
>
> Dr. Clerf seldom raised his voice, but could put the fear of God in you with just a glance...He was scholarly without being dry. He was always polite. He enjoyed a good story as well as a good drink...He was charitable both in his mind and with his pocketbook. He was a very loving man.[11]

Patients from all over the world were referred to Dr. Clerf. Among his surgical contributions was the development with Dr. Thomas A. Shallow of a unique one-stage operation for the correction of pharyngeal diverticulum. Without the benefit of antibiotics the procedure was successfully performed by Clerf and Shallow in over four hundred cases with no single instance of infection or mediastinitis.[12]

Dr. Louis H. Clerf also did pioneering work in laryngeal photography and in 1924 made the first successful pictures of the still larynx. When motion pictures and color film came into use Clerf was one of the first to photograph the larynx in action, as well as various diseased states of this organ.

Dr. Clerf was a leader on the national scene and president of the following societies: the American Broncho-esophagological Association, the American Laryngological Association, the American Laryngological, Rhinological, and Otological Society, the New York Laryngological Society, the Pennsylvania State Medical Society, the Philadelphia County Medical Society, and the Philadelphia Laryngological Society. He also served on the American Board of Examiners in Otolaryngology and the American Board of Chest Physicians, and was a governor of the American College of Surgeons.

Dr. Louis H. Clerf won the De Roaldes Medal and Newcomb Award of the American Laryngological Association, the Chevalier Jackson Award of the American Bronchoesophagological Association, the Strittmatter Award from the Philadelphia County Medical Society, the Signum Fidei Medal from La Salle College, and the Clarence E. Shaffrey, S.J. Award from St. Joseph's College. He also received honorary degrees from Villanova University, St. Martin's College, and Jefferson Medical College.

Clerf was a loyal Jeffersonian, and in the eyes of many, "a Mr. Jefferson." He served as interim dean in 1950. He was president of the alumni association in 1934. He headed the alumni contributions to the new hospital pavilion and reorganized the annual alumni giving fund. He was the first recipient of the alumni achievement award in 1964. He was chosen as the portrait honoree by the class of 1949, and the class of 1955 dedicated its yearbook to him.

The portrait of Professor Clerf was painted by Frederick Roscher in 1948 and presented in 1949. The physician is seated facing partly left, next to a desk with books. His right index finger marks his place in a book placed on his thigh, and his left hand rests on top of the other hand. His attention has been diverted and he looks up toward the viewer with a somber expression.

He wears a black academic gown with a startlingly bright, almost phosphorescent green hood, front panels, and stripes on the sleeves. The robe has deep folds and full, draped sleeves which form dramatic curving lines. The dark atmospheric background has an unusual reddish-orange glow around the sitter.

The painter Frederick Roscher was born in Weiden, Germany in 1890. He graduated from the University of Nuremberg and completed his art studies in Paris, Rome, and Florence. Before emigrating to the United States in 1921 he traveled in South America and resided briefly in Brazil.

Roscher made his American home in Philadelphia until 1926 when he purchased a four-hundred-acre tract in rural Berks County, Pennsylvania. There he designed for himself a thirty-room, white chateau popularly known as "Roscher's Castle," with extensive formal gardens and promenades dotted with statuary. Roscher maintained both indoor and outdoor studios and a gallery to showcase his work. He also favored his other home in West Palm Beach, Florida and a studio in Palm Beach's elegant Breakers Hotel.

Roscher was in demand internationally as a portraitist and was extraordinarily successful financially. He worked very quickly and it has been estimated that he completed several thousand portraits. Some of his distinguished European and South American subjects included: Pope Benedict XV (who made the artist a knight of the Order of St. Gregory the Great), Pope Pius XI, Queen Wilhelmina and Princess Juliana of the Netherlands, King Ludwig III of Bavaria, and President Washington Luis of Brazil.

Notable American subjects included: Eleanor Roosevelt, Dennis Cardinal Dougherty, Mrs. Livingston Biddle, Chief Justice of the U.S. Supreme Court Frederick M. Vinson, Governor James Duff of Pennsylvania, and Bethlehem Steel Corporation president Eugene Grace. In addition to portraits of three Jefferson physicians, Roscher also painted American College of Surgeons president Frederick A. Besley, M.D., and University of Pennsylvania surgeon Charles H. Frazier, M.D.[13]

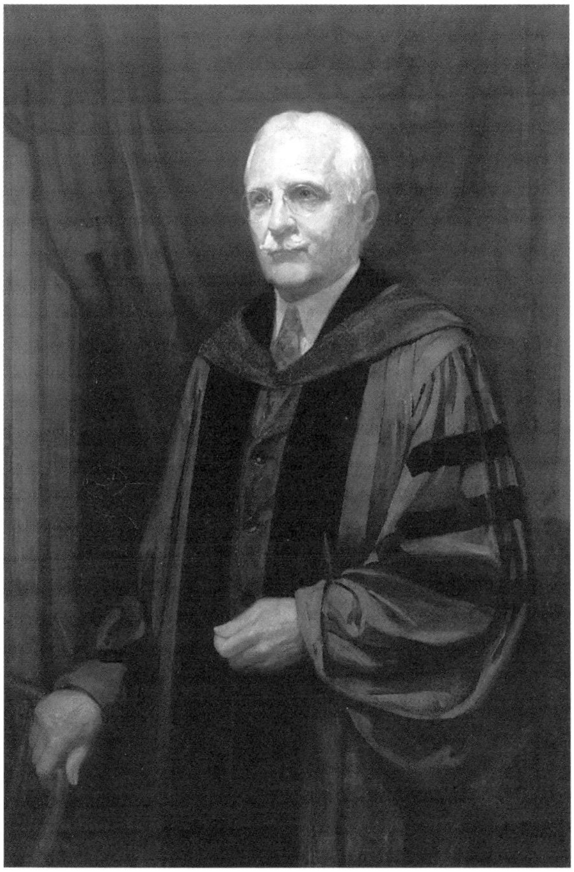

Portrait of Hiram R. Loux

HIRAM RITTENHOUSE LOUX, M.D. (1859-1930)
By William Taylor Thomson (1858-1941)

Oil on canvas
1929
54 x 38 in.

Signed lower right: "W. T. Thomson"

Given by JMC class of 1929
Accession number: 1929+e.P.02

Dr. Hiram Rittenhouse Loux succeeded Dr. Orville Horwitz as chair of genito-urinary surgery at Jefferson Medical College in 1912, and served until his sudden death in 1930.

Hiram R. Loux was born in Sellersville, Pennsylvania in 1859, a descendant of the distinguished Rittenhouse family of Pennsylvania. He worked as a schoolteacher for three years before graduating from Jefferson Medical College in 1882. Convinced by his mentor, Dr. Samuel D. Gross, to spend three years instead of taking the customary two-year course, Loux graduated with honors and received the Henry C. Lea Prize. He practiced general medicine in Souderton, Pennsylvania for the next ten years.

His desire to be associated with an active teaching staff brought him back to Jefferson in 1892 and he became an assistant to Dr. W. W. Keen. In 1893 he was appointed demonstrator of surgery and demonstrator of fractures and dislocations. In 1894 he was made chief clinical assistant to Dr. Orville Horwitz who had just become the first chairman of the department of genito-urinary diseases. Loux rose in the ranks from assistant genito-urinary surgeon in 1900 to professor of genito-urinary surgery by 1912. He was also surgeon to the Philadelphia General Hospital from 1907 until 1925.

Dr. Loux was admired by medical students who founded the Hiram H. Loux Urological Society, dedicated the 1926 yearbook to him, and chose him as portrait honoree in 1929.

In the portrait by William T. Thomson the subject is shown two-thirds length and life-sized. Dr. Loux stands in front of a maroon curtain, facing partly to the left with his right hand resting on a chair back. He is attired in a black academic robe with green mantle. His bearing is dignified and his expression serious. The planes and surfaces of his angular features, pince-nez, and thick, white mustache and hair are beautifully rendered with impasto pigment.

Portrait of Thomas C. Stellwagen

THOMAS COOKE STELLWAGEN, M.D., D.D.S. (1879-1935)
By Benedict Anton Osnis (1872-1941)

Oil on canvas
1935
62 x 41 in.

Signed and dated lower right: "B. A. Osnis/1935"

Given by JMC class of 1935
Accession number: 1935+e.P.02

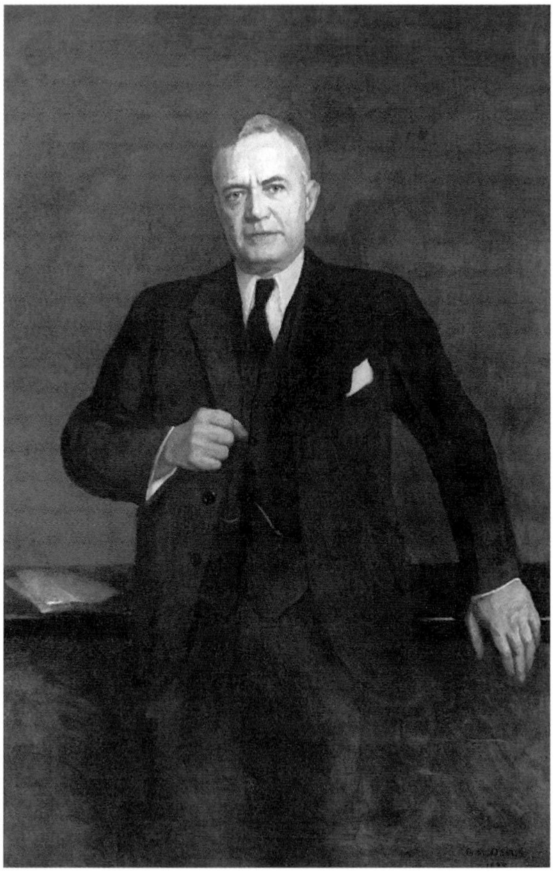

Dr. Thomas Cooke Stellwagen was the third chair of genito-urinary surgery at Jefferson Medical College. He served in the post until his premature death at the age of fifty-six in 1935.

Thomas C. Stellwagen was born in 1879 in Media, Pennsylvania, a descendant of early Delaware settlers. After graduating from Central High School in Philadelphia, Stellwagen received a doctor of dental surgery degree from the Philadelphia Dental College where his father was a faculty member. For a period Dr. Stellwagen taught physiology at the dental school. He became an honors graduate of Jefferson Medical College in 1903.

He was resident pathologist at Jefferson Hospital, and then appointed to the staff of Dr. Orville Horwitz and made chief of clinic in the outpatient genito-urinary department. Later he was named surgical assistant to Dr. J. Chalmers DaCosta and chief of the surgical outpatient department. During World War I Stellwagen served first with the British Army, then with the U.S. Army. In 1917 he was a member of the Jefferson Base

Hospital Unit, and later sent to the front in charge of a mobile unit. He was discharged with the rank of major in the Medical Corps.

Dr. Stellwagen returned to Jefferson, two years later was elected associate professor, and succeeded to the chair in 1930 upon the death of Dr. Loux. Stellwagen was also attending surgeon to the Philadelphia General Hospital and consulting surgeon to the Jewish Hospital. He was a charter member and president of the Genitourinary Society.

Dr. Stellwagen was chosen as portrait honoree by the class of 1935, and the portrait by Benedict A. Osnis was completed before the professor's death of angina pectoris on March 16, 1935. He is depicted two-thirds length and life-sized, facing front and looking straight ahead. He stands erectly in front of a long wooden shelf with papers. One hand rests on the shelf and the other is clenched into a fist held chest high. His expression is serious, almost impatient. Dr. Stellwagen's distinctive features are his rectangular-shaped face, square jaw, high cheekbones, and thick neck. His complexion is pale with ruddy cheeks. The painting's warm, brown background is mottled with red tones.

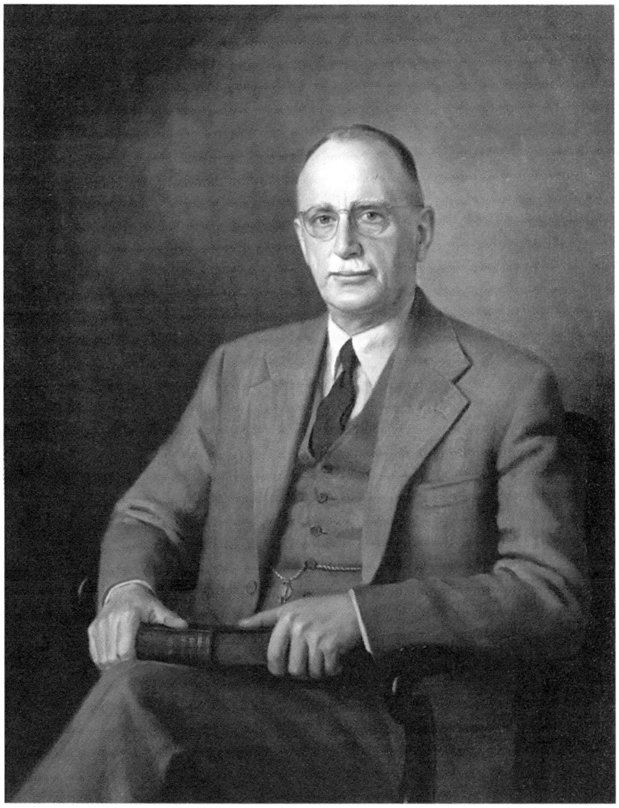

Portrait of David M. Davis

DAVID MELVIN DAVIS, M.D. (1886-1982)
By Isabella Hunner Parsons (b. 1903)

Oil on canvas
1952
40 x 32 1/4 in.

Signed lower left: "I. HUNNER PARSONS"

Given by JMC class of 1952
Accession number: 1952+e.P.01

Dr. David M. Davis was the fourth chair of genitourinary surgery at Jefferson Medical College. The renowned investigator, teacher, and clinician served from 1935 until 1951.

David M. Davis was born in Buffalo, New York in 1886, and was a graduate of Princeton University (1907) and the School of Medicine of the Johns Hopkins University (1911). After interning a year at the Baltimore City Hospital, he served as assistant in pathology at Johns Hopkins, and then as pathologist and director of research at Hopkins's Brady Urological Institute.

Dr. Davis was studying chemistry in Munich when World War I broke out, and he served as bacteriologist to the American Ambulance Hospital in Neuilly-sur-Seine, France. In 1916 he attended training camp in Plattsburg, New York and then served abroad for two years with the British Expeditionary Forces and the American Expeditionary Forces. He was discharged with the rank of major in 1919.

After the war, Dr. David M. Davis returned to the Brady Institute to work with Dr. Hugh H. Young and was coauthor of the authoritative textbook *Young's Practice of Urology, Based on a Study of 12,500 Cases* (1926). Davis also completed a two-year residency in urology during this period, and became associate editor of the *Journal of Urology*, founded in 1917.

In 1924 Dr. Davis moved to the University of Rochester's new medical school as assistant professor of surgery in charge of organizing the urology department. Four years later he returned to Baltimore as an associate of Dr. Young. In 1930 the peripatetic surgeon went to Phoenix, Arizona where he forsook academic urology for private practice for a brief period.

In 1935 Dr. David M. Davis returned to academia as chair of the department of genito-urinary surgery at Jefferson Medical College, succeeding Dr. Thomas C. Stellwagen. In 1946 Davis became the first Nathan Lewis Hatfield Professor of Urology, a chair named in memory of the father of the donor, Henry Reed Hatfield.

Dr. Davis believed that medical education should be concentrated more on laboratory sessions and patient contact, and less on textbook memorization. He instituted changes in teaching urology (the new name of the department) by reducing large didactic lectures in favor of instruction in small groups with active student participation. His quiz sections were memorable according to the student yearbook of 1952: "the Master assum[ed] an authoritative stance in front of the room wielding a long pointer to designate his victims and verbally fencing with a skillful mixture of invective and cajolery until the point was driven home."

Under Dr. Davis advanced training in urology was established in 1939 with Jefferson's first residencies in that specialty. He greatly improved the standard of care in the urology ward and outpatient clinic. Some of his ideas elicited heavy opposition at first, such as the appointment of a female head nurse in the urology ward, but he won that battle saying that she was "excellent" and the ward was "whipped into shape in no time."

Dr. Davis devised original operative procedures for correction of ureteral and uretero-pelvic obstructions and hypospadias. He was one of the first to recognize the importance of urinary system hydrodynamics. He designed a specific modification of a fluoroscopic table that bears his name. He wrote the textbooks *Urological Nursing* (1929) and *Mechanisms of Urologic Disease* (1953).

He served as president of the Medical and Surgical Association of the Southwest, the Mid-Atlantic Section of the American Urological Association, the Philadelphia Urological Society, and the American Association of Genito-urinary Surgeons. Davis was honored to be the first recipient of the Hugh Hampton Young Award of the American Urological Association in 1969.

Upon his retirement in 1951 Dr. Davis was named emeritus professor, but he remained actively engaged in practice and writing until 1968. He received an honorary doctor of science degree from Jefferson in 1972.

The portrait of Dr. Davis was presented by the Jefferson Medical College class of 1952, the year after he retired as department chair. The artist was Isabella Hunner Parsons, a Baltimore painter and designer. To date no additional information about her career has been found.

In the two-thirds-length portrait, Davis is seated in an armchair with his legs crossed, facing partly to the left. He balances a maroon-bound textbook on his knee with both hands. He is attired in a medium brown business suit and maroon tie, with his Phi Beta Kappa and Alpha Omega Alpha keys prominently displayed on a gold chain. The greenish-gray background fades to lighter shades around his head. The paint style is extremely smooth and the figure is convincingly solid and three-dimensional.

However, the sitter's facial expression is staring and blank. The whole effect is so quiet and reserved that it gives no hint of the sitter's dynamic personality in real life. Perhaps the Baltimore artist had few sittings with the subject, and was primarily dependent on photographs. Perhaps that is why the source of light is ambiguous and appears artificial rather than natural.

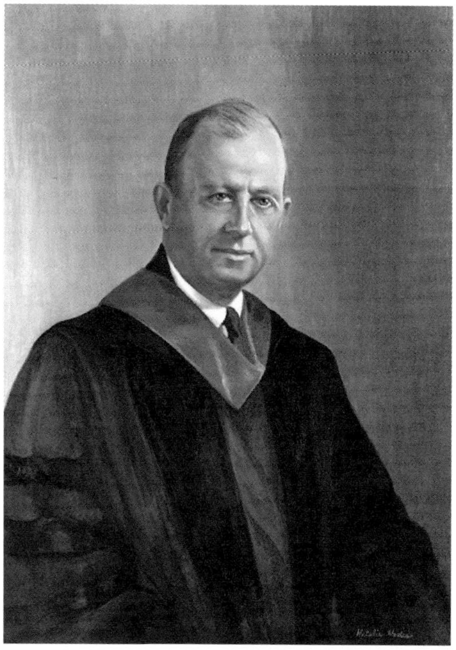

Portrait of Willis F. Manges

WILLIS FASTNACHT MANGES, M.D. (1876-1936)
By Natalie (Mrs. Philip J.) Hodes (1911-82)

Oil on canvas
1959
40 x 30 in.

Signed lower right: "Natalie Hodes"

Given in 1959 by Natalie Hodes
Accession number: 1959+e.P.03

Within a year of Wilhelm Conrad Roentgen's discovery of X-rays in 1895, the first X-ray equipment was installed in the Jefferson Hospital. Dr. Willis F. Manges was a pioneer roentgenologist who became Jefferson's first chairman of roentgenology in 1929.

Willis F. Manges was born in 1876 in Luthersburg, Pennsylvania. Before graduating from Jefferson Medical College in 1903 he had attended Gettysburg College and the Philadelphia College of Pharmacy and was an assistant in pharmacy at the Jefferson Hospital. During his internship at Jefferson he became fascinated by the rapidly expanding possibilities of the roentgen rays, and took special training under Drs. Sterrett Metheny and William M. Sweet.

Dr. Manges's career at Jefferson lasted thirty-two years from his first appointment as roentgenologist in 1904, to clinical professor of roentgenology in 1925, and professor and first chair of roentgenology in 1929, a post he held until his death in 1936. As a member of the U.S. Medical Corps during World War I he was in charge of the Camp Greenleaf School of Roentgenology at Fort Oglethorpe, Georgia. He rose to the rank of lieutenant colonel.

Dr. Willis F. Manges enlarged the scope of roentgenology by his technical contributions and by his administration of a department that saw an increase from five hundred patients in 1904 to 13,500 outpatient and hospital patients in 1935. He devised a method for accurately measuring the pelvis of pregnant women. With colleagues he discovered the roentgen signs for localizing and removing foreign bodies in the air and food passages, and for opaque, nonmagnetic foreign bodies in the eye. He introduced pyeloscopy as an adjunct and control for pyelography, and described the mechanism and significance of obstructive emphysema and atelectasis in connection with foreign bodies and endobronchial lesions.

Dr. Manges was also physician to the Bryn Mawr Hospital and Philadelphia General Hospital. He served as a founder and president of the Philadelphia Roentgen Ray Society and president of the American Roentgen Ray Society in 1918. He was instrumental in forming the section on radiology of the American Medical Association and was its chairman in 1924. He was an original member of the American Board of Radiology.

The class of 1937 erected a bronze plaque in memory of Dr. Manges who died November 24, 1936. An unsigned and undated portrait of Dr. Manges was presented about 1938 by Dr. Manges's colleague, John T. Farrell Jr., M.D. It appears to be a copy of a posthumous portrait of Manges by Benedict A. Osnis, commissioned by the Philadelphia Roentgen Ray Society in 1937 and presented to the College of Physicians of Philadelphia that same year.

A second portrait of Dr. Willis F. Manges was painted in 1959 by Natalie Hodes, wife of Dr. Philip J. Hodes, M.D., professor and fifth chairman of Jefferson's department of radiology. Mrs. Hodes had volunteered to paint the portrait in 1959 to coincide with the annual oration honoring Dr. Manges of the Philadelphia Roentgen Ray Society at which Dr. Hodes was the speaker.

The pose of Natalie Hodes's bust-length, larger-than-life-sized portrait of Dr. Manges loosely resembles the

Osnis portrait, but instead of a business suit the physician is now garbed in a black academic gown with a green mantle. His face is forcefully executed and his steely gaze is piercing. The atmospheric background is rendered in umber, green, and maroon tones.

According to family members, Natalie Hodes was trained at the Fawcett School of Fine and Industrial Arts (in northern New Jersey) and earned an M.F.A. degree at Tyler School of Art of Temple University (1959). She had many portrait commissions and taught painting at the Long Beach Island Foundation of the Arts in New Jersey, the Wallingford Art Center in suburban Philadelphia, and privately in her home.

Mrs. Hodes was also a graduate of the New Jersey Law School (now Rutgers University) and practiced law before her marriage to Dr. Hodes. She participated in religious and women's affairs and was a sought-after speaker at local churches and synagogues. The dynamic activist was a founder and first president of the Main Line Reform Temple in Wynnewood, Pennsylvania, and the first woman ever elected president of an American Reform Jewish congregation.

The Basic Scientists

Portrait of J. Parsons Schaeffer

JACOB PARSONS SCHAEFFER, M.D., Ph.D. (1878-1970)
By Lazar Raditz (1887-1958)

Oil on canvas
1932
46 x 36 in.

Signed lower right: "Lazar Raditz"

Given by JMC class of 1932
Accession number: 1932+e.P.03

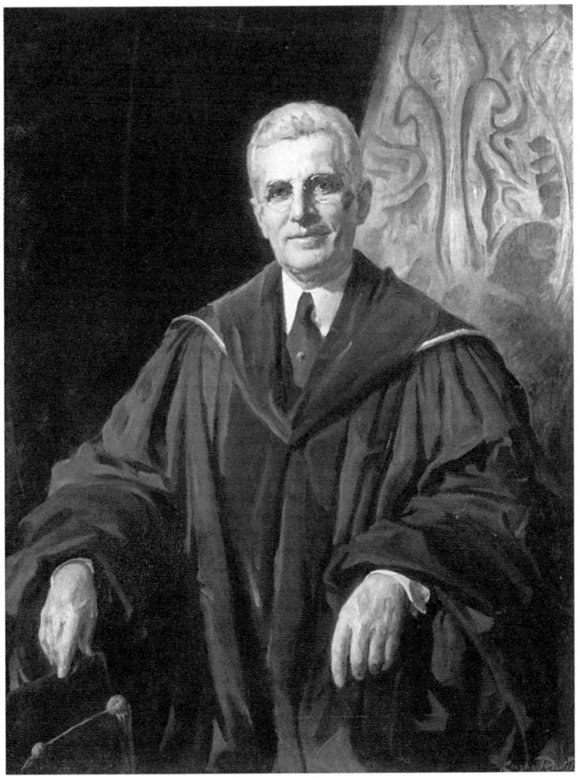

Dr. Jacob Parsons Schaeffer became the ninth chairman of the anatomy department at Jefferson Medical College in 1914. He served with great distinction for thirty-four years.

J. Parsons Schaeffer's path toward a career in medicine was particularly circuitous. He was born in 1878 in Shamokin Dam, Pennsylvania and raised on a small farm. After graduating from Central Pennsylvania College (1897), he spent a year teaching in a one-room school house. While working for an uncle who was an undertaker, Schaeffer developed a profound awe for the human body, and he was subsequently graduated from the United States School of Embalming in New York. While earning bachelor's (1901) and master's (1903) degrees at Keystone State Normal School (now Kutztown University), Schaeffer sold school books from town to town.

After three years as supervising principal of schools in East Greenville, Pennsylvania, he returned to his earlier interest in the human body and graduated from the School of Medicine of the University of Pennsylvania (1907) and took his residency at the hospital there. He pursued graduate studies in the respiratory system at Cornell University and received a master's degree (1909) and a Ph.D. degree (1910). He taught briefly at the University of Pennsylvania, Cornell University, and Yale University.

When Dr. J. Parsons Schaeffer became chair of anatomy at Jefferson Medical College in 1914, the department was reunited after having been divided between general anatomy and applied and topographic anatomy since 1905. He prevailed upon Daniel Baugh to provide research facilities in the building adjoining the Baugh Institute of Anatomy. Schaeffer's comprehensive knowledge of the subject of anatomy and his unlimited energy and personal charm attracted men of the highest caliber, to make the Baugh Institute an outstanding department.

Schaeffer said that "modern anatomy, at least in the better medical schools, is no longer restricted to a purely descriptive study and used primarily as a handmaid. Having expanded into its proper spheres, it now enjoys the dignity and importance of an independent science."[14] His own research centered on the nose, paranasal sinuses, lachrymal apparatus, and olfactory organ.

Dr. Schaeffer was the author of *The Nose, Paranasal Sinuses, Nasolacrimal Passageways, and Olfactory Organ in Man: a Genetic, Developmental, and Anatomico-physiological Consideration* (1919). He was coauthor with Drs. Henry K. Pancoast and Eugene P. Pendergrass of *The Head and Neck in Roentgen Diagnosis* (1940). He was a contributing author (sixth through twelfth editions) and editor (tenth through twelfth editions) of Sir Henry Morris's *Human Anatomy; a Complete Systematic Treatise*.

Among Dr. Schaeffer's many awards are the gold medal of the American Medical Association (awarded in 1931 jointly to Dr. Warren B. Davis and preserved today in the Jefferson archives), the Strittmatter Award, and the Clarence E. Shaffrey, S.J. Award from St. Joseph's College. He received an honorary master's degree from Yale, and honorary D.Sc. degrees from Susquehanna University and Jefferson Medical College. He was elected president of the American Association of Anatomists, the College of Physicians of Philadelphia, and the Anatomical Board of Pennsylvania. He became a member of the American Philosophical Society in 1927.

Professor Schaeffer also served as chairman of Jefferson's executive faculty for many years. When he retired in 1948 he was made professor emeritus. The J. Parsons Schaeffer Alpha Omega Alpha annual lectureship at Jefferson was conceived to honor the beloved and respected professor. The students of 1924 dedicated their yearbook to him. The Spitzka Anatomical League was renamed the J. P. Schaeffer Anatomical League in 1914, and in 1932 he was the senior class portrait honoree.

Lazar Raditz depicted Dr. Schaeffer in a life-sized, half-length pose seated in an armchair and facing slightly to the left. The subject turns his head to look directly at the viewer. His right hand balances his academic cap on his thigh. His black academic gown is decorated with green stripes on the sleeves, mantle, and front panels. An anatomical illustration of the paranasal sinuses is placed in the upper right corner.

His thick white hair and regular features with large blue eyes, straight nose, and square jaw accord with descriptions of Dr. Schaeffer's striking appearance and his dignified yet amiable personality. A memoir in the minutes of the alumni association's executive council (March 10, 1970) praised the popular professor's "personal charm and sincerity," and said, "His interest and pride in each of his students, and in their successes, was as deep and abiding as though they were his own sons."

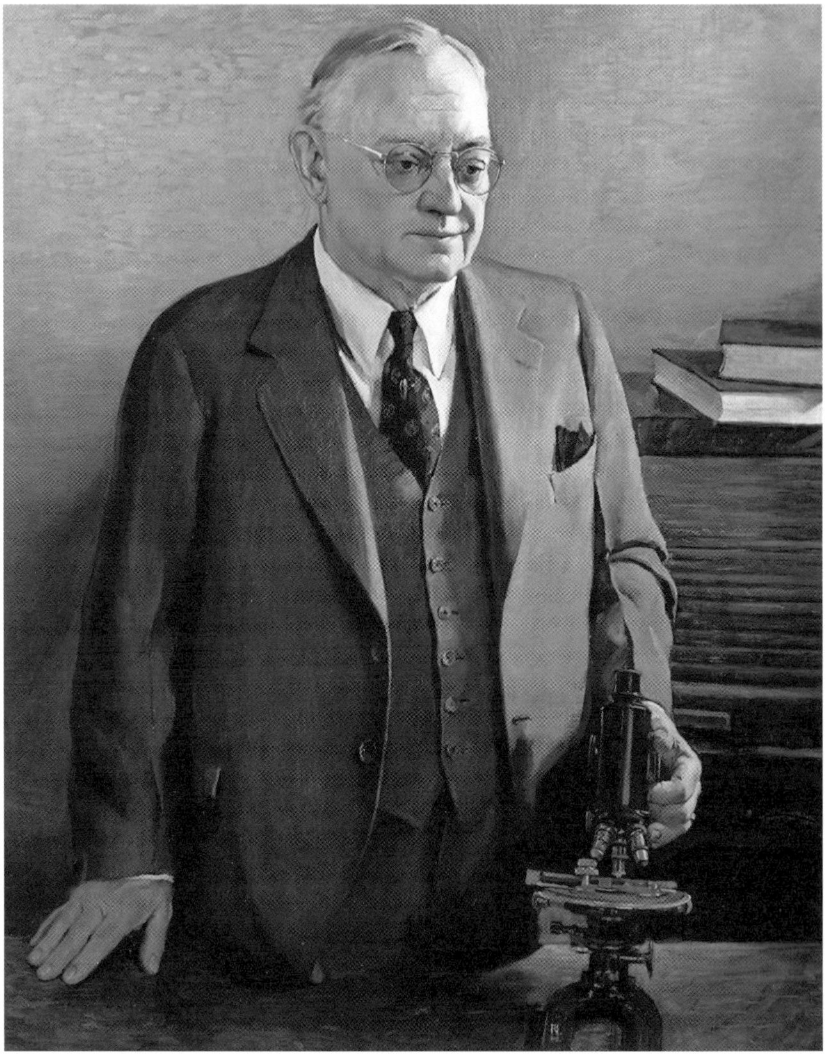

Portrait of Henry E. Radasch

(See color plate)

HENRY ERDMANN RADASCH, M.D. (1874-1942)
By Roy Cleveland Nuse (1885-1975)

Oil on canvas
1942
40 x 34 in.

Signed and dated lower center: "RN/42"

Given by JMC class of 1942
Accession number: 1942+e.P.01

Dr. Henry E. Radasch was professor of histology and embryology at Jefferson Medical College. He was a noted author of manuals on histology and anatomy and a respected and cherished teacher.

Henry Radasch, affectionately known as "Rad," was born in Keokuk, Iowa in 1874. After earning bachelor of science (1895) and master of science (1897) degrees from the State University of Iowa, he spent a year as lecturer in the College of Physicians and Surgeons in Keokuk. While earning his degree at Jefferson Medical College (1901) he served as an assistant in histology under Dr. Randle Rosenberger, and following graduation he was elected demonstrator of histology and embryology. His studies continued abroad at the zoological laboratory of the University of Leipzig, and upon his return he was promoted to associate in histology and embryology at Jefferson. In 1921 he was appointed full professor of histology and embryology, and when he retired in 1942 he was named emeritus professor.

Dr. Radasch won the admiration and affection of the thousands of students who benefitted from his concentrated series of lectures, demonstrations, and quizzes, showing his absolute knowledge of his subject and systems of study. The Jefferson student yearbook of 1925 commented, "Foremost in our fond memories will always be this jovial old friend with eyeshade and microscope who helped us out of some most trying circumstances."

Radasch contributed to the medical literature on muscular anomalies, red blood cells, acid cells of the stomach, the composition of compact bone, superfetation, and senility of bone. He was the author of *A Compend of Histology* (1905), *A Manual of Anatomy* (1917), *A Manual of Histology* (1918, known as *Practical Histology* in the second revised edition of 1924), and the section on histology in *Contribution to the Reference Handbook of the Medical Sciences: 1914-1918.*

Dr. Radasch often showed the students examples from

his extensive collections of stamps and decorative arts featuring miniature elephants and pitchers, and many former students sent him rare specimens as gifts. The class of 1932 dedicated its yearbook to him and the class of 1942 selected him as portrait honoree.

Roy C. Nuse depicted Dr. Radasch in his office. He is shown half length and life-sized, standing with one hand focusing his monocular microscope and the other hand leaning on a table. He is attired in a bluish-gray, three-piece suit with a purplish-maroon, patterned tie and pocket handkerchief. Behind the doctor is his tambour, rolltop desk with two purple-bound books on top. His expression is pensive as he looks down away from the viewer.

As in Roy Nuse's other portraits of Jefferson physicians, Dr. Radasch's body is rendered with solidity and precision, the setting and attributes suggest the subject's work, and the dramatic contrast of light and shade and the colorful brush strokes create an animated painting surface.

Portrait of Albert P. Brubaker

ALBERT PHILSON BRUBAKER, M.D., D.D.S. (1852-1943)
By William Taylor Thomson (1858-1941)

Oil on canvas
1926
40 x 32 in.

Signed and dated upper left: "W. T. Thomson-1926."

Given by JMC class of 1926
Accession number: 1926+e.P.01

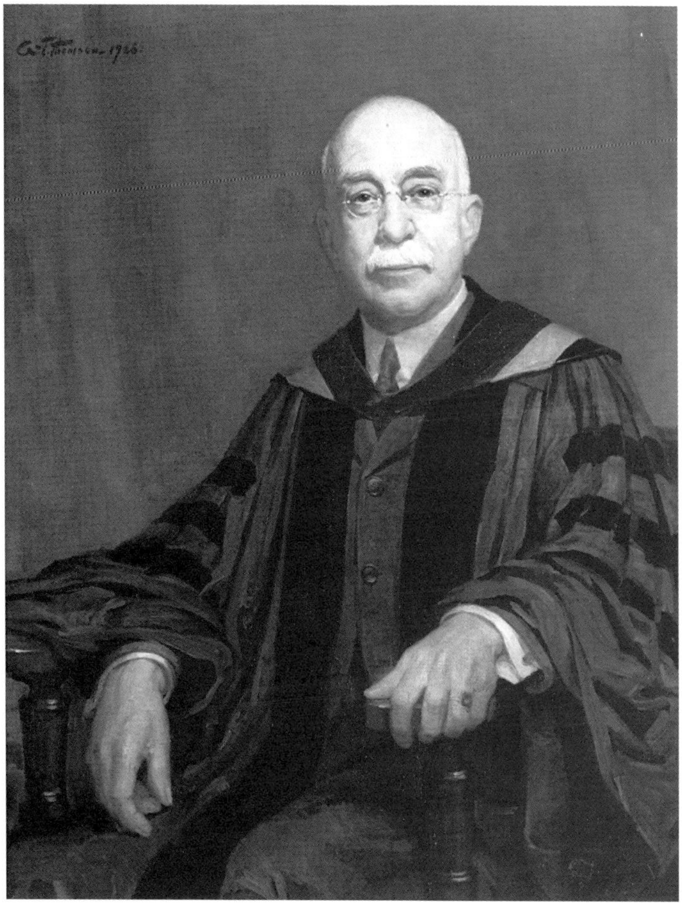

Dr. Albert P. Brubaker was another accomplished basic scientist at Jefferson Medical College. He was chair of the department of physiology and medical jurisprudence from 1909 to 1927.

Albert Brubaker was born in Somerset, Pennsylvania, the son of Henry Brubaker, M.D., a Jefferson alumnus of 1851 and a general practitioner. After graduating from Jefferson Medical College with distinction in 1874 Dr. Albert Brubaker became an assistant to Dr. James C. Wilson in Jefferson's medical clinic. He also served at clinics in the Charity Hospital and the Orthopaedic Hospital and Infirmary for Nervous Diseases.

Around 1879 he was appointed demonstrator of physiology under Dr. Henry C. Chapman who had just become chair of the institutes of medicine at Jefferson. Brubaker also held important posts at other institutions:

in 1880 he was appointed a demonstrator in physiology and pathology at the Pennsylvania College of Dental Surgery where he was made professor in 1885 and earned a dental degree in 1886; in addition, he was a lecturer in physiology and hygiene at the Drexel Institute of Science, Art, and Industry from 1892 to 1914.

Dr. Albert P. Brubaker's career at Jefferson Medical College advanced rapidly from lecturer in materia medica and therapeutics in 1891 to full professor of physiology in 1904. When Dr. Chapman retired in 1909 Dr. Brubaker was made chair of the department of physiology and medical jurisprudence. He was also elected chairman of the faculty by his peers. Although he submitted his resignation in 1926 Jefferson trustees prevailed upon Dr. Brubaker to continue as department head for another year. By then he had served the college faithfully for five decades.

Brubaker's two best-known literary works passed through many revised editions: *A Compend of Human Physiology* (1883), especially adapted for the use of medical students, and *A Text-book of Human Physiology* (1904), with a section on physiologic apparatus. He was a member of numerous medical and scientific societies including the American Philosophical Society.

Dr. Albert P. Brubaker received the Strittmatter Award from the Philadelphia County Medical Society in 1924. He also received an honorary doctor of laws degree from Franklin and Marshall College. Jefferson Medical College students organized the Albert P. Brubaker Physiological Society. In May 1927 the class of 1929 presented him with a silver loving cup upon the occasion of his last lecture. He was the portrait honoree of the class of 1926.

In William T. Thomson's depiction Dr. Brubaker is shown two-thirds length and life-sized, seated in an armchair in front of a bright, reddish-maroon drapery. He wears a black academic robe over a brown suit. His body faces partly left and his head turns to engage the viewer directly with a pleasant expression. Distinguishing features of his ruddy face are his high-domed forehead with wisps of white hair, thick nose, full white mustache, and wide mouth.

His affable countenance suggests the love and respect won from students who dedicated the 1916 yearbook to the professor they affectionately called "Daddy" Brubaker. They praised his "method of giving such lucid lectures with an entire absence of nonsense, with rare humor, with delicacy of feeling and unfailing kindness." They appreciated that his personal knowledge of physiology came from direct experimental and practical work rather than "second hand information derived from books."

Portrait of J. Earl Thomas

JACOB EARL THOMAS, M.D. (1891-1972)
By Frederick Roscher (1890-1968)

Oil on masonite
1948
48 x 36 in.

Signed center right: "ROSCHER/1948"

Given by JMC class of 1948
Accession number: 1948+e.P.01

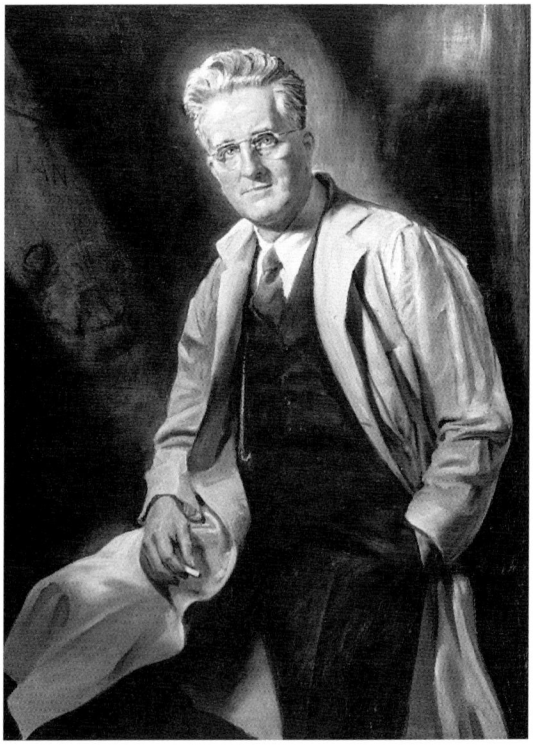

In 1927 Dr. J. Earl Thomas became Jefferson's fifth chair of physiology. He was well known for his ingenuity in instrumentation and investigations in the field of gastrointestinal physiology.

Jacob Earl Thomas was born on a homestead in 1891 in Steilacoom, Washington to parents who had migrated to the Northwest from Indiana and Kentucky. As a boy he spent summers as an apprentice in machine shops, and it is thought that this experience led to his genius for designing laboratory equipment. After attending the Free Methodist Church School (later Seattle Pacific College) and the University of Washington, he received an M.D. degree (1918) and M.S. degree (1924) from St. Louis University.

Dr. Thomas was associate professor of physiology at West Virginia University from 1920 to 1921, then returned to St. Louis University as an associate professor. In 1927 he came to Philadelphia as professor of physiology at Jefferson Medical College, succeeding Dr. Albert P. Brubaker. He held the post until 1956 when he was named emeritus professor.

Unwilling to retire from research, Dr. J. Earl Thomas then accepted a position as distinguished professor of physiology and administrative head of the department at the College of Medical Evangelists (later Loma Linda University) in California. In 1964 he relinquished the chairmanship but continued to teach and conduct research until his death in 1972.

During Thomas's tenure at Jefferson Medical College he expanded the full-time department faculty from one to three, introduced research as a student option in the new physiology laboratory, and granted fellowships for full- or part-time research or teaching. He devised several instruments and techniques that became widely used in teaching and research: the Thomas drop recorder, the Thomas wrench, the Thomas cannula, the Thomas gastric pouch, and the Thomas pancreatic fistula. He also served as chair of the executive faculty at Jefferson Medical College.

During World War II Dr. J. Earl Thomas was an advisor on problems of nutrition and appetite in combat troops. He was the author of *The External Secretion of the Pancreas* (1950). He was a member of the editorial board of the *American Journal of Physiology* and the *Journal of Applied Physiology*.

Dr. Thomas received an honorary doctor of science degree from Jefferson Medical College (1960) and the prestigious Friedenwald Medal from the American Gastroenterological Association (posthumously in 1972). Jefferson alumni established the Thomas Physiology Fund and the Thomas Physiology Library.

Professor Thomas was selected by the class of 1948 as their portrait honoree. In Frederick Roscher's depiction the physician is shown life-sized and three-quarters length in an informal pose, casually half-sitting on the edge of a table. He wears a tan laboratory coat over a brown business suit. The sitter's rectangular face is topped by thick, wavy, blond-gray hair. He tilts his head in a jaunty way, and his upward gaze is alert and lively. Frederick Roscher commented that "'Doctor Thomas has a remarkable face, in which you feel warmth, friendship, and integrity...the curiosity of one who is dedicated to establishing truth through research.'"[15]

The subject's left hand is placed in his trouser pocket, and his right hand holds a small piece of white chalk and rests on his thigh. It has been said that the object in his hand was changed from a cigarette to chalk, because Mrs. Melrose Weed, executive secretary of the Jefferson Medical College alumni association, was incensed at the depiction of a Jefferson professor smoking, and until the substitution was made refused to accept the portrait.[16]

Roscher's painting style is streaky with long, distinct brush strokes. The artist utilizes dramatic contrasts of light and dark, especially on the highlighted folds of the costume and in the spotlighted beams of light in the dark background. Just barely discernible on the left is an anatomical illustration of the pancreas and duodenum with identifying labels. In its original state the painting showed a more clearly detailed illustration of these organs labelled in German and Latin, but later the chart was almost obscured by the artist for an unknown reason.[17]

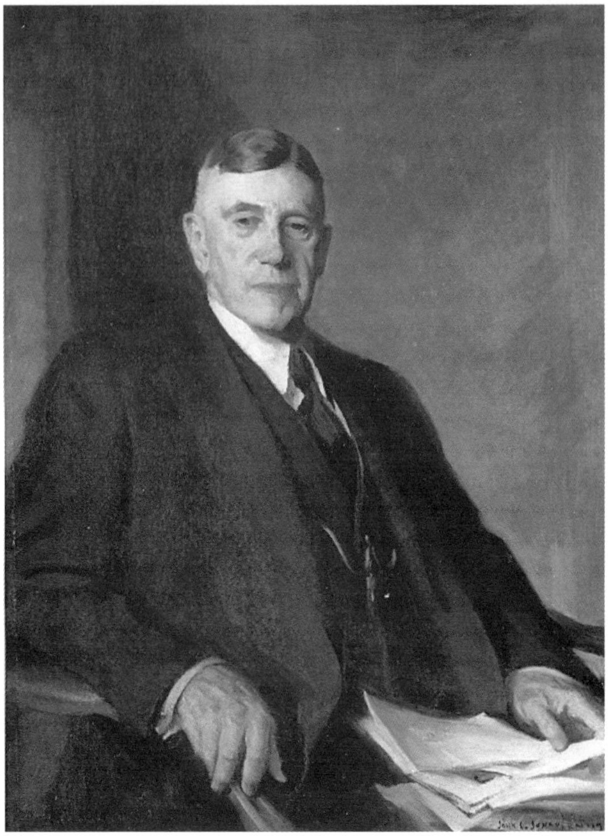

Portrait of David R. Morgan

DAVID REYNOLDS MORGAN, M.D., D.P.H. (1890-1978)
By John Christen Johansen (1876-1964)

Oil on canvas
1957
40 x 31 in.

Signed and dated lower right: "JOHN C. JOHANSEN 1957"

Given by JMC class of 1957
Accession number: 1957+e.P.01

Dr. David Reynolds Morgan was the curator of the pathological museum at Jefferson Medical College from 1923 to 1967 and a professor of pathology. He was also a highly decorated war hero.

David R. Morgan was born in 1890 in Edwardsville, Pennsylvania, a grandson of Dr. Benjamin J. B. Davis, a Jefferson alumnus of 1849. Morgan graduated from the Wyoming Seminary in Pennsylvania in 1912 and from Jefferson Medical College in 1916. He interrupted his internship at the Jefferson Hospital to volunteer for service as medical chief in the French Army. He requested discharge when the United States entered the war in 1917, and enlisted as a private with the Eighteenth Infantry Regiment of the First Division.

For his bravery at Sommerville in searching for and removing the wounded, including his commanding officer, to first aid stations while under constant fire, Morgan was awarded the Croix de Guerre and promoted to first lieutenant. During subsequent offensive actions he was severely burned with mustard gas and wounded in his right leg by shrapnel.

For his bravery on the front lines at Cantigny, Soissons, St. Michel, and the Argonne Dr. Morgan received three Palms to the Croix de Guerre, two Silver Stars, the Bronze Star, the Purple Heart, and the Distinguished Service Cross. He later was named an officer of the French Legion of Honor.

Dr. Morgan returned to Philadelphia and earned a doctorate in public health at the University of Pennsylvania (1922) and a master of science degree in surgery from the university's Graduate School of Surgery (1923). Then he accepted Dean Ross V. Patterson's offer to join the Jefferson Medical College department of pathology as assistant instructor in surgery and assistant curator of the pathology museum. He was quickly named museum curator and rose in the ranks to become professor of pathology.

Dr. David R. Morgan's special interest and great love was the museum. He added more than twelve thousand specimens stored in large ceramic crocks to the preexisting five or six thousand mounted specimens, thus constituting the second largest repository of morbid anatomical specimens in the world. Under his care the museum became a college showplace and attracted visitors from around the world.

Soon after the United States entered World War II Morgan pulled strings to return to active duty as the chief of laboratory service and assistant commanding officer at the Station Hospital in Camp Pickett, Virginia. He served a similar post in Staunton, Virginia and was discharged with the rank of colonel in 1946.

When he resumed his teaching duties at Jefferson he was heartbroken to find that one-third of the pathology museum space had been converted to offices and laboratories, and worse, the majority of the specimens in jars had dried out because of insufficient supplies of formaldehyde, a critical war material. They had to be discarded.

Dr. David R. Morgan retired as professor of pathology in 1967. In addition to his duties at Jefferson Medical College he was also director of laboratories at St. Joseph's Hospital and St. Luke's and Children's Medical Center, and medical director of the Eastern State Penitentiary.

Although he never married, Dr. Morgan took on the responsibility of raising five orphaned nieces and nephews. Although of modest means, he also aided many students in financial distress so they could complete their medical studies. "Davey" or "Colonel" Morgan was much beloved by Jefferson medical students and they dedicated the 1935 and 1941 yearbooks to him. He received the Christian R. and Mary F. Lindback Award for Distinguished Teaching in 1963.

The class of 1957 chose Dr. Morgan as their portrait honoree. In John C. Johansen's depiction the sitter is shown half length and life-sized, seated at a desk. His right hand grips the chair arm and his left hand holds a sheaf of papers. The prevailing neutral greens of the background and dark tones of the subject's black business suit are only slightly enlivened by his gold Alpha Omega Alpha key hanging from a chain. Dr. Morgan's posture is stiff and his expression is somber and dour, giving no hint of his outgoing and compassionate nature.

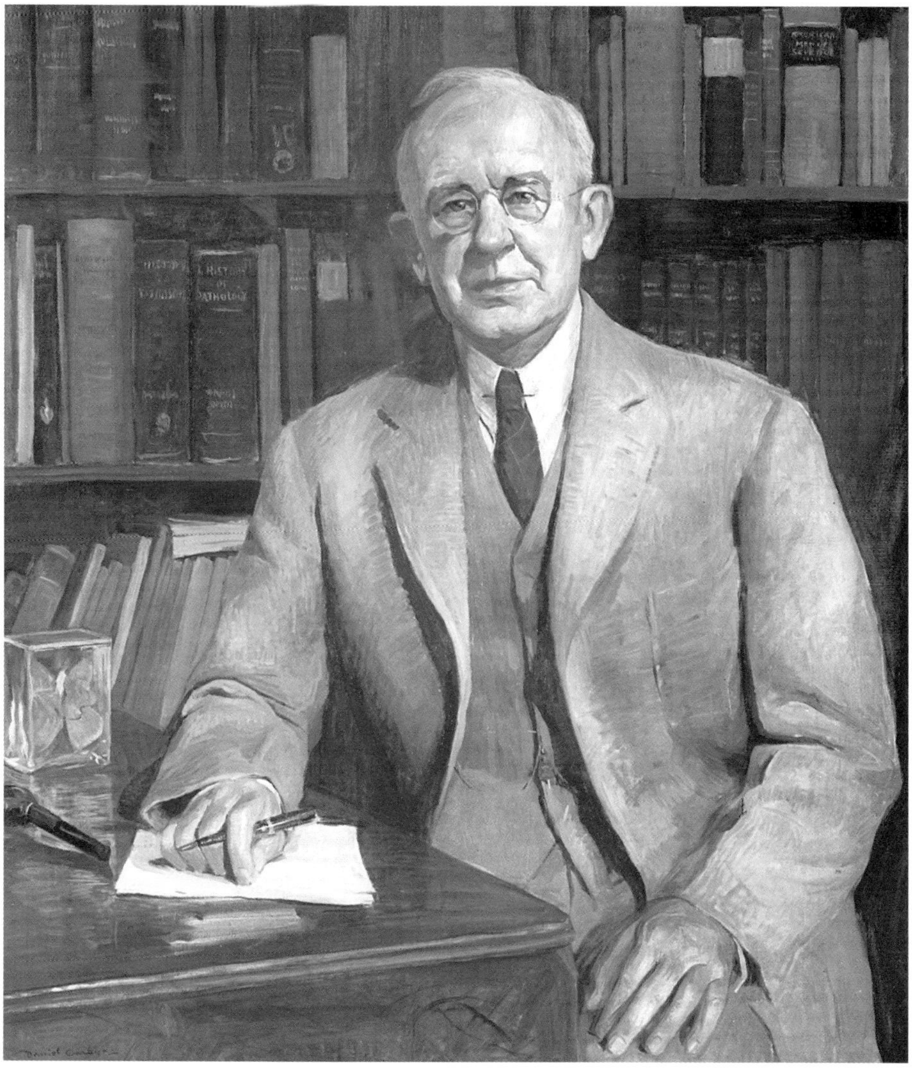

Portrait of Virgil H. Moon

VIRGIL HOLLAND MOON, M.D. (1879-1964)
By Daniel Garber (1880-1958)

Oil on canvas
1943
40 x 36 in.

Signed lower left: "Daniel Garber"

Given by JMC class of 1943
Accession number: 1943+e.P.01

Dr. Virgil H. Moon was chairman of the department of pathology at Jefferson Medical College. He was world famous for his work on the mechanism of shock and related phenomena.

Virgil Holland Moon was born in 1879 in Craig, Indiana, the son of a country doctor. He was descended from an English Quaker forbear who had originally settled in Morrisville, Bucks County, Pennsylvania adjacent to William Penn's estate. Moon's family moved to Kansas when he was a young child. He earned bachelor of arts (1910) and master of science (1911) degrees at Kansas State Teachers College, and a medical degree (1913) from Rush Medical College in Chicago. Starting in 1914 he quickly moved up the ranks at Indiana University School of Medicine to become professor of pathology and bacteriology there and chief of pathology at the Indianapolis City Hospital.

In 1927 he was appointed chair of pathology at Jefferson Medical College and remained in the post for twenty-one years. He was also director of laboratories at the Jefferson Hospital and visiting chief pathologist at Philadelphia General Hospital. After his retirement from Jefferson in 1948 he moved to Florida where he was appointed research professor of pathology at the University of Miami School of Medicine.

Dr. Moon was dedicated to his research and teaching, most notably on the mechanism, pathology, and complications of shock. His conclusions about the condition at first met with opposition, but he lived to see his work universally accepted, and applied during World War II to save countless lives. His internationally recognized monographs were: *Shock and Related Capillary Phenomena* (1938) and *Shock, Its Dynamics, Occurrence and Management* (1942). A medal from the Congress of Anesthetists meeting in Philadelphia in 1939 called the earlier book "an invaluable contribution to the salvaging of human life and the world conquest of pain and for the benefit of suffering humanity."

Jefferson students formed the Virgil Holland Moon Society of Pathology, and the Jefferson class of 1943 chose Professor Moon as its portrait honoree. In the depiction by Daniel Garber the physician is shown two-thirds length and life-sized, at work in his office or study. Seated at a desk in front of a bookcase, he holds a fountain pen in his right hand which rests on some pamphlets. He looks up from his writing as though acknowledging an unseen visitor. He is attired in a gray suit, white shirt, and maroon necktie with tie pin. The key hanging from his vest is probably his Phi Beta Kappa key. Dr. Moon's expression is friendly and open and his bright blue eyes seem to twinkle.

The bookshelves are lined with medical texts, two of which have legible titles: Esmond R. Long's *History of Pathology* (1928) and the annual biographical directory, *American Men of Science*. Two other objects on the desk allude directly or indirectly to his work: the sealed jar with a preserved wet pathological specimen, and the pipe (traditionally signifying an intellectual or thoughtful man).

Daniel Garber has situated the subject in his familiar working environment, described the unique quality of his physical features, and suggested his affable and inquiring personality. The artist's painterly style lends a freshness and appearance of spontaneity to the portrait through the rosy coloring of the sitter's skin tones; the blues, umbers, and violets worked into his gray suit; the reflections and shadows of objects on the desktop; the deep folds in the fabric of his suit; and the shadows between the multicolored bindings of the textbooks on the bookshelves.

In spite of his technical and interpretive abilities, one wonders why Daniel Garber, a celebrated landscape painter and only occasional portraitist, was commissioned. Most of Moon's contemporaries at Jefferson had chosen noted portrait specialists.

However, Dr. Moon could possibly have admired Garber's portraits of Drs. Charles W. Burr and William Zentmayer at the College of Physicians of Philadelphia. Further, although it is not known if Moon and Garber were social acquaintances, perhaps one factor was their common Bucks County and Midwestern roots. Daniel Garber was born in North Manchester, Indiana in 1880, the son of a Pennsylvania farmer from Bucks County whose Mennonite forbears had settled in Pennsylvania in the mid-eighteenth century. He moved East and forged his career near the artists' colony in New Hope, Bucks County.

Garber studied first at the Cincinnati Art Academy in 1897, and then at the Pennsylvania Academy of the Fine Arts from 1899 to 1905.[18] While at the Academy Garber won a First Toppan Prize and a Cresson traveling scholarship which enabled him to journey to England, Italy, and France for two years with his wife, Academy student Mary Franklin. Four of Garber's paintings were accepted for the Paris Salons of 1906 and 1907.

Upon their return to America the Garbers divided their time between a town house in Philadelphia and a rustic stone cottage in Cuttalossa Glen near Lumberville in Bucks County. Daniel Garber began teaching life and antique drawing classes at the Philadelphia School of Design for Women in 1904. In 1909 Garber was employed at the Pennsylvania Academy where he remained a beloved and respected faculty member teaching cast drawing, figure painting, and still life classes for four decades. He also taught landscape painting at the Academy's summer school in rural Chester Springs. When he retired from the Academy in 1950 he was elected emeritus professor.

The artist garnered prizes and honors throughout his prolific career. As early as 1909 Garber's entry won the First Hallgarten Prize at the National Academy of Design. He was elected an academician in 1913 and won four other important prizes there. He received four awards and a purchase from the Corcoran Gallery of Art. In 1911 he won the Potter Palmer Gold Medal at the Art Institute of Chicago. In 1914 he was named one of the youngest members ever to serve on a jury of awards at the Carnegie Institute, and won awards there in 1924 and 1933. He was a consistent prizewinner at the Pennsylvania Academy of the Fine Arts from 1911 through 1947.

At international expositions he won the bronze medal at Buenos Aires in 1910 and a gold medal at the Panama-Pacific fair in San Francisco in 1915. He executed a commission for a large landscape mural for the Pennsylvania Building at the Sesqui-centennial Exposition in Philadelphia in 1926. The work was lost, but decades later discovered at a school in western Pennsylvania, and installed in the Michener Art Museum in Doylestown, Pennsylvania in 1995.

Daniel Garber exhibited frequently in New York's Macbeth Gallery both alone and with other New Hope landscape painters, and he contributed to a touring exhibition of the "New Hope Group" from 1915 to 1917. Garber had one-man shows of paintings, etchings, and drawings at the Philadelphia Art Alliance, the Norfolk, Virginia Museum of Arts and Sciences, the Woodmere Gallery in Philadelphia, and the Corcoran Gallery, and major retrospective exhibitions at the Pennsylvania Academy in 1945 and 1980.

In 1948 Daniel Garber was elected to the American Institute of Arts and Letters and given a one-man show. The popular and respected artist is represented in muse ums and public institutions as well as private collections all over the country.

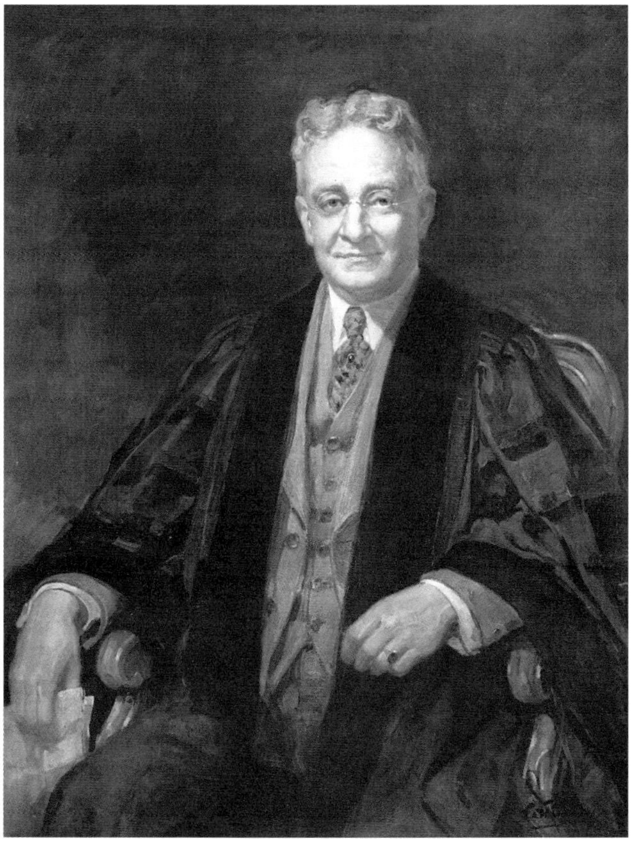

Portrait of Randle C. Rosenberger

RANDLE CRATER ROSENBERGER, M.D. (1873-1944)
By William Taylor Thomson (1858-1941)

Oil on canvas
1928
50 1/4 x 40 1/4 in.

Signed lower right: "W. T. THOMSON"

Given by JMC class of 1928
Accession number: 1928+e.P.01

Dr. Randle Crater Rosenberger was a bacteriologist and professor at Jefferson Medical College for almost three decades.

Of Pennsylvania German ancestry, Randle C. Rosenberger was born in Philadelphia in 1873. After graduating from Central High School he received a medical degree from Jefferson Medical College in 1894. That year he was made an assistant demonstrator of histology and assistant in outpatient diseases of children.

In 1898 Rosenberger was appointed demonstrator of normal histology and bacteriology and curator of Jefferson's pathology museum, and held the latter post until 1910. He rose in the academic ranks to become Jefferson's first professor of hygiene and bacteriology in 1909. This title was changed to professor of preventive medicine and bacteriology in 1924, and professor of bacteriology and immunology in 1941.

Dr. Randle Rosenberger's positions at other medical centers included: assistant pathologist to the Philadelphia Hospital, lecturer of hygiene and then professor of preventive medicine at Women's Medical College of Pennsylvania, pathologist to the Henry Phipps Institute and St. Joseph's Hospital, and director of the clinical laboratory of the Philadelphia General Hospital. His civic activities included membership on the City of Philadelphia's Milk Commission and the Pneumonia Commission, and the chairmanship of the Study of Poliomyelitis and Encephalitis. He received an honorary D.Sc. degree from the Philadelphia College of Pharmacy in 1942.

Professor Rosenberger was very proud that Jefferson students invariably made their highest marks in bacteriology in the National Board Examination, justifying his method of teaching. He held that the function of a medical school was to train physicians for general practice, and he fashioned his course in bacteriology to be of practical rather than theoretical value.

Dr. Randle Rosenberger was famous for his prodigious ability to remember names, faces, and incidents in the lives of hundreds of individuals, especially his students. The class of 1910 dedicated their yearbook to him and the class of 1928 selected him as class portrait honoree. Subscription notices to alumni inaugurating the Rosenberger Memorial Fellowship Fund in 1945 began, "Remember Rosie? He remembers you!"

The portrait by William T. Thomson shows Dr. Rosenberger two-thirds length and slightly over life-sized. He is seated in a curving, Louis XV-style, painted armchair with gold trim. The subject's arms rest on the chair arms and his right hand holds a sheaf of papers. He wears a black academic robe trimmed in green over his tannish-gray, three-piece suit. The warm maroon background color harmonizes with the dabs of reds and pinks in his ruddy complexion. His warm brown eyes look straight ahead through steel-rimmed glasses, and his expression is friendly and affable, almost conversational.

In 1963 Mrs. Randle Rosenberger bequeated another portrait of her husband to Jefferson. It was painted by Robert T. Lukens, M.D., an alumnus of 1953 and former student of Dr. Rosenberger.

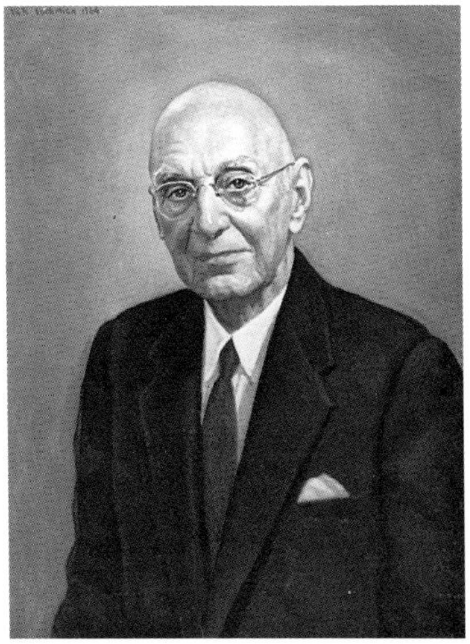

Portrait of Victor G. Heiser

VICTOR GEORGE HEISER, M.D. (1873-1972)
By Vuk Vuchinich (b. 1901)

Oil on canvas board
1964
28 x 22 in.

Signed and dated upper left: "Vuk Vuchinich 1964"

Given in 1965 by the subject
Accession number: 1965+e.P.02

Dr. Victor G. Heiser was a pioneer in public health administration and preventive medicine, an alumnus who forged his career away from Jefferson. He was remarkably influential and productive throughout his ninety-nine years.

Victor Heiser was born in 1873 in Johnstown, Pennsylvania. After graduating from Jefferson Medical College in 1897 he interned at Lankenau Hospital. He decided against private practice which he called "a retail effort," saying, "The prevention of disease on a wholesale basis appealed to me far more."[19] He joined the Marine Hospital Service (later named the U.S. Public Health Service) where he examined immigrants to the United States.

From 1903 to 1914 Dr. Heiser served as the chief quarantine officer and later the commissioner of health in the Philippine Islands. His contributions included founding a leper colony for thirty thousand patients, opening a new hospital and medical school, and introducing sanitation methods and preventive medicine procedures. He spearheaded a smallpox vaccination campaign that reduced the annual rate from forty thousand to seven hundred cases.

Starting in 1914 Dr. Heiser served as director of the East for the International Health Board of the newly created Rockefeller Foundation. For twenty years he spread medical knowledge about hookworm, dysentery, typhoid, and other intestinal diseases to Hawaii, Japan, China, Ceylon, and Siam. An autobiographical book about his experiences, *An American Doctor's Odyssey: Adventures in Forty-five Countries* (1936), was a best-seller.

While in his sixties Dr. Heiser began a new career in American industry as advisor on occupational medicine for the National Association of Manufacturers. He worked in this field until finally retiring at age ninety in 1963. His book *You're the Doctor* (1939) counseled readers on how to live longer.

Dr. Victor G. Heiser was president of the International Leprosy Association (1931-38) and received its Damien-Dutton Award (1969). He was director of the American Museum of Health and chairman of the National Malaria Committee. He received honorary degrees from Jefferson Medical College (1911), Rutgers and Temple Universities, and Thiel College. In 1968 he was awarded the Jefferson alumni achievement award.

In 1965 Jefferson Medical College was pleased to accept the gift of his portrait from Dr. Victor G. Heiser. The bust-length portrait by Vuk Vuchinich had been painted the year before when Heiser was aged ninety-one but still looked very vigorous and alert. His deeply lined face is rendered in great detail, emphasizing his bald head, steadfast gaze, hooked nose, and pursed lips. His complexion is rather dark, perhaps suggesting his long stays in the tropics. Strokes of green are seen in the eyebrows and sparse hair, and the halo effect in the atmospheric background.

Vuk Vuchinich was a sculptor, painter, and etcher born in Montenegro, Yugoslavia in 1901. He studied and forged his career in New York.

Portrait of Charles M. Gruber

CHARLES MICHAEL GRUBER, M.D., Ph.D. (1887-1974)
By Walter Stuempfig Jr. (1914-70)

Oil on canvas
1953
40 x 30 in.

Given by JMC class of 1953
Accession number: 1953+e.P.01

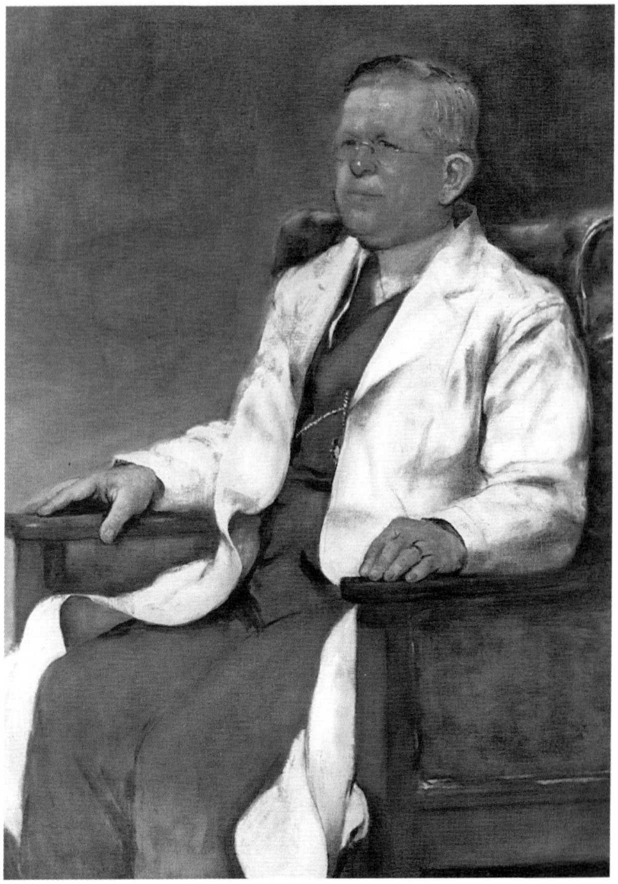

Dr. Charles M. Gruber was professor and first chair of pharmacology at Jefferson Medical College. He played a major role in the development of this field as an independent academic discipline.

Charles M. Gruber was born in 1887 on a farm in Hope, Kansas, the youngest of nine children of German immigrant homesteaders. He started his career as a physiologist with undergraduate (1911) and master of science (1912) degrees from the University of Kansas, and a Ph.D. from Harvard University (1914). He taught at the University of Pennsylvania, Albany Medical College, and the University of Colorado School of Medicine. After receiving a medical degree at Washington University in St. Louis (1921) he was associate professor of pharmacology at the university until 1932.

Dr. Gruber was appointed professor and first chairman of the department of pharmacology at Jefferson Medical College in 1932. From the very beginning of his tenure he encouraged Jefferson faculty and students to carry on research. Professor Gruber was a significant voice in developing the graduate training program in the basic medical sciences, and in 1949, the Board for the Regulation of Graduate Studies. This, in turn, led to the College of Graduate Studies of Thomas Jefferson University in 1969.

Dr. Gruber was the author of *Handbook of Treatment and Medical Formulary* (1948) and associate editor of the *Cyclopedia of Medicine, Surgery and Specialties* (1948-53). He served as president of the American Society for Pharmacology and Experimental Therapeutics and was a charter member of the American College of Cardiology.

After Dr. Charles Gruber retired and was named emeritus professor at Jefferson in 1953, a whole new career developed for him in California. He accepted an invitation to establish a new department of pharmacology at the College of Medical Evangelists in Loma Linda. His final teaching post was visiting professor of biology at the University of Redlands from 1957 until 1963. Dr. Gruber's son, Charles M. Gruber Jr., M.D., graduated from Jefferson in 1941.

The class of 1953 chose Dr. Gruber as its portrait honoree. In the three-quarters-length, smaller-than-life-sized portrait by Walter Stuempfig Jr., the subject is seated in a greenish-yellow, upholstered armchair. He wears a white lab coat over a brown vest and trousers, with a green tie and his Phi Beta Kappa key. His forearms rest squarely on the chair arms. His very narrow brown eyes gaze abstractedly into the distance through rimless glasses.

Judging from the thin paint surface and rapidly executed contours of the figure, the portrait was produced with an economy of means and with great verve. The brilliant white coat is more thickly painted and it contrasts strikingly with the otherwise neutral palette. Yet there is a conspicuous dichotomy between the freely brushed, informal paint style and the physician's pinched and tense expression and almost gnome-like body. There is no hint here of Gruber's oft-noted charm and sense of humor.

Considerable criticism of the portrait, illustrating the difficulties faced by painters of public portraits, was expressed in minutes of Jefferson executive faculty meetings. Other Jefferson documents include correspondence between Dr. Gruber and a Philadelphia law firm representing the artist. The faculty felt that the portrait was "not in keeping with the other portraits," and a request was made for it to be "retouched" or "redone." Mr. Stuempfig's reaction was that his "artistic integrity had been assailed," and he indignantly offered to take the portrait back and charge no fee.

The artist was at the height of his nationwide fame, and although his offer was apparently accepted by the faculty (with the approval of Gruber who was in California), the "rejected" portrait never did leave the Jefferson campus.

Although considered primarily a painter of naturalist landscapes and cityscapes and of poetic still lifes in a style called "romantic realism" by contemporary art critics, Walter Stuempfig also produced a number of strikingly idiosyncratic portraits. Ironically, the Gruber portrait's divergence from the conventional norms of the 1950s characteristic of full-time portrait painters, is now regarded in a more positive light.

A native Philadelphian born in 1914, Walter Stuempfig switched from studying architecture at the University of Pennsylvania to studying painting at the Pennsylvania Academy of the Fine Arts (1931-34) where he won a Cresson traveling scholarship.

The Pennsylvania Academy made its first purchase of Walter Stuempfig's work as early as 1935, and he exhibited there almost annually between 1933 and 1966. He was a professor of composition and drawing at the Academy for twenty-two years until his death at age fifty-six in 1970. Stuempfig was a consistent prizewinner at national exhibitions and his work was acquired by museums throughout the country. Besides easel paintings he executed two murals in 1964, a fantasy of Rome for the Bryn Mawr, Pennsylvania home of Mr. and Mrs. Alexander Biddle, and a view of Naples for the upscale restaurant of Helen Sigel Wilson in Philadelphia.

Stuempfig's first one-man show was at the Philadelphia Art Alliance in 1942, and he exhibited biennially at the Durlacher Brothers Gallery in New York from 1943 to 1961. Other one-man shows were held in galleries and museums in San Francisco, London, Philadelphia, Boston, Miami, Newport, Fort Worth, and Birmingham. In addition to solo shows at the Pennsylvania Academy in 1947 and 1965, he was accorded a memorial show in 1972.

Walter Stuempfig won a silver medal and the Second W. A. Clarke Prize at the Corcoran Gallery of Art in 1947. He was made an academician at the National Academy of Design in 1951, and won its Benjamin Altman Landscape Prize in 1953. In 1952 Stuempfig was one of fifteen Americans granted an award by the National Institute of Arts and Letters. In 1955 he was elected a member of New York's Century Association, and in 1963 he received a Ford Foundation grant.

In spite of Walter Stuempfig's considerable reputation, opinion was not swayed in his favor at Jefferson Medical College. As a result of the embarrassing contretemps over his portrait of Dr. Gruber, it was resolved at an executive faculty meeting of May 25, 1953 that a special committee be formed to adopt policies with regard to subject, artist, and general suitability and acceptability of portraits.

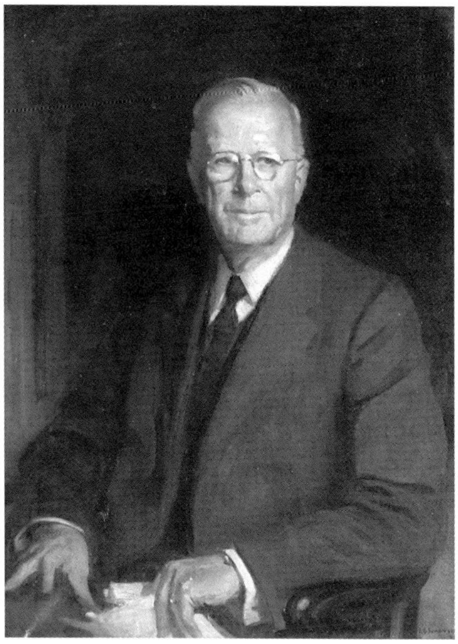

Portrait of Charles M. Gruber

CHARLES MICHAEL GRUBER, M.D., Ph.D.
By John Christen Johansen (1876-1964)

Oil on canvas
1955
35 1/2 x 37 in.

Signed and dated lower right: "J. C. JOHANSEN/1955"

Given in 1955 by JMC faculty
Accession number: 1955+e.P.02

The Jefferson faculty decided to order a second portrait of Dr. Gruber. The commission was awarded to John C. Johansen who in 1954 had completed portraits of Drs. Lewis C. Scheffey and Baldwin L. Keyes. The new portrait of Gruber was greeted with relief over its acceptability and presented in 1955. Johansen's conventional, half-length depiction lacks the verve and personality of the Stuempfig portrait, but the subject looks much more confident and accessible. Ironically both paintings are displayed today.

Portrait of Joseph J. Wilson

JOSEPH J. WILSON (1879-1957)
By Roy Cleveland Nuse (1885-1975)

Oil on canvas
1954
36 x 30 in.

Signed and dated lower left: "RN/54"

Commissioned in 1954 through a bequest by Brooke M. Anspach, M.D.
Accession number: 1954+e.P.02

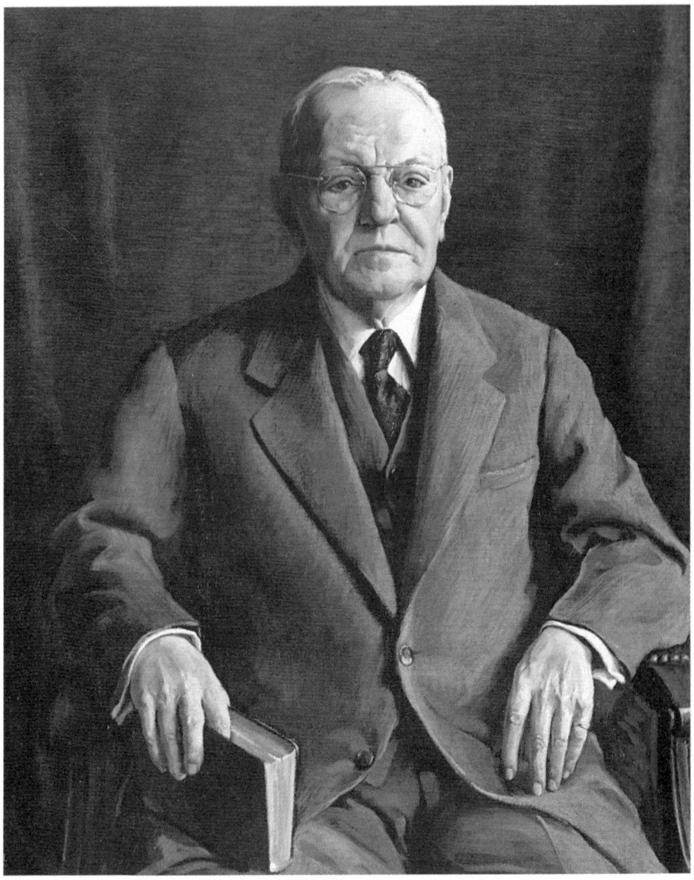

Joseph J. Wilson succeeded Charles L. Frankenberger as librarian of Jefferson Medical College in 1917. He oversaw significant expansion in the library's collection and facilities during his thirty-two years in the post.

Joseph Wilson was born in Philadelphia in 1879 and graduated from Central High School in 1896. That same year he began on-the-job training at the Free Library of Philadelphia in the cataloguing, binding, and shipping departments. He worked for many years in branch libraries before 1917 when he became the librarian at Jefferson. Wilson continued as part-time head of the overdue department at the Free Library until 1940.

When Joseph J. Wilson arrived at Jefferson the reading room and books were located in the 1898 College Building. In 1929 the library was relocated to the first floor of the new College Building where it remained until 1970. Wilson was instrumental in increasing the library's modest collection from 6,500 volumes and sixty-one journals to over twenty-seven thousand volumes and three hundred journals.

During his tenure Wilson received important donations of private libraries from Jefferson faculty Drs. Hobart A. Hare, Albert P. Brubaker, William M. L. Coplin, and Pascal B. Bland. In 1929 Jefferson Medical College received a bequest of eight thousand books and a large sum of money from Samuel Parsons Scott, Esq. for whom a new library was subsequently named.

Joseph J. Wilson performed many unofficial duties for students and faculty, and was affectionately admired and respected for his warm and friendly counsel. He even helped students find living accommodations and administered the college bookstore. He managed several student athletic teams, and acted as advisor to the student yearbook and to the faculty portrait committee.

The Jefferson Medical College alumni association commemorated his twenty-fifth anniversary as "librarian and friend" with the installation of the "Joseph J. Wilson Table" in the reading room of the library. An inscribed silver plaque was placed in the center of the handsome, round, walnut table.

In 1954 the library committee of Jefferson's executive faculty commissioned Roy C. Nuse to paint a portrait of Wilson who had retired five years earlier. It was funded by a 1951 bequest of Dr. Brooke M. Anspach who had stipulated such a painting.

The librarian is depicted half length and life-sized, seated in a leather armchair in front of a purplish-umber drapery. His position is frontal and he stares directly forward through wire-rimmed glasses. He uses his right index finger to mark his place in a book which rests on his thigh. He wears a three-piece, slate blue business suit and a dark blue necktie. The impasto surface and contrasts of light and shade emphasize the deeply creased features of the seventy-five-year-old sitter, especially above his knitted brows and around his tightly drawn lips.

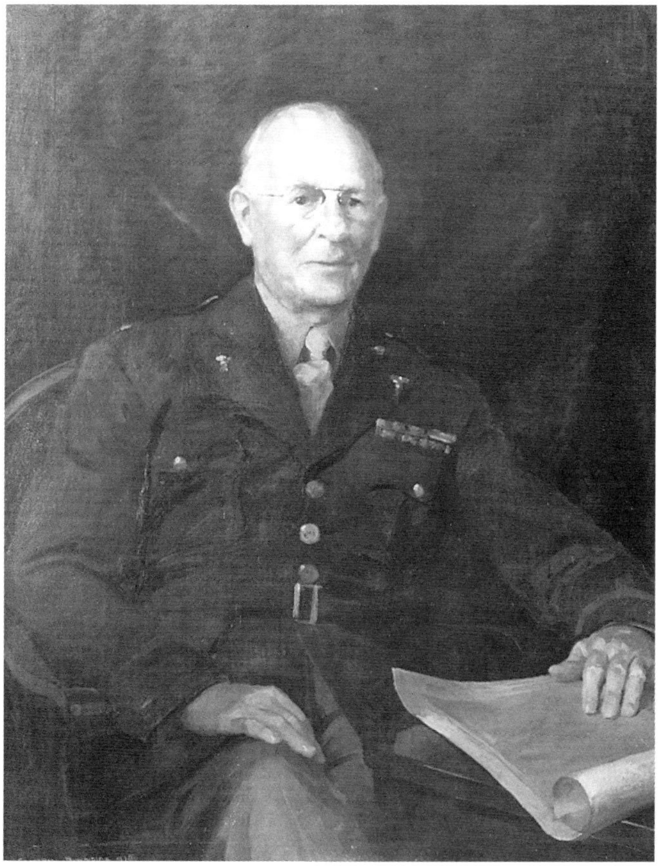

Portrait of Frederick H. Mills

COLONEL FREDERICK HUBBELL MILLS, M.D.
(1869-1955)
By Cameron Burnside (1887-1952)

Oil on canvas
1945
40 x 32 in.

Signed and dated lower left: "CAMERON BURNSIDE 1945"

Given in 1945 by friends, colleagues, and students
Accession number: 1945+e.P.02

Colonel Frederick H. Mills, M.D., Jefferson professor of military tactics and science, had the distinction of serving the United States Army as a surgeon in seven wars and conflicts.

Frederick H. Mills was born in 1869 in Leon, New York. After obtaining a bachelor's degree from Princeton (1891) and medical degree from Jefferson (1894), he pursued further training at the Niagara University Medical School and the New York Postgraduate Medical College and Hospital.

Mills's U.S. Army career began in 1898 when he was acting assistant surgeon during the Spanish-American War. He served as a contract surgeon between 1901 and 1908. He had firsthand experience with the Philippine Insurrection and the Chinese Boxer Rebellion.

In 1917 Mills became a first lieutenant in the regular army and rose to major by 1918. The versatile physician served as assistant to the chief surgeon at Fort Sam Houston, Texas, camp surgeon at Fort Knox, Kentucky, professor of hygiene and sanitation at Infantry Officers School at Camp Lee, Virginia, commanding officer at Fort Bragg, North Carolina, and eye, nose, and throat specialist at the United States Dispensary, New York City.

In 1924 Dr. Mills was appointed the professor of military tactics and science of the Jefferson Medical College Reserve Officers Training Corps unit and served until 1931. He was recalled to active duty in 1942 and again assumed the professorship at Jefferson. In 1943 he was promoted to the rank of colonel, and in 1945 he was made commanding officer of the 3,555th Service Unit—the Student Army Training Corps at Jefferson.

Students, friends, and colleagues honored Colonel Mills with his portrait in 1945. In the two-thirds-length, life-sized depiction by Cameron Burnside the officer/physician is dressed in his khaki and tan uniform. He is seated in an armchair with legs crossed at the knee. One hand rests on his thigh and the other presses down a map on a nearby table. Mills has paused in reading the map to gaze directly at an unseen visitor. The background is a maroon curtain with curving folds.

The bearing of the seventy-six-year-old colonel is formidably erect and his expression is stern. Though in need of restoration, the portrait still bears the unmistakable hand of Cameron Burnside in the loosely brushed and well formed head and hands. The austerity of pose and neutral color scheme are offset by two rows of multicolored ribbons and the gleaming brass buttons, insignia, and buckle of Mills's uniform, and the pastel-colored map.

At the portrait presentation ceremony Colonel Mills received a special certificate of commendation from the Medical Corps as a "counsellor, guide, and inspiration to his men." The presenting officer praised Jefferson's contributions to the war effort, commenting that no other medical college had more men in the army.

Thirty-eighth General Hospital

THIRTY-EIGHTH GENERAL HOSPITAL, CAMP BOWIE, TEXAS
By Walch Studio

Photograph mounted on board
1942
9 1/8 x 32 3/4 in.

Signed lower right: "Walch Studio"
Inscription below image: "38th General Hospital/Camp Bowie, Texas/July 3, 1942"

Given after 1942 by a member of the hospital
Accession number: 1942+f.Ph.01

A thirty-two-inch-long photograph shows rows of officers and nurses posed in front of the tents and barracks of Jefferson Medical College's Base Hospital Thirty-eight at Camp Bowie, Texas.

The hospital was descended from the original Base Hospital Thirty-eight organized by the Red Cross to support the American Expeditionary Forces going to

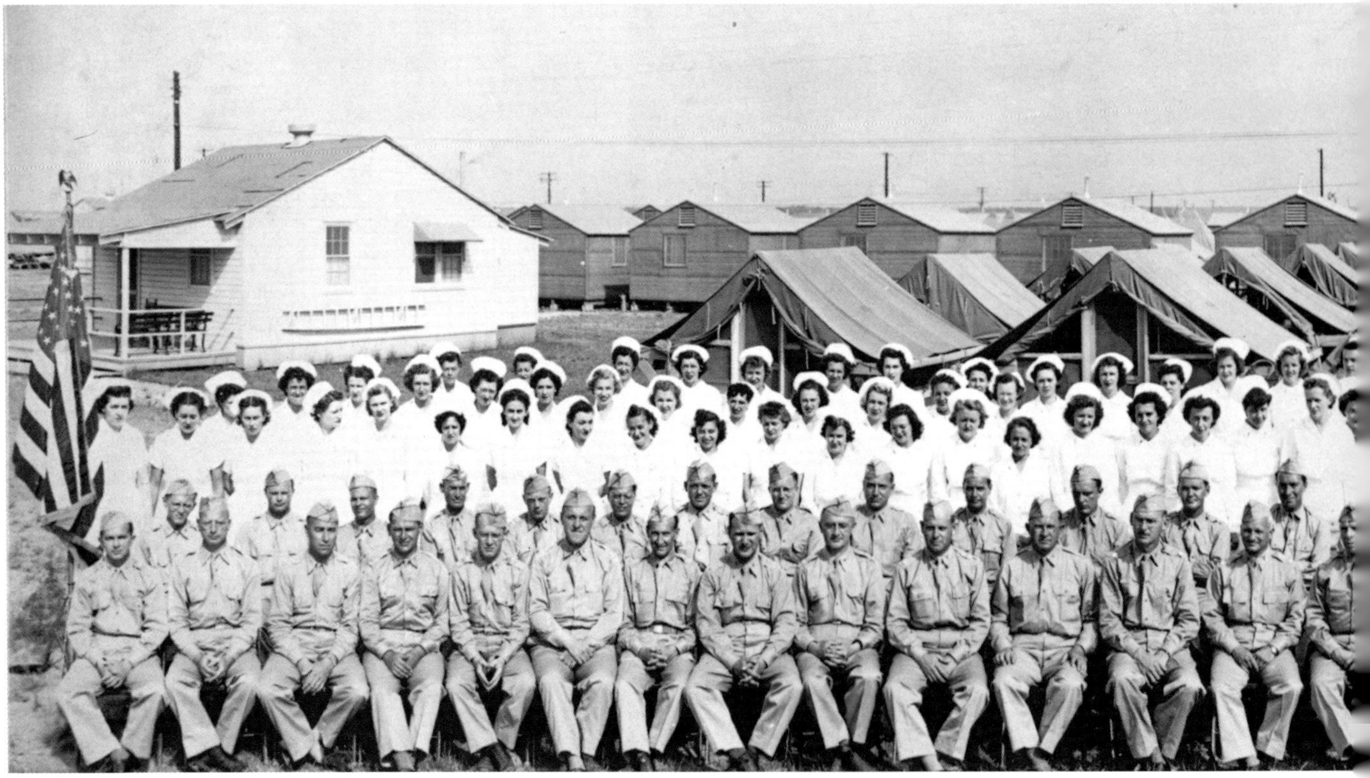

France in World War I. The hospital was reactivated at the request of the U.S. Surgeon General in 1940. The administrators were Drs. Baldwin L. Keyes, executive officer and commandant in charge of medical affairs, and Burgess L. Gordon, chief of medical services, and Major Edna W. Scott, R.N., director of nurses. The hospital unit left Philadelphia for Camp Bowie on May 15, 1942 and this photograph was taken July 3.

In late August fifty-six officers and 105 nurses left Camp Bowie for mobilization at a secret destination. They sailed from Staten Island on a refitted former British luxury liner, the *Aquitania*, to Teufik, the port of Suez located thirteen kilometers from Cairo.

The Thirty-eighth Hospital, known unofficially as "Kilo Thirteen," opened in November 1942, although construction and supplies were incomplete and desert conditions were unfamiliar to the personnel. The buildings were built of sand-mud brick so porous that sand blew through the walls during storms. Participants remember improvising bed trays out of packing cases and washing and feeding patients out of tin cans.[20]

The hospital served mainly noncombatants because the German Army's North African campaign was failing, and the anticipated Allied casualties never materialized in that region. Therefore Kilo Thirteen was reduced from one thousand to five hundred beds and most of the original staff were transferred to other posts. But the hospital was cited by the commanding general of the African-Middle Eastern Theater for "exceptionally difficult tasks and for maintenance of a high standard and discipline."

In the fall of 1941 eighty-three Jefferson Medical College students had enrolled in the Reserve Officer Training Corps and been commissioned second lieutenants in the Student Army Training Corps. After graduating from an accelerated medical program and undergoing further military training they were commissioned first lieutenants in the Medical Corps of the U.S. Army.

Almost one-third of Jefferson's living alumni served in World War II. For heroism and devotion to duty Jefferson alumni won virtually every decoration awarded. A commemorative bronze plaque in the Curtis Building bears the names of thirty-two Jeffersonians who gave their lives "in freedom's cause."

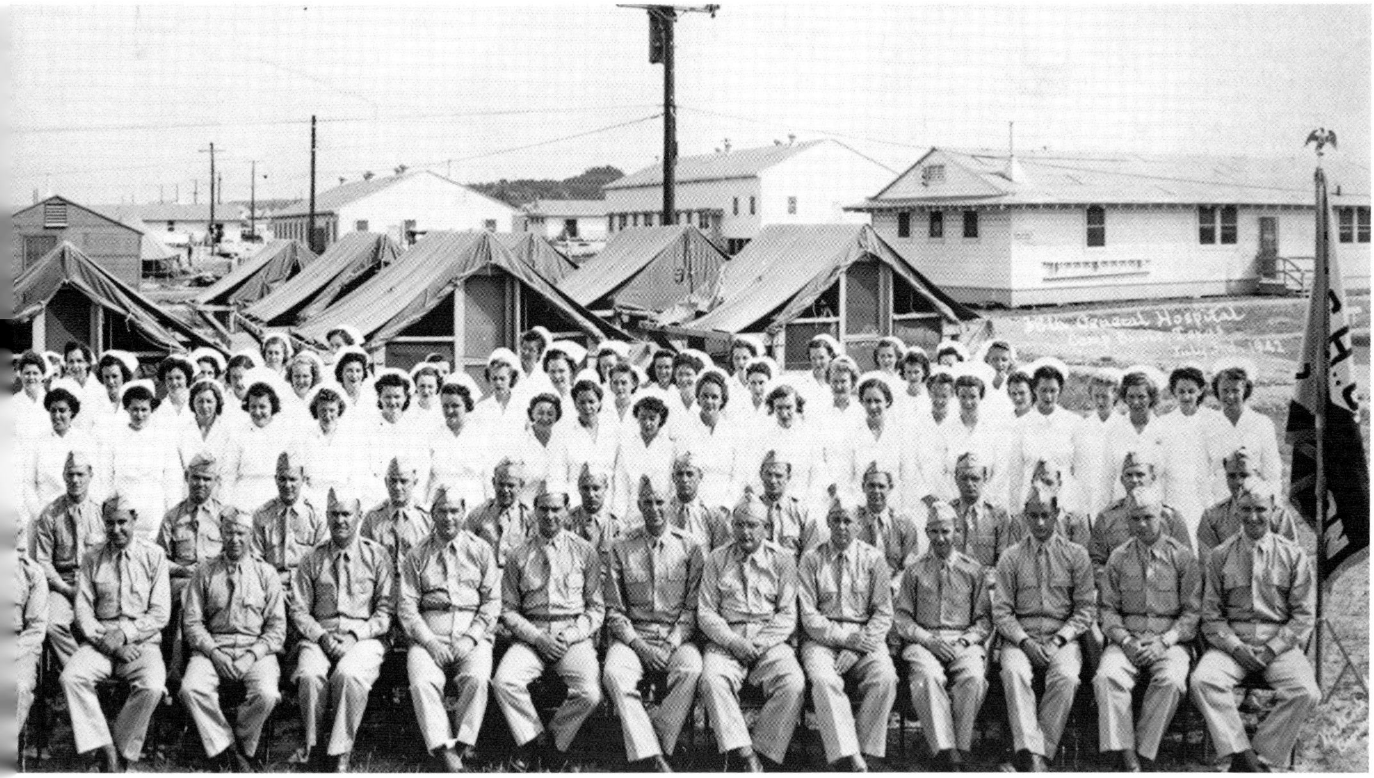

In 1982 two pairs of medical prints were donated to the Jefferson art collection by Dr. August J. Podboy, an alumnus of 1932, and Mrs. Podboy. The earlier set consisted of world-famous caricatures by the French artist Adrien Barrère. The later set was a lampoon of the Barrère originals drawn by Carl E. Miksch, a student who graduated in 1923. The group of four prints are affectionately known at Jefferson as the "Podboy cartoons."

Adrien Barrère was a caricaturist who contributed regularly to French humor magazines and who exhibited at the 1929 Salon des Humoristes in Paris. He also designed distinctive theatrical posters for a theater specializing in horror shows, and composed an album on the subject of war.

Barrère's greatest popular success was a series of six satiric chromolithographs of contemporary professors on the faculties of medicine and law in Paris. The artist himself printed the edition of physicians and lawyers, and his editor is said to have sold at least forty-two thousand copies in twenty-five years.

The second series shows a lineup of sixteen ridiculous and occasionally bemedalled and besotted French physicians.[21] The characters hold objects ranging from a severed head, a leg prosthesis, and a uterus to a large hypodermic needle, a clarinet, champagne bottles, and a windup toy dirigible. The aproned surgeon on the right with instruments held carpenter-style in his belt hovers over a nude woman lying on her back on a table. She turns her head to smile coyly at the viewer, a spoof of

Portraits Charges des Professeurs à la Faculté de Médecine (Deuxième Série)

PORTRAITS CHARGES DES PROFESSEURS À LA FACULTÉ DE MÉDECINE
By Adrien Barrère (1877-1931)

Chromolithograph
1905
Image size: 18 x 35 in. (sight size)

Signed lower right: "A. Barrère"

Given in 1982 by Dr. August J. Podboy (JMC 1932) and Mrs. Podboy

Accession number: 1982+e.Pr.04

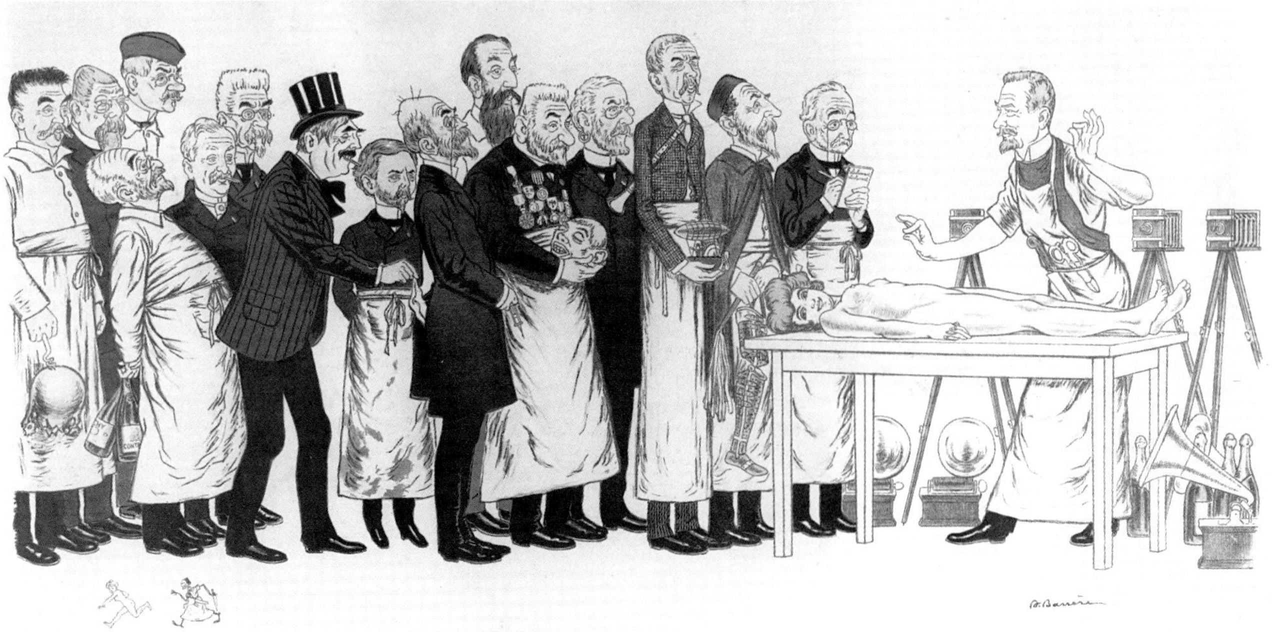

seductive odalisques in nineteenth-century French painting. The surgeon's assistant recording notes resembles a waiter taking dinner orders. The seventh man from the left wearing a top hat inches forward to pick the pocket of the man holding the hypodermic. Apparently the group will soon celebrate and memorialize the occasion with cameras, record players, and champagne. At the bottom left is a miniature figure of Death with a saw and sword chasing after a tiny nude woman.

Carl E. Miksch, M.D. was inspired by Adrien Barrère's caricatures to transpose the heads and bodies of contemporary Jefferson faculty onto the original French faculty in two cartoons made while he was a senior student at Jefferson Medical College in 1923. Later Dr. Miksch practiced general medicine and surgery in North Charleroi, Pennsylvania until his death in 1955.

Immortalized in Miksch's cartoon are the following familiar Jefferson professors, from left to right: Drs. Leighton F. Appleman, Hiram R. Loux, Fielding O. Lewis, Charles F. Nassau, Thomas E. Shea, Solomon Solis-Cohen, S. MacCuen Smith, Frederick J. Kalteyer, Willis F. Manges, Hobart A. Hare, J. Parsons Schaeffer, Edward J. G. Beardsley, Baxter L. Crawford, Chevalier Jackson, Thomas McCrae, Lucius Tuttle, and John C. DaCosta.

Miksch made amusing changes in the various organs and other objects grasped by the Jefferson professors, notably the kidneys held by Dr. Loux (a specialist in urology), the upper gastrointestinal tract held by Dr. Crawford (pathology), and the frog held by Dr. Tuttle (physiology). Dr. Kalteyer (medicine) reaches across Dr. Manges (roentgenology) to pick the pocket of Dr. Hare (therapeutics). On the far right is Dr. DaCosta (surgery) whose gestures, attire, and supercilious expression are almost identical to those of Docteur Doyen, his French counterpart.

Miksch's caricatures graced the cover of the April 27, 1970 *Journal of the American Medical Association* which reported on the centennial of the founding of the Jefferson Medical College alumni association. The cover prompted several letters to the editor which correctly identified Barrère as the source for Miksch's drawings.

Jefferson Medical College Faculty of 1923 (Second Series)

JEFFERSON MEDICAL COLLEGE FACULTY OF 1923
By Carl E. Miksch, M.D. (ca. 1901-55)

Aquatint, softground etching, etching
1923
Image size: 10 3/4 x 20 1/2 in. (sight size)

Signed lower right: "C. Miksch"

Given in 1982 by Dr. August J. Podboy (JMC 1932) and Mrs. Podboy
Accession number: 1982+e.Pr.02

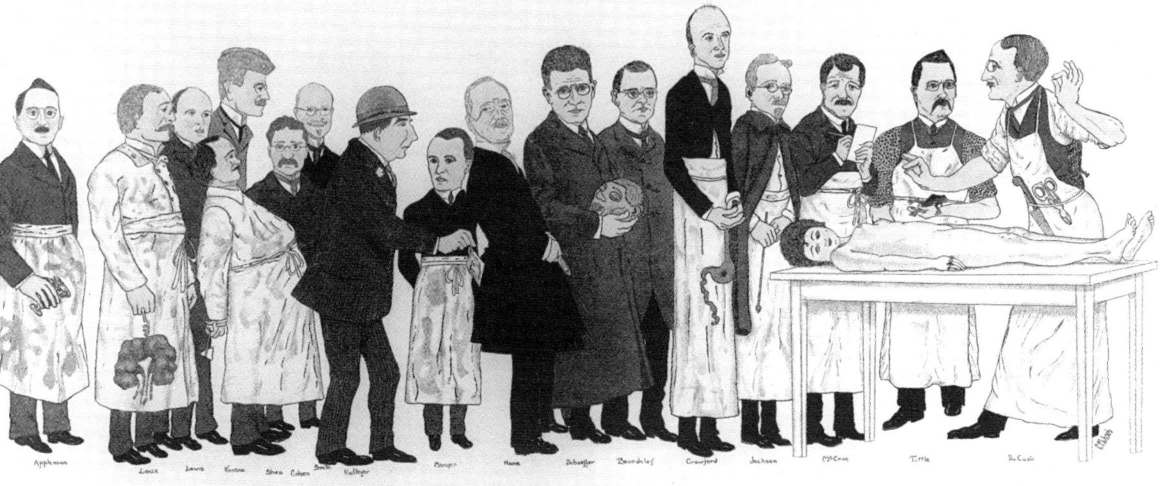

1. "The New Building to Be Added to the Jefferson Hospital," *Jefferson Medical College Alumni Bulletin* 1 (Dec. 1922): 9-10.
2. For a more complete account, see Julie S. Berkowitz, "Re-discovery of a Rare Antiquity at Jefferson," *Jefferson Medical College Alumni Bulletin* 38 (winter 1989): 4-11. Consultants included: Brunilde Sismondo Ridgway, Ph.D., the Rhys Carpenter Professor of classical and Near Eastern archeology, Bryn Mawr College; John Stephens Crawford, Ph.D., professor of the history of art, University of Delaware; Beth Cohen, Ph.D., art historian and archeologist; Donald White, Ph.D., associate curator, Mediterranean section, University Museum of the University of Pennsylvania; Claire Romano, Ph.D., coordinator of exhibitions, University Museum of the University of Pennsylvania; and Elizabeth Bartman, Ph.D., assistant professor of art history, University of Pennsylvania.
3. For details of McCrae's biography including his puzzling terminal illness, see Frederick B. Wagner Jr., M.D., "Thomas McCrae: A Life Patterned after Osler," *The Persisting Osler—II: Selected Transactions of the American Osler Society 1981-1990* (Malabar, Fla.: Krieger Publishing Co., 1994), 127-32.
4. Information courtesy of John A. Lindquist, M.D., who had invited Irene Burnside to reside in a cottage on his property until her health deteriorated and she moved to a nursing home.
5. J. Liberty Tadd was a student of Thomas Eakins at the Pennsylvania Academy of the Fine Arts intermittently between 1876 and 1881. See Maria Jo Chamberlin-Hellman, *Thomas Eakins as a Teacher* (Ph.D. diss., Columbia University, 1981) (Ann Arbor, Mich.: University Microfilms International, 1981), 541, 557.
6. John Hauschild, "*Titanic* People, Titanic Life—A Woman of the '90's—Charlotte Drake Martinez Cardeza," *The Titanic Commutator* 17 (May-July 1993): 68-70.
7. Dates for Dr. Knowles's tenure are sometimes given as 1919 to 1947.
8. Wagner, *Thomas Jefferson University: Tradition and Heritage* (Philadelphia: Lea & Febiger, 1989), 556-57.
9. Chevalier Jackson, M.D., *The Life of Chevalier Jackson: An Autobiography* (New York: Macmillan Co., 1938), 137-38.
10. A profile view of the Maraffi bust is the frontispiece of Dr. Chevalier Jackson's autobiography (1938), with a caption stating that it was presented to Jackson in 1937 by a group of his pupils and colleagues.
11. William H. Baltzell, M.D., "Louis H. Clerf, 1889-1989," *Jefferson Medical College Alumni Bulletin* 39 (fall 1989): 14.
12. Wagner, "Addendum" [to Dr. William H. Baltzell's article, "Louis H. Clerf, M.D.,'12—'Mr. Jefferson'"], *Jefferson Medical College Alumni Bulletin* 38 (fall 1988): 23.
13. Lists of portrait subjects were taken from local Berks County newspapers and from George R. Pechstein, M.D., "The Contribution of Frederick Roscher to Jefferson's Art Collection," *Jefferson Medical College Alumni Bulletin* 41 (winter 1992): 14.
14. J. Parsons Schaeffer, M.D., "Anatomy in the Modern Medical School," *Jefferson Medical College Alumni Bulletin* 2 (May 1940): 2, a summary of an address originally read to the Association of American Medical Colleges several years earlier.
15. "J. Earl Thomas, M.D., D.Sc., Emeritus Professor of Physiology," *Jefferson Medical College Alumni Bulletin* 21 (spring 1972): 29.
16. Pechstein, 14. Dr. George R. Pechstein (JMC 1948), a Jefferson radiologist, was a friend and neighbor of Frederick Roscher.
17. Pechstein, 14. Dr. Pechstein revealed the original underpainting of the Thomas portrait by using infrared black and white film, red filter, and white light.
18. For biography and career of Daniel Garber see Kathleen A. Foster, *Daniel Garber: 1880-1958* (Philadelphia: Pennsylvania Academy of the Fine Arts, 1980).
19. "A Doctor's Odyssey Revisited," *Jefferson Medical College Alumni Bulletin* 18 (spring 1968): 2-3.
20. Jacquelyn S. Mitchell, "The 38th 38 Years Later," *Jefferson Medical College Alumni Bulletin* 28 (summer 1979): 6.
21. The French physicians depicted are, left to right, Drs. Segond, Déjerine, de Lapersonne, Landouzy, Gaucher, Gariel, Brissaud, Gilbert, Reclus, Roger, Lannelongue, Le Dentu, Richet, Kirmisson, Terrier, and Doyen.

CHAPTER 8

Postwar Period through the Nineteen-sixties

After World War II Jefferson Medical College and Hospital implemented a new administrative structure to adjust to its increasingly complex business and medical affairs. On April 7, 1949 Robert P. Hooper, who had been president of the college since 1936, was inaugurated as the first chairman of the board of trustees. After serving for a year he was succeeded by Percival E. Foerderer, who was the board's dynamic leader until 1962.

On May 1, 1949 Vice Admiral James L. Kauffman, U.S.N. (Ret.) became Jefferson's first full-time president and served until 1959, when he was succeeded by William W. Bodine Jr. who energetically performed this job until 1966.

For more than two decades Jefferson trustees had been assembling nearby tracts of land for a comprehensive plan: a new hospital to accommodate the annual rise in patient admissions, expansion of crowded research laboratories, and new student housing. The New Pavilion (renamed Foerderer Pavilion in 1962) on Eleventh Street between Sansom and Walnut Streets was dedicated in 1954; the Charlotte Drake Cardeza Laboratories at 1015 Chestnut Street in 1960; and the Stein Radiation Biology Research Center at 202 South Hutchinson Street in 1965.

The James R. Martin Nurses' Residence at Eleventh and Walnut Streets was opened in 1959, and the Louis B. and Ida K. Orlowitz Residence Hall at Tenth and Walnut Streets in 1967. The last and largest building of the sixties was Jefferson Alumni Hall, a combined basic science and student commons building (1968).

The New Pavilion (Foerderer Pavilion)

THE FOERDERER PAVILION
Building by Vincent G. Kling & Associates
Erected 1954

Reproduction of architectural rendering
Original watercolor by Vincent G. Kling & Associates
Image size: 5 1/4 x 9 3/8 in.
Sheet size: 9 5/8 x 13 1/4 in.
Ca. 1952

Inscription below image: "JEFFERSON HOSPITAL"
Signed lower right: "Vincent G. Kling, architect"

Ordered in 1952 by JMC
Accession number: 1952+c.D.01

Promoted as "the hospital of tomorrow," the New Pavilion helped solve the dual problems of increasing bed capacity and modernizing and concentrating laboratories and operating rooms. The fourteen-story building connected by bridges to the adjacent Thompson Annex, and with the Old Main Hospital these buildings occupied the entire block of Sansom Street between Tenth and Eleventh Streets. By adding three hundred mainly semiprivate beds, the New Pavilion helped eliminate the long waiting list that had existed after World War II. Vacated areas in the older buildings were now utilized for modernized classrooms, demonstration rooms, postoperative recovery rooms, and a unit for psychiatric inpatients.

The building was constructed of fireproof steel and reinforced concrete and its two emergency fire towers ran the full height of the building. A new power center in the subbasement had the capacity to serve all three hospital buildings. The most advanced air conditioning system was installed. The interior was conceived in the spirit of an attractive hotel with restful decor featuring large picture windows. Patient rooms had bath and toilet facilities, telephone, oxygen equipment, and electronic communication to the nursing stations. Dual elevator systems separated visitors from patients and technical equipment. The new laundry was considered the most modern, fully mechanized, institutional laundry in Philadelphia. "Televoice" allowed doctors and nurses to transmit messages to an automatic recording station.

The ultramodern hospital had seven nursing floors including one devoted to maternity patients who had optional rooming-in privileges. Patient floors were located on the top seven stories and featured solaria and open air balconies facing south. Radiology facilities and clinical pathology and hematology laboratories were on the second and third floors, conveniently located immediately below two floors with fourteen operating rooms; the latter were provided with coaxial cable for television transmission. Another floor was reserved for gynecology and obstetrics patients. A covered roof terrace was available for convalescent patients.

The Pavilion Building is a narrow slab with a wing creating an L-shaped footprint. The salmon-colored brick facade has horizontal, flush, strip windows of dark glass. The slab visually "floats" above the ground because it is supported on rectangular concrete stilts with recessed glass between them on the first floor. The main entrance is shielded with an aluminum awning. A planted area with honey locust trees and yews faces the Walnut Street side. Projecting eaves define the skyline. The concrete section at the base with polished granite strips, big concrete globes, and flower beds is a later addition. The building won the gold medal of the American Institute of Architects in 1955.

Architect Vincent G. Kling was born in 1916, a native of East Orange, New Jersey. He received an undergraduate degree in architecture from Columbia University (1940) and a master's degree from the Massachusetts Institute of Technology (1941). The architectural firm he founded in Philadelphia in 1946, Vincent G. Kling and Associates, went through a series of restructurings until 1986 when the Kling Partnership (architects), Kling-Lindquist, Incorporated (engineers), and Kling Interior Design merged to become the Kling-Lindquist Partnership, Incorporated. Principals Vincent G. Kling retired in the mid-1980s and Fred H. Lindquist in 1991.

The architectural division has won numerous awards including: National Honor Awards of the American Institute of Architects for the Lankenau Hospital in Overbrook, Pennsylvania (1954), the Molecular Electronic Laboratory of the Westinghouse Corporation in Baltimore (1964), the Philip T. Sharples Dining Hall at Swarthmore College (1966), the Municipal Services Building in Philadelphia (1967), and the Technical Center of the Union Carbide Corporation in Tarrytown,

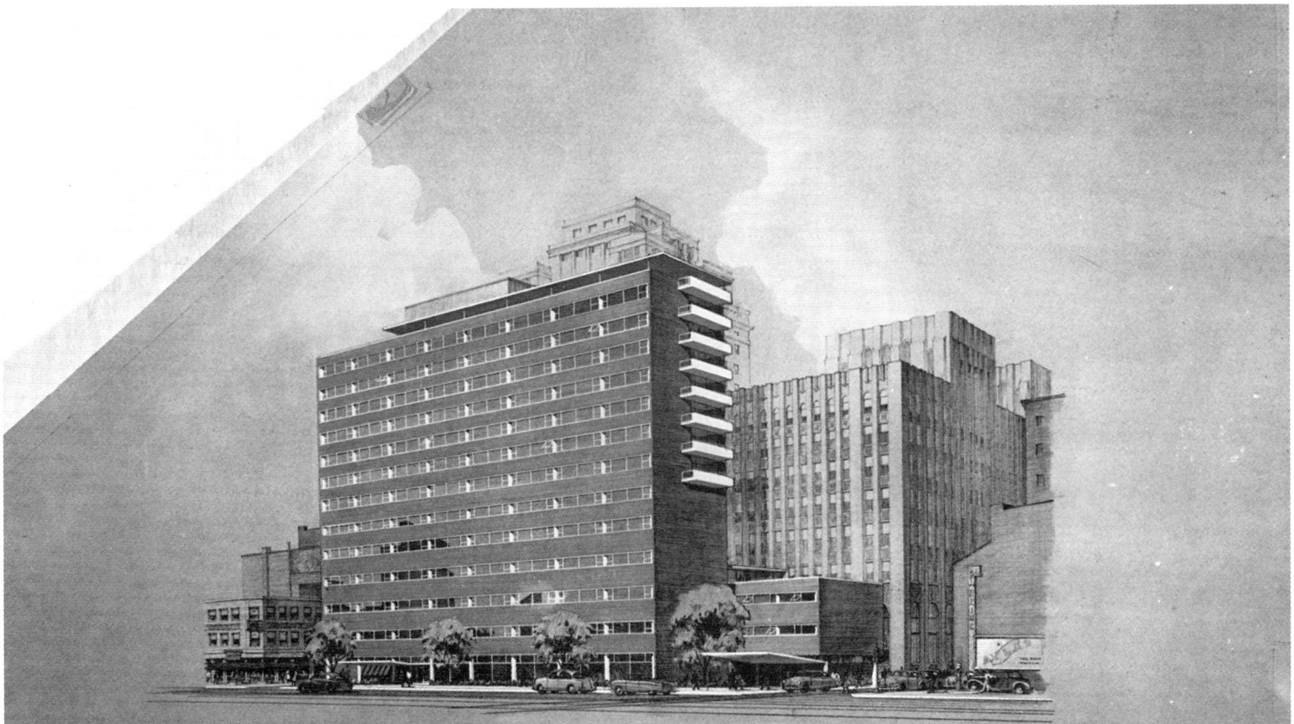

New York (1970); and Award Citations from the magazine *Progressive Architecture* for the Transportation Center, Penn Center, Philadelphia (1955), and the national headquarters of the Monsanto Company in St. Louis (1956).

Vincent G. Kling has been a trustee of Columbia University, the University of Pennsylvania, and the Episcopal Academy in Merion, Pennsylvania. He is the recipient of the Samuel F. B. Morse Medal of the National Academy of Design (1968, 1972), the gold medal and Diploma of Honor of the City Council of Quito, Ecuador (1961), and the Philadelphia Arts Festival Award in Architecture (1959). In 1965 he was president of the Philadelphia chapter of the American Institute of Architects.

Portrait of Percival E. Foerderer

(See color plate)

PERCIVAL EDWARD FOERDERER (1885-1969)
By Sir Gerald Festus Kelly (1879-1972)

Oil on canvas
1959
38 1/2 x 29 1/2 in.

Signed and dated lower right: "Kelly 1959"
Exhibition: London, *Summer Exhibition*, Royal Academy, 1959

Given in 1962 by Mr. and Mrs. Percival E. Foerderer
Accession number: 1962+e.P.02

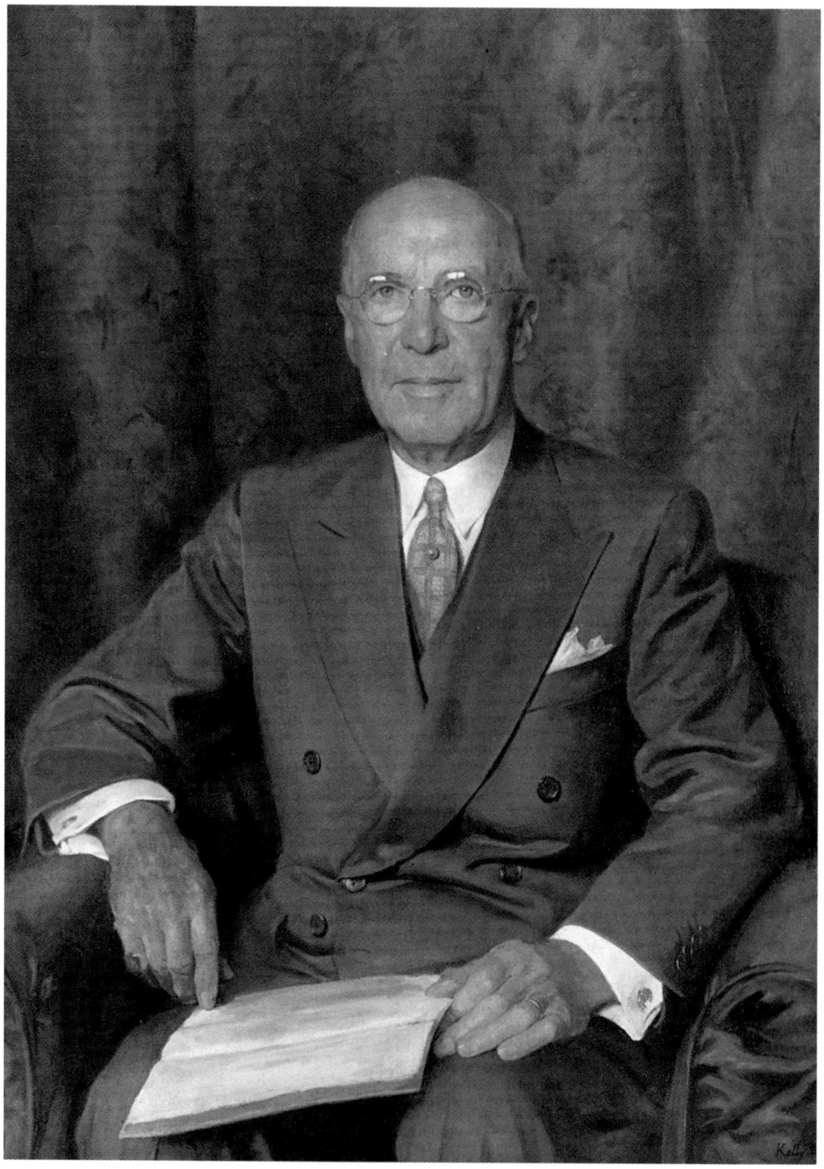

When Percival E. Foerderer resigned as chairman of the Jefferson Medical College board of trustees in 1962, other board members could think of no tangible gift that would express their appreciation for his exceptional leadership and contributions, and so decided unanimously to rename the New Pavilion in his honor.

He had been elected to the board in 1928, was chairman of the finance committee from 1932 to 1937 and chairman of the college committee from 1938 to 1950, and was named chairman of the board in 1950. Besides overseeing the architectural expansion and rehabilitation projects mentioned above and enlarging the clinical and basic research facilities, Foerderer was credited with uniting the efforts of trustees, administrators, faculty, and staff by means of his modest demeanor and warm but forthright personality.

In 1951 Jefferson awarded Foerderer an honorary doctor of laws degree. Upon his retirement in January 1962 Foerderer was presented with a silver tray signed by members of the executive faculty, and an illuminated manuscript signed by the trustees, president, dean, and medical director of the hospital. Three years later "Mr. Jefferson" received the alumni achievement award, a rare honor for a nonphysician.

The extraordinary commitment to Jefferson of the Foerderer family was amplified considerably by the creation of the Percival E. and Ethel Brown Foerderer Foundation in 1962. While this foundation also supported other Philadelphia educational, health care, social welfare, and cultural institutions, Jefferson was the primary beneficiary. Thomas Jefferson University presented its Cornerstone Award to the Foerderer Foundation in 1981 in appreciation for its generosity.

In 1994 the Foerderer Foundation transferred its assets to the endowment fund of Thomas Jefferson University. The nine million dollar gift provided perpetual endowment for three of the foundation's longstanding programs: the Foerderer fellowships in the College of Graduate Studies which support about twelve scholars annually; the annual Martin E. Rehfuss lectureship; and grants for biomedical investigations.

The foundation has also supported the Health Careers Guidance Clinic of the College of Health Professions and helps to attract and retain disadvantaged students from minority backgrounds. During a severe nursing shortage the foundation supported reorientation programs for nurses returning to the field after an absence of several years and greatly reduced the nursing turnover rate.

Percival E. Foerderer was a native Philadelphian, born in 1885. His father was a businessman and United States congressman. He was educated at the William Penn Charter School and the University of Pennsylvania. The elder Foerderer's untimely death at age forty-two forced the son to leave college after only one year to tend to family business.

But the young man had earlier worked as an assistant superintendent in his father's leather business. The company was widely known for its patent of a chrome tanning process for a product called Vici Kid, used to make shoes. He rose rapidly in the firm to become vice president in 1907, and then succeeded his uncle as president the following year. Under his administration the business prospered and become the largest factory of its kind in the country. When the business climate became unfavorable in the 1930s Foerderer dissolved the company.

He was recognized throughout the city as an industrialist, philanthropist, and civic leader, and was a trustee or director on the boards of the Pennsylvania Forge Company, the Land Title Bank and Trust Company, the Philadelphia Chamber of Commerce, and the Philadelphia Bourse. He was chairman of the Pennsylvania Mutual Life Insurance Company, the Tanners Council of America, and the Republican Finance Committee of Metropolitan Philadelphia.

Foerderer was a director of the Eastern Pennsylvania Psychiatric Institute, the Institute for Cancer Research, and the Associated Hospital Services of Philadelphia; and a trustee of the Drexel Institute of Technology, Moore Institute of Art (now Moore College of Art and Design), and Magee Memorial Hospital. During World War I he served on the Council for National Defense. He rose to the rank of lieutenant colonel in the Army Specialist Corps in World War II, and later was Philadelphia chairman of the postwar National Council for Economic Development.

Mr. and Mrs. Foerderer entertained Jefferson trustees and faculty regularly at their palatial, Spanish Revival home, "La Ronda." The 249-acre estate in Bryn Mawr, Pennsylvania was maintained by more than two dozen servants.

The family's largesse even extended to the donation of portraits of Percival and Ethel Foerderer. When the New Pavilion was renamed in 1962 Jefferson trustees discussed commissioning a sculpted portrait of Percival Foerderer for the lobby, but instead Mr. and Mrs. Foerderer generously presented an oil portrait that had been painted in 1959 by Sir Gerald F. Kelly. Their choice of the famed English portraitist assured that the portrait subject and artist were of comparable professional and social rank.

In the life-sized, two-thirds-length portrait Percival Foerderer sits in an upholstered armchair. He looks straight at the viewer with a solemn but confident expression. He is elegantly attired in a three-piece, gray, double-breasted suit and plaid necktie, a pearl tie pin, gold cuff links, and two gold rings. The green armchair contrasts effectively with the pinkish-mauve curtain which is decorated with a subtly figured pattern and arranged in graceful folds.

The sitter's beautifully rendered face and hands are solid and three-dimensional, demonstrating the artist's command of the underlying anatomy. One senses that the subject is a powerful and commanding personage, not only from his erect posture, confident expression, and elegant attire, but also from his placement on the canvas. His body authoritatively fills the width of the canvas in the foreground and confronts the viewer directly.

The subject's right index finger points to a document, the only attribute in the painting. Board of trustees minutes of February 5, 1962 explain its significance, "The painting is particularly appropriate since Mr. Foerderer holds in his hands the legal documents relating to the establishment here at Jefferson of the Strickler-Root Memorial Obstetric and Gynecologic Research Unit which papers had been mailed to him in London for signature."

Sir Gerald Festus Kelly was a self-taught portrait, figure, and landscape painter who became outstandingly successful. In spite of a bohemian life he was a member of the art establishment and a noted proponent of arts causes.[1] Among his portrait subjects were fashionable artists and writers, entertainers, socialites, and aristocrats including T. S. Eliot, Ralph Vaughan Williams, W. Somerset Maugham (eighteen portraits), and Hugh Walpole.

Kelly was born in 1879 in London and spent his boyhood in Camberwell where his father was vicar of St. Giles. He traced his ancestry back to tenth-century Ireland. His education at Eton was interrupted by illness but he took a degree in 1897 at Trinity Hall, Cambridge University. He decided to become a painter and moved to Paris in 1901. Through an introduction to the art dealer Paul Durand-Ruel he met many of the leading contemporary French and English artists. Though he studied independently rather than at an art school or artist's atelier, he met with almost immediate success and showed two early portraits at the Paris Salon of 1902.

He soon developed his own meticulous painting style and gained an influential patron, Sir Hugh Lane, an Irish collector, dealer, and critic. William Somerset Maugham became one of his closest friends and many characters in his novels bear a resemblance to Kelly. In 1904 Kelly became a member of the Salon d'Automne and he began to exhibit in London. He was a founding member of the Modern Portrait Painters Society in 1907 and the National Portrait Society in 1910.

Kelly spent a year in Burma painting landscapes and Burmese dancers after being deserted by his dancer girlfriend. He settled in London permanently in 1909 and made many study trips to Spain. He joined the intelligence department of the admiralty during World War I, and in 1920 married a young model. His usual working attire for painting and dress for lively dinner parties at his home was a "boiler suit" (overalls).

Gerald F. Kelly first exhibited at the Royal Academy in 1909. He was elected an academician in 1930 and worked as a visiting teacher at the Royal Academy Schools. As a member of the Royal Fine Arts Commission from 1938 to 1943, he offered strenuous opinions about over-cleaning of paintings in the National Gallery. In 1945 he was named the honorary surveyor of the Dulwich College Picture Gallery. In 1949 at age seventy he was elected president of the Royal Academy where he organized loan exhibitions. He became a narrator of related BBC television programs, both shocking and delighting viewers with his salty comments. He was invested as Knight Commander of the Victorian Order in 1955.

Other honors include: academician of the Royal Hibernian Academy (1914), honorary member of the Royal Society of the Arts (1950), honorary fellow of the Royal Institute of British Architects (1950), and honorary doctor of laws from Cambridge and from Trinity College, Dublin University (1950).

In 1938 he was commissioned to paint the state portraits of King George VI and Queen Elizabeth on the recommendation of Sir Kenneth Clark, Surveyor of the King's Pictures. The portraits were nine feet high and six feet wide, and intended to hang in the private apartments at Windsor Castle. They were not actually completed until 1945 when they were exhibited at the Royal Academy. Gerald F. Kelly was knighted by the king in 1945.

In a remarkably productive career he continued to turn out detailed likenesses of fashionable sitters into his seventies and eighties (including Percival Foerderer's). The Diploma Gallery of the Royal Academy held a retrospective exhibition of Kelly's portraits in 1957. His works are included in many public and private collections throughout Great Britain.

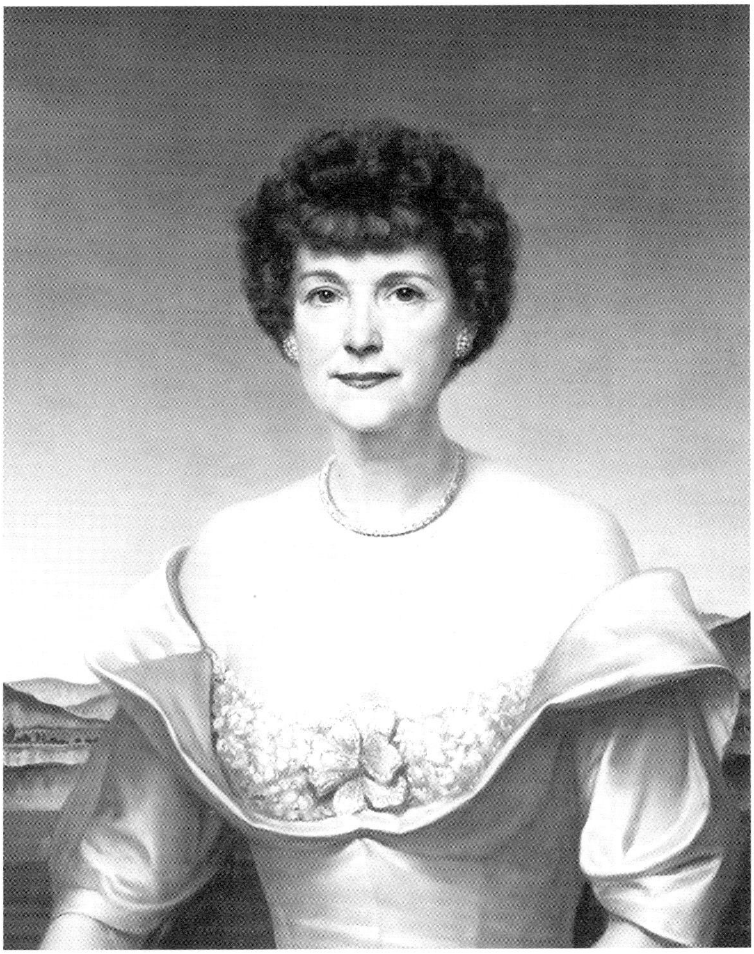

Portrait of Ethel T. B. (Mrs. Percival E.) Foerderer

ETHEL TILLYER BROWN (MRS. PERCIVAL E.) FOERDERER (1886-1981)
By Gerald Leslie Brockhurst (1890-1978)

Oil on canvas
1950
30 x 25 in.

Signed and dated lower left:
"BROCKHURST/1950"

Given in 1983 by Shirley Foerderer (Mrs. Charles) Ames, daughter of the subject
Accession number: 1983+e.P.04

Mrs. Percival E. Foerderer, the former Ethel Tillyer Brown, shared many of the ideals of her husband and was noted for civic and philanthropic works of her own.

Born in 1885 in Philadelphia, she was the daughter of a textile machinery manufacturer and traced her lineage directly to Thomas Brown who came to America from England in 1637. She was educated at Friends Select School and Miss Hill's Private School in Philadelphia and Ingleside Preparatory school at New Milford, Connecticut. She married Percival Foerderer in 1910. They enjoyed frequent trips to Europe, and she knew London and Rome as well as Philadelphia.[2] Their cosmopolitan travels probably account for their commissions of English artists to paint their portraits.

Ethel Foerderer first joined the women's board at Jefferson Hospital in 1930 and served as president from 1947 to 1952. In addition to her innovative ideas for fund-raising events, renovation and furnishing of hospital buildings, and funding for nursing scholarships, she also introduced a voice for the women's board on Jefferson's board of trustees. Her benevolence was not limited to Jefferson Hospital. Mrs. Foerderer was also active at the Hospital of the University of Pennsylvania and Bryn Mawr Hospital. During World War II she participated in affairs of the Seamen's Church Institute, the Navy League Service, and the War Finance Program.

Ethel Brown Foerderer was one of the guiding forces of the Foerderer Foundation. A resolution by Jefferson's board following her death in 1981 said that she was an "intellectually alert and inquisitive lady [by] whom the most visionary project at Jefferson was fully understood and...evaluated."

On September 26, 1983 was the dedication of Jefferson's Rehabilitation Travel/Test Solarium, a facility which provided simulated training conditions for patients with physical handicaps. It had been funded by a gift from the estate of Ethel Brown Foerderer, and a plaque to her memory was unveiled. A second event that day was the presentation of Ethel Foerderer's portrait by her daughter, Shirley Foerderer Ames. The family's only stipulation for the gift was that the portraits of Percival and Ethel Foerderer should hang together.

The portrait by Gerald L. Brockhurst is a romantic depiction of the subject in front of a stone ledge with an imaginary landscape behind, a Renaissance convention. Her body is half length and slightly smaller than life-sized, and positioned frontally. She gazes directly at the viewer with luminous brown eyes and bright red lips that impart a poised and confident expression. Her captivating features are crowned by softly curled, dark brown hair with bangs. She wears an elegant, silvery, off-the-shoulder gown with elbow length sleeves. The inset bodice with a center rose is encrusted with sequins and beads. Her costume is completed with diamond earrings and choker.

The distant landscape, low on the horizon, includes a river, shore, trees, and rolling hills. The expansive sky shades softly downward from bluish-green to a glowing, pale cream color, complementing the sitter's fair skin tones and glittering dress. The painting's meticulous surface features brush strokes that are very smooth and polished.

Gerald Leslie Brockhurst was born in Birmingham, England in 1890. He entered the Birmingham School of Art at age twelve, and continued his art training at the school of the Royal Academy in London when he was seventeen.[3] There his paintings and drawings were recognized with several prizes including the Landseer Studentship, the Armitage Medal, the British Institute Studentship, and the gold medal. A traveling scholarship allowed him to go to the Continent to study the old masters in Paris and Milan.

Although primarily self-taught in the technique of etching, he is perhaps remembered today as much for his exquisite portrait etchings executed in the 1920s and 1930s as for his oil portraits. He was elected a fellow of the Royal Society of Painter Etchers in 1921, a member of the Royal Society of Portrait Painters in 1923, and a royal academician in 1937.

In the twenties and thirties he exhibited frequently in London and at several Carnegie Institute international exhibitions in Pittsburgh. Dealers in London, New York, Philadelphia, Chicago, and Detroit promoted his etchings. In the mid-1930s exhibitions of his etchings were held at the Carnegie Institute, the Brooklyn Museum, and the Toledo Museum of Art.

Brockhurst came to the United States in 1939 for the first time to serve as a juror for the Carnegie Institute international exhibition and to attend a show of his paintings at the Knoedler Gallery in New York. This exhibition included portraits of the Duchess of Windsor and Mrs. Paul Mellon, assuring his reputation here as a painter of socially prominent women. He settled in New Jersey with his second wife and never returned to England.

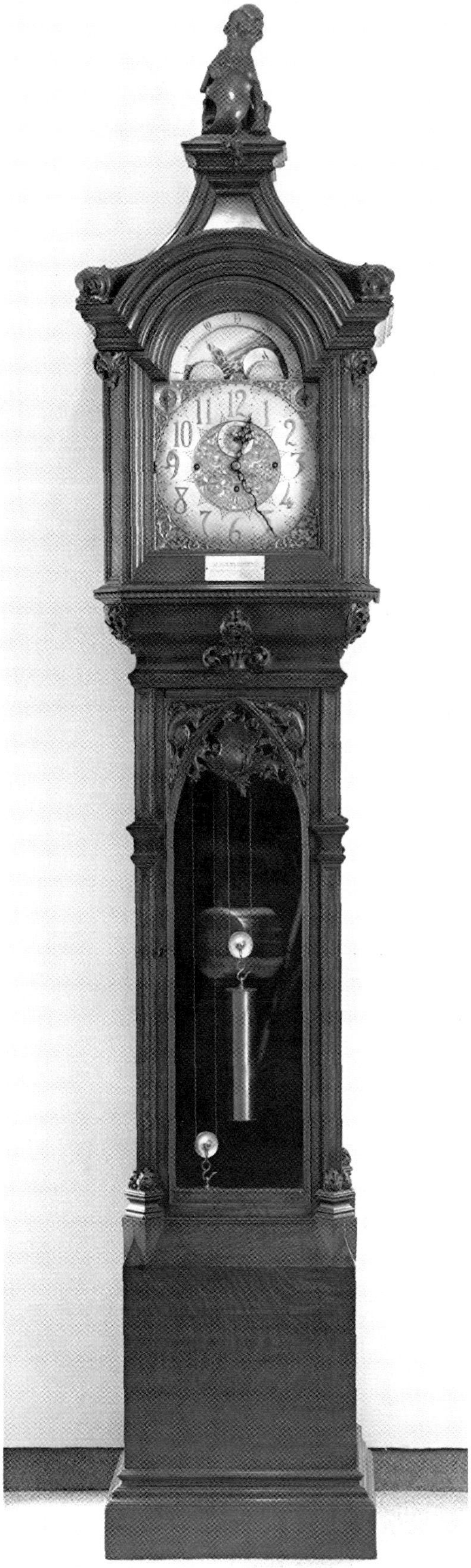

Tall Case Clock

(See color plate)

TALL CASE CLOCK
Works by Elliott of London (?)

Oak
1890-1920
115 1/2 x 24 x 20 in.

Given in 1963 by Mr. and Mrs. Percival E. Foerderer
Accession number: 1963+e.DA.02

Two prized examples of decorative arts at Thomas Jefferson University also were given by Mr. and Mrs. Percival E. Foerderer. In 1963 they gave a magnificent tall case clock which in recent years has adorned the president's office.

Stylistically eclectic, the oak clock combines elements of Gothic and Renaissance Revivals with Queen Anne. The works are probably by Elliott of London and the ornately carved case is English or American. The domical hood is surmounted by a recessed mansard plinth whose corners project out into dolphin terminals supporting a lion and shield finial. The dial is brass with a steel chapter ring and brass numerals, enclosing a chased field with a floral bouquet. The dial is surrounded by four scrolled brass spandrels of leafy vine work; the upper two contain inset registers pertaining to the Whittington and Westminster coil chimes.

The front and sides of the trunk have Gothic arch panels carved elaborately with tattered leafage. The glass front door has spandrels at the top carved with fantastic beasts flanking a ribbon and leaf motif that form a cartouche resembling the shield held by the lion above. The corners of the glass door are square pilasters with carved leafage at the bottom. The straight rectangular base is on a stepped base molding.

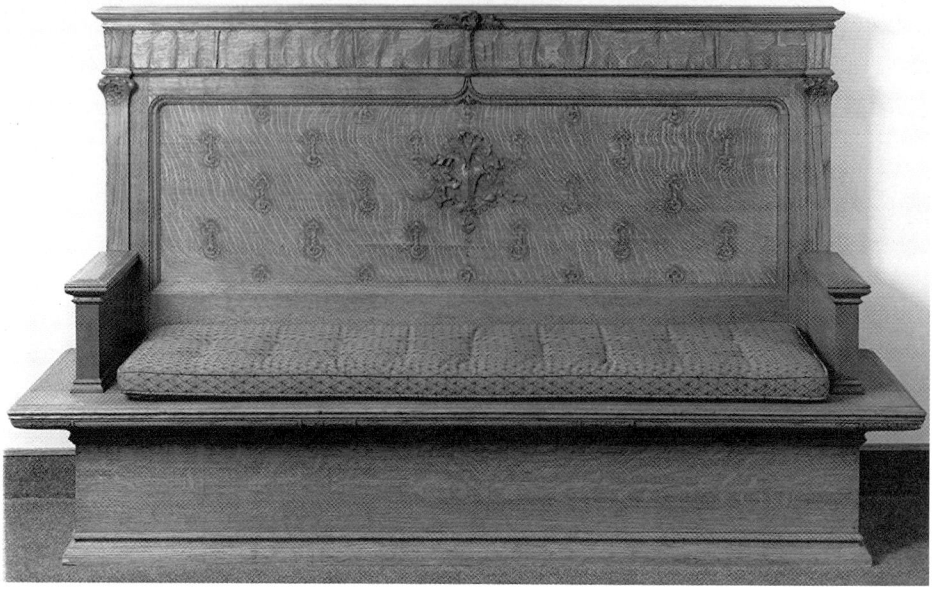

Bench

BENCH
By unknown maker

Oak
1880-90
45 1/2 x 75 1/2 x 20 3/4 in.

Received ca. 1970 from office of Percival E. Foerderer
Accession number: 1970+c.DA.01

About a year after Percival Foerderer died in 1969 a decorative oak bench was rescued from a trash heap at the Fidelity Bank Building after removal from his office at the Foerderer Foundation.[4] It was brought to the Jefferson campus by Dr. Francis J. Sweeney (JMC 1955), then medical director of the hospital. In recent years it has been located in the anteroom of the president's office.

The carved oak Victorian bench was probably made in America (or less likely England) around 1880-90. Its carving is similar to that on the Foerderer clock. The bench's straight molded cornice is centered with carved foliage above a deep frieze with planked, undulating ribbon work. The cornice is supported by pilasters with scrolling leaves. The inset back panel is carved with a center shield-form cartouche enveloped by tattered leaves and ribbon, and surrounded by a repeat pattern of key-shaped trefoils with spirals. Low straight arms flank the hinged seat lid raised on a molded straight base.

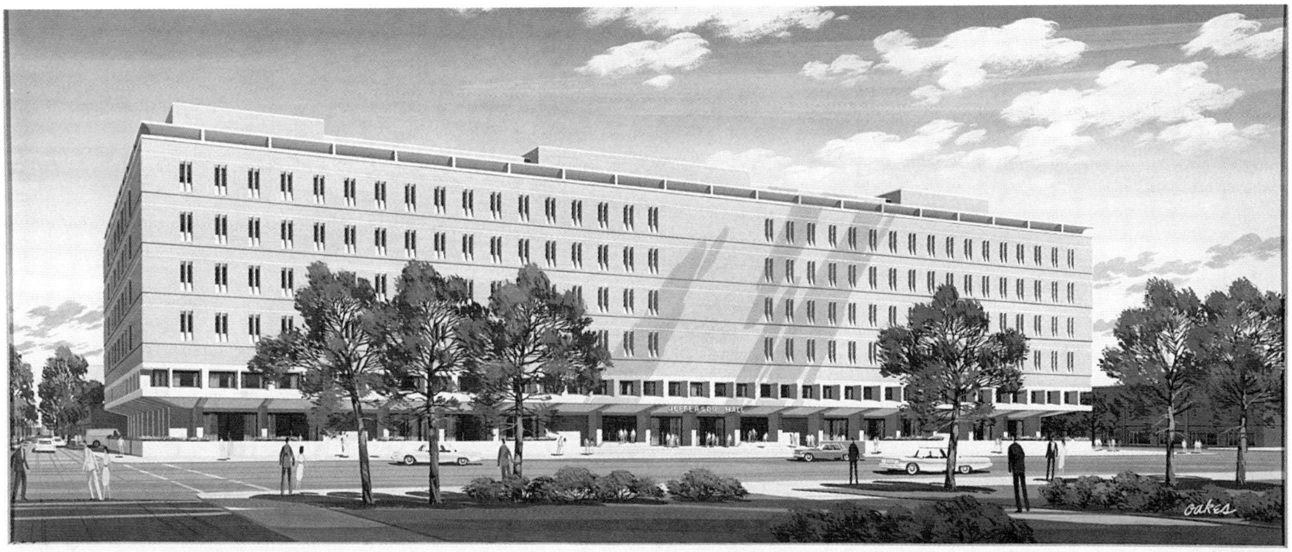

Jefferson Hall - Jefferson Medical College
Philadelphia, Pa.

Vincent G. Kling FAIA
Architect

Jefferson Alumni Hall

JEFFERSON ALUMNI HALL
Building by Vincent G. Kling & Associates
Opened 1968

Architectural rendering
By "Oakes" for Vincent G. Kling & Associates
Gouache on paper mounted on board
Ca. 1963
Image size: 14 1/2 x 33 1/4 in.
Board size: 24 x 42 in.

Signed lower right: "oakes"
Inscriptions below image: on left "Jefferson Hall-Jefferson Medical College/Philadelphia, Pa."; on right "Vincent G. Kling FAIA/Architect"

Ordered ca. 1963 by JMC
Accession number: 1963+c.D.01

Jefferson Hall was opened in time for the start of the school year in 1968, dedicated the following March, and renamed Jefferson Alumni Hall in 1971. Forming the southern boundary of the campus, the building occupies two adjoining one-acre sites on the south side of Locust Street between Tenth and Eleventh Streets. The architectural plan turns inward toward east and west open-air atria which are visible from large windows in the hallways.

The orange brick and concrete facade features a set-back ground floor with large windows and entrance stairs. The mezzanine level has large horizontal windows. The upper floors have rows of double vertical windows and overhang the entrance by concrete supporting pillars that lift the mass off the ground. The penthouse is topped by a coved roof line. Planters at the entrance and flowering pear trees at the curb soften the severe regularity of the block-long building.

Student commons facilities are located on the main and basement floors. The mezzanine floor has meeting rooms, offices, and the faculty club. The upper five floors contain teaching and research facilities for the basic sciences. Animal quarters are located in the penthouse which includes a powerful venting system. The building houses several auditoriums, and an escalator as well as an elevator.

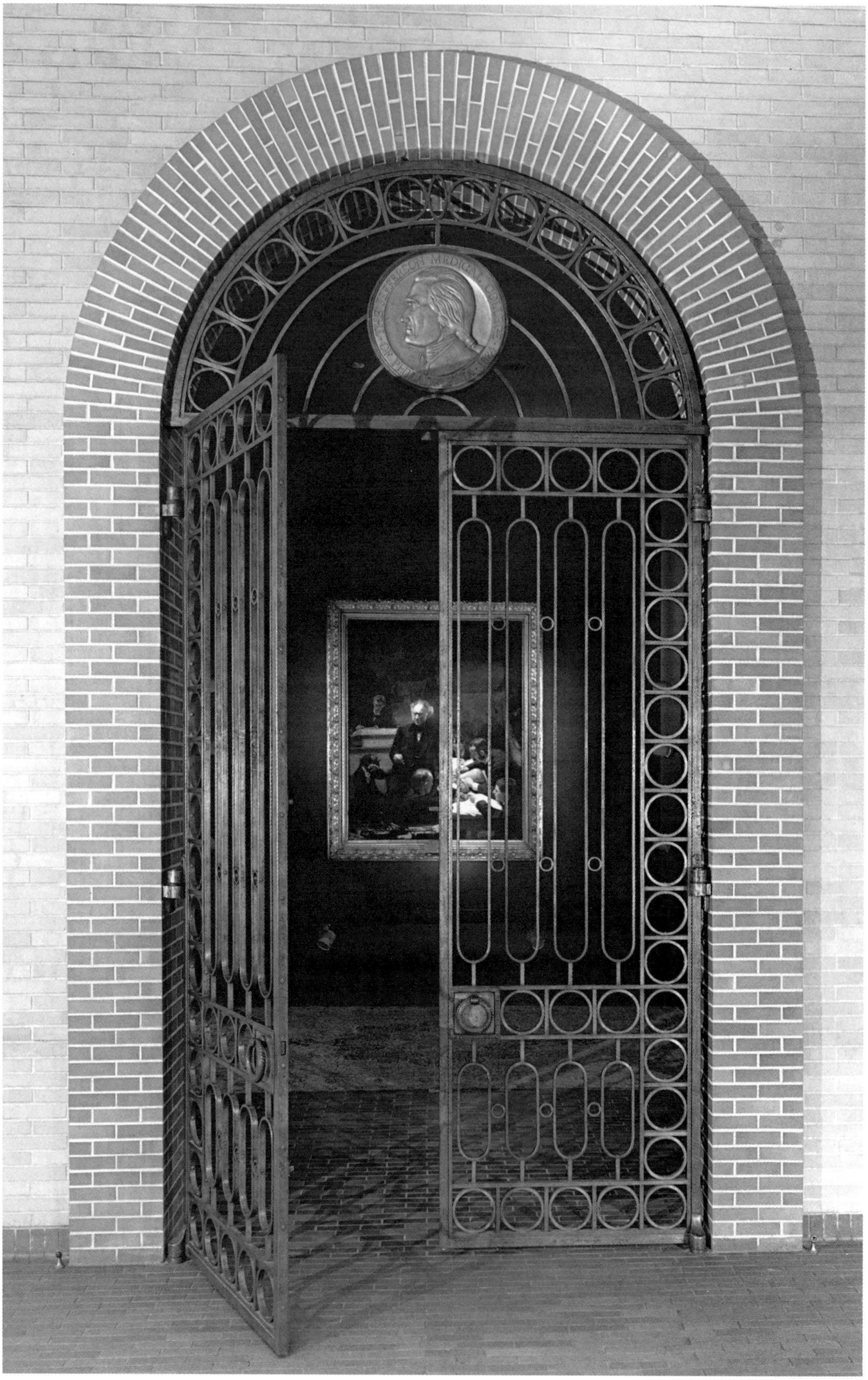

Alumni Gates of Eakins Gallery

ALUMNI GATES OF EAKINS GALLERY
By Samuel Yellin Metalworkers

Iron
1982
187 1/2 x 96 1/2 x 7 in.

Signed on back of handles: "YELLIN"

Given in 1982 by JMC alumni association
Accession number: 1982+e.DA.02

As noted above *The Gross Clinic* and other Thomas Eakins portraits were relocated to Jefferson Alumni Hall in 1968. The definitive installation of the paintings took place in 1982 in the elegant, specially designed Eakins Gallery on the west side of the ground floor.

The spacious, high-ceilinged main gallery is entered through the Alumni Gates from the Eakins Lounge, an adjoining gathering place. The stately wrought iron gates by the famed workshop of Samuel A. Yellin were a gift from Jefferson's alumni association. The artistry of Yellin's prolific and imaginative decorative ironwork and his influence with architects and patrons had been almost singlehandedly responsible for a rebirth of hand-wrought ornamental ironwork in America before World War II.

The Alumni Gates, over fifteen feet high and eight feet wide, are set into a dark orange brick archway. They are made in three sections comprised of matching rectangular doors beneath a semicircular lunette, made of unembellished, slender, square members. The open-work design repeats geometric patterns of circles, squares, semicircles, and rounded rectangles. Centered in the lunette is a large round profile medallion of Thomas Jefferson.

Samuel A. Yellin was born in Galicia, Poland in 1885 and apprenticed at age eleven to a Russian blacksmith. By the age of seventeen he was a master craftsman and spent the next five years working in Belgium, Germany, France, and England. Soon after arriving in Philadelphia in 1906, he enrolled at the Pennsylvania Museum School of Industrial Art where he so impressed the faculty that he was asked to organize classes in wrought iron and taught there until 1919. An exhibition of his metalwork was sponsored by school alumni in 1911.

About 1909 Yellin established his first small studio in a fourth-floor attic over a surgical instrument manufacturer. His first real break was winning a commission to design a small gate for the J. P. Morgan estate on Long Island in 1911. Yellin rapidly attracted so many important commissions that by the 1920s he was employing over two hundred craftsmen. They worked at sixty forges in an elegant, two-story Spanish style building in West Philadelphia. Yellin's firm was selected by many of the most prominent American architects to provide decorative gateways and doors, window grilles, balconies, fireplace screens, weathervanes, furniture, altar screens, hardware, and signposts for diverse buildings.

In addition to private homes of American industrialists, examples of public works are at the Federal Reserve Bank, the Frick Collection, and the Cathedral of St. John the Divine in New York; the Grace Cathedral in San Francisco; the National Cathedral in Washington, D.C.; Yale, Harvard, Princeton, and Northwestern Universities; and the Public Library and Institute of Arts in Detroit. Notable works in the Philadelphia area are at the Curtis Institute of Music, the Packard Building, St. Mark's Church, Bryn Mawr and Swarthmore Colleges, the University of Pennsylvania, and the Washington Memorial Chapel at Valley Forge.

In addition to Samuel Yellin's regular teaching duties as visiting professor of design and craftsmanship in the School of Fine Arts at the University of Pennsylvania, he opened his atelier to all who wanted to learn about the contemporary crafts revival.

Yellin received the Boston Architectural Award, Philadelphia's Bok Civic Award, and the Alumni Medal of the Pennsylvania Museum and School of Industrial Art, and was similarly honored by the Art Institute of Chicago, the American Institute of Architects, and the Architectural League of New York.

Samuel A. Yellin died in 1940 at the age of fifty-four. But the Samuel Yellin Metalworkers Company continued under the direction of his son, Harvey Z. Yellin, until his death in 1985, and the tradition was carried on for many years by Harvey Yellin's wife, Marian, and their daughter, Clare. In 1985 a traveling exhibition entitled *Samuel Yellin: Metalworker* was organized by the alumni association of the Philadelphia College of Art.

Lavar Kirman Rug

LAVAR KIRMAN RUG
Iranian

Wool
1880-1900
164 x 122 in.

Given in 1982 by Mrs. Thomas Laffey Jr.
Accession number: 1982+e.DA.01

In 1982 Mrs. Thomas Laffey Jr., a member of the women's board of Thomas Jefferson University Hospital, donated a late-nineteenth-century Lavar Kirman carpet to decorate the Eakins Gallery. Lavar is a town near Kirman in Southeast Iran (formerly Persia).

The rug is of low wool pile woven with "Persian" (asymmetrical) knots upon a cotton foundation ending in a close-clipped warp fringe. The ivory ground has a traditional centered medallion and surrounding foliage in bright rose, blue-green, gold, ivory, and navy colors. The curvilinear, lobed medallion has radiating palmettes anchored by large lancehead palmettes, enveloped by curving flowering branches of assorted trees and paisley designs.

The central area is framed with an ivory primary border of stylized, triple petalled flowers on an undulating vine, flanked by two pairs of guard borders comprising a pair of red secondary borders, flanked by ivory tertiary borders, all decorated with flowering vines. All are framed by a narrow red perimeter.

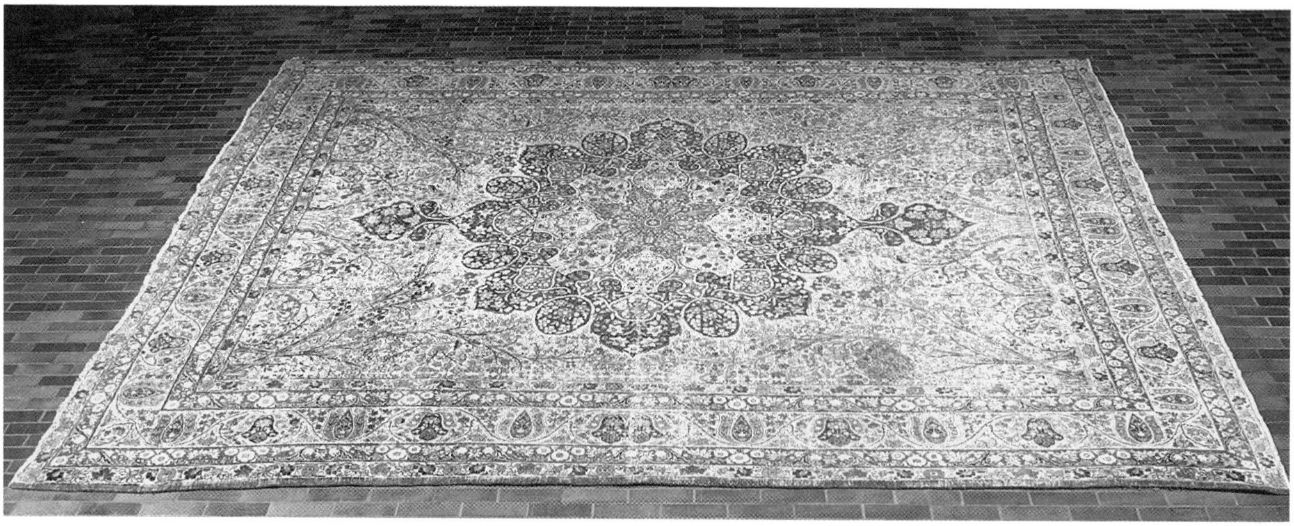

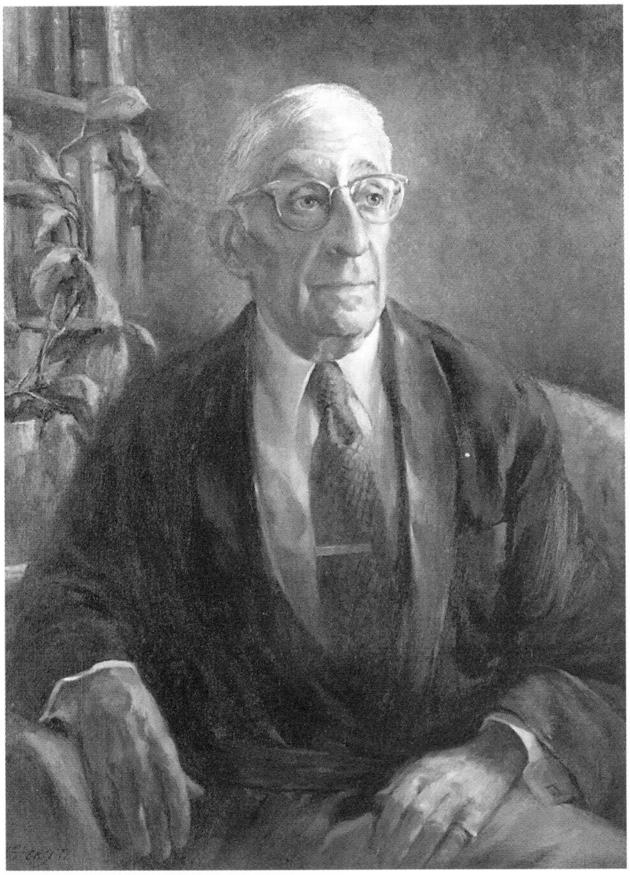

Portrait of D. Hays Solis-Cohen

DAVID HAYS SOLIS-COHEN (1887-1978)
By Katharine Shelden Ferg (b. 1914)

Oil on canvas
1971
32 1/4 x 25 1/4 in.

Signed and dated: "K. S. FERG '71"

Given in 1971 by Nelson J. Luria and the late Herbert L. Luria
Accession number: 1971+e.P.03

Another distinguished member of the Jefferson Medical College board of trustees in the postwar era was D. Hays Solis-Cohen, Esq., a trustee from 1951 until his death in 1978. For over a century family members had served the college with distinction including his father Dr. Solomon Solis-Cohen and his uncle Dr. Jacob da Silva Solis-Cohen. D. Hays's brother Dr. Leon Solis-Cohen was a member of the Jefferson class of 1912.

Descended from a pre-Revolutionary family, D. Hays Solis-Cohen was born in 1887 in Philadelphia. He attended the Wharton School of the University of Pennsylvania and obtained a law degree from the university in 1909. He became a senior partner in the prominent Philadelphia law firm of Wolf, Block, Schorr and Solis-Cohen. He was a leader in civic affairs and Jewish philanthropy. Solis-Cohen was a governor of the Philadelphia Bar Association and a director of the Lawyers Club of Philadelphia. He was a director of the Horn and Hardart Company of Philadelphia and New York, Luria Brothers and Company, Bankers Securities Corporation, Andrew James Investment Company, William Goldman Theaters, Wilkening Manufacturing Company, and the Booth and Flinn Company, Pittsburgh. He was president of Congregation Mikveh Israel, vice president of the American Council for Judaism, and devoted to the advance of Jewish education at Dropsie College and Gratz College.

Like his father and uncle before him who had received honorary degrees from Jefferson Medical College, D. Hays Solis-Cohen was awarded a doctor of laws degree in 1965. It recognized his more than twenty years of service, especially in his capacity as chairman of the board's expansion and development committee.

A permanent and tangible reminder of his contributions to Jefferson Medical College was the naming of the D. Hays Solis-Cohen Auditorium in Jefferson Alumni Hall in 1968. As early as 1967 trustees had hoped that Solis-Cohen would be persuaded to sit for a portrait. He finally relented in 1970, but the work on the painting was delayed for nearly a year because of his frail health. Portraitist Katharine S. Ferg made five trips to Solis-Cohen's home, but found the attorney too ill to pose for more than ten minutes at a time. She completed the figure with the aid of photographs and the sitter's costume in her studio.

D. Hays Solis-Cohen is depicted two-thirds length and life-sized, seated in a bluish-gray, upholstered armchair and turned slightly to the right. His large blue eyes gaze thoughtfully, almost mournfully into the distance. Although the artist made an attempt to soften the ravages of illness, the subject's unusually narrow face is marked by an aquiline nose, wide mouth with thin lips, and signs of aging throughout. However, he is fashionably dressed in a blue dressing gown, gray trousers, white shirt, red-figured tie, and jewelry including tie clip, cuff links, and pinky ring. Behind the figure are book-lined shelves and a philodendron plant in a terra cotta planter.

The portrait of D. Hays Solis-Cohen joined those of his father and uncle outside the auditorium in a dedication ceremony on September 22, 1971. The portrait had been commissioned by Jefferson trustees with funds donated by Nelson J. Luria and his father Herbert Luria, friends of the subject.

Katharine Shelden Ferg is a Moorestown, New Jersey artist who graduated from Philadelphia's Moore Institute of Art and Design (now Moore College of Art and Design) where she won the George Elkins European fellowship for study in France, Italy, and Germany. Upon her return to the United States she conducted private painting classes in Philadelphia and New Jersey. Subsequently she worked for fifteen years as an advertising designer for the W. B. Saunders/C.B.S. Medical Publishers in Philadelphia. She has also exhibited paintings in local exhibitions and executed portraits of prominent men and women from Philadelphia and southern New Jersey.

Portrait of William W. Bodine Jr.

WILLIAM WARDEN BODINE Jr. (1918-83)
By George Augusta (b. 1922)

Oil on canvas
1966
40 1/2 x 32 1/2 in.

Signed and dated upper left: "G. Augusta/'66"

Given in 1966 by JMC trustees, faculty, and friends

Accession number: 1966+e.P.01

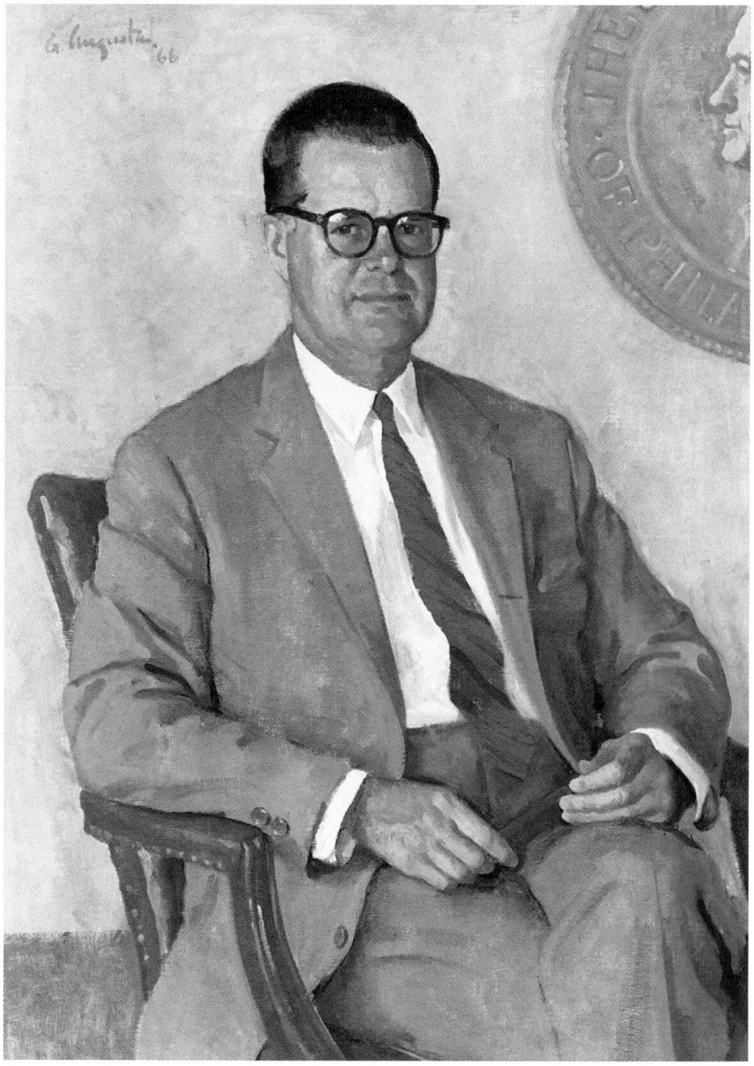

William W. Bodine Jr. was elected a Jefferson Medical College trustee in 1954 and five years later succeeded Vice Admiral James L. Kauffman as president of the college. Bodine continued in that post until 1966, was named a life trustee in 1970, and served as the fourth chairman of the board from 1970 to 1977.

At his death in 1983 sorrowful Jefferson trustees eulogized William W. Bodine, "A man of vision, he guided Jefferson Medical College into Thomas Jefferson University and was responsible for a major expansion program from 1957 to 1977."

During his association with Jefferson, construction included: the Stein Research Center, Jefferson Alumni Hall, Orlowitz Residence Hall, Scott Library Building, Edison Building, the university parking garage, Barringer Residence Hall, and the New Hospital (Gibbon Building). Unparalleled growth also included significant increases in the operating budget, total assets, and endowments. It was under Bodine's leadership that the board was expanded to admit three Jefferson alumni and one recent medical school graduate.

As early as the 1950s it was concluded that Jefferson Medical College should either seek university affiliation or develop into a university itself in order to survive increasingly complex demands and to avoid academic isolation. Although affiliation was explored with sixteen universities, most seriously with Pennsylvania State University, it was ultimately decided that Jefferson should develop university status alone.

The charter designating Thomas Jefferson University was granted by Pennsylvania's Department of Instruction in May 1969. The four divisions of Thomas Jefferson University were: Jefferson Medical College, the College of Graduate Studies (organized in 1949 in six basic science departments), the College of Allied Health Sciences, and Thomas Jefferson University Hospital.

The dynamic leader William W. Bodine Jr. was born in 1918, a descendant of an old Philadelphia family with a tradition of public service. His father was a lawyer and businessman. After graduating from St. Paul's School in Concord, New Hampshire, William Bodine attended Harvard University but left in 1940 to enlist in the U.S. Army. He followed in his father's footsteps by serving in the 108th Field Artillery and was sent to fight in Europe. As the commander of a tank-destroyer unit he and many of his men were wounded and taken prisoner at the Battle of the Bulge. Bodine escaped to the Allied lines and was hospitalized for five months after which he was assigned to General Dwight D. Eisenhower's staff as lieutenant colonel. He won several awards for heroism.

In the business world William W. Bodine was president of Arthur C. Kaufmann and Associates, a management consulting firm. Prior to that post he had been financial secretary of the Penn Mutual Life Insurance Company and assistant treasurer of the Tradesman's National Bank and Trust Company.

An obituary in the Philadelphia *Inquirer* called Bodine a superb organizer who was as enthusiastic about civic work as most men are about their sports and hobbies. He served as a board member or director of an exceptional number of institutions including: the United Fund, the Elwyn Institute, Temple University, Bryn Mawr Hospital, St. Christopher's Hospital for Children, the Mental Health Association of Southeastern Pennsylvania, the YMCA Foundation, the Philadelphia Urban Coalition, the Committee of Seventy, the Greater Philadelphia Partnership, the Chamber of Commerce of Philadelphia, the Greater Philadelphia Economic Development Coalition, WHYY-TV/Channel 12, the Philadelphia Drama Guild, the Free Library of Philadelphia, and the Smithsonian Institution in Washington, D.C.

Bodine was chairman of the board of the University City Science Center and president of the board of the Eastern Pennsylvania Psychiatric Association. He was perhaps best known to the general public as president of the World Affairs Council. Among Bodine's many awards were the Young Man of the Year of the Junior Chamber of Commerce of Philadelphia and the Good Citizenship Gold Medal of the Philadelphia Continental Chapter of the Sons of the American Revolution. He received an honorary doctor of laws degree from Jefferson in 1967.

William W. Bodine died of cancer in August 1983. In March 1987 Thomas Jefferson University dedicated a new facility at the Jefferson Hospital in his memory, the Bodine Center for Cancer Treatment, an advanced radiation therapy center.

When the Jefferson faculty proposed to commission a portrait upon Bodine's retirement in 1966, correspondence shows that he pursued the project with characteristic enthusiasm and efficiency. After receiving the pleasant news on July 7, 1966 from portrait committee chairman Dr. John H. Gibbon Jr., within five days Bodine had written to seven prominent Philadelphia area artists. He requested to see their portfolios and asked whether they could complete the portrait within six weeks in time for a reception on September 9 just prior to his departure for Europe.

The commission was not awarded to a Philadelphia artist because none whose work he admired was available on such short notice. But by July 18 Bodine reported to Dr. Gibbon that he had already reviewed the work of nine other portrait artists, and from this group had selected George Augusta of Norwood, Massachusetts and Kennebunkport, Maine. Augusta was willing to come to Philadelphia for eight sittings of two hours each and agreed to meet the September deadline.

Bodine set the artist up in an air-conditioned studio with a northern exposure in the boardroom of the Foerderer Pavilion. Bodine promised to hold his outside appointments to an "absolute minimum" for five days. He also stated that he wanted the portrait to be "informal and nonacademic." By September 1 Bodine wrote that the "mission was completed" during the week of August 15, that colleagues pronounced the portrait "a fine job," and that the painting was being photographed and framed.

William Bodine stipulated that his portrait be hung on the ground floor of Jefferson Alumni Hall after the building's projected opening in the summer of 1967. The painting then circulated around the campus for two decades and in 1987 was installed permanently in the Bodine Cancer Center.

In the two-thirds-length, life-sized portrait William W. Bodine is seated in a leather armchair with his legs crossed at the knee. His forearms rest on the chair arms and he holds a red pencil, suggesting administrative action. He wears a gray suit with white shirt and red and blue striped necktie. On the plaster wall one sees the lower left quadrant of a circular university plaque with the profile of Thomas Jefferson and some letters of the surrounding border: "THE T...OF PHILADE..."

The sitter's pleasant expression and direct gaze express confidence and accessibility. His dark hair and eyeglass frames contrast with the middle range of his warm skin tones and the bright reds of necktie and pencil. The artist has depicted a convincingly three-dimensional figure in a relaxed and engaging posture with quickly brushed and deft strokes that appear spontaneous and effortless.

George Augusta was born in Boston in 1922. He first became interested in painting during World War II while serving with the U.S. Army Signal Intelligence Service in Italy. He studied briefly in Florence and then privately from 1946 to 1950 with Boston artist Ernest Lee Major (1864-1950).

Augusta is most noted for portraits of distinguished public officials, university presidents, and prominent businessmen and their spouses including among others: Rosalynn Carter, Cyrus Vance, Warren Burger, Senator Morris Cotton of New Hampshire, Harvard University president Derek Bok, Wellesley College president Ruth Adams, Dr. and Mrs. An Wang of Wang Industries, and Henry M. Watts Jr., chairman of the board of the New York Stock Exchange.

William W. Bodine Jr. Fountain

WILLIAM W. BODINE Jr. FOUNTAIN ("OTTER FOUNTAIN")
By Henry Weber Mitchell (1915-80)

Bronze, rocks, granite, concrete, water
1978-79
79 x 178 x 178 in.

Cast at Battaglia Foundry, Milan

Commissioned in 1978 by TJU trustees
Accession number: 1979+e.S.01

The *William W. Bodine Jr. Fountain* by Henry W. Mitchell was dedicated on September 25, 1979. Located on the west side of the Scott Plaza, the sculptural fountain was created to comply with the Redevelopment Authority's one percent fine arts regulation for the newly constructed Barringer Residence Hall and the parking garage.

At the dedication ceremony Jefferson president Lewis W. Bluemle Jr., M.D., chairman of the board Frederic L. Ballard, and former chairman James M. Large credited William W. Bodine with revitalizing Jefferson with a leadership style that embodied "devotion, sound judgement, and courage, above all, courage." Bodine was presented with a bronze replica of the fountain's smallest otter.

The fountain consists of five bronze otters frolicking in streams of water rippling down the angled sides of a central pyramid of rocks set into an octagonal granite pool. One otter sunbathes at the top of the rocks, three others swim around the base, and one plays at the edge of the pool. The lithe marine mammals range in length from eighteen to thirty-nine inches. The rock formation is fifty-seven inches high. The fountain base is surrounded by two steps. On a sunny day light and shadows add to the playfulness of the construction, as does the sound of running water.

Henry Mitchell won a competition for this commission and the proposal he submitted delineated his choice of subject and his sensitivity to the Scott Plaza site:

> I have chosen otters as a subject first because of their love of fun and play, second because they are found in all latitudes and, third, because they are as at home in snow and ice as in water. Consequently, if the water must be shut off in freezing weather, they will look happy in winter.
>
> I have chosen the octagonal form as a traditional Renaissance shape to complement the lovely architecture of the Scott building. The profile has been deliberately kept low to avoid any conflict with Dr. Gross [bronze statue by Alexander Stirling Calder] and to be a pleasant surprise as one first comes over the Locust Street steps. The forty feet of wall holding the pool should provide a cool central spot for sitting or sunning.

For the five hundred guests attending the dedication Dr. Bluemle described the university's affection for the work that quickly became known as the "Otter Fountain":

> For faculty, secretaries, technicians, and others, it will be a refreshing oasis for a hurried lunch break. For relatives and friends of patients in our hospital...it may serve as a reminder that there is more to life than the pain and anguish they have recently felt...For the medical student returning late from Doc Watson's Pub after a tough biochemistry examination, it may be a place to receive consolation from a sympathetic otter.

When introduced at the dedication Henry W. Mitchell thanked the "marvelous gang of assistants who really put the whole thing together," recognizing the many individuals required to execute and install a major art work.

Best known as a sculptor of public animal monuments, Mitchell contributed more than twenty bronze works to sites in Philadelphia. His animals are abstractly simple in form and appear fun-loving, agile, and energetic, inviting interaction from viewers.

Besides the two monumental works at Jefferson, other favorite Philadelphia works include *Mother Hippopotamus, Baby Hippopotamus,* and *Leaping Impalas,* the latter a fountain sculpture, all at the Philadelphia Zoo; *Black Leopards* at Children's Hospital of Philadelphia; *Running Free,* a group of horses at Drexel University; *Hsieh Chai,* a mythical Chinese goat-dragon at the University of Pennsylvania School of Law; *Three Cats* for the Betsy Ross House Fountain; and *Courtship* for the Henry M. Phillips Memorial Fountain at the Philadelphia Museum of Art.

Henry W. Mitchell was born in Canton, Ohio in 1915 and graduated from St. George's School in Newport, Rhode Island and from Princeton University (1937). After college he returned to Canton to work as a designer of diesel engines for Hercules Motors. He served in the Coast Guard during World War II.

When a sculptor acquaintance encouraged him to

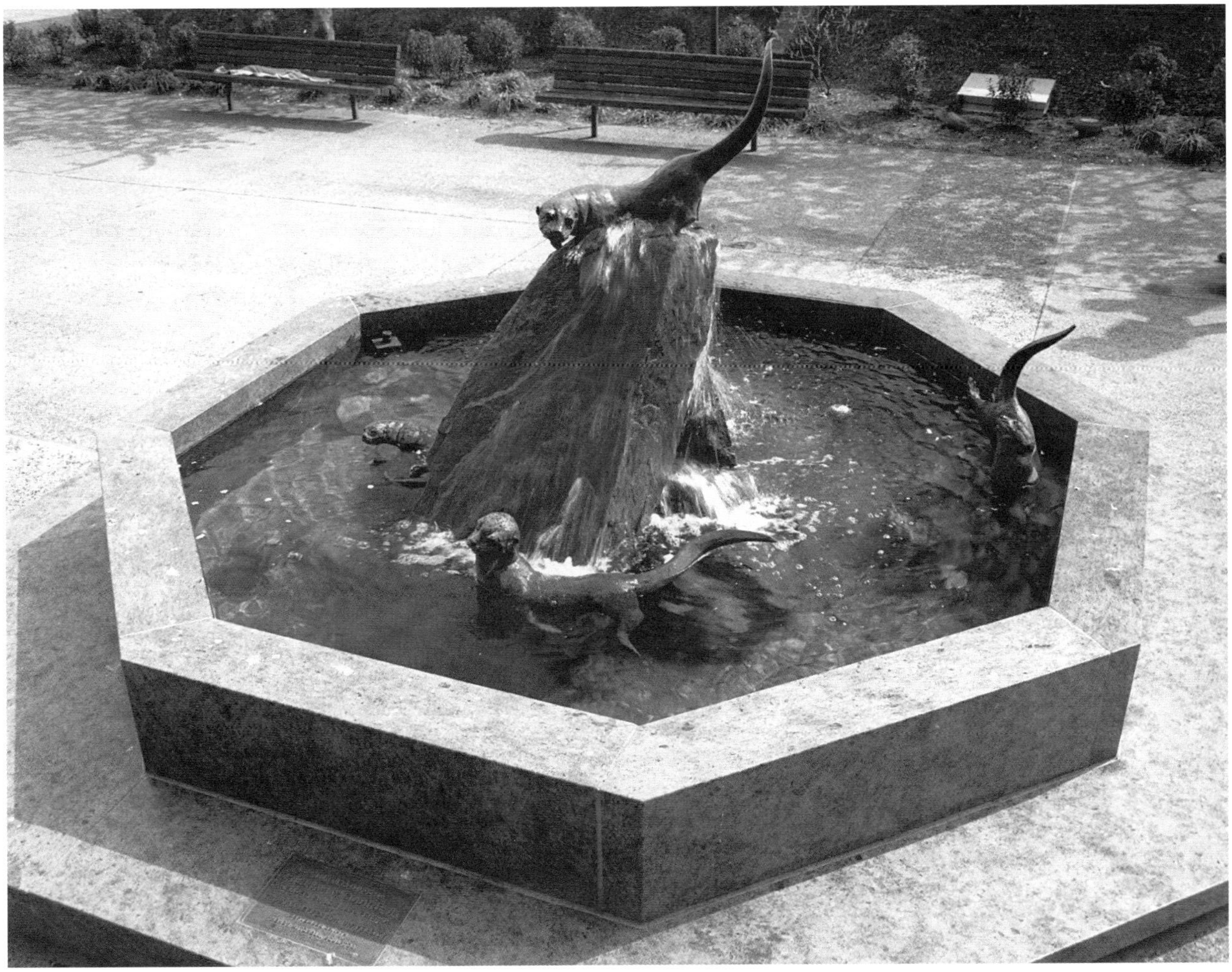

study art, and with the encouragement of his wife, art historian and museum educator Marian Mitchell, with no prior training he earned a master's degree at Tyler School of Fine Arts of Temple University in 1950. That same year he was awarded a Fulbright scholarship to study with famed sculptor Marino Marini at the Accademia di Brera in Milan (1950-52). While abroad he held an exhibition in Florence sponsored by the U.S. Information Service.

Upon returning to America the Mitchells made their home in Philadelphia, but almost every year the artist returned to Milan where many of his pieces were cast in bronze. He taught at the Philadelphia Museum College of Art and at the museum itself. Mitchell was represented by the Kraushaar Gallery in New York where he had one-man shows in 1953 and 1959. Later he dealt directly with architects and other clients.

Henry Mitchell had solo shows at the Philadelphia Art Alliance (1954), the Pennsylvania Academy of the Fine Arts (1956), the Cultural Center in Fort Lauderdale (1959), the Morris Gallery in Bryn Mawr, Pennsylvania (1962), the Provident National Bank in Philadelphia (1968), and the Performing Arts Center in Saratoga, New York (1977).

In 1980 Henry Mitchell died unexpectedly in Charleston, South Carolina where he had gone to supervise a sculpture installation. His memorial service in Philadelphia was held at Thomas Jefferson University where he had won the friendship and admiration of so many people. Mitchell's friend and fellow artist Alden M. Wicks presented a slide lecture on the sculptor's career, and President Bluemle recounted his unabashed pleasure at observing the installation of the *Otter Fountain*'s hydraulic works.

A retrospective exhibition of the artist's reliefs, sculptures, sketches, models, and casts was held in 1990 at the Goldie Paley and Levy Galleries at the Moore College of Art and Design in Philadelphia. Included were a replica of the smallest otter and an intermediate model for Mitchell's *Winged Ox*.

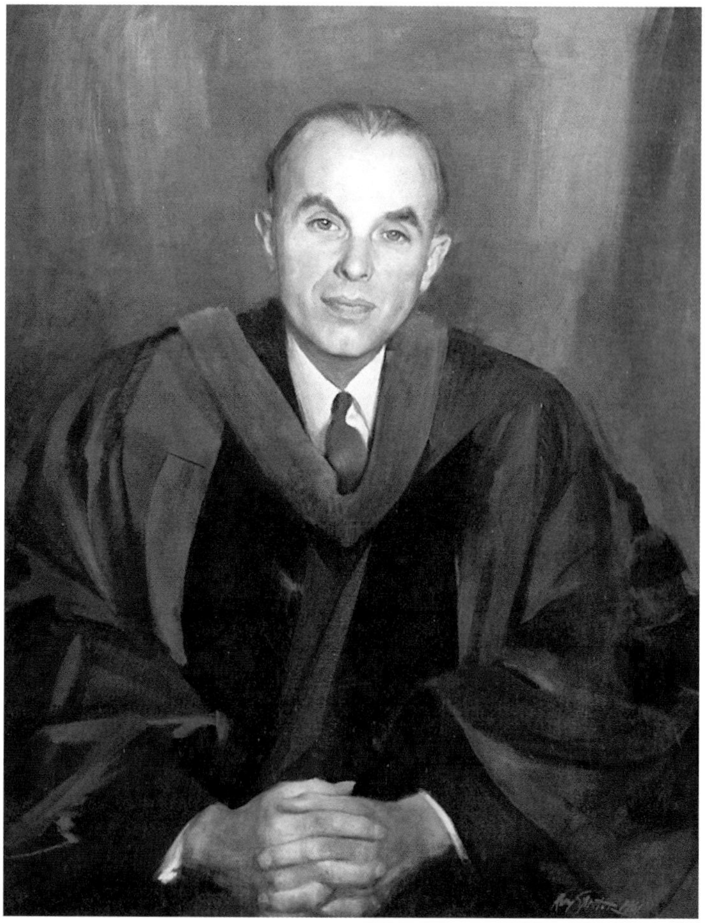

Portrait of Peter A. Herbut

PETER ANDREW HERBUT, M.D. (1912-76)
By Roy Frederic Spreter (1899-1967)

Oil on canvas
1961
34 x 28 in.

Signed and dated lower right: "Roy Spreter 1961"

Given by JMC class of 1961
Accession number: 1961+e.P.01

Peter A. Herbut, M.D. succeeded William Bodine as the third president of Jefferson Medical College in 1966, becoming in 1969 the first president of Thomas Jefferson University. He was the first faculty member to advance to the presidency and worked tirelessly to guide the transition from college to university.

Peter Herbut was born in 1912 in Edson, Alberta, Canada. After studying at the University of Alberta (1930-35) he received doctor of medicine and master of surgery degrees from the McGill University Faculty of Medicine (1937). He served one-year internships at Children's Memorial Hospital in Montreal and at Wilkes Barre General Hospital in Pennsylvania. Planning a career in surgery, he served a residency in the surgical pathology laboratory at the Medical College of Virginia but was persuaded by mentors to become a pathologist instead.

Dr. Herbut accepted an appointment at Jefferson Medical College as an assistant demonstrator in pathology, and soon was assistant director of the clinical laboratories. Known as a prodigious worker with great powers of concentration, he published seventy-five papers during his first nine years at Jefferson. During the war he almost singlehandedly carried the anatomical pathology workload for the clinical laboratories.

By 1948 at the age of thirty-six Herbut was appointed professor of pathology and chairman of the department, succeeding Dr. Virgil H. Moon. He served in this post until 1966. From 1956 to 1966 he was also chairman of the executive faculty. After his appointment as director of the clinical laboratories in 1951 the residency program was considerably strengthened and the quality and quantity of research expanded.

Dr. Herbut was known as a superb diagnostic morphologist and cytopathologist. For his investigation into the cytologic diagnosis of cancer he received the Ward Burdick Award of the American Society of Clinical Pathologists in 1950. He served on the editorial advisory board of *Acta Cytologica* and was a consultant in pulmonary cytology of the International Academy of Gynecologic Cytology. He was the author of four important textbooks: *Surgical Pathology* (1948), *Urological Pathology* (1952), *Gynecological and Obstetrical Pathology* (1953), and *Pathology* (1955).

Dr. Herbut received honorary degrees from the Philadelphia College of Pharmacy and Science and from Washington and Jefferson University. He won the Clarence E. Shaffrey, S.J. Award from St. Joseph's College. He was president of the Pathological Society of Philadelphia. In 1979 he was honored posthumously when the College Building's auditorium was named the Herbut Auditorium. The Peter A. Herbut Professorship of Pathology was established in 1985 by friends and colleagues.

The pathologist's portrait by Roy F. Spreter was presented by the class of 1961. In the half-length, life-sized depiction Dr. Herbut is seated in a frontal pose with hands tightly clasped in his lap. He wears a black academic robe with green hood. His figure fills the whole width of the canvas. The painting's mood is somewhat tense because of the subject's almost iconic pose, his head that sinks into his shoulders, and his intense gaze.

Yet in a memoir of April 6, 1976 for the Jefferson faculty's executive council Herbert A. Luscombe, M.D. wrote with obvious feeling, "Peter Herbut was a gentle man, a kind man, a humble man, and in many respects a godly man, for he tried to bring happiness to all with whom he was associated." Similarly, the student spokesman at the portrait ceremony said the class of 1961 admired him because he "explored the depths of his being to give to us a portion of his philosophy of life as well as an education."

Roy F. Spreter was born in 1899 in Chicago. He studied at the Art Institute of Chicago and worked as a freelance advertising illustrator. He was invited to come to Philadelphia around 1920 to work for the N. W. Ayer and Son agency. He also maintained a second career as a fine artist, especially as a portrait painter.

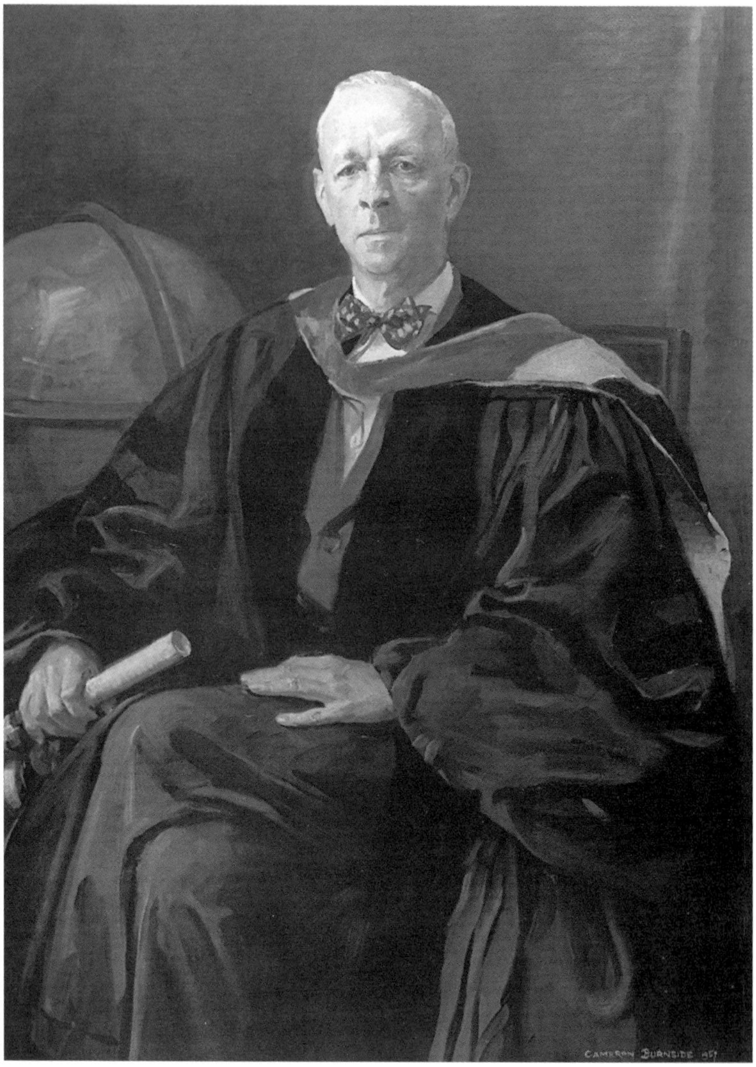

Portrait of William H. Perkins

WILLIAM HARVEY PERKINS, M.D.
(1894-1967)
By Cameron Burnside (1887-1952)

Oil on canvas
1951
50 1/4 x 36 1/4 in.

Signed and dated lower right: "CAMERON BURNSIDE 1951"
Exhibition: Philadelphia, *Cameron Burnside Memorial Exhibition*, Woodmere Art Gallery, 1953

Given in 1951 by JMC class of 1917
Accession number: 1951+e.P.04

In 1941 Dr. William H. Perkins was named dean of Jefferson Medical College, succeeding Dr. Henry K. Mohler. He was also professor and chair of the newly established department of preventive medicine. He was well known for innovations in both medical education and preventive medicine.

William H. Perkins was born in Philadelphia in 1894 and received his M.D. degree from Jefferson in 1917. After interning at the Jefferson Hospital he served as a first lieutenant in the medical corps of the U.S. Army as detachment commander to the 120th Base Hospital in Tours, France.

Upon his return to this country Perkins worked as an assistant pathologist at the Philadelphia General Hospital and as an instructor in medicine at Jefferson Medical College. He was also appointed a fellow in medical education of the Commonwealth Fund of New York. In 1926 he accepted a post offered by the Rockefeller Foundation in cooperation with the Siamese government as visiting professor at the medical school of the Chulalangkarana University in Bangkok. In recognition of his contributions to medical education during his four-year stay, he was awarded the decoration of Order of the White Elephant by the King of Siam.

When he returned to the United States in 1930 Dr. Perkins became an instructor in medicine at Tulane University School of Medicine. The following year he was appointed professor and chairman of a new department of preventive medicine, with support from the Commonwealth Fund. He established an innovative health maintenance clinic. In 1938 he published one of the first comprehensive textbooks in the field: *Cause and Prevention of Diseases*.

When Dr. William H. Perkins came to Jefferson in 1941 he again established a health maintenance clinic. A foundation of his teaching was the "disease as a process" concept which held that early detection of primary factors and avoidance of contributing factors were keys to the prevention of disability.[5]

Dr. Perkins was vice chairman of the section on public health of the American Medical Association in 1933. He was active in the planning for district health centers in Philadelphia. In 1958 the College of Physicians of Philadelphia established an annual William Harvey Perkins Award for the best essay pertaining to preventive medicine by a Philadelphia medical student. While dean at Jefferson Perkins was awarded the Sc.D. degree from Franklin and Marshall College and the LL.D. degree from Dickinson College. He received the Litt.D. from Jefferson Medical College in 1962. He was president of Jefferson's alumni association in 1945.

Failing health forced Dr. Perkins to retire as dean in 1950 but he remained professor and department chairman until 1959 when he was named emeritus professor. A lecture room in the Kellow Conference Center in the College Building was named in his honor in 1977.

The year after he retired from the deanship, fellow members of Perkins's class of 1917 decided to commission his portrait. They hired Cameron Burnside for the job, the same year he had painted the portrait of Dr. Hobart A. Reimann.

The elegant depiction shows Dr. William H. Perkins full length and life-sized, seated in an armchair with legs crossed at the knee. His face is brightly illuminated from the left, lending drama to his serious, somewhat drawn expression. He wears a black academic gown trimmed with a yellow and green mantle that undulates in a graceful curve over his shoulder. The deep folds in the voluminous sleeves are fluidly brushed.

His right hand holds a rolled paper tied with blue and black ribbons (Jefferson colors), a medical college diploma. A large globe on the left alludes to his medical missionary work in the Far East.

Though known for his scholarship and seriousness of purpose Dr. Perkins was also considered a genial man with a good sense of humor. At the presentation ceremony he described the experience of posing and commented drily on the results,

> Each time that I look at this portrait I feel as though I were frozen in time and space; that for the next hundred years or more I will be just like that. To those who think it makes me look younger, remember I was younger when Mr. Burnside started painting it. If you think it looks older, then give me time and I will grow up to it.

Portrait of George A. Bennett

GEORGE ALLEN BENNETT, M.D. (1904-58)
By Julius Thiengen Bloch (1888-1966)

Oil on canvas
1959
36 x 30 in.

Signed lower left: "Julius Bloch"

Given in 1959 by JMC board of trustees and faculty
Accession number: 1959+e.P.02

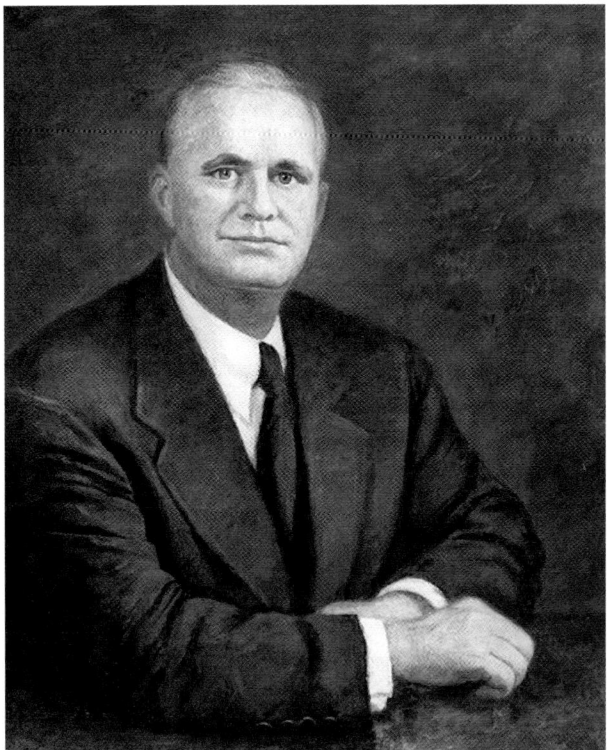

Like his predecessor Dr. William H. Perkins, Dr. George A. Bennett was dean at Jefferson Medical College and had significant academic achievements abroad. Bennett was also chair of the anatomy department.

George Bennett was born in 1904 at Water Valley, Mississippi. His interests in science and the humanities were unusually broad. After earning an undergraduate degree at Wabash College in Crawfordsville, Indiana at the age of eighteen, he received a Ben Hur scholarship to study ancient history and archaeology at the University of Athens and the University of Zurich. By 1928 he qualified in medicine at the University of Munich where he studied both philosophy and medicine.

Bennett returned to the United States that year and became an instructor in histology at Baylor University College of Medicine, and then a teaching fellow in anatomy at Harvard Medical School. In 1929 he returned to Munich for six more months of anatomical research. In 1930 he was appointed professor of histology at Georgetown University School of Medicine and acting head of the department of biology. He returned to the University of Munich again for research in dermatology and as an assistant in anatomy and thoracic surgery, and received his doctor of medicine degree *summa cum laude* there in 1937. He remained in Munich for postgraduate studies in anthropology, chemistry, and pathology until the precarious political climate forced his return to the United States in 1939.

Dr. Bennett obtained a teaching position in anatomy at Jefferson Medical College, and rose quickly in the professorial ranks until he was elected professor and department chair in 1948. Two years later he was named dean.

According to a memoir in executive faculty minutes of May 26, 1958, it was as a teacher of anatomy that Dr. Bennett "realized his greatest happiness," and that through his knowledge of surgery he was unusually well qualified to teach applied and surgical anatomy. His enthusiastic, clear, and concise lectures motivated many students to embark on academic careers in basic or clinical anatomy. The 1944 Jefferson yearbook was dedicated to him.

The executive faculty minutes also praised Dr. Bennett's anatomical research on the tongue, the eye, the thyroid, and the spleen. For his work on the effects of wear and tear on the supraspinatus muscle and shoulder joint capsule (with Drs. Anthony F. DePalma and Gerald E. Callery), Bennett was awarded the gold medal of the American Academy of Orthopaedic Surgeons in 1948.

In recognition of his accomplishments he won the honorary degrees of doctor of science from St. Joseph's College, Dickinson College, and Grove City College, and doctor of laws from Temple University. He received a Consultant's Certificate of Merit from the U.S. Armed Forces for teaching postgraduate courses to army and navy medical officers during World War II.

Dr. Bennett's untimely death occurred in February 1958, four months before he was scheduled to receive an honorary degree from Jefferson.

Minutes of executive faculty and trustees meetings show that when the board implemented the faculty's suggestion of a posthumous portrait of Dean Bennett, several artists were considered for the commission. Julius T. Bloch was selected on the recommendation of Philadelphia Museum of Art trustee R. Sturgis Ingersoll, a knowledgeable art collector, connoisseur, and close friend of the artist. The chairman of the faculty's portrait committee even went to Bloch's studio to interview the painter and see examples of his work. The selection of Bloch assured that artist and subject were well matched in academic training and professional attainments.

Dr. Bennett is depicted half length and slightly larger than life. His hands rest on a desk or table that extends across the canvas. The subject wears a dark blue suit and tie, the atmospheric background is gray-blue, and there are harmonious overtones of rust and brownish-purple throughout. The figure is very solidly rendered and the stippled surface of the painting is lively.

Compared with the original photograph provided by Mrs. Bennett, there are similarities in the sitter's earnest and pleasant expression and the thickness of his neck. However, in the painting his face seems less jowly and more square, and his shoulders look broader and more powerful. The thrusting curve of his right arm swooping across the massive table suggests forcefulness and authority. To Bloch's credit, the depiction avoids the wooden artificiality that often appears in posthumous portraits.

Julius Bloch was born in 1888 in Kehl, Germany of

Jewish parents. The family emigrated to Philadelphia when Bloch was aged five, and he remained in that city for the rest of his life. He enrolled in the Pennsylvania Museum School of Industrial Art for three years. From 1908 to 1912 he studied at the Pennsylvania Academy of the Fine Arts where he won a Toppan Prize and two Cresson traveling scholarships for study in Europe. During World War I Bloch was sent to join the Meuse-Argonne Drive in France, and after the Armistice studied at the University of Clermont-Ferrand.

Upon his return to Philadelphia Bloch took courses at the Barnes Foundation. Early in his career as a painter he concentrated on naturalistic flower paintings and portraits, and glimpses of the urban scene. Although his subject matter would change later, he continued to paint portraits including such notable sitters as art collector and educator Dr. Albert C. Barnes, singers Paul Robeson and Marian Anderson, and artists Charles Demuth and Horace Pippin.

Julius Bloch was a faculty member at the Graphic Sketch Club for a year in 1931, but his major teaching career was at the Pennsylvania Academy of the Fine Arts where he taught portraiture from 1947 to 1962. He was a regular exhibitor there for almost fifty years, and in 1962 received the Academy Fellowship's Percy M. Owens Memorial Prize. He was also an administrator of several Works Progress Administration projects in Philadelphia, including a show in a subway concourse.

In the late 1920s and 1930s Bloch embraced the egalitarian principles of socialism as a protest against racism and nationalism, and contributed lithographs to the *New Masses*. Bloch was especially sympathetic to the plight of African-Americans, the working poor, and the unemployed. His desire was to depict dignity in the human condition, regardless of class distinctions.

One of his most famous Depression-era works was *The Prisoner* (Philadelphia Museum of Art), depicting a manacled black man in a jail cell awaiting execution. In 1932 the newly organized Whitney Museum of American Art purchased Bloch's *The Lynching*. In 1934 Bloch's *Young Worker* was chosen by Mrs. Franklin D. Roosevelt as the best picture in a Public Works of Art show at the Corcoran Gallery and earmarked for display at the White House. In 1935 Bloch's *The Striker* won special attention from President and Mrs. Roosevelt at the Corcoran biennial and the painting was purchased by the gallery. Bloch's self-portrait was acquired by the Whitney in 1937. The Pyramid Club, an organization of black professionals in Philadelphia, awarded Bloch the unusual honor of a one-man show in 1940.

From the 1930s through the 1950s other solo shows in Philadelphia were held at the Little Gallery of Contemporary Art, the Edward Side Gallery, the Warwick Gallery, the Philadelphia Art Alliance, the Pennsylvania Academy of the Fine Arts, the Woodmere Art Gallery, and the Newman Gallery. Bloch also exhibited widely at national shows including the Golden Gate International Exposition in San Francisco and the New York World's Fair (1939), and the *Artists for Victory* show at the Metropolitan Museum of Art (1942).

The year after Julius T. Bloch's death in 1966 memorial exhibitions were held at the Philadelphia Art Alliance and the Little Gallery of Contemporary Art. His will stipulated that art works remaining in his studio be distributed by three executors (one of whom was Ingersoll) to museums and colleges. Groups of drawings, prints, or paintings were given to Lincoln University, the Philadelphia Museum of Art, and many others. In 1983 the Philadelphia Museum exhibited its works by Julius Bloch along with loans from other institutions and private collectors.

Bloch was a beloved, nurturing figure in the Philadelphia art world. He was not only a favorite faculty member at the Academy but continued to critique the work of former students long after their graduation. His cultivation of young artists even extended to jurying exhibitions of Philadelphia school children.[6]

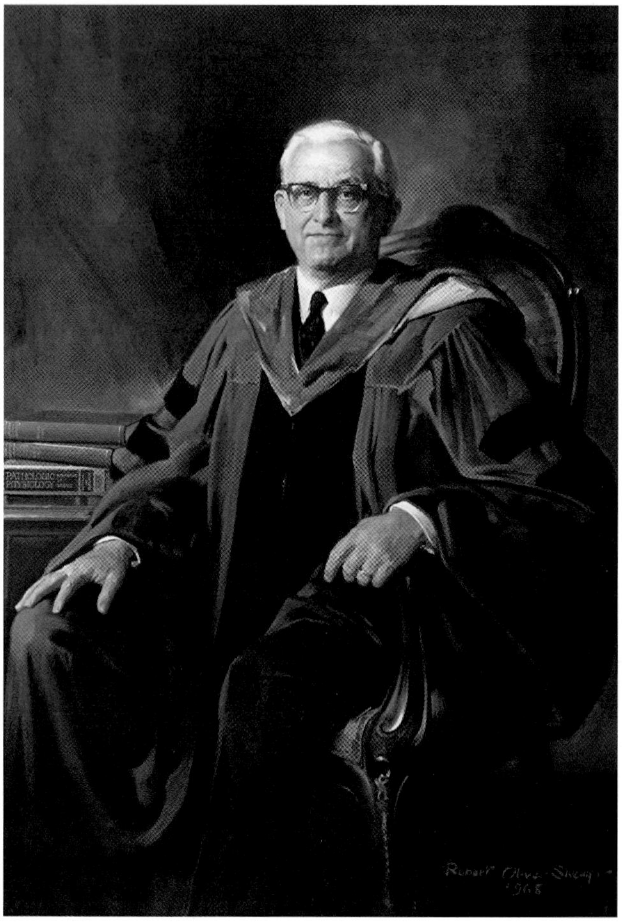

Portrait of William A. Sodeman

WILLIAM ANTHONY SODEMAN, M.D. (1906-95)
By Robert Oliver Skemp (1910-84)

Oil on canvas
1968
56 x 40 in.

Signed and dated lower right: "Robert Oliver Skemp/1968"

Given in 1968 by colleagues and friends
Accession number: 1968+e.P.03

Dr. William A. Sodeman succeeded Dr. George A. Bennett as the nineteenth dean of Jefferson Medical College in 1958. He was an outstanding educator, researcher, author, administrator, and consultant.

William Sodeman was born in 1906 in Charleroi, Pennsylvania and reared in Toledo, Ohio. He received his undergraduate (1928) and medical (1931) degrees from the University of Michigan. Following an internship in Toledo and a residency in internal medicine at Tulane University, he returned to Michigan as a Commonwealth Fund fellow in cardiology.

He spent the next two decades at Tulane University where in 1941 he was named professor and chairman of the department of preventive medicine, and later of tropical medicine and public health. He took a year's leave of absence to be a visiting professor at the School of Tropical Medicine in Calcutta, India.

In 1953 Sodeman became professor and chairman of the department of internal medicine at the University of Missouri School of Medicine. He joined the faculty at Jefferson Medical College in 1957 as Magee Professor of Medicine and chair of the department. In his single year as department chairman Sodeman moved to strengthen the subspecialties and to keep these units within the department. His energetic productiveness, political skills, and personal friendliness led to his being named dean in 1958 and vice president for medical affairs in 1962.

During Sodeman's nine-year tenure as dean he initiated or encouraged programs and reforms that markedly improved Jefferson's reputation. Changes included: admitting women medical students; encouraging research and increasing its funding base; vesting the admissions committee with the final selection of medical school applicants; introducing the National Board Examinations into the curriculum; setting up a program of continuing medical education; implementing an accelerated five-year college and medical school program with Pennsylvania State University; providing larger blocks of elective time within the medical school's core curriculum; and initiating full-time status for all heads of major departments.

Dr. Sodeman edited the authoritative *Pathologic Physiology: Mechanisms of Disease* (1950), a text that was translated into five languages and went through seven editions. He served on the editorial boards of the *Journal of Laboratory and Clinical Medicine* and the *American Journal of Cardiology*.

Dr. William A. Sodeman served as president of the American Society of Tropical Medicine, the Heart Association of Southeastern Pennsylvania, the American College of Cardiology, and the American College of Physicians. He was chair of the American Medical Association Council on Medical Education and of the Liaison Committee on Medical Education. He was a consultant to the United States Public Health Service, the National Institutes of Health, and the Surgeon General.

Sodeman was the recipient of many awards, including the Clarence E. Shaffrey, S.J. Award from St. Joseph's College, the Sesquicentennial and Distinguished Alumni Awards of the University of Michigan, and the Strittmatter Award of the Philadelphia County Medical Society. Dr. Sodeman was named a distinguished fellow of the American College of Cardiology and the emeritus president of the American College of Physicians. In 1979 he received the prestigious Distinguished Service Award from the American Medical Association. He received an honorary doctor of science degree from Villanova University and doctor of humane letters from Jefferson Medical College.

After his resignation from Jefferson Dr. Sodeman was named dean emeritus and professor emeritus of medicine. Instead of retiring, however, he remained very active in medical affairs. First he took the post of scientific director of the Life Insurance Medical Research Fund, sponsored by American and Canadian life insurance companies. Then in 1970 he became the executive director of the Commission on Foreign Medical Graduates. Three years later he became a clinical professor of medicine at the new Medical College of Ohio in Toledo.

Starting in late 1966 a group of Dean Sodeman's colleagues and friends at Jefferson decided to honor him with a portrait timed to coincide with his stepping down as dean.

In his portrait by Robert O. Skemp the physician is depicted life-sized and full length, seated in an armchair. The white-haired, bespectacled physician turns his head to look directly toward the viewer with a serious and confident expression. Over a dark suit he wears a black academic robe with black velvet stripes and a green mantle lined in blue and yellow. On a nearby table is a colorful stack of bound volumes including his own book *Pathologic Physiology*, the *Journal of Medical Education*, and the *American Journal of Cardiology*. The elaborate French Rococo Revival armchair has maroon upholstery, and is trimmed with gold braid and ormolu mounts, lending an air of elegance to the imposing depiction.

A letter dated August 9, 1968 from Dr. Andrew J. Ramsay, chairman of the Sodeman portrait committee, to Robert Skemp expressed the extremely enthusiastic reception of the dean's portrait. He mentioned that the upcoming senior class expected to raise sixteen hundred dollars for its faculty portrait and frame, and asked if Skemp would "make a concession" and agree to that fee for the class portrait that "need not be as large as that of Dr. Sodeman." Apparently the arrangement was satisfactory, and Skemp ultimately painted a total of eleven portraits for Jefferson between 1968 and 1981.

Robert O. Skemp was born in 1910 in Scottdale, Pennsylvania. He studied at the Art Students League and the Grand Central School of Art in New York. Following service in the Merchant Marines he continued his studies abroad in France and Spain. He taught at the Chicago School of Professional Art from 1937 to 1940. Some prominent portrait subjects include the art collector J. Paul Getty, Mr. and Mrs. Lowell Thomas, Treasury Secretary Donald Regan, and Admiral Richard Byrd.

Besides his reputation as a portrait painter, Skemp was also a muralist, marine painter, and freelance illustrator. He painted religious murals for the Church of Jesus Christ of Latter-Day Saints exhibit at the New York World's Fair in 1964 and the 1969 fair in Osaka, Japan. He is represented in public and private collections throughout the United States and in Canada, France, South America, and Iran.

As a young man Skemp was fascinated with ships and the sea and had firsthand experience as a foremast hand on ships bound for the Far East. Later he was an avid yachtsman and researched and painted some of the great mid-nineteenth-century clipper ships.

Portrait of Robert I. Wise

ROBERT IRBY WISE, M.D., Ph.D. (b. 1915)
By Robert Oliver Skemp

Oil on canvas
1974
36 x 30 in.

Signed and dated lower right: "Robert Oliver Skemp/1974"

Given in 1975 by friends and colleagues
Accession number: 1975+e.P.03

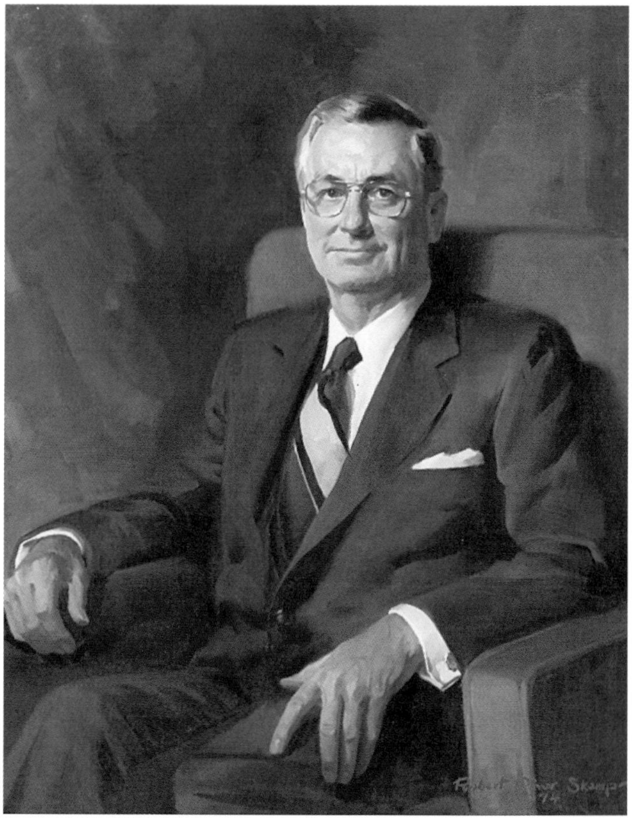

In 1959 Dr. Robert I. Wise was appointed the Magee Professor of Medicine and chair of the department, succeeding Dr. William A. Sodeman. Wise's expertise was in the field of infectious diseases and he was a nationally known authority on the control of staphylococcal infections in hospitals.

Robert Wise was born in 1915 in Barstow, Texas and received his undergraduate degree from the University of Texas in 1937. He earned the M.S. degree in 1938 and the Ph.D. degree in bacteriology in 1942 at the University of Illinois. Before receiving his medical degree from the University of Texas Medical Branch in Galveston in 1950, he worked as an assistant instructor in bacteriology at the University of Illinois and assistant professor of bacteriology in Galveston.

During his internship at the U.S. Public Health Service Hospital in New Orleans Dr. Wise became acquainted with Dr. William A. Sodeman. Following his residency at the University of Minnesota Hospitals in Minneapolis, Wise was appointed assistant professor of medicine and bacteriology there.

Dr. Robert I. Wise joined the faculty at Jefferson Medical College in 1955 as assistant professor of medicine. Four years later he was elected the Magee Professor of Medicine and chair of the department and physician-in-chief of the Jefferson Hospital. He was also assistant chief in the medical service at Philadelphia General Hospital from 1955 to 1969.

As chair of Jefferson's department of medicine his primary goal was to bring unity. He instituted an integrated approach to teaching and patient care that included nurses, nutritionists, pharmacists, and social workers, as well as physicians, as part of the teaching unit. During his tenure the number of endowed chairs increased from two to five. Existing divisions in the department were strengthened and new academic divisions were created. The rotating internship was changed to a straight intern program, constituting the first year of residency.

Dr. Wise was a member of the editorial board of *Annals of Internal Medicine*. He won the Ashbell-Smith Distinguished Alumni Award of the University of Texas Medical Branch, the Julius W. Strumer Memorial Lecture Award of the American College of Pharmacy and Science, and an honorary doctor of science degree from Thomas Jefferson University. He served on the boards of trustees of Magee Memorial Hospital, Drexel University, and the West Philadelphia Corporation.

After serving as department chair for sixteen years, he retired in 1975 and was named the Magee Professor Emeritus of Medicine. He moved to Togus, Maine to help plan the establishment of Maine's medical school and to become the chief of staff at the Veterans Administration Medical and Regional Office Center. He retired from that position in 1984.

Dr. Robert I. Wise's colleagues and friends honored him with a portrait that was painted by Robert O. Skemp in late 1974 and presented in May 1975 upon his retirement. The physician is shown life-sized and two-thirds length, seated in a blue, upholstered armchair. He turns his head to gaze directly toward the viewer. His right hand rests on the chair arm, and his left hand is placed on his thigh. The pose is almost identical to that of Dr. Sodeman, except that the hand position is reversed.

However, Dr. Wise's posture is more relaxed and his expression is more pleasant, almost smiling, compared with Dr. Sodeman's stiff and serious demeanor. Dr. Wise is attired not in an academic robe, but in a dark blue business suit. In keeping with the mood of the characterization, Wise's armchair is an unadorned club type, not the high-styled, carved chair featured in the Sodeman portrait.

Portrait of C. Wilmer Wirts Jr.

CHARLES WILMER WIRTS Jr., M.D. (1907-97)
By Alden MacMaster Wicks (1914-87)

Oil on canvas
1978
40 x 30 in.

Signed lower right: "Wicks"

Given in 1978 by friends and colleagues
Accession number: 1978+e.P.07

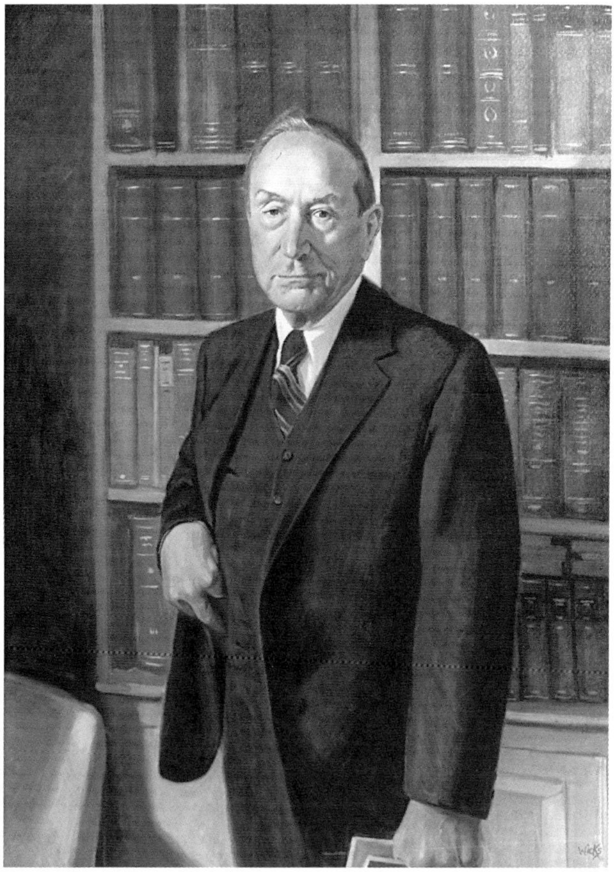

Dr. Charles Wilmer Wirts was a professor of medicine and chief of the division of gastroenterology at Jefferson Medical College. He was a pioneer in the field of gastrointestinal endoscopy.

C. Wilmer Wirts was born in 1907 in Pittsburgh, and was a graduate of Lafayette College (1930) and Jefferson Medical College (1934). After an internship at St. John's General Hospital and a pathology residency at St. Francis Hospital, both in Pittsburgh, he continued his training in Paris at the American Hospital, and worked in two endoscopic clinics there.

Dr. Wirts returned to Jefferson for an appointment as the first Ross V. Patterson fellow in gastroenterology (1940-42). He rose in the ranks from assistant professor to professor of medicine by 1972. Among other positions, Dr. Wirts was also an associate physician at Pennsylvania Hospital and gastroscopist at Philadelphia General Hospital.

In 1946 Dr. Wirts became head of the gastrointestinal clinic and developed the first division of gastroenterology at Jefferson; he served as division chief until 1966. After taking a course with Dr. Rudolf Schindler in Chicago, he introduced the use of the Schindler flexible gastroscope at Jefferson. He collaborated on numerous research projects with Dr. Franz Goldstein, and they obtained the first National Institutes of Health gastrointestinal research and training grant at Jefferson.

Dr. Wirts reached the rank of lieutenant colonel during three years of service in World War II. He served as president of the American College of Gastroenterology and the American Gastroscopic Society, and was a member of the American Board of Gastroenterology. He was named honorary professor at Jefferson in 1977 and emeritus professor five years later. Dr. Wirts continued in practice until 1985. His son Steven graduated from Jefferson Medical College in 1974.

Dr. Franz Goldstein was cochairman of the committee that commissioned a portrait of Dr. C. Wilmer Wirts in 1978. The artist selected was Alden M. Wicks, a favorite Jefferson portraitist who depicted seventeen faculty members between 1959 and 1985.

Dr. Wirts is shown life-sized and two-thirds length, standing in front of a bookcase with one arm raised, the other hanging down and holding a book. His right hand rests awkwardly in the watch pocket of his vest, and his left hand marks the place in his book. His body faces slightly left, and he turns his head to look out directly toward the viewer with a sober expression. Dramatic light and shadow on his face delineate signs of aging in his puffy lower lids and the deep creases flanking his nose and mouth. The portrait's setting and the subject's posture and expression suggest the personality traits attributed to Wirts by colleagues: incisive, deliberate, methodical, and judicious.

Alden Wicks's characteristic underlying geometric composition is evident in the arrangement of books, supports, and shelves in the bookcase and in the paneling of the wainscotting below. Another device is the play of bright primary colors in the book bindings and chair upholstery contrasted with the physician's dark blue business suit and maroon necktie.

Artist and educator Alden M. Wicks was born in Holyoke, Massachusetts in 1914. He was a Phi Beta Kappa and *magna cum laude* graduate of Princeton University (1937) where his father was dean emeritus of the University Chapel. Wicks began his teaching career almost immediately at Princeton (1937-40) and then taught for a year at Hunter College in New York. He saw active duty in the Atlantic and Pacific theaters as a lieutenant in the U.S. Navy for four years during World War II. He also studied art abroad at the Sorbonne in Paris and at the University of Munich.

After the war Wicks continued his unusually thorough education by earning a master's degree from Tyler Art School of Temple University in 1947. He taught drawing, painting, and art history there for many years, and among his students was sculptor Henry W. Mitchell. Wicks joined the faculty at Moore College of Art (now Moore College of Art and Design) in 1961 and became the associate dean of faculty the following year. He was named professor emeritus at his retirement from Moore in 1981.

Although most noted as a naturalistic portrait painter, Wicks also painted precise, symbolic paintings on biblical and medieval themes such as *The Ship of Fools*, *Jonah*, and *The Metaphysicians* (all in private collections). Wicks is very interested in the space program, and was honored to be included in the NASA art group and has made sketches during several Apollo launches at Cape Kennedy.

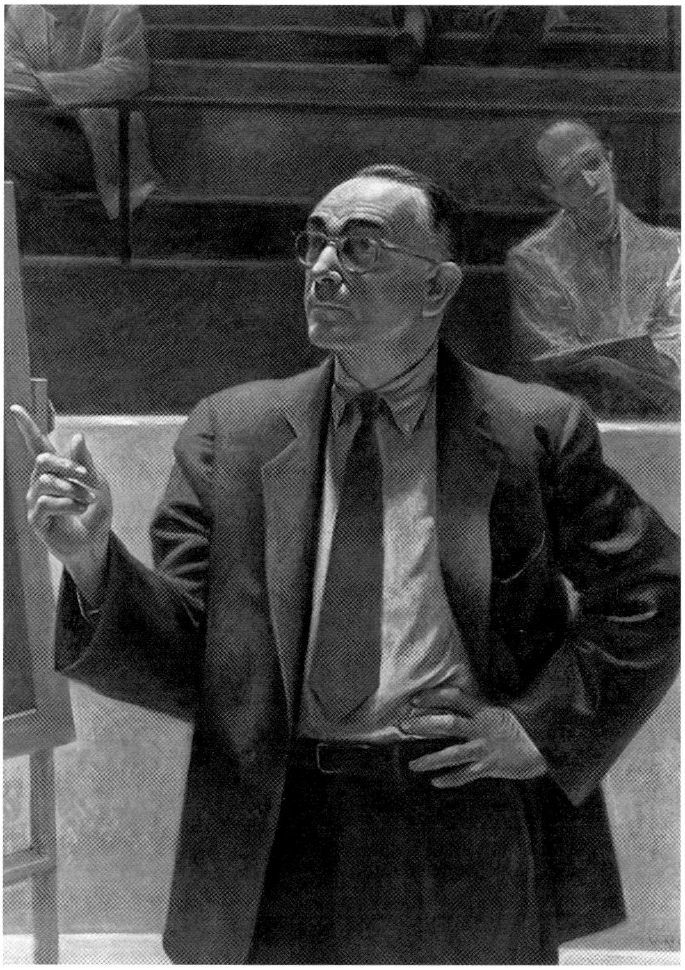

Portrait of Bernard J. Alpers

BERNARD JACOB ALPERS, M.D., D.Sc. (1900-81)
By Alden MacMaster Wicks

Oil on canvas
1959
48 1/4 x 36 1/4 in.

Signed and dated lower right: "Wicks 1959"
Exhibitions: New York, *Members Exhibition*, The Century Association, 1963; Philadelphia, Moore College of Art, 1963

Given by JMC class of 1959
Accession number: 1959+e.P.01

Dr. Bernard J. Alpers was professor of neurology and chair of the department at Jefferson Medical College from 1938 to 1965. He was a nationally recognized educator, researcher, and author.

Bernard Alpers was born in Salem, Massachusetts in 1900 and was a graduate of Harvard Medical School (1923). He received graduate training at the Philadelphia Orthopaedic Hospital and Infirmary for Nervous Disease and was a Commonwealth fellow in neuropsychiatry at the University of Pennsylvania (1925-28). A Francis Clark traveling fellowship in neurosurgery allowed him to study abroad at universities in Madrid, Hamburg, and Oxford. He earned a doctor of science degree in medicine from the University of Pennsylvania (1930). He was appointed director of the neuropathology laboratories at the University of Pennsylvania and the Institute of Pennsylvania Hospital, and was the George Harrison Frazier fellow in neurosurgery.

In 1938 Dr. Alpers joined the faculty at Jefferson Medical College as professor and chair of neurology. He served until his retirement in 1965 when he was elected emeritus professor. Under his energetic leadership the neurology department established special divisions of neurophysiology, neurochemistry, neuropharmacology, and pediatric neurology. Shortly after his arrival Alpers began to train residents in clinical neurology and neuropathology. By 1964 seven of his former residents had become heads of their own departments. Between 1944 and 1964 graduates from Jefferson Medical College ranked second in number among the diplomates of the American Board of Psychiatry and Neurology.

Dr. Alpers was the first to describe Alpers disease, a rare condition affecting the brains of children under the age of twelve. He was a major contributor to the neurology literature, especially for his research on rehabilitation for stroke patients. His most important textbooks are *Clinical Neurology* (1945, seven editions through 1971), *Management of the Patient with Headache* (with Perry S. MacNeal, M.D. and William R. O'Brien, M.D., 1957), *Vertigo and Dizziness* (1958), and *Essentials of the Neurological Examination* (with Elliott L. Mancall, M.D., 1971). Dr. Alpers was the associate editor of the *Archives of Neurology and Psychiatry.*

Dr. Alpers also was neurologist or consultant to the Pennsylvania, Wills Eye, Naval, and Kensington Hospitals, and the Institute of Pennsylvania Hospital.

He served terms as president of the American Neurological Association, the American Board of Psychiatry and Neurology, and the American Association of Neuropathologists. He was honored by the naming of the Alpers Neurology Laboratory at Hebrew University in Israel. He was awarded an honorary doctor of laws degree from Jefferson Medical College in 1968, and also received honorary degrees from Hahnemann Medical College and the Medical College of Pennsylvania. The new Alpers Neuropathology Laboratory was named in his memory at Jefferson in 1988.

Alpers was admired by generations of Jefferson students for his knowledge and eloquence and for his personal qualities of modesty, kindness, and a delightful sense of humor in the classroom. The classes of 1953 and 1958 dedicated their yearbooks to him, and he won the Christian R. and Mary F. Lindback Award for Distinguished Teaching in 1962. Students formed the Bernard J. Alpers Neurological Society in his honor.

Chosen as class portrait honoree in 1959, Alpers was the earliest Jefferson subject of Alden M. Wicks. A letter dated February 23, 1959 from the chairman of the student portrait committee to Dean William A. Sodeman, M.D. describes arrangements with the artist. Wicks agreed to present sketches of the background and the subject's face for approval by student and faculty portrait committees. He planned to observe many of Dr. Alpers's "early Saturday morning 'pits' to sketch him in action," to draw the amphitheater when empty for architectural details, and to arrange sittings at Jefferson so as not to "overburden such a busy man as Dr. Alpers." The plan was for the physician to visit Wick's studio in New Hope, Pennsylvania "at least once for final touches."

Alpers is depicted life-sized and two-thirds length, lecturing next to a blackboard in the amphitheater. He is attired in a brown suit with his customary blue shirt and Harvard crimson necktie. He stands with his left hand placed on his hip and the index finger of his right hand pointing upwards (said to be characteristic gestures). He raises his head with an inquiring expression as though quizzing a student. Portions of the bodies of three seated students in white coats are seen in the background. Light from above falls dramatically on the professor's forehead, right hand, and shirtfront, and on the white plaster wall at the base of the amphitheater steps.

Alden Wicks commented that the portrait of Dr. Alpers was among his most challenging because the setting is the same as *The Gross Clinic*, "an awe-inspiring situation for any artist." He said, "I'm working in the Eakins tradition...of a portrait as a realistic study of a man at his work."[7]

Portrait of Baldwin L. Keyes

BALDWIN LONGSTRETH KEYES, M.D. (1893-1994)
By John Christen Johansen (1876-1964)

Oil on canvas
1954
38 x 30 in.

Signed and dated lower left: "JOHN C. JOHANSEN 54"

Given by JMC class of 1955
Accession number: 1955+e.P.01

In 1942 Dr. Baldwin L. Keyes was named professor of psychiatry and first chairman of the department at Jefferson Medical College. This respected and beloved leader in Philadelphia psychiatry led a remarkable personal life.

Baldwin Keyes was born in mountain and jungle territory near Rio de Janeiro in 1893 of American parents. His father was an oral surgeon as was his paternal grandfather, a Confederate loyalist from Mobile, Alabama who had joined a colony of disaffected American southerners in Brazil. His maternal grandfather, a Philadelphia Quaker pacifist, had settled in Brazil as an antidote to melancholia brought on by guilt over purchasing the services of a substitute soldier who was killed at the Battle of Gettysburg.

Keyes's early education was with governesses in Rio and a boarding school in London, then at age ten he was dispatched to relatives in Philadelphia and attended Germantown Academy and Swarthmore Preparatory School. After one year at the dental school at the University of Pennsylvania his interest turned to medicine, and he enrolled at Jefferson Medical College and graduated in 1917.

Keyes enlisted in the medical department of the U.S. Army after graduation and the following year was

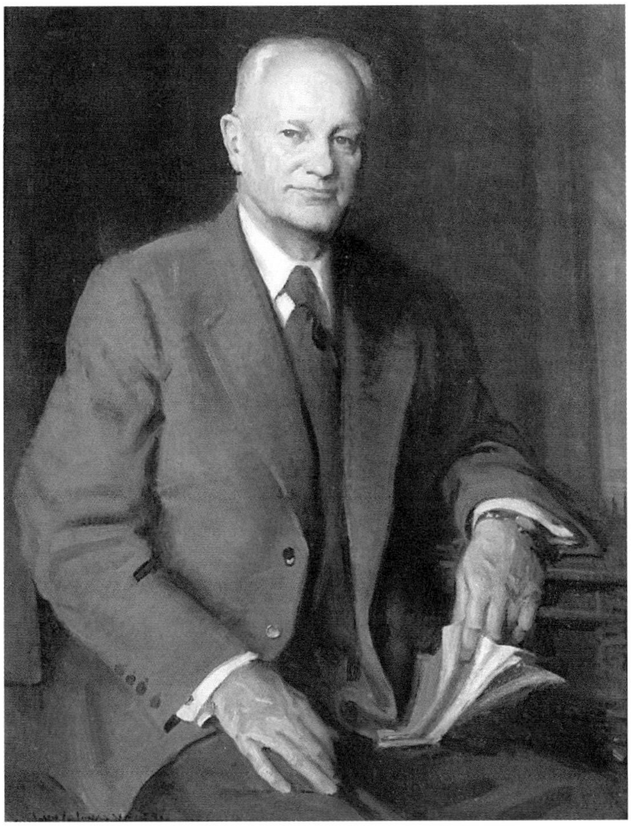

awarded the British Military Cross for Valor with four battle stars for his service in France as a combat surgeon with the British Expeditionary Forces, the Gordon Highlanders. He was recalled to the American army and made second in command at a hospital for treating soldiers wounded in frontline duty at Aix-les-Bains in the French Alps.

Upon returning to Philadelphia Keyes interned at Misericordia Hospital in 1919, then returned to Rio de Janeiro for training in tropical diseases at the Santa Casa de Misericordia Hospital. This was followed by a year of postgraduate work at the University of Pennsylvania. Drawn to the field of neurology and psychiatry he went to work for Dr. Edward A. Strecker, a Jefferson alumnus of 1891, at the Institute of Pennsylvania Hospital.

In 1926 Dr. Strecker recommended Keyes as an assistant to Daniel J. McCarthy, M.D., a clinical practitioner who was also professor of medical jurisprudence at the University of Pennsylvania's law and medical schools. Keyes became interested in forensic issues in psychiatry, especially juvenile delinquency, and later became a founder of the Medico-legal Institute of Philadelphia. Keyes conducted a neuropsychiatry private practice with Dr. McCarthy and several others from 1925 to 1931.

In 1928 Jefferson's chair of pediatrics Dr. Edwin L. Bauer asked Dr. Keyes to set up the first psychiatric clinic in a pediatric department in the United States. Soon Keyes was asked to give the psychiatry lectures for Jefferson's department of nervous and mental diseases. In 1937 he was appointed clinical professor of psychiatry in the neurology department. In 1942 Keyes was named chairman of a new separate department of psychiatry.

At the outbreak of World War II Dr. Baldwin Keyes was ordered to organize the Jefferson unit, the Thirty-eighth General Hospital near Cairo, Egypt. He was the executive officer and commandant in charge of medical affairs until he was transferred to England as a consultant to survey psychiatric institutions. After the war he was a senior consultant to the Office of the Surgeon General and the Veterans Administration and helped train hundreds of young physicians in the School of Military Neuro-psychiatry. He retired from the medical reserves in 1954 after thirty-seven years of continuous military service.

Dr. Baldwin L. Keyes was a leader in developing psychiatric facilities in Philadelphia. In 1957 he opened one of the first inpatient psychiatric programs in a general hospital on the fourteenth floor of Jefferson's Thompson Building. He was an organizer of the first psychiatric diagnostic manual by the American Psychiatric Association. He helped set up the Eastern Pennsylvania Psychiatric Institute. He participated in the 1952 revision of the Pennsylvania Mental Health Act. He was a psychiatric consultant to the Municipal Court of Philadelphia and chairman of the Medical Advisory Committee of the Philadelphia County Courts. His contributions to the literature were on subjects ranging from war neuroses, adolescent problems, and capital punishment, to alcoholism and drug addiction.

Besides his positions at Jefferson Dr. Baldwin Keyes was consultant or honorary consultant at the Veterans Administration, Philadelphia General Hospital, Chester County Hospital, Eastern State Psychiatric Institute, and the Institute of Pennsylvania Hospital. He served as president of the Philadelphia Psychiatric Society and received its Lifetime Achievement Award in 1989. He was also a founder and president of the Pennsylvania Psychiatric Society. Keyes was a trustee at the Drexel Institute of Technology, the Fairmount Farm Sanitarium (of which he was also a founder), the Philadelphia Institute for Study and Prevention of Nervous and Mental Diseases, and the Willard Foundation. Keyes received an honorary D.Sc. degree from Drexel Institute and LL.D. degree from Jefferson Medical College.

Dr. Keyes served as president of the Jefferson Medical

College alumni association in 1955 and received its alumni achievement award in 1971. He resigned as chairman of Jefferson's psychiatry department in 1958, and was named emeritus professor. He continued clinical practice until 1979 when he regretfully closed his office at the age of eighty-six. He lived to the age of one hundred.

Dr. Baldwin Keyes's portrait by John C. Johansen was presented by the class of 1955. He is depicted lifesized and two-thirds length with his back to his desk. His attention is diverted from his reading material, and he marks his place with his left index finger and gazes directly at the viewer. The expression in his bright blue eyes and wide mouth is pleasant in a bland way, but does not capture the "famous smile" referred to by a senior student at the portrait ceremony. He called that smile "the real window through which we can see into Dr. Keyes's soul."

The physician was known by students and colleagues to be positive, optimistic, understanding, and supportive. Keyes was such an outstanding role model as a teacher and clinician that during his tenure as chairman of the department an unusually high percentage of students entered the study of psychiatry.

Portrait of Leandro M. Tocantins

LEANDRO MAUES TOCANTINS, M.D. (1901-63)
By Samuel George Phillips (ca. 1890-1965)

Oil on canvas
1964
34 x 27 in.

Signed upper left: "S. George Phillips"

Given in 1964 by the Charlotte Drake Cardeza Foundation and friends and colleagues
Accession number: 1964+e.P.02

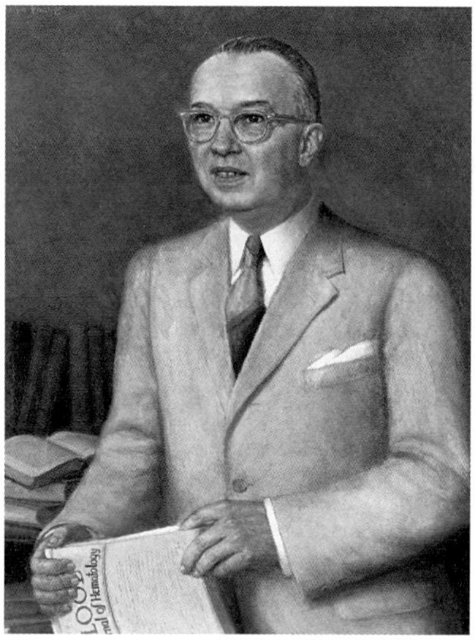

Dr. Leandro M. Tocantins was a Jefferson Medical College alumnus and professor recognized worldwide as an investigator and author in hematology.

Leandro Tocantins was born in 1901, a native of Para, Brazil. He graduated from Cornell University in 1922 and Jefferson Medical College in 1926. After an internship at Chestnut Hill Hospital in Philadelphia he entered general practice in Cleveland for three years. He returned to Jefferson in 1930 as the J. Ewing Mears research and teaching fellow. He was appointed associate in medicine in 1936 and rose in the academic ranks to become professor of clinical and experimental medicine, and acting head of the department of medicine in 1952.

Dr. Tocantins succeeded Dr. Harold W. Jones as director of the Charlotte Drake Cardeza Foundation for Research and Diseases of the Blood in 1954, and was named the Thomas Drake Martinez Cardeza Professor of Clinical Medicine and Hematology in 1959. While engaged in planning the expansion of the Cardeza Laboratories, he died suddenly in 1963.

Dr. Tocantins had also been head of the department of hematology at Pennsylvania Hospital from 1944 to 1954. He was a consultant in hematology to the Naval Hospital in Philadelphia and the National Clinical Center in Bethesda, Maryland, a member of the subcommittee on thrombosis and hemorrhage of the National Research Council, and a member of the hematology study section of the National Institutes of Health. He was a founder of both the American Society of Hematology and the International Society of Hematology, and president of the National Blood Club. He received an honorary degree from the University of Brazil in 1960.

Dr. Tocantins contributed more than two hundred papers on his investigations in blood platelets, the action of antiplatelet antibodies, prothrombin, antithromboplastin, and anticephalin, the coagulability and fluidity of blood, lipid coagulants and anticoagulants, the preservation and transplantation of bone marrow, the clinical management of hemorrhagic states, and the role of inhibitors in hemophilia. Tocantins was editor of the textbook *The Coagulation of Blood: Methods of Study* (1955), and a member of the editorial boards of *Blood: The Journal of Hematology* and the *American Journal of Physiology*.

A Jefferson executive faculty memoir of May 27, 1963 recalled that Dr. Leandro M. Tocantins was "endowed with a personality which portrayed external quiet, humility, and non-assumptuousness, yet within this same framework there burned a blue hot flame of ambition which drove him to achievements attained by but few Jeffersonians." The Cardeza Foundation library was dedicated to his memory, and Mrs. Tocantins donated her husband's impressive hematologic collection to the library.

Members of the Cardeza Foundation and other friends and colleagues commissioned S. George Phillips to paint a posthumous portrait of Dr. Leandro Tocantins in 1964. The physician is depicted half length and life-sized, standing next to a table with piles and rows of books. He wears a light gray suit and maroon and gray necktie. He holds an issue of *Blood: The Journal of Hematology* in front of his body. His left index finger marks his spot in his reading material, as he gazes eagerly to the left at some unknown interruption.

S. George Phillips was born in 1890 in Philadelphia and studied at the Pennsylvania Academy of the Fine Arts. Early in his career he was a magazine illustrator well known for a painting of Santa Claus for the Whitman Candy Company. For half a century he commuted daily from his home in Atlantic City to his Philadelphia studio where he painted portraits and occasional landscapes. In addition to prominent contemporary sitters, he had a specialty niche in ancestor portraits, painted after photographs, miniatures, and daguerreotypes.

Clinicians in the Surgical Specialties

Portrait of John H. Gibbon Jr.

(See color plate)

JOHN HEYSHAM GIBBON Jr., M.D. (1903-73)
By Gardner Cox (b. 1906)

Oil on canvas
1963
45 1/4 x 35 1/4 in.

Signed and dated lower right:
"Gardner/Cox/'63"

Given by JMC class of 1963
Accession number: 1963+e.P.01

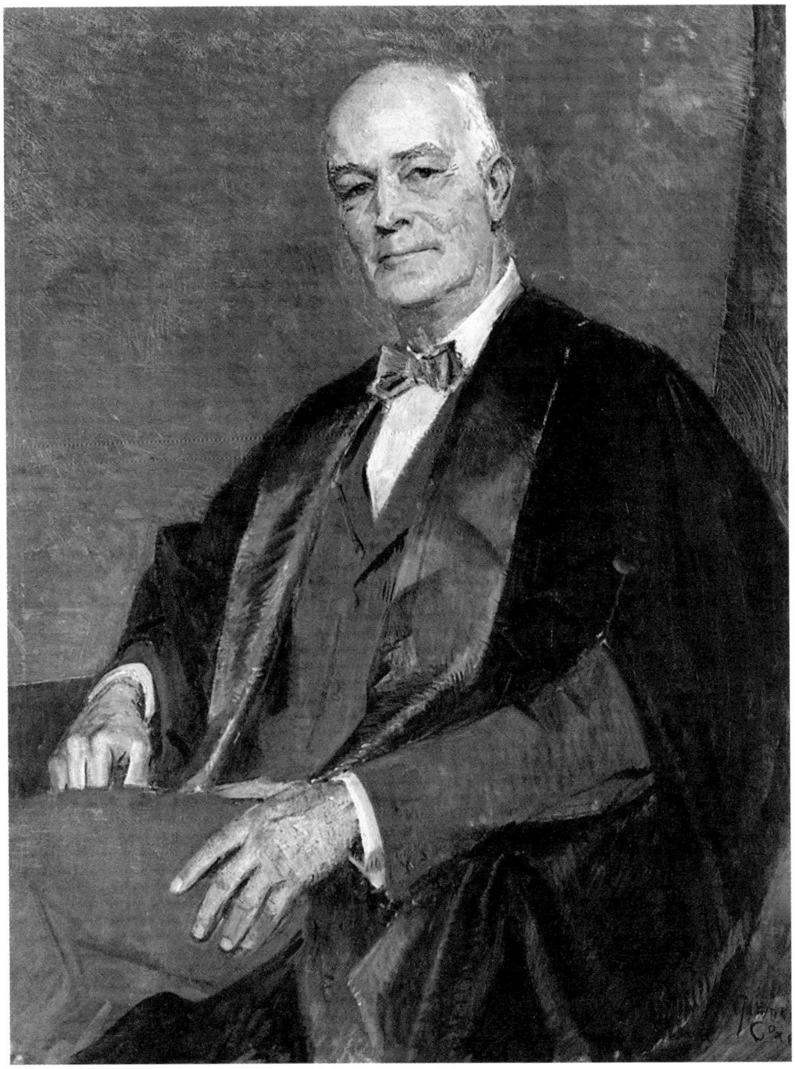

Dr. John H. Gibbon Jr. was the Samuel D. Gross Professor of Surgery and chair of the department at Jefferson Medical College. Internationally celebrated as the developer of the heart-lung machine, his pioneering investigative work paved the way for open-heart surgery including procedures for correction of congenital heart defects, repair of heart valves, coronary bypass, and heart transplants.

Dr. Gibbon carried forth longstanding family traditions as a fifth-generation physician and the third Jefferson alumnus in his family. Born in 1903 in Philadelphia, he was a graduate of

Princeton University (1923) and Jefferson Medical College (1927). After interning at Pennsylvania Hospital he was a research fellow in surgery at Harvard Medical School with Dr. Edward D. Churchill (1930-31 and 1934-35).

It was at Harvard that Dr. Gibbon first conceived the idea for a device that could perform the functions of the heart and lungs for critical short periods during emergency surgery. It was during his second fellowship at Harvard that Gibbon made the first successful attempt to use the heart-lung machine to "short-circuit" blood around a partial obstruction in the pulmonary artery of an animal (a cat).[8] In 1931 he married Mary ("Maly") Hopkinson, a laboratory technician and assistant to Dr. Churchill at Massachusetts General Hospital.

Gibbon also pursued his research at the School of Medicine of the University of Pennsylvania. He was a fellow in medicine in 1931-32 working with Dr. Eugene H. Landis to study the effects of temperature and tissue pressure on the movement of fluid through the human capillary wall. Then he was a Harrison fellow in surgical research at Penn from 1936 to 1942. Maly Gibbon continued to work alongside her husband in their experiments with a second extracorporeal device; they sought to demonstrate that the internal organs of animals suffered no damage from the device.

In 1940 Dr. Gibbon was commissioned a major in the Army Medical Reserve Corps and two years later went on active duty with the Pennsylvania Hospital Unit in the Southwest Pacific. He was promoted to lieutenant colonel in 1944 and returned to the United States where he became chief of the surgical service at Mayo General Hospital in Galesburg, Illinois.

In 1946 Gibbon accepted an offer from Dr. Thomas A. Shallow to join the Jefferson Medical College faculty as professor of surgery, director of surgical research, and attending surgeon. Shallow aimed at promoting research in the surgery department and knew of Gibbon's interest in developing a heart-lung machine.

Dr. Gibbon's more than twenty years of research culminated on May 6, 1953 with the first successful repair of an interatrial septal defect at open cardiotomy with complete support of the patient by extracorporeal circulation. This pioneering work of Gibbon's team ushered in the modern era in cardiothoracic surgery.

Another of Dr. Gibbon's major interests was the diagnosis and surgical management of lung cancer. He was also among the first to employ artificial ventilation to prevent respiratory acidosis during thoracic operations. His research laboratories developed the use of ion exchange for restoration of the normal chemical balance of bank blood. Gibbon added a period of basic research in the laboratory to Jefferson's surgical residency program, and a number of residents and fellows achieved high academic positions in their own careers.

Among Gibbon's most significant contributions to the medical literature was his authoritative textbook *Surgery of the Chest* (1962) which went through five editions. He was an editor of *Circulation Research* and *Annals of Surgery*.

In 1956 Dr. John H. Gibbon Jr. was appointed Jefferson's eighth chairman of surgery, third Samuel D. Gross Professor of Surgery, and attending surgeon-in-chief. His posts at other hospitals included Bryn Mawr Hospital, Pennsylvania Hospital, and the Veterans Administration Hospital.

Dr. Gibbon was a member of numerous learned societies including the American Academy of Arts and Sciences, and was an honorary fellow of the Royal College of Surgeons of England and of the Society of Thoracic Surgeons of Great Britain and Ireland. He was elected president of the American Association for Thoracic Surgery, the American College of Surgeons, the American Surgical Association, the Society of Clinical Surgery, and the Society for Vascular Surgery. Locally, he was president of the College of Physicians of Philadelphia, the Philadelphia Academy of Surgery, and the Jefferson Medical College alumni association.

After an early retirement from Jefferson in 1967 Dr. Gibbon was named the Samuel D. Gross Professor Emeritus of Surgery. He died in 1973 at the age of sixty-nine after suffering a heart attack on the tennis court.

A particularly incisive memoir describing Dr. John H. Gibbon's impact on Jefferson's surgery department and on the institution as a whole was written by Dr. John Y. Templeton III, a resident under Gibbon and his successor in the chair of surgery. The memoir appeared in faculty executive council minutes of March 6, 1973 and was reprinted in trustee minutes the following month:

> His advanced concepts of surgical training...his indefatigable attention to the well-being of his patients and the education and advancement of the members of his staff, created an atmosphere on his service not since seen at Jefferson and rarely encountered elsewhere...
>
> He was deeply concerned with education and his lectures to the students and his presentations of patients...were models of logical, lucid interpretation...Although he permitted [surgical residents] the latitude and responsibility that their ability and experience justified, he remained their severest critic, requiring of them performance to the same high standards that he exacted

[of] himself.

His research...remains a classic example of precise delineation of a problem, long years of careful investigational work in the laboratory and final successful application to a seriously ill human patient...

He was congenial and gregarious...A man of strong opinions of right and wrong, reasonably arrived at, he had many close friends and a few enemies. The friends he supported strongly and the enemies he fought to the best of his ability...those who were fortunate enough to be closely associated with him remember him best for his dedication to their own progress in surgery.

Dr. Gibbon's qualities of perseverance and strength of character are manifest in his depiction by Gardner Cox. He is shown two-thirds length and slightly larger than life-sized, appropriate for a surgical giant. He is seated and facing partially left, with legs crossed at the knee and large hands resting on his thighs. His head is turned and tilted to emphasize his chiseled features and square jaw. His sparkling blue eyes further enliven his alert and agreeable expression. His relaxed but erect posture exudes athletic energy. His academic gown is black with red center panels, signifying the Royal College of Surgeons. A jaunty blue bow tie and the open robe lend a note of informality and accessibility to this internationally celebrated physician. The artist's rapidly executed brush strokes contribute to a sense of the sitter's physical and mental liveliness and spontaneity.

The portrait was presented by the senior class on May 6, 1963, the tenth anniversary to the day of the first successful use of the heart-lung device. Out of admiration and affection for Gibbon, the ceremony was held in the amphitheater and not the customary auditorium. The class president explained, "Students of Dr. Gibbon know well that the walk from the back row to the center of this amphitheater is, indeed, a long one for the unprepared student. To be asked to discuss a case here is somewhat frightening, but always enlightening when Dr. Gibbon is moderator."

Gardner Cox was a noted portrait painter with impressive academic credentials and Boston connections like the portrait subject's. He was born in Holyoke, Massachusetts in 1906 and raised in Cambridge. His earliest art instruction came from his father, an architect, and his mother, a painter. His formal studies began at age seventeen in a summer art school in Provincetown, Massachusetts. While studying art at Harvard University from which he graduated in 1928, he spent summers at the Art Students League in New York and an artists' colony in Rockport, Massachusetts. After Harvard he received advanced training in painting at the Boston Museum of Fine Arts School while simultaneously studying architecture at the Massachusetts Institute of Technology.

Within a few years of his decision to devote himself exclusively to painting rather than continue working in his father's architectural firm, Gardner Cox was hailed as a portrait painter who could endow his sitters with life. Among his most celebrated subjects were Justice Felix Frankfurter, Judge Learned Hand, Robert Frost, Dylan Thomas, Robert F. Kennedy, Walter Lippman, Alfred North Whitehead, Dean Acheson, and General George C. Marshall.

Gardner Cox was head of the painting department at the Boston Museum School for two years starting in 1954. He was a member of the National Institute of Arts and Letters and the American Academy of Arts and Sciences, and a trustee of the American Academy in Rome. A selection of Cox's portraits, landscapes, and paintings of birds were shown at a one-man show at the William A. Farnsworth Library and Art Museum in Rockland, Maine in 1956. His portraits are found in many American museums and other public institutions.

Dr. John H. Gibbon Jr.'s father-in-law was Boston artist Sidney Hopkinson whose portrait of Gibbon hangs at the College of Physicians of Philadelphia. The painting was presented posthumously during a 1973 symposium cosponsored by Thomas Jefferson University and the College of Physicians to commemorate the twentieth anniversary of the first open-heart operation. Sadly, Dr. Gibbon died just three months before the planned celebration.

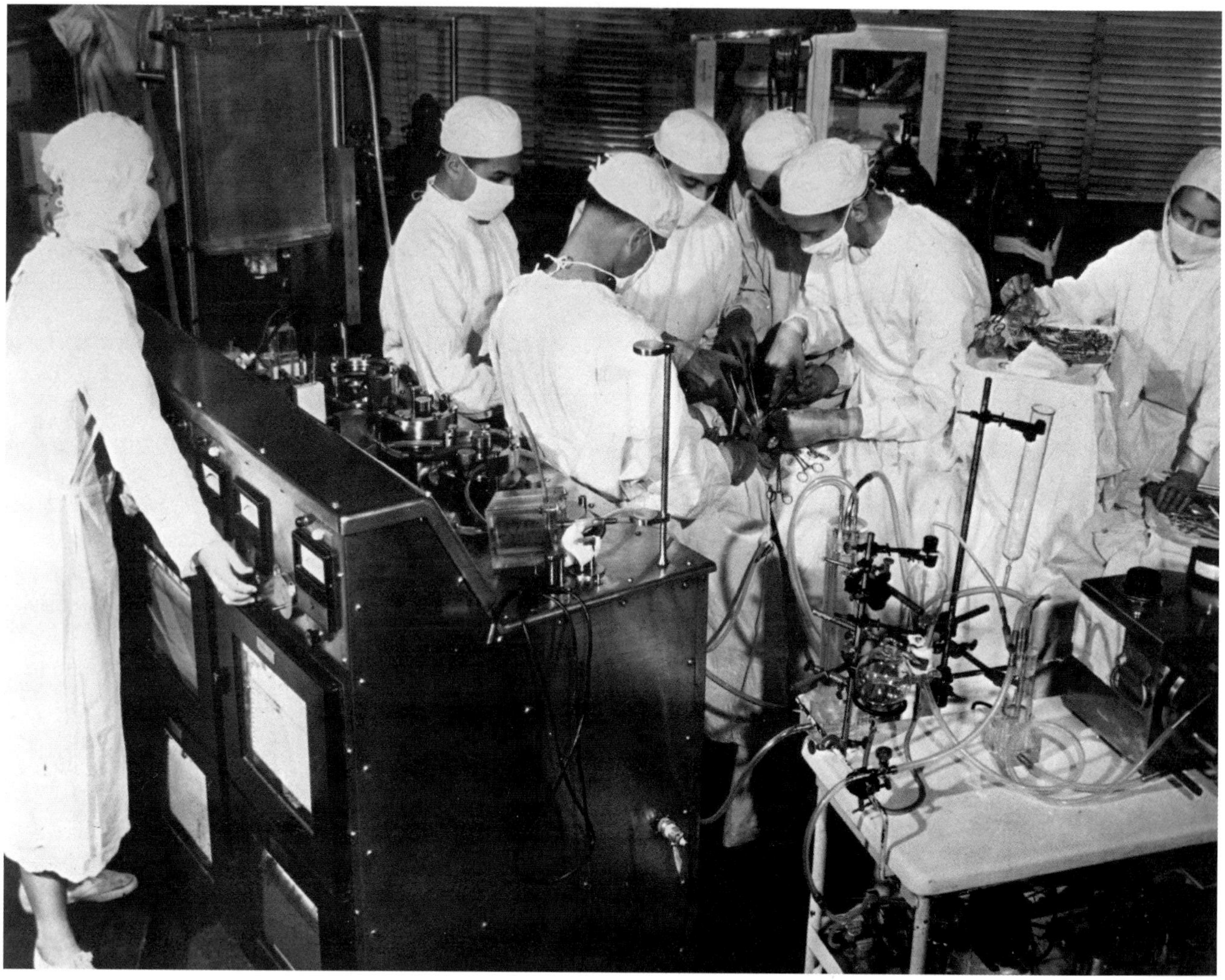

Animal Experiment on the Heart-lung Machine

ANIMAL EXPERIMENT ON THE HEART-LUNG MACHINE
Copy of original photograph
By unknown photographer

Original 1952
7 1/8 x 8 3/4 in.

Photographed for JMC
Accession number: 1952+e.Ph.01

Shortly after Dr. Gibbon arrived at Jefferson Medical College in 1946 he contacted the International Business Machines Corporation about his investigations. A close working relationship developed between personnel in Jefferson's surgical research laboratory and engineers at IBM resulting in a series of experimental heart-lung models.

Dr. Bernard J. Miller had just completed his residency when he became research associate in charge of the laboratory (1950-54). He was largely responsible for the design of electronic and other components within the extracorporeal circuit, and he conducted the research program that made the heart-lung machine practical for human use.[9] Only after the most painstaking experiments when the success rate with the screen oxygenator using medium-sized dogs had risen significantly, and the perfusion time had increased to about one hundred minutes, was the method applied to human patients.

The first successful open-heart operation using the heart-lung machine was conducted at the Jefferson Hospital on May 6, 1953 on Cecilia Bavolek, an eighteen-year-old woman from Wilkes Barre, Pennsylvania. The patient was connected to the apparatus for a total of forty-five minutes, and for twenty-six minutes all cardiorespiratory functions were maintained by the apparatus. She recovered fully.

Dr. Gibbon was assisted by Drs. Frank F. Allbritten Jr., Bernard J. Miller, and Thomas F. Nealon Jr. Experiencing relief, exhilaration, and joy, Gibbon later said that this was the first and only time that he did not write his own operative note immediately following surgery.[10]

The 1952 photograph shows members of the research team conducting an animal trial in the surgical research laboratory on the eighth floor of the College Building. Participants (kindly identified by Dr. Bernard J. Miller) are, from left to right: Anna, a technician; Steve Hudock, a technician; Dr. Richard Brown, a resident; Dr. Miller; an unidentified man; Dr. Hans Engel, a Rockefeller Research Associate at Jefferson (1953-54); and Joanne Crothers, a technician.

The technician on the left is using the manual controls for the venous pump. In the foreground are tubes leading into the collection cylinder. The pump on top of the table had been salvaged from a tachometer. Under the table is the capacitor circuit. Participants observed the dog's heart pulsating throughout the procedure.

When Dr. John H. Gibbon became professor of surgery at Jefferson, his wife, Maly, was named research assistant in Jefferson's first department of surgical research. Although Mrs. Gibbon is not present in this photograph, she continued her collaboration with the team. Jefferson awarded her an honorary doctor of science degree for her contributions in 1980.

John Scott Medal

JOHN SCOTT MEDAL (REVERSE)
By unknown designer

Bronze
1953
4 in. diameter

Inscriptions: on reverse, "AWARDED BY THE CITY OF PHILADELPHIA" along the outer border, and "PHILADELPHIA MANETO" under the coat of arms; on obverse, "THE JOHN SCOTT MEDAL TO THE MOST DESERVING" along the outer border, and "JOHN H. GIBBON, JR. B.A.M.D./FOR/THE INVENTION OF THE/HEART-LUNG APPARATUS/SEPTEMBER 18, 1953" inside the wreath

Given in 1980 by Maly (Mrs. Lovell) Thompson (formerly Mrs. John H. Gibbon Jr.)
Accession number: 1980+e.M.01

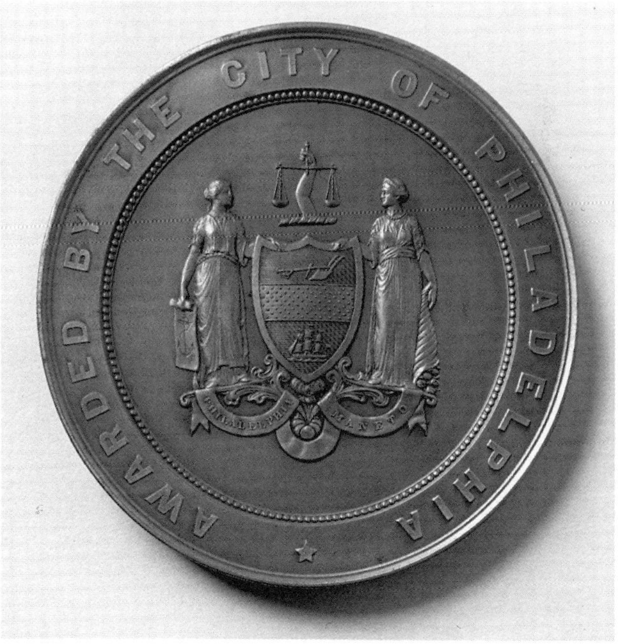

Dr. John H. Gibbon Jr. received local, national, and international awards for his achievements. His first such honor was the John Scott Medal awarded in 1953 by the Board of Directors of City Trusts of the City of Philadelphia. The medal is given annually to the most deserving man or woman whose inventions have contributed to the "comfort, welfare and happiness" of mankind. Previous recipients included Madame Curie, Thomas Edison, the Wright Brothers, Edwin Land, Jonas Salk, Glenn Seaborg, and Guglielmo Marconi.

The donor, John Scott, was an Edinburgh druggist who set up a fund in the early 1800s to honor "ingenious men or women who make useful inventions." It is not known why Scott chose Philadelphia to administer his bequest, but it is believed that he was an admirer of Benjamin Franklin.

The medal is made of bronze with a copper-colored finish. The obverse features the coat of arms of the City of Philadelphia, surrounded by a bead border. In the center is a shield with a plough and a ship in full sail, supported by allegorical figures of Abundance holding a cornucopia, on the right, and Hope holding a scroll with an anchor, on the left. The two figures stand on swags with the motto "PHILADELPHIA MANETO" ("let brotherly love continue").[11] Above the shield is an arm holding a balance. The reverse features a wreath enclosing the presentation inscription, and surrounded by a sunken bead border.

Among the distinguished surgeon's other important awards are the Rudolph Matas Award in Vascular Surgery from Tulane Univeristy, the Distinguished Service Award of the International Society of Surgery, the Gairdner Foundation International Award from the University of Toronto, the Philadelphia Award, the Research Achievement Award of the American Heart Association, the Roswell Park Medal, and the Albert Lasker Clinical Research Award.

Dr. Gibbon received honorary degrees from the University of Buffalo, Princeton University, the University of Pennsylvania, Dickinson College, Duke University, and Jefferson Medical College. Other honors at Jefferson include the Gibbon Scholar Program (a combined M.D./Ph.D. program of the Medical College and the College of Graduate Studies established in 1985) and the annual John H. Gibbon Jr. lectureship inaugurated two years later. In 1991 the "New Hospital" was renamed the Gibbon Building in his honor.

Portrait of Anthony F. DePalma

ANTHONY FREDERICK DePALMA, M.D. (b. 1904)
By Paul Froelich (1897-1968)

Oil on canvas
1962
45 1/2 x 42 1/4 in.

Signed and dated lower left: "P. Froelich/1962"

Given by JMC class of 1962
Accession number: 1962+e.P.01

Dr. Anthony F. DePalma was professor and chairman of the department of orthopaedic surgery at Jefferson Medical College. In addition to his enormously busy clinical practice, he was a dynamic teacher who stimulated many students to seek careers in orthopaedics.

Anthony F. DePalma was born in Philadelphia in 1904. He studied at the University of Maryland and received his medical degree from Jefferson Medical College in 1929. Following an internship at Philadelphia General Hospital he was a resident in orthopaedic surgery at the New Jersey Orthopaedic Hospital in Orange, and soon became orthopaedic surgeon to five hospitals in northern New Jersey. During World War II Dr. DePalma achieved the rank of commander in the United States Navy.

DePalma's first appointment at Jefferson Medical College was in 1946 as assistant professor of orthopaedic surgery. He rose quickly through the ranks, and in 1950 became the third James Edwards Professor and chairman of the department, succeeding Dr. James R. Martin. He was also chief orthopaedic surgeon at Methodist Episcopal Hospital, attending at Fitzgerald Mercy Hospital, consultant at the Veterans Administration Hospital, and a member of the rotating service at Philadelphia General Hospital.

DePalma enlarged the residency program in orthopaedics, and many former Jefferson residents later became leaders in their field. He also established the or-

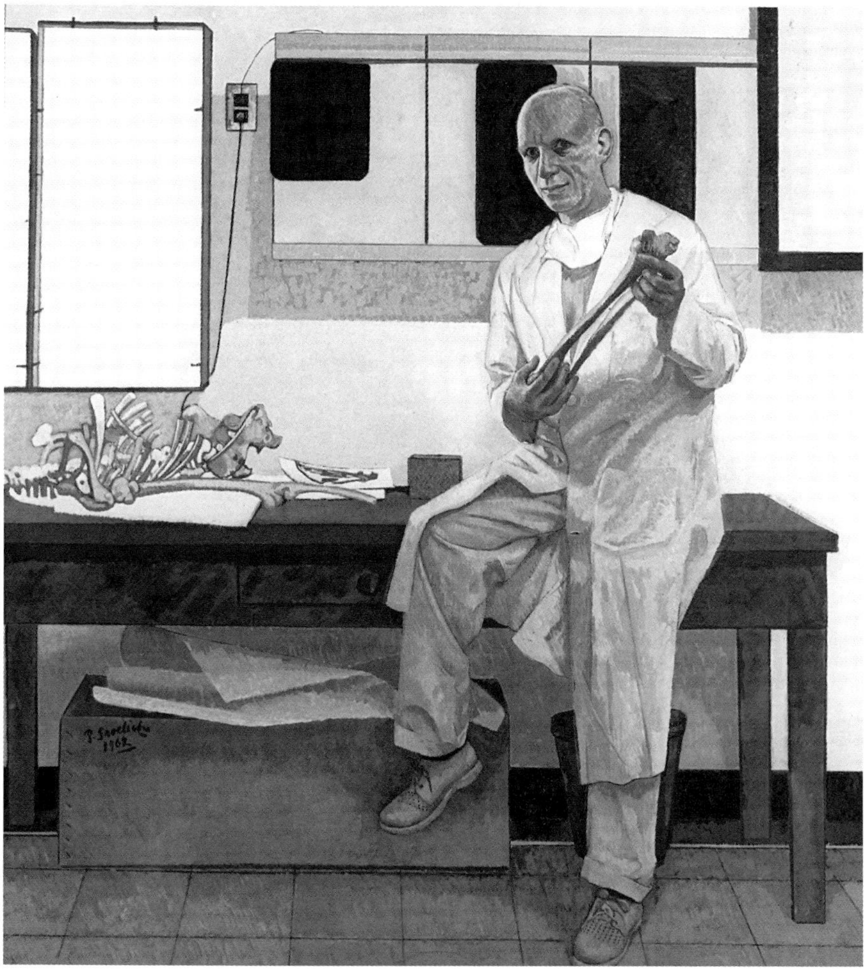

can Academy of Orthopaedic Surgeons in 1948. DePalma demonstrated his teaching and operating expertise abroad in the Dominican Republic, Japan, and Vietnam.

Dr. Anthony F. DePalma was president of Jefferson's alumni association in 1959 and received its achievement award in 1975. In 1990 the Jefferson Orthopaedic Society, a group founded by DePalma in 1960 and composed of former residents and fellows, funded renovations in the Thompson Annex's auditorium. The new facility was named in his honor and his portrait was moved there.

The Jefferson class of 1952 dedicated its yearbook to Dr. DePalma, and the class of 1962 elected him portrait honoree. In Paul Froelich's full-length, smaller than life-sized depiction, DePalma perches informally on the edge of a table, probably in an office in the orthopaedics department. Dressed for work, he wears a long white physician's coat, green scrub suit and operating shoes, and a white surgical mask dangling from his neck. He holds a human tibia and fibula in front of his body. Arranged on an adjacent table is a deconstructed skeleton including the spine, thorax, and ribs. On the yellow wall is a light box with X-rays. Below the table on the blue and green tile floor is a cardboard carton and a trash basket.

thopaedic research laboratory, and in 1965 obtained one of the first orthopaedic training grants awarded by the NIH. By the time Dr. DePalma retired in 1970 and was named emeritus professor, the department had been considerably strengthened. That same year he received the Rehabilitation Physician of the Year Award and the Christian R. and Mary F. Lindback Award for Distinguished Teaching.

Dr. DePalma was a prolific writer of classic orthopaedic texts including: *Surgery of the Shoulder* (1950), *Diseases of the Knee: Management in Medicine and Surgery* (1954), *Degenerative Changes in the Sternoclavicular and Acromioclavicular Joints in Various Decades* (1957), *The Management of Fractures and Dislocations: An Atlas* (1959), and *The Intervertebral Disc* (1970, coauthored with Richard H. Rothman, M.D.). In 1953 he was founding editor of *Clinical Orthopaedics*, a series of volumes in symposium form.

Dr. DePalma's initial research on the shoulder joint won him and his associates the gold medal of the Ameri-

The unconventional composition is geometrically composed with an overall linear design of rectangles and squares. Deep shadows and bright highlights on the physician's face and costume and a loosely brushed paint style enliven the surface. However, the subject's oversized, domelike head and deep facial creases, his unstable posture, and his piercing stare and restless expression give the viewer a feeling of unease. In addition, the brightness and acidity of the yellow, green, and blue colors add a jarring, almost irritating note.

These qualities of the painting metaphorically describe the orthopaedic surgeon's personality. Though a tireless worker in his clinical practice, in academic pursuits, and in the expansion of his department, DePalma was a controversial figure among his colleagues, considered by some to be too much of a "one-man show," and often arbitrary and brusque.[12] At the portrait presentation, the class president first expressed the students' respect and "frank awe" of Dr. DePalma, then described his contradictory effect:

> He has the ability to draw the best from his students. He has the impatience necessary to thwart his students['] need for laziness and yet the patience to allow honest mistakes—if made only once...He is arrogant enough to competitively bring out the best in his colleagues but yet honest in his praise for a job well done...
>
> A paradox of a man—one who fits no conventional pattern, who is accepted on his own terms. And it is in this mood that we chose to portray him on canvas.

Paul Froelich was born in 1897, a native Philadelphian who became noted as an advertising artist, illustrator, and painter. He studied at the Liberty Tadd School of Art and at the Pennsylvania Academy of the Fine Arts where he won two Cresson scholarships.

Froelich worked as an art director at the N. W. Ayer and the Gray and Rogers advertising firms. His work in advertising illustration may have influenced the simplified geometric forms and forceful colors of his painting. He was also associate director of the division of drawing and painting at the Philadelphia Museum College of Art which awarded him an honorary doctorate degree in fine arts in 1967.

Froelich exhibited figures, animals, and rural scenes in oils, watercolors, and prints regularly at local and national exhibitions. He had one-man shows at several Philadelphia galleries, the Philadelphia Art Alliance, and the Philadelphia Museum School of Art.

Portrait of Lewis C. Scheffey

LEWIS CASS SCHEFFEY, M.D. (1894-1969)
By John Christen Johansen (1876-1964)

Oil on canvas
1954
40 1/2 x 33 1/2 in.

Signed and dated lower left: "JOHN C. JOHANSEN 1954"
Exhibition: Pittsburgh, the Carnegie Institute, unknown date

Given by JMC class of 1954
Accession number: 1954+e.P.01

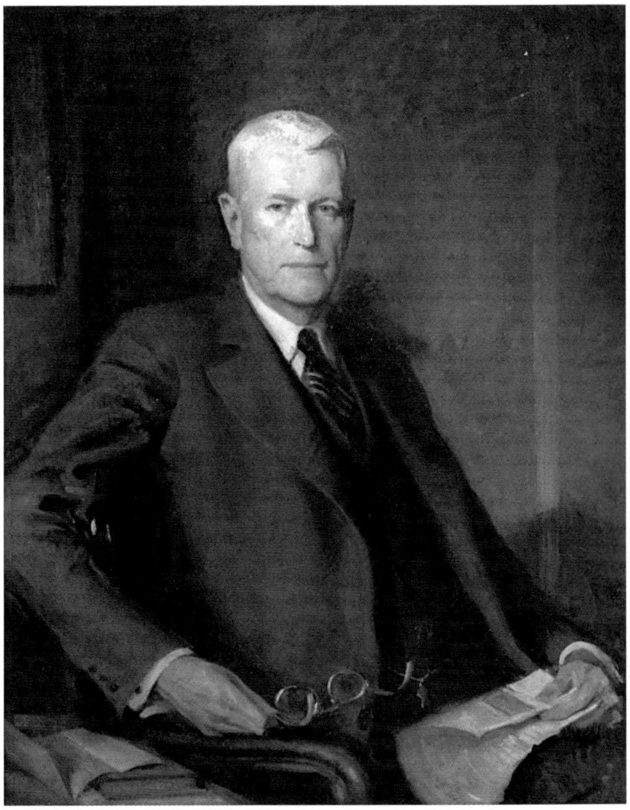

In 1940 Dr. Lewis C. Scheffey was named professor and chair of the department of gynecology. Six years later he was appointed the head of a new combined department of obstetrics and gynecology.

Lewis C. Scheffey was born in 1894 in Stamford, Connecticut and reared in Reading, Pennsylvania. He was a graduate of the Philadelphia College of Pharmacy and Science (1915) and Jefferson Medical College (1920). After serving a two-year residency at Jefferson he joined the faculty as an assistant demonstrator of gynecology and clinical assistant in the hospital. He also was a private assistant to Dr. Brooke M. Anspach and assisted in the revision of the latter's textbook, *Gynecology* (fifth edition, 1934). Scheffey rose through the academic ranks from assistant professor of gynecology in 1932 to professor and department chair in 1940, succeeding Dr. Anspach.

Under Dr. Scheffey's leadership of a unified department of obstetrics and gynecology starting in 1946, an integrated program for students and residents was developed and the teaching faculty was augmented. In 1949 a new maternity wing was opened with expanded facilities for private, semiprivate, and ward patients, and nursing facilities for full-term and premature babies.

Scheffey was recognized for his contributions to the field of pelvic cancer, especially methods for early diagnosis and treatment. An early advocate of vaginal cytology, Dr. Scheffey was a founder of the Inter-Society Cytology Council in 1951 (later known as the American Society of Cytology) and served as its president in 1956. He was also president of the Philadelphia Division of the American Cancer Society. He received the American Cancer Society's gold medal for his contributions in 1962.

He was elected president of the American Gynecological Society, the Philadelphia County Medical Society, and the College of Physicians of Philadelphia. He received an honorary doctor of science degree from Ursinus College and the Strittmatter Award of the Philadelphia County Medical Society.

Scheffey was elected president of Jefferson's alumni association in 1944. After his retirement in 1955 he was named emeritus professor. In 1979 the Lewis C. Scheffey Scholarship Fund was established at Jefferson by members of his family.

In 1954 the senior class presented a portrait of Dr. Scheffey by John C. Johansen to the college. The physician is shown life-sized and two-thirds length, seated in an armchair and facing slightly to the right. He holds his glasses in one hand and a folded paper in the other hand. He turns to look directly toward the viewer with an attentive and kindly expression. To give a sense of the surrounding space, the artist has added some books and papers on a table in the lower left corner and the edge of a framed picture in the upper left corner.

The subject's business suit is gray and the neutral palette is subdued throughout the painting. Although the portrait has undergone considerable restoration, Johansen has captured Dr. Scheffey's gentle, wise, and steadfast character, as described by speakers at his portrait presentation.

Portrait of Thaddeus L. Montgomery

THADDEUS LEMERT MONTGOMERY, M.D. (1896-1994)
By Roy Frederick Spreter (1899-1967)

Oil on canvas
1961
35 x 30 in.

Signed and dated lower right: "Roy Spreter/61"

Given in 1961 by JMC department of obstetrics and gynecology
Accession number: 1961+e.P.03

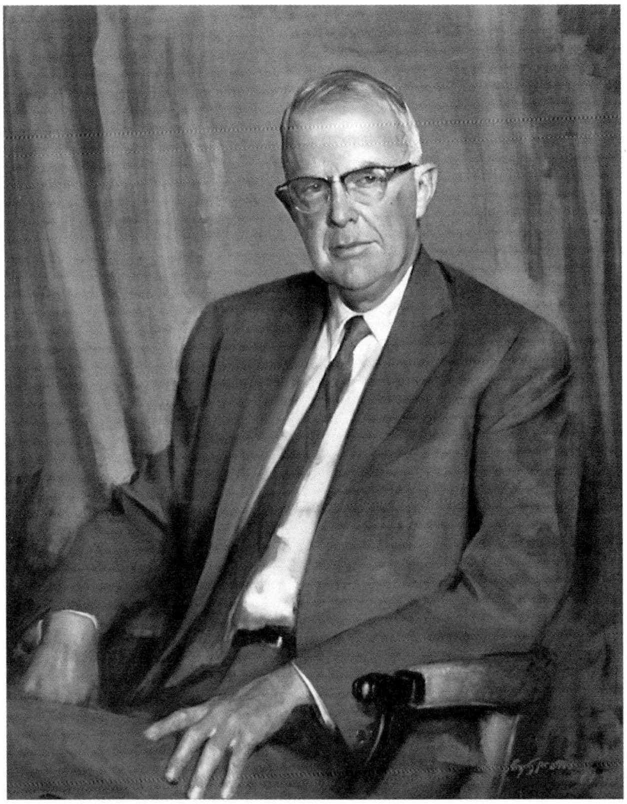

Dr. Thaddeus L. Montgomery succeeded Dr. Lewis C. Scheffey as the second chairman of the unified department of obstetrics and gynecology.

Thaddeus Montgomery was born in 1896 in Macon, Illinois and received his bachelor's degree from the University of Illinois in 1917. He graduated from Jefferson Medical College in 1920 and interned at Jefferson Hospital.

From 1922 to 1925 he held appointments at Jefferson as instructor of both anatomy and surgery, and was also an assistant to his uncle, Dr. Edward E. Montgomery, then the professor emeritus of gynecology. During the next decade Dr. Thaddeus Montgomery conducted a general practice and was assistant to Dr. Pascal B. Bland. He assisted in the work for Bland's textbook *Practical Obstetrics: for Students and Practitioners* (1932), and was coauthor of two subsequent editions.

From 1923 to 1940 Dr. Montgomery was clinical professor of obstetrics, then resigned to become the professor of obstetrics and gynecology and first head of the combined department at Temple University School of Medicine. He returned to Jefferson in 1946 as professor of obstetrics and gynecology and director of the division of obstetrics at Jefferson Medical College. He succeeded Dr. Lewis C. Scheffey as chairman of the unified department in 1955.

Montgomery was a proponent of conservative obstetrics, the "physiologic approach" to childbirth. He favored "natural childbirth" and breast-feeding, and was concerned about the overuse of drugs and instruments to speed up labor and delivery and the overuse of anesthesia and analgesia. He introduced the father participation program and the rooming-in program for mother and infant to the Jefferson obstetrics service. He contributed to the medical literature on these topics and on causes for maternal and infant mortality, and was editor of *Fetal Physiology and Distress* (1960).

Dr. Thaddeus Montgomery served as president of the American Association of Obstetricians, Gynecologists, and Abdominal Surgeons, and of the Obstetrical Society of Philadelphia. A dedicated Jeffersonian, he served as president of the alumni association. He was a recipient of the Christian R. and Mary F. Lindback Award (1961), an honorary LL.D. (1962), and the alumni achievement award (1970). The 1960 student yearbook was dedicated jointly to Drs. Thaddeus Montgomery and John B. Montgomery.

At the time of his academic retirement in 1961 Dr. Thaddeus L. Montgomery was named emeritus professor but maintained his private practice for many years. A painter and writer, he was working on a historical novel based on the family of Jesus at the time of his death in 1994.

In 1957 Dr. and Mrs. Thaddeus Montgomery with their family and friends presented an electric organ for McClellan Hall in memory of their son Richard Woods Montgomery who died in the service of his country. Dr. Montgomery's portrait, presented in 1961 by the department of obstetrics and gynecology, was placed adjacent to the organ.

Roy F. Spreter depicted the physician two-thirds length and life-sized, seated in an upholstered armchair and facing slightly left. His head is turned and tilted so that he averts his eyes from the viewer. His posture is relaxed and the figure is capably rendered in three dimensions. His blue-gray business suit has touches of warm colors that relate to the reddish drapery folds in the background. The subject's reserved demeanor scarcely hints at his affectionate nickname of "T. L.," or the humaneness, patience, and generosity admired by his patients, colleagues, and students.

Portrait of John B. Montgomery

JOHN BARRICK MONTGOMERY, M.D. (1900-87)
By Alden MacMaster Wicks (1914-87)

Oil on masonite
1965
40 x 32 in.

Signed lower left: "Wicks"

Given by JMC class of 1965
Accession number: 1965+e.P.03

Dr. John B. Montgomery was appointed professor of obstetrics and gynecology at Jefferson Medical College in 1952, capably aiding Dr. Lewis G. Scheffey in the division of gynecology. In 1961 he succeeded Dr. Thaddeus Montgomery (no relation) as chairman of the unified department.

John Montgomery was born in 1900 in Lewistown, Pennsylvania and graduated from Juniata College in 1921. After a year of graduate school at the University of Pennsylvania, he entered Jefferson Medical College where he received his M.D. degree in 1926. He interned at the Jefferson Hospital.

Dr. Montgomery became the assistant and later the

associate of Dr. Brooke M. Anspach, an alliance that lasted from 1928 to 1940. Montgomery rose through the ranks to become clinical professor of gynecology in 1940, professor of obstetrics and gynecology in 1952, and chair in 1961. Although he relinquished the chairmanship in 1965 and was made emeritus professor, he continued his career as chief of the obstetrics and gynecology service at Methodist Hospital until 1969. He retired from active practice in 1980. His son Bruce B. Montgomery, M.D. graduated from Jefferson in 1960.

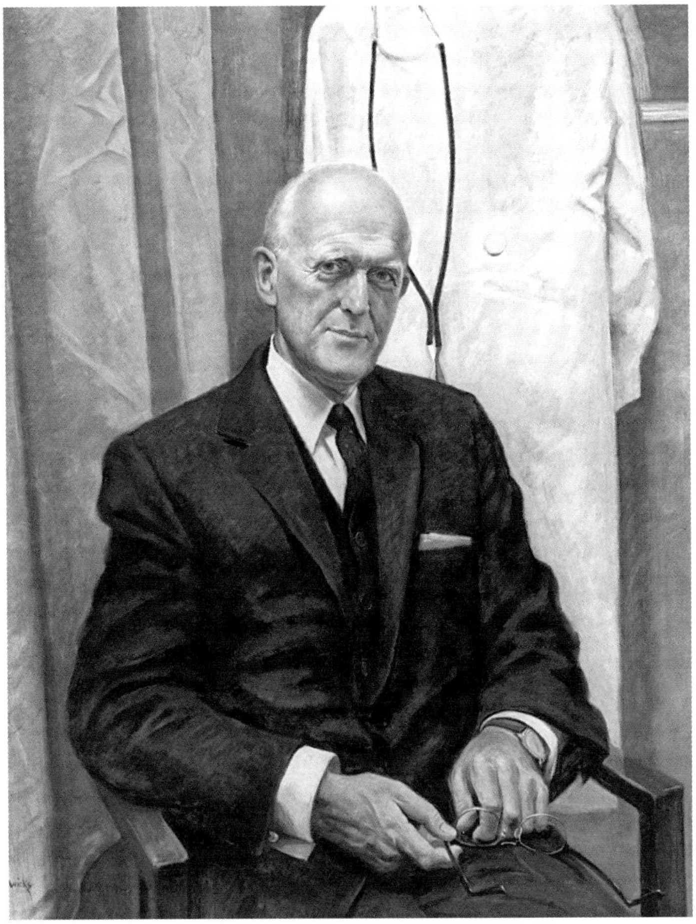

Dr. John Montgomery was president of the Philadelphia Obstetrical Society. He contributed to the medical literature on ovarian tumors, the menopause and postmenopausal bleeding, the management of uterine displacements, and urethral obstruction from pelvic lesion. He received an honorary doctor of science degree from Juniata College in 1951.

Montgomery served a term as president of the Jefferson Medical College alumni association, received its achievement award in 1979, and was awarded an honorary doctor of pedagogy degree from the college in 1972. Recipient of the Christian R. and Mary F. Lindback Award in 1964, he was regarded as a superb teacher by Jefferson students and was selected as portrait honoree by the class of 1965.

Depicted by Alden M. Wicks, Dr. Montgomery is shown two-thirds length and life-sized, seated in a plain wooden armchair. He is dressed in a dark brown business suit, and holds his reading glasses in his lap. He turns his head to gaze directly toward the viewer with an alert and confident expression.

Dr. Montgomery is located in his working environment, a patient examining room. Behind him is a white physician's coat and stethoscope hanging on a green curtain which conceals the examining table. Although the subject seated in an armchair in front of a curtain resembles the depiction of Dr. Thaddeus L. Montgomery, the portrait of "J. B." more capably suggests the subject's tireless energy and the personal interest he extended toward his patients, students, and colleagues.

Portrait of Benjamin F. Haskell

BENJAMIN FRANKLIN HASKELL, M.D. (1901-82)
By Molly Guion (b. 1910)

Oil on canvas
36 x 30 in.
1975

Signed lower right: "M. GUION"

Given in 1975 by JMC volunteer faculty association
Accession number: 1975+e.P.01

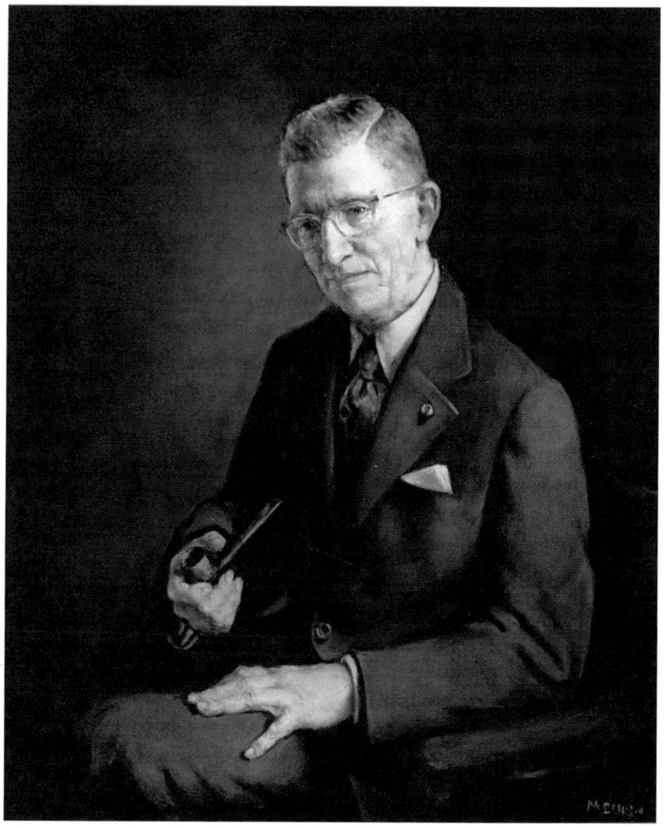

Dr. Benjamin F. Haskell, clinical professor of surgery (proctology), was one of the most beloved and respected clinicians of his era at Jefferson Medical College. He maintained a private practice in Philadelphia for fifty-six years and was known as the dean of Philadelphia proctologists.

Born in 1901 in Norfolk, Virginia, Benjamin Haskell took a premedical course at Temple University and graduated in the class of 1923 at Jefferson Medical College. After an internship at the Jefferson Hospital and a residency in pathology, he was appointed a clinical assistant in the department of proctology, and in 1938, chief clinical assistant. He rose in the academic ranks from assistant professor in 1946 to clinical professor of proctology in 1952. He was elected honorary professor in 1966.

Exceptionally active in Jefferson Medical College's alumni association, Dr. Haskell was its president in 1963, and was instrumental in initiating the alumni achievement award, of which he was the recipient in 1978. His contributions to college and hospital affairs included founding the Parents' Day program for sophomore students, and helping to develop the volunteer faculty association of which he was the second president. The Benjamin F. Haskell lectureship was established in his honor in 1981.

In addition to his posts at Jefferson, Dr. Haskell was also attending proctologist at Mt. Sinai Hospital for ten years. In 1956 he was president of the Pennsylvania Proctologic Society. His wife Gertrude has long been a devoted member of Jefferson Hospital's women's board, and their son David S. graduated from Jefferson in 1960.

The volunteer faculty association presented Dr. Haskell's portrait in 1975. Depicted by Molly Guion, the physician is shown two-thirds length and life-sized, seated in an armchair and turned partly left. His right hand holds a pipe, an attribute once commonly used to denote contemplation; Dr. Haskell's serious expression and downward gaze augment the suggestion of someone deep in thought.

His dark blue business suit and maroon dotted necktie contrast with the bright green background and intense flesh tones. His lined face and strong hands are spotlighted from the right, and delineated in minute dabs of pinks, reds, maroons, yellows, and blues.

A resident of Rye, New York, Molly Guion was born in 1910 and studied at the Grand Central Art School, the Art Students League, and privately. She has participated in group shows throughout the country and had a one-person show at the Seattle Art Museum. An exhibition of her British portraits toured the United States and Canada. Her two portraits of Queen Elizabeth hung in the mess hall of the British Royal Navy in Portsmouth, England and at the British Consulate in New York. She had a private showing at Buckingham Palace and was elected a fellow of the Royal Society of Arts.

Molly Guion's two portraits of Governor Thomas E. Dewey hang at Columbia University and the New York State Capitol in Albany. Among her awards are the Ellerhusen Memorial Prize of the Allied Artists of America and gold medals from the National Art Club and the American Artists Professional League.

Portrait of Fred Harbert

FRED HARBERT, M.D., D.Sc. (Med.) (1905-90)
By Ben Solowey (1900-78)

Oil on canvas
1978
40 x 32 in.

Signed and dated lower right: "Ben Solowey/1978"

Given in 1978 by friends and colleagues
Accession number: 1978+e.P.02

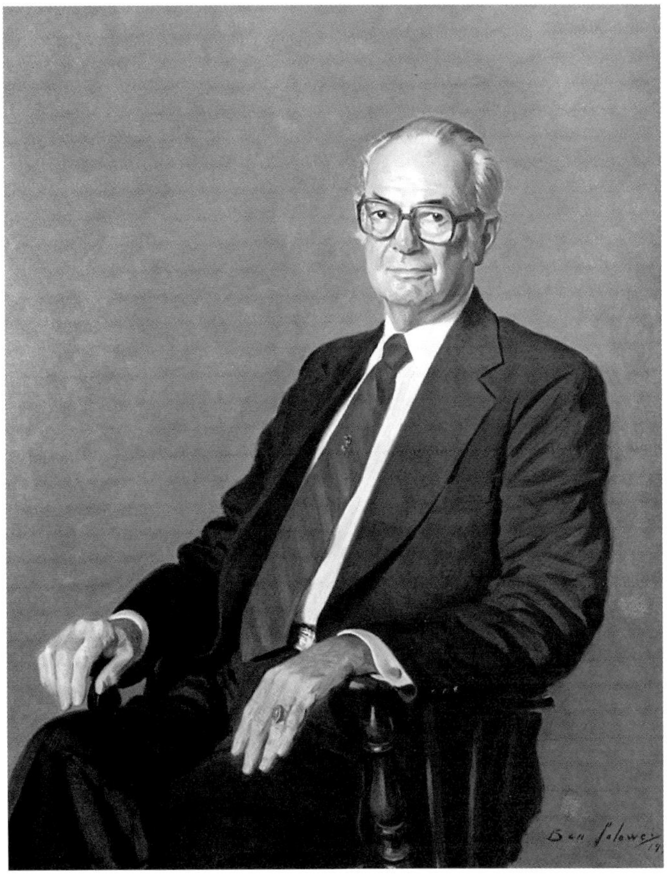

Dr. Fred Harbert was appointed professor and head of the department of otology at Jefferson in 1951. Three years later he was elected the first professor and chair of a new department of otolaryngology which combined otology with rhinology, laryngology, and bronchoesophagology.

Fred Harbert was born in 1901 in Detroit and received his bachelor of arts and bachelor of medicine degrees in 1928 from Wayne State University. He enlisted in the U.S. Navy and after serving a year's internship at the Philadelphia Naval Hospital, he received his doctor of medicine degree at Wayne State University School of Medicine (1929).

Harbert also received an M.S. degree (1940) and a D.Sc. degree (1942) in otolaryngology at the Graduate School of Medicine of the University of Pennsylvania. He completed a residency in ophthalmology at the Illinois Eye and Ear Infirmary in 1943. He returned to Penn to teach following the war.

Harbert's naval career before World War II included tours of duty in China and the Philippine Islands. During the war he served as chief of the EENT department on hospital ships and the battleship U.S.S. *Alabama*. Between 1947 and 1954 Dr. Harbert supervised residency training programs in otolaryngology at naval hospitals in Philadelphia and Bethesda, Maryland. He retired from the service with the rank of captain in the U.S. Navy Medical Corps in 1954.

After Dr. Fred Harbert became chair of otolaryngology at Jefferson Medical College in 1954 he fulfilled his primary goal of attracting and training a large number of high quality residents who appreciated his reputation as an exacting taskmaster. Harbert was also a consultant to the Philadelphia General Hospital and the U.S. Naval Hospital in Philadelphia. He was a visiting lecturer in otolaryngology at the University of Pennsylvania School of Medicine from 1952 to 1967.

Dr. Harbert had terms as president of the American Otorhinologic Society for Plastic Surgery, the Philadelphia Laryngological Society, and the Neurotology Group. He received Distinguished Service Citations from Wayne University Medical College (1967) and its alumni association (1968). He was elected emeritus professor upon his retirement from Jefferson in 1970. He died in 1990 and was interred at Arlington National Cemetery with full military honors.

Dr. Fred Harbert's portrait by Ben Solowey was presented in 1978 by his many friends and colleagues. He is shown three-quarters length and life-sized, seated in an armchair and facing slightly left. His posture is erect but relaxed. He looks directly at the viewer with a serious but pleasant expression on his square-shaped face. Dr. Harbert was known to be very kind to patients and charitable toward colleagues.

The painting's atmospheric background is a warm gray, contrasting with the sitter's dark blue business suit and maroon necktie. The artist's paint style is fluid and quickly brushed, especially on the sitter's face and hands.

Ben Solowey was a noted painter, sculptor, and cartoonist of stage and screen personalities. Born in Warsaw, Poland in 1900 he spent his early years in St. Petersburg, Russia where his father was bootmaker in the

Czar's court. Fearing conscription into the Russian army the family emigrated to Philadelphia in 1914.

As a youth Solowey studied art in free courses at the Graphic Sketch Club and at the Spring Garden Institute, and then won a three-year scholarship to the Pennsylvania Academy of the Fine Arts. In 1924 he financed a study trip abroad by working as a ship's steward. Upon his return to Philadelphia Solowey opened a studio where he worked as a commercial artist for interior decorators and furniture stores, while honing his skills as a portrait painter.

In 1928 he decided to forge his career in New York where for several months he was employed by newspapers to make theatrical pastel portraits after photographs. The next year he was assigned to sketch actress Ethel Barrymore in her dressing room. The notable picture by the nervous young artist was published in the April 7 edition of the *New York Times* and established his reputation as a portraitist. It was the first of more than five hundred live sketches of the theatrical "Who's Who." Among his subjects were Laurence Olivier, Cornelia Otis Skinner, Spencer Tracy, Jimmy Durante, Ethel Merman, Katherine Hepburn, Al Jolson, Noel Coward, Gertrude Lawrence, Claudette Colbert, and John Gielgud.

In 1936 Solowey and his wife moved to a farm in Bedminster, Bucks County, Pennsylvania and his studio soon became a gathering place for local artists, writers, and patrons. His watercolors and oils of still lifes and rural landscapes won several awards including the Dawson Memorial Medal of the Philadelphia Water Color Club and the gold medal of the Pennsylvania Academy's Fellowship. He produced many private as well as public portraits.

Ben Solowey taught painting at the Philadelphia Museum School of Art, the Fleisher Memorial Foundation, the Allen's Lane Art Center, and the New Hope Fine Arts Workshop. In 1958 there was a retrospective exhibition of his work at the Woodmere Art Gallery.

Portrait of Daniel C. Baker Jr.

DANIEL CLIFTON BAKER Jr., M.D., D.M.Sc. (1909-74)
By Molly Guion (b. 1910)

Oil on canvas
1974
40 x 30 in.

Signed lower right: "M. GUION"

Given in 1974 by the artist
Accession number: 1974+e.P.01

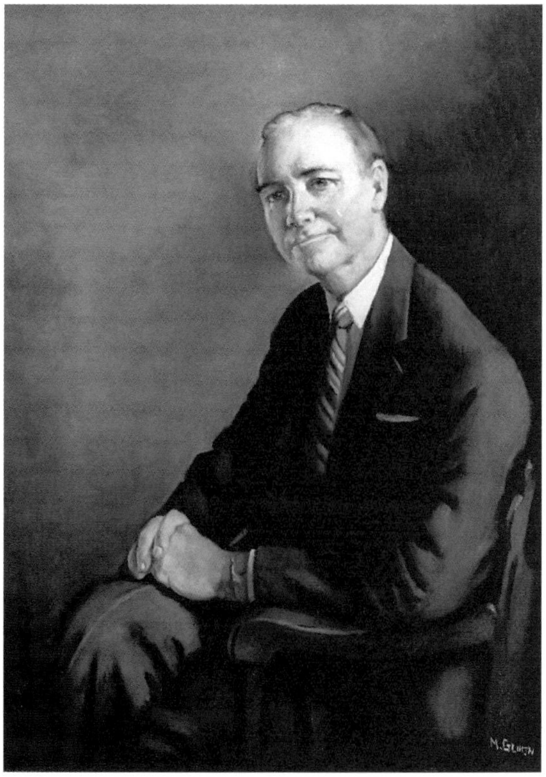

Dr. Daniel C. Baker Jr. was a native Philadelphian and Jefferson Medical College alumnus who became a nationally known otolaryngologist. He forged his career at the College of Physicians and Surgeons of Columbia University.

Daniel Baker was born in 1909 and graduated from the University of Pennsylvania (1929) and Jefferson Medical College (1933). While an intern and resident at Jefferson he attracted the attention of Dr. Louis H. Clerf, whom he strove to emulate. Dr. Baker later received a doctorate in medical science in otolaryngology from the College of Physicians and Surgeons of Columbia University (1939).

After wartime service as a lieutenant commander at the National Naval Medical Center in Bethesda, Maryland Dr. Baker joined the faculty at Columbia as an assistant professor in 1946. In 1964 he was appointed professor and chairman of the department of otolaryngology and director of the otolaryngology service at Presbyterian Hospital.

Dr. Baker was a director of the American Board of Otolaryngology and president of the American Broncho-esophagological Association, and delivered many named lectures for local and national otolaryngological societies. He was president-elect of the American Laryngological Society (whose Newcomb Award he had received in 1971) when he died in 1974.

Sadly, his death occurred just days before he was to have received Jefferson Medical College's alumni achievement award. The silver plaque was accepted by his son, Daniel C. Baker III, M.D., and his widow who had graduated from Jefferson's School of Nursing.

One month after the award presentation, Molly Guion graciously presented to Thomas Jefferson University a copy of her 1971 portrait of Dr. Baker in the possession of his family.

The physician is depicted two-thirds length and life-sized, seated in an armchair. His hands are tightly clasped, resting on his thigh. He looks toward the viewer with an attentive and pleasant expression. The turn and tilt of the subject's head call attention to the elongation of his neck and the steep, diagonal slope of his shoulder, eccentric traits of Molly Guion portraits.

The hues of the sitter's dark blue suit and striped necktie are repeated and heightened in the cool green, purple, and blue-black colors of the atmospheric background. The pigments are laid on with thickly brushed, energetic strokes throughout.

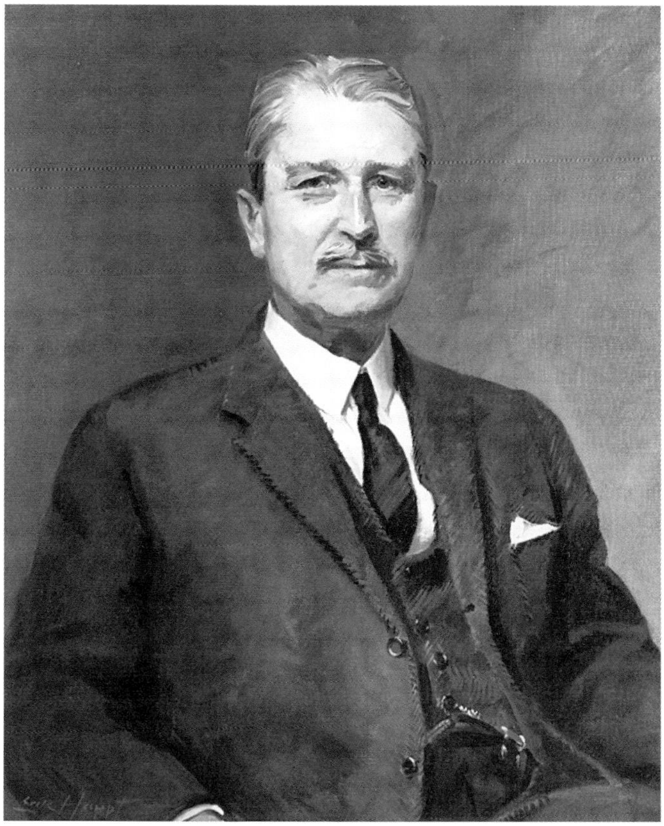

Portrait of George J. Willauer

GEORGE JACOB WILLAUER, M.D. (1896-1977)
By Erik Guide Haupt (b. 1891)

Oil on canvas
1965
30 x 25 in.

Signed lower left: "Erik Haupt"

Given in 1965 by former surgical residents and friends
Accession number: 1965+e.P.04

Dr. George J. Willauer, a clinical professor of surgery at Jefferson Medical College, was a nationally recognized pioneer in vascular surgery and inventor of a number of surgical instruments.

George Willauer was born in 1896 in Stockertown, Pennsylvania and received degrees from Franklin and Marshall College (1917) and Jefferson Medical College (1923). He served in the cavalry of the U.S. Army during World War I.

Following an internship at Jefferson Hospital Dr. Willauer studied abroad for a year in Vienna and

Munich. He returned to Jefferson for further training at the Daniel Baugh Institute of Anatomy (1927-34). He rose from assistant professor of surgery in 1938 to clinical professor by 1952, and was director of anesthesia. He was named honorary clinical professor in 1961.

He was director of surgery at Methodist Hospital from 1948 to 1961 as well as president of the medical staff and director of the department of anesthesia. He was also director of the department of surgery at Eagleville Sanatorium in Eagleville, Pennsylvania from 1928 to 1964.

Dr. George Willauer became expert in the surgical treatment of pulmonary tuberculosis and massive trauma to the thorax. He pioneered the use of continuous spinal anesthesia for thoracoplasty. He was one of the first surgeons in Philadelphia to remove a patient's lung successfully. His designs of surgical instruments include the Willauer modification of the Deaver retractor and the Willauer dissecting clamp.

Dr. Willauer was a founder of the American Association for Thoracic and Vascular Surgery, and president of the Pennsylvania Association of Thoracic Surgery and the Philadelphia Academy of Surgery. He was also a founder and president of the Laennec Society. He received an honorary D.Sc. degree from Franklin and Marshall College and an honorary LL.D. degree from Jefferson Medical College. Other Jefferson honors accorded Dr. Willauer include his service as president of the alumni association (1962), and his selection for the alumni achievement award (1972) and alumni representative to the board of trustees (1968-71).

A portrait of Dr. George Willauer by Erik G. Haupt was presented to the college in 1965 by former residents and friends. The physician is shown half length and life-sized, seated and turned slightly to the right. He looks directly toward the viewer with a lively and attentive expression. The artist's command of the figure and his rapid brushwork convey the forcefulness and confidence of the subject. The dashing appearance of the mustached figure with chiseled features is enhanced by his well tailored, bluish-gray, three-piece suit and striped necktie, pocket handkerchief, and gold watch chain.

Though he was known as a "drill sergeant" teacher with exacting standards, his explanations of technical material were often colorfully delivered with the skill of an actor. Among his close friends he was known as a dramatic storyteller and he enjoyed their camaraderie during hunting, fishing, and camping trips.

Portraitist Erik G. Haupt was born in Cassel, Germany in 1891. His studies at the Royal Academy in Munich and the Julian Academy and Colarossi Academy in Paris were followed by graduate work at the Maryland Institute in Baltimore. He exhibited nationally and had one-man shows at the Pittsfield, Massachusetts Museum and the National Arts Club. He was an instructor in drawing at the Maryland Institute. Haupt's portraits have entered many private and public collections including Johns Hopkins and Yale Universities, Vassar College, and the U.S. Supreme Court.

Portrait of William H. Kraemer

WILLIAM HENRY KRAEMER, M.D. (1879-1962)
By Mary Stevenson (Mrs. Melrose E.) Weed (d. 1956)

Oil on canvas
1944
42 x 30 in.

Signed lower right: "M. STEVENSON WEED"

Given in 1944 by the Elizabeth Storck Kraemer Memorial Foundation for Cancer Research

Accession number: 1944+e.P.01

Dr. William H. Kraemer was an associate professor of surgery (oncology) at Jefferson Medical College. He was the founder and director of the Elizabeth Storck Kraemer Foundation, a pioneering center for chemotherapy research.

William H. Kraemer was born in 1879 in Schwieberdingen, Germany. His family emigrated to West Virginia when Kraemer was aged five. Although his only prior formal education was at a rural elementary school, he nonetheless pursued self-education with such zeal that he ultimately achieved degrees from the College of Pharmacy of New York (1901) and Jefferson Medical College (1906).

Dr. Kraemer entered general practice in Wilmington, Delaware, and was also physician to the Black Powder Division of the E. I. duPont de Nemours Company. In the 1920s Kraemer became interested in the

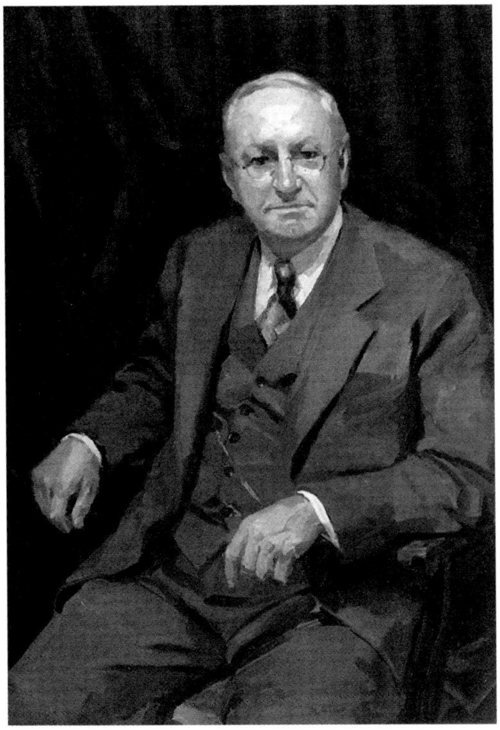

possibility of curing cancer with chemotherapeutic agents. This work caught the attention of Pierre S. duPont, a grateful patient. In 1928 duPont proposed the development of the Elizabeth Storck Kraemer Memorial Foundation for Cancer Research (named for Dr. Kraemer's second wife who had died of cancer). The foundation was supported by the duPont family and the Longwood Foundation.

Kraemer was made director of research at the Kraemer Foundation, a post he filled from 1929 until his death in 1962. The tumor clinic division (Jefferson's division of neoplastic diseases) and the biological laboratory (in the department of pathology) were located at Jefferson Medical College. The chemical division was located at the duPont experimental station in Wilmington.

The Kraemer Foundation published more than twenty papers on experimental cancer by Dr. Peter A. Herbut, the majority of which were coauthored by Dr. Kraemer. By 1959 four thousand chemicals had been screened for antitumor properties and one thousand cancer patients had received chemotherapy.

Dr. Kraemer served as president of Jefferson Medical College's alumni association in 1931 and was awarded an honorary doctor of science degree by the college in 1961. He was also cited by the American Cancer Society for distinguished services in 1958.

In 1944 the foundation presented to the college a portrait of Dr. William H. Kraemer painted by Mary Stevenson Weed. The subject is shown two-thirds length and life-sized, seated in an armchair. He looks straight out toward the viewer with an earnest expression. Dr. Kraemer wears a three-piece, brown business suit and striped necktie. A dark maroon drapery is the background. Although the painting shows deterioration in the blotchy face and hands, it does communicate a certain vibrancy.

Portrait of Philip J. Hodes

PHILIP J. HODES, M.D., D.Sc. (1906-95)
By Agnes Allen (b. 1897)

Oil on canvas
1971
44 x 32 in.

Signed lower right: "Agnes Allen"

Given in 1971 by friends and colleagues
Accession number: 1971+e.P.02

Dr. Philip J. Hodes was professor of radiology and chairman of the department at Jefferson Medical College. He was internationally recognized in his field.

Philip Hodes was born in 1906 in New York City and reared in Orange, New Jersey. He earned all his academic degrees at the University of Pennsylvania: bachelor of science (1928), doctor of medicine (1931), and doctor of medical science in radiology (1940). He was also an intern and fellow in radiology at the Hospital of the University of Pennsylvania.

During World War II Dr. Hodes served as chief of radiology with the Twentieth General Hospital (the University of Pennsylvania unit) and achieved the rank of colonel in the U.S. Army Medical Corps. He was a professor of radiology at Penn's School of Medicine from 1952 to 1958.

When Dr. Philip Hodes joined the Jefferson faculty in 1958 as professor and chair of radiology he already was

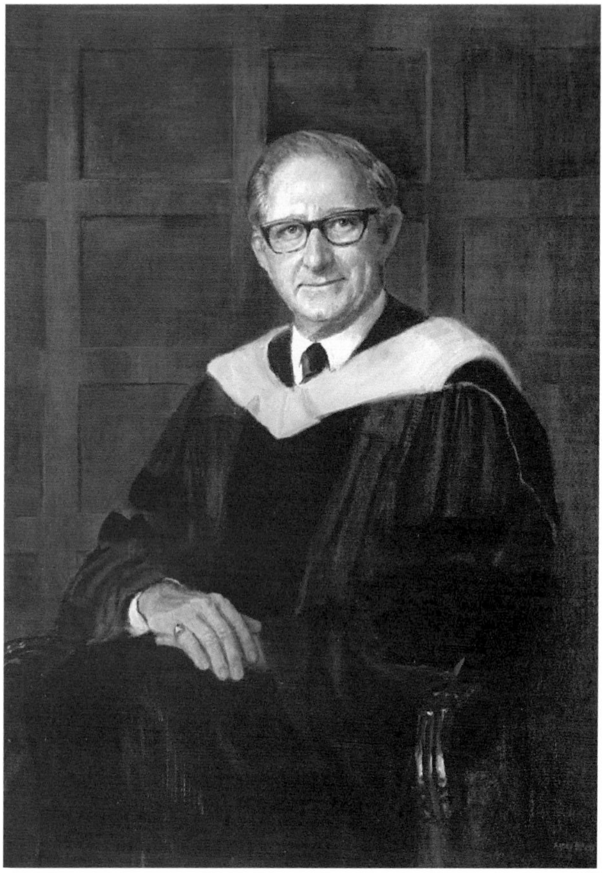

regarded as a dynamic leader in teaching, research, and humanitarian pursuits. He brought with him a stellar team of academic radiologists from the University of Pennsylvania. By the time of Dr. Hodes's retirement in 1971 Jefferson's department of radiology had been completely revitalized. It had quadrupled its numbers of residents and staff, many of whom went on to their own illustrious academic careers. Among his achievements was the establishment of the Stein Radiation Biology Research Center in 1965.

Dr. Hodes was a consultant-lecturer at the U.S. Naval Hospital in Philadelphia, the Walter Reed Army Hospital, and the Armed Forces Institute of Pathology. He served as president of the Philadelphia Roentgen Ray Society and the American Cancer Society, Philadelphia Division. He was equally well known south of the border and was an active participant and officer in several inter-American congresses. He delivered endowed lectureships at the Minnesota Medical Society, the University of Minnesota, the Medical Society of St. Louis, and the Detroit Radiological Society.

Dr. Hodes was coauthor with Drs. Eugene P. Pendergrass and J. Parsons Schaeffer of *The Head and Neck in Roentgen Diagnosis* (second edition, 1956), and coauthor with Dr. Jack Edeiken of another classic text, *Roentgen Diagnosis of Diseases of Bone* (1967). He was editor-in-chief of the *Atlas of Tumor Radiology* and chairman of the editorial commission of *Acta Radiologica Americana*.

Further recognition of Dr. Hodes's contributions to radiology included gold medals for distinguished service awarded by the Radiologic Society of North America, the American Roentgen Ray Society, and the American College of Radiology. He received the Humanitarian Award of the American Cancer Society in 1971. He was a chancellor of the American College of Radiology which designated him a "Living Legend" in 1986.

Dr. Hodes retired from Jefferson in 1971 when he was named emeritus professor. He was honored in 1988 with the first annual Philip J. Hodes lecture. In 1995 the Hodes Memorial Research Fund was initiated to endow a research laboratory within the department of radiology.

After having built departments at the University of Pennsylvania and Jefferson Medical College, in 1971 Dr. Hodes accepted a new challenge to build a radiological diagnostic division for the New Jersey College of Medicine in Newark. His last position was as distinguished professor of radiology at the University of Miami School of Medicine. Dr. Hodes's wife was artist Natalie Hodes and their son Barton L. Hodes graduated from Jefferson in 1966.

Dr. Philip J. Hodes's portrait by Agnes Allen was presented in conjunction with a daylong scientific program commemorating his retirement from Jefferson. The event was attended by friends and colleagues from all over the country.

Dr. Hodes is depicted three-quarters length and life-sized, seated in an armchair in front of a panelled wall. His body faces slightly left and his hands rest comfortably in his lap. He turns toward the viewer with an expression radiating confidence, alertness, and affability. He wears a black academic robe with a brilliant yellow hood edged in red. The warm highlights and impasto surfaces of the sitter's face and hands, costume, and carved chair arms contrast effectively with the neutral, small rectangles of the background wall.

An insight into the selection of Agnes Allen as portraitist was revealed during the presentation ceremony. It was mentioned that Dr. Hodes was a violinist and a friend of Eugene Ormandy, music director of the Philadelphia Orchestra. Agnes Allen was Hodes's sole choice because he so admired her portrait of Ormandy which was prominently installed at Philadelphia's Academy of Music.

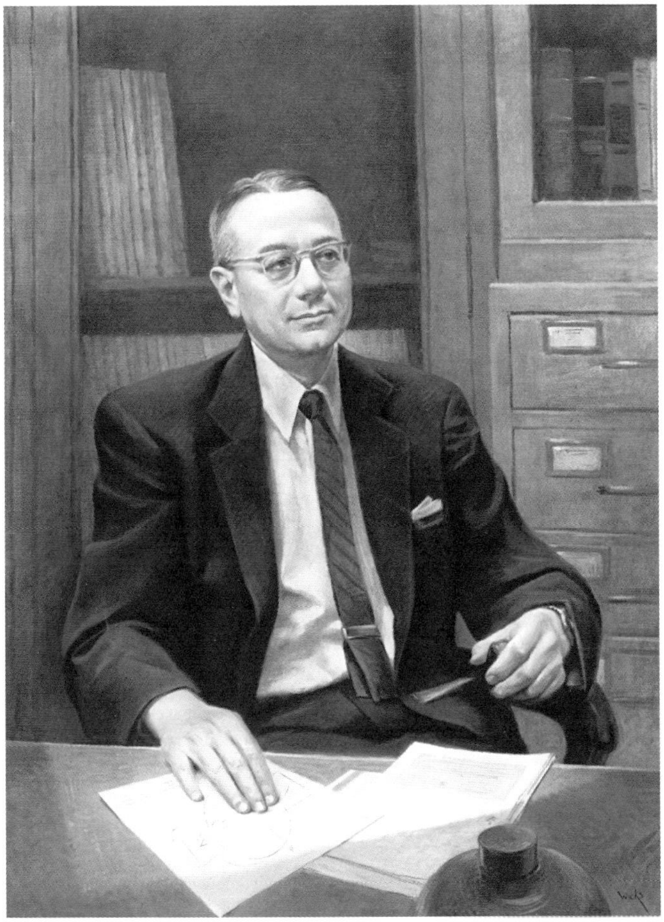

Portrait of Abraham Cantarow

ABRAHAM CANTAROW, M.D. (1901-79)
By Alden MacMaster Wicks (1914-87)

Oil on canvas
1960
48 x 36 in.

Signed lower right: "Wicks"

Given by JMC class of 1960
Accession number: 1960+e.P.01

Dr. Abraham Cantarow was named professor of biochemistry and chairman of the department at Jefferson Medical College in 1945. He served in that post until his retirement in 1966 when he was named emeritus professor.

Abraham Cantarow was born in 1901 in Hartford, Connecticut and followed in the footsteps of his family's many physicians: his father, grandfather, and two uncles. While pursuing undergraduate work at Trinity and Tufts Colleges the multitalented student also took advanced training in violin at the New England Conservatory of Music. He graduated from Jefferson Medical College in 1924, and while there played the violin in a medical student dance orchestra. He spent his entire career at Jefferson.

He rose in the academic ranks from assistant demonstrator in the department of medicine in 1929, to associate professor of biochemistry in 1939, and professor and chairman of the department in 1945. He was biochemist to the hospital from 1931 to 1945.

Cantarow's appointment as chair of biochemistry was in line with a national trend in the 1940s to treat biochemistry as an independent discipline separated from clinical chemistry, and he gradually modernized the department. The department accepted graduate students and offered special seminars in advanced biochemistry as well as a course in chemistry for Jefferson's diploma nursing students.

Dr. Abraham Cantarow was the author of five widely used textbooks: *Calcium Metabolism and Calcium Therapy* (1931), the first monograph on this subject; *Biochemistry in Internal Medicine* (1932), coauthored with Dr. Max Trumper, with second to sixth editions known as *Clinical Biochemistry*; *Lead Poisoning* (1944), coauthored with Dr. Max Trumper; *Biochemistry* (1954), coauthored with Dr. Bernard Schepartz; and *Clinical Endocrinology* (1954), coauthored with Drs. Karl E. Paschkis and Abraham E. Rakoff. Cantarow was also a member of the editorial board of the journal *Metabolism*.

Dr. Abraham Cantarow was one of only six American representatives invited to an international African Congress on Liver Cancer in 1956. He was awarded a silver medal from the Finnish government for his assistance in reorganizing the department of chemistry at the University of Helsinki in 1963.

Dr. Cantarow was a loyal and dedicated Jeffersonian. He was president of the alumni association and recipient of its alumni achievement award in 1968. He was awarded an honorary doctor of science degree in 1969 and named alumni representative to the board of trustees the following year. After his retirement from Jefferson in 1966 Cantarow was appointed associate chief of program analysis at the National Cancer Institute in Bethesda, Maryland.

Cantarow was admired by thousands of students for the clarity and organization of his lectures and for his approachability outside the classroom. The classes of 1943 and 1959 dedicated their yearbooks to him, and the class of 1960 chose him as portrait honoree.

In the painting by Alden M. Wicks the physician is shown working in his office. He is depicted half length and life-sized, seated behind a gray desk. He wears a dark gray suit complemented by a gray and maroon striped necktie. He looks up from his work with a warm and welcoming expression. His right hand rests on a yellow paper bearing a biochemical diagram and his left hand holds a pipe. Behind the physician are glass-enclosed bookshelves with journals and a green filing cabinet below a row of multicolored books.

This is one of Alden Wicks's finest portraits among the seventeen Jefferson physicians he depicted—the figure is solidly rendered and engagingly alert, the geometric composition of the room and its objects is compellingly arranged, and the angular patterns of colors and light and shade on the figure and desk are artfully disposed.

Portrait of Samuel S. Conly Jr.

SAMUEL STINGER CONLY Jr., M.D. (b. 1919)
By Alden MacMaster Wicks

Oil on canvas
1983
36 x 30 in.

Signed lower left: "Wicks"

Given in 1983 by friends and colleagues
Accession number: 1983+e.P.02

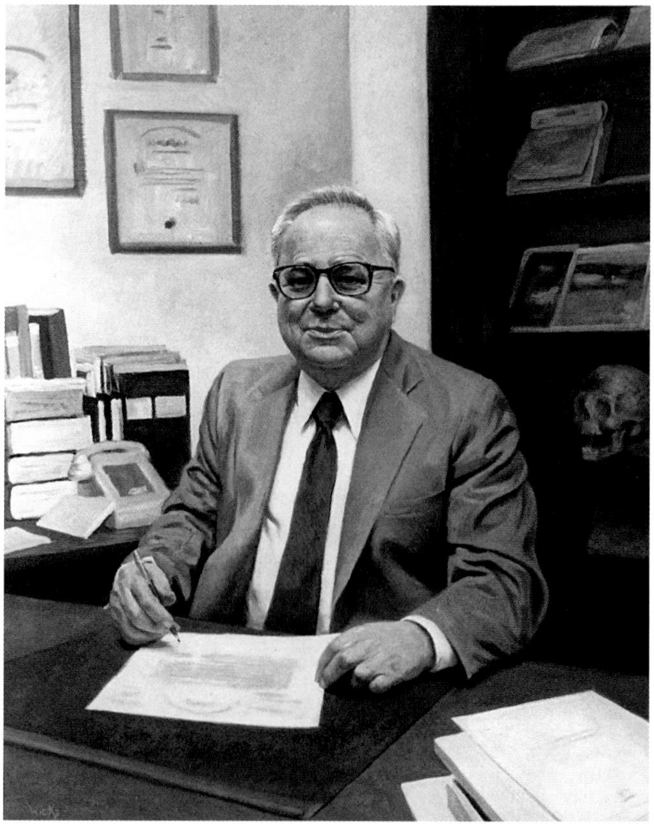

Dr. Samuel S. Conly Jr. was associate dean and director of admissions at Jefferson Medical College and an associate professor of physiology. He retired in 1983 after thirty-three years of service to the college.

Samuel Conly was born in 1919 in Philadelphia, and graduated from Lafayette College (1941) and Jefferson Medical College (September 1944). As the United States was about to enter World War II the curriculum at Jefferson was modified to graduate two classes a year, and Conly along with most junior students entered the Army Student Training Program as privates. After an abbreviated internship at Bryn Mawr Hospital, Conly served in the U.S. Marine Corps from 1945 to 1947.

Upon his return to civilian life Dr. Conly joined Jefferson's department of physiology from 1947 to 1950. After spending the next three years in private practice, he returned to Jefferson as assistant professor of physiology and by 1955 was appointed associate professor. The following year Dr. George Bennett offered Conly a joint appointment as assistant to the dean. He was promoted to assistant dean in 1960 and was associate dean from 1965 until 1983.

As director of admissions for sixteen years Dr. Samuel Conly was praised for his integrity and compassion. The versatile administrator was also the faculty advisor to the Student Council, the first student financial aid officer, and a member of faculty committees on student problems and postgraduate medical education.

"Let Sam do it" was the theme of a *Jefferson Medical College Alumni Bulletin* article (spring 1986) about Conly when he assumed the alumni association presidency. He had chaired numerous college committees. He was also chair of the Philadelphia coordinators of MEND (Medical Education for National Defense), a program that extended his interest in aviation physiology.

Dr. Conly was named emeritus associate dean and honorary associate professor of physiology upon his retirement in 1983. On this occasion his portrait was presented to the university by his friends and colleagues. In recognition of his contributions Conly was the first recipient of the Dean's Medal.

In Alden Wicks's depiction, Dr. Samuel S. Conly is shown half-length and slightly smaller than life-sized. As in the portrait of Dr. Abraham Cantarow, the subject is seated at a desk in his office surrounded by the accoutrements of his academic work. Conly glances up toward the viewer while holding a pen poised over a letter on a blue blotter. The expression on his rotund face is engaging, almost whimsical. He wears a pearl gray business suit with a royal blue necktie. A pile of papers and books on the desk awaits his attention. The walls, shelves, and table in his office are laden with books, journals, files, framed documents, and even a skull.

In accepting the portrait for the university, Dr. Lewis W. Bluemle Jr. praised the artist's ability to render a convincing likeness of the sitter and to capture Dr. Conly's personality, especially his "impish smile which suggests he knows something that you don't or that he's got a plan in mind that he will tell you about very shortly."

Portrait of M. H. F. Friedman

MOE HEGBY FRED FRIEDMAN, Ph.D. (1909-98)
By Alden MacMaster Wicks

Oil on canvas
1974
36 x 30 in.

Signed upper right: "Wicks"

Given in 1974 by friends and colleagues
Accession number: 1974+e.P.04

Dr. M. H. F. Friedman joined the Jefferson Medical College faculty in 1941 as an associate in physiology. He advanced to professor of physiology in 1954 and department chairman in 1957.

Friedman was born in Montreal in 1909. His degrees were earned at McGill University (B.Sc. in 1930 and Ph.D. in 1937) and the University of Western Ontario (M.A. in 1932). His early posts were: at McGill demonstrator in zoology, research associate in physiology, and fellow in gastric secretions; at Western Ontario demonstrator in zoology; and at Wayne State University School of Medicine research associate.

In 1941 Dr. Friedman acquitted himself favorably at a meeting of the Federation of American Societies for Experimental Biology in Chicago. On the basis of his presentation he was offered a position in Jefferson's physiology department by chairman Dr. J. Earl Thomas.

Friedman collaborated with members of Jefferson's clinical departments in his research on gastrointestinal physiology, experimental ulcer therapy, the autonomic nervous system, the physiological effect of hypothermia, and cardiovascular physiology. Dr. Friedman worked to develop a method of isolating pure secretin from pig intestine, a method ultimately utilized by Wyeth Laboratories in the first commercially successful method in America of obtaining secretin; it was this preparation that Drs. J. Earl Thomas and Joseph O. Crider utilized in their pioneering studies of pancreatic physiology.[13]

Friedman served a term as president of the Physiological Society of Philadelphia. He was a fellow of the American Association for the Advancement of Science and an honorary foreign member of the Belgian Gastroenterological Society. He was editor of the *American Journal of Digestive Diseases* and the proceedings of *Functions of the Stomach and Intestine*, a symposium cosponsored by Jefferson's department of physiology and the Physiological Society of Philadelphia in 1975.

Upon his retirement in 1974 Dr. M. H. F. Friedman was named emeritus professor, and his portrait by Alden Wicks was presented to the college by friends and colleagues. Typical of Wicks's portraits of Jefferson professors the subject is shown in his working environment, here teaching in a lecture room.

Dr. Friedman is depicted half length and slightly smaller than life-sized, standing in front of a blackboard. The silver-haired professor faces the unseen audience holding a pointer in his right hand, with the clenched fist of his left hand hanging over the lectern. His expression is serious, almost grim as he points to an illustration of the gastrointestinal tract on the blackboard to explain how the stomach empties when the pressure gradient is higher than the pressure in the intestine.

Friedman wears a white doctor's coat with his name and department embroidered in blue over a mustard-colored shirt and patterned necktie. The only other bright colors in this essentially neutral painting are the tiny red, blue, and green tips of the pens in his uniform pocket.

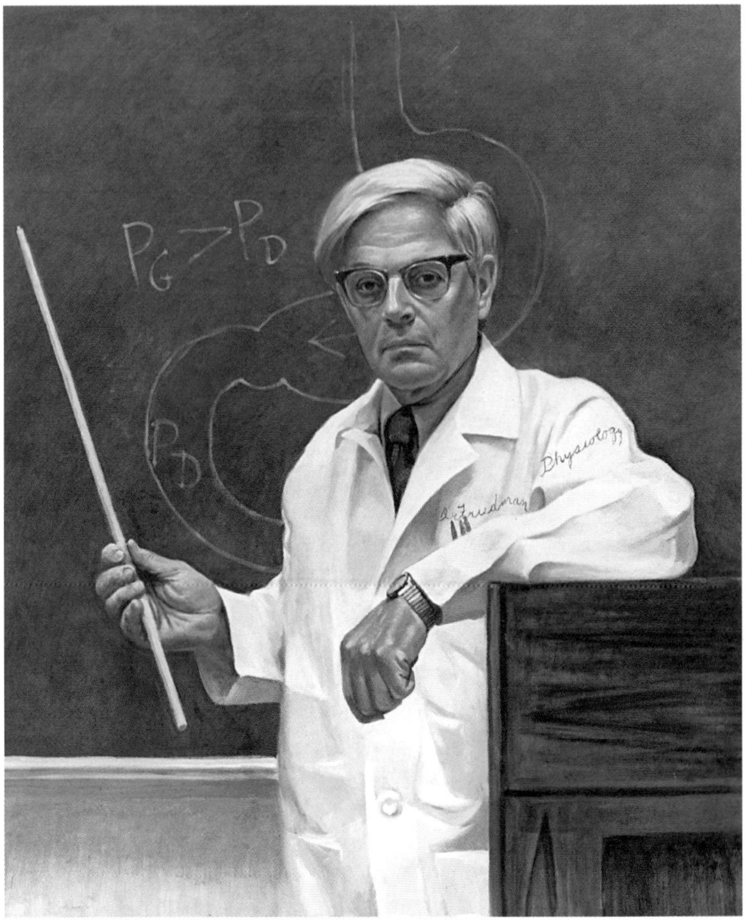

Portrait of M. H. F. Friedman

Portrait of Kenneth Goodner

KENNETH GOODNER, Ph.D. (1902-67)
By Alden MacMaster Wicks

Oil on canvas
1968
36 x 30 in.

Signed lower right: "Wicks"

Given by JMC class of 1968
Accession number: 1968+e.P.02

Dr. Kenneth Goodner was an internationally known investigator of infectious diseases when he accepted the position as second chair of the department of bacteriology and immunology at Jefferson Medical College.

Kenneth Goodner was born in 1902 in McCune, Kansas and received his undergraduate and master's degrees at the University of Kansas. He earned a Ph.D. at Harvard University in 1929 and spent the next year as instructor in bacteriology and immunology in the School of Public Health at Harvard. During the following decade he was on the staff at the Rockefeller Institute, studying immunity to pneumococci and developing a type-specific antipneumococcal rabbit serum. In 1940 he became a member of the Field Staff of the International Health Division of the Rockefeller Foundation where he began his participation in the investigation of infectious diseases throughout the world.

Dr. Kenneth Goodner joined the Jefferson faculty as chair of bacteriology and immunology in 1946, succeeding Dr. Randle Rosenberger. Goodner introduced the principles of scientific research into the curriculum and helped to develop a program of graduate education, while attracting outstanding faculty to the department. After serving for twenty-one years Goodner retired and was named emeritus professor, just two months before his death.

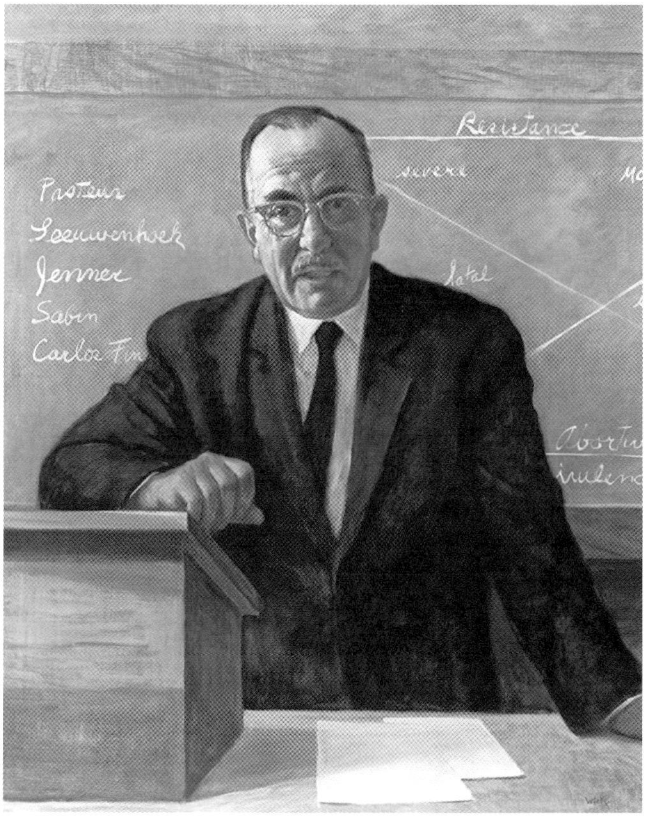

A moving memoir about Dr. Goodner's contributions to bacteriology was composed by his former colleague Dr. Theodore E. Woodward, professor of medicine and chair of the department at the University of Maryland School of Medicine:

> Each member of the cholera family hurts over the loss of Ken Goodner...Since 1958 his personal investigative talents were directed toward clarification of the mysteries of pathogenesis, detection and control of the ancient scourge, Asiatic cholera. His laboratory teemed with vibrios; through his efforts collections of valuable strains were culled from the world over. Laboriously he prepared valuable typing sera which he generously shared and distributed to fellow associates...Never one to shun work, he pressed his tired but willing body over the globe, to Africa for study of yellow fever, to Madagascar and problems of plague, and during the last decade to the Asian subcontinent and Pacific Far East for cholera. Ken was one of the major architects of the SEATO Cholera Research Laboratory and continued to provide fuel toward its success until the time of his death...
>
> Ken was occasionally sensitive and subject to abrasion when his points of view were ignored; always he emerged a little scathed, never beaten. Often he took the opposite stand mainly to avoid acceptance of superficial or ill-conceived answers to difficult problems. He was usually right.

Though even Dr. Goodner's admirers occasionally dubbed him "irascible" or "unpredictable," no Jefferson faculty members doubted the devotion of "K. G." to students and young scientists. He sparked their enthusiasm and developed their thought processes, and was always available for counsel. He nonetheless adamantly refused the attempts of six senior classes to have his portrait painted. After his sudden death in 1967 the next class succeeded in preserving his image by commissioning a posthumous depiction by Alden M. Wicks.

Dr. Goodner is shown teaching in the lecture room in a portrait that is conceptually similar to that of Dr. M. H. F. Friedman. Goodner is depicted half length and smaller than life-sized standing in front of a chalkboard, with one clenched fist on the lectern and the other hand leaning on a table. However, instead of a laboratory coat he is attired in a dark brown suit and necktie. He faces the audience intently with eyebrows raised and his mouth slightly open, as though speaking to a student.

The papers on the table are probably his lecture notes. A diagram and list of great immunologists, "Pasteur, Leeuwenhoek, Jenner, Sabin, Carlos Fin[lay]," are inscribed in white chalk on the green board. The bright light streaming in from the left betrays the photographic source for Wicks's portrait.

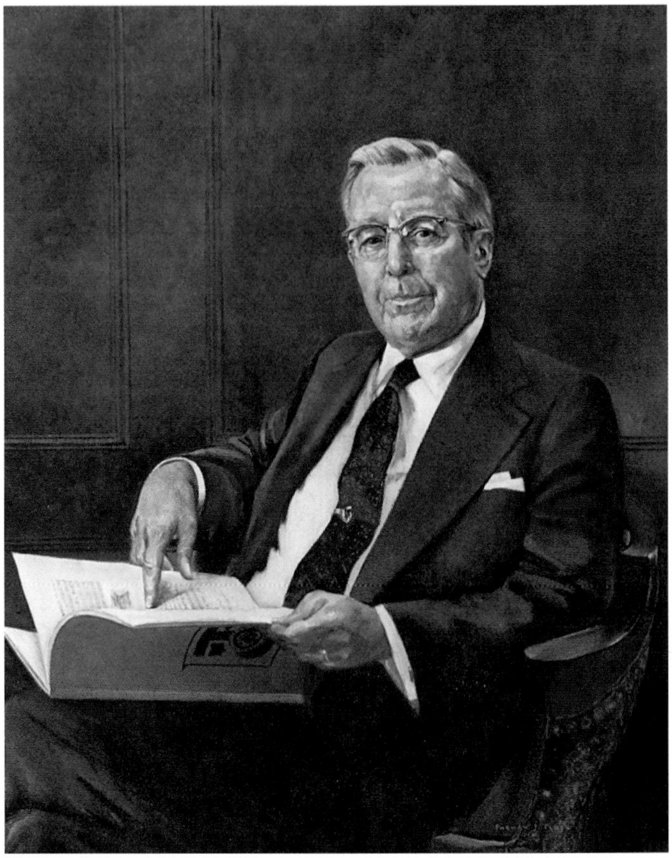

Portrait of Julius M. Coon

JULIUS MOSHER COON, M.D., Ph.D. (b. 1910)
By Furman J. Finck (1900-97)

Oil over tempera on canvas
1976
36 x 30 in.

Signed lower right: "FURMAN J. FINCK"
Exhibition: Philadelphia, *Furman J. Finck: A Retrospective,* Woodmere Art Gallery, Nov. 15-Dec. 16, 1980

Given in 1976 by friends and colleagues
Accession number: 1976+e.P.01

Dr. Julius M. Coon was professor and chairman of the department of pharmacology for twenty-three years, succeeding Dr. Charles M. Gruber in 1953. Like several of his mid-twentieth-century colleagues at Jefferson, Coon's roots were in the Midwest.

Julius Coon was born in 1910 in Liberty, Missouri. He received his undergraduate degree at Indiana University in Bloomington in 1932. In the midst of graduate studies in biochemistry at the University of Chicago, he switched to pharmacology and received his Ph.D. in 1938. He rose from instructor to associate professor in pharmacology at Chicago between 1939 to 1953, but with interruptions for war service and a medical degree earned in 1945 from the University of Illinois.

During the war Dr. Julius Coon conducted research on the toxicology of chemical warfare agents at the University of Chicago's toxicity laboratory established by the U.S. Office of Scientific Research and Development. From 1948 to 1953 he was director of this laboratory (renamed the U.S. Air Force Radiation Laboratory) which continued research on the toxicology of insecticides that were chemically related to compounds proposed as chemical warfare agents and which became food contaminants. This research led to interests in food additives, chemical changes in foods due to processing, and the natural chemical constituents of food.

Professor Coon served on advisory panels and committees of the National Academy of Science's National Research Council, the National Institutes of Health, the Food and Drug Administration, the U.S. Department of Agriculture, the Environmental Protection Agency, the World Health Organization, and the Food and Agriculture Organization. He was on the editorial boards of the *Journal of Pharmacology and Experimental Therapeutics*, *Toxicology and Applied Pharmacology*, and *Clinical Medicine*.

After Dr. Coon's appointment as professor and chairman of pharmacology at Jefferson Medical College in 1953, toxicologic issues gradually became a substantial part of the research and graduate training activities of the department, well supported by government training and research grants. Under Coon's leadership forty-two students received their Ph.D. degrees in pharmacology.

After his retirement in 1976 Dr. Coon served on expert panels or advisory boards for numerous scientific and industrial concerns. He received the Merit Award (1978) and the Education Award (1983) of the Society of Toxicology.

Friends and colleagues presented a portrait of Dr. Julius M. Coon to Jefferson Medical College in 1976, shortly before his retirement and election as emeritus professor. Furman J. Finck depicted him two-thirds length and life-sized, seated in an upholstered armchair with legs crossed at the knee, in front of a panelled wall. Dr. Coon looks up from reading and marks his place on the page with his right forefinger. The cover of the slim tan volume features a partial view of the Thomas Jefferson University logo.

Finck's ability to consolidate individual facial features into a naturalistic and animated likeness draws the viewer's attention to the sitter's silvery hair, creased forehead and cheeks, metal-rimmed glasses framing the steady gaze of his clear blue eyes, high-bridged nose, and thin mouth with pursed lips. The energy of the composition continues in the undulating contours, folds, and shadows of the sitter's blue business suit, patterned necktie, and white shirt.

The artist's lively palette consists of short strokes of pinks, reds, violets, blues, and greens in the skin tones, and maroons, browns, grays, reds, and sienna in the background panelled wall. He even contrasts the highlighted brass nail heads with the green upholstery of the armchair. Finck's painstaking technique consists of first rendering the composition in tempera in shades from dark to light over a red ground, followed by an overlay of oil colors.

Portrait and figure painter Furman J. Finck was an artist and educator with a national reputation. Born in Chester, Pennsylvania in 1900, he was introduced to art by his father, a lithographer and engraver from Alsace. He studied at the Pennsylvania Academy of the Fine Arts where in 1924 he won a Cresson traveling scholarship. He continued his studies in Paris at the Académie Julian and the École des Beaux-Arts.

Furman Finck has depicted such acclaimed public figures as Dwight D. Eisenhower, Harry S. Truman, Bishop John N. Neumann, Pablo Casals, Helen Hayes, and Julie Harris. He is probably best known for his portraits of men and women of science, including Drs. Michael DeBakey and Emily H. Mudd. His *Babcock Surgical Clinic*, a large mural at Temple University School of Medicine, is a commemorative group portrait in the operating room of Dr. W. Wayne Babcock with past and present professors, deans, chairmen, and surgeons on the Temple faculty. Finck also worked on a large series of portraits of pharmacy school deans commissioned by Wyeth Laboratories.

In 1968 Furman Finck was named emeritus professor after more than forty years on the drawing and painting faculty at Tyler School of Art of Temple University. He was also visiting professor at the American Academy in Rome.

Furman Finck was the author of several books on art education and portrait painting. He won the Carnegie Prize and the First Altman Prize of the National Academy of Design, and the Popular Award of the Worcester Museum. He received an honorary doctor of fine arts degree from Muhlenberg College. A retrospective exhibition was held at Philadelphia's Woodmere Gallery in 1980.

Portrait of Charles P. Kraatz

CHARLES PARRY KRAATZ, Ph.D. (b. 1910)
By Furman J. Finck

Oil on canvas
1970
44 1/4 x 36 1/4 in.

Signed lower right: "FURMAN J. FINCK"

Given by JMC class of 1970
Accession number: 1970+e.P.01

Dr. Charles P. Kraatz was a member of the department of pharmacology at Jefferson Medical College for twenty-three years. He joined the faculty in 1947 as assistant professor and was named professor in 1955.

Charles Kraatz was born in Rochester, New York in 1906 and received his undergraduate degree from Berea College (1926), master's degree in zoology from the University of Kentucky (1932), and doctorate in zoology from the University of Cincinnati (1936). Between 1936 and 1943 he was a faculty member of the department of pharmacology and physiology at the University of Chicago School of Medicine. During World War II Charles Kraatz was an aviation physiologist in the U.S. Navy working in the low pressure chamber and with night vision training. Upon his discharge he became an assistant professor of physiology at Oklahoma A. and M. College.

At Jefferson Dr. Kraatz became chairman of the interdepartmental seminar, chairman of the pharmacy subcommittee of the hospital, and briefly the acting director of medical college admissions. His research centered on the mode of actions of the botulinum toxin, the actions of phenothiazines at the cellular level, the actions of barbiturates on the muscle and neuromuscular systems, and the ionic changes related to electrical changes in frog muscles.

When the class of 1970 selected Dr. Kraatz as portrait honoree it was the first time a portrait subject had been elected by formal ballot. The pharmacologist's viewpoint that teaching medical students was his "number one job" had earned him the students' respect and affection.

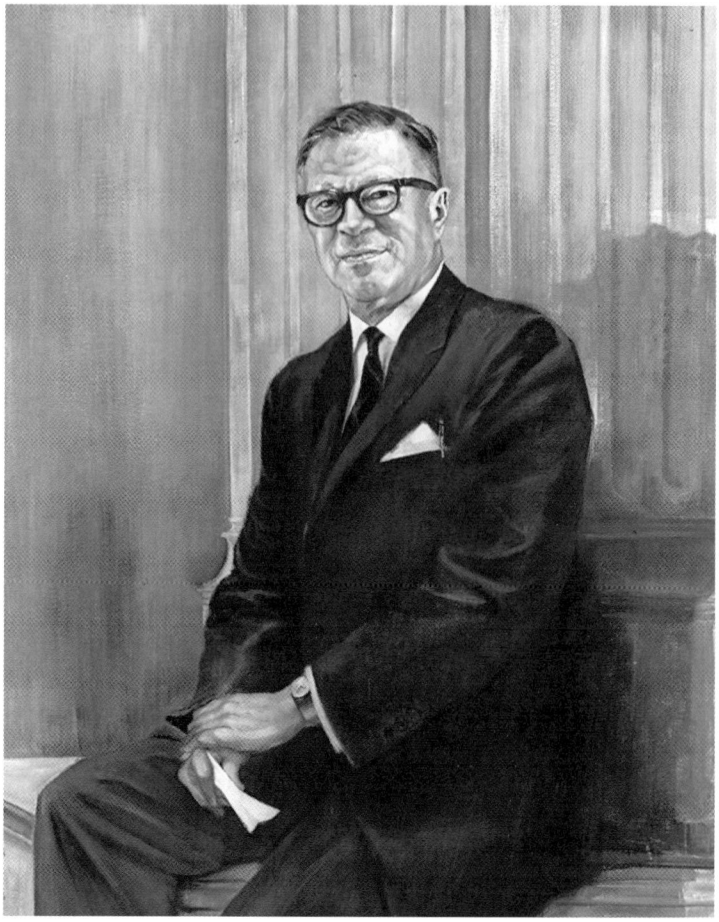

The portrait by Furman J. Finck shows the subject two-thirds length and life-sized, seated on a stone platform in front of a wide, fluted column of gray stone. His hands hold a sheet of paper and rest on his lap. The most arresting feature of his jowly face are the brown, almond-shaped eyes that stare penetratingly through heavy, dark-framed glasses. The artist's use of small strokes of reds, pinks, and grays in the sitter's skin tones, the contrast of the sitter's dark brown suit against the light column, and the dramatic shadow on the column are effective stylistic elements.

However, the formal, austere, and non-Jefferson architectural setting and the subject's stiff posture and almost pugnacious expression give little hint of Dr. Kraatz's warm, outgoing, and humorous personality. During lectures he often called on his extracurricular interests in the theater, photography, gourmet cooking, ballroom dancing, construction, and winemaking to enlist the students' attention and counter their resistance to learning facts by rote.

Portrait of Nicholas A. Michels

NICHOLAS ALOYSIUS MICHELS, D.Sc. (1891-1969)
By John Christen Johansen (1876-1964)

Oil on canvas
1958
51 3/4 x 36 1/2 in.

Signed and dated lower right: "J. C. JOHANSEN/'58"

Given by JMC class of 1958
Accession number: 1958+e.P.01

Dr. Nicholas A. Michels had received unusually extensive scientific training and academic appointments before joining the Jefferson Medical College faculty as associate professor of anatomy. He was known for his investigations in hematology.

Born in 1891 in St. Paul, Minnesota, Nicholas A. Michels graduated from St. Thomas College there in 1914, and received an S.T.B. degree from Catholic University and an M.A. degree in hematology from the University of Minnesota. He continued his studies abroad, first receiving a doctor of science degree, *maxima cum laude*, from the University of Louvain in Belgium in 1922, followed by further work at the Sorbonne in Paris and the University of Siena in Italy.

Upon his return to the United States, he taught biology at St. Thomas College, conducted research at the

University of Chicago, and then moved East to work at New York University and Bellevue Hospital. He taught briefly at St. Louis University School of Medicine, and the Creighton University School of Medicine in Omaha, Nebraska.

In 1929 Dr. Michels was appointed associate professor of anatomy at Jefferson Medical College and full professor in 1948. The colorful professor had taught gross anatomy to more than five thousand students by the time of his retirement in 1962 when he was elected emeritus professor.

Michels's early interest in hematology resulted in numerous publications on erythrocytes, mast cells, plasma cells, and other elements of the connective tissue and hemopoietic series. Dr. Michels was belatedly honored for his early work at the International Congress on Mast Cells in 1962. His original monograph, "The Mast Cell in the Lower Vertebrates" (published in *La Cellule*, volume 33, 1923), was reprinted in the proceedings compiled by the New York Academy of Sciences the following year.

Dr. Michel's best-known text was *Blood Supply and Anatomy of the Upper Abdominal Organs; with a Descriptive Atlas* (1955). For this he was elected chairman of anatomy in the allied science section of the International College of Surgeons. He was also a fellow of the International Society of Hematology.

Although his professorial manner could be gruff and intimidating, Jefferson students responded to "Bull" Michels's sincere love for teaching. His lectures were unusually animated and sometimes included extraneous props for emphasis, but almost always incorporated learned references to the history of medicine and anatomy.

Students honored Dr. Michels as dedicatee of the 1946 yearbook, recipient of the Christian R. and Mary F. Lindback Award for Distinguished Teaching in 1962, and subject of the class portrait in 1958.

In the two-thirds-length and life-sized portrait by John C. Johansen Dr. Michels is garbed in the brilliant red, gray, and white academic robe of the University of Louvain

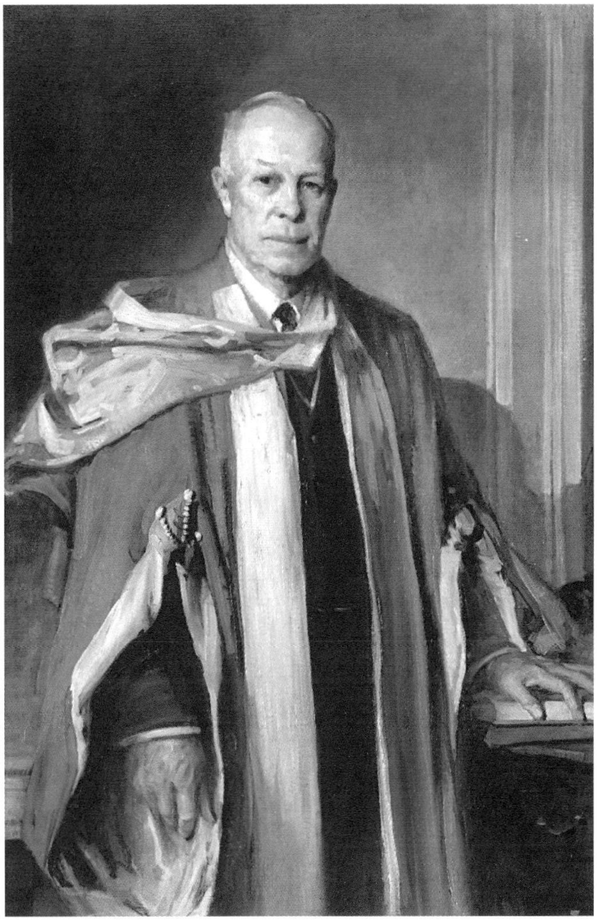

that he customarily wore during Jefferson academic processions. He stands next to a desk with his left hand resting on some books. His expression is serious as he gazes directly toward the spectator. The background panelled wall includes a fluted pilaster and chair rail.

The depiction is unusually animated for a portrait by John C. Johansen. The paint style is loose and free without sacrificing a sense of the figure's mass, and the flesh tones pick up reflections from the red gown. The bright colors and flowing forms of the robe add considerable energy to the painting.

Portrait of Andrew J. Ramsay

ANDREW JACKSON RAMSAY, Ph.D. (1907-91)
By Alden MacMaster Wicks (1914-87)

Oil on canvas
1966
40 x 30 in.

Signed lower right: "Wicks"

Given by JMC class of 1966
Accession number: 1966+e.P.03

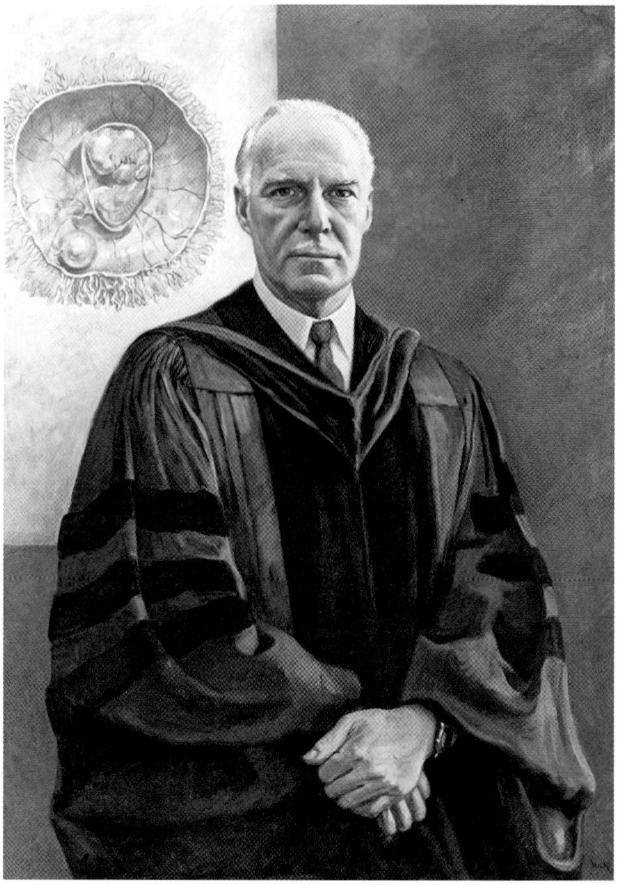

Dr. Andrew J. Ramsay was professor and chair of the department of anatomy and director of the Daniel Baugh Institute of Anatomy at Jefferson Medical College. He was later named the first Daniel Baugh Professor of Anatomy for his distinguished service to the department and to the university.

Andrew Ramsay was born in 1907 in Angola, Indiana and graduated from DePauw University in 1930. He earned a Ph.D. degree in anatomy at Cornell University in 1934, and remained in Ithaca for postdoctoral study and a post as instructor in histology and embryology.

Dr. Andrew J. Ramsay accepted a position as associate in histology and embryology at Jefferson Medical College in 1936. He advanced through the ranks to become full professor by 1948. Ten years later he succeeded Dr. George A. Bennett as chair of anatomy. Upon his retirement in 1972 Ramsay was named emeritus professor and received an honorary degree of doctor of science.

As department chair Dr. Ramsay achieved his goals of strengthening the laboratory and classroom teaching programs and fostering diversified research. He assembled a teaching collection of lantern slides, charts, models, and other teaching aids. He introduced the use of electron microscopy for image amplification, and developed the first controlled optical lighting apparatus for color photomicrography, a technique he continued to teach even after retirement. He was a member of the Electron Microscopy Society of America and the Royal Microscopy Society. Through his initiative Jefferson's first centralized division of audiovisual services was created in 1972 under the direction of Theresa Powers.

Under the aegis of Dr. Ramsay, closed-circuit television demonstrations in anatomy and histology became an integral part of student laboratory studies and continuing education of physicians in outlying areas. He was chairman of the board of the Council on Medical Television of the Institute for the Advancement of Medical Communications, and a member of the National Association of Educational Broadcasters and the National Audiovisual Association.

Dr. Ramsay contributed to the medical literature in the fields of in utero development and embryogenesis. His work in transplanting embryonic anlagen in mammals helped to initiate the new field of experimental mammalian embryology. His study of lymph flow was an important factor in understanding the metastasis of cancer cells.

Dr. Ramsay was head of the faculty portrait committee, and was appointed by Dr. Herbut as the first chairman of the newly formed university art committee in 1971. Ramsay photographed the portrait collection and delivered slide talks on Jefferson history. In 1958 he was made an honorary member of the alumni association. In 1981 at the ceremony commemorating Ramsay's election as the first Daniel Baugh Professor of Anatomy, there was a rededication of Lazar Raditz's portrait of Daniel Baugh with his two grandsons, *The Three Daniels*.

As an accomplished athlete, sportsman, and photographer, Dr. Ramsay recognized the importance of recreational facilities for the beleaguered medical student, and he was chairman of the student commons planning committee. The Jefferson classes of 1965 and 1975 dedicated their yearbooks to the popular teacher and the class of 1966 chose him as portrait honoree.

Alden M. Wicks depicted the physician half-length and life-sized, with his hands clasped close to his body. He is garbed in a black academic gown with a blue and red mantle. His patrician features are enhanced by his neat white mustache and hair. On a wall behind the anatomist is an illustration of a developing embryo. The gentlemanly professor is appropriately dignified in manner, but his posture appears stiff and his expression severe. The artist said that Dr. Ramsay requested a formal, robed portrait because of his role as marshal at Jefferson academic processions, and that "adding an embryo was incongruous but I liked it."[14]

Portrait of Franz X. Hausberger

FRANZ XAVER HAUSBERGER, M.D. (1908-98)
By Alden MacMaster Wicks

Oil on canvas
1967
40 x 30 in.

Signed lower right: "Wicks"

Given by JMC class of 1967
Accession number: 1967+e.P.02

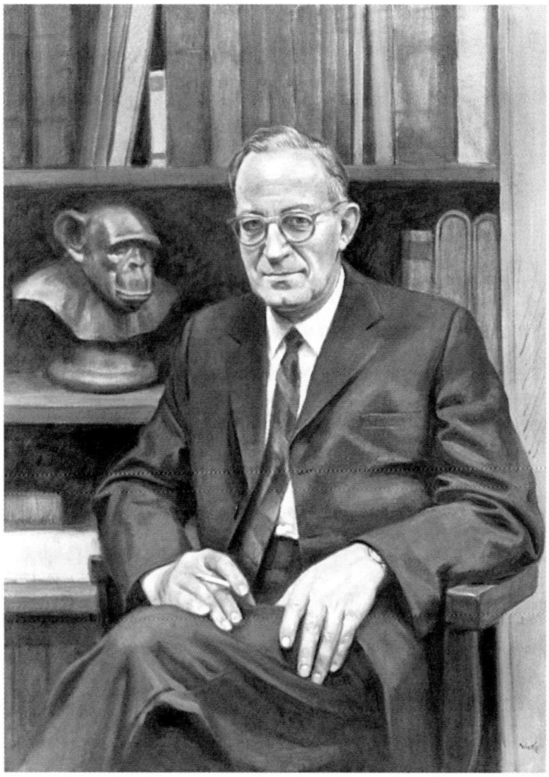

Dr. Franz X. Hausberger was professor of anatomy and head of the division of gross anatomy at Jefferson Medical College.

Franz Hausberger was born in 1908 in Muhldorf, a small Bavarian town near Munich. After receiving a medical degree in 1935 at the University of Munich he was appointed an assistant in anatomy there. The next several years were spent in clinical medicine and research at hospitals in Berlin, Koeslin, and Erlangen.

Dr. Hausberger was drafted into the German army during World War II and assigned to head the internal medicine division of a large military hospital in eastern Germany. Four years later he was captured by the invading Russian army and put in charge of the medical care of a huge prisoner-of-war camp. To avoid being transported to Russia and almost certain death, he daringly escaped from the camp by cutting through the barbed wire. After the war he became chief of the endocrine division of the University of Erlangen Medical School Hospital.

Dr. Hausberger emigrated to the United States in 1948. Two years later he was appointed assistant professor of anatomy at Jefferson through Dr. George A. Bennett whom he had known in prewar Munich. He was promoted to full professor in 1963 and served until 1975 when he retired and was made emeritus professor.

Hausberger was acclaimed for his basic research on adipose tissue: its structure, development, and function in both health and disease, especially diabetes. The American Physiological Society's volume on adipose tissue in its 1965 *Handbook of Physiology* was dedicated to Dr. Hausberger, known as "the founding father of adipose tissue research."

A gifted and dedicated teacher, Dr. Franz Hausberger won the Christian R. and Mary F. Lindback Award in 1965. He received an honorary doctor of science degree from Jefferson in 1978.

Dr. Hausberger was voted portrait honoree by the class of 1967. Alden M. Wicks depicted the anatomist two-thirds length and life-sized, seated in an armchair in front of a bookcase in the anatomy department's library. His legs are crossed in a relaxed posture and he holds a cigarette. He looks directly toward the viewer through his horn-rimmed glasses. The physician's slight trace of a smile suggests an amiable, almost conversational mood.

In addition to rows of books on the shelves is a plaster bust of a gorilla. Commenting about this attribute at the portrait presentation, Dr. Hausberger said, "I asked Mr. Wicks to include in the picture this remote relative of ours from some twenty million years ago, not only as a remembrance of our old dear DBI [Daniel Baugh Institute of Anatomy] building, but also as a humble reminder of our human beginnings."

1. For biographical information on Kelly see Derek Hudson, *For Love of Painting: The Life of Sir Gerald Kelly, K.C.V.O., P.R.A.* (London: Peter Davies, 1975).
2. For biographical information about Percival and Ethel Foerderer, see Frederick B. Wagner Jr., M.D., *Percival E. Foerderer: A "Mr. Jefferson"* (privately printed for Thomas Jefferson University, 1997).
3. For biographical information on Brockhurst see Marilyn F. Symmes, "Gerald F. Brockhurst's Portraits of Henry Rushbury," *Print Review* 17 (1983): 51-62.
4. I thank Catherine Tomeo, assistant to former President Lewis W. Bluemle Jr., M.D., for this information.
5. Wagner, *Thomas Jefferson University: Tradition and Heritage* (Philadelphia: Lea & Febiger, 1989), 423.
6. Patricia Likos, "Julius Bloch: Portrait of the Artist," *Philadelphia Museum of Art Bulletin* 79 (summer 1983): 21.
7. Elizabeth Landreth, "Alden Wicks: Whales, Nudes and Angels...and Doctors," *Jefferson Medical College Alumni Bulletin* 21 (summer 1972): 9.
8. For biographical details and reliable chronology on Dr. Gibbon see Ada Romaine-Davis, *John Gibbon and His Heart-Lung Machine* (Philadelphia: University of Pennsylvania Press, 1991).
9. Wagner, *Jefferson*, 590.
10. Romaine-Davis, 122.
11. Joseph Jackson, *Encyclopedia of Philadelphia* (Harrisburg: National Historical Association, 1931), 139-40.
12. Wagner, *Jefferson*, 660.
13. Wagner, *Jefferson*, 171.
14. Landreth, 13.

CHAPTER

9 The Seventies to the Mid-eighties

The period of the nineteen-seventies to the mid-nineteen-eighties saw significant architectural expansion at Thomas Jefferson University. In 1977 Frederick L. Ballard, Esq. succeeded William W. Bodine Jr. as chairman of the board of trustees and he served until 1984. Also in 1977 Dr. Lewis W. Bluemle Jr. was appointed the new president of the university.

Two major additions to the campus were the Scott Library and Administration Building and the "new" hospital (now the Gibbon Building). Other new structures were the Barringer Residence Hall at the southeast corner of Tenth and Walnut Streets, and the university parking garage with separate entrances flanking the Scott Plaza on Tenth and Eleventh Streets. The Edison Building at Ninth and Sansom Streets was also acquired and renovated.

Scott Library and Administration Building

SCOTT LIBRARY AND ADMINISTRATION BUILDING
By Harbeson Hough Livingston & Larson
Erected 1970

Architectural rendering
By "Oakes" for Harbeson Hough Livingston & Larson

Gouache on paper mounted on board

1966
Image size: 15 1/4 x 24 3/4 in.
Board size: 24 x 32 3/4 in.

Signed and dated lower left: "oakes/9/30/66"
Inscription below image: "THE SCOTT LIBRARY-ADMINISTRATION BUILDING/Jefferson Medical College and Medical Center/Philadelphia, Pennsylvania/HARBESON HOUGH LIVINGSTON & LARSON ARCHITECTS"

Ordered in 1966 by the trustees
Accession number: 1966+e.D.01

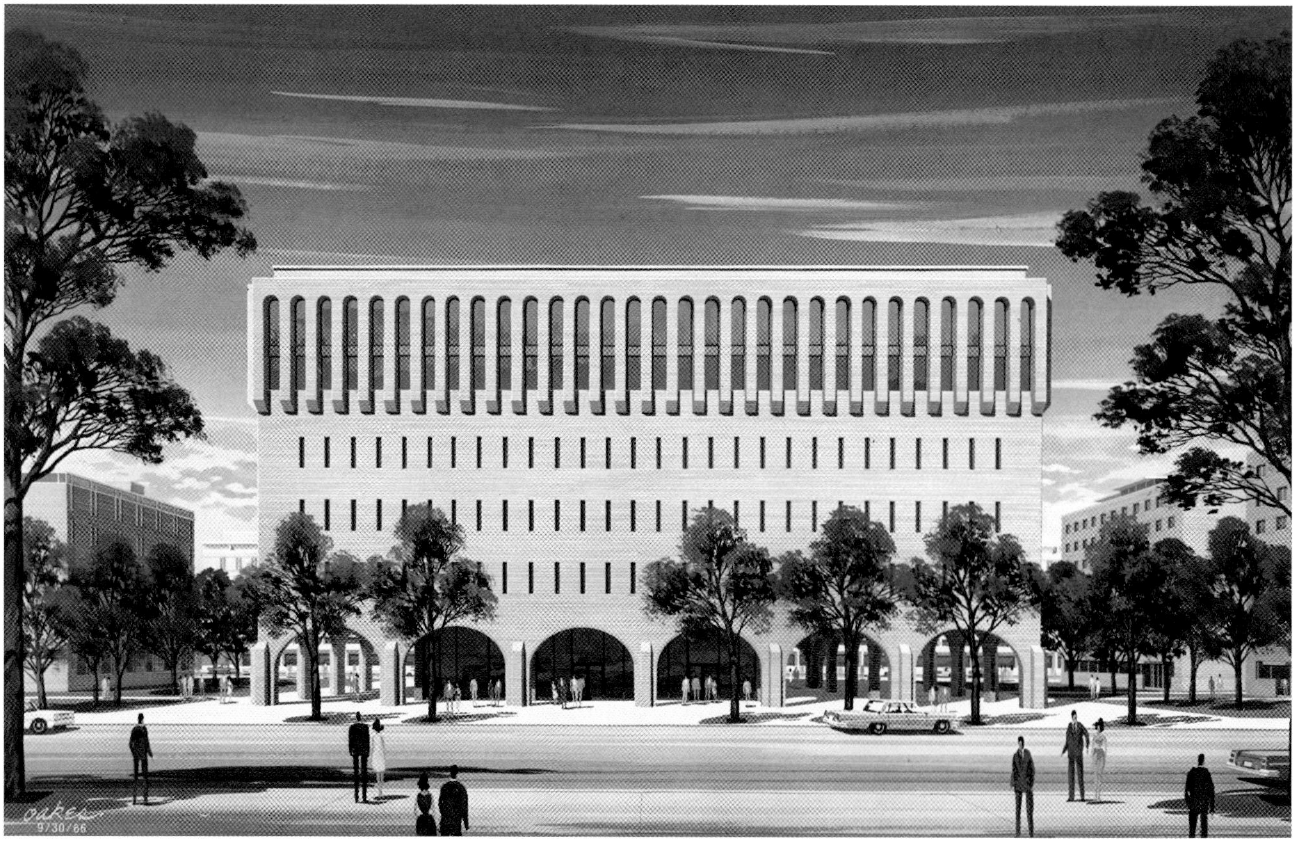

Before Jefferson's first freestanding library building was erected in 1970, libraries had been located in the 1898 and 1929 College Buildings. By the 1960s an acute shortage of space for the library's expanding collections coincided with a need to centralize the university's scattered administrative offices. The two functions were combined in the Scott Library and Administration Building which opened in late 1970 in the heart of the Jefferson campus. The building occupies about two-thirds of the south side of Walnut Street between Tenth and Eleventh Streets.

The library's facilities take up the first four floors and the university's corporate offices the upper two floors. The library moved toward automation in the late 1970s and was soon fully computerized with state-of-the-art facilities and training for students and staff. Of singular interest to this author is the library's special collections and archives.

By 1931 the library's official name had become the Samuel Parsons Scott Memorial Library in gratitude for a bequest of over eight thousand books and accompanying endowment made in 1925. Samuel P. Scott was an Ohio attorney and author who said he had been cured of a chronic respiratory condition by a Jefferson professor he had met serendipitously on a train ride.

The variegated brick building is reminiscent of Romanesque fortresses and Italian medieval palaces. It also responds to the historicizing ornamentation on the College and Curtis Buildings across Walnut Street. Arched loggias at ground level on all four sides provide protection from the elements and congenial gathering places. The horizontality of the design is further emphasized by three rows of tall, narrow windows on the lower levels and the corbeling effect creating tall, arched windows on the top two levels. The building won a silver medal from the Pennsylvania Society of Architects.

The Scott Building is set back from Walnut Street. To the south lies the Scott Plaza's open space with its trees, benches, and large containers for seasonal flowers. Besides its daily use as a quiet respite from the stress of professional duties and urban bustle, the plaza hosts events ranging from health fairs to con-

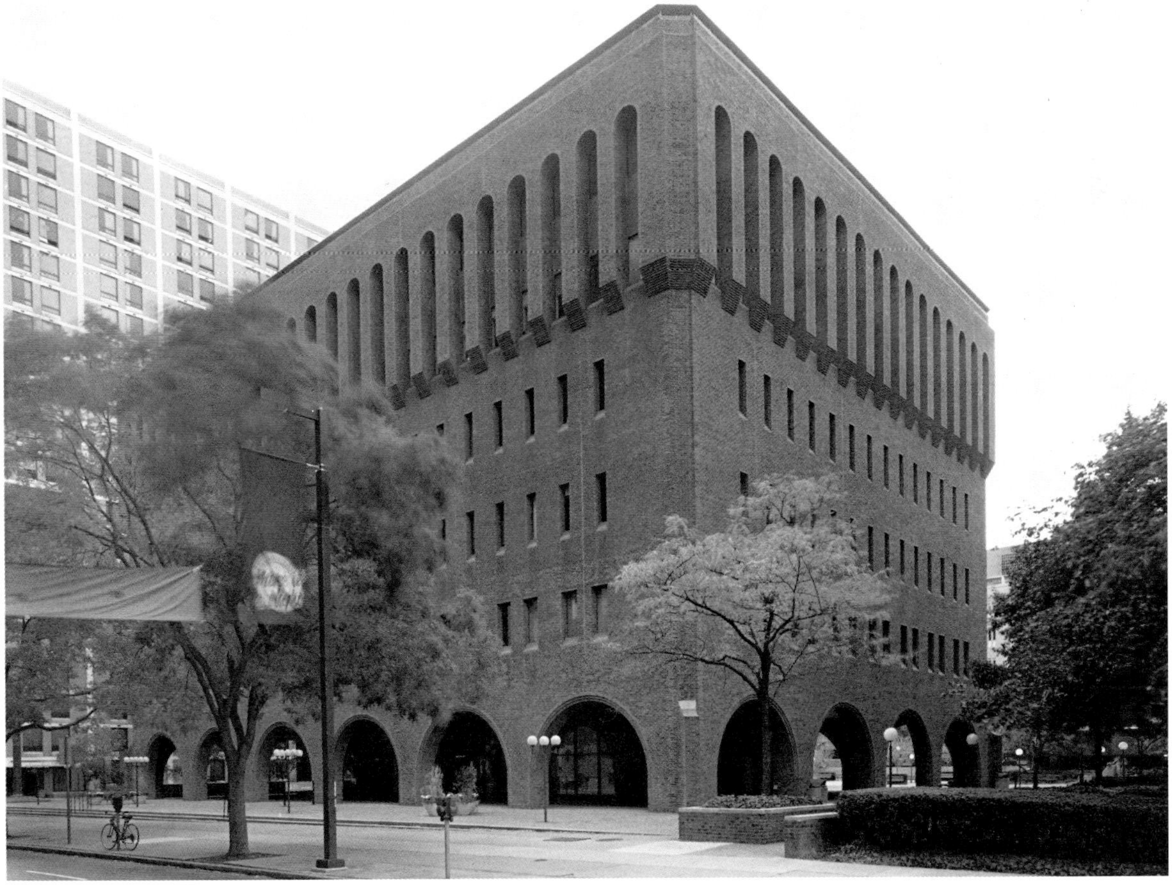

Scott Building in Recent Years

certs and neighborhood restaurant bazaars.

The Harbeson Hough Livingston and Larson architectural firm played a major role in the evolution of the Jefferson campus in the 1960s and 1970s by developing a master plan and acting as supervising architects. Besides the Scott Building the firm designed the Gibbon Building and the university's twin parking garages. It made renovations to the Edison Building, the "Old Main" Hospital, and clinical units throughout the campus.

The firm is descended from that founded by Paul Philippe Cret (1876-1945), a distinguished architect of eclectic designs. A native of Lyons, France, Cret came to Philadelphia to teach at the University of Pennsylvania in 1903 and he remained on the faculty until 1937.

Cret's Philadelphia buildings include the former Federal Reserve Bank at 925 Chestnut Street, most of which is now occupied by Jefferson personnel.

Among Cret's most famous designs are the Pan American Union Building, the Federal Reserve Board Building, and the Folger Shakespeare Library all in Washington, D.C. Other courthouses, museums, libraries, and college buildings can be found in Detroit, Indianapolis, West Point, Annapolis, Austin, and Dallas.

In the Philadelphia area Cret made the first design for the Benjamin Franklin Parkway, and designed the Barnes Foundation Gallery, the Rodin Museum, the 2601 Parkway Apartments, and the Washington Memorial Arch at Valley Forge Historical Park, and was consulting architect for several bridges.

His professional honors include gold medals from the Architectural League of New York and the American Institute of Architects, the Philadelphia Award, the Distinguished Award of the Washington Society of Architects, and the Prize of Honor at the Fifth Pan-American Congress of Architects. He received an honorary doctor of science degree from the University of Pennsylvania in 1913 and an honorary doctor of arts degree from Harvard University in 1940.

Four of Cret's students at the University of Pennsylvania later became partners in his firm: John F. Harbeson, William J. H. Hough, William H. Livingston, and Roy F. Larson. After Cret's death in 1945 the firm was renamed Harbeson Hough Livingston and Larson, and subsequently H_2L_2 Architects/Planners. Some local projects include the Philadelphia Electric Company Headquarters, the Children's Hospital, the Radnor Corporation, the Philadelphia Bourse, and the SmithKline Beckman World Headquarters Building.

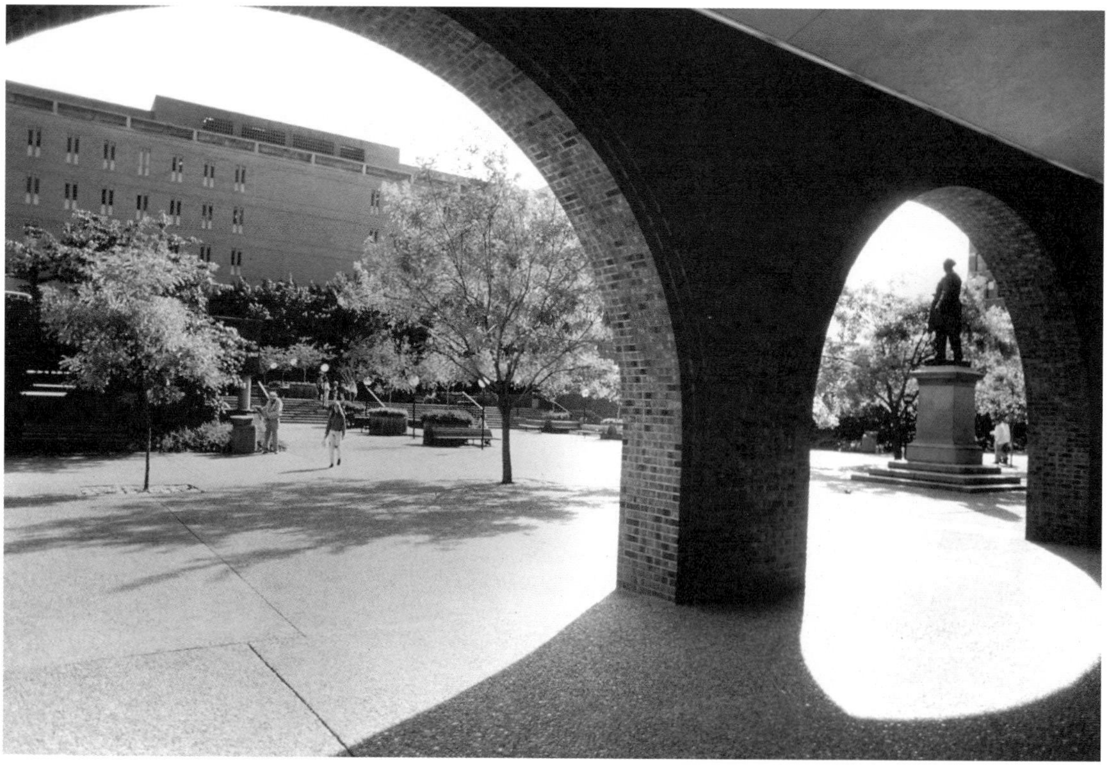

View of Scott Plaza (Photograph by Bob Neroni)

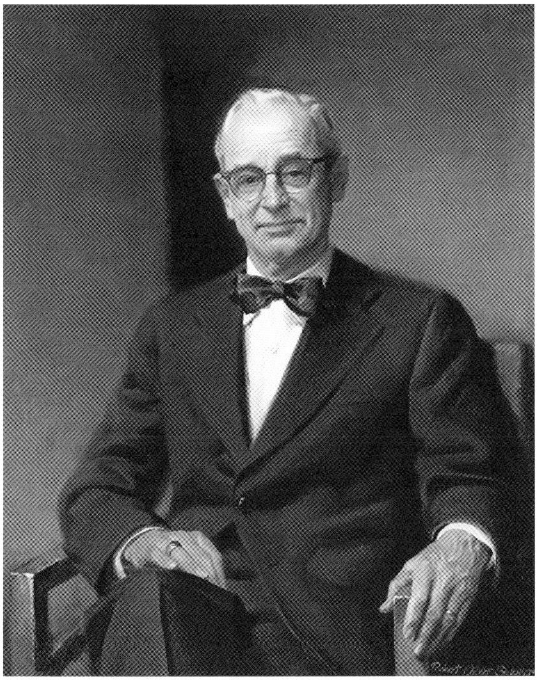

Portrait of Robert T. Lentz

ROBERT T. LENTZ (1910-98)
By Robert Oliver Skemp (1910-84)

Oil on canvas
1975
36 x 30 in.

Signed and dated lower right: "Robert Oliver Skemp/1975"

Given in 1975 by friends and colleagues
Accession number: 1975+e.P.02

Robert T. Lentz spent a long and fruitful career as the librarian and archivist of Jefferson Medical College. Generations of students benefitted from Lentz's teaching of medical bibliography and the effective use of library resources.

Born on a farm in Thorofare, New Jersey in 1910, Robert Lentz attended secretarial school in Philadelphia. He came to Jefferson in 1931 as a clerk-typist, and received training in cataloguing, classification, reference work, and other library skills from head librarian Joseph J. Wilson. While working at Jefferson Lentz took classes part-time, and received a bachelor's degree in education from Temple University (1948) and a master's degree in library science from Drexel Institute of Technology (1951).

During World War II Lentz spent three years in the medical department of the U.S. Army, including eighteen months in the European theater. Marjorie Kirby Lentz substituted for her husband as assistant librarian during his absence and continued working for a time as reference librarian after his return.

Robert Lentz succeeded Joseph Wilson in 1949. His valuable contributions to education were recognized when he was named Jefferson's first professor of medical bibliography and library science in 1965. He was appointed emeritus librarian and emeritus professor in 1975, but stayed on to organize the library's first archives and served as part-time archivist until 1986. Lentz also taught medical bibliography at Drexel's Graduate School of Library Science from 1959 to 1974.

Under Lentz's leadership a building program was planned and implemented for the new Scott Memorial Library. He was successful in gaining a construction award from the Federal Medical Library Assistance Act, a resource grant from the National Library of Medicine, and a grant from the Pennsylvania State Library for charter membership in the national On-line Computer Library Center with access to the holdings of two thousand libraries nationally, including two hundred health science libraries. Under Lentz's tenure the library expanded substantially in collections, services, staff, and space.

Robert Lentz was a founding member of the Philadelphia chapter of the Medical Library Association and served as its national president. He won the Drexel University Library School's distinguished alumni award in 1973, and received an honorary D.Sc. degree from Thomas Jefferson University in 1980.

Robert T. Lentz's portrait by Robert O. Skemp was presented in 1977 by friends and colleagues. The librarian is depicted two-thirds length and life-sized. He is seated in a blue, upholstered armchair and faces the viewer frontally. He wears a dark brown suit, white shirt, and jaunty bow tie. His friendly and accessible expression is set off by twinkling brown eyes and dimples, and he seems barely able to suppress a broader smile.

The Winged Ox

THE WINGED OX
By Henry Weber Mitchell
(1915-80)

Bronze
1975
305 x 123 x 91 in.

Signed on integral base:
"Mitchell"

Commissioned in 1975 by TJU
Accession number: 1976+e.S.01

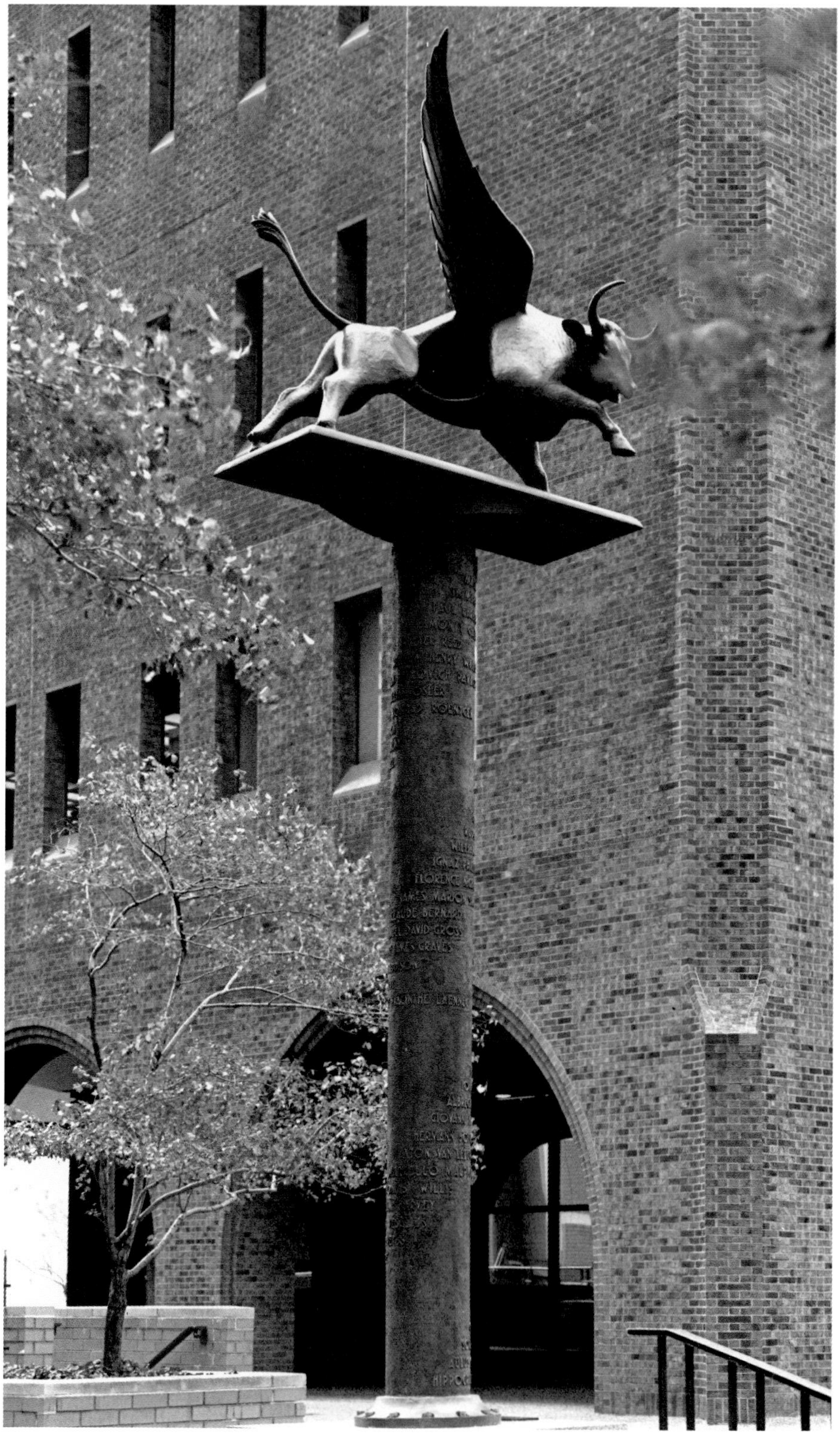

The Winged Ox has become a landmark in Philadelphia since its erection in 1975 on the southwest corner of Tenth and Walnut Streets. The tall bronze sculpture is Jefferson's fulfillment of the Redevelopment Authority's One Percent Fine Arts Program to enhance the nearby Scott Library and Administration Building and the Orlowitz Residence Hall.

Unlike the same sculptor's more whimsical and playful *Bodine Fountain*, Mitchell's submission to this competition attempted a more lofty goal: in essence a history of medical achievement through the ages. The competition's jury awarded the commission to Mitchell, and the sculpture was cast at the Battaglia Foundry in Milan where the sculptor lived for many years.

The Winged Ox was installed in November 1975 and dedicated amidst lively celebrations the following May.

The sixteen-and-one-half-foot column of the bronze sculpture rises dramatically from its base of granite steps and terminates in a stylized winged ox with a span of eight and one-half feet. The beast is poised for flight with wings spread, tail raised, head turned, mouth opened, and right front leg bent and lifted. Though monumental in size and weight, the ox appears light because of its hollowed out,

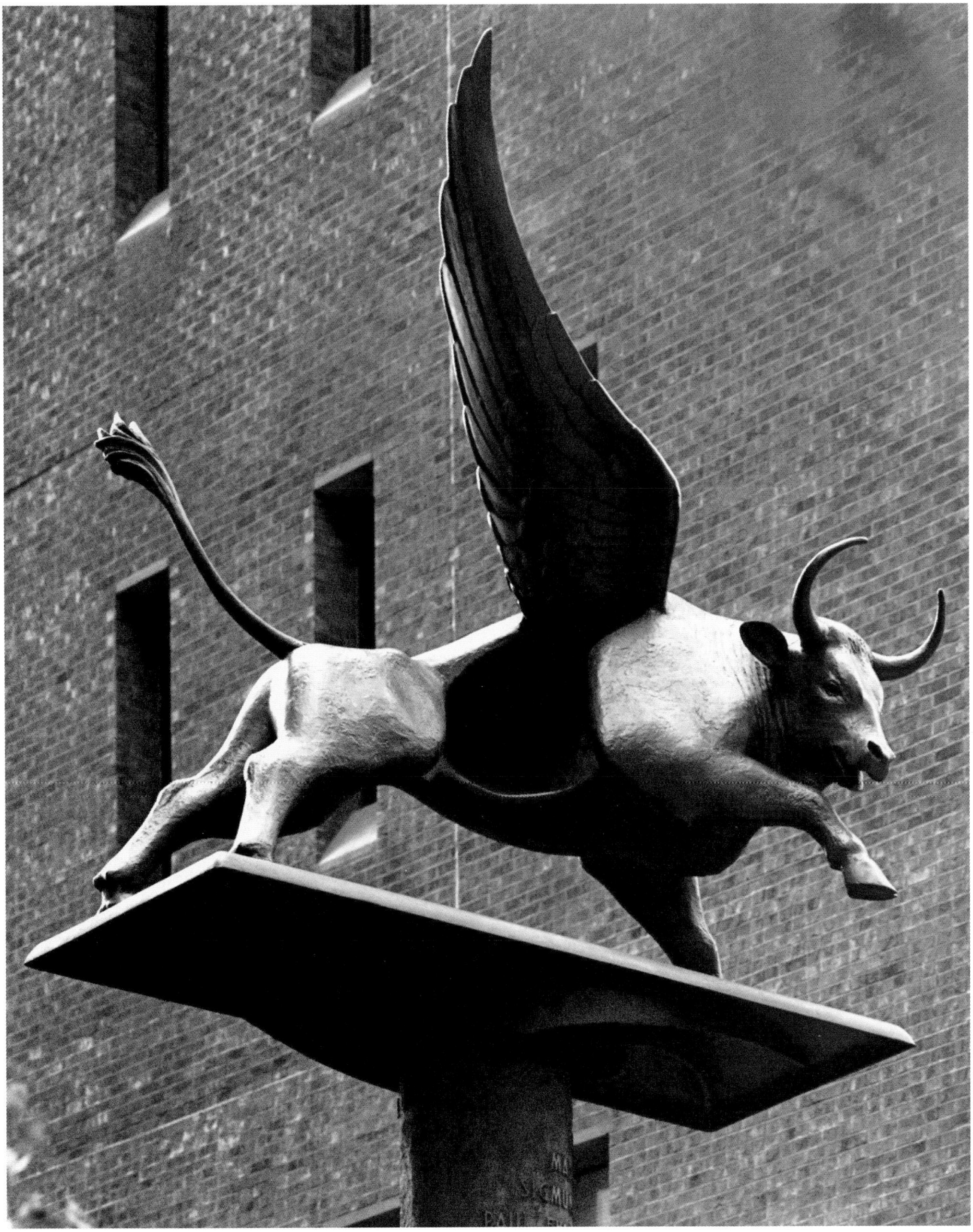

Detail: Closeup of the Ox

concave stomach. The winged creature radiates a sense of alertness and vitality as it prepares to take off from its supporting platform.

The ox is the attribute of the evangelist St. Luke, known as the "beloved physician" who became the patron saint of physicians and painters. Through the ages the four evangelists were often represented as winged beasts. Luke, whose gospel is concerned with the sacrificial death of Christ and begins with the sacrifice of the priest Zacharias, was symbolized as an ox, the sacrificial animal.

The medical theme is advanced by a list of fifty celebrated individuals in the history of medicine. The raised letters of their names spiral around the column like the coiling snakes of the physician's winged caduceus. Beginning with Hippocrates and ending with Dr. John H. Gibbon Jr., the names include four other Jefferson alumni: Drs. Samuel D. Gross, Carlos Finlay, J. Marion Sims, and Chevalier Jackson.[1]

Ceremonial Mace of Thomas Jefferson University

CEREMONIAL MACE OF THOMAS JEFFERSON UNIVERSITY
By Eugene Zweigle
1986

Solid silver, sterling silver, ebony, lapis lazuli
49 x 10 1/4 x 9 in.

Signed and dated underside of ox: "GENE ZWEIGLE PHILA/1986"; marked "J. E. CALDWELL CO" on rim underneath base

Commissioned in 1986 by TJU
Accession number: 1986+e.DA.01

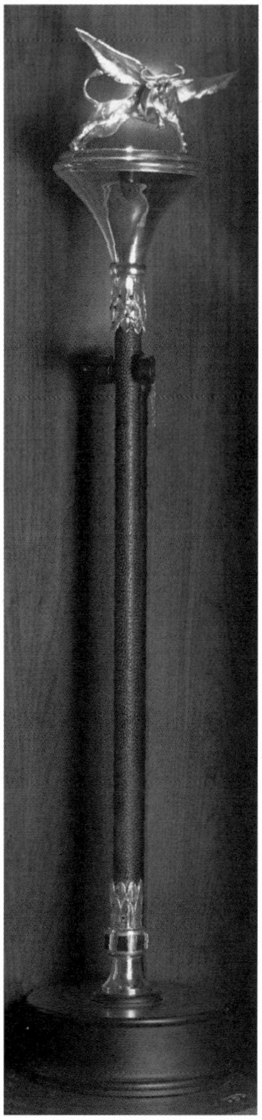

The Winged Ox soon became so integrated into the university's consciousness that in 1986 a miniature replica (eight and three-quarters inches wide) was crafted to ornament the shaft of a new ceremonial mace used in formal academic processions.

The ox is cast in pure and solid silver, and supported on a sterling silver, funnel-shaped form with a sterling silver sleeve of stiff leaves embellished with small lapis lazuli cabochons. This arrangement surmounts a thirty-four-inch-long ebony shaft terminating in a sleeve of stiff silver leaves over a band of rectangular lapis cabochons resting on a splayed sterling silver base. The Thomas Jefferson University seal is mounted on the base of the staff.

Ebony and lapis lazuli were selected because black and blue are the official Jefferson colors. The mace was first carried by microbiology professor Robert J. Mandle, Ph.D., grand marshal at the commencement exercises held at the Academy of Music on June 6, 1986. During ceremonies it rests in its own specially made stand. The mace is displayed in the Eakins Gallery when not in use.

Production of the mace was coordinated by the J. E. Caldwell Company of Philadelphia. It was designed by Howard Serlick and made by Philadelphia craftsmen Eugene Zweigle, silversmith, and Michael Copeland, woodturner.

Smaller bronze replicas of *The Winged Ox* and gold lapel pins bearing its image are awarded to contributors of distinguished service or generous donations to Thomas Jefferson University. The cast bronze replicas have been provided by and generously donated to the university by Mrs. Henry Mitchell, the sculptor's widow. The lapel pins signify membership in the Winged Ox Society, a high level of giving in the President's Club.

Gibbon Building

GIBBON BUILDING
By Harbeson Hough Livingston & Larson
Erected 1978

Photograph of architects' wooden model
(whereabouts unknown)
Ca. 1976

Ordered by TJU
Accession number: 1976+c.Ph.01

After more than a decade of arduous planning and fund-raising, ground was broken for the new Thomas Jefferson University Hospital on April 7, 1975. The building covers the entire block between Chestnut and Sansom Streets and Tenth and Eleventh Streets.

The planners' goal was "to provide both the total range of patient care and the educational experience in one facility...by integrating the three general aspects of patient care: inpatient units; diagnostic and therapeutic facilities; and physicians' offices."[2] The facility opened five months ahead of schedule and was dedicated on June 9, 1978. In 1990 the "New Hospital" was renamed the Gibbon Building in honor of Dr. John H. Gibbon Jr., the distinguished alumnus and pioneering cardiothoracic surgeon.

Plans called for inpatient units with a total of 411 beds to be grouped by medical condition with related diagnostic, therapeutic, nursing, and administrative services on the same floor—mini-hospitals in effect. Physicians' of-

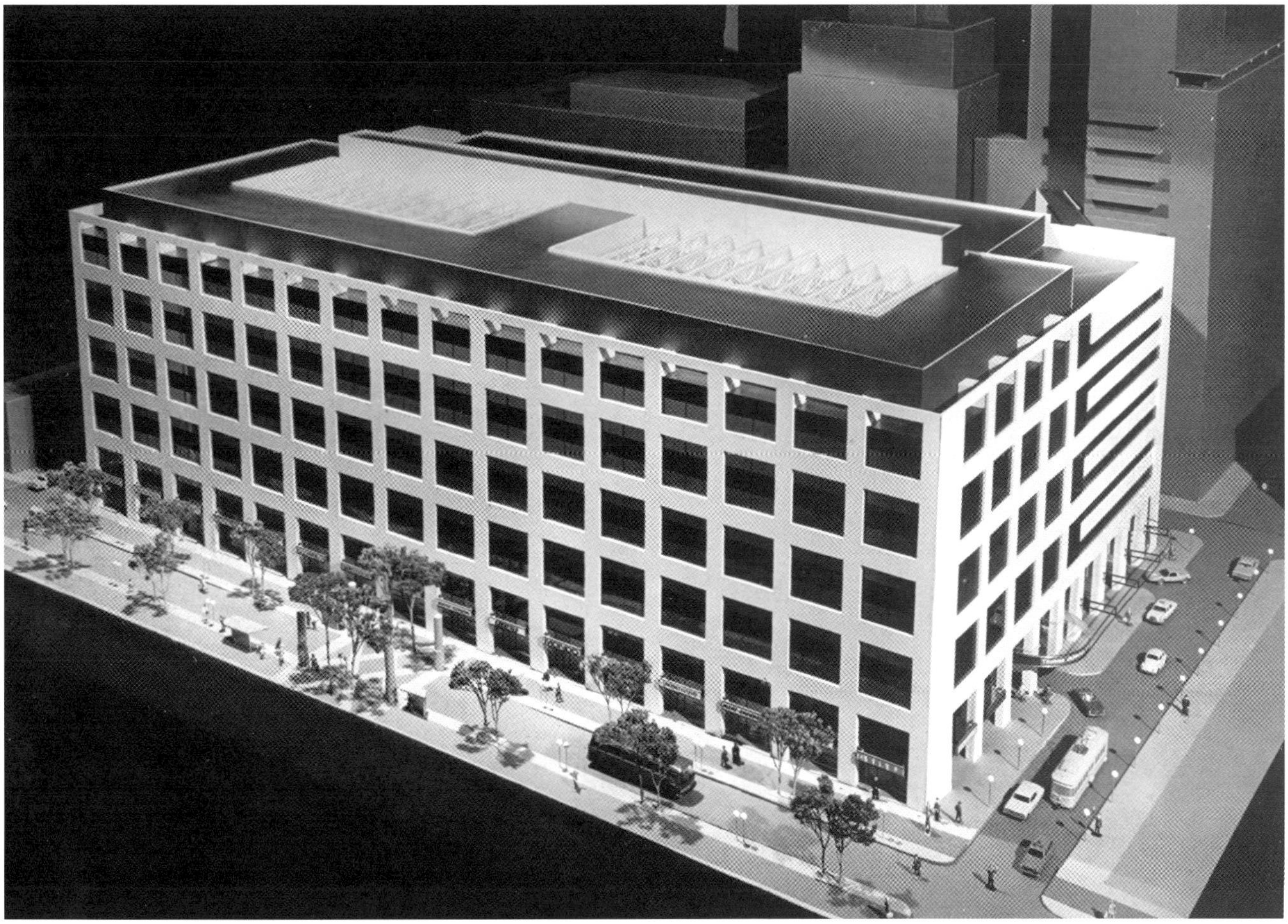

fices for ambulatory patients would be located on alternate floors. Bridges on seven levels across Sansom Street would connect the hospital to the newly renovated Foerderer Pavilion. The new hospital was the first in the city to place the majority of patients in private rooms.

The main entrances of the nine-story "hospital of tomorrow" are located on Tenth and Eleventh Streets, and the remaining street frontage is occupied by commercial retail stores. The smooth orange brick exterior is punctuated by recessed vertical windows that correlate with the windows of the adjoining Foerderer Pavilion. The Eleventh Street entrance has a drive-through area for vehicles, with a projecting, curved sign above.

The interior is built around two enclosed, skylighted atria. The huge, airy light wells contain cafeterias for 240 patrons, with interior landscaping and suspended rainbow banners and mobile cutouts of floating clouds.

Portrait of Lewis W. Bluemle Jr.

LEWIS WILLIAM BLUEMLE Jr., M.D. (b. 1921)
By Nelson Shanks (b. 1937)

Oil on canvas
1990
42 1/2 x 34 1/2 in.

Signed lower left: "Nelson Shanks"

Given in 1990 by TJU board of trustees, friends, and colleagues
Accession number: 1990+e.P.01

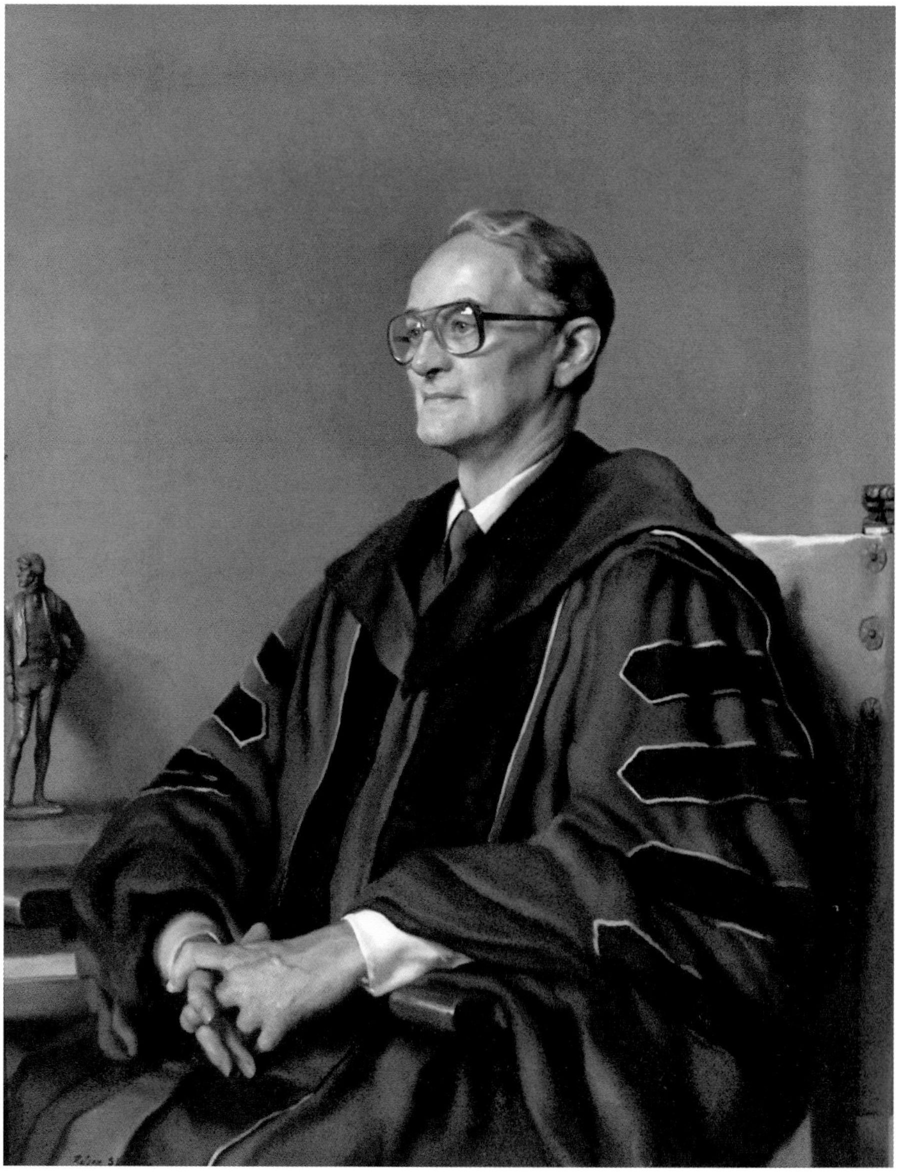

In 1977 Dr. Lewis W. Bluemle Jr., a distinguished scholar, educator, and administrator, was inaugurated as the second president of Thomas Jefferson University. He succeeded the interim president, George M. Norwood Jr., who served following the unexpected death of Dr. Peter A. Herbut. "The Bluemle era" lasted until his retirement in 1990 when he was named professor emeritus and president emeritus.

"Bill" Bluemle was born in Williamsport, Pennsylvania in 1921 and received both his undergraduate degree (1943) and medical degree (1946) from Johns Hopkins University. After a rotating internship and residency in internal medicine at the Hospital of the University of Pennsylvania, he was a fellow in the chemical section of the university's department of medicine and then a faculty member of the department where he rose to associate professor by 1961. An outstanding researcher and teacher, he was a Markle Scholar in Academic Medicine (1955-60), and received the Christian R. and Mary F. Lindback Award for Distinguished Teaching (1966).

Between 1961 and 1968 Dr. Bluemle organized and was director of the clinical research center at the hospital. He was associate dean at Penn's School of Medicine from 1966 to 1968. He also established the renal dialysis unit and was its chief from 1951 to 1968. He was internationally known for his numerous research publications on fluid and electrolyte metabolism, collaborative studies on diuretics, and the changes in body composition in different disease states. With the help of Penn's chemical engineering department Dr. Bluemle's work in designing and modifying the early artificial kidney apparatus was awarded several patents. He performed the first successful kidney dialysis in Philadelphia, third in the nation.

Dr. Bluemle was a charter member and president of the American Society for Artificial Internal Organs. He was a consultant to the National Institute of Health's artificial kidney/chronic uremia program, and consultant to the Bureau of the Budget's study group on treatment of chronic renal disease.

In 1968 Dr. Bluemle was appointed president of the Upstate Medical Center of the State University of New York, a post he held until 1974. Then he moved to Portland, Oregon to become president of the University of Oregon Health Sciences Center.

A decision by the largest search committee ever formed at Thomas Jefferson University culminated in the appointment of Lewis W. Bluemle Jr., M.D. as president in 1977. Two years later when writing about the university at the millennium, Bluemle stressed two important factors upon which Jefferson's future depended: one, financial stability and economic soundness because of rising costs and shrinking government support for education and patient care, the areas being studied by the task force on university planning; and two, the "ability to attract and nurture truly gifted people, the charismatic teacher, the brilliant researcher, the model clinician, and above all, intellectually curious students."[3]

By 1990 the university's endowment fund had tripled, research funding had doubled every two years since 1984, and the sixty-five-million-dollar 1980s Decade Fund far exceeded its goal. The president's academic, research, and clinical appointments had attracted top professionals, and the Jefferson Institute for Molecular Biology was established.

Besides new faculty and administrative staff, new construction and renovation projects, and new programs in the College of Allied Health Sciences and College of Graduate Studies including the Gibbon Scholars M.D./Ph.D. seven-year integrated program, affiliations were established with the Alfred I. duPont Institute in Wilmington, Magee Rehabilitation Hospital, Wills Eye Hospital, and the Geisinger Medical Center. Emergency and trauma services were expanded so that Jefferson was now recognized as a Level One Trauma Center and a Regional Spinal Cord Injury Center. A number of new hospital services were provided including a liver transplant program and the only extracorporeal membrane oxygenation program in the region.

The 1989 board of trustees annual report attributed much of Jefferson's progress during Bluemle's term to his "quiet, collegial style, always trying to develop a consensus among the major parties to any significant decision." That Dr. Bluemle's objectives were realized is attested to in the citation of his honorary doctorate of humane letters awarded by Johns Hopkins University in 1990, which stated in part:

> You are one of the leading lights of professional health education in the United States. As president of Thomas Jefferson University for the past twelve years, you have nurtured an institution that today has a national reputation as a center of excellence in research and clinical care...
>
> You have been a magnet for research and clinical talent in almost every department, you have brought Jefferson Hospital to one of the soundest fiscal positions in the region and you have increased dramatically the university's public and private research support.
>
> An individual of imagination and originality, you have been called a craftsman of science and enduring relationships.

Dr. Bluemle's professional and civic appointments ranged across scientific, urban, educational, business, and cultural affairs. He was on the board of directors or trustees of the Association of Academic Health Centers, the University City Science Center, the Urban Affairs Partnership, Narco Scientific, the Girard Company and Girard Bank, Mellon Bank (East), Teleflex, Incorporated, the Greater Philadelphia First Corporation, and the Citizens' Crime Commission of Delaware Valley.

He served as president of the College of Physicians of Philadelphia, chairman of the steering committee of the Greater Philadelphia Organization for Clinical Trials, member of the advisory board of the Philadelphia Chapter of the Physicians for Social Responsibility, member of the Philadelphia Commission on AIDS, and a member of the board of overseers of the Law School of the University of Pennsylvania. He was also a member of the Orchestra Council of the Philadelphia Orchestra Association and the Mayor's Business Roundtable, and cochair of the Urban Affairs Partnership and the City of Philadelphia's Solid Waste Advisory Council.

In 1981 Dr. Lewis W. Bluemle Jr. was made a fellow of the Royal College of Physicians of Edinburgh. Among his other honors are the Distinguished Philadelphian Award of the Chestnut Street Association, the Maimonides Award of the Anti-defamation League of B'nai B'rith, the Strittmatter Award of the Philadelphia County Medical Society, the Magee Hospital Humanitarian Award, and the Distinguished Service Award of the Pennsylvania State Medical Society. He received honorary doctor of science degrees from the Philadelphia College of Pharmacy and Science and the Medical College of Pennsylvania, and an honorary doctor of humane letters degree from Washington and Jefferson College.

At a celebration marking Dr. Bluemle's tenth year as president of Jefferson the trustees presented him with a wood lathe and a set of turning tools. These distinctive personal gifts reflect his interest and ability in craftsmanship. Bluemle formed close bonds with several Jefferson artists, and attended meetings of the university art committee whenever his schedule allowed. Though not an alumnus, Bluemle was proud of the university's traditions and contributions, and appointed Jefferson's first university historian, university archivist, and university art historian.

When Dr. Bluemle retired in 1990, the university arranged a festive farewell dinner attended by over four hundred friends, colleagues, and family members. There it was announced that the new research building scheduled for completion in 1991 would be named the Bluemle Life Sciences Building. Guests viewed the first airing of *Legacy of Excellence*, a videotape of interviews and photographs relating to Dr. Bluemle's accomplishments. Another highlight of the evening was the unveiling of the honoree's portrait by Nelson Shanks. The painting was later installed in a sun-filled corner of the entrance lobby of the Bluemle Life Sciences Building.

Shanks depicted the subject seated in an armchair in a three-quarters view turned left, gazing into the far distance. His hands are clasped with fingers loosely entwined in front of his body. His flowing, black presidential robe has voluminous sleeves and a green hood bordered with a thin, yellow edge. Black velvet front panels and stripes on the sleeves are edged in light blue. Next to the figure is a table with four books and a small bronze replica of Lloyd Lillie's sculpture of Thomas Jefferson.

Dr. Bluemle's angular features are accentuated by the high forehead and cheekbones, thin lips, and jutting jaw line, all modeled in sculptural forms and planes, testimony to the artist's knowledge of the underlying anatomy. Because the subject's body and head are turned away from the viewer, and his serious and pensive expression suggests preoccupation with inner thoughts, some friends and colleagues have found the depiction aloof and lacking in the subject's customary warmth.

However, the austerity of the introspective mood is countered by the graceful and elegant surface achieved by the artist. Nelson Shanks is noted for the superb craftsmanship of his rich, meticulously rendered, smooth surfaces, uncommon color schemes, and unusual attention to textures and shadows. The square-backed, orange velvet, Renaissance-style armchair (a studio prop) is studded with bronze rosettes and has carved wooden finials. The modulated, atmospheric background of neutral greenish-umber has quiet overtones of some of the brighter colors seen elsewhere. Highlights and shadows throughout the painting create a lively surface, especially on the subject's face and glasses, and the rippling folds of his presidential robe.

Nelson Shanks is an internationally known artist who was born in 1937 in Rochester, New York, and descended from Scottish forbears who had emigrated to Virginia in 1702. He was reared in Wilmington, Delaware. After beginning his studies in architectural engineering at the University of Kansas, he switched to art at the Kansas City Art Institute, and after one semester relocated to New York where he studied at the Art Students League and the National Academy of Design. Aided by successive grants from the Elizabeth T. Greenshields Memorial Foundation and the John F. and Anna Lee Stacey Memorial Foundation he went abroad for travel and study at the Accademia di Belle Arti in Florence.

Upon his return to the States, the faltering career of the discouraged young artist was rescued by a portrait commission received through a family connection in Memphis, Tennessee. He completed the portrait and stayed there to teach at the Memphis Academy of Art. In 1977 a "friend of a friend" invited him to live and paint at the American Embassy in Paris where his traditional and refined style attracted favorable attention.

While abroad he was commissioned to paint a portrait of Queen Juliana of the Netherlands. Over the years he has painted portraits of other notable European sitters including Diana, Princess of Wales, Lady Margaret Thatcher, Luciano Pavarotti, and King Gustav and Queen Silvia of Sweden.

Other teaching posts have been at the National Academy of Design and the Art Students League in New York, the Art Institute of Chicago, the Princeton Art Association, the University of the Arts in Philadelphia, and George Washington University. In 1993 he was awarded an honorary doctor of fine arts degree from Beaver College in Glenside, Pennsylvania. Famed portrait and figure painter Bo Bartlett, who studied privately with Shanks after graduating with numerous awards from the Pennsylvania Academy of the Fine Arts, said unabashedly, "I learned how to paint from Nelson Shanks."[4]

Nelson Shanks has also rendered portraits of such renowned Americans as Ronald Reagan, C. Everett Koop, M.D., Katharine Graham, J. Carter Brown (former director of the National Gallery of Art), and Robert Wood Johnson Jr. He has exhibited portraits, nudes, symbolic works, and still lifes in galleries and museums throughout the United States, including a one-man show at the Pennsylvania Academy of the Fine Arts in 1996.

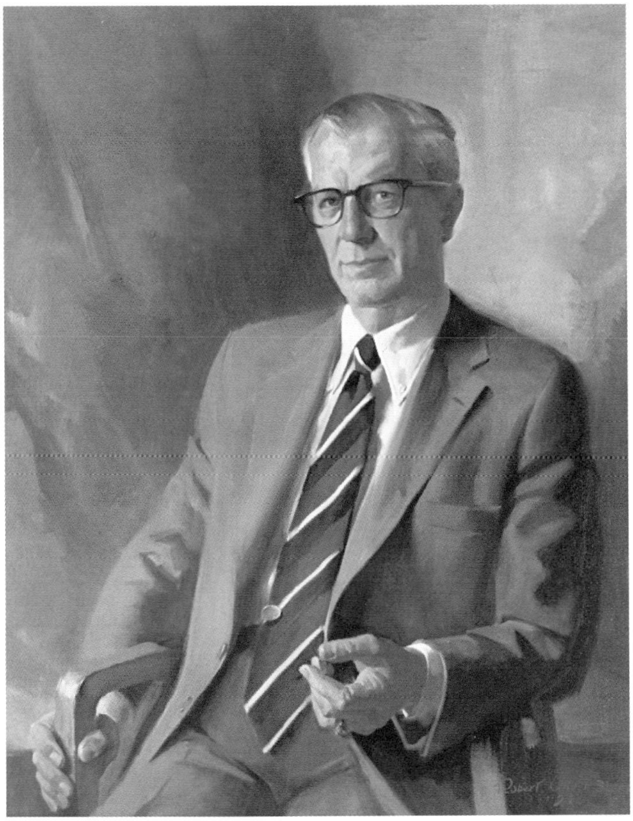

Portrait of Francis J. Sweeney

FRANCIS J. SWEENEY, M.D. (1925-90)
By Robert Oliver Skemp (1910-84)

Oil on canvas
1978
36 x 30 in.

Signed and dated lower right: "Robert Oliver Skemp/1978"

Given in 1978 by friends and colleagues
Accession number: 1978+e.P.05

Dr. Francis J. Sweeney served as medical director of the Jefferson Hospital and vice president for health services at Thomas Jefferson University. He was also a faculty member in Jefferson's division of infectious diseases.

A native Philadelphian, Francis J. Sweeney was born in 1925. He enlisted in the navy before graduating from the University of Virginia in 1947 and Jefferson Medical College in 1951. His medical residency at Jefferson was interrupted by service as medical officer aboard the U.S.S. *Rehoboth* during the Korean War.

After returning to Jefferson to complete his residency, he was appointed to the faculty in the department of medicine. Well regarded by students, he won a Christian R. and Mary F. Lindback Award for Distinguished Teaching in 1963. He rose to professor of medicine in

1979. He was appointed director of the university's hospital in 1967 and five years later he became vice president for health services. He held his academic and administrative posts until his resignation in 1984.

As a hospital administrator in the early 1970s Dr. Sweeney was a guiding force in the planning and financing for the new Thomas Jefferson University Hospital, and for the adoption of "one level of care," ending the distinction between ward and private care. He also oversaw changes in cost reimbursement involving Medicare and third-party payment programs. He advocated such initiatives as the hospital's helicopter pad and short-procedure units.

Sweeney's research interests were in infectious diseases, and during the late 1950s he performed epidemiological studies of staphylococcal infections at the Norristown State Hospital with Dr. Robert I. Wise, in collaboration with Dr. Robert Mandle. In 1959 he was a member of the Jefferson Medical College/U.S. Public Health Service Cholera Study Team in Thailand. He was also a consultant in infectious diseases at Chestnut Hill Hospital, Philadelphia General Hospital, and Eagleville Sanitarium for Consumptives.

Dr. Sweeney served as chairman of the board of regents of the American College of Physicians from 1983 to 1985. His numerous board memberships included the Joint Commission on Accreditation of Hospitals, the National Health Council, the Hospital Utilization Project of Pennsylvania, the Health Systems Agency of Southeastern Pennsylvania, the Board of Health of the City of Philadelphia, and the Philadelphia Association for Clinical Trials. He was chairman of the Blue Cross Joint Provider Plan Committee.

Among Sweeney's many awards from the American College of Physicians are the Special Presidential Citation, Laureate Award Medal, and Alfred Stengel Memorial Award. He also received the Clarence E. Shaffrey, S.J. Award of St. Joseph's University. He won Jefferson's alumni achievement award in 1983 and the Winged Ox Award the following year.

In 1984 Dr. Sweeney left Jefferson to become vice president of the Temple University Health Sciences Center. In 1986 he moved to Mercy Catholic Medical Center as vice president for professional affairs and medical director.

Dr. Frank J. Sweeney's portrait by Robert O. Skemp was presented by Jefferson friends and colleagues in 1978. He is shown half length and life-sized, seated in a low-backed, office type of armchair. The curled fingers of his left hand suggests a conversational gesture, but his facial expression is not particularly animated. He looks straight ahead rather sternly through his square-shaped, tortoise-shell glasses.

The portrait's color scheme is mainly neutral, especially the sitter's gray suit and the broadly brushed, grayish-green, atmospheric background. A startlingly bright note is Dr. Sweeney's red, white, and blue, diagonally striped necktie.

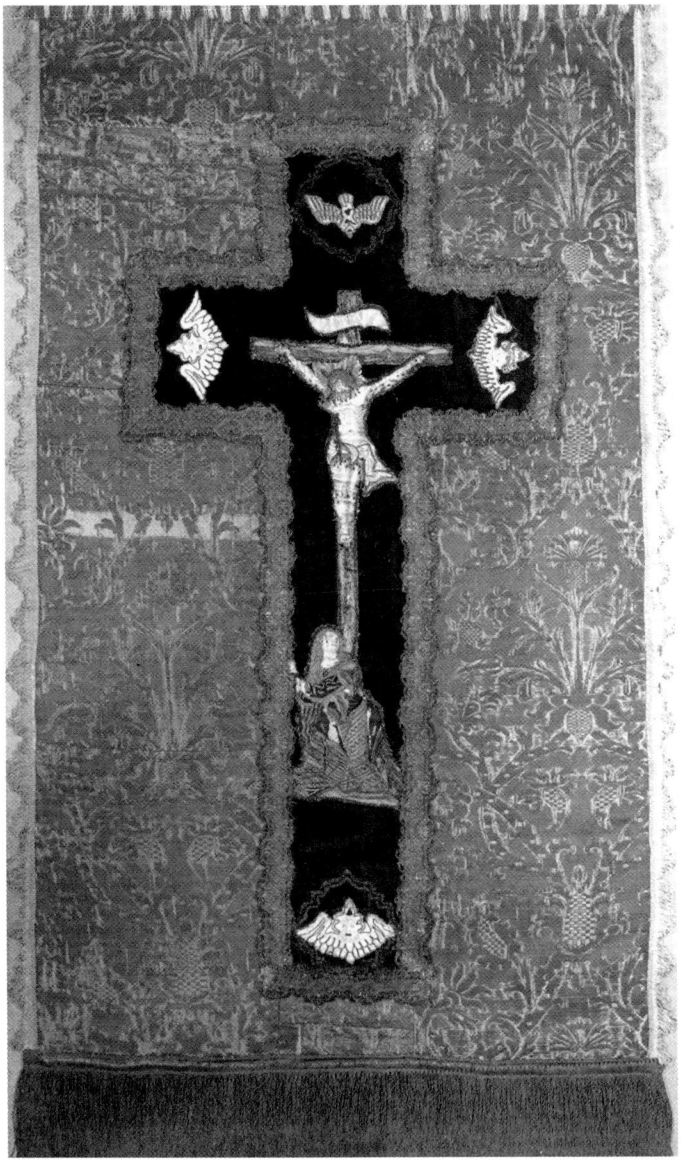

Crucifixion Textile Panel

CRUCIFIXION
By unknown English craftsman

Silk, velvet, gold, silver
Ca. 1840
55 x 31 1/2 in.

Given 1956-71 by Florence Foerderer (Mrs. William) Tonner in memory of Ida Hubacher
Accession number: 1956-1971.DA.01

In 1956 the House Committee of the Women's Board donated a "meditation room" to the Foerderer Pavilion. The chairman of the committee was Mrs. William T. Tonner, the former Florence Foerderer who was a sister of trustee Percival E. Foerderer. In 1981 the chapel was relocated to the ninth floor of the new hospital by Dr. Francis J. Sweeney Jr. and his family and friends, "in loving memory of Helen Drueding Sweeney," Dr. Sweeney's wife who had died in 1979.

Among other objects the chapel contains three religious textiles donated by Mrs. Tonner, a collector of antique art, decorative arts, and religious objects. Upon her death in 1971 she deeded her valuable collection and the seventeen-acre family estate, Glen Foerd, to the Lutheran Church.

Subjects of the tapestries are a Crucifixion, Ivanhoe, and saints. Created in mid-nineteenth-century England, the textiles resemble Venetian or Spanish embroideries of the sixteenth to early eighteenth centuries.

The Crucifixion is made of green velvet with embroidered silk figures including a weeping Virgin and four angels. The background of the scene is made of dark red, silk damask decorated with joined palmettes and leafy vines. Its broad borders are made of couched metallic (spun gold and silver) thread. The top and bottom fringed borders are probably original, while the side borders may be later additions.

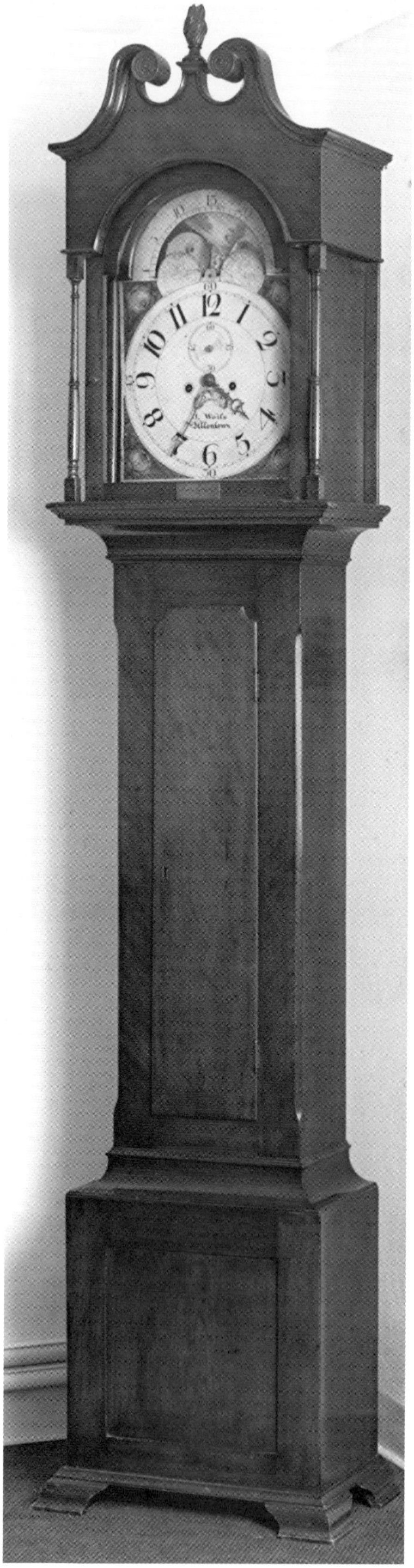

Tall Case Clock

(See color plate)

TALL CASE CLOCK
Works by Joseph Weiss (1802-63)

Cherry
1830s-1840s
95 x 21 x 11 in.

Signed on clock face below calendar register:
"J. Weifs/Allentown"
Inscription on plaque below dial: "CHILDREN'S HEART HOSPITAL/1972"

Given before 1932 by William Anderson to Children's Heart Hospital, and given in 1972 to TJU
Accession number: 1972+e.DA.01

An antique tall case clock now in the Jefferson Hospital had originally been given sometime before 1932 to the nurses' home at Children's Heart Hospital in Philadelphia by one of its founders, William M. Anderson. His son, James, approved the relocation of the clock to the office of Dr. Francis J. Sweeney in 1972, and it can still be found in the Jefferson Hospital's administrative offices.

Children's Heart Hospital had been incorporated in 1927 to care for children with rheumatic fever and rheumatic heart disease. When the number of heart patients decreased after the introduction of sulfa drugs and penicillin in the 1930s and 1940s, the hospital expanded its mission to care for children with other chronic conditions. In 1970 Thomas Jefferson University agreed to assume the hospital's operational and clinical responsibilities, and in 1986 the name was changed to Children's Rehabilitation Center and was relocated to the fourth floor of the nearby Jefferson Park Hospital (a special affiliate of the university since 1987).

The works of this American clock were made in the 1830s or 1840s by Joseph (sometimes called Joshua) Weiss of Allentown, Pennsylvania, the last clock maker of note from Lehigh County. The case was probably made at about the same time and place, but not necessarily by Weiss. Typical of provincial Pennsylvania clocks of the period, it mixes Chippendale and Federal forms.

The hood has slender columns supporting the cornice which terminates in steep swan's neck volutes flanking a flame finial. The painted iron face has a dial painted white with black Arabic numerals, a chapter ring enclosing a seconds dial, and a calendar register. These elements are surrounded by spandrels decorated with polychromed roses with foliage over a gold background. The lunette is fitted with polychromed moon phases. The waisted trunk beneath chamfered corners is hinged with a pendulum door which conceals the weights and pendulum. The paneled base is raised on ogee bracket, splayed feet.

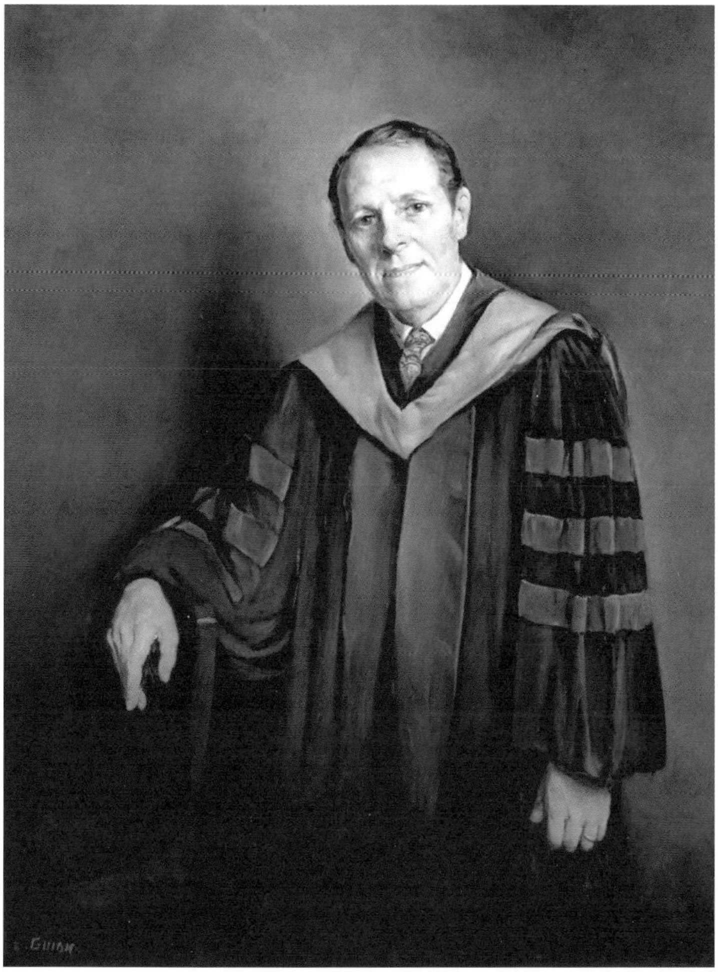

Portrait of William F. Kellow

WILLIAM FRANCIS KELLOW, M.D. (1922-81)
By Molly Guion (b. 1910)

Oil on canvas
1978
50 1/4 x 40 1/4 in.

Signed lower left: "M. GUION"

Given in 1978 by JMC alumni, friends, and colleagues
Accession number: 1978+e.P.04

Dr. William F. Kellow was appointed dean, professor of medicine, and vice president at Jefferson Medical College in 1967. His distinguished accomplishments and leadership ability brought him gratitude and esteem by his colleagues as well as many awards from the medical profession.

Born in Geneva, New York in 1922 "Will" Kellow received his undergraduate degree from the University of Notre Dame (1943) and his medical degree from the Georgetown University School of Medicine (1946). He was a medical intern and resident at the District of Columbia General Hospital and then assistant surgical resident at Georgetown and Walter Reed Hospitals. During the Korean War he served as chief of the medical service at Beale Air Force Base Hospital in California.

Dr. Kellow's academic career began as clinical instructor in both surgery and medicine at Georgetown. This was followed by a move to the University of Illinois College of Medicine where he became associate professor of medicine and associate dean by 1959. In 1961 Kellow accepted positions as dean and professor of medicine at Philadelphia's Hahnemann Medical College where he guided successful building programs and increased teaching affiliations.

His accomplishments at Hahnemann brought him to the attention of Jefferson Medical College which appointed him professor, dean, and vice president in 1967. Dean Kellow was an outstanding administrator and motivator, and a prudent fiscal manager. He instituted many new programs such as the medical practice plan, the department of family medicine, the office of minority affairs, and the office of medical education. Kellow democratized faculty participation by forming a general faculty and professorial faculty and opening membership on college committees to the faculty at large, not just chairmen.

To respond to a physician shortage the Jefferson enrollment increased by more than twenty percent without compromising quality of education, and to aid in the better distribution of future physicians a Physician Shortage Area Program in conjunction with Indiana University of Pennsylvania was begun. Kellow concluded formal agreements with affiliated hospitals, and began a new partnership with the Delaware Institute of Medical Education and Research, funded by the legislature of the State of Delaware (which has no medical school), to provide access to Jefferson Medical College for up to twenty qualified Delaware students.

Dr. Kellow was a board member or regent of the American College of Physicians, the National Institutes of Health's General Research Support Program Advisory Committee, and the Regional Comprehensive Health Planning Committee of the City of Philadelphia. He was chairman of the American Medical Association's Advisory Committee on Undergraduate Medical Education and the Council on Medical Education, and chairman of the Liaison Committee on Medical Education of the American Medical Association and the Association of American Medical Colleges.

Dr. William F. Kellow received honors from many institutions including the Centennial of Science Award from the University of Notre Dame, Mastership in the American College of Physicians, and the Clarence E. Shaffrey, S.J. Award from St. Joseph's University. He was awarded honorary doctor of science degrees from St. Joseph's University and Georgetown School of Medicine, and a doctor of humane letters from Hahnemann Medical College.

The Jefferson classes of 1968 and 1971 dedicated their yearbooks to the popular dean. He served until November 16, 1981 when grave illness forced his retirement and he was named emeritus dean and emeritus professor. He received two special honors at a quiet ceremony at his home: the alumni achievement award (as an honorary alumnus) and the first Winged Ox Award for distinguished service to Jefferson. In addition, a remodeled suite of classrooms and conference rooms in the College Building was designated the Kellow Conference Center. He died on December 3 and an honorary doctorate of laws was awarded posthumously the following year.

Dr. William F. Kellow's portrait by Molly Guion had been presented in 1978 by the alumni association, friends, and colleagues. Breaking with college tradition, the portrait was unveiled by his five daughters rather than a professional associate. Family members say that he was already ill when he sat for his portrait.

Dr. Kellow is depicted two-thirds length and life-sized, standing almost frontally with his right arm leaning heavily on the back of a nearby chair. His tilted head juts forward, but he looks straight ahead toward the viewer with a neutral expression. His features are distinguished by his square jaw and cleft chin, and tightly pursed lips.

He wears a black academic gown with green front panels and green stripes on the sleeves. The V-shaped yellow mantle adds a note of bright yellow against the prevailing dark colors of his robe and the atmospheric background. The ruddy complexion of his face and hands is more thickly and loosely painted than the smoother costume and background.

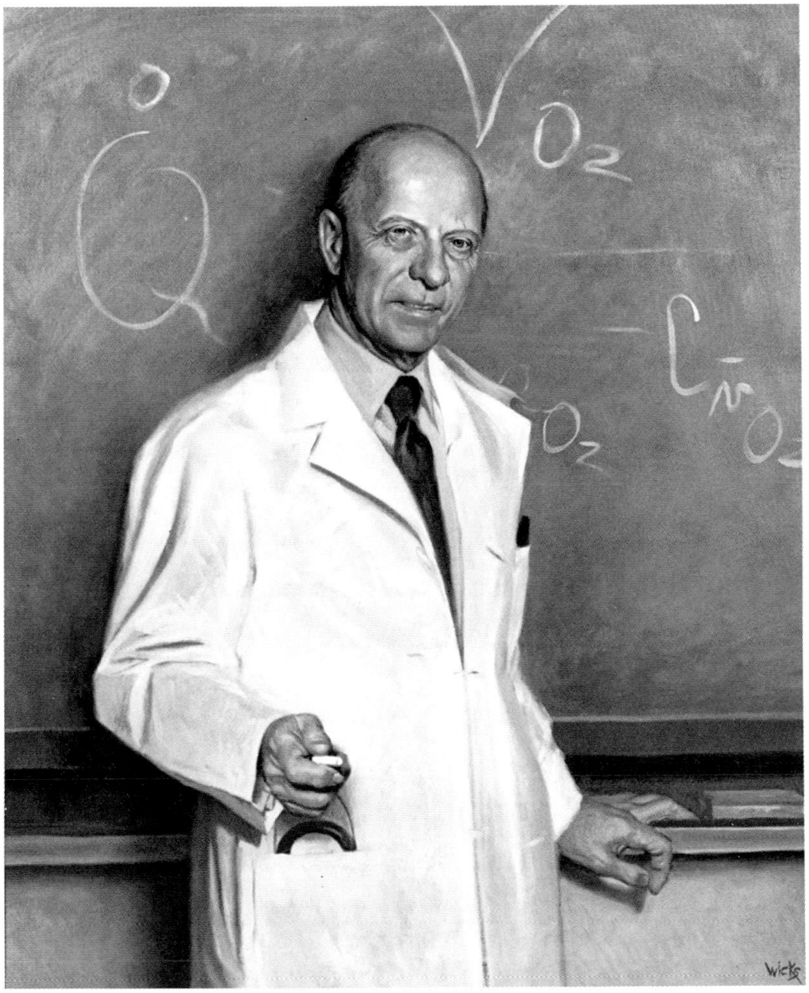

Portrait of Frank D. Gray Jr.

FRANK DAVIS GRAY Jr., M.D.
(1916-97)
By Alden MacMaster Wicks
(1914-87)

Oil on canvas
1982
36 x 30 in.

Signed lower right: "Wicks"

Given in 1982 by JMC department of medicine

Accession number: 1982+e.P.03

Dr. Frank D. Gray Jr. was Jefferson's Magee Professor of Medicine and fourteenth chairman of the department, serving from 1976 to 1981. Upon his retirement he served as interim dean briefly until a permanent successor to Dr. William F. Kellow was appointed.

Frank D. Gray was born in 1916 in Marshall, Minnesota, the son of a surgeon. He graduated from Northwestern University (1938) and the Columbia University College of Physicians and Surgeons (1943). After a year as intern and assistant resident at Bellevue Hospital in New York, he spent two years on active duty with the U.S. Army Medical Corps, including the landing at Normandy and the Battle of the Bulge, as an infantry battalion surgeon. He was made regimental surgeon and rose in rank to major by 1946. By the time he retired from the reserves in 1971 he had reached the rank of colonel.

After the war Dr. Gray became an assistant in surgery at Johns Hopkins University. He received further training as an assistant resident at the Grace-New Haven Community Hospital, and research fellow in medicine at Yale University. At Yale he rose to associate professor of medicine in 1957, with positions as director of the section on chest diseases and director of the cardiopulmonary laboratory at the Yale-New Haven Medical Center, and director of the cardiac and chest clinics at the Grace-New Haven Hospital.

In 1968 Dr. Gray moved to Philadelphia to fill the position as director of the division of medicine and program director of the medical residency at the Lankenau Hospital in suburban Philadelphia. In 1976 he joined the Jefferson faculty as Magee Professor and chairman of the department of medicine at Jefferson. Gray's other hospital appointments included Magee Rehabilitation Hospital, Lankenau Hospital, and Wills Eye Hospital.

In addition to numerous articles and chapters on pulmonary and heart diseases, Dr. Gray was the author of *Pulmonary Embolism* (1966) and served on the editorial board of *Diseases of the Chest*. He served the American College of Chest Physicians as a member of the executive council and board of regents, and vice chairman of the board of governors.

In the late 1960s and 1970s Dr. Gray became certified in courses at special management schools, including management sciences at the Institute for Advanced Technology at the Center for Disease Control in Washington, D.C., and the executive program in health policy and management for chiefs of clinical services at the Harvard School of Public Health.

Dr. Gray was named professor emeritus in 1982 and the department of medicine presented his portrait shortly after he retired. Alden M. Wicks has shown the physician two-thirds length and life-sized. He is standing in a lecture room in front of a chalkboard, and gesturing with his right hand which holds a piece of chalk. Apparently he is explaining the formulas written on the board pertaining to cardiac and respiration physiology.

The professor's blue eyes look straight ahead toward his unseen audience of students, and the expression on his deeply creased face is attentive and communicative. A stethoscope emerges from the pocket of his brilliant white coat which is opened at the neck to reveal his blue shirt and red necktie. Wicks's characteristic geometric design is attained by dividing the background into rectangles by means of the molding and ledge of the gray chalkboard above the pale green wall.

Portrait of Allan J. Erslev

ALLAN JACOB ERSLEV, M.D. (b. 1919)
By Alden MacMaster Wicks

Oil on canvas
1972
40 x 30 in.

Signed lower right: "Wicks"

Given by JMC class of 1972
Accession number: 1972+e.P.02

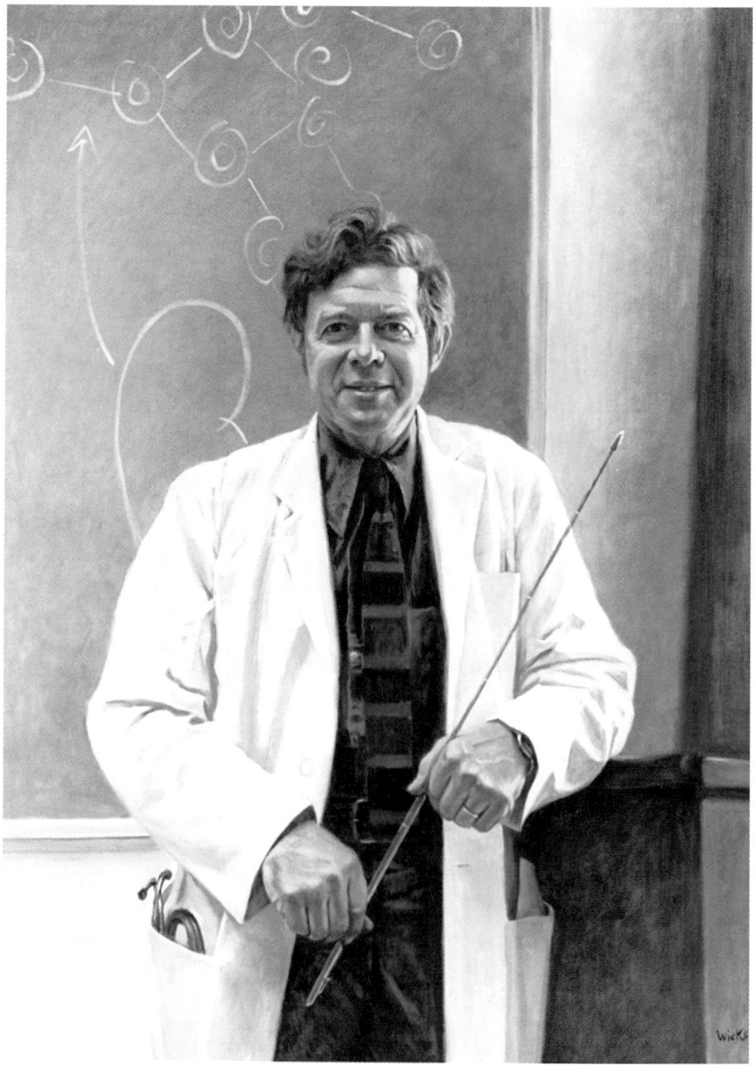

Dr. Allan J. Erslev was internationally recognized for his discovery of the renal hormone erythropoietin. He worked for more than three decades at Thomas Jefferson University, and was one of a select few to be named Distinguished Professor.

A native of Copenhagen, Allan Erslev was born in 1919. He received both his undergraduate and medical education in Denmark at the University of Copenhagen (1937-45) and served his internship at the Copenhagen County Hospital. He emigrated to New York in 1946 for successive fellowships at the Sloan-Kettering Institute for Cancer Research, followed by a postgraduate course in internal medicine at the Cornell Division of Bellevue Hospital.

He moved to New Haven where he was a resident, Damon Runyon research fellow, and instructor at the Yale University School of Medicine (1948-53). There he identified a case of aplastic anemia as being caused by chloramphenicol and published the second case of this association. He wrote widely on the subject of untoward hematologic drug reactions over the next two decades.

It was also in New Haven that he first became interested in erythropoiesis suggesting the possible presence of a hemopoietin stimulating red blood cell production, and he published his first paper in 1953. A fact sheet in connection with a lectureship in his honor held four decades later at Jefferson summarized the important contributions he eventually made in this field:

> Dr. Erslev's pioneer work in the identification of an erythropoietic hormone led to the concept that a feedback mechanism controls red cell production and firmly established the role of erythropoietin as the main regulator of erythropoiesis. His visionary concept of treating patients with anemia of renal disease with exogenous erythropoietin has finally flourished, as recombinant erythropoietin is now successfully used for the prevention and treatment of anemia in renal patients. This early success with erythropoietin has led to the clinical use of other hematopoietic growth factors and is producing a revolutionary change in the management of hematologic diseases.

Dr. Allan J. Erslev was committed to pursuing his career in the United States soon after his arrival, and he became a naturalized citizen in 1949. He served as a captain in the U.S. Army Medical Corps at Fort Devens, Massachusetts. After his training in New Haven he worked in Boston between 1954 and 1959 as a research associate at the Thorndike Memorial Laboratory and as an assistant professor of medicine at Harvard Medical School.

When Dr. Erslev was recruited by Jefferson Medical College in 1959 he was named associate director of the Cardeza Foundation for Hematologic Research and associate professor of medicine. After the sudden death of Dr. Leandro M. Tocantins in 1963, Erslev was appointed director of the Cardeza Foundation and the Thomas Drake Martinez Cardeza Research Professor of Medicine. Throughout his tenure he attracted new investigators and expanded federal funding for research.

When Dr. Erslev stepped down as director of the division, a symposium entitled *Erythropoiesis, 1985* was held on the occasion of his retirement. He was named Distinguished Professor Emeritus of Medicine in 1989. Another tribute, the annual Allan J. Erslev distinguished lectureship, was instituted at Jefferson in 1991.

Dr. Erslev authored or coauthored over three hundred fifty abstracts, reviews, and articles. He was coauthor of *Pathophysiology of Blood* (1975), and coeditor of *Hematology* (1972) and *Erythropoietin: Molecular, Cellular, and Clinical Biology* (1991). He was also a contributing editor of the journals *Acta Haematologica* and *Stem Cells*, and a member of the editorial board of *Hematologic Pathology*.

Dr. Erslev's additional honors include a Guggenheim fellowship, the first William B. Castle lecture at Boston University, the Fogarty fellowship award, and the annual Hagedorn Medal and Prize from the Danish Society of Internal Medicine. He was made a fellow of the American Association for the Advancement in Science in 1987. Erslev served as president of the National Blood Club and as a member of several hematology study sections of the National Institutes of Health.

Despite all his personal achievements, Dr. Erslev is most proud of the numerous Jefferson students and fellows who have been coauthors of his publications and who are becoming leaders in hematology around the world. In accepting his honorary doctor of science degree from Jefferson in 1989, Dr. Erslev described his satisfaction from educating not only students and house staff, but also patients:

> For me, the care of patients has been a joy and a rewarding experience...Educating patients as to the cause and manifestations of their disease, and getting their cooperation and participation in its treatment are major and often time-consuming commitments. I always send a copy of my consultation report to the patient. After all it is his disease and he should know as much about it as the referring physician.

Dr. Erslev was very moved at being selected by students of the class of 1972 for the annual class portrait. Alden M. Wicks depicted the hematologist two-thirds length and life-sized, teaching in a lecture room. The composition is strikingly similar to that of Dr. Frank D. Gray's portrait. Erslev, too, stands in front of a chalkboard addressing unseen students. Here the board has an illustration of a kidney and the model of the feedback system of erythropoietin.

The professor rests his left arm on a podium and holds a pointer in both hands while he looks engagingly toward his audience. A slight smile animates his intent expression, and his full cheeks and thick, wavy brown hair add to the dynamic effect. A stethoscope shows in the pocket of his white lab coat, which is unbuttoned to show his informal attire underneath. He wears a dark blue sport shirt with a long pointed collar and a scattered green pattern, brown trousers, and a necktie with multicolored, horizontal stripes. Rather than the usual neutral background found in many portraits, here the colorful green chalkboard, yellowish wall, and red curtain on the right edge add momentum to the energetic mood of the depiction.

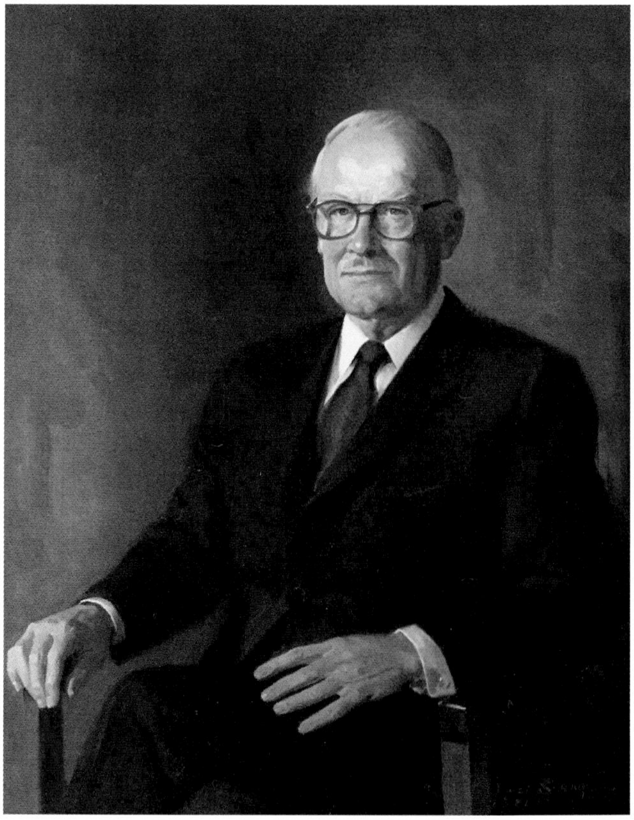

Portrait of John H. Hodges

JOHN HENDRICKS HODGES, M.D. (b. 1914)
By Robert Oliver Skemp (1910-84)

Oil on canvas
1981
36 x 30 in.

Signed and dated: "Robert Oliver Skemp/1981"

Given in 1981 by friends and colleagues
Accession number: 1981+e.P.04

Dr. John H. Hodges was the Ludwig A. Kind Professor of Medicine and the first director of the division of general medicine at Jefferson Medical College. He spent almost his entire career at Jefferson and was the recipient of many of its honors and awards.

The son of a physician, John H. Hodges was born in Harper's Ferry, West Virginia in 1914. He received his undergraduate degree from Catholic University of America in Washington, D.C. (1935) and his medical degree from Jefferson Medical College (1939). After an internship at Philadelphia General Hospital he went into general practice in West Virginia for a year. He returned to Jefferson for a residency in medicine and was a Ross V. Patterson fellow in medicine under Dr. Hobart A. Reimann. In 1943 he was a Mary Markle Foundation fellow in tropical medicine at the Walter Reed Army Medical Center in Washington, D.C. and in Central America.

Hodges rose through Jefferson's academic ranks, from assistant in medicine in 1942 to professor in 1964 when he was appointed the first Ludwig A. Kind Professor of Medicine. This named professorship was instituted by Ludwig Kind's widow who requested that Dr. Hodges occupy the chair because he had been so effective as their physician. Dr. Hodges held this title until his retirement in 1979 when he was named emeritus professor.

For almost three decades he directed the Laboratory of Clinical Medicine course. Dr. Hodges stressed that the laboratory was not just a place to send specimens, but a place to correlate clinical findings about the patient with the laboratory studies on him.[5] In addition he was the director of the division of general (internal) medicine from 1969 to 1977 and an associate member of the Cardeza Foundation of Hematology from 1969 to 1979.

Medical students considered Hodges a superb teacher who had the ability to bridge the gap between the basic sciences and clinical material. The classes of 1951 and 1962 dedicated their yearbooks to "Clinical John" Hodges. He received the Christian R. and Mary F. Lindback Award for Distinguished Teaching in 1966. Though known for surprise oral quizzes "that miss nary a man," the physician was also praised for his warmth, kindness, and patience.

Dr. John Hodges had a very active clinical practice, and in 1955 was asked to establish the first private outpatient offices for both regular and volunteer faculty; he directed the Mohler Physicians Offices until 1975. He also chaired a committee that established the first intensive care unit in the department of medicine.

Dr. Hodges's other hospital appointments were at Inglis House, the Veterans Administration Hospital in Philadelphia, and the Lankenau Hospital. He was a trustee at the Children's Rehabilitation Hospital, Mercy Catholic Medical Center, and Magee Rehabilitation Hospital. He received the alumni achievement award in medicine from Catholic University in 1969.

Dr. Hodges was president of Jefferson's alumni association in 1972. He served two terms as alumni trustee on the board between 1978 and 1984, and was named a trustee emeritus. In 1989 he received the Dean's Medal, and the following year the alumni achievement award.

The portrait of Dr. John H. Hodges was presented by friends and colleagues in 1981. He is depicted by Robert O. Skemp two-thirds length and life-sized, seated in an office-type armchair. His posture is relaxed, and he looks directly out toward the viewer with a neutral expression. His most dominant features are his neat gray-blond hair and mustache and his square jaw and cleft chin. He wears a dapper, dark blue business suit, white shirt, and maroon necktie. The large brush strokes of the atmospheric background range from soft green to umber.

At the portrait presentation ceremonies Dean William F. Kellow, M.D. praised Hodges's qualities as a practicing physician,

> I have heard it said many times that one of the highest tributes that a doctor can have paid to him by another doctor is being asked to take care of the doctor's family... At Jefferson he is known as the doctors' doctor. He has taken care of me, my wife, Stella, and every one of our children. I would dare say that there is probably not a person in this room who has not had John Hodges's care at some time.

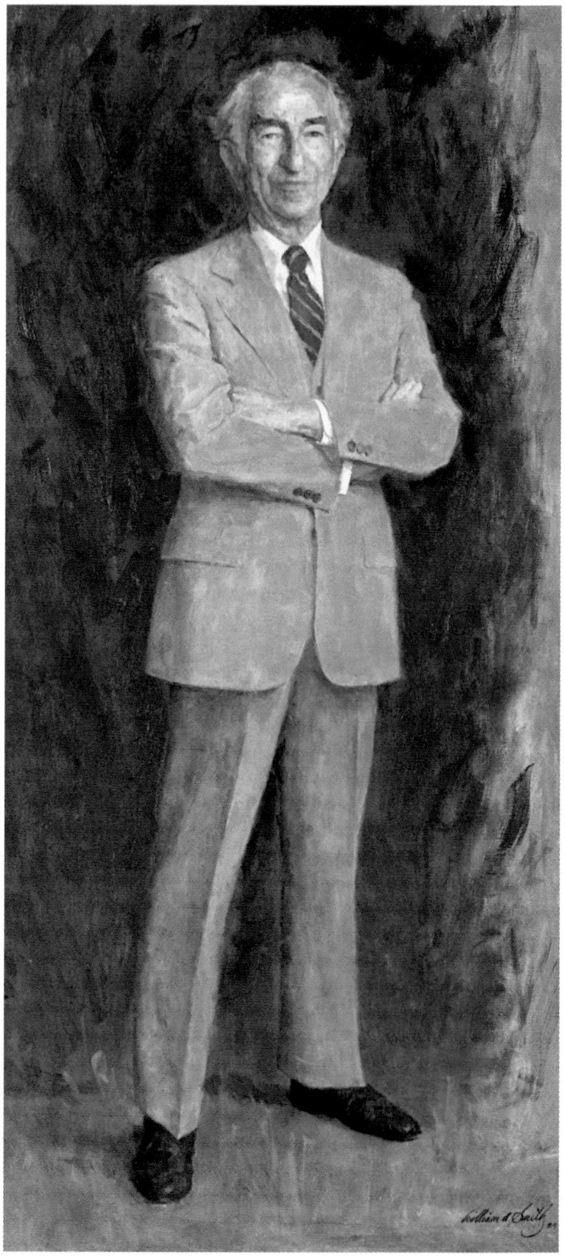

Portrait of Harold L. Israel

HAROLD LOUIS ISRAEL, M.D. (1909-96)
By William Arthur Smith (1918-89)

Oil on canvas
1984
62 3/4 x 30 in.

Signed and dated lower right: "William A. Smith/84"

Given in 1984 by friends and colleagues
Accession number: 1984+e.P.02

Dr. Harold L. Israel was an internationally recognized expert in the field of pulmonary medicine, especially sarcoidosis. The professor of medicine was associated with Jefferson for more than two decades as clinician, researcher, and teacher.

Harold Israel was born in Boston in 1909 and graduated from Amherst College in 1930 and Jefferson Medical College in 1934. He interned at Philadelphia General Hospital and took his residency training at the Henry Phipps Institute of the University of Pennsylvania where he performed epidemiologic research. He also received a master's degree in public health from the university in 1942. During three years of service in World War II he attained the rank of major in the army.

Dr. Israel was chief of pulmonary medicine and associate professor of medicine at the Graduate Hospital of the University of Pennsylvania from 1939 to 1959, and chief of the Graduate School medical service at Philadelphia General Hospital. He was also associate professor of medicine at Women's Medical College from 1947 to 1950.

Dr. Harold L. Israel joined the Jefferson faculty in 1959 as clinical professor and chief of Jefferson's medical service at Philadelphia General Hospital. He was named professor of medicine in 1972. Medical students, interns, and residents all benefitted by his diagnostic acumen at the sarcoidosis clinic he pioneered, and at his hospital rounds which were unusually thorough and unhurried. Many colleagues called him the "primary physician's primary physician." Israel was named professor emeritus upon his retirement in 1982 at which time he was awarded the Dean's Medal. His son Daniel is an alumnus of the class of 1967.

Dr. Israel's research on the clinical and immunologic aspects of sarcoidosis, and in the fields of tuberculosis, pneumonia, and pulmonary embolism was aided by grants from the National Institutes of Health, the American Trudeau Society, and the National Lung Institute. He published nearly two hundred scientific papers on his investigations.

He was chairman of the Panel on Granulomatous Lung Disease of the National Heart and Lung Institute's Task Force on Respiratory Diseases, and assistant director of the Tuberculosis Division of the Philadelphia Department of Health. Recognition from several foreign societies included fellowship in the Royal Society of Medicine, and honorary membership in the British Tuberculosis and Thoracic Association and the Société Française de la Tuberculose et des Maladies Respiratoires.

The portrait of Dr. Israel was presented by his friends and colleagues in 1984. The painting by William A. Smith is composed on an unusually long and narrow canvas. The physician is depicted full length and lifesized, standing with his arms folded tightly in front of his body. He is turned very slightly to the right, and his widespread, diagonal stance plants his weight firmly on the ground. His bushy gray hair encircles his dark, thick eyebrows, narrow blue eyes, and bulbous aquiline nose. His full lips are pressed tightly together. Deep creases in his cheeks and neck add to the striking physiognomy of the seventy-four-year-old physician.

Dr. Israel is wearing a khaki-gray business suit, white shirt, and blue and khaki striped necktie. The large strokes of the very freely brushed, atmospheric background provide subtle notes of deep purples and pale mauves to the prevailing neutral tones of the composition.

The subject's almost supercilious expression, combined with the physical barrier of his folded arms, suggests a commanding and somewhat distant personality. A 1977 profile of Dr. Israel called him a man "who never seems unsure" and "opinionated but loveable," but in the final analysis, "so bright and so knowledgeable that his opinions are almost always proven right."[6] The artist has achieved a notably interpretive and artistic portrait of a strong medical personality.

William A. Smith was a noted painter, illustrator, photographer, and graphic artist. Because of international acclaim and leadership in their respective fields, artist and sitter seem unusually well matched, and they became friends during the portrait sittings.

Smith was born in 1918 in Toledo, Ohio where he studied art as a teenager at the Theodore Keane Art School. An outstanding draftsman, he won three nationwide competitions for high school students at age fourteen and worked as a courtroom artist for the San Francisco *Examiner*. He also studied briefly at the University of Toledo where he later received an honorary master's degree.

In 1937 Smith moved to New York where he established a studio, studied at the Art Students League, and taught at the Grand Central School of Art. He also did advertising and illustration for such magazines as *McCalls*, *Good Housekeeping*, and *The Saturday Evening Post.* He became fascinated with Chinese culture and was commissioned to illustrate Pearl S. Buck's *The Chinese Children Next Door*, and two volumes of Chinese folk tales. Good notices about his drawings led to his recruitment by the Office of Strategic Services in China from 1944 to 1945 for intelligence work and "morale operations."

After the war Smith moved to Paris and studied at the École des Beaux-Arts and the Académie de la Grande Chaumière. His many activities abroad in postwar years included lecturing at the Academy of Fine Arts in Athens, the University of Santo Tomas in Manila, and the Academy of Fine Arts in Warsaw. He became active in the International Association of Art, an affiliate of UNESCO which represented artists from seventy nations, and he was president of its U.S. committee in the 1970s. While serving as an official delegate to the USSR under the Cultural Exchange Agreement in 1958, he formed lasting ties with many Soviet artists. In 1964 the U.S. State Department invited him to lecture and exhibit his paintings on a world tour to Europe and the Far East as a cultural ambassador.

In 1956 Smith relocated from Manhattan to Bucks County, Pennsylvania where he became very active in local affairs, joining Pearl Buck's Welcome House and founding the Gallery Ten in New Hope for works by international artists. Long after he stopped teaching at the Grand Central Art School in New York and at the Pratt Institute in Brooklyn, he continued to give private art classes.

Smith was president of the American Water Color

Society in 1956, and a frequent recipient of its major prizes between 1948 and 1973. During this period he also won the Adolf and Clara Obrig Prize for Oil Painting, the American Artists Group Prize for Lithography at the Society of American Graphic Artists, the Knobloch Prize, the Winslow Homer Memorial Prize, and the American Patriots Medal. He was one of the youngest full academicians of the National Academy of Design, served on its council, and won its watercolor awards in 1949 and 1951.

The artist's most public art works were a thousand-square-foot mural about Maryland history commissioned for an information and recreational center operated by the state, and a series of eight U.S. postal stamps depicting events leading to the American Revolution. His Boston Tea Party stamp won the Postal Commemorative Society Prize.

Smith was honored with numerous one-man exhibitions throughout America, Asia, and Europe. His work is included in many public and private collections including the Metropolitan Museum of Art, the Los Angeles County Museum of Art, the National Portrait Gallery, and the Library of Congress. One of his most notable sitters was his friend Carl Sandburg who responded with a poem called "Bill Smith":

Flowers and promises,
   rocks and rookeries,
Horses of galloping anxiety
and houses whose walls hide
characters in search of themselves,
faces of gnomes saying
much of history is an alley crap game,
Shadow feet moving toward fables
just around the next corner,
gnarled fingers feeling in pockets
for a time-table and bus-fare,
   people and meditations
placed in a quiet whispering gallery
   —these linger with me
   from the graphic art
   of my friend Bill Smith.

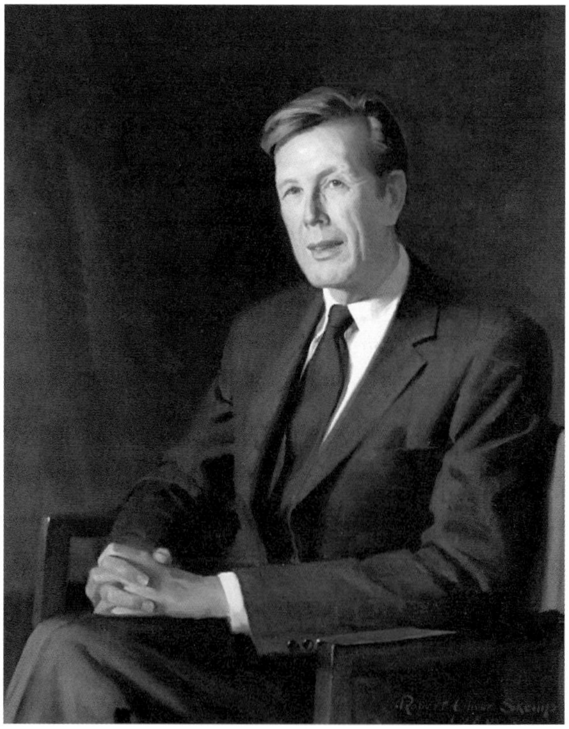

Portrait of Nathan M. Smukler

NATHAN M. SMUKLER, M.D. (b. 1922)
By Robert Oliver Skemp (1910-84)

Oil on canvas
1980
36 x 30 in.

Signed and dated lower right: "Robert Oliver Skemp/1980"

Given in 1980 by friends and colleagues
Accession number: 1980+e.P.03

Dr. Nathan M. Smukler is a professor of medicine and was the first full-time head of the rheumatology division at Jefferson Medical College.

Nathan Smukler was born in Philadelphia in 1910, the son of Maximilian E. Smukler, M.D. who graduated from Jefferson in 1910. Nathan Smukler received his undergraduate degree from the University of Pennsylvania in 1943 and his medical degree from Jefferson in 1947. After interning at Mount Sinai Hospital in Philadelphia and Kings County Hospital in New York, he returned to Mount Sinai for his residency. As a first lieutenant in the U.S. Army he was stationed at Aberdeen, Maryland for two years. Following military service he completed a fellowship in the arthritis section at the University of Pennsylvania School of Medicine, after which he was appointed an associate in medicine there.

In 1959 Dr. Nathan Smukler joined the faculty at Jefferson Medical College as assistant professor, and rose through the academic ranks to become professor of medicine in 1974. As chief of the rheumatology division from its formation in July 1959 until 1980, Dr. Smukler was a highly regarded teacher and clinician. Twice he won the Medical Residents Award for Excellence in Bedside Teaching. A quarter century later in 1998 he was the recipient of the Leon A. Peris Memorial Award for excellence in clinical teaching and superior patient care.

Dr. Smukler's research interests included the suspected role of psychological disorders in rheumatoid arthritis and other systemic inflammatory rheumatic diseases. He also investigated spinal arthritis, the neuroanatomy and neurophysiology of pain, and systemic vasculitis. Smukler served as president of the Philadelphia Rheumatism Society and the Eastern Pennsylvania chapter of the Arthritis Foundation. He was a member of the President's Commission on Aging.

The portrait of Dr. Nathan Smukler by Robert O. Skemp was presented by friends and colleagues in 1981. It shows the physician two-thirds length and life-sized, seated in an office armchair and turned to the left. His hands are folded tightly and rest on his lap. His head is tilted slightly and turned to the right, so that his narrow blue eyes are directed upward. He wears a gray suit, white shirt, and maroon necktie, and the dark atmospheric background is a neutral gray-green.

His slightly open mouth and upraised eyes suggest uncertainty more than inspiration. Though the portrait was appreciated as a good likeness of the professor, his unexplained facial expression offers little evidence of Dr. Lewis W. Bluemle Jr.'s characterization at the portrait ceremony of Dr. Nathan Smukler as the personification of "kind, intelligent concern for others, the most noble quality of our profession."

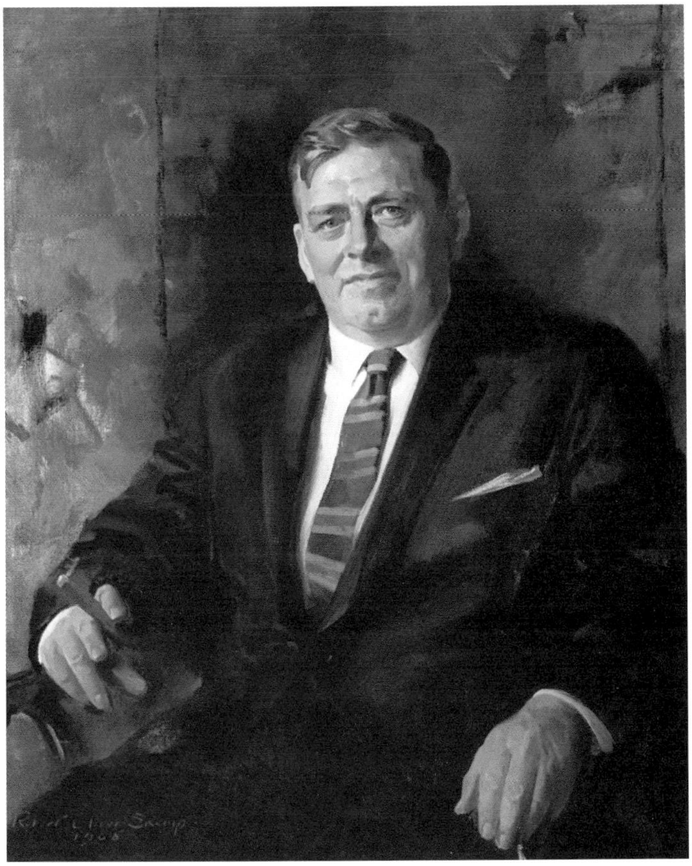

Portrait of Joseph J. Rupp

JOSEPH J. RUPP, M.D. (b. 1915)
By Robert Oliver Skemp

Oil on canvas
1968
36 x 30 in.

Signed and dated lower left: "Robert Oliver Skemp/1968"

Given by JMC class of 1969
Accession number: 1969+e.P.01

Dr. Joseph J. Rupp forged his entire career at Jefferson Medical College where he was a professor of medicine, director of the division of endocrinology, and assistant director of continuing medical education.

Joseph Rupp was born in 1915 in Scranton, Pennsylvania and graduated from the University of Scranton in 1937. He was an alumnus of Jefferson Medical College (1942) and took his internship there. From 1943 to 1946 he served with the U.S. Infantry in Italy and was awarded a Silver Star, Bronze Star, and Purple Heart.

He returned to Jefferson for a residency and fellowship training in endocrinology, medicine, and oncology. He rose from assistant in medicine in 1951 to full professor in 1972. Dr. Rupp was the director of the division of endocrinology and metabolic diseases from 1961 until 1969. His investigations in endocrinology were particularly productive on the effects of thyroid hormone on protein metabolism. He was coauthor with Drs. Abraham E. Rakoff and Abraham Cantarow of the third edition of *Clinical Endocrinology* (1967).

In 1969 Dr. Rupp took on new responsibilities as assistant director of continuing medical education. He planned symposia and courses on recent developments in various medical fields held at Jefferson, and also delivered lectures at community hospitals throughout Pennsylvania and Delaware. Upon his retirement in 1981 he was named professor emeritus.

Dr. Rupp was greatly esteemed by the students and received the Christian R. and Mary Lindback Award for Distinguished Teaching in 1964. He was chosen to administer the Hippocratic Oath at commencement four times between 1967 and 1981, and was class day speaker in 1970.

The class of 1969 elected Dr. Rupp as senior portrait honoree. Robert O. Skemp has depicted the physician two-thirds length and life-sized, seated in an armchair. His head is turned to look directly at the observer and his right hand holds a lit cigar. He is attired in a navy blue business suit, white shirt and pocket handkerchief, and a necktie with green, blue, and tan stripes.

The loosely brushed, free, painting style of figure and background further animate the sitter's pleasant, almost convivial expression. His ruddy complexion, wayward lock of hair on his forehead, bright blue eyes, and cleft chin, combined with his powerful neck, hands, and torso, and topped off with his smoking cigar, all contribute to a depiction that is unusually vivid and engaging for portraitist Skemp.

The portrait captures the amiable personality of the teacher so well liked by students. He encouraged questions on complex concepts and occasionally even abandoned a prepared lecture to pursue a point raised by a student. The 1968 student yearbook commented neatly about Rupp, "Questions, a puff on a fat cigar, and a concise explanation constitute his favorite teaching method."

Portrait of Carla E. Goepp

CARLA ELISABETH GOEPP, M.D. (b. 1939)
By Robert Oliver Skemp

Oil on canvas
1981
36 x 30 in.

Signed and dated lower right: "Robert Oliver Skemp/1981"

Given by JMC class of 1981
Accession number: 1981+e.P.03

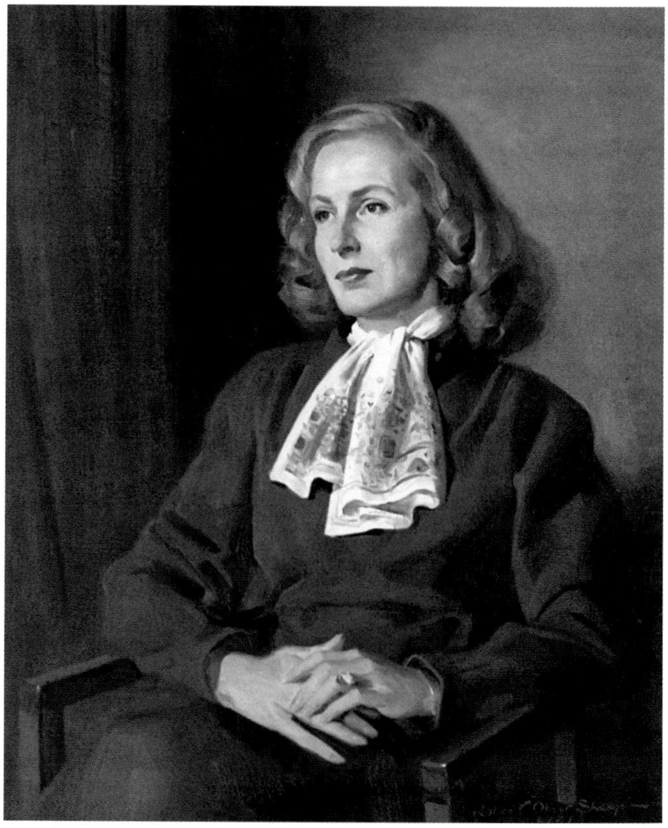

Dr. Carla E. Goepp's career at Jefferson Medical College included teaching, clinical, and administrative work. She was clinical professor of medicine, attending physician, and associate dean at the time she left active practice in 1993.

Carla Goepp was born in 1939 in Philadelphia and reared in New Castle, Delaware and the Washington, D.C. area. Her grandfather was R. Maximilian Goepp, M.D., a Jefferson faculty member who worked closely with Dr. Solomon Solis-Cohen. Carla Goepp graduated from the College of New Rochelle, New York (1960) and Georgetown University School of Medicine (1964).

One of only seven women in her medical school class, she was awarded the Mollari Medal for outstanding performance in microbiology. Her subsequent postgraduate training included an internship at Jefferson, a two-year fellowship in oncology and cytogenetics at the National Cancer Institute, and a residency in internal medicine at Jefferson.

The environment for women residents was marginal at best when Dr. Goepp arrived at Jefferson. According to an account by Dr. Francis J. Sweeney, a speaker at Goepp's portrait presentation, the first women had been admitted but not yet graduated from the medical school when Goepp arrived. She was the first woman to go through Jefferson's medical residency from a straight medical internship. Sweeney said that the women's house staff quarters, which held a maximum of four people and were not air conditioned, were located next to the pediatric wards in the old hospital right next to the infection ward. There was only one ladies' rest room in the entire building. Dr. Sweeney continued, "Carla in her effective, quiet way made it quite clear to the Director of the house staff program that the quarters were totally unacceptable, particularly as the male house staff quarters were completely air-conditioned and had been recently refurbished."

Dr. Carla Goepp rose in the academic ranks from her position as instructor in 1968 to clinical associate professor of medicine in the divisions of medical oncology and genetics in 1978. She was the first woman to be a clinical associate professor at Jefferson. In 1989 she was appointed clinical professor, and at her retirement in 1996 she was named honorary clinical professor.

Dr. Goepp coordinated the Approach to the Patient and Introduction to Clinical Medicine courses for freshmen and sophomores from 1973 to 1984. She was the recipient of the Christian R. and Mary F. Lindback Award for Distinguished Teaching in 1976, and a National Endowment for the Humanities fellowship in 1978. She was named associate dean of student affairs, student counseling, and career planning in 1984.

Besides her appointment at Jefferson, Dr. Goepp was attending at Our Lady of Lourdes Medical Center in Camden, New Jersey, and consultant to the Fox Chase Cancer Center in Philadelphia. She was a board member of the Philadelphia Professional Standards Review Organization, the American Heart Association, and the Philadelphia Division, American Cancer Society. She was a member of the American Association for the Advancement of Science.

Dr. Carla Goepp was particularly honored to be the first woman selected as class portrait honoree in 1981. In the two-thirds-length, life-sized portrait by Robert O. Skemp she is shown seated in a plain office chair. Her hands rest calmly on her lap and she gazes away from the observer into the distance. Her striking appearance is dominated by ash-blond, shoulder-length hair, large brown eyes, high cheek bones, and crimson lipstick. She wears a dark red, long-sleeved dress accented by a silk scarf with a green, red, and umber pattern on a white background. The atmospheric background shades from light to dark green.

Dr. Goepp's expression, posture, and costume exude a kind of personal confidence and strength of purpose. She was very supportive of students and their needs, and arranged for counselors in the student affairs office to provide coverage twenty-four hours a day. At the portrait ceremony she commented on the class's exceptional spirit and performance, and expressed pride in her portrait with a quotation from Shakespeare, "Silence is the perfectest herald of joy: I were but little happy, if I could say how much."

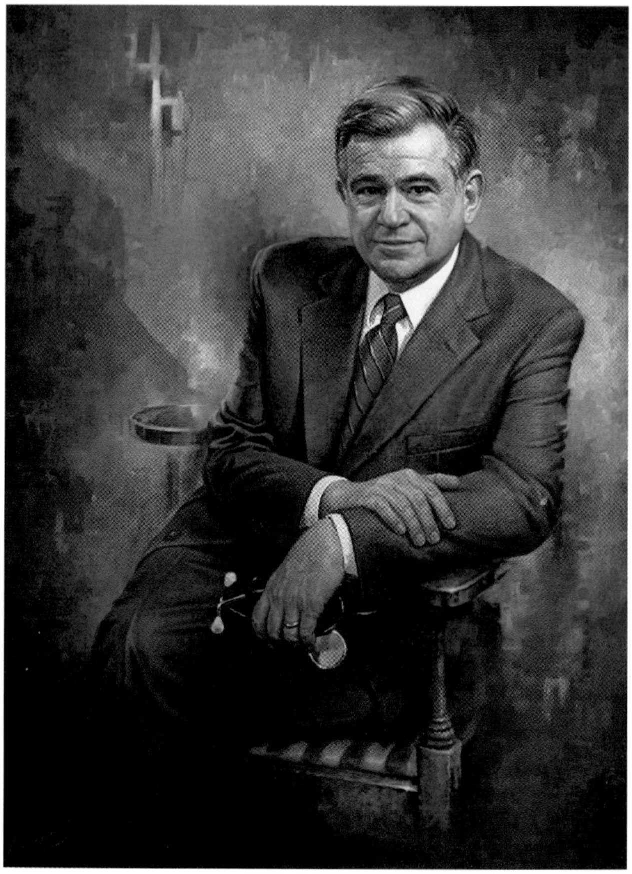

Portrait of Warren P. Goldburgh

WARREN PEARLMAN GOLDBURGH, M.D. (b. 1927)
By Dean L. Paules (b. 1931)

Oil on canvas
1987
44 x 34 in.

Signed and dated lower left: "PAULES/4-87 A.P.S.C."

Given in 1987 by friends and colleagues
Accession number: 1987+e.P.01

Dr. Warren P. Goldburgh was a clinical professor of medicine at Jefferson Medical College and a devoted and respected teacher and clinician. He was known as "the physician's cardiologist."

Warren Goldburgh was born in 1927 in Philadelphia. His father was Dr. Harold L. Goldburgh, a Jefferson graduate in 1915 and a professor of medicine. After earning his bachelor's degree at Franklin and Marshall College in 1948, Warren Goldburgh graduated from Jefferson Medical College in 1952.

Between his internship and residency at Jefferson Dr. Goldburgh took a cardiology fellowship at Philadelphia General Hospital. By 1979 he had risen in the academic ranks from clinical assistant in medicine to clinical professor of medicine. He was director of the cardiac clinic from 1965 until it closed in 1975. Goldburgh was an active member of the executive committee of the medical staff and served a term as its president. He was chairman of the hospital's credentials committee, and president of the volunteer faculty association. In 1989 he departed from Jefferson and was named honorary clinical professor of medicine.

Goldburgh's teaching ability was recognized when he received the Christian R. and Mary F. Lindback Award for Distinguished Teaching in 1973 and the Medical Residents Award in 1972 and 1979. He also won the Leon A. Peris Memorial Award in 1989. For three years he served on the board of governors of the American Heart Association.

Friends and colleagues presented Dean Paules's portrait of Dr. Warren Goldburgh in 1987. The physician is depicted three-quarters length and life-sized, seated in an armchair with blue and gray striped upholstery. His left hand holds a stethoscope. The expression on his round face is pleasant and accessible, highlighted by warm brown eyes which gaze directly toward the viewer, and wrinkles in his forehead, under his eyes, and around his mouth. He wears a gray suit with a faint plaid pattern, a white shirt, and red necktie with black and yellow diagonal stripes. The busy atmospheric background has large reddish, blue, and umber brush strokes which distract the viewer's attention.

At the portrait presentation ceremony, colleagues repeatedly praised Dr. Goldburgh's warm and gentlemanly manner and added that he was their personal cardiologist. The honoree said proudly that there had been a

Dr. Goldburgh at Jefferson for seventy-six years. He vividly remembered waiting in the hospital lobby as a child for his father to "complete those endless, endless rounds, so was filled with the Jefferson spirit from the very beginning." He credits his father with being a role model and imparting the enjoyment of practicing medicine, the essence of a good teacher.

The portrait of Dr. Warren Goldburgh was the first of more than twenty portraits by Dean Paules to enter the Jefferson collection. Paules was born in 1927 in New Freedom, Pennsylvania. After studying electronics at the Rehrig Technical School in Baltimore, he worked for the Bendix Corporation in that city, and then returned to New Freedom where he was vice president for Crescent Industries for more than thirty years. Even while working in industry he was honing his skills as an artist. He was almost entirely self-taught except for occasional workshops with other artists.

He gradually turned away from painting landscapes to concentrate on portraiture. In a short period his ability to create a vivid likeness became known and his services were sought after by scientists, business executives, and religious, military, and political figures. Some notable sitters include Nobel laureate Dr. George Hitchings, North Carolina governor Dan K. Moore, chancellor of North Carolina State University Dr. Bruce Poulton, major league baseball commissioners Peter Uberroth and A. Bart Giamatti, and vice chairman of the Joint Chiefs of Staff General Richard Ellis.

In 1985 Dean Paules was awarded American Portrait Society Certification and he often writes "A.P.S.C." next to his signature on paintings. In 1991 he received the John Howard Sanden Award for Excellence at the National Portrait Seminar. In 1996 his portrait of Jeffersonian Dr. Robert L. Brent won honorable mention at the National Portrait Competition.

A keen observer will notice a cross shape blended into the atmospheric background in the portrait of Dr. Goldburgh and some other early portraits. Usually a small fish insignia appears next to the artist's signature, and often "A.M.D.G." is written on the back of the canvas. The fish is an early Christian symbol for Christ and the four initials stand for the phrase, "To the greater glory of God." In a promotional brochure about his portraiture Dean Paules wrote, "How marvelous that the last creative act of God—His crowning piece of handiwork—was mankind. Immortality—set in motion by the Creator."

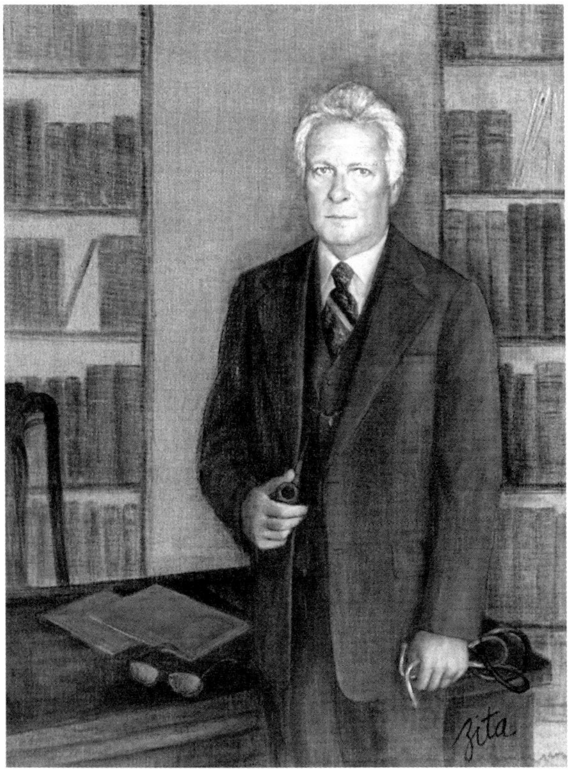

Portrait of Joseph Medoff

JOSEPH MEDOFF, M.D. (1913-88)
By Zita Davisson

Oil on canvas
1976
46 x 36 in.

Signed lower right: "Zita"

Given in 1976 by the Hobart Amory Hare Honor Medical Society and friends, colleagues, and patients
Accession number: 1976+e.P.03

Dr. Joseph Medoff was a clinical professor of medicine at Jefferson Medical College and a noted gastroenterologist and expert on diseases of the liver. He was also a devoted teacher and faculty advisor.

Joseph Medoff was born in 1913 in Philadelphia, and was a graduate of Villanova University (1935) and Jefferson Medical College (1939). After service in the U.S. Army during the war, Dr. Medoff joined the Jefferson faculty in 1947 and rose through the ranks to become clinical professor of medicine in 1970. Dr. Medoff was a member of the gastrointestinal clinic staff from 1946 until 1960. Upon his retirement in 1978 he was named emeritus clinical professor of medicine.

The type of clinical teaching most rewarding to Dr. Joseph Medoff was the preceptorship in internal medicine, a one-to-one relationship between physician and student he considered ideal because the student participates in the total care of the patient. Dr. Medoff was the first Jefferson professor to be asked to be a preceptor in 1957 and after that trained a junior student every six weeks and a resident every month. He was admired for his wealth of clinical knowledge and the clarity of his lectures on liver disease. In a profile of Medoff in the summer 1969 *Jefferson Medical College Alumni Bulletin*, one preceptee said, "It seemed like he had a book of differential diagnosis in his head."

Medoff was the recipient of the Christian R. and Mary F. Lindback Award for Distinguished Teaching in 1967, and won a teaching award from residents in 1971. He established two prizes: the Philip and Bella Medoff Memorial Prize in memory of his parents, and the Alexander and Lottie Katzman Award in Gastroenterology in memory of his in-laws.

Dr. Medoff had a special relationship with Jefferson's Hare Society, having revitalized it from almost defunct status in 1960. During his sixteen years as faculty advisor it became the most active student society at Jefferson and the sponsor of many prestigious speakers. In 1976 student members of the society initiated a portrait commission to honor Dr. Medoff. Other subscribers included friends, colleagues, and former patients.

In the portrait by Zita Davisson, the physician is shown two-thirds length and life-sized, standing in his office in front of a desk. He looks directly toward the viewer with a somber, tight-lipped expression. His most arresting feature is his thick white hair. He holds a pipe in his right hand and a stethoscope in his left hand. Journals and his glasses lie on the green desktop. The background wall is framed by shelves lined with multicolored groups of books.

The most unusual aspect of this portrait is the unconventional colors of his apparel: the three-piece suit is burgundy-maroon, the shirt is pink, and the striped and patterned necktie is purple and pink. The paint application of the flat depiction is thin and patches of canvas are visible throughout. No information about the artist has been found.

Portrait of Robert C. Mackowiak

ROBERT C. MACKOWIAK, M.D. (1938-84)
By Robert Oliver Skemp (1910-84)

Oil on canvas
1980
36 x 30 in.

Signed and dated lower right: "Robert Oliver Skemp/2/14/80"

Given by JMC class of 1980
Accession number: 1980+e.P.02

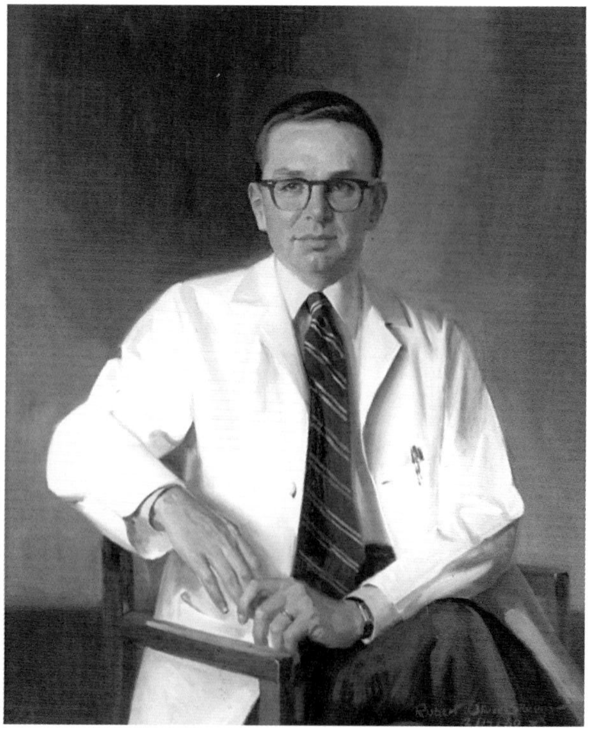

Dr. Robert C. Mackowiak was a clinical professor of medicine at Jefferson Medical College with a special interest in cardiology. This promising teacher and student affairs administrator died suddenly in 1984 at the age of forty-six.

Robert Mackowiak was born in 1938 in Hazleton, Pennsylvania. An outstanding student, he was a *cum laude* graduate of the University of Pennsylvania (1960), Jefferson Medical College (1964), and a member of the Phi Beta Kappa, Sigma Xi, and Alpha Omega Alpha honor societies. After a year's internship at Methodist Hospital in Philadelphia, he returned to Jefferson as an instructor in physiology and published a total of nineteen papers on different aspects of the cardiovascular system. After a residency at Mercy Catholic Medical Center he joined the Jefferson faculty and rose in the academic ranks to become clinical professor of medicine in 1982.

Always a dedicated teacher and interested in the welfare of the medical students, Dr. Mackowiak won the Christian R. and Mary F. Lindback Award for Distinguished Teaching early in his career in 1968. The very next year he was designated "Outstanding Basic Science Lecturer" by the medical student council. He served as associate dean and director of student affairs, then director of allied programs and continuing education.

Mackowiak was a founding member of the American Academy of Cardiology, a charter member of the Bioengineering Society, and a member of the Field Studies Coordinating Committee of the National Board of Medical Examiners.

Dr. Robert Mackowiak was selected for the class portrait in 1980. Student speakers at the presentation ceremony called him a "trusted counselor and friend," who was chosen for his "accessibility to students" and "uncompromising commitment to total student welfare."

Robert O. Skemp has depicted the physician two-thirds length and life-sized, seated in an office armchair. His upper body is frontal, and his lower torso is turned to the right with legs crossed at the knees. His brown eyes gaze directly at the viewer through horn-rimmed glasses, and his expression is serious and forthright. His white lab coat contains pens in the outer pocket and is open to reveal the subject's blue shirt, blue striped necktie, and gray trousers. The modulated atmospheric background is a neutral green, contrasting with the brightness of the white coat.

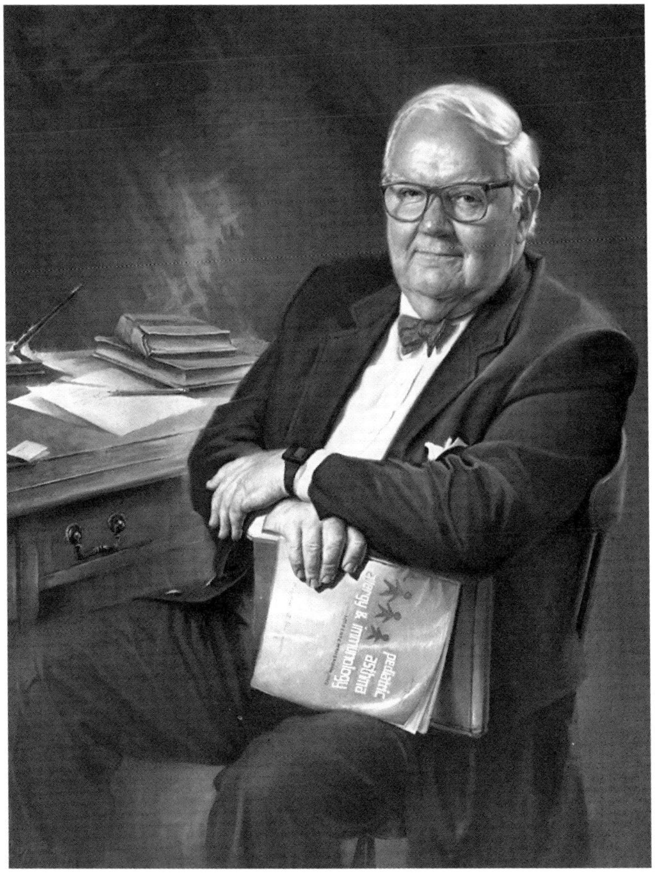

Portrait of Herbert C. Mansmann Jr.

HERBERT C. MANSMANN Jr., M.D. (b. 1924)
By Dean L. Paules (b. 1931)

Oil on canvas
1991
40 x 32 in.

Signed and dated lower left: "PAULES/12-91"

Given in 1992 by friends and colleagues
Accession number: 1992+e.P.01

Dr. Herbert C. Mansmann Jr., professor of pediatrics and associate professor of medicine at Jefferson Medical College, is nationally recognized for his clinical and research contributions to pediatric allergy and immunology.

Herbert Mansmann was born in Pittsburgh in 1924 and attended the University of Pittsburgh. He left to join the infantry during the war, returned to complete his college degree (1949), and then graduated from Jefferson Medical College (1951).

His extensive postdoctoral training included an

internship at St. Francis Hospital in Pittsburgh and a pediatric residency at Children's Hospital of Pittsburgh; a research fellowship in medicine at Massachusetts General Hospital and Harvard University; and a research fellowship in microbiology at New York University College of Medicine and a public health fellowship at the National Microbiological Institute in New York.

From 1956 to 1959 he was a senior research fellow in pathology at the University of Pittsburgh School of Medicine. He was a faculty member in the department of pediatrics at Pittsburgh from 1952 until 1968. During this period he developed an active private practice and was on the staffs of St. Francis Hospital, Magee-Women's Hospital, St. Margaret's Memorial Hospital, and Children's Hospital where he was director of the allergy and immunology research and service laboratories.

In 1968 Dr. Herbert C. Mansmann Jr. joined the Jefferson Medical College faculty as professor of pediatrics and associate professor of medicine. He was the founder of the division of allergy and clinical immunology which he directed until 1989, and director of the pediatric pulmonary program. Dr. Mansmann is particularly gratified by the changes in the scientific basis for allergy research since his entry into the field, and is proud at having trained over seventy fellows at Jefferson. He was also the medical director and director of the asthma/pulmonary disease program at Children's Rehabilitation Hospital.

Dr. Mansmann has made significant contributions to the literature in allergy, asthma, and related fields. He was coeditor of *Cutis, Special Issue: Pediatric Allergy* (1974) and *Immunopharmacology, Proceedings of the Conference on Immunopharmacology* (1976). In 1987 he was the founding editor of *Pediatric Asthma, Allergy & Immunology*. He has also served on the editorial boards of the *Journal of Asthma, Annals of Allergy, Pediatric Pulmonology*, and the *American Journal of Rhinology*.

Mansmann was also a leader in professional societies. He was a founding director and for more than twenty years the executive secretary of the American Board of Allergy and Immunology. He was a board member of the Association of Convalescent Homes and Hospitals for Asthmatic Children, the Care Association of America, the Learning Disabilities Foundation, and the Board of Pediatric Allergy of the American Board of Pediatrics. He was president of the Association for the Care of Asthma. He has also served on several advisory committees of the Food and Drug Administration. He was elected president of the Pittsburgh Allergy Society, and the Philadelphia and Pennsylvania Allergy Associations.

His many honors include the Recognition Award of the Puerto Rico Medical Association, the Lawrence F. Flick, M.D. Award of the American Lung Association, and the Bret Ratner Award in Allergy of the American Academy of Pediatrics. He was the John McGovern lecturer at the American College of Allergy and Immunology in 1993.

The portrait of Dr. Mansmann by Dean Paules was presented in 1992 by his friends and colleagues. At the ceremony the painting was unveiled by his children, including Kevin and Paris who graduated from Jefferson in 1981 and 1984 respectively.

Their father is depicted two-thirds length and life-sized, seated at his desk. He turns away from his books and papers to gaze directly toward the viewer. The expression on his round face is warm and affable, engaging and accessible to the viewer. His folded arms rest on an issue of *Pediatric Asthma, Allergy and Immunology*, with his name clearly printed on the cover.

Dr. Mansmann wears a navy blazer, blue shirt, dark gray slacks, and a jaunty, red polka dot bow tie. His convincingly robust and sturdy figure hints at his athletic prowess as a skier, hunter, fisherman, and former college football star. The paint application on his ruddy, almost glowing face is deliberate and finicky compared with the more broadly painted costume. Unlike the figure which is convincingly solid, his desk seems weightless, is crowded into the corner, and fades inexplicably into the background.

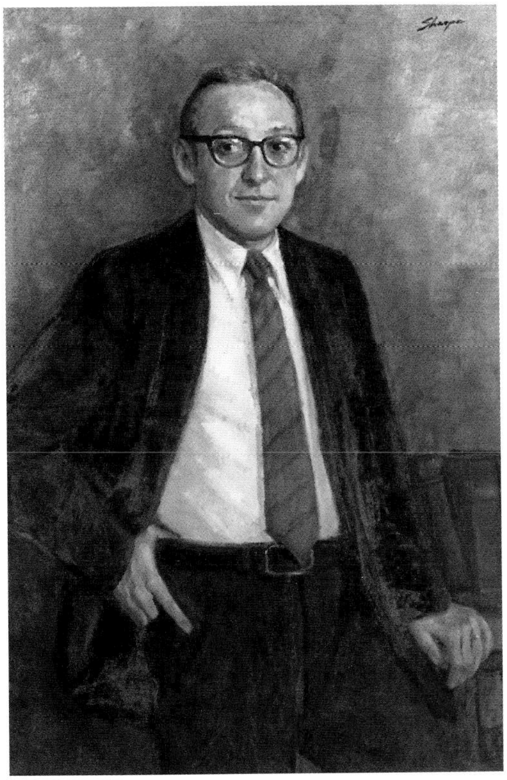

Portrait of Irving J. Olshin

IRVING J. OLSHIN, M.D. (b. 1927)
By Marion Potter Sharpe

Oil on canvas
1973
48 x 34 in.

Signed upper right: "Sharpe"

Given by JMC class of 1973
Accession number: 1973+e.P.03

Dr. Irving J. Olshin was a professor of pediatrics and director of pediatric education services. He was respected by students for both his scholarship and personal warmth.

Irving Olshin was born in 1927 in Philadelphia and received his undergraduate (1950) and medical degrees (1954) from the University of Pennsylvania. After an internship at Meadowbrook Hospital in Hempstead, New York he served his residency there and at Long Island Jewish Hospital.

During the ensuing years he was a National Foundation for Infantile Paralysis fellow in virology at Children's Hospital of Philadelphia, and then worked as coordinator of the newborn follow-up program of the National Institutes of Health cerebral palsy study at Pennsylvania Hospital. He had appointments at the latter two hospitals and also as instructor in pediatrics at the University of Pennsylvania School of Medicine.

After brief stints on the pediatrics faculty at Jefferson Medical College and Temple University School of Medicine, he was named chairman of pediatrics at Meadowbrook Hospital in 1964. Three years later he returned to Jefferson as associate professor of pediatrics and was named professor the following year. For many years he was director of pediatric medical education services and director of the division of student health in the office of student and employee health. When Olshin retired after two decades at Jefferson he was named honorary professor of pediatrics.

Admired by students for his clinical and teaching prowess, humanistic values, and sense of humor, Dr. Olshin was the recipient of the Christian R. and Mary F. Lindback Award for Distinguished Teaching in 1969. The class of 1973 chose him as portrait honoree.

He was depicted by Marion Potter Sharpe, a faculty member of the Portland School of Fine Arts and the Albany Institute of History and Art. She was a resident of Kennebunkport, Maine.

Dr. Olshin is shown two-thirds length and life-sized, looking solemnly to the left through dark, horn-rimmed glasses. Noted for his informality, Dr. Olshin stands in a rakish pose with one hand hooked into his belt and the other hand leaning on a low bookcase. The colors of the book bindings and the subject's blue sport coat, blue shirt, dark gray trousers, and red and green striped necktie are repeated in the mottled background. The thin painting surface is very loosely brushed.

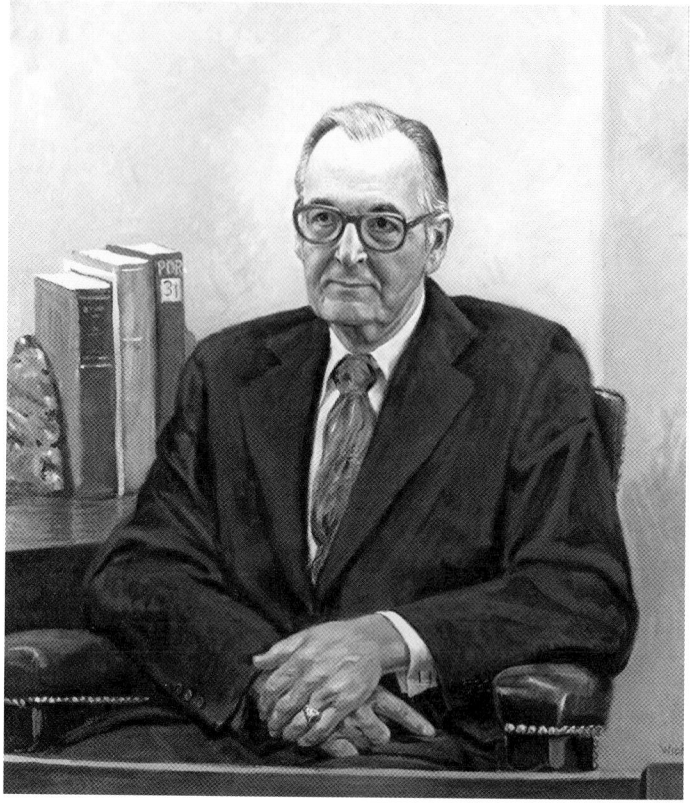

Portrait of Herbert A. Luscombe

HERBERT A. LUSCOMBE, M.D. (b. 1916)
By Alden MacMaster Wicks (1914-87)

Oil on canvas
1977
30 x 26 in.

Signed lower right: "Wicks"

Given in 1977 by friends and colleagues
Accession number: 1977+e.P.02

Dr. Herbert A. Luscombe was a professor of dermatology and chairman of the department at Jefferson from 1959 to 1986, the longest-held chairmanship of any dermatology department in the United States. Under his leadership significant progress was made in modernizing the department.

Herbert Luscombe was born in 1916, a native of Johnstown, Pennsylvania. He was a graduate of St. Vincent's College in Latrobe, Pennsylvania (1936) and Jefferson Medical College (1940). During the war he was stationed at the Fort Meade Reception Center and then spent eighteen months as a captain attached to the 115th General Hospital in Europe. He returned to Jefferson for his residency in dermatology and received further training at the University of Pennsylvania Graduate School of Medicine.

Dr. Luscombe was appointed to the Jefferson faculty in 1949 and within ten years was named professor and chairman of the department. During his long tenure the residency program became a fully accredited three-year program, and students received the option of electing a clinical clerkship in dermatology as a special rotation.

Dr. Luscombe's clinical practice also included a post as consultant in dermatology at Wills Eye and Lankenau Hospitals. He served as president of the Philadelphia Dermatological Society as well as president of the medical staff of Thomas Jefferson University Hospital. He received national recognition when he won the Dermatology Foundation's Clark W. Finnerud Teacher of the Year Award in 1981. Among other contributions to the literature, Dr. Luscombe is coauthor of *Color Atlas of Difficult Diagnoses in Dermatology* (1993).

A loyal and dedicated Jeffersonian, Luscombe served a term as president of the alumni association in 1971 and received its achievement award in 1997. The dermatology department initiated the annual Herbert A. Luscombe visiting lectureship in 1984. He was named emeritus professor of dermatology in 1987.

Friends and colleagues honored Dr. Luscombe with his portrait in 1977. In a depiction by Alden M. Wicks, the physician is shown half length and life-sized, seated in a red leather, brass-studded armchair. His hands are crossed in front of his body, and he looks slightly to the left with a serious expression. Distinctive features are his long nose, thin lips, and square jaw. He is wearing a dark blue suit, white shirt, and necktie with patterns in red, blue, and orange.

Although his demeanor seems reserved and almost withdrawn in the portrait, his large hands crossed in front of his body suggest strength and energy. Dr. Luscombe was described at the portrait ceremony as being a superb role model, articulate and cultivated, soft-spoken but with the authority that comes from experience and command of his subject.

At the portrait presentation Dr. Lewis W. Bluemle Jr. said humorously that by choosing Dr. Luscombe for their own health care, Jefferson doctors "paid him a great honor but not that much money." He continued, "If we were to recognize properly all of the care which Dr. Luscombe has given freely...we would be obliged to hang multiple portraits of him in every building on campus." He had also treated a dozen Jefferson trustees and Bluemle noted wryly, "There is only one way to treat a trustee and that is successfully. Doctor Luscombe has done just this, and consistently."

Bluemle also enumerated the Jeffersonians in Dr. Luscombe's family: his wife Sally graduated from the School of Nursing in 1942; his children, Herbert and Susan, graduated from the medical college in 1968 and 1975 respectively; his daughter Jill graduated from the College of Allied Health Sciences in 1978 (and from the University of Pennsylvania School of Veterinary Medicine almost twenty years later).

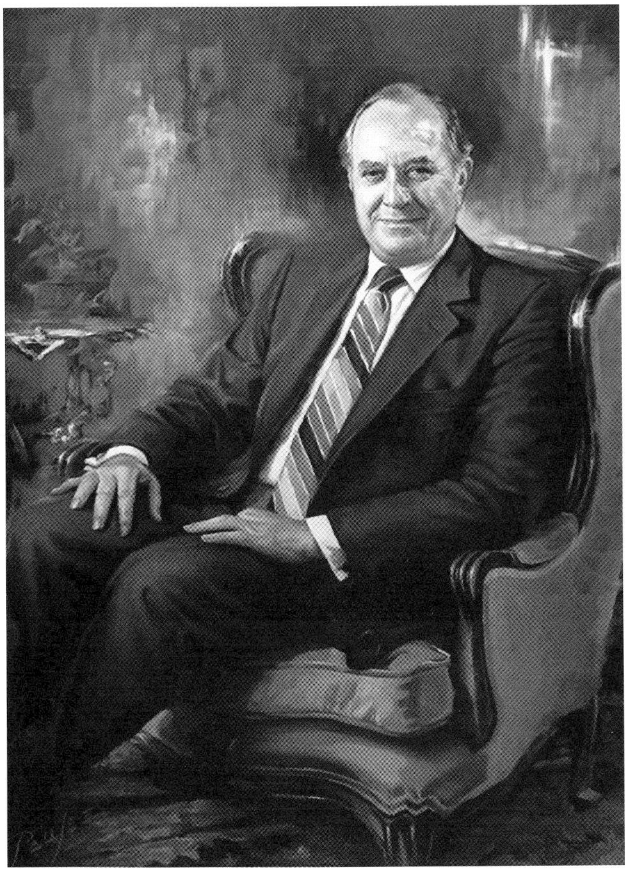

Portrait of Daniel Lieberman

DANIEL LIEBERMAN, M.D. (b. 1919)
By Dean L. Paules (b. 1931)

Oil on canvas
1987
44 x 34 in.

Signed lower left: "PAULES"

Given in 1987 by friends and colleagues
Accession number: 1987+e.P.03

Dr. Daniel Lieberman was a professor of psychiatry and human behavior, and interim chair of the department at two points. His organizational, curricular, and clinical contributions strengthened the department significantly.

Daniel Lieberman was born in 1919 in Gunnison, Utah and reared on a ranch in the San Fernando Valley of California. He received his undergraduate degree at the University of California at Santa Barbara (1942) and medical degree from the University of California at San Francisco (1946). After an internship and rotating residency at the U.S. Marine Hospital in San Francisco, he was a resident in radiology at the Army and Navy General Hospital in Hot Springs, Arkansas, and a captain at the Scott Air Force Base Regional Hospital in Illinois. While taking his residency in psychiatry on a half-time basis at the Langley-Porter Neuropsychiatric Institute in San Francisco (1949-54) he was chief of hospital services and then assistant superintendent of medical services at Sonoma State Hospital.

Subsequent public health positions were as superintendent and medical director of Mendocino State Hospital, and chief deputy director and then director for California's State Department of Mental Hygiene. During this decade he had teaching appointments as assistant clinical professor in neuropsychiatry at the University of California School of Medicine and visiting lecturer at the School of Public Health at the University of California at Los Angeles.

When Dr. Lieberman relocated to the East Coast in 1964, he continued his administrative career by organizing and serving as first commissioner of Delaware's Department of Mental Health, a post he held until 1967. He organized and directed activities that resulted in a long-range plan for mental health services in Delaware for children and adults.

He joined the Jefferson faculty in 1965 as assistant professor in clinical psychiatry. Two years later Dr. Lieberman was the force behind planning, fund-raising, and establishing the Jefferson Community Mental Health/Mental Retardation Center, of which he was director until 1974. He became associate professor in the department of psychiatry and human behavior in 1967 and professor the following year. He was interim chairman of the department in 1974-76 and 1983-88.

Lieberman also served as director of the Division of Consultation/Liaison Psychiatry and Psychosomatic Medicine (1976-83) and director of the Pain Treatment Center (1978-83). Under his leadership the psychiatry department also established a day treatment center, crisis treatment center, family therapy service, expanded child psychiatry service, psychosomatic clinic, and biofeedback program. He developed a new program called Medicine and Society that introduced psychiatry lectures to freshman and sophomore medical students.

Dr. Lieberman was active in city mental health boards, was chairman of the Delaware Institute of Human Behavior, and was a member of the National Institute of Mental Health's Task Force on Continuing Education in Community Mental Health. He was elected president of the Philadelphia Psychiatric Society and received its Lifetime Achievement Award in 1994. He was a charter fellow of the American College of Psychiatrists. He was an editorial advisor of the *World Journal of Psychosynthesis* and a member of the editorial review board of the *Journal of Pain Management.*

After twenty years as professor at Jefferson, Dr. Lieberman went on active emeritus professor status in 1988. An endowed chair in his name was established in 1990 to recognize his contributions. From 1991 to 1994 he was corporate medical director of the AGCA/ MEDCO Behavioral Care Corporation. He then continued his consulting psychiatric practice.

A further recognition of Dr. Daniel Lieberman's leadership and contributions was a portrait presented by his colleagues and friends at Jefferson in 1987. Dean Paules depicted the physician life-sized and almost full length, seated in an upholstered wing chair. His body faces partly left, and his head turns to look directly toward the viewer. His smiling, almost conversational expression is achieved by means of his sparkling brown eyes, wide upturned mouth, and creases in his cheeks.

The subject's attire is a brown business suit, white shirt, and necktie with brown, tan, blue, and gray stripes. Shades of these colors, as well as oranges, maroons, and pinks are strewn about the thickly painted and randomly arranged, brush strokes of the overly busy background.

However, the artist's ability to record the subject's likeness with his characteristic warm expression was well received. It accords with the description at the portrait ceremony by Dr. Lewis W. Bluemle Jr. of Lieberman as a "gentle Rock of Gibraltar" for his "powerful force for stability and moving ahead in critical times," and his leadership ability that was exerted "in a very gentle, kind, and wise way."

Portrait of Richard G. Berry

RICHARD GEORGE BERRY, M.D. (b. 1916)
By José Fernandez Marcote (b. 1950)

Oil on canvas
1977
52 x 44 in.

Signed and dated lower right: "MARCOTE/77"
Exhibition: Birmingham, Ala., *The Art of Healing: Medicine and Science in American Art*, Birmingham Museum of Art, 1981

Given by JMC class of 1977
Accession number: 1977+e.P.01

For sixteen years Dr. Richard G. Berry served Jefferson Medical College as a respected neuropathologist.

Richard Berry was born in 1916 in Bethel, Connecticut. He graduated from Wesleyan University in 1937 and spent a year there as research assistant in psychology before earning his medical degree from Albany Medical College in 1942. After an internship at the U.S. Naval Hospital in Newport and a residency in neurology at Jefferson Medical College he spent the next six years as staff neurologist at naval hospitals in Philadelphia and Bethesda, Maryland and held teaching posts in neurology at Georgetown University School of Medicine and the U.S. Naval Medical School in Bethesda.

Dr. Richard Berry joined the faculty at Jefferson in 1954 as associate professor of neurology and was promoted to full professor of neuropathology in 1959, and then professor of neurology (neuropathology) in 1968. He was director of the neuropathology laboratory from 1954 to 1983 and vice chairman of the neurology department from 1967 to 1982. Upon his retirement in 1984 he was appointed emeritus professor of neurology.

Berry was the coordinator of neurosciences for freshmen students, the teacher of sophomore neuropathology, and the coordinator for the senior neuroscience elective. In 1975 he received the Christian R. and Mary F. Lindback Award for Distinguished Teaching.

Dr. Berry's best-known contributions to the literature concerned his research on cerebrovascular disease, pituitary disease, intracranial arterial anatomy, and syringomyelia. He was president of the Philadelphia Neurological Society and vice president of the American Association of Neuropathologists.

During the course of his career Dr. Berry held positions as consultant in neurology or neuropathology at the New Jersey State Hospital at Ancora, the U.S. Naval Hospital in Philadelphia, the Eastern Pennsylvania Psychiatric Institute, Philadelphia General Hospital, and Wilmington Medical Center.

In 1977 the senior class elected Dr. Richard G. Berry as portrait honoree. José F. Marcote's painting is one of the most unusual depictions of a professor in his working environment in the entire Jefferson art collection.

Dr. Berry is shown full-length and slightly smaller than life-sized, standing off-center to the left. With weight on his forward foot, he leans casually against a countertop in his neuropathology laboratory, holding his ever present pipe. He rivets the viewer with an intense stare and sober expression. His most notable feature is his thick, gray, flat-topped hair.

Complementing the informal posture is his unassuming attire. Wearing neither suit jacket nor lab coat, he is dressed in a white shirt loosened at the neck and with sleeves rolled up to the elbows, and with two pens emerging from the pocket.

The horizontal format of the large scale canvas allows the artist to depict an array of scientific specimens and apparatus in a laboratory setting. The most noticeable object is the isolated brain and spinal cord on a tray in the center of the countertop, awaiting gross examination. According to Dr. Berry, other specimens in jars nearby on the counter and on shelves above are either awaiting examination or "in storage until the case is completed."

Balancing the figure on the left are glaring flood lamps in the center and right. They shine brightly on the photography stand at the far right, to which the specimen will soon be moved for photography. Dr. Berry observed that the stand is covered by blue glass for background color contrast, and that the lights on the right are clipped to a music stand for maneuverability.

The bright lights also shine on the green cabinet, yellow wall, and the right side of the subject's head and shirt. The figure casts shadows on the floor and cabinet behind him. Marcote's photorealist style is smooth and almost glasslike, and all objects are described in solid, three dimensional volumes.

When first submitted to the senior portrait committee the depiction caused such consternation that a letter was written to the artist complaining that Berry's skin tones were too dark, the likeness "inaccurate," the physique "too thin," and his legs "abnormally foreshortened, producing a rather grotesque effect." The record shows that the artist did comply with some requests for changes. The committee's letter continued with a philosophical statement of what a portrait should convey:

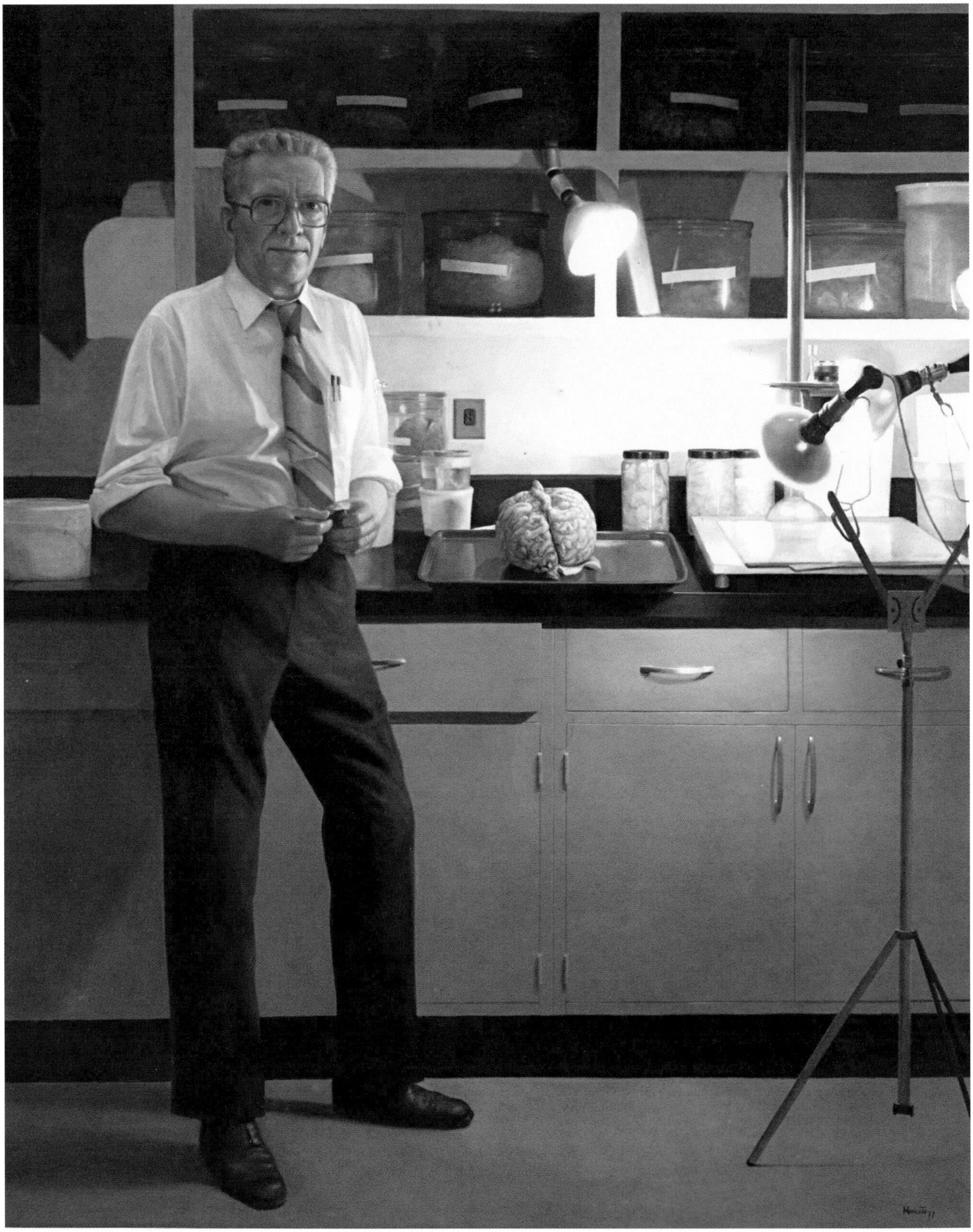

While it is true that Dr. Berry is more comfortable while dealing with the specimens and artifacts of his specialty, we must keep in mind that the purpose of this portrait is to honor the man, as a human being and a patient teacher, rather than to honor his contributions to medicine, per se. As painted, the portrait now focuses more on the work than on the man. Were this a monument to neuroanatomy more than to a man, the portrait might be acceptable.

The setting of the Berry portrait may indeed eclipse the nominal subject, not unlike the situation in Thomas Eakins's *Portrait of Dr. Benjamin H. Rand.* However, the statement glosses over the fact that Berry must have approved the concept. He told me that he had invited Marcote to his laboratory so that the artist could observe and photograph his "usual routine in the gross examination." One can applaud the physician's courage in allowing a depiction that emphasizes his working environment at the expense of usual portrait conventions and personal vanity. Many viewers react positively to the informal pose and attire, and feel that Dr. Berry is in command of his laboratory and probably eager to return to work.

This portrait was among the five Jefferson portraits chosen for an important *ars medica* exhibition, *The Art of Healing: Medicine and Science in American Art*, at the Birmingham Museum of Art in 1981. (The other selections were the three Eakins portraits and the Samuel B. Waugh portrait of Dr. Samuel D. Gross.)

José F. Marcote was born in 1950 in Salvatierra, Spain and spent his childhood in Vitoria. It was while working in a bookstore that he discovered painting through reading the shop's inventory of art books. He studied painting at the School of Fine Arts of San Fernando in Madrid from 1966 through 1971. He married a woman from Philadelphia, and in 1973 the couple moved to New York where Marcote continued to paint realistic figure subjects.

Marcote said that they relocated to the "idyllic" medieval town of Cuenca, Spain after having experienced New York's "excitement and misery," and then moved again to Vitoria. The artist has had six one-man and numerous group shows in galleries in New York and Los Angeles, as well as Madrid and other Spanish cities. Public institutions that own his work include several museums in Spain and the Chrysler Museum in Norfolk, Virginia.

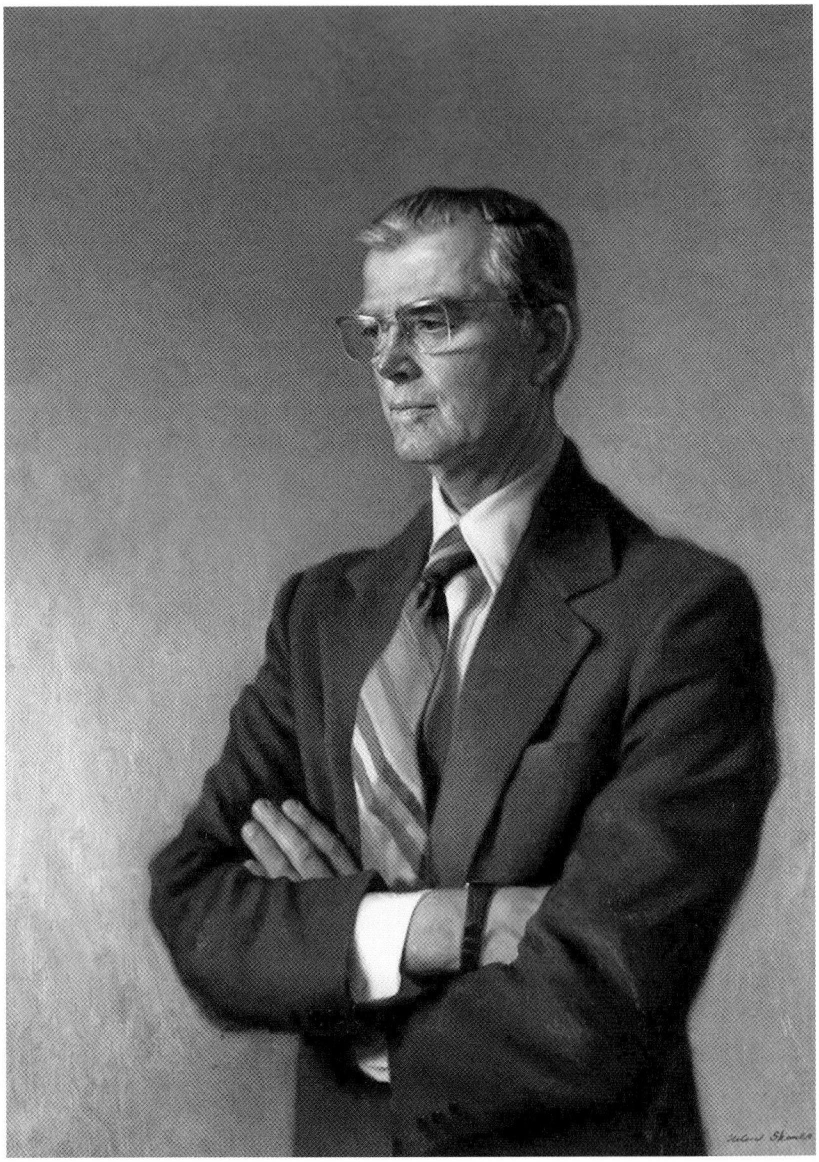

Portrait of John Y. Templeton III

(See color plate)

JOHN YOUNG TEMPLETON III, M.D.
(b. 1917)
By Nelson Shanks (b. 1937)

Oil on canvas
1982
40 x 30 in.

Signed lower right: "Nelson Shanks"

Given in 1982 by friends and colleagues
Accession number: 1982+e.P.06

Dr. John Young Templeton III, at first a protégé of Dr. John H. Gibbon Jr., became in his own right an acclaimed pioneer in the field of cardiovascular surgery. He was a professor of surgery at Jefferson and served briefly as the ninth chair of the department.

John Templeton was born in 1917, a native of Portsmouth, Virginia. He was reared in Mooresville, North Carolina and graduated from Davidson College in Virginia in 1937. Four years later he graduated from Jefferson Medical College where there were family connections: his father, John Y. Templeton Jr., and brother, Thomas B. Templeton, were members of the class of 1913 and 1955, respectively; and his wife, Dorothy, graduated from the School of Nursing in 1941. After interning at Jefferson Dr. Templeton served in the Army Medical Corps from 1942 to 1946, reaching the rank of major.

Dr. John Templeton's surgical career began auspiciously with his residency from 1946 to 1950 under John H. Gibbon Jr., for whom he was the first resident to work in the laboratory on the heart-lung machine. He continued his training at Jefferson the next two years as an American Cancer Society fellow and Damon Runyon fellow. He was appointed instructor on the Jefferson faculty in 1950 and rose rapidly to become clinical professor in 1957, all the while working closely with Dr. Gibbon in his laboratory and clinical practice. Templeton left in 1964 to become professor of surgery at the University of Pennsylvania School of Medicine and Graduate School of Medicine, and chief of surgery at Pennsylvania Hospital.

Dr. Templeton returned to Jefferson in 1967 to succeed Dr. Gibbon as the Samuel D. Gross Professor of Surgery and chair of the department. When he tendered his resignation as chair for personal reasons effective January 1, 1969, considerable disappointment was registered by colleagues, residents, nursing staff, and students who revered the prominent surgeon. However, he remained as professor of surgery and carried on an outstanding clinical practice until his retirement in 1987 when he was named emeritus professor. In 1977 Templeton won the Golden Scalpel Award from the division of cardiothoracic surgery.

Over the years the innovative and prominent cardiac surgeon was also consultant to hospitals that included Philadelphia General, Chestnut Hill, Lankenau, the Polyclinic Hospital in Harrisburg, and the Delaware Medical Center in Wilmington.

Dr. Templeton was extremely active academically and professionally. He wrote over eighty articles on basic and clinical research in pulmonary, vascular, gastrointestinal, and cardiac surgery. He was a member of the editorial board of *American Practitioner and Digest of Treatment*.

He served on the board of governors or as committee chairman of more than fourteen national and international surgical, cardiothoracic, and vascular societies. He was president of the Philadelphia County Medical Society and received its Strittmatter Award in 1992. He was also president of the Philadelphia Academy of Surgery, the Laennec Society, the Pennsylvania Association for Thoracic Surgery, and the Pennsylvania State Medical Society. He received an honorary D.Sc. degree from Davidson College in 1987.

A dedicated Jeffersonian, Dr. John Templeton served as president of the alumni association and of the hospital's medical staff, and acted as alumni trustee. The institution bestowed many honors on Templeton including the alumni achievement award (1981), the Winged Ox Award (1987), and an honorary doctor of laws degree (1987). The annual John Y. Templeton III lectureship was established in 1980 by Dr. Benjamin Bacharach (JMC 1956) and Mrs. Bacharach, in memory of their fathers, Gunard O. Carlson and Jack Paul Bacharach. The first lecturer was the internationally known surgeon Dr. Denton A. Cooley, founder of the Texas Heart Institute.

In 1980 Dr. Templeton's former residents and colleagues arranged for his portrait to be presented. It was painted by a self-taught artist who was a Jefferson alumnus and former resident. Misunderstandings between him and the portrait committee resulted in the painting being returned to the artist. A new portrait by the acclaimed Nelson Shanks was successfully unveiled at the annual Templeton lecture in 1982.

Shanks's imposing depiction shows the physician life-sized and half-length, standing at an angle to the picture plane. His posture and expression are somewhat austere, with arms folded close to his body, and somber gaze directed down into the distance. The square outline of his face and jaw is repeated by the lenses of his rimless glasses. His well-defined features are crowned by his full head of silver hair. The subject wears a dark blue business suit, white shirt, and necktie with blue, yellow, umber, and purple stripes. The dappled, soft, atmospheric background is cool gray and green.

The artist's smoothly modulated tones ranging from deep shadows to bright highlights sculpt the planes of the figure's face and hands. Volumetric forms are also applied to elements of his costume: the necktie swells away from his body and leaves its shadow on his shirt, and the fabric of his suit has deep folds and irregular contours. Bright pinks and reds in the spotlighted skin tones of his face and highlights on his glasses contrast effectively with the dark, almost silhouetted costume and the middle range of tones in the background. The portrait's unusual format, coupled with the spacious background that surrounds the figure, suggests the august prominence of the subject.

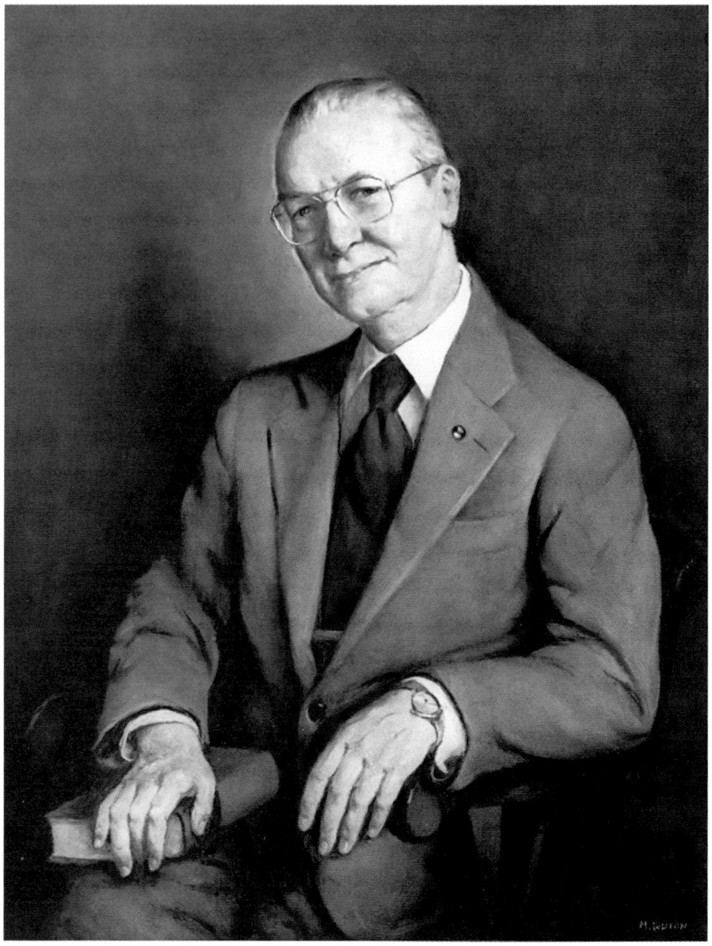

Portrait of Frederick B. Wagner Jr.

FREDERICK BALTHAS WAGNER Jr., M.D. (b. 1916)
By Molly Guion (b. 1910)

Oil on canvas
1978
40 x 30 in.

Signed lower right: "M. GUION"

Given in 1978 by friends and colleagues
Accession number: 1978+e.P.06

The contributions of Dr. Frederick B. Wagner Jr. to Thomas Jefferson University are unique for their diversity and longevity over a period of more than fifty years. A busy clinical surgeon, he was named the second Grace Osler Revere Professor of Surgery. As the university historian he is the editor or coauthor of three authoritative books on Jefferson history.

Frederick B. Wagner was born in Philadelphia in 1916. He won a full scholarship to the University of Pennsylvania where he graduated *summa cum laude* in 1937. Equally outstanding in the class of 1941 at Jefferson Medical College, he won the obstetrics and ophthalmology prizes, the W. B. Saunders Prize, the William Potter Memorial Prize, and the Alumni Prize for highest overall average. His wife Jean, a graduate of the School of Nursing in 1941, became an obstetrical nurse at Jefferson and Pennsylvania Hospitals.

After his internship and surgical residency at the Jefferson Hospital he was a Ross V. Patterson research fellow from 1945 to 1946. He accepted the invitation to become the private assistant of Dr. Thomas A. Shallow, known as "the boss" or "the last of the Geheimrats." Wagner's demanding duties during a ten-year period, recounted in *Jefferson Medical College: Legend and Lore*, are illustrative of a bygone era: he was first assistant at every operation, gave the spinal anesthesias, supervised the pre- and postoperative care of thirty-five to fifty private patients, performed all night and weekend emergencies, and did the fundamental research and literary work on scientific papers.

Dr. Wagner rose in the academic ranks to become clinical professor of surgery in 1955, a position he held until 1978. He was attending surgeon at the Jefferson Hospital from 1965 until 1985. Wagner was noted for operations of the gastrointestinal tract, breast, thyroid, parathyroid, and the peripheral venous system. A pioneer in vascular surgery and arteriography, "Fearless Fred" Wagner performed the first abdominal aortigram in Philadelphia and the first abdominal aneurysm surgery at Jefferson. In addition to his posts at Jefferson, Dr. Wagner was director of surgery at the William B. Kessler Memorial Hospital in Hammonton, New Jersey

(1963-72), and consultant in vascular surgery at St. Mary's Franciscan Hospital in Philadelphia (1963-65).

In 1977 Wagner was offered the post of acting chairman of Jefferson's surgery department to "heal old wounds and create harmony" in the demoralized department. At Wagner's portrait presentation the following year Dean William F. Kellow, M.D. recounted the surgeon's surprise at this administrative opportunity, noting that "proud men ask to be honored, but...a man like Wagner with the comparatively rare virtue of humility receives tributes because of the real respect friends and colleagues feel for him." Wagner proved an effective leader during his thirteen-month term. In 1978 the new chairman, Dr. Francis E. Rosato, appointed Dr. Wagner the Grace Revere Osler Professor of Surgery, the first to hold that title since Dr. George P. Muller. Upon his retirement in 1982 Wagner was named emeritus professor with the same designation.

He was a founding member of the American College of Angiology and served a term as president of the Philadelphia Academy of Surgery. He was also a member of the board of trustees of Children's Rehabilitation Hospital. He was author of *Preoperative and Postoperative Care* (1947).

Dr. Wagner's activities on behalf of Jefferson are almost unsurpassed. He was president of Jefferson's alumni association in 1975. He was an alumni member of the board of trustees from 1985 to 1991 and was invited to continue attending meetings after his term was completed. It was through his leadership that the Gross Conference Room in the surgery department offices and the Eakins Gallery and Eakins Lounge in Jefferson Alumni Hall were funded and erected, the latter with the help of Dr. Thaddeus L. Montgomery. Wagner also spearheaded the alumni effort to prevent the proposed sale of *The Gross Clinic* during the administration of President Peter A. Herbut, M.D.

His interest in medical history resulted in the book *The Twilight Years of Lady Osler* (1985), and membership in the exclusive American and Japanese Osler Societies. At the conclusion of his surgical career he began an entirely new vocation as the first Thomas Jefferson University Historian with the mission of preserving the legacy of the university. An exhaustive trilogy of books was published in seven years: *Thomas Jefferson University: Tradition and Heritage* (edited by Dr. Wagner, 1989); *Thomas Jefferson University: A Chronological History and Alumni Directory, 1824-1990* (with coauthor Dr. J. Woodrow Savacool, 1992); and *Jefferson Medical College: Legend and Lore* (also with Dr. Savacool, 1996). In 1997 Wagner resolved the confusing identity of the last residence of Jefferson founder George McClellan, M.D. at 912 Walnut Street, and arranged for a plaque designating the site.

A noted church organist, Dr. Wagner played at a ceremony in 1957 dedicating the Hammond organ in McClellan Hall to the memory of Richard Woods Montgomery, son of Dr. and Mrs. Thaddeus L. Montgomery. Since then Wagner was invited to play the organ at the annual Rehfuss lectures and at almost every portrait presentation through 1996.

Thomas Jefferson University thanked Dr. Wagner for his manifold contributions with the Samuel D. Gross Distinguished Service Award in 1980, the Dean's Medal in 1987, and the alumni achievement award in 1990. At the 1996 Jefferson commencement Dr. Wagner received an honorary doctor of humane letters degree.

In 1985 friends and colleagues commissioned a portrait of Dr. Frederick Wagner painted by Molly Guion. The surgeon is depicted two-thirds length and life-sized, seated in an armchair. A surgery textbook is balanced on his right thigh. His head is tilted sharply to the right and he looks directly toward the spectator. His most prominent features are his square jaw, cleft chin, broad mouth, and blue eyes behind metal-rimmed glasses. He engages the viewer with a kindly and attentive expression, reminding friends of his optimistic and generous personality.

The subject is wearing a gray business suit with white shirt, maroon necktie, and the Jefferson President's Club lapel pin. The atmospheric background is very dark except for the greenish halo effect around the sitter's head. The paint style is smooth except for the choppy brush strokes of pinks, greens, yellows, and blues in the well defined face and hands.

Portrait of Charles Fineberg

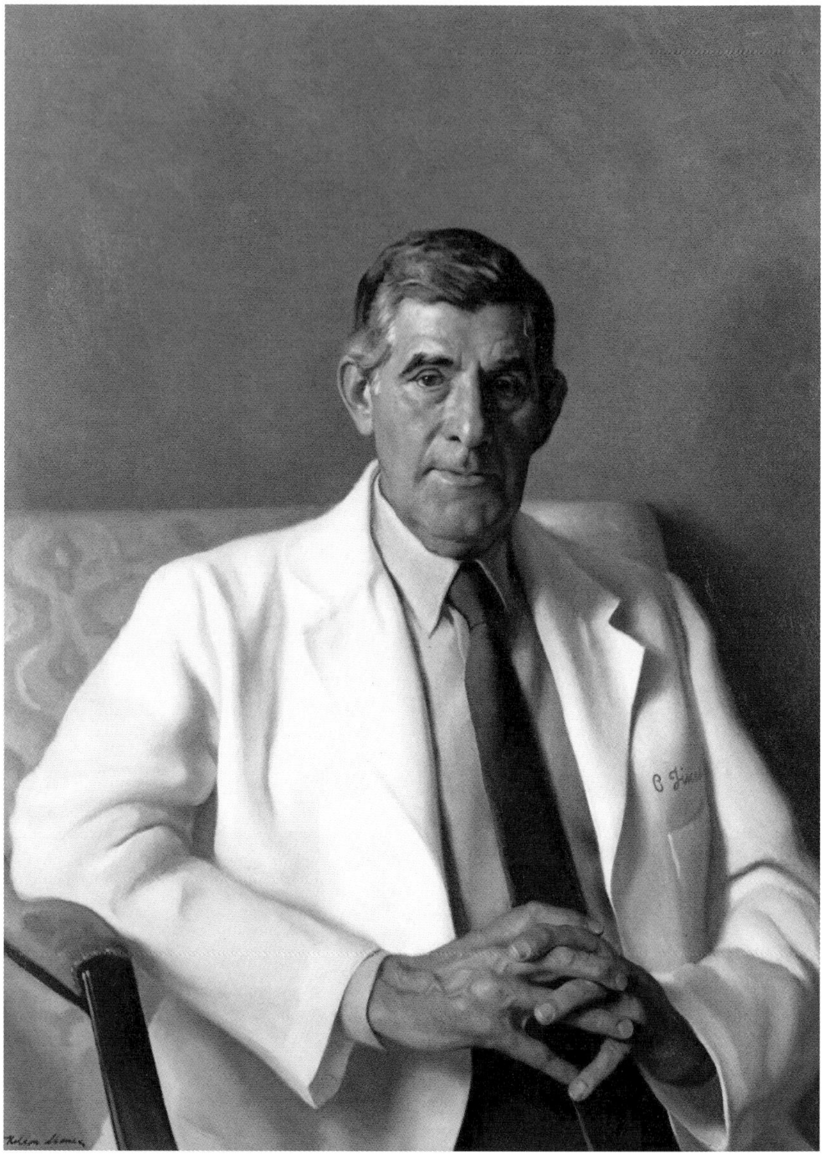

CHARLES FINEBERG, M.D. (1921-94)
By Nelson Shanks (b. 1937)

Oil on canvas
1983
40 x 30 1/2 in.

Signed lower left: "Nelson Shanks"

Given in 1983 by friends and colleagues
Accession number: 1983+e.P.03

Dr. Charles Fineberg was a noted professor of surgery at Jefferson. Fineberg had been a surgical resident who operated with Dr. John H. Gibbon Jr. and worked with him on the development of the heart-lung machine like his colleague Dr. John Templeton.

Charles Fineberg was born in Philadelphia in 1921 and reared in New York. He graduated in 1941 from Wake Forest University where he played varsity basketball, baseball, and football on an athletic scholarship. Immediately after graduation he entered the Coast Guard Academy and spent four years on active duty commanding ships in the South Pacific and the North Atlantic rescuing men whose vessels had been torpedoed. Although before the war he had signed to play baseball in the New York Yankees farm system, he opted for a career in medicine instead, and graduated from Hahnemann Medical College in 1950.

Dr. Fineberg interned at Mount Sinai Hospital in Philadelphia, and took a residency and surgical research fellowship at Jefferson, followed by a fellowship at the National Cancer Institute of the U.S. Public Health Service. He rose through the faculty ranks at Jefferson from assistant in surgery in 1955 to professor of surgery in 1972. He was chairman of the executive cancer committee at Jefferson Hospital. He also served as director of vascular and thoracic surgery at the Samuel H. Daroff Division of Albert Einstein Medical Center from 1968 to 1987.

In addition to his work on the heart-lung machine, Dr. Charles Fineberg's research included experimental myocardial revascularization. Fineberg was chairman of the surgical advisory committee of the American College of Surgeons and a member of the scientific advisory board of the National Foundation for Ileitis and Colitis. Among other societies he was a fellow of the Royal Society of Medicine.

"Chuck" Fineberg had been a respected surgeon, teacher, and scientist at Jefferson for over thirty years when friends and colleagues presented his portrait to the university in 1983. Painted by Nelson Shanks, the subject is shown half length and life-sized, seated in an upholstered armchair. His head is turned to look directly out toward the viewer. He has thick, steel gray hair, black eyebrows atop his piercingly dark eyes, and a tightly clamped mouth. The long fingers of his powerful hands are interlaced in front of his body.

The subject wears a white doctor's coat over a blue shirt and red necktie. His embroidered name is partially visible over the coat pocket: "C. Fineb." The pearl gray upholstered chair has a delicate paisley pattern and the modulated, atmospheric background glides from umbers and grays to pale salmon. As usual with portraits by Nelson Shanks, the painting surface is very smooth and meticulously rendered. The solid figure is described so sculpturally that one has a palpable sense of his presence in real space. Even the white coat has an undulating surface with folds in deep shadow contrasted with brightly highlighted areas.

The viewer is struck immediately by the physical strength of the subject: the muscularity and large size of his face and hands which are visually connected by the red necktie, and the expansive width of his shoulders. The perception of forcefulness also arises from the closeup placement of the figure at the bottom edge of the canvas, and the fact that his head rises above the chair back but well below the top edge of the canvas. Fineberg was known as a man of strong principles and a stern taskmaster, but his almost pugnacious expression does not suggest the qualities of compassion and dedication to his patients for which he was also noted.

Portrait of John J. Gartland

JOHN J. GARTLAND, M.D. (b. 1918)
By Alden MacMaster Wicks (1914-87)

Oil on canvas
1981
36 x 30 in.

Signed lower left: "Wicks"

Given in 1981 by friends and colleagues
Accession number: 1981+e.P.02

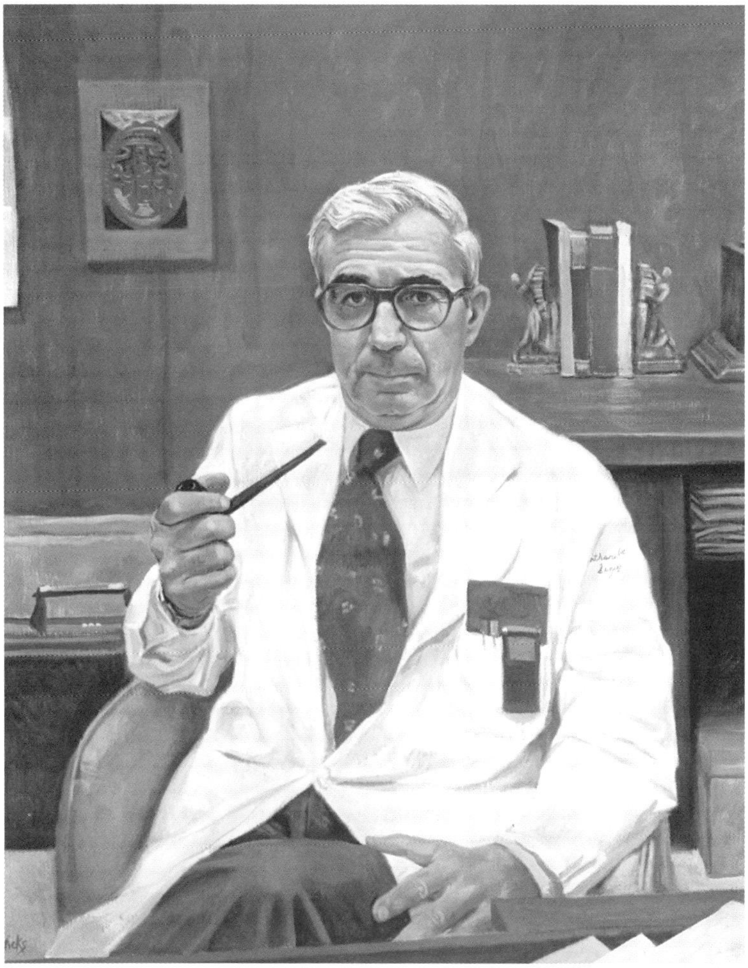

Dr. John J. Gartland was the James Edwards Professor of Orthopaedic Surgery at Jefferson and chairman of the department. After his retirement from clinical practice he has served the university in numerous capacities including trustee.

A native Philadelphian, John J. Gartland was born in 1918 and graduated from Princeton University (1941) and Jefferson Medical College (1944) where he served his internship. After two years of service in the U.S. Army, he completed his residency in orthopaedic surgery at Jefferson and the New York Orthopaedic Hospital, Columbia-Presbyterian Medical Center. At Jefferson he rose from instructor in orthopaedic surgery in 1952 to associate professor in 1967. He became the James Edwards Professor of Orthopaedic Surgery in 1970 and chair of the department, a post he held until 1985. He was named emeritus professor of orthopaedic surgery in 1989.

Appointments at other hospitals before his chairmanship at Jefferson included: attending orthopaedic surgeon at Fitzgerald Mercy Hospital, chief orthopaedic surgeon at the Methodist and Lankenau Hospitals, and chief of the lower extremity service at the Pennsylvania State Hospital for Crippled Children in Elizabethtown. While orthopaedist-in-chief at Thomas Jefferson University Hospital from 1970 to 1985, he was also consultant in orthopeadic surgery at the Methodist, Cooper, Lankenau, and Bryn Mawr Hospitals.

During Dr. Gartland's tenure the orthopaedics department was considerably strengthened. He increased the number of full-time faculty to complement the volunteer faculty, and restructured the residency program. New divisions included hand surgery and pediatric orthopaedics. The affiliated orthopaedic departments at Methodist, Bryn Mawr, and Lankenau Hospitals, as well as the Alfred I. duPont Institute and the Wilmington Veterans Administration Hospital were made available for graduate education. Further opportunities were provided by cooperative programs with Jefferson's own divisions of rheumatology and rehabilitation medicine. The department began the *Jefferson Orthopaedic Journal* in 1972, and it continues publication today.

Dr. Gartland is the author of *Fundamentals of Orthopaedics* (1965) and *Medical Writing and Communicating* (1993). He has written over one hundred articles on specific orthopaedic conditions and treatments including his research on methyl methacrylate at a basic laboratory level, the influence of hyaluronidase on experimental bone repair and fracture healing, and the McKee-Farrar total hip replacement prosthesis anchored with methacrylate bone cement. Other articles include considerations of governmental intervention in medicine, the practice and future of orthopaedic surgery, and medical technology and communications. His movies on posterior tibial transplant for recurrent club foot and the technique of McKee-Farrar total hip replacement are available in the permanent film library of the American Academy of Orthopaedic Surgeons.

Dr. Gartland's extensive literary background includes service on the editorial boards of the *Journal of Bone and Joint Surgery* and *Medical Communications* (the former *Journal of the American Medical Writers Association*). He has earned credits in scientific writing at the University of Minnesota and was certified in editing by the American Medical Writers Association. He is currently university medical editor at Jefferson, assisting faculty and staff in their professional papers and case reports, research protocols, and grant applications.

Dr. Gartland was president of the Jefferson Orthopaedic Society, the Philadelphia Orthopaedic Society, the Pennsylvania Orthopaedic Society (also chairman of its scientific research committee), the American Academy of Orthopaedic Surgeons, and the Council of Medical Specialty Societies. He was visiting professor at fifteen universities in America, the University of Athens, and Hebrew University in Jerusalem. He was the speaker at endowed lectures at Columbia-Presbyterian Medical Center, the University of Iowa, the University of North Carolina in Chapel Hill, the University of Connecticut, and Jefferson.

Dr. John Gartland served as president of Jefferson's alumni association in 1974, received the alumni achievement award in 1989, and in 1996 was elected an alumni trustee of Thomas Jefferson University. His portrait by Alden Wicks was presented by friends and colleagues in 1981.

The subject is depicted two-thirds length and life-sized, seated with legs crossed behind a desk. He looks directly toward the viewer and holds a pipe in his right hand. He wears a white doctor's coat over a blue shirt, a dark blue tie with a yellow pattern, and dark gray trousers. A small notebook, pager, and pens fill his coat pocket. The words "Orthopaedic Surgery" are embroidered on his left sleeve.

The subject's steely look of determination and commitment is enhanced by his iron gray hair, raised black eyebrows over horn-rimmed glasses, deep creases in forehead and cheeks, and lips that are tightly pressed together. Wicks's characteristic geometric organization of the office space includes objects referring to the sitter's academic work: a briefcase, books and pamphlets, files, and a replica of the presidential medal of the American Academy of Orthopaedic Surgeons.

Conceding that he was touched and honored in remarks at the presentation ceremony, Dr. John Gartland said incisively, "It has been said about me that I am dedicated...We are in the business of making tomorrow—tomorrow's science, tomorrow's preventive medical care, and tomorrow's doctors. That is what I hope our dedication is all about."

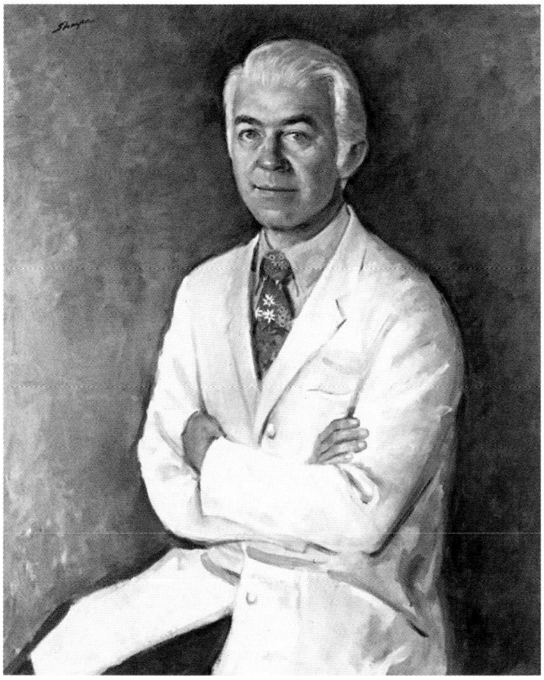

Portrait of John J. Dowling

JOHN JOSEPH DOWLING, M.D. (b. 1923)
By Marion Potter Sharpe

Oil on canvas
1974
46 x 38 in.

Signed upper left: "Sharpe"

Given by JMC class of 1974
Accession number: 1974+e.P.03

Dr. John J. Dowling was a clinical professor of orthopaedic surgery at Jefferson and became chief of orthopaedic surgery at Lankenau Hospital.

Born in Johnstown, Pennsylvania in 1923, John J. Dowling attended Notre Dame University before receiving his degree from Jefferson Medical College in 1947. During a rotating internship he seriously considered psychiatry or obstetrics and gynecology until his training with Dr. Anthony DePalma inspired him to enter orthopaedics. He completed his residency at Jefferson and joined the faculty in 1955. He received the coveted Christian R. and Mary F. Lindback Award for Distinguished Teaching at Jefferson in 1971. By 1973 he had risen in the ranks to clinical professor of orthopaedic surgery. In 1984 Dowling was elected president of Jefferson's alumni association.

Since 1970 Dowling was also chief of orthopaedic surgery at Lankenau Hospital, succeeding Dr. John Gartland. Other posts were at Misericordia Hospital and the State Hospital for Crippled Children in Elizabethtown. He is the author of *Musculoskeletal Disease: Staged for Rapid Comprehension* (1985).

In 1974 Dr. John Dowling won the Thomas Foster Bright Award of the Main Line Junior Chamber of Commerce for his years of service as attending surgeon to St. Edmond's Home for Crippled Children in Rosemont. Dowling brought third-year Jefferson students there for lectures on spina bifida and cerebral palsy and to experience the full impact of the home's environment. His activities on behalf of these children led to a papal knighthood, the Order of St. Gregory the Great, awarded by John Cardinal Krol of Philadelphia in 1982. In 1983 he received St. Edmond's Man of the Year Award.

The class of 1974 chose Dr. John J. Dowling as its portrait honoree. Marion P. Sharpe depicted the physician two-thirds length and slightly larger than life-sized. He is seated with arms folded tightly against his body. His large blue eyes gaze directly toward the viewer, and his expression is friendly. His thick white hair is echoed by the brightness of the white doctor's coat. He wears a blue shirt and an unusually colorful necktie decorated with yellow, white, and blue flowers on a red background. The portrait's yellowish-brown atmospheric background is loosely painted.

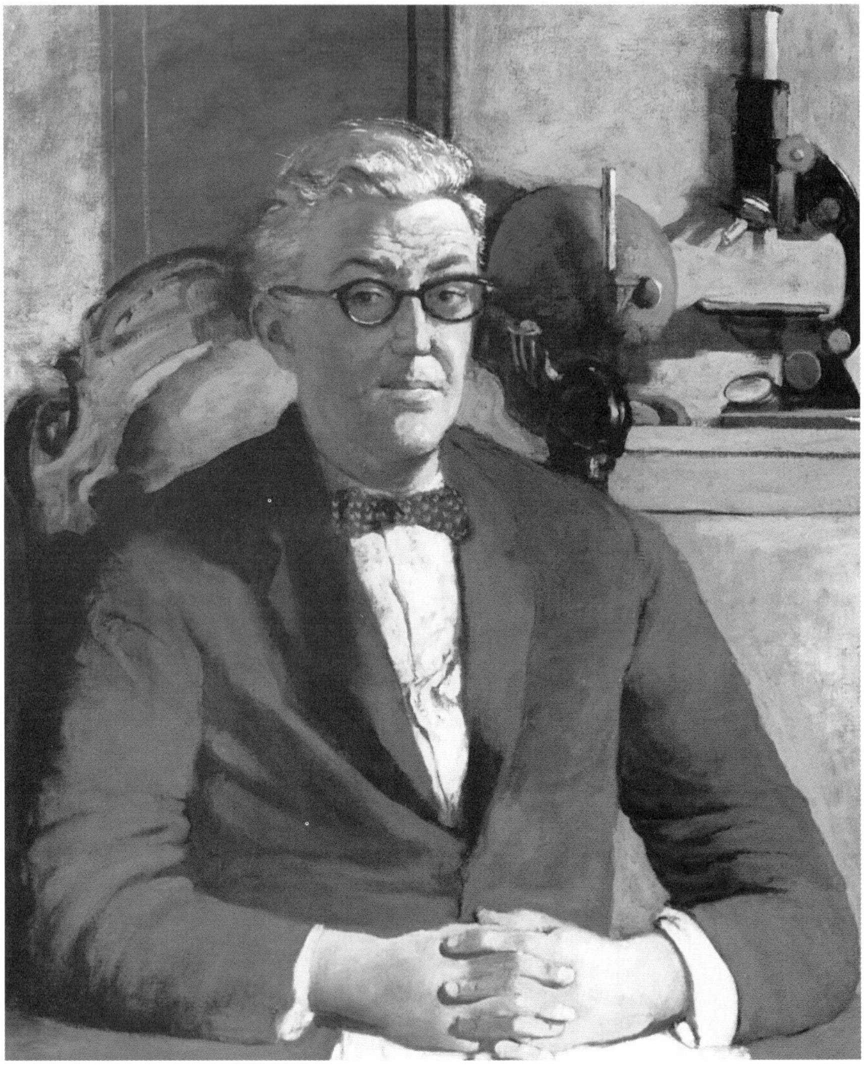

Portrait of Abraham E. Rakoff

ABRAHAM EDWARD RAKOFF, M.D. (1913-81)
By Walter Stuempfig Jr. (1914-70)

Oil on canvas
1964
30 x 26 in.

Given by JMC class of 1964
Accession number: 1964+e.P.01

Dr. Abraham E. Rakoff was an internationally acclaimed reproductive endocrinologist who forged his entire career at Jefferson.

Abraham Rakoff was born in 1913 in Philadelphia, and graduated from the University of Pennsylvania (1933) and Jefferson Medical College (1937) where he won the obstetrics award. Shortly after receiving his medical degree he published the first paper on the combined use of estrogen and progesterone to help salvage threatened abortions. After an internship at Frankford Hospital he returned to Jefferson as a research fellow in the department of obstetrics and gynecology and was appointed to the faculty.

Dr. Rakoff rose through the academic ranks to become professor of obstetrics and gynecology (endocrinology) in 1960, and received a secondary appointment as professor of medicine (endocrinology) in 1965. He was the first head of reproductive endocrinology, a division which was created in 1972. He was named honorary professor of medicine in 1978 and emeritus professor of obstetrics and gynecology in 1980.

Dr. Rakoff had joined with Drs. Karl Paschkis and Abraham Cantarow in 1940 to form an endocrine outpatient facility, an endocrine laboratory, and an informal research group. By 1948 Jefferson trustees formalized the interdepartmental group as the division of endocrine and cancer research. Dr. Rakoff's research in gynecologic endocrinology developed procedures for increasing the sensitivity of the pregnancy test, the bioassay of pituitary and chorionic gonadotropins, and the assessment of the pituitary-ovarian-adrenal function in infertility and hirsutism.

Dr. Rakoff trained more than sixty residents in reproductive endocrinology, and many forged their own illustrious careers at other universities. His clinical reputation was worldwide and infertile couples came from afar to seek his counsel. He was known for kindness to his patients and for investigating their problems in the laboratory as well as the library.

Besides his posts at Jefferson Dr. Abraham Rakoff was also visiting lecturer in gynecic endocrinology at the Graduate School of Medicine of the University of Pennsylvania, consultant at the U.S. Naval Hospital, and on the courtesy staff at Methodist and Pennsylvania Hospitals.

Rakoff was the author of chapters in twenty-two textbooks, and coauthor of *Clinical Endocrinology* (with Karl E. Paschkis and Abraham Cantarow, 1954) and *Vaginal Infections, Infestations, and Discharge* (with J. B. Bernstine, 1953). He was on the editorial boards of *Acta Cytologica* and *Fertility and Sterility*.

His leadership in professional societies led to posts as president and chairman of the editorial committee of the Inter-Society Cytology Council, board member of the American Cancer Society, founding member of the International Academy of Gynecologic Cytologists, and president of the Philadelphia Endocrine Society. He was a member of the American Association for the Advancement of Science.

A loyal Jeffersonian, Dr. Abraham Rakoff was president of the alumni association during its centennial year in 1971. On the first anniversary of this respected physician's death, Rakoff's family voiced their gratitude in the *Jefferson Medical College Alumni Bulletin* of summer 1982 to the more than one thousand friends, patients, and colleagues who expressed their condolences through a bountiful "avalanche" of letters, gifts, flowers, and contributions in his memory.

The Abraham E. Rakoff memorial scholarship was established in 1983. For the first time in its history the alumni association bestowed its achievement award posthumously to Dr. Rakoff in 1984. At the presentation ceremony Dr. Burton L. Wellenbach recalled moments of crisis when his mentor and friend was "chosen to either lead the group or personally intervene in someone's behalf," as best exemplified by his election as first president of the volunteer faculty, "when our university needed a respected, responsive, and altruistic leader." Wellenbach also praised Dr. Rakoff's empathy with all segments of the medical community.

The senior class had selected Dr. Abraham Rakoff as portrait honoree in 1964. As depicted by Walter Stuempfig Jr., the physician is shown half length and life-sized, seated in an upholstered armchair. His clasped hands rest on papers on the desktop. His wavy, silver hair, horn-rimmed glasses, and pursed lips are his most salient features. His unfocused eyes and quizzical expression scarcely hint at the sitter's impressive intellect, energy, and personal warmth.

Dr. Rakoff is wearing a brown suit, white shirt, and jaunty maroon bow tie with yellow polka dots. A microscope rests on a shelf behind the yellow back of his ornately carved, Baroque Revival chair. The background walls are pale blue, and his silver hair is streaked with the same blue color. The most unusual feature of the impasto surface is the sharp contrast of light and shade on the subject's face and costume, with few transitional middle tones. It is as though the room were bathed in some sort of mysterious, direct sunlight. It is well to remember that Walter Stuempfig was best known as a landscape artist.

Portrait of Paul A. Bowers

PAUL APPLEGATE BOWERS, M.D. (b. 1911)
By Nelson Shanks (b. 1937)

Oil on canvas
1982
40 1/4 x 28 1/4 in.

Signed lower right: "Shanks"

Given in 1982 by friends and colleagues
Accession number: 1982+e.P.01

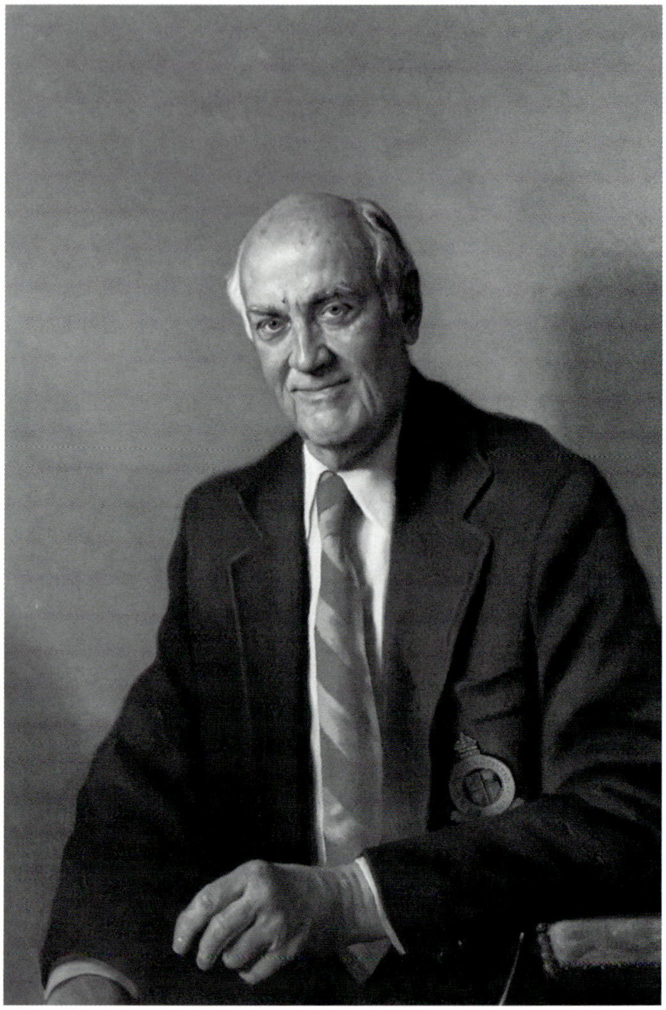

Dr. Paul A. Bowers was a professor of obstetrics and gynecology at Jefferson. He was a forward-thinking clinician who developed a widespread practice of devoted patients.

Paul Bowers was born in 1911 in Big Run, Pennsylvania, and graduated from Bucknell University (1933) and Jefferson Medical College (1937). After an internship at the Jefferson Hospital, he became a resident in obstetrics and gynecology at the Lying-In Hospital of the University of Chicago.

His residency was interrupted by war, and he saw four years' service in the Medical Corps of the U.S. Army in the continental United States and the Pacific. While stationed in Hawaii he met his future wife, Eloise Bechtel, a member of the Nursing Corps of the U.S. Army.

After twenty-seven years Dr. Bowers reached the rank of colonel in the Army Reserves. For his loyal and outstanding service he was decorated with the Military Award for World Wars and the Outstanding Civilian Service Medal.

After World War II Dr. Paul Bowers returned to Jefferson to join Dr. Thaddeus L. Montgomery in the development of the newly combined department of obstetrics and gynecology, and they remained partners for over thirty years. When Montgomery presided at his partner's portrait presentation, he outlined their "pioneer efforts" to "preserve the physiological concepts of labor," including natural childbirth, the husband's presence in the delivery room to participate in the birth, and the rooming-in of child and mother, when such procedures were "looked upon askance in the ivory halls of medical pedagogy."

Bowers rose from clinical assistant in the outpatient department in 1946 to professor of obstetrics and gynecology in 1971. He was named emeritus professor in 1979. In addition to his posts at the Jefferson Hospital, he was consultant at the Veterans and Germantown Hospitals in Philadelphia, the Valley Forge General Hospital, the Pottstown Hospital, and St. Mary's Hospital in Langhorne, Pennsylvania. At Philadelphia General Hospital he served as president of the medical staff and chairman of the department of obstetrics and gynecology, Division A.

Bowers served as president of the Obstetrical Society of Philadelphia. He was chairman of District III of the American College of Obstetricians and Gynecologists, and received the society's Outstanding Service Award in 1985. He also won the Physicians Recognition Award of the American Medical Association and Bucknell University's alumni achievement award in 1959.

Dr. Bowers was president of the Jefferson alumni association in 1973 and served as an alumni trustee. He won the university's Winged Ox Award in 1985. The establishment of the Paul A. and Eloise B. Bowers Professorship in Obstetrics and Gynecology was announced in 1995. Mrs. Bowers has been an active participant in Jefferson community service activities, including terms as president of the faculty wives club and the Jefferson Hospital women's board.

A portrait of Dr. Bowers was commissioned by friends and colleagues and painted by Nelson Shanks in 1982. The subject is shown half length and slightly larger than life-sized. His oval-shaped face is dominated by the high domed forehead with fringes of silver hair, alert blue eyes, and a wide smile that deepens the creases in his cheeks and under his eyes. The subject turns toward the viewer and leans forward energetically, gesturing with his left hand as though in conversation.

Dr. Bowers is wearing a dark blue jacket with a crest, a white shirt, and a red and gray striped tie. The red, white, and gold crest indicates his membership in the British Officers Club, an honor won for participating in the medical treatment of British military personnel in the Pacific during World War II. The pearl gray atmospheric background suggests deep space by the curving shadows behind the sitter.

The viewer's positive response to Dr. Bowers's direct and engaging manner brings to mind his warm and considerate personality and concern for the human relationships in medicine. In a profile in the spring 1969 *Jefferson Medical College Alumni Bulletin*, Bowers credited the satisfactions of contributing to family life and working with an "agreeable group of patients" as reasons for choosing the practice of obstetrics, even with its twenty-four-hour, unpredictable schedule. He said that in many cases women patients are easier to deal with than men: "They follow recommendations. They don't expect miraculous cures. They are understanding, appreciative, gentle. And you are dealing with a young group of people at a happy time."

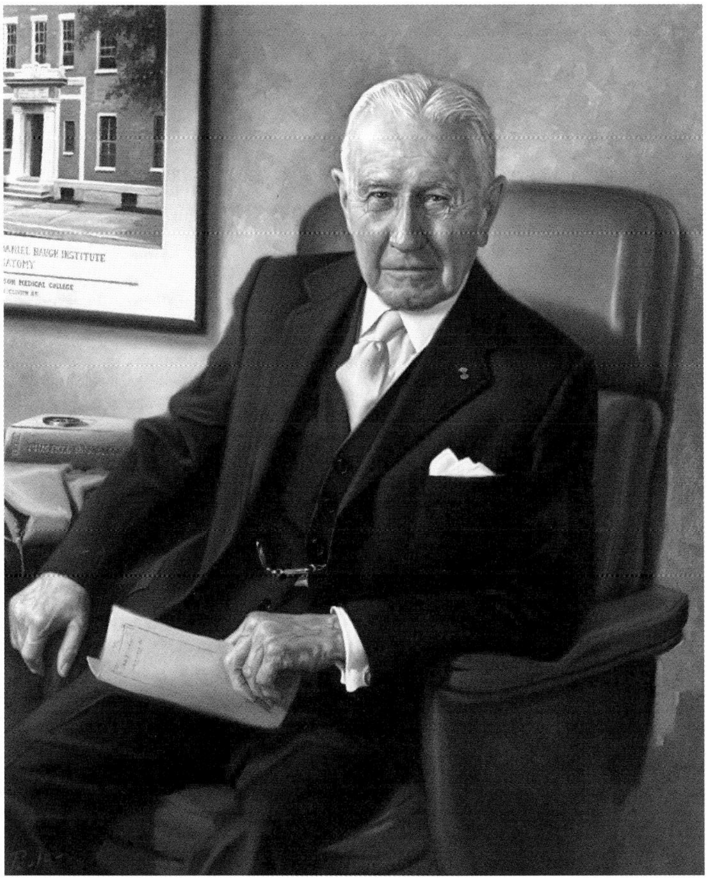

Portrait of Joe Henry Coley

JOE HENRY COLEY, M.D. (b. 1907)
By Dean L. Paules (b. 1931)

Oil on canvas
1995
38 x 32 in.

Signed and dated lower left: "Paules/3-95"

Given in 1995 by JMC alumni association
Accession number: 1995+e.P.03

Affectionately known as "Mr. Jefferson" or "Mr. Alumnus," Dr. Joe Henry Coley has received almost every award Thomas Jefferson University can bestow upon a dedicated alumnus. He has combined a career in obstetrics and gynecology with generous civic involvement.

Joe Henry Coley was born in 1907 in Alexander City,

Alabama, the son of Dr. Andrew Jackson Coley (JMC 1880) who practiced medicine until age eighty-nine. The elder Coley moved his family to Oklahoma City in 1909. Joe Coley received his bachelor's degree from Oklahoma City University in 1930 and his medical degree from Jefferson Medical College in 1934. He interned at St. Luke's Hospital in Bethlehem, Pennsylvania and received further training in obstetrics and gynecology at the University of Oklahoma.

He opened a private practice in Oklahoma City, and in 1937 he joined the faculty of obstetrics and gynecology at the University of Oklahoma School of Medicine. He was also on the staffs of Children's Memorial Hospital of the University of Oklahoma and Presbyterian Hospital. He was named emeritus professor at his retirement from the faculty about forty-five years later.

Dr. Coley was called to active duty during World War II and he retired with the rank of commander. He served with the U.S. Marine Corps in the South Pacific and later with the Navy in San Diego and Washington, D.C. He was a founder or charter member of numerous organizations in his home state. Among his civic endeavors he served as chairman of the Oklahoma Medical Board for Teachers' Retirement for twenty-five years.

Geographic distance never interfered with Dr. Coley's efforts on behalf of his alma mater. He served the alumni association as a class agent, member of the executive committee, and chair of the alumni division during the successful sesquicentennial fund drive. He served for six years as alumni trustee, not minding the commute to the board's regular meetings.

Marking the occasion of the hundredth anniversary of his father's graduation from Jefferson in 1880, Dr. Joe Henry Coley received an honorary doctor of science degree in 1980. Two years later he was the recipient of the alumni achievement award. In 1984 he won the Cornerstone Award at the President's Club dinner for his generosity to the university. The next year he won the Dean's Medal. In 1993 the Joe Henry Coley lectureship was established.

His portrait by Dean Paules was commissioned by the alumni association and presented to the university as part of the graduation and reunion week festivities in 1995.

The physician is depicted two-thirds length and life-sized, seated in a maroon leather armchair and holding an unidentified pamphlet. His head is turned so that he stares directly toward the viewer through narrowed blue eyes. The intense and penetrating gaze is softened by his snowy white hair and fair complexion, cleft chin, and slight trace of a smile, as well as his relaxed posture. As usual with portraits by Dean Paules the facial details are smoothly rendered in ultra-sharp detail to create an astonishing likeness.

The sitter's elegant attire includes a dark blue suit with vest and white pocket handkerchief, a white shirt, an almost iridescent pastel pink tie, gold cuff links and watch chain, and a Jefferson lapel pin. The atmospheric background is more loosely painted in warm neutral tones. The framed picture on the wall depicts the Daniel Baugh Institute of Anatomy and resembles a pastel painting by Dr. Hobart A. Reimann that was donated to Jefferson by Dr. and Mrs. Coley in 1981. Other medical attributes on the nearby table are Dr. Pascal B. Bland's textbook *Practical Obstetrics*, a bronze medallion that could be the Dean's Medal, and some yellow and black material that probably represents a folded academic gown.

At the portrait ceremony Dr. Coley reminisced engagingly about the history of the Daniel Baugh Institute of Anatomy and the "indelible impression" of his professors, especially Dr. J. Parsons Schaeffer teaching anatomy there:

> When Dr. Schaeffer appeared before the freshman class every afternoon dressed in a long black dissection gown, his steel gray hair immaculately combed, his silver-rimmed glasses on, and in his hand a long pointer that tapered to a sharp end, he was a commanding figure and made a fearsome and lasting impression. This instrument of terror, the pointer, he used in interrogating his students. The back seats of the amphitheater were filled first, each student hoping to be beyond the reach of his pointer. Dr. Schaeffer started the interrogation by calling the student's number and then he would fire a question, and while the student talked Dr. Schaeffer would begin to move the pointer in his direction and as the student's reply began to falter, he would push the pointer a little closer to him and say, "Yes, yes, doctor, what else, what else, come, come, surely you know this?" This was quite a lesson and quite an experience.

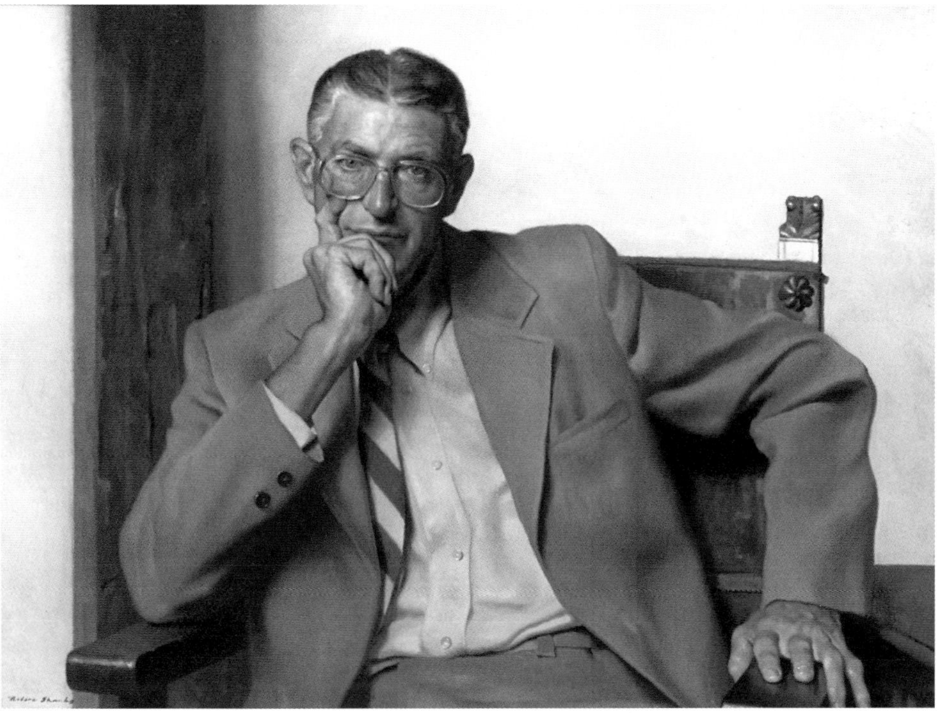

Portrait of Thomas D. Duane

(See color plate)

THOMAS DAVID DUANE, M.D., Ph.D. (1917-93)
By Nelson Shanks (b. 1937)

Oil on canvas
1982
30 1/4 x 40 1/4 in.

Signed lower left: "Nelson Shanks"

Given in 1982 by ophthalmology staffs at Wills Eye and Thomas Jefferson University Hospitals and former Jefferson ophthalmology residents

Accession number: 1982+e.P.02

Dr. Thomas D. Duane was recognized nationally for his clinical, research, and administrative contributions. He was a professor of ophthalmology and chairman of the department at Jefferson, and ophthalmologist-in-chief at Wills Eye Hospital.

Thomas Duane was born in 1917 in Peoria, Illinois, the son of an ophthalmologist. He graduated from Harvard University in 1939 and from Northwestern University Medical School in 1943. He completed an internship at Evanston Hospital Association while simultaneously earning a master's degree in physiology at Northwestern. He completed a residency in ophthalmology at Iowa State University and also received a Ph.D. for a thesis on the metabolism of the cornea.

Dr. Duane moved to a farm in Bethlehem, Pennsylvania where he opened a private practice. While working as a flight surgeon during the Korean conflict Dr. Thomas Duane conducted research on the cause of blackout, finding that it was retinal hypoxia rather than cerebral ischemia. Upon his return to civilian life he relocated to a farm in Bedminster, Bucks County, and combined private practice with research at the School of Medicine of the University of Pennsylvania.

In 1962 Dr. Duane assumed his posts as professor and chairman of the department of ophthalmology at Jefferson. Under his supervision a modern clinical facility in the Curtis Building was constructed in 1964, replacing the original eye clinic that dated to 1931. He was a pivotal contributor to the implementation of changes in the medical school curriculum at Jefferson. He retired from the chairmanship in 1981 and was named emeritus professor in 1988.

Dr. Duane was also ophthalmologist-in-chief at Wills Eye Hospital from 1973 until 1981. Established in 1834, Wills was the first hospital in the Western Hemisphere to be devoted to the eye. Duane became a driving force behind plans for a new Wills Hospital at Ninth and Walnut Streets, and worked tirelessly to create an affiliation between Wills and Jefferson. The staffs were amalgamated in 1980, and the agreement preserved the autonomy and identity of both hospitals.

Dr. Duane's three-year, comprehensive survey of American ophthalmological research (*Ophthalmic Research, U.S.A.*) was instrumental in the establishment of the National Eye Institute as part of the National Institutes of Health in 1968. Duane was appointed to the Eye Institute's National Advisory Eye Council and chaired its planning subcommittee and its melanoma task force. He was also a board member of the American Academy of Ophthalmology, the American Board of Ophthalmology, and the Association of University Professors in Ophthalmology.

When Dr. Duane retired from his chairmanships in 1981 he continued as professor of ophthalmology at Jefferson and consulting surgeon at Wills Eye and other hospitals. The Thomas David Duane Professorship in Ophthalmology was established at Jefferson in 1987, and he was named emeritus professor the following year.

In more than seventy scientific papers Dr. Thomas Duane reported his findings on microwave cataracts, the G force origin of blackout, Valsalva retinopathy, and the histopathology of white-centered hemorrhages, among other topics. He was the editor of *Clinical Ophthalmology* (1976) and *Biomedical Foundations of Ophthalmology* (with Dr. Edward A. Jaeger, 1982). The latter became a standard text.

Duane was honored to receive the Howe Award of the American Ophthalmological Society in 1981 and the Distinguished Service Award of the American Academy of Ophthalmology in 1985.

In 1982 Dr. Duane's portrait by Nelson Shanks was commissioned by the ophthalmological staffs at Wills Eye and Jefferson Hospitals joined by the Ex-Jefferson Ophthalmology Residents Society. The portrait presentation took place at Wills Eye Hospital on September 28, 1982 in conjunction with the hospital's 150th anniversary. The painting was presented to Thomas Jefferson University, but has been located in the auditorium at Wills Eye Hospital on "temporary display" ever since.

The physician is depicted half length and life-sized, leaning toward one side of his armchair and looking toward the viewer. His curious twisting posture implies two different mindsets: his right hand supports his chin in a traditional meditative pose, but his left elbow juts out sharply and his hand pushes against the chair arm, suggesting momentary action. This left arm is unnaturally attenuated.

Duane's knitted brows, tightly pressed lips, and penetrating gaze suggest thoughtfulness and reflection, but his posture suggests that a decision has just been reached. His khaki-colored suit and blue shirt are set off by a blue and white necktie with wide stripes. His personal energy is deftly echoed by elements of his costume in motion: the curving tie has moved off-center and is partially tucked under his jacket front, and the front placket of his shirt seems to undulate.

The painting's unconventional horizontal shape allows for the subject's unusual posture and for a close-up, almost iconic image. A vertical wooden beam in the background divides the silvery wall into two rectangular shapes, augmented by the low, horizontal back of the seventeenth-century-style, carved armchair (the same studio chair upholstered in reddish-orange fabric seen in Nelson Shanks's portrait of Dr. Lewis W. Bluemle Jr.).

Portrait of Thomas Behrendt

THOMAS BEHRENDT, M.D. (b. 1933)
By Eric van der Vlugt (b. 1955)

Oil on board
1978
40 x 32 in.

Signed and dated lower right: "Eric van der Vlugt/'78"

Given by JMC class of 1978
Accession number: 1978+e.P.01

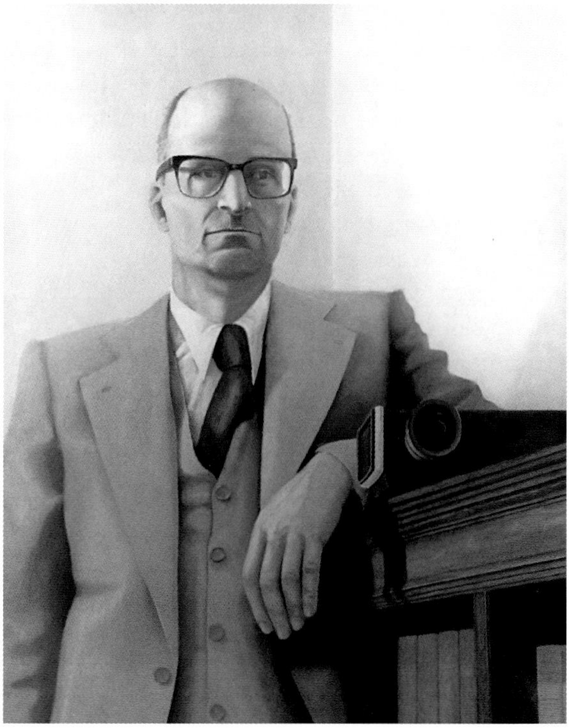

Dr. Thomas Behrendt had dual appointments as professor of ophthalmology and clinical associate professor of family medicine at Jefferson Medical College. The multitalented physician was a student of physical mathematics and spoke six languages.

Thomas Behrendt was born in Berlin, Germany in 1933 and reared in Brazil. He graduated from the Government Model School in Porto Alegre and the State University Medical School (1956) in the same city. He received general medical and ophthalmological training at the latter institution and served a preceptorship with his father, Dr. Rudolf Behrendt, former associate of the University of Berlin and director of the Elizabeth Stifft Eye and Ear Hospital in Berlin.

Between 1957 and 1962 Dr. Thomas Behrendt was eye surgeon and clinical ophthalmologist for the Clinica do Olhos Santa Efigenia and ophthalmic consultant to the Medical School of the University of Rio Grande do Sul in Porto Alegre. He was invited to join the Jefferson faculty in 1963 as assistant professor of ophthalmology and director of ophthalmic research. He rose in the academic ranks to professor of ophthalmology in 1971, and associate professor of family medicine in 1975. Behrendt was also staff ophthalmologist at Wills Eye and Fitzgerald Mercy Hospitals, and consultant at Magee Rehabilitation and Bryn Mawr Hospitals.

Dr. Behrendt was author of numerous ophthalmological articles, notably on the subjects of instruments of measurement and nonsurgical aspects of the retina. Jefferson students were exposed to his dynamic teaching methods in all four years, from freshmen introductory lectures to senior preceptorships. His interest in biophysics led to the development of a course in biomedical instrumentation. In 1977 and 1978 Behrendt was course director for "Ophthalmology for Non-ophthalmologists" at the American Medical Association conventions.

The senior class selected Dr. Thomas Behrendt as the portrait honoree in 1978. The commission was awarded to a young Philadelphia artist, Eric van der Vlugt, who was then a senior student at the Philadelphia College of Art and a friend of a Jefferson student in the class of 1978.

The stark and stylized depiction shows the physician half length and larger than life-sized, facing forward. His left arm rests on top of a bookcase and his elongated left hand hangs over the edge. His forearm is hidden by a slide projector on top of the bookcase. This machine was central to Behrendt's teaching technique, and students marveled at the clarity of his lectures which used as many as three projectors simultaneously.

His balding, bespectacled, square-jawed, thick-necked, hook-nosed, thin-lipped visage transmits a morose, almost forbidding expression. He appears pushed into a corner of the room and his downward stare avoids eye contact with the viewer. Equally unusual is the color scheme: the pale silver-yellowish walls are reflected on the subject's ashen face and his light gray suit; in striking contrast are his superbright, red necktie and the turquoise-bound books. The artist's command of the smooth surface is augmented by his use of geometrical internal shapes, extremely sharp contours, and contrast of dark shadows and strong highlights.

Eric van der Vlugt was born in Rotterdam, the Netherlands in 1955 and studied at the École des Beaux-Arts in Brussels. He graduated from the Philadelphia College of Art in 1978. In addition to oil painting, he is also a freelance illustrator and advertising artist. He has taught design at the Philadelphia College of Art and printmaking at the Maryland Institute of Art.

Portrait of Paul D. Zimskind

PAUL DONALD ZIMSKIND, M.D., Ph.D. (1931-76)
By Peggy Peplow (Mrs. William) Gummere

Oil on canvas
1983
44 x 34 in.

Signed lower right: "Peggy Peplow Gummere/'83"

Given in 1983 by family, friends, and colleagues
Accession number: 1983+e.P.08

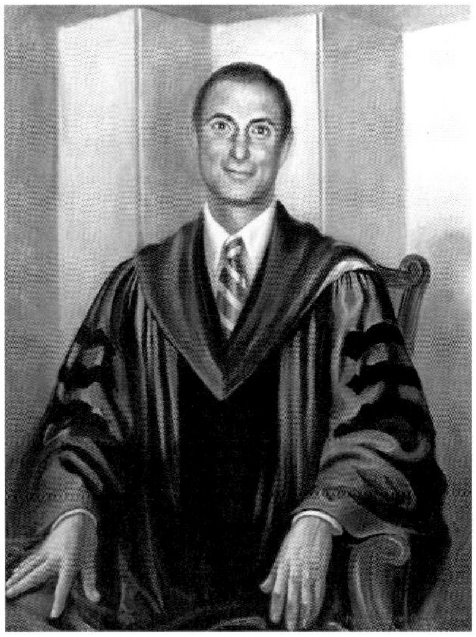

Dr. Paul D. Zimskind was one of the youngest physicians ever to head a medical department at Jefferson Medical College. He was appointed the Nathan Lewis Hatfield Professor of Urology and head of the department in 1967 when aged thirty-six.

Paul D. Zimskind was born in 1931 in Trenton, New Jersey, the son of Joshua N. Zimskind (JMC 1927). A *magna cum laude* graduate of Princeton University, he received his medical degree from Jefferson in 1957, followed by an internship and residency in general surgery and urology. Next he was a National Institutes of Health postdoctoral fellow in the department of physiology and earned his Ph.D. degree in 1964, while still a research associate in the urology department. He was the abstracting editor for *Urological Survey* and in 1963 received an award of merit from the American Medical Association for a urology exhibit.

In 1964 he was appointed assistant professor of urology and placed in charge of the urology research laboratories. Two years later he was honored to be selected as a John and Mary R. Markle Scholar in Academic Medicine, one of only twenty-five chosen nationally. His research in the urodynamics laboratory centered on the dynamics of normal and abnormal urinary conduction, renovascular hypertension, and enhancing the preservation of functional renal and ureteral tissue for future organ transplantation.

Tragically, the honored teacher and researcher died from a sudden illness in 1976. He had already published more than forty scientific papers and made over seventy presentations worldwide.

When Dr. Joshua Zimskind returned in 1982 for his fifty-fifth Jefferson reunion, he admired the portrait collection and discussed with his classmates the possibility of presenting a posthumous portrait of his son to the university. Through the efforts of Dr. S. Grant Mulholland who succeeded Dr. Paul Zimskind as chair of urology, a committee was formed to commission a portrait. The painting was presented in 1983 at a departmental ceremony and hung in the newly refurbished urology conference room.

For their son's portrait, Dr. and Mrs. Joshua Zimskind chose Peggy Peplow Gummere, a portrait and marine painter from Trenton. She depicted the subject half length and life-sized, seated in an armchair in front of a pale blue, folding screen. He gazes directly forward with a wide-eyed and amiable expression. He wears a black academic gown with green mantle over a white shirt and blue and white striped necktie. It is regretted that this portrait, albeit posthumous, has failed to convey the sitter's prodigious intelligence or hint at Dr. Paul Zimskind's vivaciousness and artistic gifts. He was also an accomplished violinist, thespian, photographer, and athlete.

Portrait of Jay J. Jacoby

JAY JOSHUA JACOBY, M.D., Ph.D. (b. 1917)
By Charles Diletto (1911-89)

Oil on canvas
1975
40 x 32 in.

Signed lower left: "Charles Diletto/1975"

Commissioned by JMC class of 1975, and given in 1992 by Henry A. Gerlach who received it from the artist's widow
Accession number: 1975+e.P.04

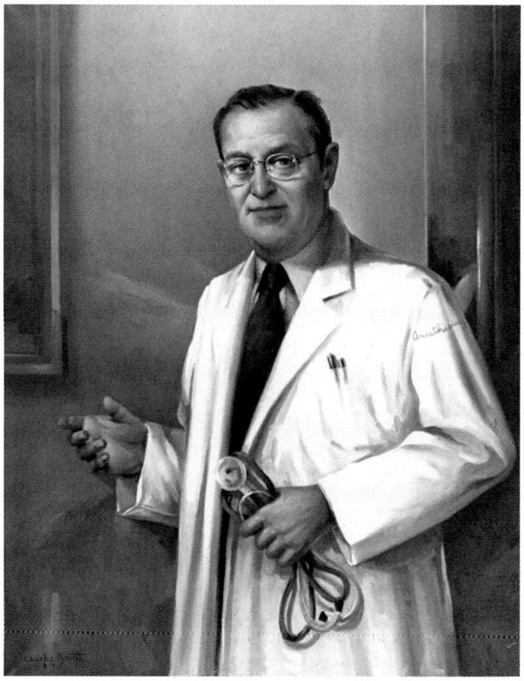

Dr. Jay J. Jacoby was professor of anesthesiology and served as second chairman of the department at Jefferson Medical College from 1965 to 1984.

A New York native, Jay J. Jacoby was born in 1917 and received both his undergraduate (1939) and medical (1941) degrees from the University of Minnesota. After interning at Kings County Hospital in New York, he served in the U.S. Army Medical Corps as anesthetist at bases ranging from Baffin Island near the North Pole to South Wales, and in hospitals in England, France, and Germany.

After the war he took a residency in anesthesiology at the University of Chicago-Billings Hospital while simultaneously earning a Ph.D. degree in pharmacology. From 1947 to 1959 he was a faculty member at Ohio State University and was appointed professor and chairman of the anesthesia department. He left for Marquette University Medical College where he was professor and chairman of anesthesia.

In 1965 the peripatetic physician was appointed to his posts at Jefferson. During his tenure as department chair the staff of physician anesthesiologists expanded from four to seventeen, and the residency program from two to thirty. When the nurses' training program was closed eleven nurse anesthetists remained as permanent staff members. An effective role model and communicator, the indefatigable physician recruited a number of students to his specialty. His graduates have yielded many professors and at least two chairmen of academic departments. Jacoby continued on the hospital staff as a practicing anesthesiologist after his retirement in 1984. He was named emeritus professor in 1988.

Jacoby authored at least one hundred articles and several book chapters on anesthesia topics. He was internationally known for his work on blind nasal intubation. He developed transtracheal resuscitation and did pioneer work on air embolism during surgery. He originated the Code Blue system of resuscitation in hospitals. He contributed the "Jefferson solution," a balanced mixture of ingredients familiarly known as "Jacoby's soup." Dr. Jacoby was a board member of the American College of Anesthesiologists and the American Society of Anesthesiologists.

Dr. Jay Jacoby's honors at Jefferson include the Christian R. and Mary F. Lindback Award for Distinguished Teaching. In 1975 the senior class chose him as portrait honoree and Charles Diletto was selected as artist.

The physician is depicted two-thirds length and life-sized, standing at an angle. His head is turned so that he looks off to the right with a slightly bemused expression, not making eye contact with the viewer. His left hand holds a stethoscope and his right hand gestures toward an unseen object. One wonders if the partial view of a frame could enclose a blackboard and the physician is meant to be teaching.

Jacoby wears a starched, white doctor's coat with the word "Anesthesiology" embroidered in red, and two pens emerge from his coat pocket. His shirt is bright blue and his necktie maroon, and the background wall is pale green. His face and hands are tightly and carefully brushed, while the costume and background are loosely brushed and rapidly executed.

Although the subject was esteemed at Jefferson, his portrait endured a disconcerting chain of events until it was restored to its rightful place in the portrait collection.

Records show that the painting was presented to and accepted by the university, to the satisfaction of the senior class portrait committee and to Dr. Jacoby whose hobby was painting. In fact, at the portrait ceremony Dr. Jacoby accepted the honor on behalf of the whole department of anesthesiology and invited all staff members to join him on the stage to "share the acclaim."

However, discontent with the likeness was expressed by the university art committee and some of Jacoby's family and friends. But Charles Diletto was insulted at their request to make substantial alterations or redo the portrait entirely. The painting remained with the artist until it was fortuitously returned to Jefferson for a five hundred dollar "rescue fee" in 1992 by Henry A. Gerlach, a local antique dealer and friend of the artist who had purchased the contents of Diletto's studio after his death.

Charles Diletto was born in Philadelphia in 1911 and studied at the Pennsylvania Academy of the Fine Arts, the Philadelphia College of Art, and the Graphic Sketch Club. Early in his career he supplemented his meager income by working on interior decorating projects in Catholic churches and by teaching. The latter pursuit he continued even through successful times.

Initially he concentrated on still lifes, landscapes, and seascapes, especially summer scenes from Gloucester and Rockport, Massachusetts painted in a loose, representational manner. Later he studied portrait painting privately with Robert Susan, and among his subjects were Secretary of the Treasury John A. Volpe, Philadelphia mayor Richardson Dilworth, and Philadelphia police chief Frank Rizzo.

Charles Diletto was president of Philadelphia's Da Vinci Art Alliance and conservator of portraits at the Philadelphia Sketch Club. He had more than a dozen one-man shows and crafted many of his frames by hand. In 1981 he won the Sketch Club's certificate of merit. The painter was also an accomplished baritone with the Philadelphia Operatic Society.

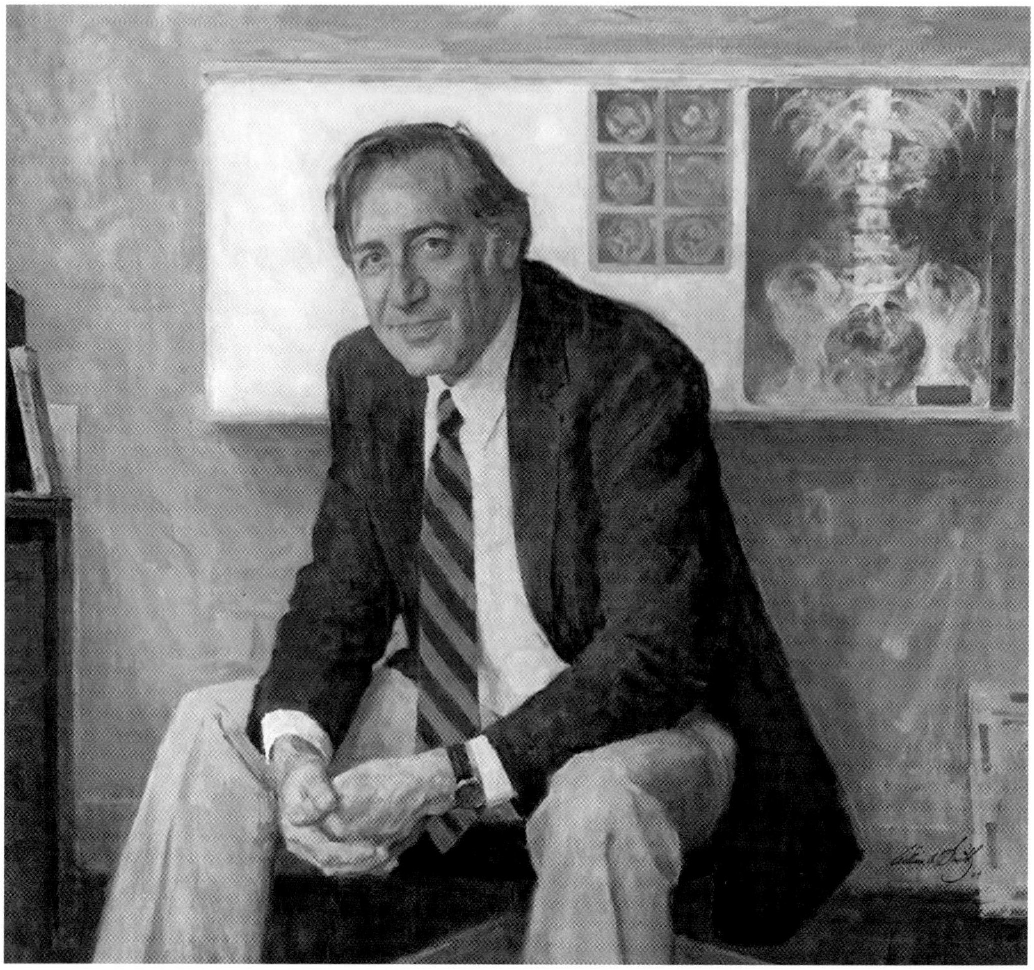

Portrait of Jack Edeiken

JACK EDEIKEN, M.D.
(b. 1923)
By William Arthur Smith (1918-89)

Oil on canvas
1984
36 x 38 3/4 in.

Signed and dated lower right: "William A. Smith/84"
Exhibition: Doylestown, Pa., *William A. Smith: A Retrospective,* James A. Michener Art Museum, Apr. 13-July 7, 1996

Given in 1984 by friends and colleagues
Accession number: 1984+e.P.01

Dr. Jack Edeiken was professor of radiology and chairman of the department at Jefferson from 1971 until his retirement in 1985. He was an internationally recognized authority on skeletal radiology.

Jack Edeiken was born in 1923 in Philadelphia, and graduated from Villanova College (1943) and the School of Medicine of the University of Pennsylvania (1947). After an internship at Mount Sinai Hospital in Philadelphia and a radiology residency at the Hospital of the University of Pennsylvania, he was a fellow at the National Cancer Institute from 1949 to 1951. He was on active duty for two years with the U.S. Army as chief of radiology at the 34th General Hospital in Orleans, France. He returned to the University of Pennsylvania School of Medicine as instructor, then assistant professor of radiology.

Dr. Jack Edeiken joined the faculty of Jefferson Medical College as assistant professor in 1958 and rose through the ranks to become full professor in 1967. He was serving as chief of radiologic diagnosis when he was appointed department chairman in 1971. During his tenure the department expanded programs in diagnostic ultrasonography, mammography, gastrointestinal radiology, thoracic radiology, head and neck radiology, and genitourinary radiology. Two of Edeiken's important research projects were on bone densitometry and the evaluation of thermography in mass screening for breast cancer. Shortly after his retirement in 1985 he was named emeritus professor, and moved to Houston's M. D. Anderson Cancer Center at the University of Texas.

Dr. Edeiken was the author of more than seventy articles and the textbooks, *Roentgen Diagnosis of Diseases of Bone* (with Philip J. Hodes, 1967) and *Roentgenologic Atlas of the Hand and Wrist in Systemic Disease* (with Morrison E. Kricun, 1973). He served as coeditor of *Critical Reviews in Clinical Radiological Sciences*, editor-in-chief of *Skeletal Radiology*, consultant editor of *Radiology* and *American Journal of Roentgenology*, consultant to *Computerized Tomography*, and coordinator of radiological topics for the *Journal of the American Medical Association.*

Among other honors, Dr. Edeiken was a visiting lecturer at the Mayo Clinic and the presidential lecturer of the American Academy of Orthopaedic Surgeons. He won the Special Lecturer Award of the Albert Einstein College of Medicine and the Malcolm B. Hanson Memorial Lecture Award of the University of Minnesota. He also received the gold medal of the Phi Lambda Kappa Medical Fraternity founded by his father, Louis Edeiken, M.D.

Dr. Edeiken was cofounder and president of the International Skeletal Society. He served as trustee of the American Board of Radiology and chairman of the commission on diagnostic radiology of the American College of Radiology. He was a consultant to the Surgeon General of the U.S. Air Force, the U.S. Public Health Service, the Veterans Administration Hospitals in Philadelphia and Wilmington, and the M. D. Anderson Cancer Center at the University of Texas.

When associates and friends decided to honor Dr. Jack Edeiken with his portrait in 1984, the presentation ceremony was arranged to coincide with the Philadelphia meeting of the International Skeletal Society, so that colleagues from all over the world could attend. At the ceremony President Lewis W. Bluemle Jr. congratulated Dr. Edeiken for giving his department an international distinction and for putting Thomas Jefferson University "on the world map in radiology."

Another speaker was Dr. Harold Jacobson, a distinguished colleague from Montefiore Medical Center, who said that Dr. Edeiken was a superb clinical radiologist with a "prescience for what's on the film." He added that Edeiken has trained "countless scientific progeny in whom he can take enormous pride." Dr. Morton G. Murdock, chairman of the portrait committee, spoke of his colleague's many extracurricular activities: "I knew Jack the chess master who wanted to challenge Bobby Fisher, Jack the skiing champion, Jack the skeet shooting champion, Jack the wizard of Wall Street, and smiling Jack the aviator." Another colleague characterized Edeiken as "outspoken, blunt, and direct; he tolerates fools, dishonest people, and charlatans badly; and he lets you know!"

The portrait by William A. Smith captures many of these personality traits. One notices immediately the burly physique of a former basketball and football player, his informal posture and slightly disheveled appearance, impressively large and strong hands, and alertness and energy.

The horizontal format best accommodates his unusual pose. Instead of the familiar armchair, he is seated on a stool and leans forward with hands clasped between his widespread legs. His body faces slightly left and he turns his head to engage the viewer. His square face with its chiseled features bears a pleasant and receptive expression. Long strands of brown hair fly away from his head. He is wearing a white shirt, dark blue unbuttoned blazer, gray trousers, and a striped gray, blue, and red necktie that dangles away from his body.

Behind the radiologist are light boxes with X-rays: a large one of the lumbar spine and pelvis, and six smaller ones that are computer tonograms of the spine. To the left is a cabinet with books and on the floor to the right rests a hospital chart. Dr. Edeiken seems eager to leap up from his stool and return to work.

The plaster walls of his office are loosely painted in gray, blue, green, and violet tones. The various elements of the painterly composition contribute to an allover, subtle harmony of cool tints.

Since William Smith was unable to attend the portrait ceremony, the articulate artist sent a videotaped message. He showed preliminary sketches of his portrait subject lecturing, teaching residents, and examining films. The artist tried to capture the movements and underlying physical tension of the athletic physician, and even interviewed associates and secretaries about his personality. Smith confessed to an earlier abandoned canvas that failed to communicate these qualities, although he said the original head was a very good likeness. The artist was pleased with the final version.

Portrait of Simon Kramer

SIMON KRAMER, M.D. (b. 1919)
By Charles F. Ellis

Oil on canvas
1983
40 x 30 in.

Signed and dated lower right: "Charles F. Ellis 1983"

Given in 1983 by friends and colleagues
Accession number: 1983+e.P.05

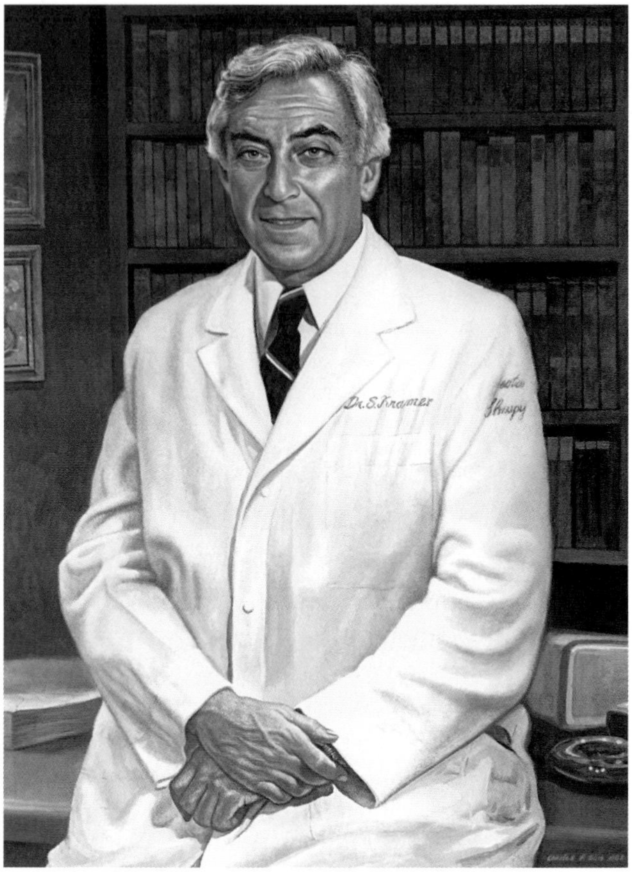

Dr. Simon Kramer was the first chairman of Jefferson's department of radiation therapy and nuclear medicine. The celebrated radiotherapist was honored in 1983 as the university's first Distinguished Professor.

A native of Chisinau, Rumania, Simon Kramer was born in 1919 and educated in London. He graduated from King's College and in 1943 from King's Hospital Medical School of the University of London. After serving with the British Medical Corps in Italy from 1943 to 1947, he was an intern at King's College Hospital and then a resident and fellow at the Meyerstein Institute of Radiotherapy, Middlesex Hospital, University of London. In 1952 he was a senior assistant at the Royal Cancer Hospital in London, then in 1954 he accepted positions as director of radiotherapy at Saint Boniface Hospital in Winnipeg, Canada and lecturer in radiotherapy at the University of Manitoba.

Dr. Simon Kramer joined the Jefferson faculty in 1956 as associate professor of radiology and rose in the academic ranks to professor in 1960. He served as chief of the division of radiation therapy and clinical radioisotope laboratories from 1956 to 1969, and chairman of the department of radiation therapy and nuclear medicine from 1969 to 1983. Under his leadership the department became known internationally for a ten-year study to determine the patterns of care in cancer management, thereby establishing national benchmarks and a method of quality assessment for radiation therapy. This was the first such study anywhere.[7]

Dr. Kramer was deeply involved in national and international activities relating to cancer and radiation therapy. He was president of both the American Society of Therapeutic Radiologists and the American Radium Society. He chaired the National Cancer Institute's patterns of radiation therapy care study and the Radiation Therapy Oncology Group, the latter a nationwide group of university departments. He was chairman of the committee on patterns in radiation therapy of the American College of Radiology. He was a member of advisory councils or panels of the Association for Brain Tumor Research, and the American Joint Committee task forces on head and neck tumors and central nervous system tumors.

Dr. Simon Kramer was the author of more than 190 publications and abstracts, with important contributions in the fields of head and neck tumors, brain and pituitary gland tumors, and breast cancer. He was on the editorial boards of the *International Journal of Radiation Oncology, Biology, Physics*, the *American Journal of Clinical Oncology/Cancer Clinical Trials*, the *Journal of Neuro-oncology*, and *Cancer Treatment Reports*.

Dr. Kramer was named a fellow of the Royal College of Radiologists and the British Institute of Radiology. He was the recipient of the Grubbe Award from the Chicago Radiological Society, and gold medal awards from the Fletcher Society at M. D. Anderson Hospital and Tumor Institute, the American Society of Therapeutic Radiologists, and the American College of Radiology. He delivered endowed lectures at the University of California San Francisco, the Radiological Society of North America, and the Roswell Park Memorial Institute.

In commemoration of a particularly notable career in

which he brought Jefferson to the forefront of radiation therapy, the first annual Simon Kramer lecture and symposium were inaugurated on Simon Kramer Recognition Day, November 4, 1983. An integral part of the celebration was the presentation of his portrait by friends and colleagues. During the ceremony President Lewis W. Bluemle Jr. announced that Dr. Simon Kramer had been named the first Distinguished Professor at Thomas Jefferson University. He saluted Kramer as a "legend in his own time" and a "warmhearted physician" who has made Jefferson a "better place to be." Dr. Kramer's children have followed in their father's footsteps at Jefferson: David was a member of the class of 1983, and Naomi the class of 1987.

Modestly acknowledging the day's festivities, Dr. Kramer expressed gratitude for having lived in an era of enormous change in medicine. When he began his career, apart from surgery there was little intervention in medicine. He determined "to do something for the patient" and became enormously impressed with the earliest interventional capability of radiation therapy. He felt extremely gratified by today's multidisciplinary approach to treatment of the cancer patient.

Kramer's portrait was painted by Philadelphia artist Charles Ellis. The physician is shown half length and life-sized, seated frontally with hands folded close to his body. The sitter's pleasant expression exudes eagerness and energy. He is wearing a white doctor's coat over a white shirt and dark blue necktie with narrow red and white stripes. Red embroidery on the pocket and sleeve of his coat reads "Dr. S. Kramer" and "...iation Therapy." The subject's skin tones are almost bronze colored, with tiny dots of reds, oranges, and neutrals contrasting with very bright highlights. The more smoothly brushed coat has cool blues, greens, and violets mixed in with the prevailing white tones.

The artist has emphasized certain anatomic details such as the differentiated strands of the sitter's gray hair and black eyebrows, creases in his forehead and cheeks, and the protruding veins of his hands. Office details include book-lined shelves, a stack of papers and an intercom speaker on his desk, and partial views of framed sailing and music pictures on the wall, alluding to Kramer's outside interests.

Portrait of Martha Southard

MARTHA SOUTHARD, M.D. (1922-79)
By Charles F. Ellis

Oil on canvas
1979
30 x 24 in.

Signed and dated lower right: "Charles F. Ellis 79"

Given in 1979 by friends and colleagues
Accession number: 1979+e.P.02

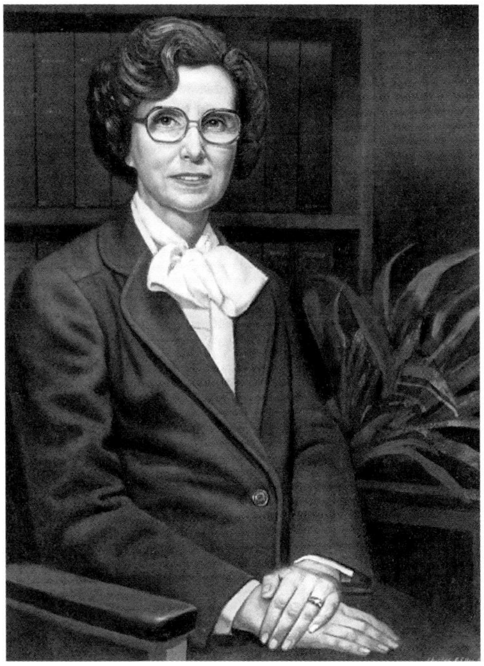

In 1969 Dr. Martha Southard, professor of radiology, was named head of the clinical division of the department of radiation therapy and nuclear medicine at Jefferson. She was appointed by Dr. Simon Kramer who later referred to her as his "right-hand person."

Born in 1922 in Columbus, Ohio, Martha Southard was the daughter, niece, and granddaughter of physicians. She graduated from Ohio State University in 1943 and the university's medical school in 1947. She spent two years as an intern in medicine and surgery at University Hospital in Columbus to prepare for a career in radiology. Her residency was at University Hospital in Columbus and at Cincinnati General Hospital. She was an assistant professor of radiology at Cincinnati and director of the cancer detection clinic.

Dr. Southard decided to practice radiation therapy full-time because she wanted greater interaction and involvement with patients. She pursued a fellowship in radiation therapy at the Hospital for Bone and Joint Diseases in New York, followed by positions as radiologist and associate professor of radiology at Temple University Hospital in Philadelphia.

In 1964 she joined the Jefferson faculty as chief of the radiation therapy department's clinical division and associate professor of radiation therapy. This was the year before Jefferson Medical College first conferred medical degrees on women. In 1968 she was promoted to professor of radiology, Jefferson's first woman full professor. She was also consultant to the Veterans Administration Hospital in Philadelphia and Cooper Hospital in Camden, New Jersey. Her clinical research in gynecological malignancies and lymphoma resulted in numerous papers and chapters in two textbooks.

Dr. Martha Southard died prematurely in 1979. She is best remembered for her humanitarian qualities. Written and oral recollections make repeated references to her compassionate care of patients, selfless devotion to duty, and inspiring teaching. She was particularly proud of training residents, including five women who became heads of their own departments of radiation therapy. With her thoughtfulness and kind, gentle manner, Dr. Martha Southard was said to have left behind a "legacy of love."

Her portrait by Charles F. Ellis was presented by friends and colleagues in celebration of her fifteenth year at Jefferson, just four months before her death. It was the first portrait of a female physician to enter the Jefferson collection.

She is depicted half length and life-sized, seated in an office armchair with hands resting calmly on her lap. Her head is turned to gaze directly and pleasantly toward the viewer. Her lips are parted but do not result in a genuine smile. She wears a dark blue suit and white blouse with a bow at the neck, and no jewelry except her wedding rings. Her businesslike attire, conventional pose, and open but reserved expression attest to a natural sense of modesty.

Book-lined shelves behind the figure and a dracaena plant on a table in the lower right corner complete the background elements. It is not uncommon in this era to find potted plants or flowers as a "softening" agent in portraits of professional women who have achieved success in male-dominated fields.

The Basic Scientists

Portrait of Gonzalo E. Aponte

GONZALO ENRIQUE APONTE, M.D. (1929-79)
By Robert Oliver Skemp (1910-84)

Oil on canvas
36 x 30 in.
1971

Signed and dated lower right: "Robert Oliver Skemp/1971"

Given by JMC class of 1971
Accession number: 1971+e.P.01

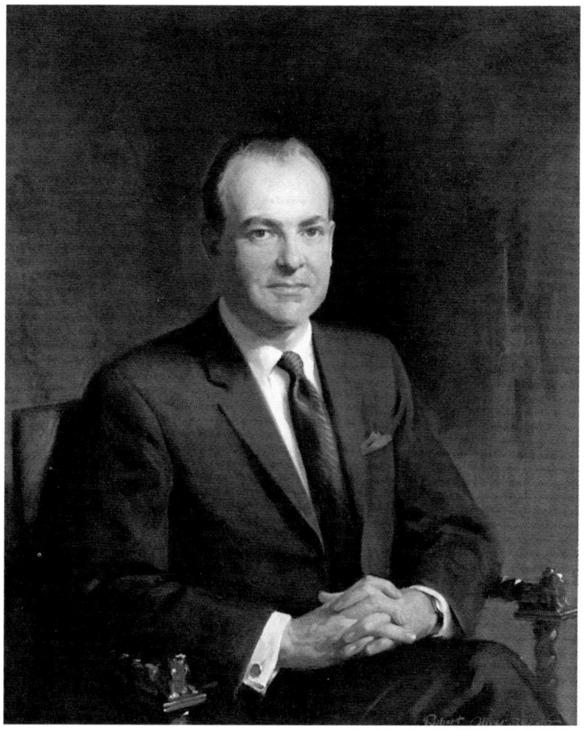

Dr. Gonzalo E. Aponte was an outstanding educator and chairman of the department of pathology, one of the youngest professors ever to head a Jefferson department.

A native of Santurce, Puerto Rico, Gonzalo Enrique

Aponte graduated first in his class from Georgetown University (1948) and from Jefferson Medical College (1952) where he was the winner of eight academic awards. From 1953 to 1957 he was an intern and resident in anatomical and clinical pathology at Jefferson Hospital, and a research fellow at the National Cancer Institute. After two years of service as chief of laboratories at the U.S. Naval Hospital in Guam, he returned to Jefferson as assistant professor of pathology in 1959.

From 1961 to 1966 Dr. "Henry" Aponte combined his clinical interests and teaching abilities as coordinator of oncologic teaching, followed by three years as assistant director of the cancer training program. In 1967 Aponte succeeded Dr. Peter A. Herbut as professor and chairman of the pathology department and director of the clinical laboratories. His interests centered on teaching and expanding the residency program.

His lectures, called "masterpieces" by appreciative students, were revised yearly to include the latest clinical data and were delivered with intelligence, energy, and an estimable stage presence. Aponte served on several student committees, and was chosen repeatedly to administer the Hippocratic Oath at commencement exercises and to address the sophomore class's Parents Day.

Dr. Aponte was a brilliant and honored scholar and educator. He was the first Jeffersonian to receive the Markle scholarship in medical science in 1960. He also received the Christian R. and Mary F. Lindback Award for Distinguished Teaching in 1962, and was named Clinical Scientist of the Year by the Association of Clinical Scientists in 1967. In 1977 he was elected president of Jefferson's alumni association.

His most noted publications concerned radiation-induced tumors and renal pathophysiology. He was president of the Pathology Society of Philadelphia and served on the editorial board of the *Annals of Clinical and Laboratory Science*. He was a member of the Educational Council of Foreign Medical Graduates. The Gonzalo Aponte Foundation was established in 1974 to sponsor Puerto Ricans and other Latin Americans in pathology fellowship programs at Jefferson.

Dr. Henry Aponte's sudden, untimely death on June 15, 1979 at age forty-nine from cardiac arrythmia occurred at the peak of his career. Board of trustee minutes of September 10 recorded a posthumous tribute with his appointment as the first Peter A. Herbut Professor of Pathology. Hundreds of devoted friends, colleagues, family, and students raised funds to endow the Gonzalo Enrique Aponte Chair of Pathology. His generous bequest to the department of pathology included all of his medical books, journals, slides, and literature.

When the senior class chose him as portrait honoree in 1971, he was one of the youngest professors so honored. He responded to the warm encomiums and standing ovation at the presentation by describing his joy, "I feel this happy event far beyond what you could imagine. Computers could not analyze it; nor could I describe it if I tried with all my might."

Robert O. Skemp depicted the pathologist two-thirds length and life-sized, seated in an armchair with folded hands. He gazes directly toward the sitter with soft, dark brown eyes under thick eyebrows and a high forehead topped with black hair. His pleasant expression seems restrained compared with the open grin or hearty smile displayed on many contemporary photographs. Dr. Aponte's natural vitality also extended to passionate extracurricular interests in poetry, theater, sports, and the history of medicine.

Unlike his customary, more flamboyant apparel, Dr. Aponte's attire in the portrait is suavely elegant, but relatively sedate. He wears a dark blue suit, a white shirt with gold cuff links, a navy and lavender striped necktie, and a red pocket handkerchief. His armchair is not the mundane office type, but an ornate, seventeenth-century-style chair carved with rope-twist arms and lion head grips. The upholstery is green, as is the atmospheric background.

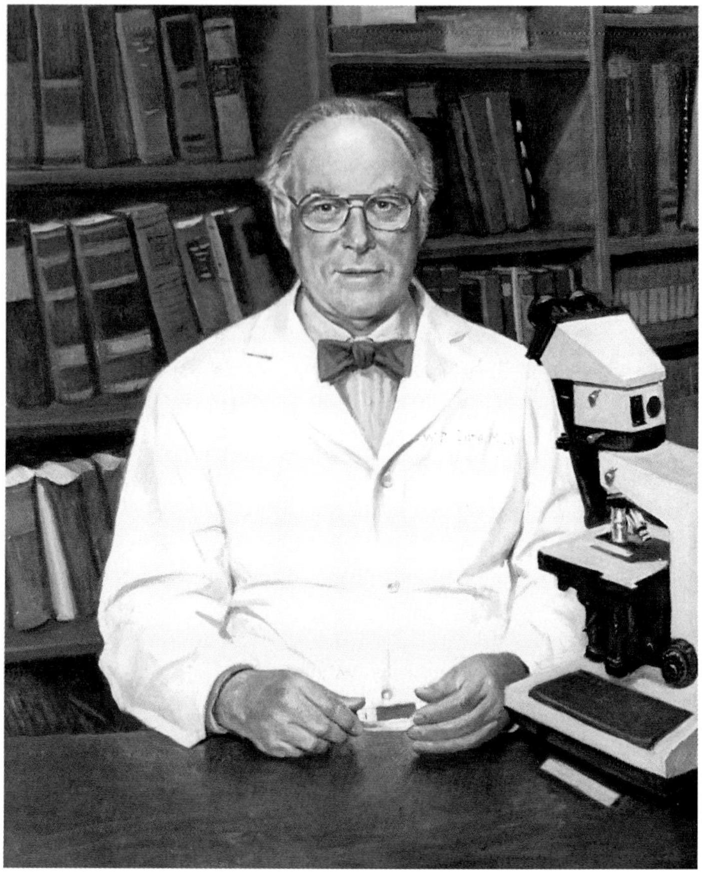

Portrait of Warren R. Lang

WARREN REICHERT LANG, M.D. (1918-87)
By Alden MacMaster Wicks (1914-87)

Oil on canvas
36 x 30 in.
1985

Signed lower left: "Wicks"

Given by JMC class of 1985
Accession number: 1985+e.P.01

After twenty years of practicing obstetrics and gynecology at Jefferson, Dr. Warren R. Lang's interest in cytopathology led him to take a second residency in pathology. He was later appointed chairman of the department of pathology and named the first Gonzalo E. Aponte Professor of Pathology.

Born in Philadelphia in 1918, Warren Lang graduated first in his class both from Temple University (1939) and Jefferson Medical College (1943) where he won seven awards. After internship and residency in obstetrics and gynecology at Jefferson, he served two years with the U.S. occupation forces in Korea as an artillery battalion surgeon. He returned to Jefferson as assistant to Dr. Lewis C. Scheffey and maintained a busy private practice, while rising through the academic ranks to become full professor in 1963.

Lang was a founding fellow of the American College of Obstetricians and Gynecologists. He was among the first in this country to reintroduce colposcopy and served as president of the American Society for Colposcopy and Colpomicroscopy. He was nationally recognized for his research and writing in vaginal biology, cytology, and diseases of the cervix.

When Dr. Lang decided to switch specialties he took training in pathology first under Dr. Gonzalo E. Aponte and then continued his residency at Case Western Reserve University. He returned to Jefferson as assistant professor of pathology in 1971. He was made associate professor in 1977 and named acting chairman of the department in 1979 upon the death of Dr. Aponte. In 1984 he was proud to be appointed the Gonzalo E. Aponte Professor of Pathology and chairman of the department, and served until his retirement in 1986.

From 1973 to 1982 Lang had been a professor of cytotechnology in the school of cytotechnology in Jefferson's College of Allied Health Sciences, and he became director of the school in 1982. In 1984 he was elected president of the American Society for Cytology and also received its George N. Papanicolaou Award that same year. Dr. Lang was a prolific author and editor of *Benign Lesions of the Cervix* (1963) and *Gynecology of the Woman over Sixty-five* (1967), both for *Clinical Obstetrics and Gynecology*.

Two years after his death in 1987 Thomas Jefferson University announced his bequest of one and one-half million dollars to the department of pathology. One of the largest gifts ever received from an alumnus, the bequest endowed the Warren R. Lang Professorship of Pathology and Cell Biology. In 1989 the Warren R. Lang lectureship was established jointly by members of Jefferson's departments of obstetrics and gynecology and of pathology and cell biology.

Dr. Warren R. Lang received the Christian R. and Mary F. Lindback Award for Distinguished Teaching in 1977. Students recalled that he often said, "Trust your Uncle Warren," and indeed, they trusted the man and his personal interest in their welfare and revered his scholarship and dedication to teaching. He could be alternately caring or stern toward students while impressing upon them the necessity of studying hard. His lively lectures were punctuated with jokes and puns (compiled in a little black book), admonishing aphorisms like "loose lips sink ships," exhortative acronyms like "SWEAT" ("study with enthusiasm and tenacity"), references to his personal interests in opera, professional wrestling, and classical languages, and the use of a whistle to command attention.

The class of 1985 chose Dr. Warren R. Lang as portrait honoree. Depicted by Alden M. Wicks, the physician is shown half-length and slightly smaller than life-sized, seated behind a desk. He looks directly toward the observer with a friendly and patient expression. He is wearing a white doctor's coat, maroon bow tie, and blue shirt. His name is embroidered in blue on his coat pocket. He has paused in his work to acknowledge an unseen visitor, and then will study the slide he holds in the microscope on the right.

Behind the figure are shelves crammed with colorfully bound medical books of varying sizes. The allover loose paint style, coupled with the slanted direction and asymmetrical arrangement of the books, contributes to an energetic composition alluding to the dynamic personality of the sitter.

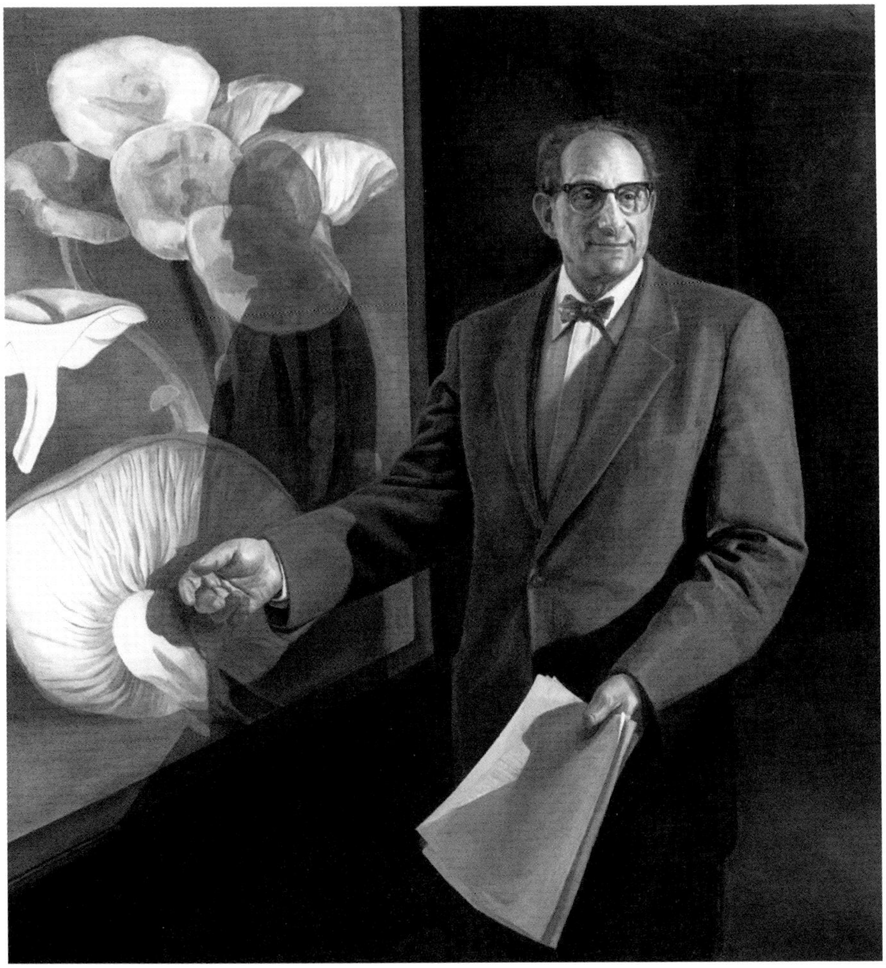

Portrait of Robert J. Mandle

ROBERT J. MANDLE, Ph.D.
(1919-95)
By Rebecca Louise Williams
(b. 1957)

Oil on canvas
1984
55 1/2 x 53 1/2 in.

Signed and dated lower right:
"BEKI WILLIAMS 1984"

Given by JMC class of 1984
Accession number: 1984+e.P.03

Dr. Robert J. Mandle was a professor of microbiology who spent thirty-three years on the Jefferson faculty. An accomplished biologist with many interests, he taught bacteriology, mycology, cell biology, and plant pathology.

"Bob" Mandle was born in 1919 in New York and reared in northern New Jersey. He was influenced in his choice of career by reading Paul de Kruif's *Microbe Hunters* as a youth. After graduating from Lebanon Valley College in Annville, Pennsylvania (1942), he served in the South Pacific at a mobile hospital in Samoa and as a medical corpsman on a U.S. Navy minesweeper. After his discharge he worked as a technician at the Rockefeller Institute for three years, then earned a doctorate in microbiology at the University of Pennsylvania in 1951.

That same year Dr. Mandle was appointed instructor in microbiology at Jefferson Medical College. He rose through the academic ranks until his appointment as professor in 1965. An inspiring teacher, Dr. Mandle formed close relationships with students in the small laboratories that he advocated, and served as a "stern but fatherly mentor" to students who needed tutoring. He brought his enthusiasm for identifying and photographing plants, especially cacti, orchids, wildflowers, and mushrooms, into the laboratory and the lecture hall. He received the Christian R. and Mary F. Lindback Award for Distinguished Teaching in 1979. He served as chairman of the university art committee from 1972 until 1986 when he retired and was named professor emeritus.

Dr. Mandle was an active faculty member of a master's program in clinical microbiology, and many of his doctoral students embarked on significant careers in academic microbiology. He also participated in a Jefferson program to inspire students from South Philadelphia High School to enter scientific careers. Outside the university he was a dedicated scout master who helped more than twenty young men reach the rank of Eagle Scout.

Dr. Mandle's scientific interests centered on the microbiology and epidemiology of staphylococci, organisms of the gut, and mycology. In 1974 he received the William H. Rorer Award of the American College of Gastroenterology. In 1992 he was awarded the medal of Jefferson's College of Graduate Studies to honor his years of teaching, research, and service. He was a councilor of the American Society for Microbiology.

In 1980 he had received a Fulbright-Hays Award, granted by the Council for International Exchange of Scholars, to teach diagnostic mycology at the Pontifica Universidad Catolica in Quito, Ecuador. He also acted as consultant to the school's clinical laboratories, set up a mycology laboratory, and stimulated the faculty to teach and do research in the field. In summarizing the semester's experience, Mandle was most proud that "important bridges had been built between the university, the community, and the U.S."

Students in the class of 1984 chose Dr. Robert J. Mandle as portrait honoree. The depiction is as daring and unconventional as that of Dr. Richard Berry, though in different ways. Mandle conceived the complex composition with its dual depiction of him as teacher and as "mushroomer," and awarded the commission to a promising but unknown young artist, Rebecca L. Williams.

The microbiologist had a lifelong interest in wild mushrooms: the mycorrhizal or parasitic relationship with trees, the microscopic morphology of spores for identification, and the toxicities of some classes. He was also interested in mushrooms as a gourmet food source, and his photographs show that he was keenly aware of their beauty.

In the portrait Dr. Mandle is shown two-thirds length and life-sized, teaching in a lecture room. He stands off-center to the right gazing toward an unseen audience and gesturing with an open hand toward a projected slide of mushrooms. Superimposed on the brightly lit screen is a profile shadow of his figure. His head and the sheaf of lecture notes in his left hand are partially spotlighted by the projector's beam of light.

Mandle's distinguishing features such as receding and close-cropped dark hair, high forehead, hooded eyes behind large glasses, long nose, wide mouth, and thin lips, accord with contemporary photographs as does his amiable, yet forceful expression. His unusual attire consists of a wide-shouldered, bright maroon sport jacket combined with a white shirt, a trademark red, patterned bow tie, and brown trousers. Completing the uncommon color scheme, the mushrooms are drawn in shades of bright yellow, white, orange, and brown.

At the portrait presentation ceremonies, Jussi J. Saukkonen, M.D., dean of the College of Graduate Studies, commended Dr. Mandle as the "conscience" of the faculty, always ready to help solve "thorny" problems. President Lewis W. Bluemle Jr. praised Mandle's "immense contributions to the quality of life" at Jefferson: his "stewardship" of Jefferson culture, its professional values, its art, and its human relationships and common courtesies.

"Beki" Williams was born in 1957 in Canton, Ohio. She attended Kent State University before and after graduating from the Pennsylvania Academy of the Fine Arts in 1982. She said that she studied scientific illustrations of mushrooms for many weeks in order to satisfy Dr. Mandle's requirements for botanical accuracy and artistry in his portrait. Williams also painted portraits of two deans at Temple University School of Medicine before moving to San Francisco where she has been teaching figure drawing and painting at an art academy.

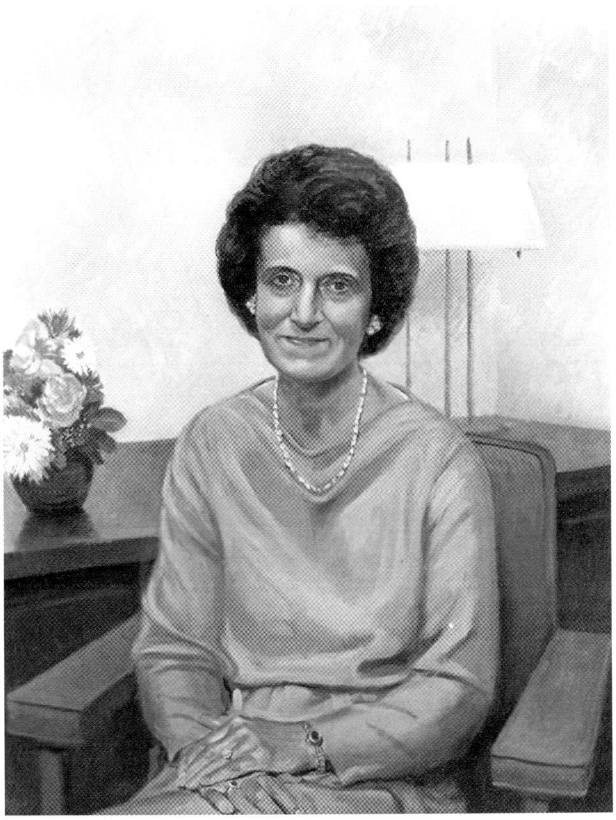

Portrait of Doris E. Bowman

DORIS E. BOWMAN, R.N., M.S. (Ed.) (1920-97)
By Alden MacMaster Wicks (1914-87)

Oil on canvas
1980
28 x 22 in.

Signed lower left: "Wicks"

Given by the Diploma School of Nursing class of 1980
Accession number: 1980+e.P.01

Doris E. Bowman, R.N. was director of the Jefferson Hospital School of Nursing from 1958 to 1982. She served with distinction during tumultuous and transitional times for the nursing profession.

Doris Bowman was born in 1920 in Hanover, Pennsylvania, and graduated from the Jefferson Hospital School of Nursing in 1942. During World War II she served at the thousand-bed General Hospital of Unit Thirty-Eight outside Cairo, Egypt. In 1953 she earned a master of science degree in education at the University of Pennsylvania and taught in New Jersey briefly.

Doris Bowman joined the nursing faculty at Jefferson the following year as an instructor in pediatrics. In 1956 she was named associate director of the nursing school, and two years later she succeeded Mable Prevost as director. Bowman served as director for twenty-four years until her retirement in 1982. She was named emeritus professor, the first member of the College of Health Professions faculty and the first woman in Thomas Jefferson University history to be so honored. She died in 1997 and was interred in Arlington National Cemetery, Washington, D.C.

One of Doris Bowman's major achievements was the attainment of the long-sought designation of full accreditation from the National League of Nursing in 1960, a seal of approval that was voluntary but invaluable in attracting the highest quality students and faculty. An advisory committee was formed in 1958, chaired by Dr. Baldwin Keyes and comprised of representatives from the board of trustees, medical staff, hospital administration, and nurses' alumnae association, in addition to the nursing school director, a clergyman, and other community educators. Other innovations during Doris Bowman's tenure were the teaching of basic nursing techniques by closed circuit television, and the launching of a new, one-year school of practical nursing.

In 1968 the school of nursing was absorbed into the newly organized School (later College) of Allied Health Sciences (now College of Health Professions). In 1972 a baccalaureate (B.S.N.) program in nursing was introduced in which students entered as juniors after completing the first two years of undergraduate study elsewhere. Male students were admitted starting in 1973.

At this time Jefferson was supporting three nursing

programs, each with its own faculty, facilities, and programs: baccalaureate, diploma, and practical. In 1979 an ad hoc committee was formed to evaluate conflicts among the three groups, and after much soul-searching it was decided to phase out diploma and practical nursing in favor of the baccalaureate program over a three year period.

Doris Bowman was deeply touched at the unveiling of her portrait at the 1980 nursing commencement, a surprise planned by the graduating class. Portraitist Alden M. Wicks must have worked from photographs. The subject is depicted two-thirds length and slightly smaller than life-sized, seated in a leather armchair with hands resting on her lap. She faces the viewer with a warm and engaging smile under bright eyes and full, dark brown hair. She is attired in a bright blue, long-sleeved, cowl-neck dress, complemented by a pearl necklace and cluster earrings, a watch, and two rings. On the sideboard behind her are a vase of fresh flowers and a table lamp.

The portrait of Doris Bowman, along with that of an earlier Jefferson nurse, the formidable Clara Melville, hang in McClellan Hall with portraits of other Jefferson administrators. The depiction of the relaxed and smiling Miss Bowman wearing street attire is infinitely softer and more approachable than the representation of the dour Miss Melville, standing rigidly at attention in her starched white uniform.

Jefferson School of Nursing: Three Nursing Uniforms

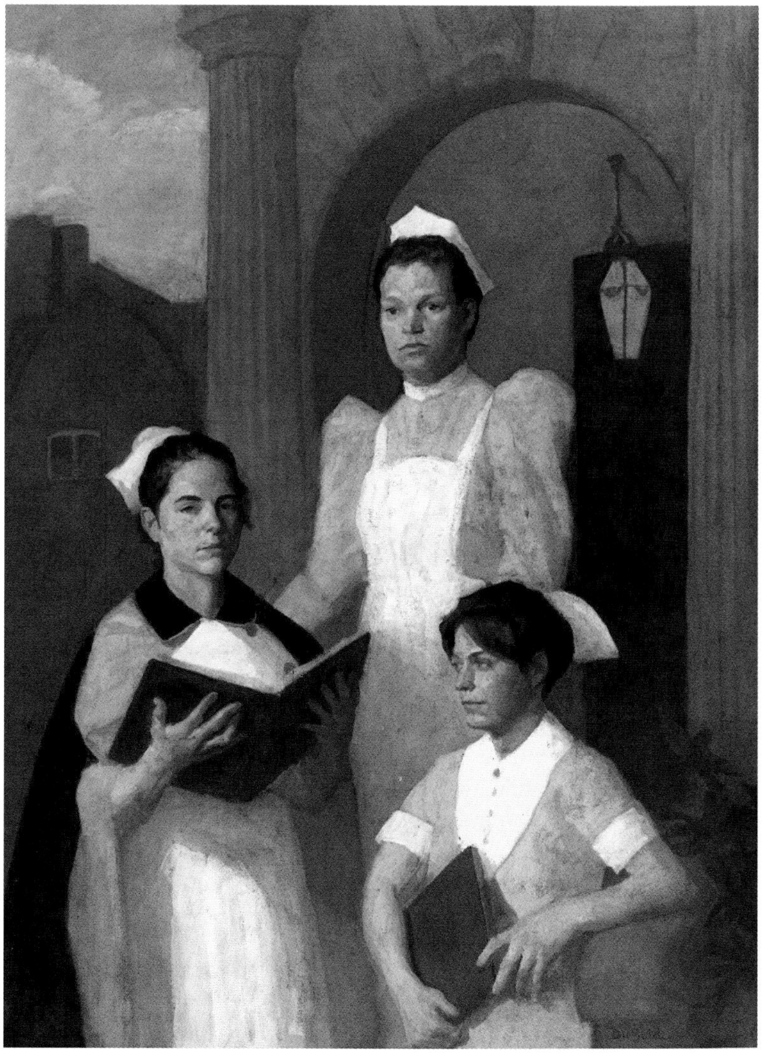

JEFFERSON SCHOOL OF NURSING: THREE NURSING UNIFORMS
By Paul DuSold (b. 1963)

Oil on canvas
1992
40 x 30 1/4 in.

Signed lower right: "DuSold"

Commissioned in 1992 by Jefferson School of Nursing class of 1942 in honor of their fiftieth graduation and in memory of their deceased classmates

Accession number: 1992+e.P.02

At the initiative of emeritus professor of nursing Doris E. Bowman, the Jefferson School of Nursing class of 1942 commissioned a painting depicting three student nursing uniforms in 1992. The painting was in honor of the class's fiftieth anniversary and in memory of their deceased classmates.

The origin for the painting was the commencement of 1982, the last class to graduate from the School of Nursing, when three students modeled uniforms from the past and present. Photographs of the event and archival information were provided to artist Paul DuSold.

The figure in the center wears a pink uniform from the 1890s with bishop's collar, ankle-length skirt, and white apron. The figure on the left is dressed in the white uniform of the late 1930s to the late 1950s. It retains the bib and apron, but the collar is open and the skirt is a bit shorter; a dark blue cloak has been added. The figure on the right wears the modern one-piece, wash-and-wear, pink uniform with short skirt and no apron, worn from 1959 through 1982. All three students wear starched white caps and the two in front hold books.

The figures are standing on the steps leading to the 1907 Jefferson Medical College Hospital, with its distinctive entrance of an arch flanked by columns. Above the door is a glowing yellow lantern, possibly a reference to the attribute seen in many portrayals of Florence Nightingale.

Although the painting was unveiled to everyone's initial delight at the fiftieth anniversary dinner, a moment later there was a group shouting as one voice, "That hair has got to go!" The artist had put shoulder length hair on the student representing this class's era (on the left), and the painting was summarily returned to the artist to correct this infraction of the rules.[8] A letter from an alumna in the class of 1942 complained about the figures' facial expressions. She said, "Would you want to be cared for by a nurse looking so somber?" She surmised that the artist must have been related to someone on the committee or the board of trustees.

Actually the noted artist Paul DuSold had already portrayed the university art committee chairman, Russell W. Schaedler, M.D., who recommended him to the nurses. DuSold was born in 1963 and was a native of Chicago. He studied fresco painting privately in 1980 with B. F. Long in Glendale Springs, North Carolina. He graduated from the Pennsylvania Academy of the Fine Arts in 1985, and then studied again with Long in Paris in 1987.

Paul DuSold has had one-man shows at Meredith College in Raleigh, North Carolina in 1986, the Giannetta Gallery in Philadelphia in 1988, and the Wayne Art Center in suburban Philadelphia in 1998. He won the Mary Beaumont Prize in 1987 at the Philadelphia Sketch Club.

Among DuSold's notable Philadelphia portrait subjects are Nancy Brewster Grace, Benita Valente, Edmund N. Bacon, and Robert Montgomery Scott. His portraits are found in the following Philadelphia institutions and firms: the Franklin Institute, Pennsylvania Hospital, the Provident Mutual Life Insurance Company, the Kling-Lindquist Partnership, the Union League of Philadelphia, and the Crown, Cork and Seal Company.

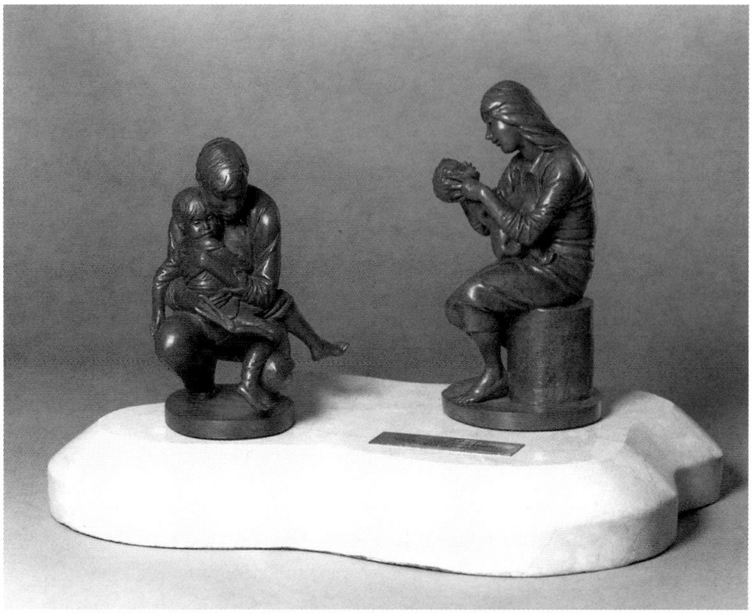

Family Group

FAMILY GROUP
By Bruno Lucchesi (b. 1926)

Bronze, marble
1976
11 1/2 x 19 x 13 1/8 in.

Signed on integral base of each group: "B. LUCCHESI"

Given in 1976 by Gustav W. Anderson (JMC 1946) in memory of his wife, Helen Dick Anderson (JMC Nursing 1945)
Accession number: 1976+e.S.02

A small, bronze figural group was donated to Jefferson's School of Nursing in 1976 by Gustav W. Anderson, M.D., a 1946 Jefferson Medical College alumnus, in memory of his wife, the former Helen Dick, a 1945 Jefferson nursing school alumna.

The works were sculpted by Bruno Lucchesi, and originally issued as separate sculptures by the Franklin Mint in 1976. Now mounted together on a marble base, the smoothly carved, intertwining figures are tender and universal images of parenthood.

Mother and Child depicts a mother holding a baby and sitting on a tree stump. The nude child faces the young woman with its legs straddling her waist and its head cradled in her hands. The mother wears a long-sleeved dress, her long hair is parted in the center, and her feet are bare. *Father and Son* depicts a father crouching on his heels holding tightly to a wriggling young boy on his lap. Both have bare feet and are dressed in shirt and trousers. The young father holds a book in his free hand, as though attempting to read to the unreceptive child.

Bruno Lucchesi was born in 1926 to a family of farmers and shepherds in the Italian village of Fibbiano Montanino in the province of Lucca. His education at the local monastery was paid for by produce from the farm. His early attempts at wood carving were encouraged and in 1947 he enrolled at the Lucca Art Institute. In 1950 he moved to Florence where he continued to study and worked in a factory that produced ceramic religious figurines. He also became a part-time assistant professor of ornamental objects at the Art Academy's school of architecture, and received occasional commissions for sculpted decorations and ceramic murals for buildings.

In 1957 Lucchesi moved to New York with his American wife who had been studying art in Florence. At first he worked in a factory making manikins. When his little terra cotta figures displayed in his father-in-law's Greenwich Village frame shop began to sell quickly, he decided to devote himself fulltime to sculpture.

Lucchesi's subjects are archetypal folk shown in the intimate details of everyday life, ranging in size from just a few inches to larger than life. From the artist's humble beginning his figurative sculptures in bronze and terra cotta have entered collections at the Whitney Museum, Brooklyn Museum, Hirshhorn Museum and Sculpture Garden, National Academy of Design, Dallas Museum of Fine Arts, Ringling Museum of Art, Pennsylvania Academy of the Fine Arts, and many university galleries. Since 1961 Lucchesi has had numerous one-man shows at the Forum Gallery in New York and at galleries throughout the country.

Among Lucchesi's commissions were an altar with four friezes for the Cathedral of San Martino in Lucca, an award sculpture for the American School of Ballet in New York, and art works for numerous banks and companies in the New York area. He enjoyed teaching at the New School for Social Research and at the National Academy of Design, and collaborated on three books about the craft of sculpting with Margit Malmstrom.

Bruno Lucchesi has won a Guggenheim fellowship and four medals from the National Academy of Design. He received gold medals from the National Arts Club in 1963 and the National Sculpture Society in 1977. He was particularly honored to win a medal from the City of Lucca in 1976 and the Italian Cultural Society's Lion of San Marco Award in 1981.

---

1. The selection was made by Jefferson's interim president George M. Norwood Jr., with the research assistance of librarian Robert T. Lentz. The names inscribed on *The Winged Ox* are: Hippocrates, Aulus Cornelius Celsus, Soranus of Ephesus, Galen, Rhazes, Maimonides, Paracelsus, Ambroise Paré, Michael Servetus, Andreas Vesalius, William Harvey, Thomas Willis, Marcello Malpighi, Anton van Leeuwenhoek, Hermann Boerhaave, Giovanni Battista Morgagni, Albrecht von Haller, John Hunter, John Morgan, Philippe Pinel, Benjamin Rush, Edward Jenner, René Théophile Hyacinthe Laennec, Richard Bright, Thomas Addison, Robert James Graves, Samuel David Gross, Claude Bernard, James Marion Sims, Florence Nightingale, Ignaz Philipp Semmelweis, William Thomas Green Morton, Rudolph Virchow, Louis Pasteur, Jean Martin Charcot, Lord Joseph Lister, Silas Weir Mitchell, Carlos Juan Finlay, Robert Koch, Wilhelm Konrad Roentgen, William Osler, Ivan Petrovich Pavlov, William Henry Welch, Walter Reed, Santiago Ramón y Cajal, Paul Ehrlich, Sigmund Freud, Marie Curie, Harvey Cushing, and John H. Gibbon Jr.

2. "TJU's New Hospital: Integrating Medical Education with a Total Range of Patient Care," *Jefferson Medical College Alumni Bulletin* 25 (winter 1976): 4.

3. Lewis W. Bluemle Jr., M.D., "Thomas Jefferson University, A.D. 2000," *Jefferson Medical College Alumni Bulletin* 28 (spring 1979): inside front and back covers.

4. Jack Smith, "Painting It Like It Is," *Philadelphia Inquirer*, Dec. 11, 1988, magazine section.

5. Cynthia J. T. Clendenin, "An Interview with John H. Hodges, '39," *Jefferson Medical College Alumni Bulletin* 41 (spring 1992): 5-7.

6. "Profile," *Jefferson Medical College Alumni Bulletin* 26 (winter 1977): 24.

7. Frederick B. Wagner Jr., M.D., *Thomas Jefferson University: Tradition and Heritage* (Philadelphia: Lea & Febiger, 1989), 750.

8. "Class of '42—Fiftieth Anniversary," *Nurses Alumni Association Bulletin* (fall 1992): 14.

CHAPTER 10

Late Eighties through the Nineteen-nineties

There were significant architectural additions to the campus and administrative changes at Thomas Jefferson University in recent years. New structures included the Bluemle Life Sciences Building and the Medical Office Building. In addition, a new Emergency and Trauma Center in the Main and Thompson Buildings was opened in 1990, tripling the previous capacity; it is one of only four facilities in the United States to be both a Level One Regional Resource Trauma Center and a federally designated Spinal Cord Injury Center.

A successful Decade Fund of the Eighties far surpassed the original goal of sixty-five million dollars to "attract the best possible new faculty leadership, to encourage research, and to offset imminent decreasing external support by government and third-party payors."[1] The Jefferson 2000 Fund of the 1990s is raising two hundred million dollars to fulfill these and other goals in preparation for the unprecedented changes occurring in health care delivery and medical education.

In 1984 Edward C. Driscoll succeeded Frederic L. Ballard as chairman of the board of trustees. Driscoll served until 1990 when James W. Stratton was elected chairman. In January 1995 Stratton was succeeded by Jack Farber.

In August 1995 Thomas Jefferson University and the Main Line Health System signed an agreement establishing a new nonprofit, corporate entity known as the Jefferson Health System, an integrated health care delivery system. It includes Thomas Jefferson University Hospitals, Incorporated, Bryn Mawr Hospital, Bryn Mawr Rehabilitation Hospital, Lankenau Hospital, and Paoli Memorial Hospital. Thomas Jefferson University, a separate entity composed of Jefferson Medical College, the College of Graduate Studies, and the College of Health Professions, is the primary academic affiliate of the Jefferson Health System. Dr. Paul C. Brucker, president of the university, became chairman of the board of the Jefferson Health System, and Douglas S. Peters was named the organization's president and chief executive officer. The late 1990s witnessed the addition of other established institutions to the Jefferson Health System, including Frankford Health Care System and the Albert Einstein Healthcare Network.

Bluemle Life Sciences Building

BLUEMLE LIFE SCIENCES BUILDING
By the Kling-Lindquist Partnership
Completed 1991

Photograph by Dave Super

Groundbreaking ceremonies for the eleven-story life sciences building were held on July 24, 1989, at Locust between Ninth and Tenth Streets. By the time of its formal dedication on October 7, 1991 the building had been named in honor of Emeritus President Lewis W. Bluemle Jr., M.D. The senior design principal for the project was Eric Chung of the Kling-Lindquist Partnership.

The first building dedicated to basic science since the erection of Jefferson Alumni Hall in 1968, the Bluemle Life Sciences Building is an architecturally bold, state-of-the-art facility.[2] It houses the departments of biochemistry and molecular biology, microbiology and immunology, dermatology, and the research division of rheumatology, as well as the Jefferson Institute of Molecular Medicine and the Jefferson Cancer Institute (now the Kimmel Cancer Institute).

The ground floor contains three multipurpose conference/lecture rooms, and the second through tenth floors contain laboratories, offices, library/seminar rooms, lounges, animal rooms, and service spaces. The building's mechanical and electrical systems and laboratory services meet the most exacting requirements for air circulation, fume exhaust, containment, limited vibration, and safety. Flexibility of design allowed scientists to choose the configuration best suited to their laboratories. "Interaction" lounge spaces are comfortably furnished to foster informal discussion among the scientists.

The brick-faced edifice is made of cast-in-place rein-

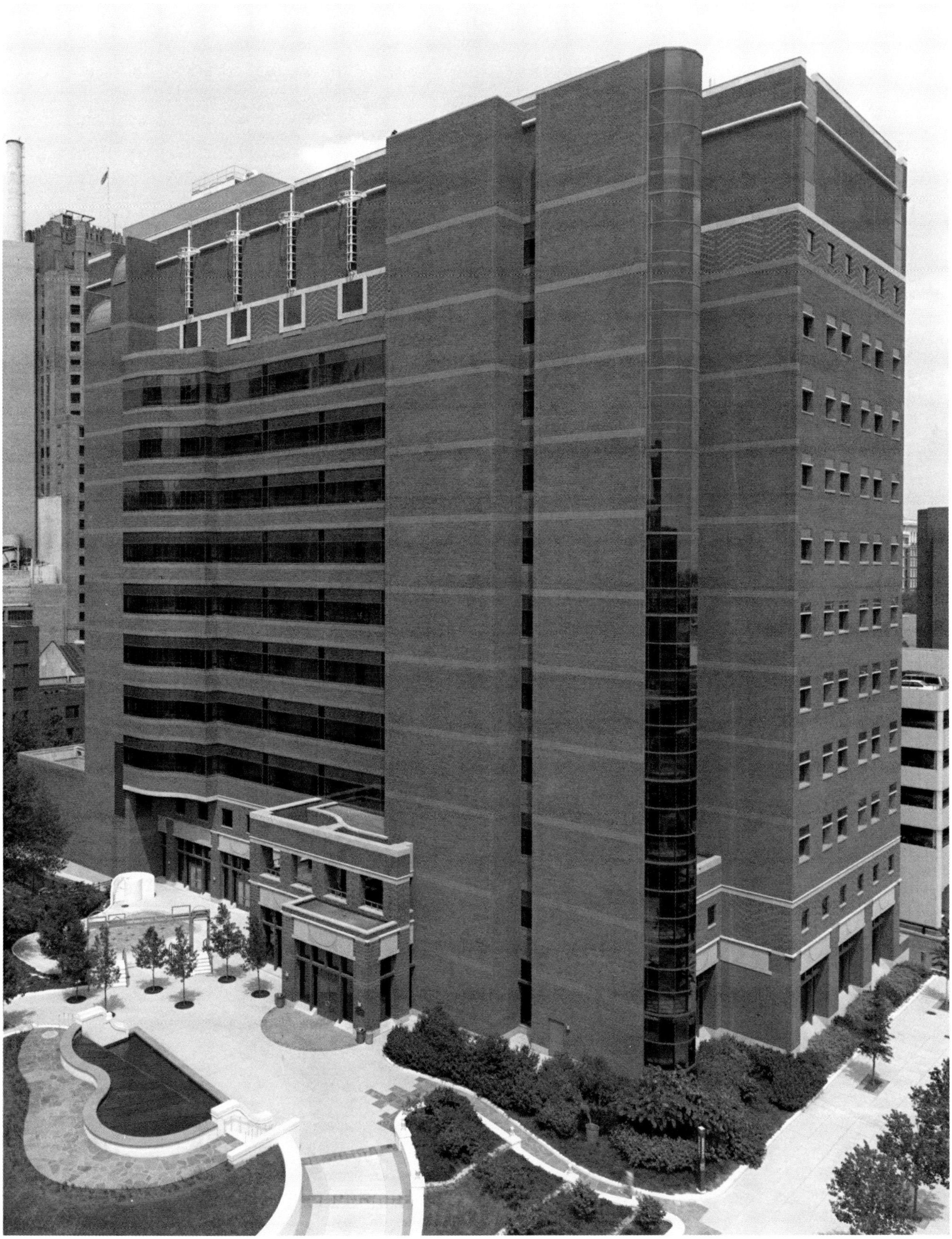

forced concrete, beam-and-slab construction. The entrance front on Tenth Street is faced with reddish-orange brick punctuated with horizontal rows of dark ribbon windows edged in smooth stripes of lighter orange. The smooth slab is interrupted by vertical elevator towers, by recessed windows, and most interestingly, by curved bays. A double "piano" curve in the facade runs from the second floor nearly to the roof. The curved corner stairwell appears as an elongated cylinder. Tan cast stone and patterned brick emphasize the divisions of space with moldings, string courses, and cornice.

Daylight streams into the building in novel, yet functional ways. The bulk of the laboratories are in the center of each floor; glass panels and doors open from them onto a sun-drenched perimeter corridor which provides views to the outside. Laboratories facing north and south have outside walls. The spectacular Center City skyline can be seen both from the glass-walled corridors and from the walls of windows in the stairwell in the southwest corner. Such views encourage researchers seeking relief from the intensity of their work to relax by walking the steps and regarding the city below them.

The Roundabout

THE ROUNDABOUT
By Alice Adams (b. 1930)

Stone, steel, water, trees, plants
1991
220 ft. north-south x 160 ft. east-west

Commissioned by TJU
Photographs by Dave Super

The Bluemle Life Sciences Building overlooks a large, parklike plaza known as the *Roundabout*. This striking example of landscaped public art by Alice Adams was installed to comply with the Philadelphia Redevelopment Authority's requirement that one percent of construction costs be allocated to a public display of art.

The *Roundabout* is an environmental work inspired by the concentric paths known as "roundabouts" at Thomas Jefferson's Virginia estate, Monticello. A second symbolic element at the site recalls the doorway-

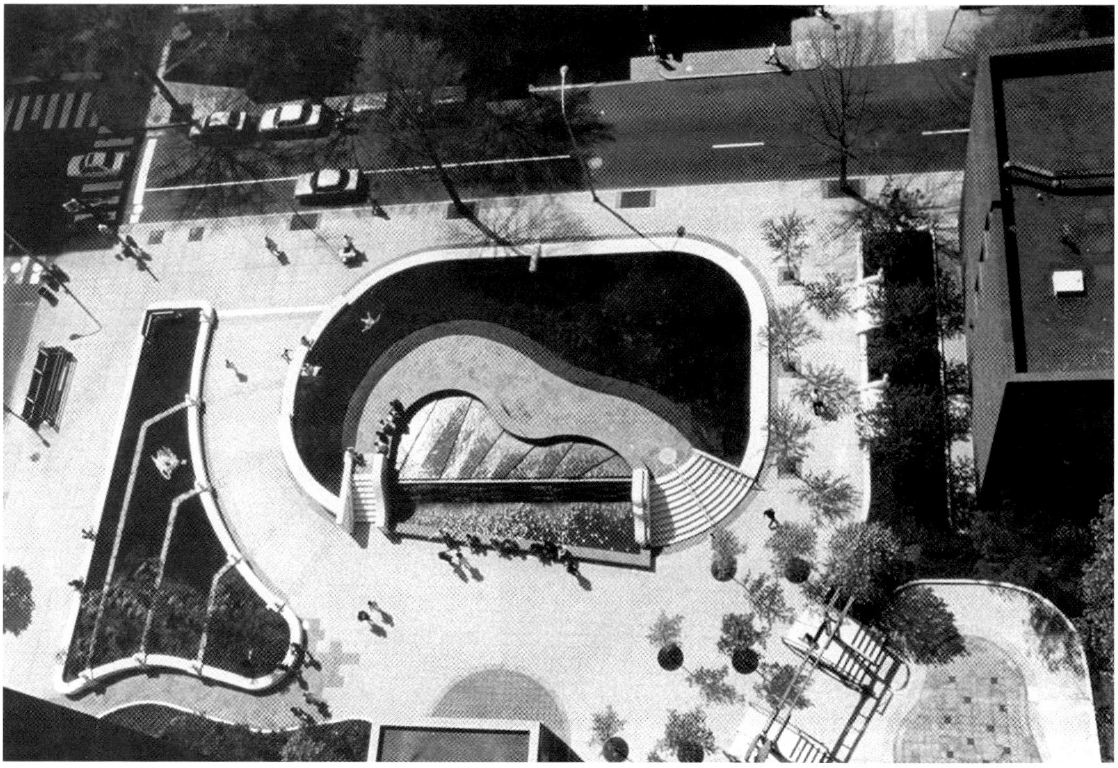

and-stoop elements of brick row houses in the adjoining Philadelphia neighborhood.

The landscaped forecourt consists of curving paths that connect various focal points providing a variety of areas for conversation or contemplation. At the center is an asymmetrical, eight-foot, grassy central mound suggesting Monticello, itself a tiny rounded mountain. A green granite "wall of water" is set into the east side of the mound, so that its waterfall and lower pool face the entrance to the Bluemle Building. The pools' curves echo the piano curve in the facade of the building. Stairways on either side lead to a flagstone path on top of the mound where there is a bluestone seating wall.

A more secluded area in the northeast corner functions like an outdoor reception room. It consists of a stylized doorway-and-stoop frame of painted steel through which one passes into an area paved with green, pink, and white granite in the shape of the Great Lawn at Monticello. Imbedded in the paving stones are bronze tablets engraved with images of medicinal plants reflecting Thomas Jefferson's research into botany and horticulture. Planting beds contain digitalis, bloodroot, vinca, may apple, and witch hazel.

The "Thicket" in the site's southeast corner contains layers of shrubs, understory trees, ground covers, and a roughhewn flagstone path that winds up from the street. An "Orchard" joining the paved outdoor room at the front contains callery pear trees, and a more formal, little garden north of the mound has boxwood hedges, holly, day lily beds, vinca, and an allée of red maple trees.

Elements of both building and forecourt are lighted

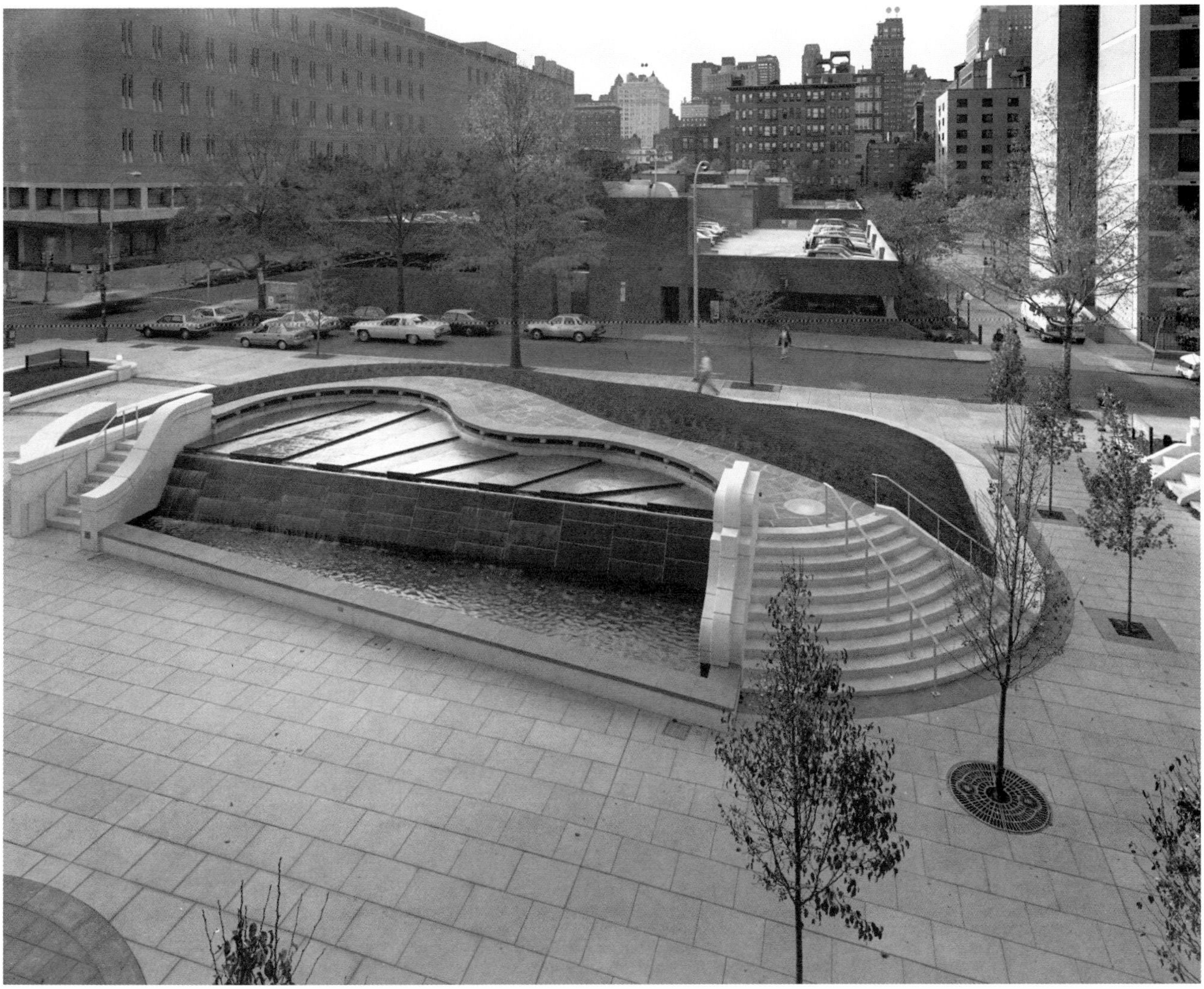

Detail: the Central Mound

Detail: the Wall of Water

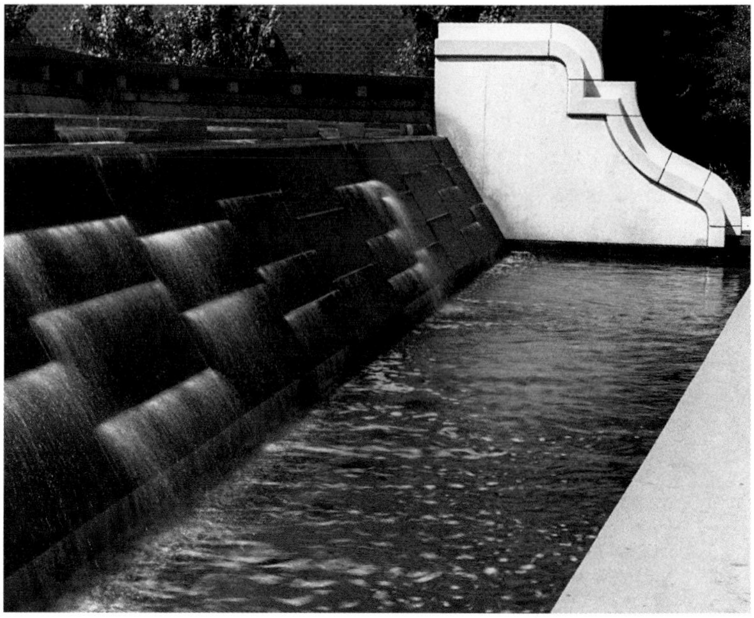

at night to great aesthetic effect: white lights on the small windows of the building's penthouse, interior lights from the horizontal band of windows underneath and from the corner stairwell, and a row of lights set into the bottom of the polished granite pool to illuminate the flowing water.

The designer of the *Roundabout* is Alice Adams. Originally a painter and weaver, she developed into a well known sculptor, construction artist, and architectural sculptor.

Adams was born in 1930 in New York and graduated from Columbia University in 1953. She continued her education on a French government fellowship and Fulbright travel grant to L'École Nationale d'Art Decoratif in Aubusson, France, a center of tapestry manufacturing since the sixteenth century. In 1966 Adams spent a summer at the prestigious MacDowell Artists Colony in New Hampshire.

She went to Aubusson because of an early interest in weaving and tapestry making. Her own weavings soon "came off the wall" to stand free in the room, and she slowly evolved into an artist of fiber sculptures. Desiring more substantial materials, she shifted to industrial fibers like flexible steel cable and tubing.

Alice Adams had always aimed to integrate the decorative arts into architectural design, and her studio work in the 1970s consisted of architectural fragments and large wall pieces in many media. Her commissions for outdoor, site-specific works in wood and metal often incorporated natural elements. Painstakingly crafted with mortise and tenon technique, her abstract architectural sculptures gradually became more complex with layers of associative meanings.

Adams's site-specific commissions can be found at the University of North Carolina at Greensboro, Wilson College in Chambersburg, Pennsylvania, Princeton University, the Dag Hammarskjold Plaza in New York, parks and gardens in Omaha, Nebraska and Dayton and Toledo, Ohio, and the Bathgate Industrial Park in the Bronx. Adams was also a member of the design teams for the Downtown Seattle Transit Project, the "Worker's Place" park and promenade in Lawrence, Massachusetts, and the Metro-Link Transit System in St. Louis, Missouri.

Since 1973 Alice Adams has had seven one-person exhibitions in galleries mainly in New York. Her sculptures in public collections are at the University of North Carolina, Rutgers University, the Hertz Corporation and the Chase Manhattan Bank in New York, and the Haags Gemeentemuseum in The Hague, The Netherlands.

Adams taught sculpture at Manhattanville College in Purchase, New York for twenty years, starting in 1960. She was also a faculty member at California State College in Los Angeles, and the Pratt Institute and the School of Visual Arts in New York. She has lectured widely at other universities and museums across the country.

Recipient of numerous awards, Alice Adams won artist's fellowships from the National Endowment for the Arts (1972 and 1976), a short-term fellowship in the humanities from Princeton University (1980), a Guggenheim Foundation fellowship (1981), and an American Academy and Institute of Arts and Letters Award in Sculpture (1984).

Heriz Rug

HERIZ RUG
Iranian

Wool, cotton
1940s
152 1/2 x 121 in.

Purchased in 1991 by TJU
Accession number: 1991+e.DA.01

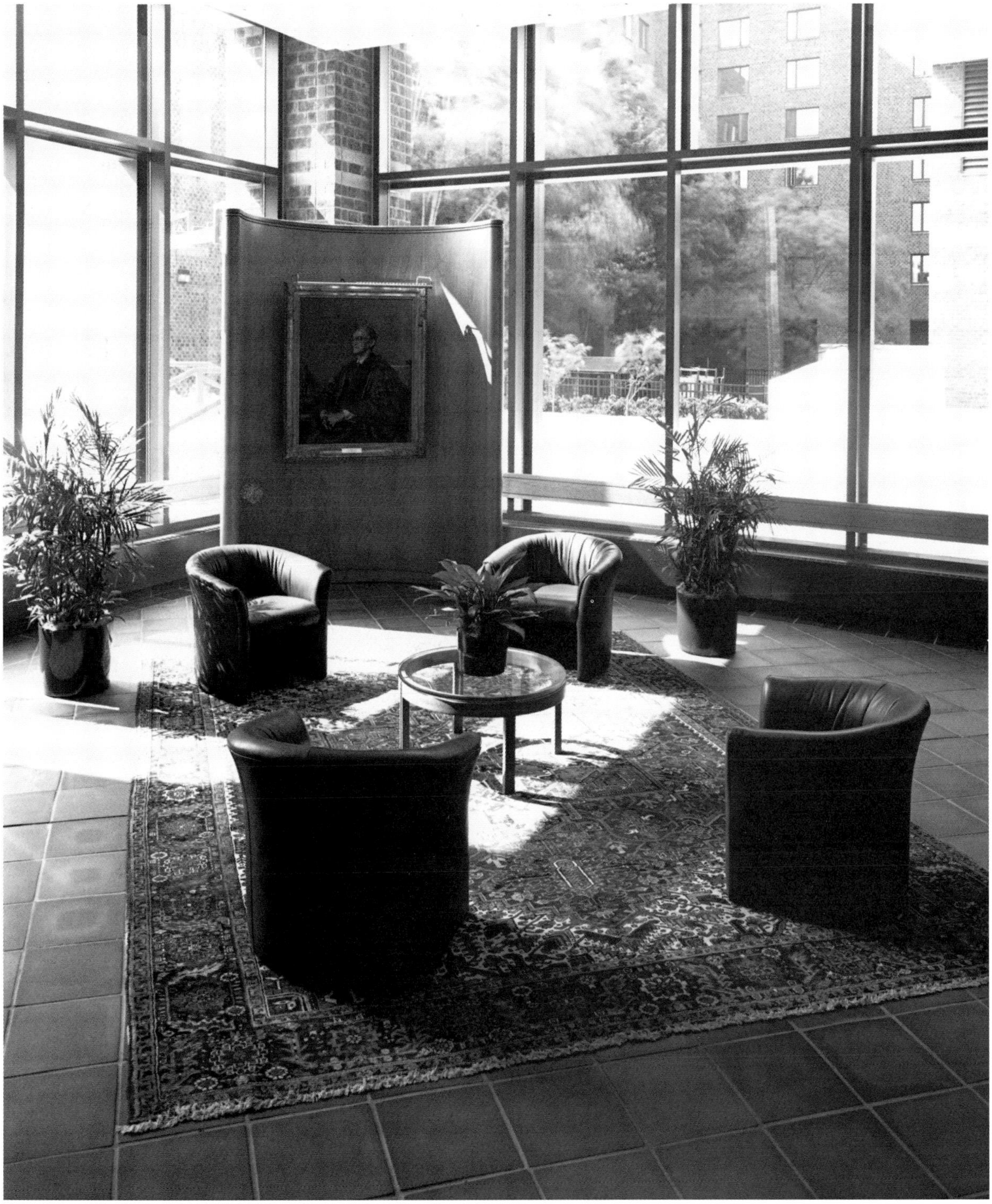

Heriz Rug Installed with Portrait in Bluemle Life Sciences Building

The light-filled lobby of the Bluemle Life Sciences Building features an attractive, corner installation of the portrait of Dr. Lewis W. Bluemle Jr., juxtaposed with a colorful Heriz rug. The portrait is mounted on a free-standing, curving wooden wall that echoes the curves of the building's facade.

The rug originated in the Heriz district of the Azarbaijan province of northwestern Iran. This district comprises sixty-two villages all with lengthy traditions of weaving rugs. Virtually all of the villages employ the same two-layer knotting technique (Turkish or symmetrical knotting with a density of two hundred knots per square inch), and decorate their rugs with the same large central medallion. General features of Heriz rugs are a complex and heavy construction with rather large knots, robustness, and durability. Differences lie in secondary features of style, color, and yarn quality.

The semi-antique, wool rug in the Bluemle Building's lobby is of the rarest grade because it comes from the village of Heriz proper, and is considered a "true Heriz." The characteristic rectilinear design is woven in shades of red, rust, navy, cobalt, bright green, ivory, and gold. The rug has a subtle rust background and features a large red, lobed medallion with radiating palmettes, anchored by massive lancehead palmettes between ivory spandrels, framed by a navy blue primary border decorated with vines and flowers, and flanked by bright blue guard borders.

In addition to the Bluemle Life Sciences Building, the Medical Office Building was also developed in the 1980s. The "MOB" is located on the southwest corner of Eleventh and Walnut Streets and was designed by Mirick Pearson Batcheler Architects. This firm also built the Bodine Center for Cancer Treatment (1986) and the award-winning Emergency and Trauma Center (1990).

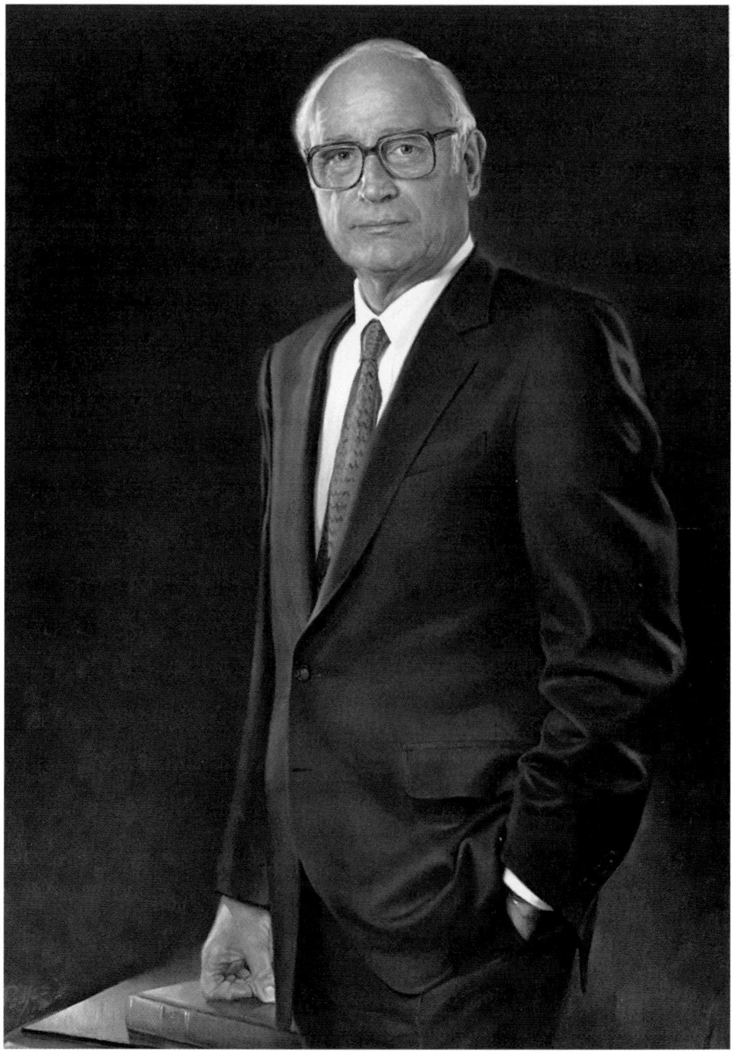

Portrait of Edward C. Driscoll

EDWARD CARROLL DRISCOLL (b. 1929)
By Dean L. Paules (b. 1931)

Oil on canvas
1992
43 1/2 x 31 1/2 in.

Signed and dated lower left: "Paules/5.92"

Given in 1992 by friends and colleagues
Accession number: 1992+e.P.05

Edward C. Driscoll was elected a Thomas Jefferson University trustee in 1974 and served vigorously as chairman of the board from 1984 to 1990. Previously he had chaired the finance and health affairs committees and was a member of the capital projects committee responsible for the construction of the Gibbon Building and renovations to the Foerderer Pavilion and the Thompson Building. He is credited with ensuring the success of the 1980s Decade Campaign Fund and for bringing several new members to the board of trustees. He was among the original members of Jefferson's Winged Ox Society.

Born in 1929, Edward Driscoll is a native Philadelphian and graduated from the University of Pennsylvania in 1951. He served as a lieutenant with the U.S. Navy's amphibious forces in the Atlantic and Pacific fleets during the Korean War. After his discharge he became a trainee at the Philadelphia management construction firm of L. F. Driscoll, founded by his father in 1931. He rose through the ranks until he became president/CEO in 1969 and then chairman of the board/CEO in 1975.

In addition to the Bluemle Life Sciences Building and others on the Jefferson campus, the Driscoll firm has constructed numerous other hospitals, schools, office buildings, research buildings, and hotels in the Philadelphia area. These include the Hershey Hotel, the Graduate Hospital, the SmithKline Beckman Research Building, the Pennwalt Building, One Liberty Place, and the Spectrum II.

Among Edward Driscoll's many civic and community responsibilities, he has been a trustee or director of the Children's Heart Hospital, the Library Company of Philadelphia, the International House, Raven Hill and Gwynedd Mercy Academies, and the University of Pennsylvania Center for the Study of Aging, and a member of the advisory council of Wills Eye Hospital. He has also been a director of the Chief Executives Organization, the Provident National Bank, the General Building Contractors' Association, and an arbitrator of the American Arbitration Association.

Edward Driscoll's portrait by Dean Paules was presented in 1992, two years after he stepped down as chairman of the board. He is depicted two-thirds length and life-sized, standing next to a table. He turns his head to engage the viewer directly. His most prominent features are white hair and high forehead, blue eyes behind horn-rimmed glasses, wide mouth, and angular jaw line. The knuckles of one hand rest on a red book lying on the table, and his other hand is concealed inside his trouser pocket. He wears a dark blue suit, a white shirt, and a red and blue figured necktie.

Driscoll's erect posture, sober gaze, and confident expression emanate authority and forcefulness, despite the informality of his hand-in-the-pocket pose. His white hair and shirt contrast effectively with the dark gray, atmospheric background. Both background and figure of the portrait are smoothly painted in an elegant and restrained manner.

At the portrait presentation President Emeritus Lewis W. Bluemle Jr., M.D. praised Edward Driscoll as a "builder par excellence not only of attractive, state-of-the-art structures, but a builder of the competitive, winning spirit which is the hallmark of Jefferson and also the hallmark of Driscoll." Bluemle proposed the new term, a "Driscoll," to mean the "minimal quantum of energy required to cut through an administrative problem with the least delay and trouble."

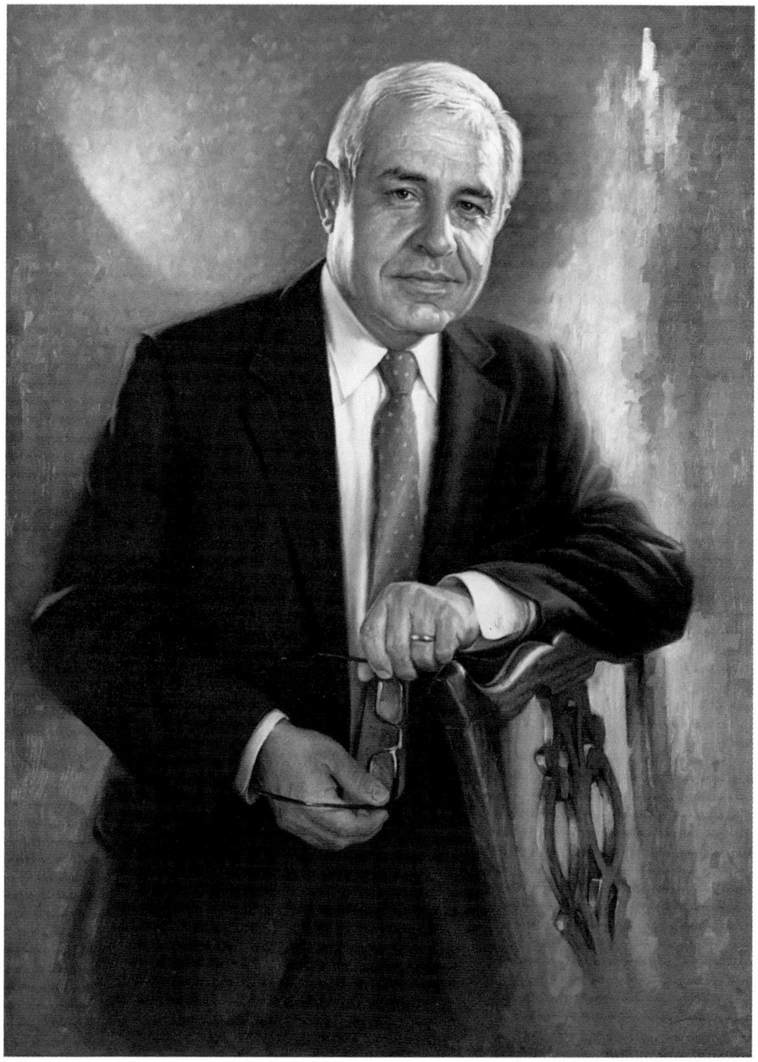

Portrait of Paul C. Brucker

PAUL C. BRUCKER, M.D. (b. 1931)
By Dean L. Paules

Oil on canvas
1989
40 x 30 in.

Signed and dated lower right: "PAULES/1-89"

Given in 1989 by friends and colleagues
Accession number: 1989+e.P.03

In 1990 Dr. Paul C. Brucker was selected as president to lead Thomas Jefferson University into the twenty-first century. Chairman of the board James W. Stratton declared, "We sought a leader—and a humanist. In Paul Brucker, we found both. I cannot imagine a better chief executive, because Dr. Brucker brings a great sense of humanity to his decision-making."

At his inaugural speech Brucker addressed issues to be incorporated into a long range strategic plan: cost containment and the factors contributing to runaway health care costs, the importance of selecting and focusing on important research areas, new opportunities and challenges in caring for the elderly, and medical education's need to attract students who "care about people" as well as academic and technological concerns.

Upon the integration of the Thomas Jefferson University Hospital with the Main Line Health System in 1995, Dr. Brucker was appointed chairman of the board of the resultant Jefferson Health System.

Paul Brucker is a native Philadelphian born in 1931. He received his undergraduate degree *summa cum laude* from Muhlenberg College in 1953 and his medical degree from the University of Pennsylvania in 1957. After an internship at Lankenau Hospital and a residency in family medicine at Hunterdon Medical Center in Flemington, New Jersey, he took further training in internal medicine at Lankenau.

In 1960 Dr. Brucker joined a group family practice in Ambler, Pennsylvania, and remained there until 1973. He was attending physician at Abington Memorial Hospital and Chestnut Hill Hospital. He was also a preceptor to medical students from Jefferson, Temple University, and the University of Pennsylvania from 1962 to 1972.

In 1970 Dr. Paul Brucker was appointed an instructor in Jefferson's new division of family medicine in the department of community and preventive medicine. A year later formal arrangements were made to establish a separate department of family medicine, and on January 1, 1973 Brucker was appointed its first chairman and the

Alumni Professor of Family Medicine. He also rose in the ranks of the department of medicine and has been a clinical professor since 1981.

Under his leadership the department of family medicine recruited outstanding faculty for the newly established undergraduate, graduate, and postgraduate programs, outpatient and inpatient facilities, research programs, affiliations, and satellite activities. From humble beginnings the department of family medicine soon reached national prominence, and the percentage of Jefferson graduates entering family practice residencies is considerably higher than the national average.

Brucker's past contributions to Thomas Jefferson University standing committees and special committees are too many to enumerate individually, but he has chaired or served on almost every major college or hospital committee for education, physician practice, and patient care. He has also been an active participant in local and national professional and civic organizations.

On the national scene Paul Brucker has served as president of the American Board of Family Practice, and was chair of both its research and development committee and its 1990 geriatric CAQ (certificate of added qualifications) examination committee. He was a board member of the Society of Teachers of Family Medicine and a trustee of its foundation. He was instrumental in forming the liaison between the American Board of Family Practice and the American Board of Internal Medicine that is responsible for fellowship training and certification in geriatrics. He is chairman of the board of the Nicholas J. Pisacano, M.D. Memorial Foundation which provides funding for accomplished students and physicians in the field of family practice.

In 1992 Dr. Brucker was appointed to the National Council on Graduate Medical Education and chaired its Workgroup on Physician Competencies in Managed Care. He has been a member of the executive committee of the National Board of Medical Examiners and chair of its Preventive Medicine and Public Health Test Committee, and in 1995 was appointed chairman of its United States Medical Licensing Examination Step II Committee.

Locally Dr. Brucker has been a board member of the Pennsylvania Academy of Family Physicians and the American Heart Association, Southeastern Pennsylvania Chapter. He is a director of Mellon Bank PSFS, the Greater Philadelphia Urban Affairs Coalition, and a member of the executive committees of Greater Philadelphia First and the Greater Philadelphia Chamber of Commerce. He is also a board member of Muhlenberg College, Gwynedd-Mercy College, the World Affairs Council, and the Philadelphia Orchestra.

Dr. Brucker has served on the editorial boards of the *Journal of the American Board of Family Practice* and the *Journal for Recertification in Family Medicine*, the editorial review board of the *Journal of Family Practice*, and the editorial advisory board of *Hippocrates Magazine*.

Dr. Paul Brucker has been the recipient of many honors during his distinguished career. In 1983 he was the Leland B. Blanchard memorial lecturer of the Society of Teachers of Family Medicine. In 1990 he received the John G. Walsh Award of the American Academy of Family Physicians. He was awarded an honorary doctor of science degree from Muhlenberg College in 1991, and inducted into Muhlenberg's Alumni Physicians Hall of Fame in 1993. An annual Brucker lectureship sponsored by Jefferson's department of family medicine was established in 1993. He was elected to membership in the Institute of Medicine of the National Academy of Sciences in 1994. In 1997 he received the F. Marian Bishop Leadership Award of the Society of Teachers of Family Medicine Foundation.

In 1989 Dr. Brucker was honored by friends and colleagues at Jefferson with the presentation of his portrait. As depicted by Dean Paules, the physician is shown two-thirds length and life-sized, standing at ease and facing the viewer. His left arm leans on the cresting rail of a carved Chippendale chair, and he holds his glasses between his hands. Highlights bathe both sides of his solidly rendered face and gray-white hair. Bright eyes under dark brows and a warm smile animate his expressive face and engage the viewer. One senses a caring man who takes pride in his complex role as clinician, educator, and administrator.

The subject is wearing a dark blue suit, white shirt, and reddish tie with a small pattern. His face and hands are painted in an extremely detailed manner, with multiple dabs of cool and warm colors superimposed over flesh tones. The lower parts of both figure and chair evaporate into the misty background which is dramatically lighted and dotted with tones of blues, purples, whites, tans, and maroons.

In his remarks at the portrait ceremony Dr. Paul C. Brucker focused on his role as physician, and expressed the joys and responsibilities of patient care:

> Appreciate the wonderful privilege it is to be involved with patients who want and need help, patients with whom you can laugh and at times cry, patients who appreciate you for your nonjudgmental approach to their problems, and above all, patients with whom you can develop a mutual trust and friendship.

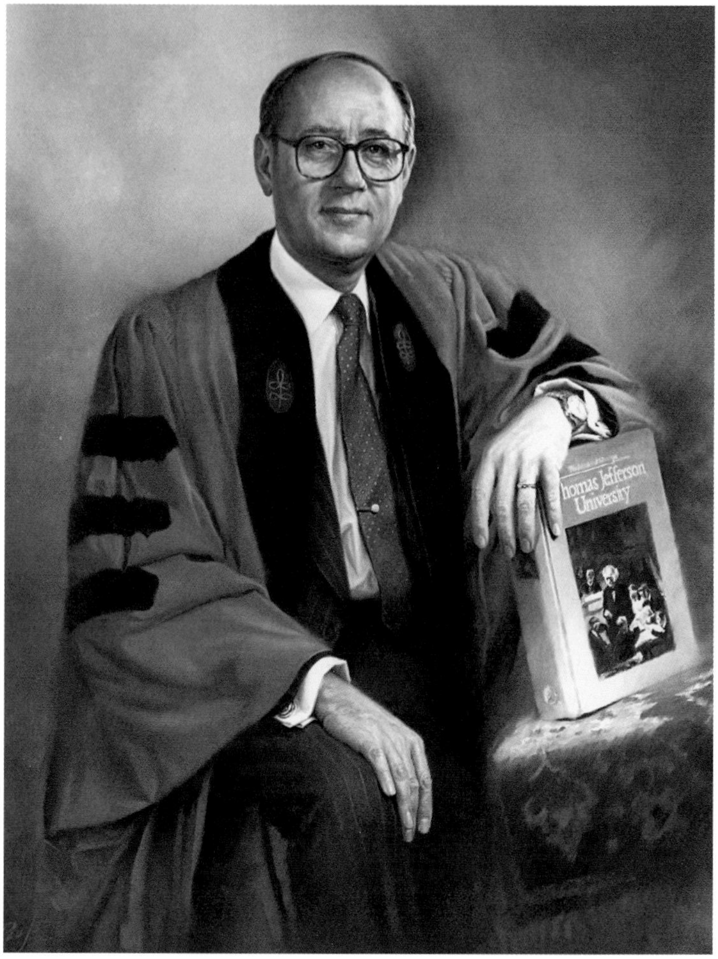

Portrait of Joseph S. Gonnella

JOSEPH SALVATORE GONNELLA, M.D.
(b. 1934)
By Dean L. Paules

Oil on canvas
1991
48 x 38 in.

Signed and dated lower left: "Paules/91"

Given in 1991 by JMC faculty
Accession number: 1991+e.P.02

Dr. Joseph S. Gonnella is dean of Jefferson Medical College and senior vice president for academic affairs of Thomas Jefferson University. He is internationally prominent in the fields of undergraduate and graduate medical education.

"Joe" Gonnella was born in 1934 in Pescopagano, Italy, a small town southeast of Naples, and moved to the United States with his family at age twelve. He was a *summa cum laude* graduate of Dartmouth College in 1956 and a Rufus Choate Scholar there. He attended Dartmouth Medical School and received his degree from Harvard Medical School in 1959.

His postgraduate training included an internship and residency in internal medicine at the University of Illinois Research and Educational Hospitals in Chicago (1959-65). Following his residency he spent a year at the University of Illinois College of Medicine as an American Heart Association fellow. For two years he served as captain in the Medical Corps of the U.S. Army.

In 1966 Dr. Gonnella moved to Philadelphia to join the faculty at Hahnemann Medical College as assistant professor of medicine and assistant dean, under Dr. William F. Kellow (whom he had known at Illinois). The following year he accepted Dean Kellow's offer to become assistant dean and assistant professor of medicine at Jefferson Medical College. Gonnella rose through the academic ranks to become professor of medicine in 1977.

By 1969 Dr. Gonnella had also progressed administratively to become associate dean and director of academic programs, as well as director of the newly established Office of Medical Education. In 1983 he was named dean for educational programs and acting dean later in the year. He was appointed dean and vice president of the university in 1984, and named the senior vice president for academic affairs in 1989. For many years Dr. Gonnella continued as attending physician in the hospital in order to maintain direct contact with students and residents at the patient's bedside.

Under Gonnella's leadership, the Center for Research in Medical Education and Health Care (which grew out of the Office of Medical Education) pioneered the Jefferson Longitudinal Study which achieved national and international prominence.[3] Believing that the effectiveness of medical education should be judged by its outcome, i.e. the quality of care rendered to patients, the long-term study evaluated clinical performance in the postgraduate period of students who entered medical school between 1964 and 1991. The categories analyzed were: academic progress, satisfaction with education, competence soon after graduation, competence at later stages of a career, and career choice. This tracking system was cited by the Liaison Committee on Medical Education on its 1993 survey as a model for other medical centers.

Dean Gonnella has contributed to the recruitment of outstanding faculty and to the development of new facilities. He has fostered regular curriculum evaluation aimed toward a closer integration of basic science material and clinical applications.

Since the six-year accelerated program with Pennsylvania State University was introduced in 1963, Jefferson has added several new combined programs during Gonnella's tenure. The seven-year M.D./Ph.D. Gibbon Scholars program was established for students interested in careers in academic medicine and medical research. The Medical Scholars program is a joint venture with the University of Delaware that prepares physicians to be health policy leaders and planners. The M.D./M.B.A. five-year program in health administration was introduced in cooperation with Widener University in Chester, Pennsylvania.

Dr. Joseph Gonnella's extensive extramural medical activities reflect his wide-ranging interests. In 1995 he was appointed cochair of the Liaison Committee on Medical Education, the accrediting body sponsored jointly by the American Medical Association and the Association of American Medical Colleges.

The dean has served as a committee member, chairman, or consultant to the following organizations: the Alliance for Continuing Medical Education, the American Board of Medical Specialties, the American Medical Association, the Association of American Medical Colleges, the Department of Health and Human Services, the Educational Commission for Foreign Medical Graduates, the Joint Commission on Accreditation of Hospitals, the National Board of Medical Examiners, and the World Health Organization.

His achievements culminated in his receiving the AAMC's most prestigious honor, the Abraham Flexner Award, in 1998.

Dean Gonnella has served on the editorial boards of the *Journal of Medical Education* and *Quality Review Bulletin*. He was coeditor of *Assessment Measures in Medical School, Residency, and Practice: The Connections* (1993), and editor of *Clinical Criteria for Disease Staging* (1983). Disease staging, an alternative to the DRG (diagnosis related groups) classification, is an evaluation system of the severity of disease complications used to assess the quality of health care and analyze the use of medical resources and costs.

For his outstanding leadership and achievements Dr. Gonnella was awarded a Presidential Medal from Dartmouth College, and the Founders Award from the American College of Medical Quality (1991). In the Philadelphia area, he became the first recipient of the Founders Award of the Hepatitis B Foundation, and also won the Clarence E. Shaffrey, S.J. Award from St. Joseph's University in 1997.

Dean Gonnella received honorary degrees in medicine from the University of Chieti in Italy and the SoonChunHyang University in Seoul, Korea. He was made an honorary professor at the Tianjin Medical College in China. He is an honorary member of the National Academy of Medicine in Buenos Aires and the National Academy of Medicine of Mexico. He received the Noguchi Award of the Noguchi Medical Research Institute of Philadelphia and Tokyo for contributions to international medical exchange in 1991. He received the Order of Civil Merit, the Dongbaeg Medal, conferred by the president of the Republic of Korea in 1992.

Special honorary titles include Commendatore nell'Ordine della Stella della Solidarietà Italiana, conferred by the president of Italy in 1979, and Grande Ufficiale of the Order of Merit of the Republic of Italy, bestowed upon him by the president of Italy and presented by the Italian consul in Philadelphia in 1996.

In 1989 Dr. Gonnella received Thomas Jefferson University's Presidential Citation. Two years later the Jefferson faculty honored him with his portrait. At the presentation ceremony, chairman of the board James W. Stratton recounted Gonnella's remark that his goal was to be dean of the finest medical college in the United States. Stratton turned the remark around to say, "In Joe Gonnella we have the finest dean of a medical college in the United States."

Dean Paules depicted the physician three-quarters length and slightly larger than life-sized. He is seated next to a small table and turned slightly to the right. His left hand supports a book standing on its edge: *Thomas Jefferson University: Tradition and Heritage* by Dr. Frederick B. Wagner Jr. Significantly, the book's cover features a clearly visible reproduction of *The Gross Clinic*.

The sitter's oval-shaped face is dominated by his high-domed forehead, dark brown eyes behind horn-rimmed glasses, and trace of a smile. He makes eye contact with the viewer, and his expression is pleasant and open. Underneath his brilliant red academic gown decorated with black velvet panels and stripes, the dean wears a dark gray, pin-striped suit, white shirt, and red necktie decorated with a small gray and white pattern.

The predominant color of this dramatic painting is red: the cherry red robe, the necktie, the red and olive tapestry covering the table, and of course, crimson red in the Eakins portrait of Dr. Gross. The atmospheric background also contains glowing reddish and purple tones. As is customary with Paules portraits, the surface is very smoothly brushed and the subject's hands and face are revealed in great detail.

In a lighter moment of his response at the portrait ceremony, Dean Gonnella said that his happiness had lasted about five minutes when notified about his selection as portrait honoree, and then his "Roman" genes had spoken up, "Why only a portrait? Certainly a statue! Marble! I am going to give you a chance. Think about it, really!"

Portrait of Joseph S. Gonnella

JOSEPH SALVATORE GONNELLA, M.D.
By Marvin Levitt (b. 1925)

Bronze
1996
17 1/8 x 13 3/4 x 11 3/4 in.

Signed rear center:
"M. LEVITT"

Given in 1996 by Dr. and Mrs. Robert L. Brent
Accession number: 1996+e.S.01

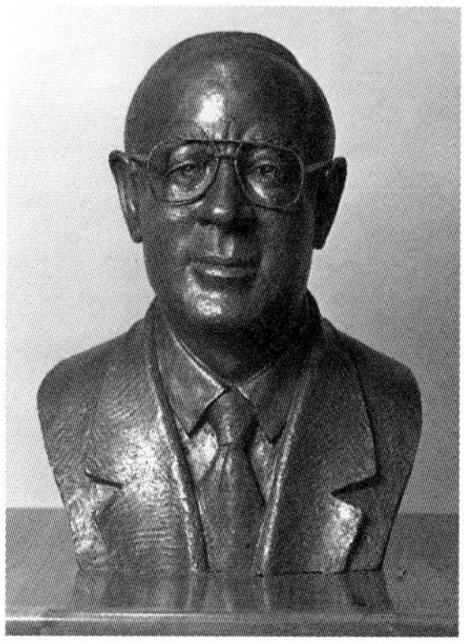

In 1996 a statue of Dean Joseph S. Gonnella, M.D. *was* presented. The occasion was the alumni banquet at graduation weekend when a bronze bust of the dean was donated to the university by Dr. and Mrs. Robert L. Brent. The life-sized sculpture by Marvin Levitt shows the subject dressed in shirt, necktie, and coat and wearing glasses. His demeanor is relaxed and he wears a slight smile. The irregular bronze surface is etched with raised lines to make a lively texture.

Marvin Levitt, a sculptor, painter, and printmaker, was born in Philadelphia in 1925. He received three degrees from Tyler School of Art of Temple University. He won a Fulbright fellowship to study bronze foundry work at the Istituto Statale d'Arte in Florence. For twenty-five years Marvin Levitt taught art enrichment courses in the Princeton Regional School System and was artist-in-residence there in a program funded by the New Jersey Council for the Arts. Among his commissions are sculptures for the Churchville Nature Center in Bucks County, Pennsylvania, and stained glass windows, memorial plaques, and sculptures for Beth Shalom Synagogue in suburban Elkins Park.

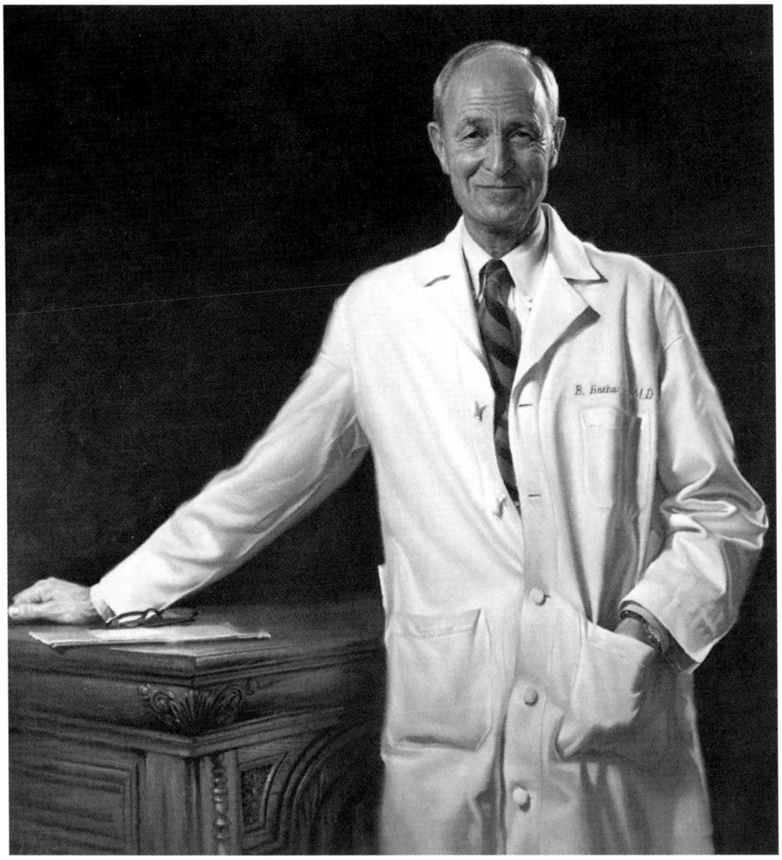

Portrait of Benjamin Bacharach

BENJAMIN BACHARACH, M.D. (b. 1930)
By Dean L. Paules (b. 1931)

Oil on canvas
1993
42 x 40 in.

Signed and dated lower left: "PAULES/4-93"

Given by JMC class of 1993
Accession number: 1993+e.P.01

Dr. Benjamin Bacharach, associate dean for admissions and chairman of the committee on admissions at Jefferson Medical College, is also clinical professor of surgery and vice chairman of the department.

"Bud" Bacharach was born in 1931 in Atlantic City, New Jersey and earned degrees at Muhlenberg College (1952) and Jefferson Medical College (1956). After interning at Atlantic City Hospital he took his residency in general surgery under John H. Gibbon Jr., M.D. at Jefferson Hospital, followed by a fellowship in cardiothoracic surgery at Pennsylvania Hospital. His training was interrupted by two years of military service as a lieutenant in the U.S. Navy Medical Corps.

Following his fellowship Dr. Bacharach joined Dr. John Y. Templeton III in clinical practice, an association that lasted over twenty years. They were joined by Dr. Stanton N. Smullens (JMC 1961) in 1971.

Bacharach's earliest surgical appointments in the 1960s were at the Henry R. Landis State Tuberculosis Sanitarium of Philadelphia, Pennsylvania Hospital, and the University of Pennsylvania School of Medicine. He was appointed attending physician at Jefferson Medical College Hospital in 1967 and was codirector of the surgical section of the coronary care unit from 1971 to 1980. He was also attendant in surgery at Our Lady of Lourdes Hospital in Camden, New Jersey.

Dr. Bacharach's faculty appointments at Jefferson advanced steadily from clinical assistant professor of surgery in 1969 to clinical professor in 1983. He served on the department's advisory committee from 1975 to 1990, and was named vice chairman of the department in 1984. He succeeded Dr. Samuel S. Conly Jr. as associate dean for admissions in 1983.

Dr. Bacharach has been a member of the admissions subcommittee of AAMC/NEGSA since 1986. He was a founding member of the Philadelphia Academy of Cardiology and is a member of the American Association for the Advancement of Science. He was honored as a Shankweiler fellow at Muhlenberg College's Alumni Physicians Hall of Fame in 1994.

Dr. Bacharach has followed in a family tradition of community involvement and generosity, notably by his grandfather and two great-uncles who founded the Betty Bacharach Rehabilitation Hospital in 1924. The home was named after their mother and was originally located in Longport, New Jersey. Since 1958 Dr.

Bacharach has been vice president of the hospital's board of governors.

Other civic activities include service on the boards of the Industrial Valley Bank and the G.O.C., Incorporated Stainless Steel Corporation, and as vice president of the board of the G. B. Carlson Foundation.

Dr. Bacharach is equally dedicated to Jefferson Medical College affairs. He is a longtime member of the executive committee of the alumni association and was elected president in 1981. He was an organizer and chairman of the President's Club. He and Mrs. Bacharach have established a lectureship honoring Dr. Templeton. Bacharach was Jefferson's distinguished honoree at the National Philanthropy Day celebration of the National Society of Fund-raising Executives in 1995.

Dr. Bud Bacharach's portrait was presented by the graduating class of 1993. At the ceremony he was warmly praised by students for his involvement in the selection of every applicant to Jefferson. He greets students on their first day at Jefferson and accompanies many through the various processing lines. His open door policy and compassionate support continue through Match Day, the culminating event of their student years. At the portrait presentation Dean Joseph S. Gonnella, M.D. called Bacharach "the best director of admissions of any medical school in the country."

Dr. Benjamin Bacharach's warmth and ready humor shine through in his portrait by Dean Paules. He is shown two-thirds length and slightly smaller than life-sized. He stands frontally and gazes directly toward the viewer with a broad and welcoming smile. His elongated right arm makes a sweeping, diagonal gesture toward the nearby desk, and his hand rests near a pamphlet and reading glasses. His left hand is placed in the pocket of his white doctor's coat.

The high-domed forehead of Dr. Bacharach's long and crinkly, oval-shaped face is crowned with grayish blond hair. His angular features are emphasized by high cheekbones, aquiline nose, and thin lips. Underneath his coat he wears a blue shirt and diagonally striped blue, red, and ocher necktie. The portrait's flat, dark, atmospheric background contrasts with the three-dimensional likeness of the subject and the beautifully sculpted and highlighted folds of his white coat.

Portrait of Joseph F. Rodgers

JOSEPH FRANCIS RODGERS, M.D. (1931-99)
By Dean L. Paules

Oil on canvas
1997
44 x 34 in.

Signed and dated lower left: "Paules/7-97"

Given in 1997 by friends and colleagues
Accession number: 1997+e.P.03

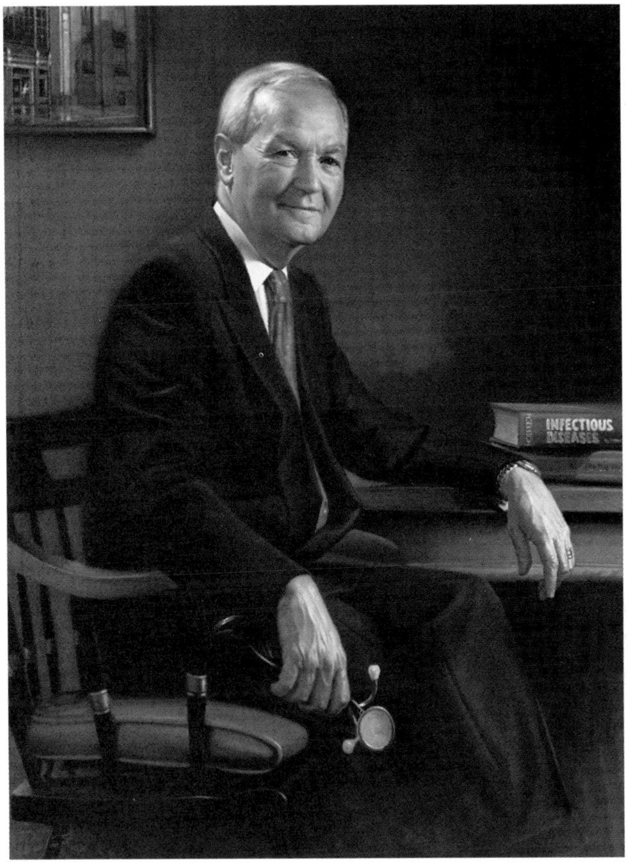

Dr. Joseph F. Rodgers was a clinical professor of medicine, and after 1984 an associate dean at Jefferson Medical College for the affiliated hospital and residency programs.

Joseph Rodgers was born in 1931, a native of Chester, Pennsylvania. He earned a bachelor of science degree at Mount St. Mary's College in Emmitsburg, Maryland in 1953. He received his medical degree from Jefferson in 1957 and interned at Chester Hospital. He was a medical resident at the Mary Fletcher Hospital of the University of Vermont Medical College and then returned to Jefferson as a fellow in infectious diseases. He completed his residency in internal medicine at the Jefferson Hospital. His wife, Adrienne Marasco Rodgers, graduated from Jefferson's School of Nursing in 1955.

In 1962 Rodgers was appointed instructor in medicine and a member of the division of infectious diseases. In 1964 he was the first full-time director of the new division of home care which he continued to supervise until 1966. Now called the Jefferson Home Health Care Program, this division treats patients with chronic diseases and helps students recognize the various medical and social problems in the management of patients in a home setting.

In 1967 Dr. Rodgers joined Dr. Warren Goldburgh in the practice of medicine, an association that lasted for ten years. Rodgers became known as a skilled diagnostician with an unusual depth of knowledge, and for being a caring and empathetic physician. He was an effective teacher both at the bedside and at conferences and rounds in the department of infectious diseases. He rose in the academic ranks from clinical assistant professor of medicine in 1970 to clinical professor of medicine in 1987, and served as president of the volunteer faculty association.

In 1984 Dr. Rodgers was appointed associate dean for affiliations and residency programs. At the portrait presentation Dr. Francis E. Rosato said, "He has been a vigilant dean in protecting the quality of residency programs and he has also been...a defender of the rights and needs of the resident staff." Rosato particularly praised Rodgers's introduction of the concept of practice management and the development of teaching and leadership skills, as well as a stress reduction program.

Dr. Rodgers's portrait by Dean Paules was presented by friends and colleagues in 1997. He is shown three-quarters length and life-sized, in an armchair parallel to his desk. He holds a stethoscope in his right hand. He turns his head to gaze toward the viewer with friendly brown eyes and an affable expression, heightened by his round-shaped face, silvery hair, and wide, smiling mouth. He is attired in a dark blue suit and a patterned tie with a reddish background. The atmospheric background of the smoothly painted portrait ranges from dark green and purple to lighter green and umber around the sitter's head. His head and hands are delineated in ultra realistic detail.

In addition to the stethoscope several other objects allude to the subject's profession and to Thomas Jefferson University. The uppermost book on the desk is *Infectious Diseases* by Paul D. Hoeprich, M.D. A framed reproduction of Ben Eisenstat's 1965 oil painting of the College Building hangs in the upper left corner.

Portrait of Willis C. Maddrey

WILLIS CROCKER MADDREY, M.D. (b. 1939)
By Dean L. Paules

Oil on canvas
1990
46 x 36 in.

Signed and dated lower left: "PAULES/A.P.S.C./4-90"

Given by JMC class of 1990
Accession number: 1990+e.P.07

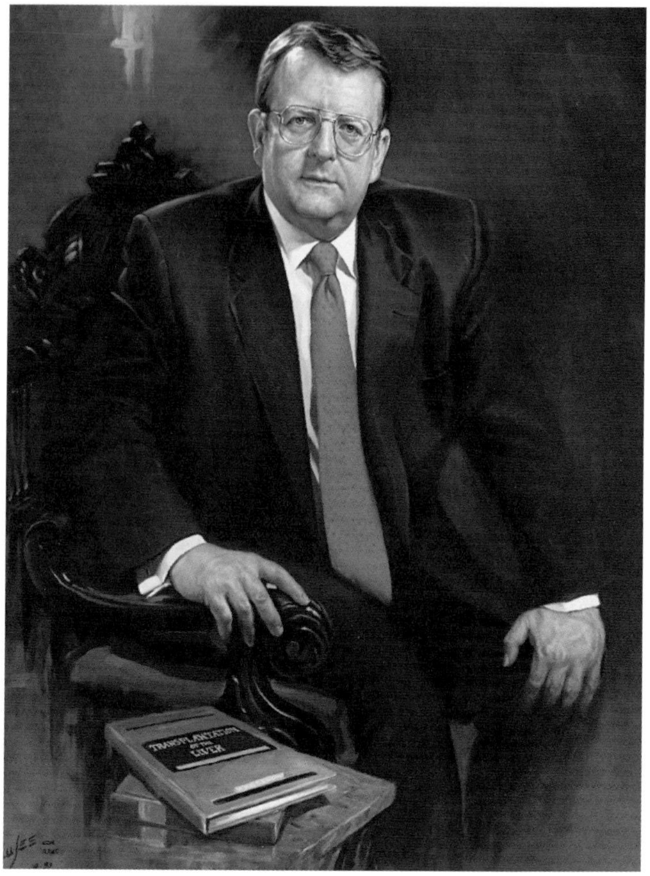

Dr. Willis C. Maddrey was the Magee Professor of Medicine and chairman of the department from 1982 until 1990. He is internationally known for his research on drug-related liver disease and alcoholic liver disease. He is also an authority on hepatic venous occlusion and granulomatous liver disease.

Willis Maddrey was born in 1939 in Roanoke Rapids, North Carolina to a family whose English and Welsh forbears had come to America in the late eighteenth century. His father, Milner Crocker Maddrey, M.D. was a surgeon who had graduated from Jefferson Medical College in 1931.

Dr. Willis Maddrey graduated *summa cum laude* from Wake Forest University in 1960 and Johns Hopkins University School of Medicine in 1964. His internship and residency in medicine at Johns Hopkins Hospital were interrupted by two years of military service in Calcutta, India with the U.S. Public Health Service. In 1970 he was a fellow in liver disease at the Yale University School of Medicine.

The following year he returned to Johns Hopkins as assistant professor of medicine. In 1975 he was named associate professor of medicine and assistant dean for postdoctoral programs and faculty development. He rose to associate director, associate physician-in-chief, and professor of medicine. He was honored to receive the Henry Strong Denison Award in the Medical Sciences in 1963 and the George Stuart Outstanding Teacher Award in 1970.

Dr. Willis Maddrey joined the Jefferson faculty in 1982 as the Magee Professor of Medicine and chairman of the department. His goals included strengthening the clinical research base, while expanding the educational and patient care programs. He recruited many talented new faculty members to achieve these goals, and by 1986 the department had grown to thirteen distinct divisions. Research funding increased markedly.

It was largely through Dr. Maddrey's initiative, in conjunction with the department of surgery, that the first liver transplant in the Philadelphia area was performed at Jefferson Hospital on May 31, 1984. Later that year a permanent liver transplant center was established. By early 1998 the program had performed its three hundredth case.

Dr. Willis C. Maddrey was a gifted teacher and he relished his contacts with students on hospital teaching rounds. He was honored with the Christian R. and Mary F. Lindback Award for Distinguished Teaching in 1986. The Jefferson medical residency continued to grow rapidly in popularity, and Maddrey was a stimulating moderator at the reorganized, weekly grand rounds. Dr. Maddrey resigned in July 1990 to become vice president for clinical affairs at the University of Texas Southwestern Medical Center in Dallas.

Among his offices in professional societies, Dr. Maddrey has been a regent and chairman of the educational policy committee of the American College of Physicians, president of the American Association for the Study of Liver Diseases, president of the Council of Subspecialty Societies, and a founder and board member of the American Liver Foundation.

Dr. Maddrey has presented endowed lectures at the Cleveland Metropolitan Hospital, the American College of Nutrition, George Washington University, Cornell University, and the Southern Medical Association. He has been visiting professor at hospitals and medical schools throughout the United States and at the University of New South Wales in Sydney, Australia.

Dr. Willis Maddrey is the author of more than one hundred articles and twenty book chapters on liver-related problems. He is the coauthor of *Liver* (with Roger Williams, 1984), editor of *Transplantation of the Liver* (1988), and author of *The Liver* (1996). Equally noted for his editorial contributions, he was associate editor of *Medicine*, consultant to the *American Journal of Medicine*, editorial board member of *Viewpoints in Digestive Diseases*, *Hepatology*, and *Gastroenterology*, and a member of the international advisory board of *Alimentary Pharmacology and Therapeutics*.

Dr. Willis C. Maddrey was selected as portrait honoree by the class of 1990 before his departure for Texas had been announced. Dean Paules depicted the physician three-quarters length and life-sized, seated in an armchair and facing partly to the right. His steely blue eyes behind metal-rimmed glasses gaze intently at the viewer. His authoritative expression suggests that he is making an emphatic point to an unseen visitor.

Rather than recline against the back of the chair he sits at an angle and leans forward, one hand grasping the chair arm and the other braced on his knee. His forceful posture and confident expression embody his reputation for remarkable analytical ability, powers of concentration, and energy.

Dr. Maddrey is wearing a black suit with a pale linear design, white shirt, and red patterned necktie. A copy of *Transplantation of the Liver* lies on a marble table next to the elaborately carved, Rococo Revival chair which is upholstered in a purplish material. His legs disappear into the misty, multicolored atmospheric background. The glowing blue cross in the upper left corner and the Christian symbol of the fish next to the artist's signature are hallmarks of Dean Paules's portraits in this period.

Portrait of Edward C. Bradley

EDWARD CHARLES BRADLEY, S.J., M.D. (b. 1928)
By Dean L. Paules

Oil on canvas
1991
40 x 34 in.

Signed lower left: "Paules"

Given by JMC class of 1991
Accession number: 1991+e.P.01

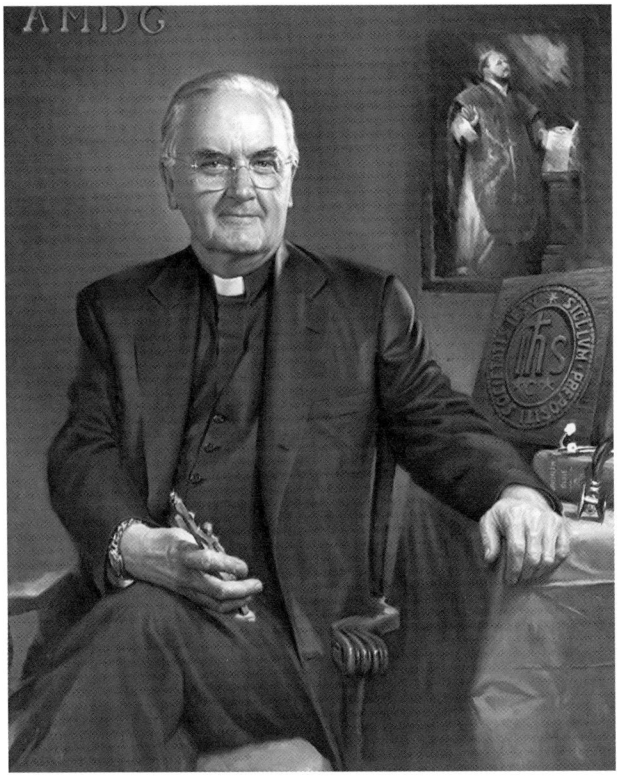

"Father Doctor" Edward C. Bradley, S.J., M.D. is an ordained priest in the Jesuit order and a clinical associate professor of medicine and Special Counselor in Residence at Jefferson Medical College. He is cherished by the Jefferson community as advisor, physician, and friend.

Edward C. Bradley was born in Philadelphia in 1928. After graduating from St. Joseph's College (1951) and Jefferson Medical College (1955) he interned at Lankenau Hospital. He trained at the U.S. Navy School of Aviation Medicine in Pensacola, Florida to become a flight surgeon and rose to the rank of lieutenant commander. Between 1959 and 1962 he completed a residency in internal medicine at Pennsylvania Hospital, Jefferson Medical College Hospital, and Lankenau. He completed fellowships in cardiology at the University of Göteborg in Sweden and in cardiovascular research at the University of Southern California School of Medicine.

Dr. Bradley was invited to join the USC faculty in 1964. He was made assistant professor in 1966 and was coinvestigator of the circulatory shock unit. For a research paper on vasoactive amines he was named one of ten finalists in the American College of Cardiology's nationwide competition for young investigators. He also received a patent for the first handheld calculator to compute cardiac output by dye dilution.

At about this time Dr. Bradley learned of a Jesuit priest in Vietnam who was in dire need of medical supplies and assistance. Bradley responded by gathering equipment and traveling to two Vietnamese villages. He opened the first clinics and became especially concerned about the ravages of tuberculosis and polio. Failing to secure additional help, Bradley appealed to President Richard Nixon who arranged for enough supplies and personnel to inoculate eight thousand villagers. Follow-up studies reported that polio was soon eradicated from the villages.

From then on Dr. Bradley pursued two callings simultaneously. In 1974 he resigned his tenured position as associate professor of medicine to become a novice in the Society of Jesus, Novitiate of St. Isaac Jogues in Wernersville, Pennsylvania. This was not a sudden conversion, for Dr. Bradley had studied there briefly after high school.

In 1975 he received an appointment at Jefferson Medical College as associate professor of medicine in the nephrology division. He was ordained in the priesthood in the Jesuit order of the Roman Catholic Church in Baltimore in 1979. He received a Master of Divinity degree from the Jesuit School of Theology in Berkeley, California in 1980. While at Berkeley, he received appointments at St. Mary's Hospital in San Francisco and at the University of Southern California/Los Angeles County Hospital.

Fr. Dr. Bradley returned East and opened a medical practice in North Philadelphia to care for the poor. He joined the Jefferson faculty as associate clinical professor of medicine in 1981. At the invitation of Dean Joseph S. Gonnella, M.D. in 1987 he moved into Orlowitz Hall as Special Counselor in Residence, and was available twenty-four hours a day to counsel members of the Jefferson community. In addition to teaching and patient responsibilities, he served as a member of the admissions committee.

Fr. Dr. Bradley was selected as portrait honoree by the class of 1991. Dean Paules depicted the physician three-quarters length and life-sized, seated in a carved, upholstered armchair. His legs are crossed at the knee, and his upper body and head are almost frontal. He gazes directly and encouragingly toward the viewer. His kindly smile is enhanced by sparkling blue eyes behind rimless glasses, dimples, square jaw, and silver hair. He wears a black clerical suit with white round collar. His right hand holds a crucifix and his left hand rests on the front corner of the adjoining table. The loosely brushed background wall is backlighted with alternating tones of glowing blues and pale oranges.

Except for a stethoscope on the table, all the other attributes in the painting are religious rather than medical. Fr. Bradley's small, wooden crucifix is a special "vow crucifix" obtained at the seminary. On the table is a *Jerusalem Bible* given by his mother and the first Bible he ever owned. The wooden plaque with the motto was carved by Bradley during his third year at the seminary, and is a replica of the Jesuit order's first seal.

In the upper right corner of Bradley's portrait is a reproduction of Peter Paul Rubens's painting of St. Ignatius of Loyola (ca. 1616, Norton Simon Museum, Pasadena, California), founder of the Society of Jesus. In the upper left corner is the inscription "AMDG" (Ad Majorem Dei Glorium, "To the Greater Glory of God"), the opening words of the Jesuit Rule. The date of Fr. Bradley's portrait was of particular significance because 1991 was the five hundredth anniversary of the birth of St. Ignatius and the 450th anniversary of the Society of Jesus.

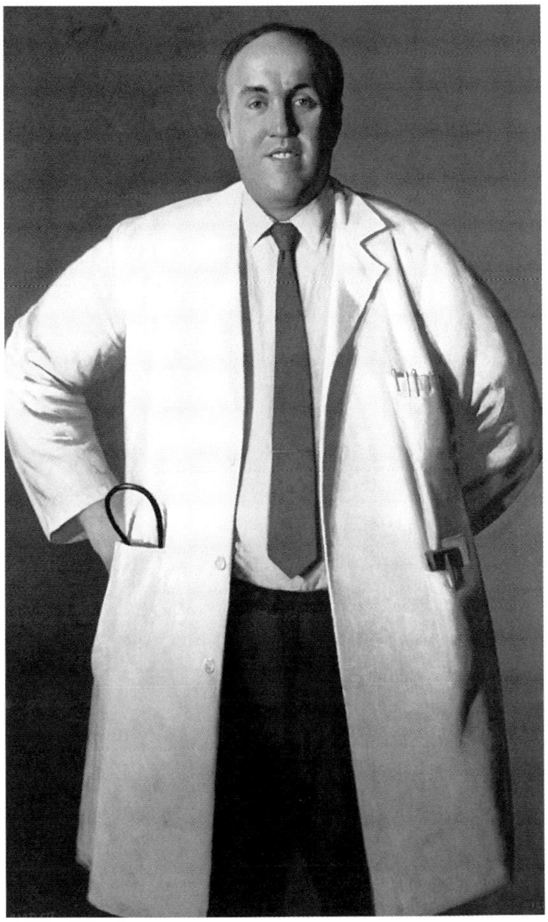

Portrait of Joseph F. Majdan

JOSEPH F. MAJDAN, M.D. (b. 1948)
By James W. ("Bo") Bartlett III (b. 1955)

Oil on canvas
1986
56 x 36 in.

Signed lower left: "BARTLETT/IGN"

Given by JMC class of 1986
Accession number: 1986+e.P.02

Dr. Joseph J. Majdan was a clinical assistant professor of medicine and cardiologist at Jefferson Medical College. He was honored repeatedly for outstanding teaching.

Joseph Majdan was born in 1948 in Hackensack, New Jersey and graduated from La Salle College in 1971. He began his medical education at the Autonomous University of Guadalajara, Mexico and received his M.D. degree from the University of Pennsylvania in 1976. He was an intern and resident at the Presbyterian/University of Pennsylvania Medical Center, and a fellow in cardiovascular diseases at Thomas Jefferson University Hospital.

Dr. Majdan joined the Jefferson faculty in 1981, and was named clinical assistant professor of medicine in 1986. For many years he contributed to the Medicine in Society course for freshmen and sophomore students, and taught the Practice of Cardiology course to seniors. He made bedside auscultation rounds three times weekly, and was teaching attending for six week blocks.

Dr. Majdan was appreciated for relating to students and house staff on a personal and caring basis. He regarded teaching as an honor and a solemn duty to impart knowledge and instill a desire to learn, not merely to impress students with one's own knowledge. He has said, "Teaching is what I was put on this earth to do."[4] He received the Christian R. and Mary F. Lindback Award for Distinguished Teaching in 1984. He won the Distinguished Teaching Award of the Thomas Jefferson University Hospital medical residents four times between 1981 and 1991. He also won Jefferson's Alpha Omega Alpha Teaching Award in 1989.

Majdan was one of seven recipients nationwide of the American Heart Association's Distinguished Teacher Award in 1985. In 1996 he was awarded La Salle University's Holroyd Award for distinguished contributions by a medical alumnus. He resigned his faculty appointment at Jefferson in January 1997.

Dr. Joseph Majdan was selected as portrait honoree by the graduating class of 1986, the youngest faculty member to receive this honor to date. The imposing portrait by James W. ("Bo") Bartlett III shows the physician two-thirds length and slightly larger than life-sized. He stands in a totally frontal position with legs apart and arms akimbo, occupying the full width and almost the full length of the canvas. He wears a white doctor coat over a blue shirt, gray trousers, and a bright red tie with a green and gold scattered pattern. Emerging from his coat pockets are some tools of his trade: stethoscope tubing, pens, papers, and a long-range pager.

His round face is dominated by a high forehead, flat nose, small mouth, and long jaw. He looks directly toward the viewer with a toothy and engaging smile. The physician's brilliant white coat billows out in a pyramidal shape, both concealing and emphasizing his physical mass. His face and the coat are painted dramatically with strong highlights and deep shadows. In contrast, the atmospheric background is smoothly painted in neutral, putty-colored tones.

Bo Bartlett's absolute control of shape, color, shadows, and contours contributes to an arresting characterization. The solidly rendered iconic figure exudes tremendous energy, verve, and warmth. One feels an immediate, almost physical connection with the portrait subject.

Bartlett's large-scale figure paintings are often allegorical in content and some have religious or biblical undertones. The initials "IGN" are found below the artist's signature on Dr. Majdan's portrait and on many of his other paintings. This monogram stands for "In God's Name" and is particularly apt, for it was mentioned during the presentation ceremony that the physician is an observant Catholic and once considered entering the seminary. The artist and subject are well matched spiritually.

Bo Bartlett was born in Columbus, Georgia in 1955. He began his art studies in 1974 working privately with Ben F. Long IV in Florence, Italy. Bartlett continued briefly at the Philadelphia College of Art and then transferred to the Pennsylvania Academy of the Fine Arts which he attended from 1976 to 1981. He was honored repeatedly by winning the Packard Prize, the Charles Toppan Prize, the Cecilia Beaux Memorial Portrait Prize, the Thouron Prize, the Consolidated/Drake Press Award, the Eleanor Gray Still Life Prize, and the Cresson traveling scholarship.

While earning a Pennsylvania Academy degree, he simultaneously studied painting privately with Nelson Shanks, attended liberal arts classes at the University of Pennsylvania, and studied anatomy at the Philadelphia College of Osteopathic Medicine. In 1986 the unusually gifted artist also earned a certificate in filmmaking at New York University.

In 1987 he received the Philadelphia Museum of Art Award at the Academy's *Fellowship Show*, and was named "Best Artist in Philly" by *Philadelphia Magazine*. He was awarded a grant by the Pew fellowship in the arts in 1994.

Bo Bartlett has exhibited in numerous important group shows and has had solo exhibitions at galleries in Philadelphia, New York, Los Angeles, San Francisco, Columbus, Georgia, and Greenville, South Carolina. In addition to private collections throughout the country, Bartlett's portraits and other figurative paintings can be found in public collections in the Philadelphia area at the Academy of Music, Beaver College, Aramark, Incorporated, Children's Hospital, the College of Physicians of Philadelphia, the Curtis Institute of Music, Fidelity Bank, the Franklin Institute, La Salle University, Old Pine Church, Pennsylvania Hospital, St. John's Episcopal Church, the Merion Cricket Club, the United States Mint, the Wistar Institute, and the Philadelphia Convention Center.

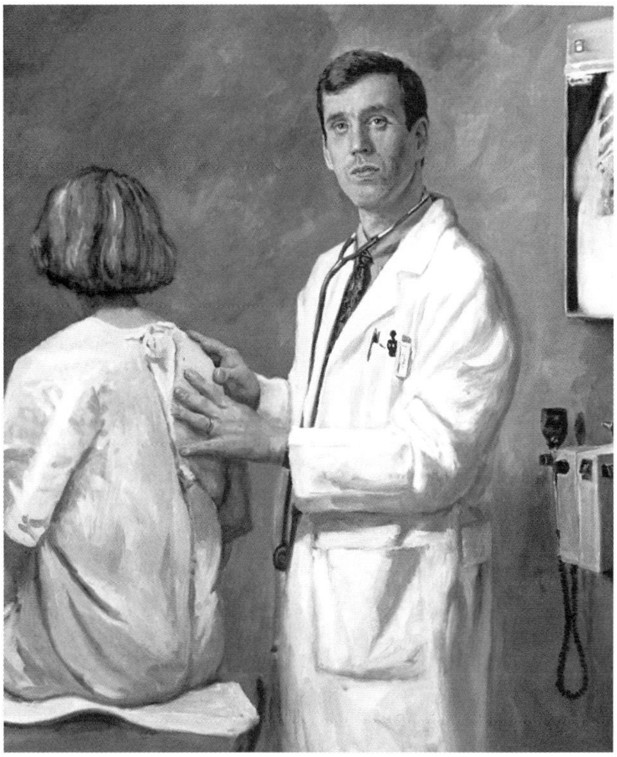

Portrait of Gregory C. Kane

GREGORY C. KANE, M.D. (b. 1961)
By Dean M. Larson (b. 1957)

Oil on canvas
1997
40 x 34 in.

Signed and dated lower right: "Dean M. Larson 1997"

Given by JMC class of 1997
Accession number: 1997+e.P.01

Dr. Gregory C. Kane is an assistant professor of medicine at Jefferson Medical College. He is board certified in pulmonary disease and critical care medicine.

Gregory Kane was born in Delaware County, Pennsylvania in 1961. He graduated from the University of Notre Dame in 1983 with high honors in engineering, and received his medical degree from Jefferson in 1987. He served his internship and residency at Lankenau Hospital.

Kane returned to Jefferson for the Alfred W. Dubbs fellowship in medicine and was made an assistant professor of medicine in 1993. He has been codirector of the pulmonary/critical care training program since 1993, and director of the medical respiratory intensive care unit since 1994.

The young physician has already made his mark as a dedicated and respected teacher and as a clinician. He won the Teaching Attending Award from junior medical house staff on the "value of humanistic care" in 1995, the Chief Residents Distinguished Teaching Award, Department of Medicine in 1996, the Dean's Award for Distinguished Teaching in a Clinical Science in 1996, and the Christian R. and Mary F. Lindback Award for Distinguished Teaching in 1998. He has written several articles and chapters on lung inflammation, new therapies for asthma, and the effect of collagen and vascular diseases on the lungs.

Speakers at the portrait ceremony consistently cited Dr. Gregory Kane's devotion to his students and compassion for his patients. Students appreciate his deep interest in the role that third- and fourth-year students play in the care of the medical patient. He has also volunteered his time treating the homeless in Philadelphia in the company of students.

At age thirty-five Dr. Gregory C. Kane was the youngest honoree ever of the senior class portrait (two years younger than Joseph F. Majdan, M.D.). Dean Larson has depicted the physician at work in a patient examining room. He is shown three-quarters length and life-sized, standing next to a seated female patient with her back to the viewer. His hands are placed on her back and shoulder and he turns away momentarily to look attentively toward the viewer. The patient was modeled by his wife, Jean, and she wears a bluish-green examining gown.

Dr. Kane is wearing a white medical coat and a stethoscope around his neck. Objects in the physician's coat pocket include a pen, calipers, and a yellow radiation exposure badge. A lateral view of a chest X-ray is visible on the screen, and an otoscope and ophthalmoscope are attached to the wall.

Dr. Kane was adamant that the portrait should include a patient and his medical instruments. At the portrait ceremony he exhorted the class to retain traditional humanistic values, even in the current changing medical environment:

> You'll note that I've chosen to be portrayed with a patient to emphasize that in this era of competition and medicine as business, we must remember it is our patients whom we serve—and our patients who must remain the focus of our educational efforts.
>
> We have tried to teach this here at Jefferson: from bedside teaching of physical diagnosis, to sessions in clinical ethics, to lessons in clinical care that emphasize connecting with your patients.

Dean M. Larson was born in 1957 in Norway, Michigan and reared in Palmer, Alaska. He received an undergraduate degree from Willamette University in Salem, Oregon in 1980 and a master's degree in art education from Towson State University in Maryland in 1984. He also received a diploma from the Schuler School of Fine Arts in Baltimore the following year.

In addition to his more "polished" portraits, Larson also paints light-filled landscapes, architectural scenes, and colorful still lifes in a spontaneous, painterly technique. He has had solo exhibitions in Washington, D.C. and Baltimore, and other cities in Alaska, Maryland, and Oregon. He won the John and Anna Lee Stacey Competition in 1984 and 1992, and was a finalist in *Artist's Magazine* national portrait competition. He received an individual artist grant from the Maryland State Arts Council in 1996.

Larson is represented by galleries and portrait representatives in Washington, San Francisco, Philadelphia, and Portland, Oregon. In addition to schools, banks, and corporate headquarters, his work can be found at Johns Hopkins University, the University of Pennsylvania School of Law, the University of Texas in Austin, the Alaska State Capitol in Juneau, and the Kuwaiti Embassy in Washington, D.C.

Portrait of Edward H. McGehee

(See color plate)

EDWARD HENDERSON McGEHEE, M.D.
(b. 1921)
By José Fernandez Marcote (b. 1950)

Oil on canvas
1976
60 1/2 x 48 in.

Signed and dated lower right: "MARCOTE 76"

Given by JMC class of 1976
Accession number: 1976+e.P.02

Dr. Edward H. McGehee was a professor of family medicine and a clinical associate professor of medicine at Thomas Jefferson University, a beloved clinician for more than four decades.

Edward McGehee was born in 1921 in Mobile, Alabama. He received his undergraduate degree from the University of Pennsylvania in 1942 and his medical degree from Jefferson Medical College in 1945. His brother, John, is a Jefferson alumnus from the class of 1952, and his father and another brother are also physicians.

Dr. Edward McGehee served his internship at City Hospital in Mobile, followed by two years in the U.S. Navy. His extensive postgraduate training included: the Ross V. Patterson fellowship in pathology at Jefferson Medical College, a research fellowship in hematology and a residency in medicine at Pennsylvania Hospital, and the Thomas McCrae fellowship in medicine of the Pennsylvania Hospital's exchange fellowship with Guy's Hospital in London.

Upon his return to Philadelphia in 1953 Dr. McGehee enjoyed a busy private family practice in the Chestnut Hill section of Philadelphia for twenty years. He was attending and then senior attending physician at Chestnut Hill Hospital from 1954 to 1973, and director of the department of medicine there from 1966 to 1970. He was also hematologist and physician to Pennsylvania Hospital from 1956 to 1966.

In 1974 Dr. Edward McGehee was the first full-time faculty member to be recruited by Dr. Paul C. Brucker, chairman of Jefferson's new department of family medicine. McGehee's affable personality and compassion for his patients were honored spectacularly when he retired from private practice to join the Jefferson faculty: over five hundred appreciative but sorrowful patients attended a surprise going-away party!

McGehee's new titles at Jefferson were professor in the department of family medicine, associate in the Cardeza Foundation for Hematological Research, and clinical associate professor of medicine (secondary faculty appointment). In 1984 he was named the first Ellen M. and Dale W. Garber Professor of Family Medicine, and was acting chairman of the department from 1990 to 1992. In 1989 Dr. McGehee was named director of the Jefferson/Kendal-Crosslands fellowship in geriatrics.

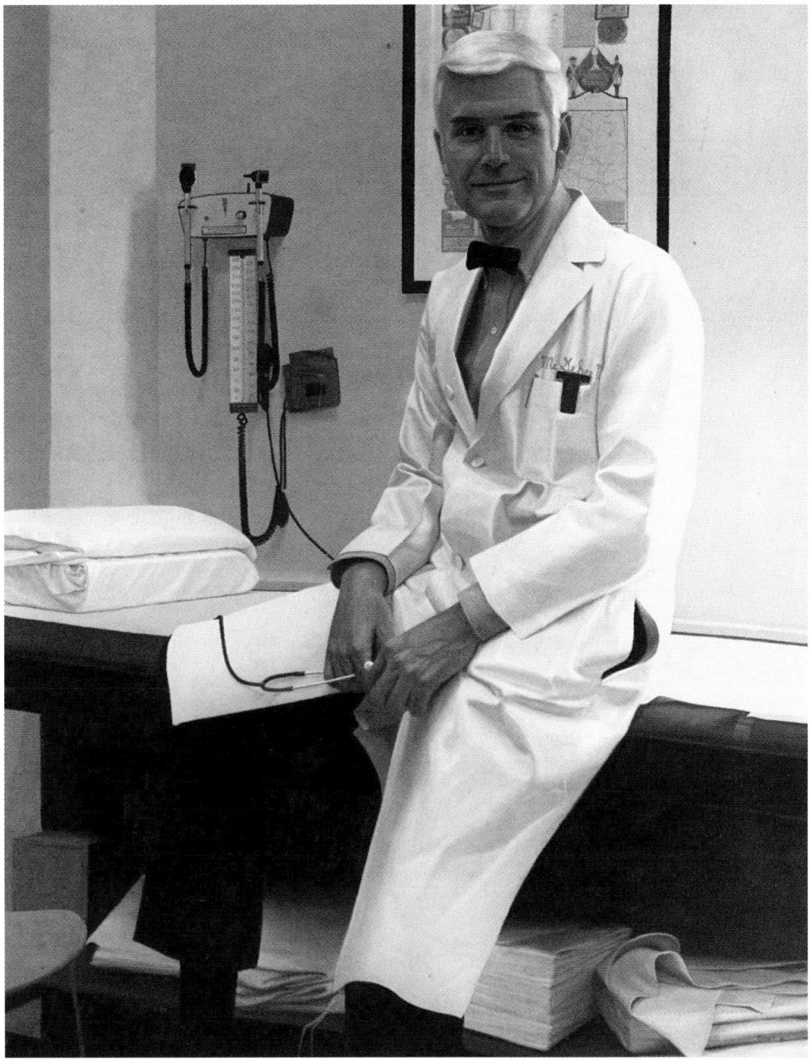

Dr. McGehee has been an enduring and strong role model for generations of medical students, as well as a dedicated primary care physician. He received the Christian R. and Mary F. Lindback Award for Distinguished Teaching in 1977, only three years after his arrival. In 1996 the McGehee Loan Fund was established in his honor to assist third- and fourth-year medical students who plan to practice family or internal medicine. Funds were donated by grateful, longtime patients Anne Banse and her late husband, Robert L. Banse.

Dr. McGehee helped develop a widely used, self-assessment examination for practicing physicians under the aegis of the Philadelphia County Medical Society and the American College of Physicians. He has been active in hospital and college committees and in professional organizations. He served two terms as president of the Philadelphia Society of Hematology in 1963 and 1977, and was president of Jefferson's alumni association in 1995. He received the Distinguished Service Award of the Committee of the Chapel of the Four Chaplains in 1980, and was Laureate of the Pennsylvania Chapter, American College of Physicians in 1987.

When elected senior portrait honoree in 1976, McGehee chose a new artist for the Jefferson collection, the talented young Spaniard José F. Marcote. The artist's wife, the former Joan Sauvion, is a native Philadelphian and her parents are patients of Dr. McGehee.

José Marcote's impressive, large-scale painting situates the subject in his working environment, as in his depiction of Richard G. Berry, M.D. which was created the following year. But here Dr. McGehee is in an examining room, not a laboratory; and unlike the Berry portrait, McGehee is centrally located in a close-up view, and is shown full length and somewhat larger than life-sized.

He is seated in a relaxed posture with legs hanging over the edge of an examining table. He holds a stethoscope between his fingers. His head turns to look directly at the viewer. His oval-shaped face and thick white hair are accented by dark eyebrows and brown eyes, straight nose, and wide, smiling mouth. His warm and engaging expression suggests an accessible personality. Perhaps he is awaiting his next patient.

The physician is dressed in a crisp white coat with "McGehee" stitched in blue thread over the pocket, a blue shirt, and black trousers and bow tie. Besides his stethoscope, other medical instruments include an otoscope, ophthalmoscope, and sphygmomanometer attached to the rear wall. Additional elements in the room are the starched white linens on the table and stacks of folded sheets below; the partial view of a low stool; and a framed antique map of Philadelphia's historic Germantown on the pale yellow wall.

The convincing likeness of the subject and his personable expression and easy posture, as well as the painting's underlying geometric design and dramatic contrasts of light and dark, all contribute to an unusually effective composition.

Dr. McGehee spoke of his longstanding philosophy about compassionate handling of patients when his portrait was presented at Senior Class Day:

> Think for a moment each day: "Am I caring about these folks?"...Take a minute to find out a bit about a patient's work, family, or background. What we hear frequently generates admiration and understanding, and builds a lasting bridge.
>
> Part of most physicians' jobs is tending the seriously ill. Never think, "I can't do anything for him so I won't go by to see him." The doctor is as important as the remedy. Visit the sick.
>
> Share a little of your own life, your family, your kid, your own illness or that of someone in your family, if it is somewhat related to your patient's problem. This evidence of humanity in the doctor reassures the patients and improves their view of the whole medical profession. Similarly, doctors can shed a tear at the death of a patient without loss of esteem. Go to funerals and speak a few appropriate words at memorial services for your patients. You will have seen them suffer and know how they handled the most trying of experiences. Your words will be helpful to family and friends.

Portrait of Robert L. Perkel

ROBERT LOUIS PERKEL, M.D. (b. 1950)
By Lauren A. Henick

Oil on canvas
1987
36 1/4 x 32 1/4 in.

Signed lower right: "Lauren A. Henick"

Given by JMC class of 1987
Accession number: 1987+e.P.04

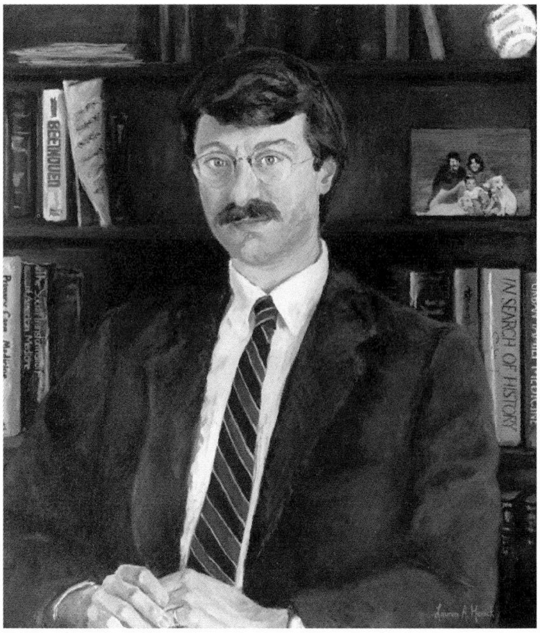

Dr. Robert L. Perkel is a clinical professor of family medicine and an instructor in medicine at Jefferson Medical College.

Robert Perkel was born in 1950 in Jersey City, New Jersey. He was a history graduate of Yale University (1972), and after two additional years of premedical study at Yale, attended Rutgers University Medical School and then transferred to Albert Einstein College of Medicine where he received his degree (1978).

Dr. Perkel served a residency in family medicine at Jefferson and joined the department in 1981. He rose in the ranks to become a clinical professor in 1996.

Among his social and humanitarian concerns, Dr. Perkel is especially interested in the medical needs of handicapped, elderly, and indigent urban patients. He has been medical director of the hospital's department of home health care, chairman of the HIV-AIDS caregivers committee, and chairman of the ethics committee. He is a member of the professional advisory committee of Judicare, a legal agency for the poor.

In the department of family medicine Dr. Perkel has been director of the Urban Home Visit Program and project director of the Geriatric Home Assessment Treatment Program in the Ludlow community. He has coordinated the freshman course in Ethics and Medicine and the sophomore course on Medicine and Society. He founded the Literature and Medicine seminar series.

Dr. Perkel has also taught third- and fourth-year students in the family medicine clinical rotation and served as advisor to many class members. In 1991 he won the Christian R. and Mary F. Lindback Award for Distinguished Teaching. In 1994 he was Class Day faculty speaker and received a special faculty award from family medicine residents.

Dr. Robert L. Perkel was a young assistant professor of family medicine when he was chosen as senior portrait honoree in 1987. He selected a youthful artist, Lauren A. Henick, for the depiction. He is shown half-length and slightly larger than life-sized, seated in front of a bookcase. He looks straight toward the viewer with an earnest expression, and perhaps a hint of inquisitiveness. His most notable features are his thick brown hair and mustache and blue eyes looking through wire-rimmed glasses. He is wearing a brown suit coat, white shirt, and necktie with red, yellow, and blue stripes.

The carefully chosen objects on the shelves reflect his professional and personal interests. Legible book titles include *Primary Care Medicine, The Social Transformation of American Medicine, Urban Family Medicine, Beethoven,* and *In Search of History*.

Dr. Perkel is an accomplished clarinetist and athlete, and his portrait also displays some unidentified sheet music and a scuffed baseball teetering on the edge of the top shelf. A family photograph shows Dr. Perkel, his wife Madeline who is a nurse, their young daughter, and two Labrador retrievers.

Portrait of Robert L. Brent

ROBERT LEONARD BRENT, M.D., Ph.D. (b. 1927)
By Neil Kosh (b. 1926)

Oil on canvas
1989
38 1/14 x 32 1/4 in.

Signed and dated lower right: "Neil Kosh/1989"

Given in 1989 by friends and colleagues
Accession number: 1989+e.P.02

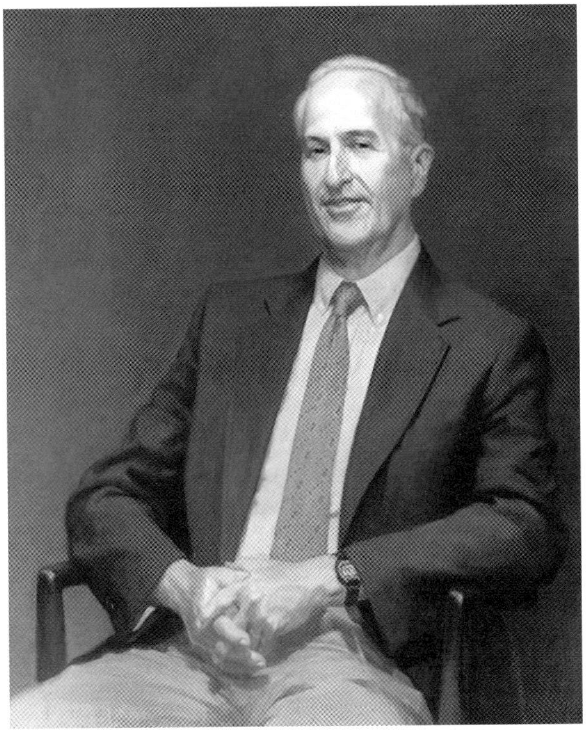

Dr. Robert L. Brent is a longtime Jefferson leader in pediatrics, radiology, and pathology, anatomy, and cell biology, and he is one of only four faculty members ever to be designated Distinguished Professor. He is an international authority on congenital malformations and developmental biology, and the effects of radiation on the embryo.

Robert Brent was born in 1927, a native of Rochester, New York. His degrees were earned at the University of Rochester: bachelor of arts (1948), doctor of medicine (1953), and doctor of philosophy in radiation biology and embryology (1955). During this period of training he was a research fellow of the National Foundation for Infantile Paralysis at Rochester, and a clinical fellow at Massachusetts General Hospital where he interned in pediatrics.

While at the University of Rochester Brent worked as a research associate on an atomic energy project in the department of genetics and embryology, concentrating on birth defects and genetic changes in development due to exposure to radiation. From 1955 to 1957 he was chief of the radiobiology section and assistant chief of pediatrics at the Walter Reed Army Institute of Research, where he developed human risk standards for radioiodine use during pregnancy.

Dr. Robert L. Brent joined the Jefferson faculty in 1957 as associate professor of pediatrics. When he became professor of pediatrics in 1961 at age thirty-three, he was the youngest full professor ever named at Jefferson. He was appointed chairman of the department in 1966 and remained in the post until 1995. He directed the Stein Research Center from 1964 to 1989, and in 1985 was named the Louis and Bess Stein Professor of Pediatrics. He was appointed professor of radiology (radiation biology) in 1962 and professor of anatomy in 1971.

In 1957 Dr. Brent had founded the clinical teratology and radiation biology division at the Stein Research Center. Under his direction animal studies were performed on the effects of high energy radiation on the developing embryo, placenta transport, embryonic nutrition, developmental immunological studies, biochemical embryology, and various techniques of embryo culture. The development and expansion of investigative research in the pediatrics department was "largely attributable to his efforts."[5] For over three decades Dr. Brent's research was funded uninterruptedly by the National Institutes of Health.

In 1991 Brent reported that since 1962 research for the Developmental Biology Research and Training Program had yielded over five hundred publications and has resulted in the training of numerous medical students, graduate students, fellows, and visiting scientists. Outstanding funded projects were generated in the divisions of neonatology, neurology, genetics and teratology, allergy and immunology, and general pediatrics.[6]

Under his direction the pediatric medical education of students and house staff was improved and broadened, and outstanding patient care programs were developed in the pediatric subspecialties. Jefferson has had strong affiliations in pediatrics with the Children's Rehabilitation Hospital, the Geisinger Medical Center, Mercy Catholic Medical Center, the Medical Center of Delaware, and most recently the Alfred I. duPont Institute and Children's Hospital in Wilmington. The latter has become the largest of Jefferson's academic pediatric programs and evolved into a full-service hospital.

Dr. Robert L. Brent is author or coauthor of almost 550 articles, abstracts, films, and book chapters. He is editor of *Prevention of Embryonic, Fetal and Perinatal Disease* (with Maureen L. Harris, 1976), *Clinics in Perinatology* (with David A. Beckman, 1986), and *Teratogen Update: Environmentally Induced Birth Defect Risks* (with John L. Sever, 1986).

Brent was a founding member of the Teratology Society, its president in 1968, and three-time editor of the journal *Teratology*. He has been a member of the editorial boards of *Fetal Medicine*, *Pediatrics*, and *Fetal Therapy*. He was a member of the editorial advisory board of the Institute for Scientific Information.

Dr. Brent has been an active committee member, advisory council member, or panelist of the Food and Drug Administration, the American Academy of Pediatrics, the National Science Foundation, the National Institutes of Health, the Society for Experimental Biology and Medicine, and the National Council on Radiation Protection and Measurements. He is also a trustee of the Health and Environmental Sciences Institute.

Dr. Brent has been the recipient of numerous American and foreign awards and honors. He has presented endowed lectures to the Radiological Society of North America, the New York Roentgen Society, the Teratology Society, the Puerto Rico Medical Association, and hospitals and universities throughout the country. He was the Royal Society of Medicine traveling fellow at Cambridge University in 1971-72, and received traveling lectureships sponsored by the Japanese Ministry of Health with the Japanese Teratology Society in 1983, and the Bureau of Health of the People's Republic of China with the World Health Organization in 1986.

Dr. Robert L. Brent was the keynote speaker at the International Conference on the Prevention of Congenital Malformations in Strasbourg, France in 1981, and at the International Society for Biomedical Research on Alcoholism at the University of Bristol, U.K. in 1992. He received the Lady Davis Scholar Award of Hadassah Medical Center at Hebrew University in 1983, and the Landauer Award of the Health Physics Society in 1994. He received an honorary doctor of science degree from the University of Rochester in 1988. In 1997 he was elected a member of the Institute of Medicine of the National Academy of Sciences.

Dr. Brent's honors for teaching and distinguished service to Thomas Jefferson University include the Christian R. and Mary F. Lindback Award for Distinguished Teaching in 1968, the Winged Ox Award for Distinguished Service in 1986, and the Burlington Northern Foundation Faculty Achievement Award in 1990. His title of Distinguished Professor of Pediatrics was announced at his portrait ceremony in 1989.

The portrait by Neil Kosh was presented by Dr. Brent's friends and colleagues. It shows the physician two-thirds length and slightly larger than life-sized, seated in an office armchair. His body is turned slightly to the left and he looks directly toward the viewer. His chiseled features include a high forehead, thin nose, strong jaw, and angular chin. His lips are slightly parted in a pleasant and straightforward expression.

He leans back comfortably in a relaxed pose. His arms rest on the chair arms and his hands are clasped with fingers interlaced. He is wearing a dark blue blazer, blue shirt, tan trousers, and an umber necktie with blue dots. The atmospheric background is maroon. Neil Kosh's painting style is smooth and fluid, and he has achieved a convincingly lifelike figure.

Almost all speakers at the ceremony stressed Dr. Brent's humanitarian concerns and compassion with patients and their families. A particularly eloquent address was given by the subject's oldest son, David A. Brent, M.D., a 1974 Jefferson graduate and associate professor and chairman of the division of child psychiatry at Western Psychiatric Institute and Clinic of the University of Pittsburgh Medical School. He said that his father

> demonstrated through his own example that life is a precious gift, not to be squandered in pettiness or self-absorption, but to be cherished and celebrated through daily acts of loving and helping others...His acts of goodness and love, of consideration, scholarship, and charity...form his most meaningful and enduring portrait.

Another son, Lawrence H. Brent, M.D., graduated from Jefferson Medical College in 1979. His daughter, Deborah Brent Foster, received a B.S. in nursing from Jefferson's College of Allied Health Sciences in 1980.

Painter Neil Kosh was born in 1926 in St. Clair, Pennsylvania. He attended Oberlin College and transferred to Tyler School of Art of Temple University where he received undergraduate and master's degrees between 1947 and 1956. He served as a naval aviation cadet during World War II, and a clinical psychology technician with the U.S. Army during the Korean War.

Neil Kosh's teaching career has always been at Tyler, where he began as an instructor in drawing and painting in 1957. He chaired the art department from 1963 to 1982, and directed the Temple University Program Abroad at the Villa Caproni in Rome from 1973 to 1975. He won the Certificate of Honor of Temple's general alumni association in 1973.

Kosh is best known as a figure painter, and his public portraits can be found in the permanent collections of Temple University, Hahnemann University, the College of Physicians of Philadelphia, and Rolling Hill Hospital, among others. He has exhibited widely in group shows throughout the country, and has had one-man shows at the Woodmere Gallery, Pearl Fox Gallery, and the Paley Cultural Center at Temple University.

Portrait of Robert L. Brent

(See color plate)

ROBERT LEONARD BRENT, M.D., Ph.D.
By Dean L. Paules (b. 1931)

Oil on canvas
1996
50 x 38 in.

Signed and dated lower left: "Paules/2-96"
Exhibition: New York, *National Portrait Competition*, Portrait Institute, 1996

Portrait of Lillian H. (Mrs. Robert L.) Brent

LILLIAN H. (MRS. ROBERT L.) BRENT (b. 1928)
By Dean L. Paules

Oil on canvas
1996
50 x 38 in.

Signed and dated lower left: "Paules/2-96"

Both portraits commissioned in 1996 by TJU
Accession numbers: 1996+e.P.02, 1996+e.P.03

The pendant portraits of Dr. and Mrs. Robert L. Brent are the only portraits ever commissioned by Jefferson of a faculty member and his spouse, and only the third couple in the collection painted by the same artist. Portraits of two other couples were painted by different artists.[7]

The occasion for the double portrait presentation on April 8, 1996 was the dedication of the Lillian and Robert Brent Auditorium on the mezzanine level of Jefferson Alumni Hall. On that same day an announcement was made of a new endowed chair at Jefferson Medical College, the Robert L. Brent Professorship of Pediatrics.

A symposium was also held on April 8, "Brent Day," and featured several of Dr. Brent's colleagues and trainees who delivered papers that would be published in *Reproductive Toxicology* as a Festschrift in his honor. Overflow crowds attended both the symposium and the portrait presentation.

Also an educator, Lillian H. Brent graduated from the University of Rochester in 1950 and earned a master's degree in education from Temple University in 1963. Until her retirement in 1992 she has taught at Temple's Laboratory School and at public and parochial suburban schools. Lillian Brent was described by President Bruck-

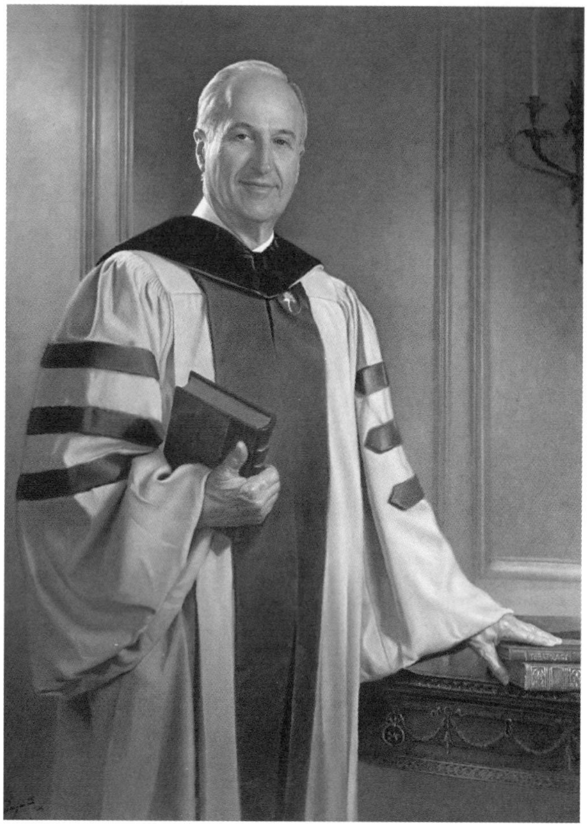

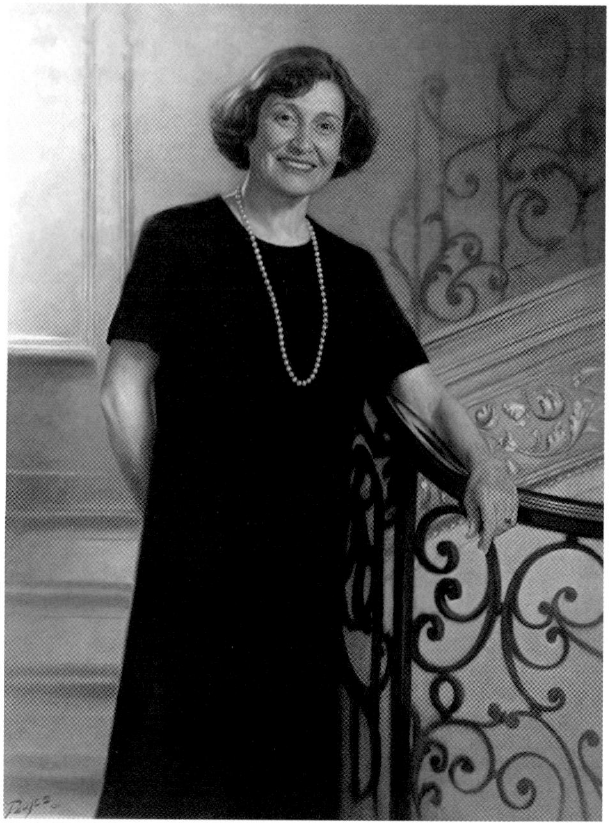

er and others at the dual portrait presentation as being an uncommon complement to Bob during his long career at Jefferson.

"Medicine, an Excuse from Living" is a lecture presented to first year students since 1966. It was written originally by Robert and Lillian Brent as part of the course Medicine and Society. It strives to take medicine off its pedestal and to strike down the notion of the overcommitted physician's "being in service" as an excuse for neglect of responsibilities toward spouse, children, parents, and friends.

The lecture was expanded into an innovative and popular sophomore elective course, Personal and Professional Problems of Physicians, and the course materials developed into a thick book of advice ranging from practical financial and legal issues to dealing with difficult life experiences.

At the ceremony Herbert C. Mansmann Jr., M.D. presented Dr. Brent with a surprise gift: a watercolor portrait bust of the honoree by pediatrician Gary Carpenter, M.D. The ceremony also included the announcement of an annual performance at Jefferson by talented young musicians from the Curtis Institute of Music, in memory of another son, James, an accomplished musician who died in 1979.

The imposing life-sized, almost full-length portraits by Dean Paules show both subjects in the morning room at the duPont mansion on the grounds of the A. I. duPont Institute. Lillian Brent stands on a winding staircase with a brass and wrought iron balustrade, before a pale green paneled wall. She wears an elegant, short sleeved black dress accompanied by a strand of opera length pearls. Her left arm rests on the curving banister and she looks straight ahead. Her dimpled smile is warm and ingratiating as though she might be receiving guests.

Dr. Robert L. Brent wears a strikingly brilliant, yellow academic gown from the University of Rochester, accented with a royal blue hood, front panels, and stripes on the full sleeves. He, too, smiles engagingly toward the viewer. His right hand holds a leather-bound book and his left hand rests on books on an adjoining carved table. A wrought iron sconce is seen on the green panelled wall above the table.

In October 1996 Dean Paules won an honorable mention for the portrait of Dr. Brent at the *National Portrait Competition* held at the Portrait Institute in New York. The painting was shown in color in an exhibition review in the December issue of *American Artist*.

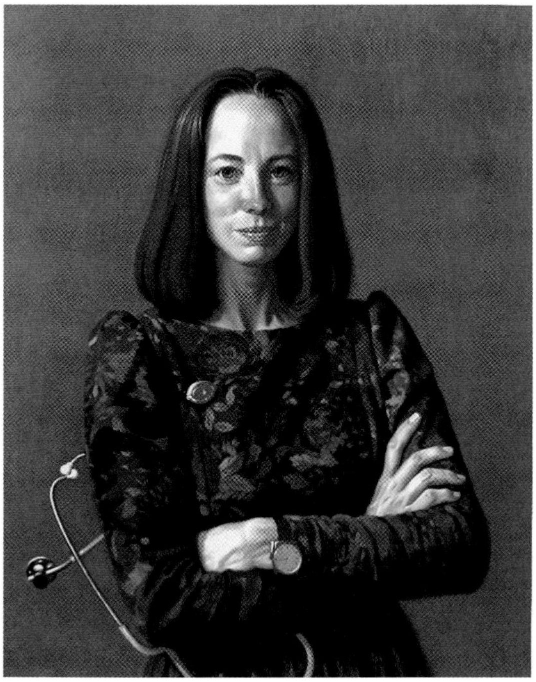

Portrait of Clara A. Callahan

CLARA A. CALLAHAN, M.D. (b. 1951)
By Stephen S. Kennedy (b. 1953)

Oil on canvas
1992
36 1/4 x 30 1/4 in.

Signed and dated lower right: "Stephen Kennedy/'92"

Given by JMC class of 1992
Accession number:1992+e.P.03

Dr. Clara A. Callahan is the associate dean for student affairs at Jefferson Medical College and a clinical associate professor of pediatrics.

Born in 1951, Clara Callahan is a native of Phillipsburg, Pennsylvania. She was a *cum laude* graduate of Wayne State University in Detroit in 1973, and winner of the pediatrics and child psychiatry awards at Medical College of Pennsylvania where she graduated in 1977. She was a resident in pediatrics at Medical College of Pennsylvania Hospital and Thomas Jefferson University Hospital. She was the first Charles E. Culpepper fellow in ambulatory pediatrics at Jefferson, and also attending pediatrician at Booth Maternity Hospital.

Dr. Callahan joined the Jefferson faculty as assistant professor of pediatrics in 1984, and has also been pediatric consultant at Wills Eye Hospital since that date. She became the assistant dean for student affairs in 1987. She was promoted to clinical associate professor of pediatrics in 1991 and associate dean for student affairs the following year.

In addition to her administrative duties in the dean's office, Dr. Callahan has been a clinical preceptor for freshman students, taught a ten-week seminar on ethical issues in medicine for sophomore students, and held a teaching conference on nutrition and immunizations for third-year students.

Dr. Clara Callahan has served as chair of the pediatric bioethics committee, and served on task forces for student life, the joint Delaware-JMC program, and primary care. She was a member of the visiting faculty in Japan sponsored by the Noguchi Medical Research Institute and the Japan-North America Medical Exchange Foundation in 1994. She won the pediatric residents' Award for Excellence in Teaching in 1987. Her impact on Jefferson students as administrator, advisor, and teacher has been significant, and she was elected senior portrait honoree in 1992.

The striking portrait by Stephen S. Kennedy shows the physician half length and life-sized, standing with arms folded in front of her body. She holds a stethoscope in her left hand. She gazes intently toward the viewer while appearing to suppress a smile at the same time. The distinctive features of her long, heart-shaped face include high forehead, large and expressive blue eyes, high cheekbones, tipped nose, full mouth, and dimples. Her sleek, thick brown hair is shoulder length. She wears a silver pin and a large, utilitarian wrist watch.

Two objects in the portrait have special meaning for Dr. Callahan. The pediatric stethoscope was a gift from her late father-in-law, David H. Goodman, M.D., a graduate in Jefferson's class of 1935. The pin was a 1987 gift from student council members in gratitude for her support of their activities.

The beautifully modulated color of this smoothly painted portrait includes the subject's pinkish skin tones, her long-sleeved, floral print dress in shades of turquoise, green, and purple on a dark ground, and the warm pinkish-brown atmospheric background. Effective use of light on the sitter's face and hands helps to reveal their sculpted forms.

At the portrait ceremony Dr. Clara Callahan was universally described as a dedicated, warm, generous, compassionate, and resilient person, an excellent role model for students and house staff. "She can make a smile grow on anyone's face, even in a dreary situation," according to the speakers, and "She's managed to tread the line between helping students overcome problems, and maintaining the guidelines of the society they must work within." Dr. Callahan comes across as innately modest, which might explain the somewhat awkward and self-conscious gesture of folded arms in the portrait.

Painter Stephen S. Kennedy was born in 1957 in Utica, New York and reared in Rochester where his father was an advertising manager and his mother an amateur artist. After one year studying theater at Catholic University in Washington, D.C., Kennedy became an apprentice illustrator for a publishing firm. During this uncertain period he took his first painting course at night with Diana Dawson in Markham, Virginia and soon became her apprentice, performing house and studio work in return for board and art training. He transferred to the studio of Nelson Shanks where he spent four more years as an apprentice painter. In addition to instruction in painting and art history Shanks provided Kennedy with models, still life setups including his prized antiques, and a rural farm setting for landscape painting.

Almost as soon as Kennedy opened his own studio in Philadelphia he has attracted portrait clients through word of mouth and eventually through an agent. His realistic portraits are known for rich color, sensitive lighting, and attention to detail. Presently his studio is located in Fort Washington, Pennsylvania and he teaches figure painting at the Princeton Art Association. His work can be found in numerous private collections and at the Academy of Natural Sciences, the Philadelphia Athenaeum, the Campbell Soup Company, and the Philadelphia Club, among others.

Portrait of John F. Ditunno Jr.

JOHN F. DITUNNO Jr., M.D. (b. 1932)
By Dean L. Paules (b. 1931)

Oil on canvas
1997
44 x 34 in.

Signed and dated lower left: "Paules/5-97"

Given in 1997 by friends and colleagues
Accession number: 1997+e.P.02

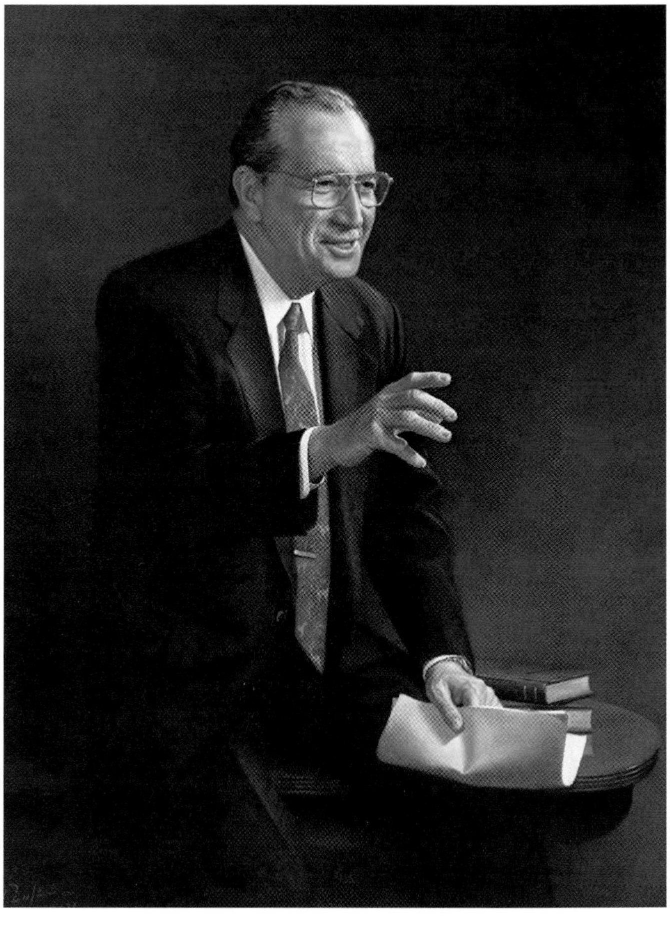

Dr. John F. Ditunno Jr. is a professor of rehabilitation medicine, and was for many years the Jessie B. Michie Professor and chair of the department at Jefferson. He also served as director of the Regional Spinal Cord Injury Center of the Delaware Valley, and is nationally renowned in this field.

Born in 1932 in Philadelphia, John F. Ditunno Jr. is a graduate of St. Joseph College (1954) and Hahnemann Medical College (1958). He served his internship and residency at Hahnemann, and worked briefly in general practice in Hot Springs, North Carolina. He pursued further postgraduate training in physical medicine and rehabilitation at Jacobi Hospital of Albert Einstein Medical School and the Hospital of the University of Pennsylvania.

Ditunno's early posts were as chief of the section of physical medicine and rehabilitation at Hahnemann Medical College, and then as director of clinical management in the division of physical medicine and rehabilitation at Temple University School of Medicine. He was appointed professor and first chair of rehabilitation medicine at Jefferson in 1969, when the division (which had been included in internal medicine) was established as a separate department. In 1987 Ditunno was appointed the first Jessie B. Michie Professor of Rehabilitation Medicine.

Starting in 1978 Dr. Ditunno was the project director of the multidisciplinary Spinal Cord Injury Center of the Delaware Valley, a cooperative program of patient care and research between Thomas Jefferson University where patients receive acute care and rehabilitation, and Magee Rehabilitation Hospital where patients are transferred for ongoing rehabilitation and lifetime follow-up. There are only thirteen government-funded regional spinal cord centers in the country, and the Jefferson facility is one of four that are also designated Level One Trauma Centers.

Dr. Ditunno was project director of Jefferson's National Rehabilitation Research and Training Center for Neural Recovery and Functional Enhancement in Spinal Cord Injury from 1988 to 1993. He has also been consultant at Lankenau Hospital, the Medical Center of Wilmington, Albert Einstein Medical Center, Crozer-Chester Medical Center, and Wills Eye Hospital. Ditunno served as chairman and editor of *International Standards for Neurological and Functional Classifications of Spinal Cord Injury* which provided a universal language for classification of injuries, now accepted throughout the world.

One of the nation's foremost experts in his field, Dr. Ditunno has served as president of the American Academy of Physical Medicine and Rehabilitation, the American Spinal Injury Association, the Association of Academic Physiatrists, the Eastern Section of the American Congress of Rehabilitation Medicine, the Philadelphia Society of Physical Medicine and Rehabilitation, and the Pennsylvania Academy of Physical Medicine. He was also chairman of the American Board of Physical Medicine and Rehabilitation, and served on advisory committees and panels for the National Institutes of Health, the Centers for Disease Control, and the Department of Health and Human Services.

Dr. Ditunno has been honored to deliver many named lectureships, including: the Licht lectureship at the University of Minnesota, the Lewis A. Leavitt memorial lectureship at Baylor College of Medicine, the Prince visiting professorship at Northwestern University Medical School, the Sidney Licht visiting professorship at Ohio State University, the Heiner Sell lectureship at the American Spinal Injury Association, and the first William Erdman lectureship at the Association of Academic Physiatrists.

Other special honors accorded Dr. Ditunno include the Presidential Award of the American Academy of Physical Medicine and Rehabilitation in 1982, the Clarence E. Shaffrey, S.J. Award of St. Joseph's University in 1994, and the Burlington Foundation Faculty Achievement Award at Jefferson Medical College in 1992.

Dr. Ditunno's friends and colleagues at Jefferson presented his portrait as one of several events marking his retirement as department chair in 1997. Dean Paules has depicted the physician two-thirds length and life-sized, seated on the edge of a table. His body and head are turned to the right, and he smiles cheerfully as though in animated conversation. The presence of an unseen visitor is suggested by Ditunno's dramatic gesture. He thrusts his right hand forward into space with the fingers spread apart. His lowered left hand holds some folded papers and rests quietly next to books.

The subject is wearing a dark blue suit, white shirt, and bright red patterned necktie. His hand, face, and other elements of the painting are illuminated in bright light entering from the right. The very dark, atmospheric background is smoothly painted in neutral umber and khaki tones.

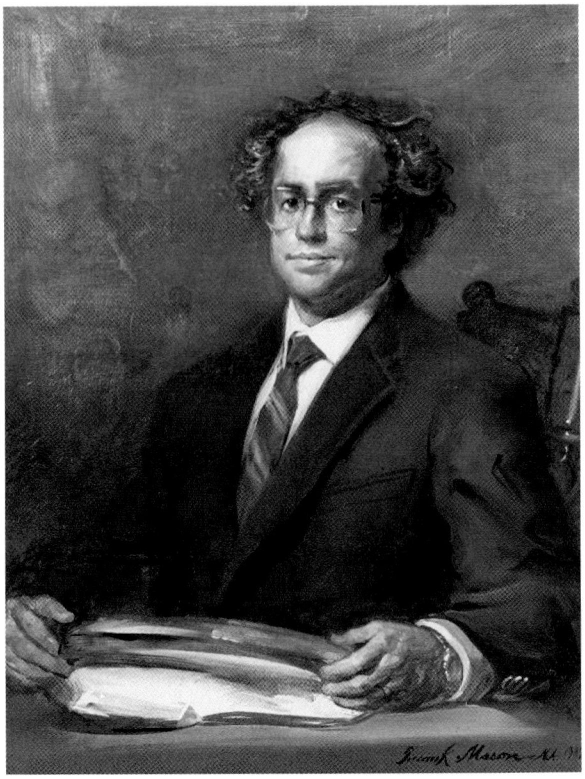

Portrait of George C. Brainard

GEORGE CURWIN BRAINARD, Ph.D. (b. 1950)
By Frank Herbert Mason (b. 1921)

Oil on canvas
1989
33 1/2 x 26 1/2 in.

Signed and dated lower right: "Frank Mason N.A. 1989"

Given by JMC class of 1989
Accession number: 1989+e.P.01

Dr. George C. Brainard is a professor of neurology and professor of biochemistry and molecular pharmacology at Jefferson. He is recognized worldwide for pioneering research in treating patients suffering from seasonal affective disorder with light therapy.

George Brainard was born in 1950, a native of Youngstown, Ohio. He earned his undergraduate degree at Wesleyan University (1973), a master of arts degree in psychology at Goddard College (1978), and a doctorate in anatomy at the University of Texas Health Science Center (1982). He was a postdoctoral fellow at Oregon Health Sciences University (1982) and at Jefferson Medical College (1983).

Dr. Brainard joined the Jefferson faculty in 1984 as assistant professor of neurology and four years later received a secondary appointment as assistant professor of pharmacology. He advanced to full professor of neurology in 1994, and received a secondary appointment as professor of biochemistry and molecular pharmacology in 1997. He has been course director of both advanced neuroscience and graduate and medical neuroscience, and codirector of the sophomore seminar on complementary medicine. He has also lectured on advanced graduate endocrinology and graduate pharmacology at Jefferson, and advanced mammalian physiology at the University of Delaware.

In 1986 after only two years on the Jefferson faculty Dr. George Brainard received the Christian R. and Mary F. Lindback Award for Distinguished Teaching. The well liked educator was chosen as Parents Day speaker by the sophomore class nine times between 1985 and 1996.

Much of Dr. Brainard's scientific investigation is concerned with the way in which light in the environment affects humans and other animals biologically, by stimulating not only the visual system, but also the immune system, hormonal system, the brain, and ultimately behavior and consciousness. Brainard is a director of a Jefferson study designed to learn how light can improve the moods of patients suffering from seasonal affective disorder, a kind of depression. It is known that decreased sunlight is a major contributing factor to the illness, and some scientists feel that melatonin or serotonin may be involved.

While the causes are still being debated, patients to Jefferson's SAD clinic are being treated with light boxes, portable head-mounted light devices, and similar therapies. In addition to being principal investigator or co-principal investigator of numerous research grants, Dr. Brainard was awarded a patent for a "portable light unit for stimulating the neuroendocrine system and achieving phototherapy for depression."

Brainard edited the section "Non-visual Effects of Radiant Energy" for the eighth edition of *Illuminating Engineering Society Lighting Handbook* (1993), and was consulting general editor of *Biology* (1990). He has been a reviewer for a dozen journals including the *American Journal of Physiology, Journal of Pineal Research, Journal of Biological Rhythms, Brain Research,* and *Photobiology and Photochemistry.*

Since 1987 Dr. George Brainard has contributed his expertise to the lighting design of NASA's space shuttle, space station, and space laboratory. He has been a consultant in experimental light therapy for the Psychobiology Branch of the National Institute of Mental Health, and has been plenary speaker at numerous national and international meetings.

Dr. Brainard's range of interests is indicated by other institutions where he has been an invited lecturer, including the Department of Energy Melatonin Summit, the U.S. Army Aeromedical Research Laboratory, the U.S. Army Environmental Hygiene Agency, the American Institute of Architects, the General Electric Lighting Institute, the Electric Power Research Institute, the Audubon Society, and Scientists Concerned for Animal Welfare.

In 1989 Dr. George C. Brainard was selected as class portrait honoree. Frank H. Mason depicted the physician half length and life-sized, facing slightly left and seated behind a desk. His broad features and large, square glasses are surmounted by unusually thick and curly brown hair that flairs out horizontally away from his face. The professor's large brown eyes look directly toward the viewer, and his animated expression is both intense and quizzically engaging. He holds two prisms between his hands, a curved one on top and a smaller, straight one below, resting on white papers. He is wearing a white shirt, gray suit, and maroon and tan striped necktie.

Even though Mason employs a freely brushed style, he has created a meticulous likeness of the subject. The prisms suggest Dr. Brainard's research into light and color. They create a rainbow effect of primary hues which are reflected in the figure's glowing, ruddy face and hands with blue-green shadows, the green desktop, and the bluish-pink atmospheric background.

At the portrait presentation ceremony Dr. Brainard predicted a strategic change in indoor illumination in the next two decades "to enhance the well-being of all humans inhabiting the environment." He also spoke movingly of the urgent need to eradicate the metaphorical darkness of global starvation and illiteracy.

Frank H. Mason is well matched to his portrait subject in terms of activist spirit. Mason was born in 1921 in Cleveland to artistic parents, his father a painter, actor, and minister, and his mother a painter and musician. After the family moved to New York, Frank's early art work was brought to the attention of Mayor Fiorello La Guardia, and the twelve-year-old boy was soon apprenticed to Manuel Reyes, a Spanish painter and poet at the New York City Music and Art High School.

At age sixteen he transferred briefly to the National Academy of Design and then to the Art Students League where he studied with the academic painter Frank Vincent DuMond. Mason continued to study with DuMond until his mentor's death in 1951 when the young artist succeeded him on the faculty. Mason has taught for more than three decades at the league, and has also taught at a summer art school in Vermont near his vacation home and studio.

In the 1950s he explored Renaissance oil glazing and other old master techniques. Throughout his career Mason has eschewed prepared art materials and ground his own pigments, prepared his own painting medium, constructed his own painting stretchers, and primed his own canvas.

In addition to portraits, genre paintings, and landscapes of the American West, Mason is perhaps best known for his commissions for large scale figure paintings of religious and allegorical subjects. In 1964 his series on the life of St. Anthony of Padua was installed at the eleventh-century church of San Giovanni di Malta in Venice.

In 1972 Mason's monumental painting of the Resurrection of Christ was hung behind the main altar at Old St. Patrick's Cathedral in New York. The painter devoted much of 1980 in researching the history of the Saudi Arabian navy for a commission of three mural-size panels hung at the King Faisal Naval Base in Jidda.

Frank Mason's celebrated portrait subjects include W. Averell Harriman, John Cardinal Wright, Prince Giacomo Colonna of Venice, Louis Auchincloss, Colonel Earl "Red" Blaik, and Thomas Wolfe. His works are owned by the Butler Institute of American Art in Youngstown, Ohio, the U.S. War Department, and the American Embassy in London. Mason was elected an academician at the National Academy of Design, and served as vice president of the National Society of Mural Painters. He is a member of the Royal Society of Arts.

Frank Mason is a socially conscious and outspoken participant in artistic and environmental debates. He is an adviser to the New York Drawing Association (dedicated to preserving and promulgating traditional drawing techniques). He is a passionate advocate of the preservation of national parks and other areas of the American Southwest, and of old master paintings. In 1976 Mason led a demonstration of artists and students in front of the Metropolitan Museum of Art rallying against what he called the museum's "overzealous" painting conservation policies which "skinned" the entire surface glazing. Some of their signs read, "Van Dyke Has Been Vandalized" and "Who Massacred Manet?"

Frank Mason was elected president of the International Institute of Conservation of Historic and Artistic Works. In 1987 he and a group of artists affiliated with the institute lobbied against the controversial restoration of Michelangelo's frescoes in the Sistine Chapel in Rome.

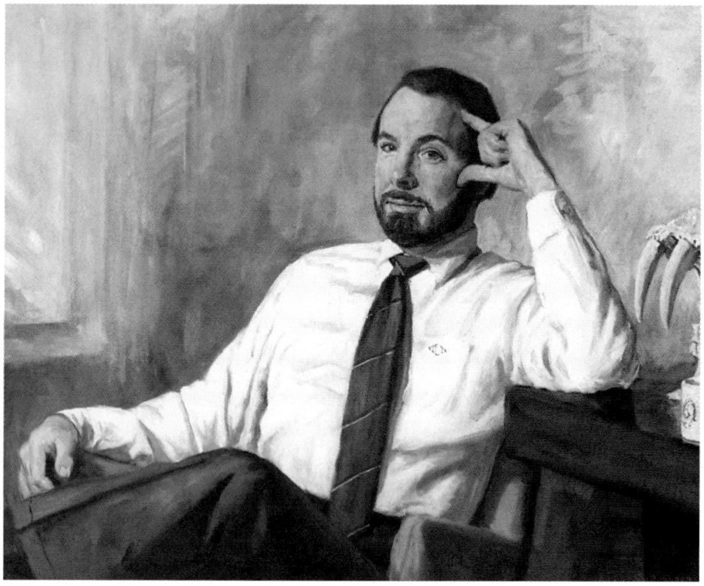

Portrait of Troy L. Thompson II

TROY L. THOMPSON II, M.D. (b. 1946)
By Dean M. Larson (b. 1957)

Oil on canvas
1995
30 x 38 in.

Signed and dated lower right: "Dean M. Larson/1995"
Given by JMC class of 1995
Accession number: 1995+e.P.01

Dr. Troy L. Thompson II is a professor in the department of psychiatry and human behavior at Jefferson Medical College.

Troy Thompson was born in 1946 in Little Rock, Arkansas, and subsequently lived in Kansas and Georgia. He earned his bachelor's (1968) and medical (1973) degrees from Emory University, where he received a behavioral science fellowship in 1971. He served his psychiatry residency at Yale University School of Medicine.

In 1977 Troy Thompson moved to Denver to serve as assistant professor of psychiatry and medicine at the University of Colorado School of Medicine where he was codirector of the residency program in general internal medicine, director of the medical-psychiatric outpatient clinic, and director of the division of consultation-liaison psychiatry. He was named associate professor in 1983.

Dr. Troy Thompson joined the Jefferson Medical College faculty in 1988 as the Daniel Lieberman Professor, and was chair of the department of psychiatry and human behavior until 1997. He has also been a faculty member of the Philadelphia Psychoanalytic Institute since 1991. He received considerable recognition for his research as principal investigator in the largest double-blind controlled study of a medication to control Alzheimer's disease, and as coprincipal investigator of a National Institutes of Mental Health research grant to improve primary care physicians' care of patients with depressive symptoms.

On the national scene Dr. Thompson has been president of the Association for Academic Psychiatry and the Academy of Psychosomatic Medicine. He was chair of the American Psychiatric Association's Committee on Consultation-liaison Psychiatry and Primary Care Education. He received the Lifetime Achievement Award of the New York Society for Liaison Psychiatry, the Distinguished Professor Award of Florida Hospital in Orlando, the Exemplary Psychiatrist Award of the National Alliance for the Mentally Ill (all in 1992), and the Nancy C. A. Roeske Certificate of Recognition for Excellence in Medical Student Education of the American Psychiatric Association (1993). He has also delivered named lectureships and been visiting professor at medical centers throughout the country.

Among the books Dr. Thompson has edited are *The Education of the General Internist* (with Richard L. Byyny, 1982), *Research Advances in Consultation-liaison Psychiatry* (1991), and *Medical-surgical Psychiatry: Treating Psychiatric Aspects of Physical Disorders* (1993). He was been an editor or editorial board member of *Psychosomatics*, *International Journal of Psychiatry in Medicine*, *Psychiatric Medicine*, and *Journal of the American Psychoanalytic Association*.

Thompson was a founder and codirector of Jefferson's Life Cycle course for freshmen students. The course teaches the biological, psychological, and social factors that both affect normal growth and development and also contribute to the emergence of pathology in each stage. The course's "doctoring" section explores the doctor-patient relationship and sociocultural issues arising in medical practice. At Dr. Thompson's portrait ceremony a student eloquently described the benefits of the course:

> There was almost a magical quality about those afternoons, as if time had stopped as we spent hours together exploring the human condition as it relates to medicine...We felt your vitality, we thrived on your energy...There were times of great stress that year, times when we needed some perspective on the pressures we were dealing with. You defused our anxiety and made time for us...We thank you for providing a forum to express our concerns and for respecting our role as students and treating us as future physicians.

In 1993 Dr. Thompson received the Distinguished Teacher in Clinical Departments Award and the Christian R. and Mary F. Lindback Award for Distinguished Teaching. In 1995 he was the portrait honoree elected by the graduating class.

As depicted by Dean M. Larson, the physician is two-thirds length and slightly smaller than life-sized, shown in his working environment. One is struck immediately by the informality of his costume and posture: he is dressed in shirtsleeves and seated in a philosopher's pose. His head leans against his left hand and his arm rests on a nearby table. His face is framed by dark brown hair, mustache, and beard, and his expression is genial. He seems totally engaged with an unseen visitor, as though he might be listening to a patient or consulting with a student.

He is wearing a white shirt with a monogram on the pocket, a blue necktie with narrow white and red stripes, and dark blue trousers. There is a hint of a picture frame in the loosely brushed, multicolored, light background.

On the table are two disparate objects: an ordinary coffee mug with the university logo and an uncommon model of a saber-toothed tiger's skull. The presence of the skull is an unsettling and unexplained ornament in his office. In fact, it was a present from his young son, and Dr. Thompson likes the object as a reminder of a creature that "did the best it could" even though now extinct.

In a private conversation, Dr. Thompson noted that a portrait describes how the sitter will be represented "to the ages," and so he deliberately chose the informal costume and a pose of attentive thinking and listening to avoid what he considered a too grand or powerful image.

Portrait of Francis E. Rosato

FRANCIS ERNEST ROSATO, M.D. (b. 1934)
By Charles Harkless Cecil (b. 1945)

Oil on canvas
1996
62 1/2 x 47 in.

Signed lower right: "CHC"

Given in 1996 by friends and colleagues
Accession number: 1996+e.P.05

Dr. Francis E. Rosato is the sixth Samuel D. Gross Professor of Surgery and chair of the department. The surgeon was among the "Best Doctors in America" named in March 1996 by *American Health,* a consumer health magazine.

"Frank" Rosato was born in 1934 in Philadelphia, the son of a busy general practitioner in the city, Ernest L. Rosato, M.D. At his portrait presentation ceremony, Dr. Frank Rosato proudly credited the professional ethics of his father and a rigorous education by nuns and Jesuits as contributing factors to his own capacity for hard work and discipline.

These family values have been handed down to the next generation as well. Dr. Frank Rosato's son, Ernest ("Gary") L. Rosato, M.D., is also a Jefferson surgeon and an alumnus of the class of 1990. His daughter Ann graduated from Jefferson in 1997, and son Francis E. Jr. is a member of the class of 1999.

Frank Rosato graduated from St. Joseph's University in 1955 and Hahnemann Medical College in 1959. After a residency in general surgery at the Hospital of the University of Pennsylvania, he became an instructor in surgery there, and a postdoctoral fellow in the biochemistry department. He returned briefly to Hahnemann as a senior instructor in surgery.

Dr. Rosato rejoined the faculty at the University of Pennsylvania School of Medicine in 1967, and rose quickly in the academic ranks to become professor of surgery in 1972. During this period he was chief of the hospital's solid tumor program and codirector of the neoplastic chemotherapy clinic. He was also a consultant in surgery at the Veterans Administration Hospital.

In 1975 Dr. Frank Rosato left Philadelphia to accept the challenge of establishing a surgery department at the new Eastern Virginia Medical School in Norfolk, Virginia. He was attending surgeon at the Norfolk General Hospital and DePaul Hospital in Norfolk, and consultant in surgery at nearby naval, veterans, and public health service hospitals.

With the new department at Norfolk successfully launched by 1978, Dr. Rosato returned to the city of his birth to accept his appointment as chair of surgery at Jefferson. In addition to being chief of surgery at the Jefferson Hospital, he is also on the consulting staffs at the Veterans Administration Hospital in Wilmington, and the Bryn Mawr, Wills Eye, and Chestnut Hill Hospitals.

When Dr. Rosato came to Jefferson he had already contributed more than 125 scientific articles on basic and clinical research to prestigious surgical journals. One of his priorities was to reinvigorate surgical investigation in the surgery department. He succeeded in appointing several outstanding researchers and acquiring new laboratory facilities and outside funding, especially in the areas of clinical nutrition, trauma, prosthetic grafts, colorectal surgery, and kidney, liver, and heart transplantation.

Under his leadership, the department now has divisions in cardiothoracic, colorectal, transplantation, and trauma surgery, and divisions of research and emergency medicine. A high point in Rosato's administrative career was his involvement in the Delaware Valley's first liver transplant at Jefferson in 1984.

Both undergraduate surgical training and the residency program have been considerably strengthened. Dr. Rosato is an outstanding teacher and twice the recipient of the Christian R. and Mary F. Lindback Foundation Award for Distinguished Teaching: in 1968 at the University of Pennsylvania when he was only thirty-four years old, and in 1983 at Jefferson Medical College.

Dr. Rosato was coauthor of *Postmastectomy Breast Reconstruction* (with Charles E. Horton and G. Patrick Maxwell, 1980), coeditor of *Surgery of the Breast* (with Jan O. Strombeck, 1986), and coauthor of *Atlas of General Surgical Technique* (with Donna J. Barbot, 1992). He has served as editor-in-chief of *Contemporary Surgery for Residents.*

He has served locally as the president of the Philadelphia Academy of Surgery and the Philadelphia County Medical Society. Nationally he has been a governor of the American College of Surgeons and chairman of its committee on continuing education, chairman of the

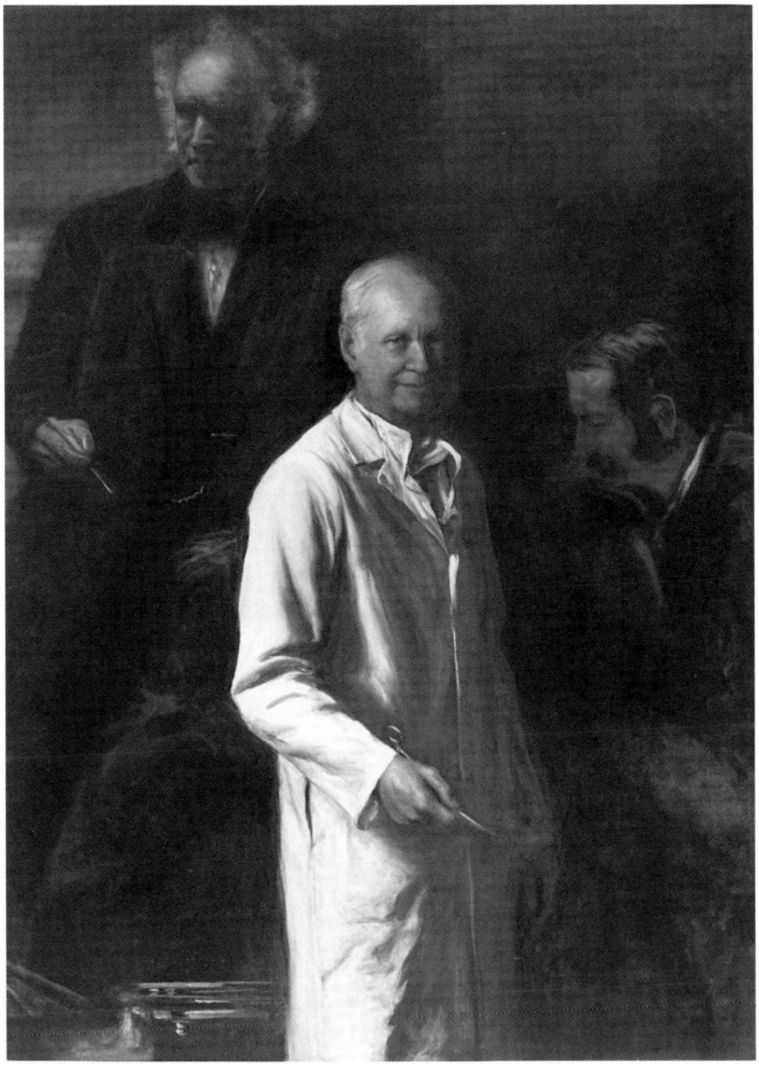

lish the Francis E. Rosato Professorship in Surgical Oncology. The conception for the large-scale portrait is astonishingly bold and must have evoked considerable discussion and planning between the sitter and the artist, Charles H. Cecil.

Dr. Rosato is depicted standing in front of *The Gross Clinic*. Details from the Eakins painting include Dr. Gross's leonine head and hand with scalpel, his clinic assistants Drs. Charles D. Briggs and James M. Barton, as well as a partial view of the surgical instruments and the reddish color of the tunnel.

Dr. Rosato is shown three-quarters length and very slightly smaller than life-sized, facing slightly to the right. The position of his arms are similar to that of Dr. Gross: Rosato's right hand hangs at his side and his left hand holds a surgical instrument, a long Kelly hemostat (not a scalpel). Dr. Rosato is wearing a white doctor's coat and a surgical mask that hangs loosely around his neck, unlike Dr. Gross and his assistants who operated in business clothes.

Dr. Rosato has a high forehead and sparse white hair, hazel eyes which gaze firmly toward the spectator, straight nose and wide mouth. His facial expression bespeaks dignity and pride. Strong light from the left illuminates his brilliant white coat and one side of his face.

Test Committee of the National Board of Medical Examiners, and a member of the steering committee of the Association of Program Directors in Surgery. He has also been a director of the American Division of World Fellowships and of the Israeli Medical Association, and a board member of St. Joseph's University.

Dr. Frank Rosato received the Clarence E. Shaffrey, S.J. Award in 1981, the Shield of Loyola Award in 1988, and Alumnus of the Year Award in 1992 (all from St. Joseph's University), and a doctor of humane letters honorary degree from Holy Family College in 1989. He was honoree, along with his brother Ernest, a professor of surgery at the University of Pennsylvania, of the Sons of Italy Grand Lodge of Pennsylvania in 1991. Frank received the Man of the Year Award from the Jewish National Fund in 1992.

Dr. Rosato's portrait was presented in 1996 at the same ceremony in which the surgeon announced a second honor, the official kickoff of a campaign to estab-

Charles Cecil has managed to interpolate the contemporary figure of Dr. Rosato into a section of Eakins's earlier painting while still keeping them separate and independent. While emulating the earlier work in its tonalities, contrasts between light and shadow, and naturalistic figures, the portrait of Dr. Rosato is unmistakably contemporary in its verve.

The portrait is a sincere homage to the great nineteenth-century professor and his depiction in *The Gross Clinic*. By explaining his rationale at the portrait ceremony, Dr. Rosato hoped to obviate some expected criticism of his personal reference to Jefferson's cherished painting:

> I was afraid that people might think me presumptuous to include in my portrait such a giant as Dr. Gross, but the idea of continuity both in surgical history and art history coming together in this picture made sense. I am honored to share my portrait with one of the most vital and important figures in the history of Jefferson. I hope Dr. Gross feels the same. I hope he doesn't mind. I'd like

to think he sees it as an expression of appreciation of the long tradition that makes this such a special place.

Charles H. Cecil was born in 1945 in Kansas City, Missouri. He graduated from Haverford College in 1967 and did postgraduate work in art history at Yale University with a grant from the National Education Defense Act. Between 1969 and 1973 he was funded by three grants from the Elizabeth Greenshields Foundation to study painting, first with R. H. Ives Gammell in Boston and then with Gammell's pupil, Richard F. Lack, in Minneapolis.

A fellowship from the John F. Stacey Foundation provided funds for him to study and paint in Europe for eighteen months, and then he returned to Minneapolis. His landscapes of Italian hill towns won the Julius Hallgarten First Prize for oil painting in 1979, and the Benjamin Altman Second Prize for landscape at the National Academy of Design in 1980.

Cecil has resided primarily in Florence since 1978. After teaching painting at the Rosary College's Graduate Studio of Fine Arts, he became codirector of the Cecil-Graves Studio in 1983, and director of the Charles H. Cecil Studios since 1991.

His school, which receives support from the R. H. I. Gammell Studios Trust, is housed in the historic Church of San Raffaello Arcangelo which was converted into a sculptor's studio in the early nineteenth century. It offers training to an international group of students in the classical techniques of drawing and painting, with a curriculum that stems from ateliers of nineteenth-century Paris.

Charles H. Cecil received several portrait commissions of Philadelphia-area surgeons through professional acquaintances of his uncle, Dr. Henry S. Cecil, a pediatrician associated with the Children's Seashore Home, Children's Hospital, and the University of Pennsylvania School of Medicine. In addition to his uncle's portrait, Charles Cecil depicted Dr. Elmer Grimes (at Our Lady of Lourdes Hospital in Camden, New Jersey) and Dr. Jonathan E. Rhoads (at the American Philosophical Society).

Portrait of Herbert E. Cohn

HERBERT E. COHN, M.D. (b. 1930)
By Dean L. Paules (b. 1931)

Oil on canvas
1990
50 x 40 in.

Signed and dated lower left: "PAULES 5-90"

Given in 1990 by friends and colleagues
Accession number: 1990+e.P.02

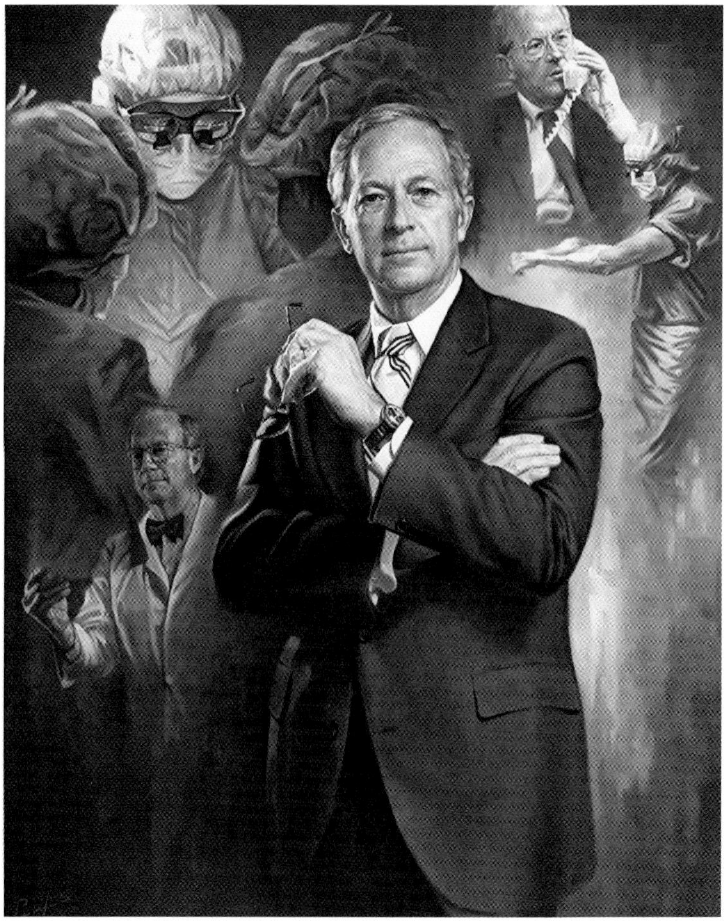

Dr. Herbert E. Cohn is a professor of surgery and vice chairman of the department at Jefferson. He is a pioneer in renal transplantation.

Herbert Cohn was born in 1930 and reared in the Philadelphia and Atlantic City areas. He graduated from Rutgers University (1951) and

Jefferson Medical College (1955), where he was first in his class and winner of eight awards. After an internship at Atlantic City Hospital, his residency in surgery at Jefferson under Dr. John H. Gibbon Jr. was interrupted by two years of military service as an Air Force captain in Fort Worth, Texas.

Dr. Cohn returned to Jefferson as an American Heart Association trainee and an American Cancer Society trainee, followed by three years as a Public Health Service trainee in cardiovascular surgery (1962-65). Dr. Cohn was named an assistant professor of surgery in 1965, and rose in the academic ranks to be professor in 1978. He won the Christian R. and Mary F. Lindback Foundation Award for Distinguished Teaching in 1981. He was named the first Anthony E. Narducci Professor of Surgery in 1998.

Dr. Cohn has been attending surgeon at the Thomas Jefferson University Hospital since 1962. In addition he was attending surgeon at Albert Einstein Medical Center-Daroff Division (1972-76), Rolling Hill Hospital (1972-85), and Albert Einstein Medical Center-Northern Division (1972-86).

Dr. Herbert E. Cohn is credited with laying the groundwork for transplantation capability at Jefferson, along with Dr. James E. Clark and others. Their combined effort resulted in a renal dialysis unit accessible to all Delaware Valley kidney patients. After several years of investigating methods to improve dialysis and inspecting transplant centers across the country Cohn performed the first transplant of a cadaver kidney in Philadelphia in 1965. Just seven years later in 1972 Cohn performed Jefferson's first successful renal transplant in which the donor kidney came from an identically matched sibling.[8]

Dr. Cohn has been director of graduate medical education in the department of surgery since 1979, and vice chairman of the department since 1985. He also led a planning effort to set the department's course to the year 2000. He served as chair of Jefferson Medical College's faculty affairs committee and was president of the volunteer faculty association. He was president of the hospital's medical staff from 1985 to 1987 and also chaired the following committees: faculty affairs, quality assurance, operating room, executive, credentials, advisory, committee, and bylaws.

Nationally, Dr. Cohn served on the continuing education committee of the American College of Surgeons from 1982 to 1992. He has been chairman of the Physicians and Surgeons Division of the Jewish National Fund, and was named its Man of the Year in 1987. He has been president of the American Division, World Fellowship, of the Israel Medical Association, and a board member of its college of continuing medical education.

Dr. Herbert Cohn's portrait by Dean Paules was presented by friends and colleagues in 1990. The artist's preparation included observing and photographing the surgeon for a full day at the Jefferson Hospital, both in and out of the operating room. This most unusual portrayal depicts the subject performing multiple activities for which he wears different clothes.

The large figure of Dr. Cohn standing authoritatively in the foreground is two-thirds length and life-sized. He presides over the action with arms folded close to his body, holding his glasses in his left hand. His expression is serious and thoughtful as he gazes toward the viewer. He is dressed in a dark blue suit, white shirt, and cream-colored necktie with narrow blue stripes.

Vignettes in the background appear like stop-action movie shots of the busy surgeon, from lower left to upper right: examining an X-ray, operating with two assistants, conferring on the telephone, and extending arms to receive gloves after scrubbing for surgery. The figures in the surgical scene are larger than the others, and the surgeons are garbed in greenish-blue scrub suits, caps, masks, and magnifying lenses.

At the portrait ceremony Dr. Francis E. Rosato praised Dr. Cohn's skill, warmth, and dedication to both house staff and patients, and added a humorous note:

> He is known to be sensitive and supporting to residents, but...intolerant of laziness, sloppiness or failure of attention to detail...an accurate and omnipresent observer, which is probably why the residents affectionately refer to him as 'the shark.'

Two of Dr. Herbert Cohn's three sons are physicians and alumni of Jefferson Medical College: Jeffrey B. graduated in 1980 and David B. graduated in 1986.

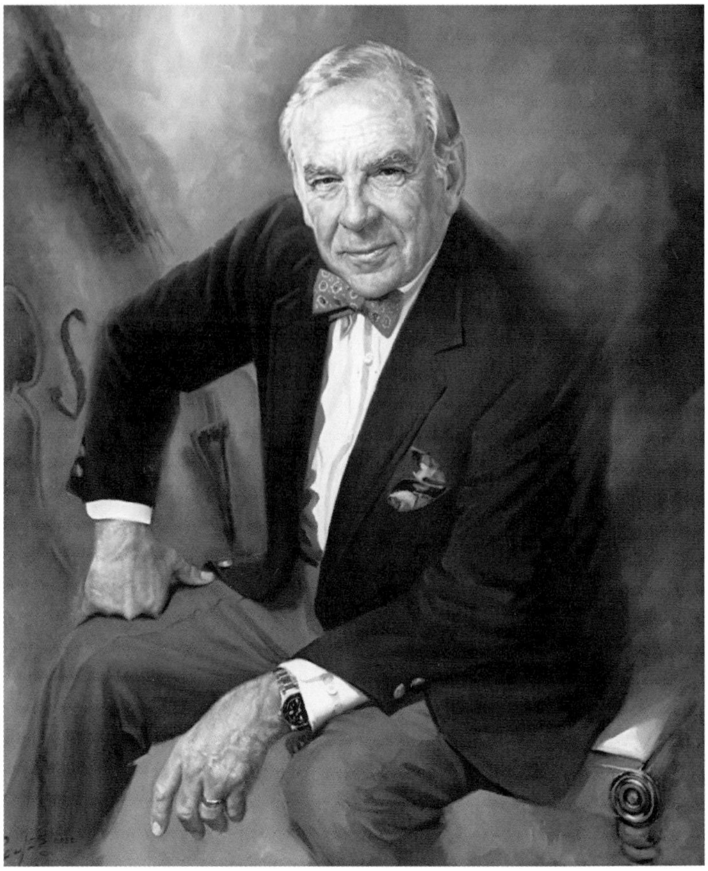

Portrait of James M. Hunter

JAMES M. HUNTER, M.D. (b. 1924)
By Dean L. Paules

Oil on canvas
1990
40 x 34 in.

Signed and dated lower left: "PAULES A.P.S.C./1-90"

Given in 1990 by friends and colleagues
Accession number: 1990+e.P.05

Dr. James M. Hunter is an internationally acclaimed hand surgeon and a Distinguished Professor of Orthopaedic Surgery at Jefferson. He is the inventor of the Hunter Active Tendon Implant, used in the staged reconstruction of damaged flexor tendons.

James Hunter was born in 1924 in Merchantville, New Jersey. He served in the U.S. Medical Corps as a staff sergeant before entering college. He graduated from Dickinson College in 1949 and Jefferson Medical College in 1953. After an internship and residency in orthopaedic surgery at the Jefferson Hospital, he became the first fellow in hand surgery at Columbia-Presbyterian Hospital in New York.

Hunter returned to Philadelphia and established himself as the first orthopaedic surgeon in the city to confine his practice to surgery of the hand. He rose in the Jefferson academic ranks to become a professor of orthopaedic surgery, and in 1989 was named the Distinguished Professor of Orthopaedic Surgery in recognition of his scientific contributions, only the fourth faculty member to be so designated. Upon retirement he was elected emeritus professor of orthopaedic surgery.

In 1962 Dr. Hunter was named associate attending orthopaedic surgeon in the division of hand surgery at Jefferson's hospital and was coordinator of the house staff education program from 1964 to 1978. Among other clinical appointments he was chief of the child amputee research clinic at Elizabethtown Hospital and Rehabilitation Center, and a consultant in hand surgery at the Chestnut Hill Hospital, the Philadelphia Naval Hospital, Valley Forge General Hospital, and the Compensation Hand Clinic for Philadelphia employees at Philadelphia General Hospital. In 1989 he was appointed to the visiting teaching staff of Albert Einstein Medical Center-Northern Division.

The Hunter Tendon Prosthesis, the first synthetic tendon for reconstructing a severely damaged hand, was announced in 1964. The two-stage reconstruction method of using passive and active implants became standard in repairing damaged flexor tendons in the hand. Hunter has played a national and international role in efforts to rehabilitate injured and diseased hands.

Dr. Hunter and his associates constituted the division of hand surgery and rehabilitation in the department of orthopaedic surgery at Jefferson. The Hand Rehabilitation Center was formed in 1972, and moved to larger quarters at 901 Walnut Street in 1980. Medical students, residents, and fellows receive their education in hand surgery from the center's surgeons, and physical and occupational therapists. The nationally prominent facility sponsors the annual Rehabilitation of the Hand Symposium and Workshop which has trained thousands of additional doctors and therapists.

Dr. James Hunter has edited the following textbooks which have become standards in the field: *Rehabilitation of the Hand* (with Lawrence H. Schneider, Evelyn J. Mackin, and Anne D. Callahan, 1978); and *Tendon Surgery in the Hand* (with Schneider and Mackin, 1987).

In 1994 Dr. James Hunter received the Hand Rehabilitation Foundation's Recognition Award for Teaching and Surgery. He was honored as a Pioneer in Hand Surgery by the International Federation of Societies for Surgery of the Hand in 1995, for whom he chaired the committee on rehabilitation and allied health. Hunter has been honored with membership in French, Pan-Pacific, Caribbean, Columbian, Australian, and Japanese orthopaedic and hand societies. He was the recipient of Jefferson's alumni achievement award in 1993.

Dr. James Hunter's portrait by Dean Paules was presented in 1990 by friends and colleagues. The surgeon is depicted three-quarters length and life-sized, seated on a bench and turned slightly to the left. He bends forward with his right arm akimbo. The sitter's face is described in literal detail to construct a startling likeness. His forward-leaning, almost restless pose is intensified by his tightly pursed lips, riveting gaze, and probing expression.

Dr. Hunter's casually elegant attire includes a navy blue blazer with brass buttons and a multicolored pocket handkerchief, a white shirt, gray slacks, and a patterned red bow tie. His hands are disproportionately large, probably to emphasize his professional and avocational interests. The knuckles of his right hand press on his thigh, with the first and fifth fingers tensely spread apart. His left hand is outstretched in a more relaxed position with fingers curled under.

In contrast to the minute details and solid colors of the figure and costume, the background is loosely brushed in blended shades of blue, brown, maroon, ochre, and lavender. A further softening element is the curving form of a double bass, alluding to another interest of this versatile man. He is ardently interested in Dixieland jazz and plays the bass in a band called the Red Peppers. Dr. Hunter was also an accomplished oarsman.

Portrait of Jerome M. Cotler

JEROME M. COTLER, M.D. (b. 1928)
By Dean L. Paules

Oil on canvas
1994
43 1/2 x 34 in.

Signed and dated lower left: "Paules/11-94"

Given in 1994 by friends and colleagues
Accession number: 1994+e.P.05

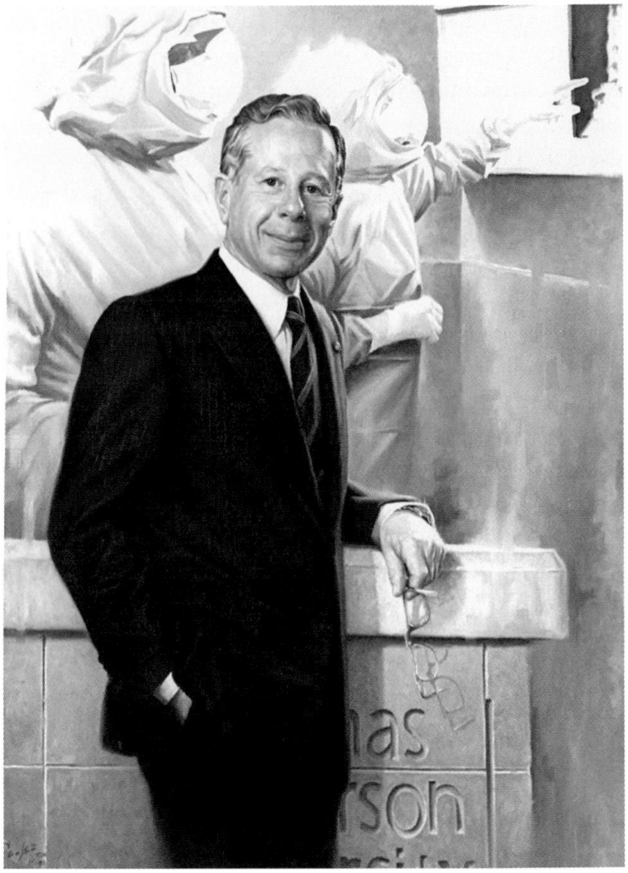

Dr. Jerome M. Cotler is the Dr. Everett J. and Marian Gordon Professor of Orthopaedic Surgery at Jefferson. He is recognized nationally for his work in spinal surgery.

Jerome Cotler was born in 1928 in Bridgeton, New Jersey and graduated from Ursinus College in 1948 and Jefferson Medical College in 1952. He continued his postgraduate training at Jefferson as an intern, surgical resident, and orthopaedic resident. After returning to Bridgeton in 1957, he practiced orthopaedic surgery there until 1973 and was active on the staffs of several southern New Jersey hospitals. He was chief of the hip service and president of the medical staff at Elizabethtown Hospital for Crippled Children and Youth during the 1970s.

In 1973 Dr. Cotler joined the full-time faculty in orthopaedic surgery at Jefferson. He became a full professor in 1981, and was named the Dr. Everett J. and Marian Gordon Professor in 1991. He was vice chairman of the department of orthopaedic surgery from 1987 to 1995, and head of the service at the Jefferson Hospital from 1986 to 1995.

Dr. Jerome Cotler was a founder of Jefferson's Regional Spinal Cord Injury Center of the Delaware Valley, along with Drs. John F. Ditunno Jr., Jewell L. Osterholm, and William E. Staas Jr. Dr. Cotler was co-associate director of the center from 1979 to 1995. He has also been a consultant at Wills Eye Hospital and Magee Rehabilitation Hospital.

Dr. Cotler has brought national recognition to his department by his many professional activities. He was president of the American Board of Orthopaedic Surgery, vice president of the American Orthopaedic Association, and chair of the undergraduate medical education committee of the Academic Orthopaedic Society. He was chairman of the board of councilors of the American Academy of Orthopaedic Surgeons, and a board member of the Orthopaedic Research and Education Foundation and the American Spinal Injury Association.

Dr. Cotler has contributed numerous articles, chapters, abstracts, book reviews, movies, and videotapes to the medical literature. He coedited the books *Spinal Fusion: Science and Techniques* (1990) and *Spinal Instrumentation* (with Howard S. An, 1992). Coeditor of the former book is his son Howard B. Cotler, M.D. who graduated from Jefferson in 1979.

Cotler has been a dedicated teacher on the undergraduate and graduate levels. He earned the Christian R. and Mary F. Lindback Award for Distinguished Teaching in 1979, and was selected by orthopaedic residents for the first John J. Gartland Award. He was president of Jefferson's alumni association in 1993-94.

Dr. Cotler's portrait by Dean Paules was presented by friends and colleagues in 1994. Conceptually similar to Paules's portrait of Dr. Herbert E. Cohn (1990), the Cotler portrait also includes accessory figures participating in a related activity in a different time frame.

Dr. Cotler is shown two-thirds length and slightly smaller than life-sized, standing in front of a low stone wall, and facing slightly to the right. His right hand is placed casually in his pocket, and his left arm rests on top of the wall, holding his glasses. His head is turned to gaze out directly to the observer. His broad smile and twinkling blue-hazel eyes affirm his reputation as a warm teacher, compassionate physician, affable friend, and devoted family member.

Dr. Cotler is attired in a dark gray, pin-striped business suit, blue shirt, and striped necktie, but there are several elements that identify his profession and whereabouts. Behind the wall are two figures garbed in blue operating room gowns, masks, hats and gloves, preparing for surgery. The figure pointing to an X-ray of a spine represents Dr. Cotler and the other figure is an operating room technician. The locale of the portrait is identified by the last few letters of the words "Thomas Jefferson University" incised into the pinkish-orange stone wall. Viewers knowledgeable about university paraphernalia will recognize Dr. Cotler's President's Club lapel pin.

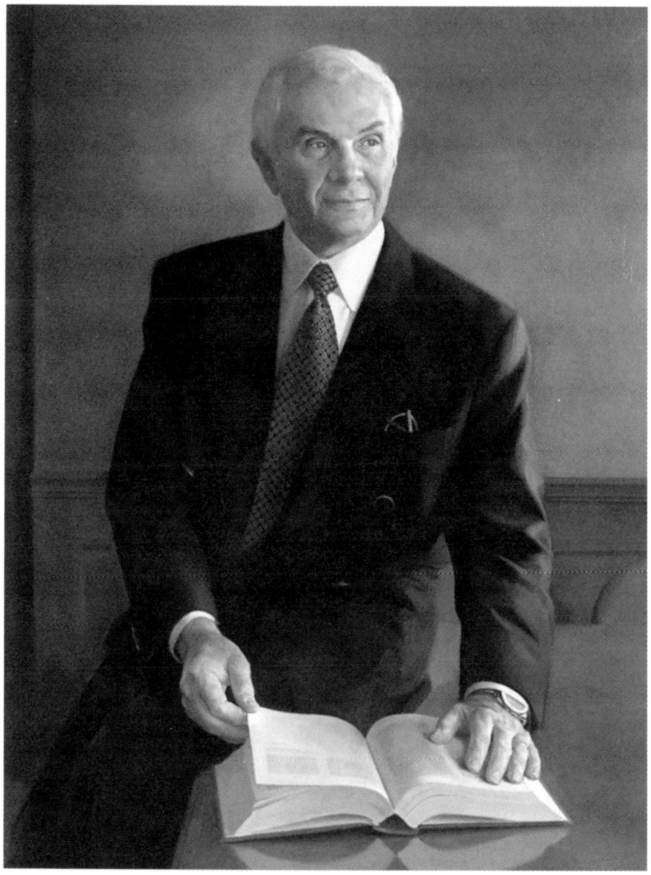

Portrait of Jewell L. Osterholm

(See color plate)

JEWELL L. OSTERHOLM, M.D. (b. 1929)
By Mark Elliot Skolsky (b. 1957)

Oil on canvas
1995
42 x 32 in.

Signed and dated upper left: "M. Elliot Skolsky/'95"

Given in 1995 by friends and colleagues
Accession number: 1995+e.P.04

Dr. Jewell L. Osterholm is professor of neurosurgery and former chairman of the department at Jefferson. He is widely acclaimed for his research on the treatment of stroke.

Jewell L. Osterholm was born in White Sulphur Springs, Montana in 1929. He is an alumnus of Montana State University (1953) and the Washington University School of Medicine (1957) in St. Louis. He stayed at the latter institution for his internship and a year of residency in general surgery, followed by a year as a Cerebral Palsy fellow in neuropathology at the Montreal Neurological Institute at McGill University. He completed his residency in neurosurgery in Montreal.

In 1963 Dr. Osterholm moved to Philadelphia to join the division of neurosurgery at Hahnemann Medical College and Hospital where he rose in the ranks to become professor of surgery by 1971. He was director of Hahnemann's division of neurological surgery, program director of the new neurosurgery residency program, and director of the Spinal Cord Injury Center and Research Laboratories. He received the Golden Apple Award as best teacher of the year in 1965, and was made an honorary Hahnemann alumnus in 1973.

In 1974 Dr. Osterholm moved to Thomas Jefferson University to succeed Dr. Philip D. Gordy as professor of neurosurgery and chair of the department. Under his leadership, the neurosurgical residency program was greatly accelerated and improved, laboratory research branched out and numerous grants were obtained, and patients were afforded the most modern methods of neurosurgical therapy.

The Regional Spinal Cord Injury Center of the Delaware Valley opened in January 1979 under the aegis of the department of rehabilitation medicine in conjunction with the departments of neurosurgery and orthopaedic surgery. At the time of admission patients are evaluated by a neurosurgeon, orthopaedist, and physiatrist. With about 150 admissions per year, this center has became the benchmark for spinal cord injury units in the United States, and the team approach has made a substantial contribution to medical practice.

Dr. Osterholm is the holder of seventy patents in America and abroad related to the oxygenation and nutritional support of ischemic neurologic tissue. His patented system to deliver a new drug, the Oxygenated Fluorocarbon Nutrient Emulsion (OFNE), throughout the brain several hours after a major stroke showed in preclinical testing that the brain can be resuscitated and severe stroke effect reversed. The premise of the drug therapy is that OFNE can perform the function of the blood whose flow is interrupted by a stroke.[9]

Dr. Osterholm was recognized for his work in oxygenated fluorocarbons with the Inventor of the Year Award in 1984 by Intellectual Property Owners, Incorporated (an association of people holding patents, trademarks, and copyrights), and the grand prize of the Cerebral Resuscitation Award in 1995 by the National Association of Emergency Medical Service Physicians. In addition to numerous scientific articles and presentations, he is the author of *The Pathophysiology of Spinal Cord Trauma* (1978).

The portrait of Dr. Jewell Osterholm was presented by friends and colleagues in 1995, and is the first in the Jefferson collection by New York artist Mark Elliot Skolsky.

The physician is depicted two-thirds length and lifesized, seated on the edge of a conference table with his right hand poised to turn the page of an open textbook. He looks up slightly to the right as though pausing in his reading to acknowledge the presence of an unseen visitor. His square-shaped face is punctuated with arched dark eyebrows and crowned with smooth white hair. His expression is pleasant and thoughtful, almost soulful.

Dr. Osterholm is attired in a dark blue, double-breasted suit, white shirt, and a necktie with geometric red and blue patterns. His glasses are visible in his breast pocket. The background shows panelled wainscotting below a pinkish-mauve wall and two round-backed chairs pushed under the table. The tabletop has such a high gloss that it reflects the curving pages of the thick textbook.

Mark Skolsky's paint style is very smooth and meticulous throughout. Light pouring in from the right creates dramatic shadows on the subject's face, hands, and clothing, all of which are solidly rendered in three dimensions. The difficult foreshortening of the subject's left hand resting on the book is beautifully executed.

Speakers at the portrait ceremony lauded Dr. Osterholm's open, supportive, and generous manner that is totally "without rancor or jealousy," and praised the surgeon as having the "head of a scholar, hands of an artist, and heart of a lion." In response to the accolades, Dr. Osterholm told the audience modestly, "In medicine there are no longer personal successes as much as collaborative ones, not individual stars as much as teamwork." A pious individual and devoted family man, Dr. Osterholm quoted Shakespeare to express his feelings, "My crown is in my heart, not on my head...my crown is called content."

Portraitist Mark E. Skolsky was born in 1957 in Long Island, New York and educated at the Rhode Island School of Design in Providence from 1975 to 1978. He received further training in dance and drawing the human figure in motion at the Erick Hawkins Dance Foundation in New York in the 1980s.

Skolsky worked in various fields of illustration from about 1978 to 1988. He was a book cover artist for Simon and Schuster, Time, and other publishers; illustrator for the magazines *Science Digest*, *Fortune*, *Parents*, and *Guideposts*; and advertising illustrator for MCA-Universal and Warner Brothers studios and the NBC-TV network.

Mark Skolsky has participated in illustration and painting shows at museums and galleries in Philadelphia, Baltimore, Boston, New York, Richmond, and Boca Raton, Florida. He received Certificates of Merit from the Society of Illustrators exhibitions in 1980 and 1983, and a Certificate of Distinctive Merit from the Society of Publication Designers in 1983.

Since the late 1980s Mark Skolsky has concentrated on oil portraits of sitters from diverse milieus including: Zubin Mehta, music director of the New York Philharmonic; Mrs. Gordon A. Auchincloss II of New York and Massachusetts; David Ingalls, director of the Cleveland Museum of Natural History; William Fisk Harrah of Harrah's Casinos in Atlantic City; Abraham Cohen, a founder of the Duane Reade Corporation; and Alton G. Marshall, chairman and president of Lincoln Savings Bank in New York.

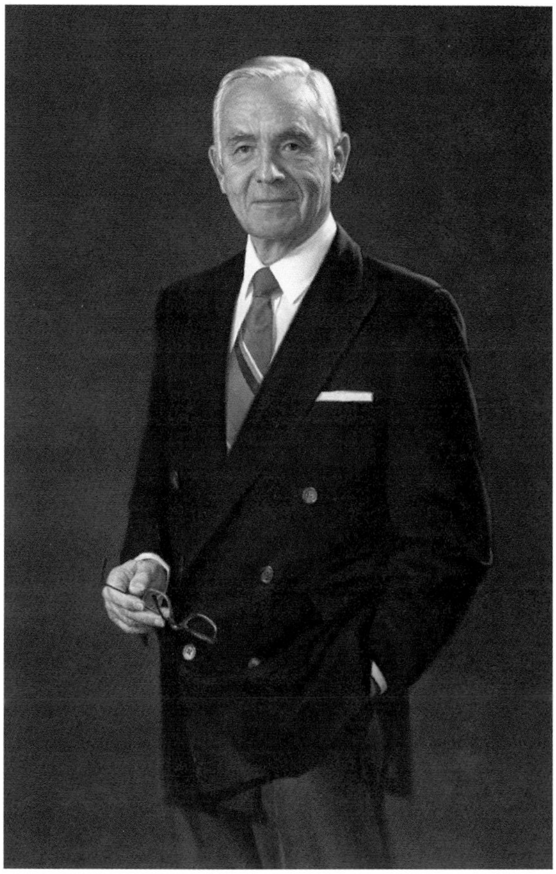

Portrait of Burton L. Wellenbach

BURTON L. WELLENBACH, M.D. (b. 1919)
By Dean L. Paules (b. 1931)

Oil on canvas
1993
44 x 30 in.

Signed and dated lower left: "Paules/4-93"

Given in 1993 by friends and colleagues
Accession number: 1993+e.P.02

Dr. Burton L. Wellenbach is a clinical professor of obstetrics and gynecology at Thomas Jefferson University. A leading practitioner and teacher, he has been very active in medical staff and medical college affairs.

Burton L. Wellenbach was born in 1931 in Philadelphia. He was introduced to medicine and to Jefferson Medical College by Jacob W. Walker, M.D., an uncle who graduated in 1913 and was an associate professor of obstetrics and gynecology at Jefferson. Dr. Wellenbach is an alumnus of Villanova University (1940) and Jefferson Medical College (1944). His accelerated, wartime internship and residency in internal medicine were taken at Jewish Hospital in Philadelphia.

After deciding to switch to obstetrics and gynecology he began a residency at Beth Israel Hospital in New York. This training was interrupted by service in the U.S. Army, one year in Japan during the Occupation and a second year at Valley Forge General Hospital. After discharge he completed his residency in obstetrics and gynecology at the Jefferson Hospital.

Dr. Wellenbach's chief mentor during his early years at Jefferson was Dr. Abraham E. Rakoff, the professor of obstetrics and gynecology whom he joined in practice following his residency. Over the course of his career he has also been associated in practice with several other physicians.

Dr. Wellenbach joined Jefferson's volunteer faculty in 1963 as an associate in obstetrics and gynecology, and rose in the ranks to clinical professor in 1982. He has lectured widely on his main areas of clinical interest: marriage counseling and sexual education, toxemia of pregnancy, and new concepts in population control. He was the first recipient of the Leon A. Peris Award for Distinguished Teaching and Patient Care in 1988.

A leader in Jefferson Medical College and Hospital affairs, Wellenbach initiated a course on human sexuality in 1964 and founded the ethics committee in 1985, when each was a rarity in American medical schools and hospitals. The hospital's ethics committee is composed of physicians and representatives from the arenas of social work, nursing, law, and hospital administration. Its mission is threefold: to educate medical students, house staff, physicians and the community at large; to develop general guidelines and policies; and to serve as a consultative body in particularly controversial cases.[10]

Dr. Wellenbach was also an active member of the executive committee of the medical staff, and has served as chairman of the impaired physicians committee, the ambulatory care center, and the University Committee on Portrait Standards. He was president of Jefferson's alumni association in 1984 and chaired its 125th anniversary celebration committee in 1995.

Dr. Burton Wellenbach's portrait by Dean Paules was presented by friends and colleagues in 1993. The physician is depicted two-thirds length and slightly smaller than life-sized. He stands facing slightly left, with his head turned to gaze at the observer directly. His right hand holds his glasses and his left hand is placed in his trouser pocket. The atmospheric background is painted smoothly in various dark, neutral tones.

The silver-haired physician is tall and distinguished looking, immaculately groomed and elegantly attired. He wears a double breasted, navy blue blazer, gray trousers, a white shirt and pocket handkerchief, and a red striped necktie. His natural self-confidence and warm affability are communicated by his engaging, almost shy smile.

Speakers at the portrait ceremony emphasized how esteemed Dr. Wellenbach is by his colleagues and how beloved by his patients. The honoree's response paid tribute to some earlier Jefferson giants of obstetrics and gynecology who had profoundly influenced his career: Drs. Lewis C. Scheffey, Abraham E. Rakoff, Thaddeus L. Montgomery, and John B. Montgomery. Not coincidentally, these physicians had also been honored with portraits in the Jefferson collection.

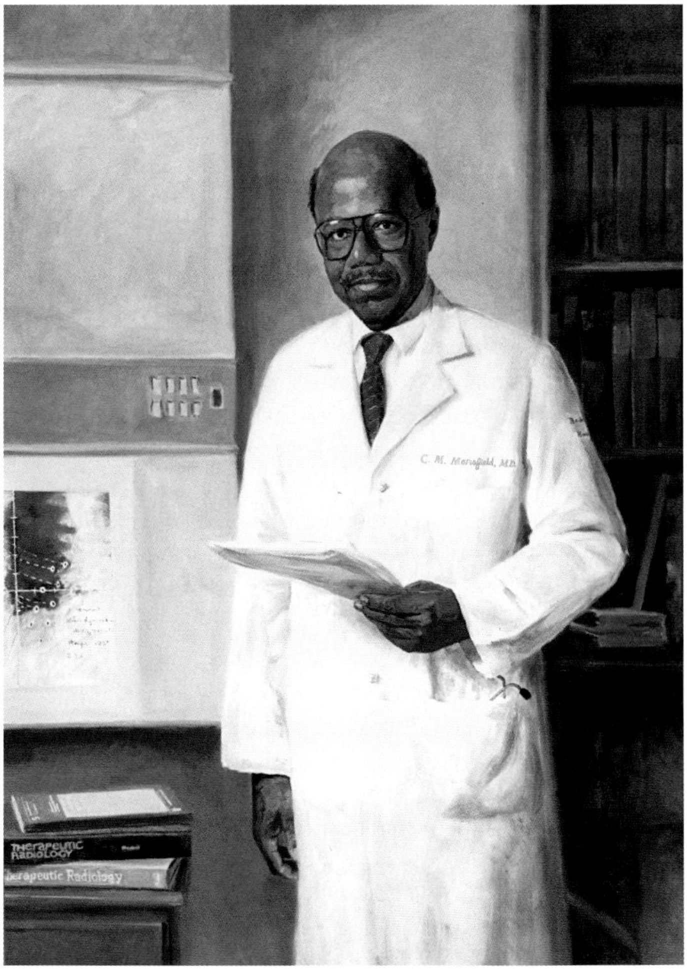

Portrait of Carl M. Mansfield

CARL M. MANSFIELD, M.D. (b. 1928)
By Dean M. Larson (b. 1957)

Oil on canvas
1994
44 x 32 in.

Signed and dated lower right: "Dean M. Larson 1994"

Given in 1994 by friends and colleagues
Accession number: 1994+e.P.04

Dr. Carl M. Mansfield was professor of radiation oncology and nuclear medicine and chairman of the department at Jefferson. The distinguished physician is internationally known for his use of intraoperative radiation therapy for breast cancer.

Carl Mansfield was born in 1928 in Philadelphia, and

is an alumnus of Lincoln University (1951) and Howard University College of Medicine (1956). After his internship and a year of residency in radiology at Episcopal Hospital in Philadelphia, he was a captain in the U.S. Air Force and chief of the department of radiology at Offutt Air Force Base in Nebraska.

Upon discharge from the service, Mansfield continued his residency in radiation therapy and nuclear medicine and radiology at Jefferson Hospital and Episcopal Hospital, respectively. His unusually thorough postgraduate training included a year as an NIH fellow in radiation therapy and nuclear medicine at Jefferson, and an additional year as an NIH postdoctoral fellow in radiation therapy at Middlesex Hospital and Medical School in London.

In 1964 Dr. Mansfield returned to Jefferson as instructor in radiology and chief of the division of nuclear medicine at Jefferson Hospital. Two additional fellowships at the Jefferson Hospital included the Chernicoff fellowship in pediatric radiation therapy and the advanced clinical fellowship of the American Cancer Society.

In 1967 Dr. Mansfield was appointed assistant professor of radiology. In 1970 he was promoted to associate professor in the department of radiation therapy and nuclear medicine, and was chief of the section of ultrasound. He took a sabbatical leave to work on the quantitative assessment of the delivery of radiation treatments at the Meyerstein Institute of Radiotherapy at Middlesex Hospital and Medical School.

In 1974 Dr. Mansfield's posts at Jefferson were professor in the department of radiation therapy and nuclear medicine, chief of the division of nuclear medicine, and chief of the section of ultrasound. At this time he was also a lecturer in radiology at the University of Pennsylvania School of Medicine, Division of Graduate Medicine.

Mansfield was now recognized nationally as a physician, researcher, and academician. In 1976 he accepted the challenge to build a new department at the University of Kansas Medical Center, and was named professor and chairman of the department of radiation therapy. He remained in Kansas City until 1983 when he was invited back to Jefferson to succeed his mentor, Dr. Simon Kramer, as professor and chairman of the department of radiation oncology and nuclear medicine.

Dr. Carl M. Mansfield maintained a continuing interest in radiation management of breast cancer and actively pursued tumor predictor research in breast cancer patients. The Bodine Center for Cancer Treatment, which had first been conceived in 1983, was built under his direction. It was formally dedicated in March 1987 and was one of the most up-to-date facilities in the country. The center was equipped with new facilities for hyperthermia, intraoperative radiation therapy, a dedicated CT scanner, and four new linear accelerators, as well as a day hospital for patients to receive combined modality therapy.

Mansfield was also an attending physician at Methodist Hospital and on the consulting staffs at Chestnut Hill Hospital, the Wills Eye Hospital, the Veterans Administration Hospital of Wilmington, and the Albert Einstein Medical Center, Daroff Division.

Dr. Carl Mansfield has written more than 120 scientific papers. He is author of *Early Breast Cancer: Its History and Results of Treatment* (1976) and editor of *Therapeutic Radiology: New Directions in Therapy* (1982). He has been a member of the editorial boards of: *Journal of the National Medical Association, CA: A Cancer Journal for Clinicians, International Journal of Radiation Oncology, Biology, Physics*, and *American Journal of Clinical Oncology*.

Dr. Mansfield was president of the American Radium Society in 1988, and chairman of the radiation therapy program committee of the Radiological Society of North America. He has also been an examiner for the American Board of Radiology, and a reviewer for the radiation study section of the division of research grants of the National Cancer Institute. He has been a director-at-large of the national board of directors of the American Cancer Society, and chairman of its professional education work/study group on radiation therapy technology training.

Dr. Mansfield was chairman of the medical and scientific committee of the Philadelphia Division, American Cancer Society in 1988, and president of the division the following year. In 1994 the division's executive vice president, William Barlow, told the audience at Mansfield's portrait presentation that the physician has worked tirelessly for the poor. In 1987 Mansfield founded the American Cancer Society's Underserved Initiative, providing cancer education and screening in communities without adequate health resources.

Another speaker at the ceremony was Dr. Luther Brady, professor and chairman of radiation oncology at Hahnemann University. He related that in 1990 when Philadelphia was selected as a test market for a new cigarette targeted toward African-American smokers, Dr. Mansfield spearheaded a grass-roots effort that took immediate action. His efforts ultimately forced a giant tobacco company to abandon the new product in Philadelphia and elsewhere.

In 1991 Carl M. Mansfield was awarded the National Bronze Medal of the American Cancer Society for community work. In 1995 the ACS created the Carl Mansfield Award presented to the group or program that demonstrates unique or successful outreaches to the underserved community. Earlier he had received volunteer achievement awards from the society's Philadelphia Division and from its Keys to Living Unit.

Lincoln University named Dr. Mansfield as recipient of its distinguished alumnus award, and in 1990 awarded him an honorary doctor of science degree. Howard University College of Medicine conferred on him its outstanding alumnus award. Mansfield was also the recipient of the Outstanding Achievement Award of the Radiology Section of the National Medical Association, and the Mercy-Douglas Lectureship Award of the Eastern Pennsylvania Medical Society.

Dr. Mansfield stepped down as chairman at Jefferson in 1994. The following year he was named adjunct professor at Jefferson after his appointment as associate director of the Division of Cancer Treatment of the National Cancer Institute in Bethesda, Maryland, with responsibility for the radiation research program.

Dr. Carl Mansfield's friends and colleagues at Jefferson presented his portrait in 1994 upon his retirement. Dean Larson depicted the physician three-quarters length and slightly smaller than life-sized, standing in an X-ray reading room. He looks directly out toward the viewer, as though just interrupted from reading the sheaf of papers in his hand. The sitter's gaze is warm and friendly and the trace of a smile is enhanced by his trim mustache. A warm, glowing light that falls on his high-domed forehead is also reflected on the lenses of his large, horn-rimmed glasses.

The subject wears a white shirt and striped necktie under his gleaming white doctor's coat with its identifying inscription embroidered over the pocket: "C. M. Mansfield, M.D./Rad.../Nu..." To the left of the figure is a large light screen with an illuminated image. Below the screen is a small table with a pile of books including two editions of Mansfield's text, *Therapeutic Radiology*. Behind the figure on the right are shelves lined with multicolored books.

Dean Larson's expressive paint style is loosely brushed but maintains control over anatomical forms and contrasts of light and shade. The doctor's coat is described in subtle variations of cool and warm white tones, and there is an allover silvery harmony of the architectural elements.

During the portrait presentation ceremony Mansfield movingly expressed his gratitude to others who "gave him a chance," starting with his mother and grandmother who helped "lift him over the obstacles of oppressive segregation" to "instill a sense of pride and faith in himself." William Barlow described Dr. Carl M. Mansfield as a quiet and unassuming man, but a physician with a passionate belief that health care is a right for all Americans, not a privilege for some.

Portrait of Esmond M. Mapp

ESMOND McDONALD MAPP, M.D. (1928-91)
By Daniel V. Cavaliere (b. 1928)

Oil on canvas
1992
25 x 20 in.

Signed lower left: "Dan Cavaliere"

Given in 1992 by TJU department of radiology
Accession number: 1992+e.P.04

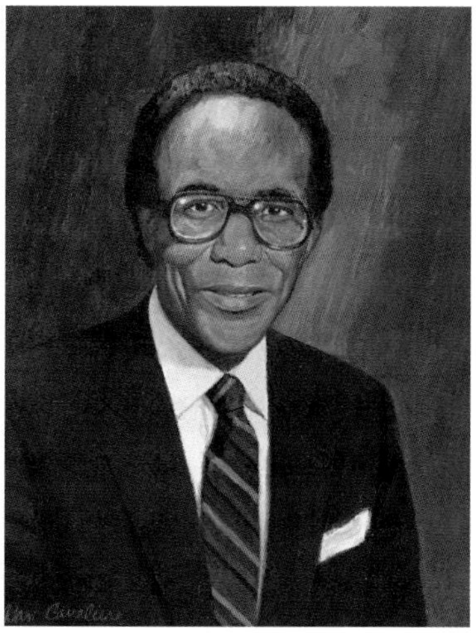

Dr. Esmond M. Mapp was professor of radiology at Jefferson. He was an outstanding teacher and known nationally for his contributions to gastrointestinal radiology.

Esmond Mapp was born in 1928 in Port-of-Spain,

Trinidad, the West Indies. He was educated at Howard University where he earned his bachelor's degree in 1953, was an NIH fellow in cardiovascular-renal physiology in 1955, and received his medical degree in 1958. After his internship at the District of Columbia General Hospital in Washington, he spent two years as captain in the U.S. Navy Medical Corps.

Dr. Mapp served a residency in radiology at the Graduate Hospital of the University of Pennsylvania from 1961 to 1964. His early faculty appointments were as assistant professor of radiology at Women's Medical College and Emory University School of Medicine, and then associate professor of radiology at Temple University School of Medicine.

After joining the Jefferson faculty in 1976 as associate professor of radiology, Dr. Mapp was promoted to clinical professor in 1980 and professor in 1983. He was attending physician at Jefferson Hospital, and a consultant at St. Agnes and West Park Hospitals in Philadelphia and at the U.S. Naval Regional Medical Center in Bethesda, Maryland.

Among his services to organized medicine, Dr. Mapp served as national chairman of the section on radiology of the National Medical Association, guest examiner for the American Board of Radiology, chairman of the Radiological Devices Panel of the U.S. Food and Drug Administration Center for Devices and Radiological Health, and member of the executive committee of the Intersociety Commission of the American College of Radiology. He was a faculty member of the postgraduate course on colon and rectal surgery at the American College of Surgeons Annual Clinical Congress in 1980.

Locally, Dr. Mapp served as treasurer and a director of the Pennsylvania Radiological Society. He initiated a joint program for radiologists and technicians between Thomas Jefferson University and Trinidad's Mount Hope Medical College at the University of the West Indies. Before his death in 1991 Dr. Esmond Mapp was chosen to receive the first annual Outstanding Educator Award of the Philadelphia Roentgen Ray Society.

In addition to many scientific presentations and visiting lectureships at hospitals and universities in the United States, Mapp lectured at the Association of Radiologists of West Africa annual conference in Monrovia, Liberia (1974), and at the Yokohama City University Hospital in Yokohama, Japan (1980). He also lectured on adrenal venography at the University College Hospital in Ibadan, Nigeria (1974).

Dr. Esmond Mapp died in 1991 after an eleven month battle with colon cancer. Dr. David C. Levin, chairman of the department of radiology at Jefferson, wrote in a memorial biography of his colleague:

> Beneath his quiet demeanor lurked a sly sense of humor and he was loved by virtually everyone in the department. He taught an entire generation of Jefferson residents how to perform and interpret barium studies, but perhaps the most unforgettable lesson he taught was how to face a grim personal prognosis with courage, determination, dignity, and the willingness to work full-time until virtually the very end.

The department of radiology commissioned a posthumous portrait of Dr. Esmond Mapp by Dan Cavaliere. The physician is depicted bust length and life-sized, gazing straight ahead through horn-rimmed glasses. His dimpled smile engages the viewer directly. The subject is wearing a black suit, white shirt and pocket handkerchief, and a multicolored, striped necktie. The atmospheric background is loosely painted in shades of olive, brown, and tan.

Daniel Cavaliere was born in 1928 in Bala Cynwyd, Pennsylvania and graduated from the Philadelphia Museum School of Art in 1951 when he won the Illustration Award. His father, Raphael J. Cavaliere, was a well known illustrator, and his son, Jamie Cavaliere, is also an illustrator and painter.

Dan Cavaliere served in Japan and Korea as a combat artist for the *Pacific Stars and Stripes* from 1951 to 1953, and worked behind the lines with news correspondents. Until 1980 he freelanced for Philadelphia advertising agencies, and painted covers and story illustrations for many publications. He won several Awards of Excellence at Philadelphia Art Directors annual shows. More recently Cavaliere has concentrated on painting historical and contemporary scenes of Philadelphia. The Rittenhouse Hotel awarded him commissions for a fifty-foot mural of Boat House Row and sixteen other paintings of the city.

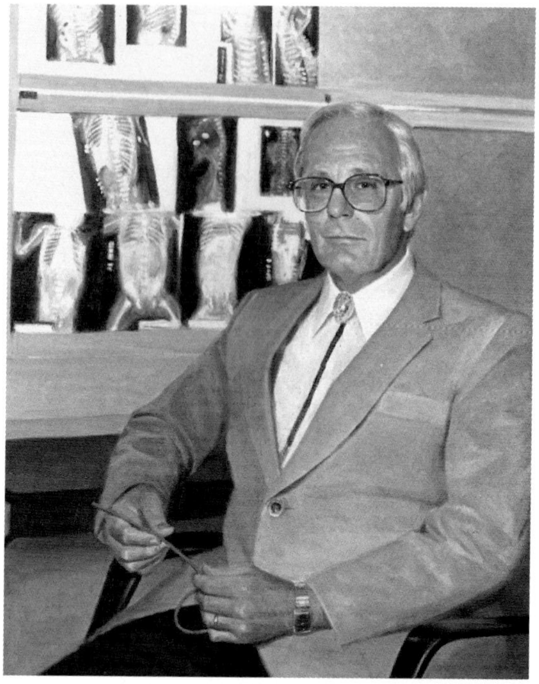

Portrait of A. Edward O'Hara

ALBERT EDWARD O'HARA, M.D. (b. 1922)
By M. Lucien LeBreton

Oil on canvas
1986
30 x 24 in.

Signed lower right: "Lucien LeBreton"

Given in 1986 by TJU departments of radiology and pediatrics
Accession number: 1986+e.P.05

Dr. Albert Edward O'Hara was a professor of radiology at Jefferson, with a secondary appointment as professor of pediatrics. His expertise was in pediatric radiology.

A. Edward O'Hara was born in Weston, West Virginia. He earned a bachelor's degree from West Virginia Wesleyan in 1944, and after two years at the West Virginia University School of Medicine transferred to the University of Pennsylvania School of Medicine where he graduated with the class of 1948.

Following his internship at Allegheny General Hospital in Pittsburgh, he took a residency in radiology at the Hospital of the University of Pennsylvania. From 1955 to 1958 he was an instructor in radiology at the Graduate School of Medicine of the University of Pennsylvania and was an associate radiologist at Children's Hospital. He met his wife, a former Jefferson nurse anesthetist, at the latter institution.

Dr. O'Hara joined the Jefferson faculty in 1958 and rose to professor of radiology in 1968. He was the first pediatric radiologist at Jefferson and developed the division of pediatric radiology within the radiology department. In 1966 he won the Christian R. and Mary F. Lindback Award for Distinguished Teaching. When he retired in 1986 he was named honorary professor of radiology and honorary professor of pediatrics.

That same year friends and colleagues in the two departments seized the opportunity to honor Dr. A. Edward O'Hara with a portrait. The painting was executed from photographs supplied by the university to Lucien M. LeBreton, an artist who specialized in this service. He was employed by Portrait Specialists, Incorporated in New York.

Dr. O'Hara is shown half length and slightly smaller than life-sized. He is seated in an armchair facing partly to the left. His ruddy face is framed by silver hair and a square jaw. He looks up toward the viewer through heavy horn-rimmed glasses with a neutral expression. In contrast to the bland expression his attire is rather rakish: a camel-colored sport jacket, black trousers, and a bola tie of gold and leather. The physician holds a section of bright orange, rubber catheter tubing between his fingers.

Dr. O'Hara appears comfortably situated in the X-ray reading room. A view box shows three rows of frontal and profile X-rays of newborn babies in the intensive care nursery. The red chair back provides another bright note in the painting.

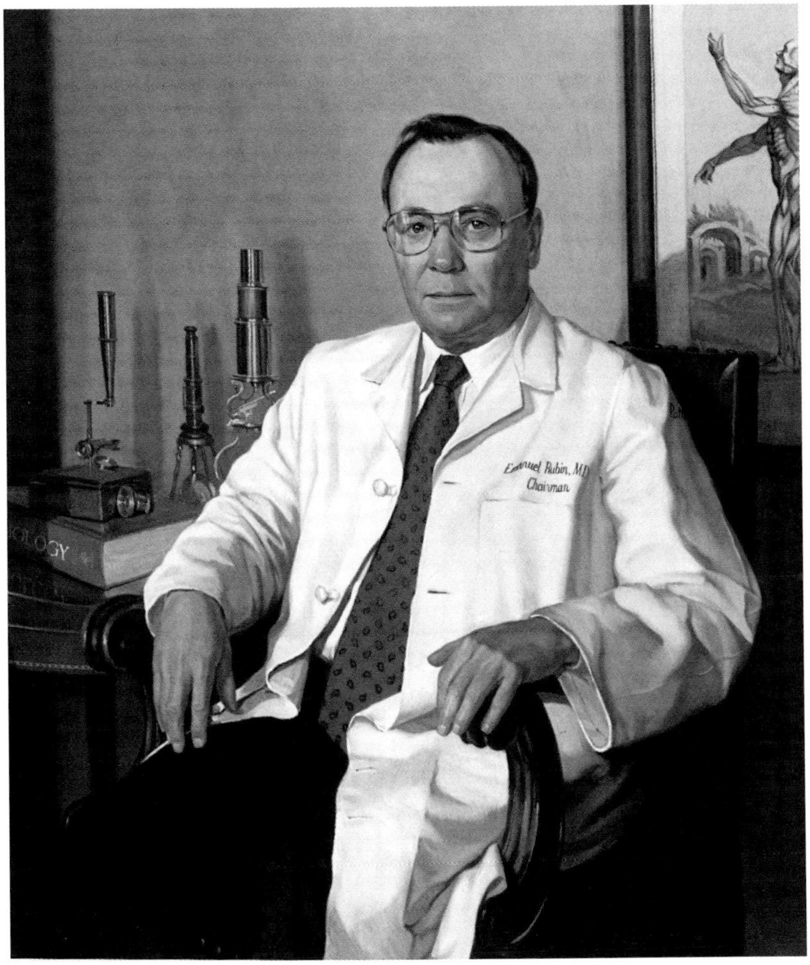

Portrait of Emanuel Rubin

(See color plate)

EMANUEL RUBIN, M.D. (b. 1928)
By Russell W. Recchion (b. 1954)

Oil on canvas
1996
42 1/4 x 36 1/4 in.

Signed and dated lower right: "RECCHION '96"

Given in 1996 by friends and colleagues
Accession number: 1996+e.P.04

Dr. Emanuel Rubin is the Gonzalo E. Aponte Professor of Pathology and chairman of the department of pathology, anatomy, and cell biology at Jefferson. He has conducted landmark studies on the effects of alcohol on the liver, heart, and membranes.

Born in 1928 in New York City and reared in Atlantic City, "Manny" Rubin received his undergraduate degree from Villanova University in 1950 and his medical degree from Harvard Medical School in 1954. After interning at Boston City Hospital he was a lieutenant in the U.S. Navy for two years, and then took a residency at Children's Hospital of Philadelphia. Fellowships at Mount Sinai Hospital in New York included the Dazian research fellowship in pathology (1958-60) and the American Cancer Society advanced clinical fellowship (1960-62).

With successive promotions on the Mount Sinai staff, he advanced to become the hospital's pathologist-in-chief by 1971. In 1966 he had been named professor of pathology at the Mount Sinai School of Medicine of the City University of New York, and in 1972 was appointed the Irene Heinz and John LaPorte Given Professor and chair of the department.

In 1977 Dr. Emanuel Rubin moved to Philadelphia to assume the professorship and chair of the department of pathology and laboratory medicine at Hahnemann University School of Medicine. During this period he was also adjunct professor of biochemistry and biophysics at the University of Pennsylvania School of Medicine.

In 1986 he joined the Jefferson faculty as the Gonzalo E. Aponte Professor of Pathology and chairman of the department of pathology and cell biology, and in 1994 this department merged with the department of anatomy. As department chair Dr. Rubin has gathered together an illustrious group of basic investigators and clinical faculty. He is principal investigator and scientific director of the Jefferson Alcohol Research Center, supported by the NIAAA. It is regarded as one of the best centers of its type in the nation.

Dr. Rubin has been a consultant to the NIAAA's biomedical research review committee, HEW's National Task Force for Alcohol and Health, and the medical advisory council of the Alcoholic Beverage Medical Research Foundation. He has also been a representative of the Association of Pathology Chairmen to the Council of Academic Societies.

His many contributions to the medical literature include more than 160 scientific articles. He has edited the following textbooks: *Advances in the Biology of Disease* (with Ivan Damjanov, 1984), *Alcohol and the Cell* (1987), *Pathology* (with John L. Farber, 1988), *Essential Pathology* (with Farber, 1990), and *Molecular and Cellular Mechanisms of Alcohol and Anesthetics* (with Keith W. Miller and Sheldon H. Roth, 1991). *Pathology* was awarded first prize in the physician's category of the American Medical Writers Association's Medical Book Awards Competition in 1989.

Dr. Rubin's journal editorships are equally as extensive. He was editor-in-chief of *Laboratory Investigation* for over twelve years. He has been field editor of *Quarterly Journal of Studies in Alcohol*, assistant editor of *Addiction Biology*, and an editorial board member of *Laboratory Investigation, Human Pathology, Gastroenterology, American Journal of Alcohol and Drug Abuse, Substance and Alcohol Abuse, Médecine et Chirurgie Digestives, Alcohol and Alcoholism*, and *Alcohol Health and Research World*.

Since 1987 Dr. Rubin has been honored to present numerous named lectures throughout the United States, including the Maude L. Menten centennial lecture at the University of Pittsburgh School of Medicine, the Whipple lecture at the University of Rochester Medical Center, the Jack M. Layton lecture at the University of Arizona School of Medicine, and the Donald Svoboda memorial lecture at the University of Kansas Medical School. He has also made keynote presentations in Sweden and Israel.

Among other honors, Dr. Rubin received an honorary doctoral degree from the University of Barcelona in 1994, and the F. K. Mostofi Distinguished Service Award of the U.S.-Canadian Academy of Pathology in 1996.

His portrait was presented to Thomas Jefferson University by friends and colleagues in 1996. Painted by Russell W. Recchion, Dr. Emanuel Rubin is depicted three-quarters length and life-sized. He is seated in an armchair in his office surrounded by various medical objects. His body faces slightly left but his head turns to look directly toward the viewer. His face is noticeably square with its high, wide forehead and angular jaw line. His hazel eyes gaze intently through metal-rimmed glasses and his wide mouth with narrow lips is firmly set.

The physician is wearing a white shirt, red necktie with a green foulard pattern, dark trousers, and a white doctor coat with "Emanuel Rubin, M.D. Chairman" clearly embroidered over the pocket. The background objects allude to his academic interests: on the table are three antique brass microscopes and his own acclaimed textbook, bound in red and with the title partly visible: "...THOLOGY;" on the rear wall is a framed illustration taken from Andreas Vesalius's *De Humani Corporis Fabrica* (q.v.).

Russell Recchion's paint style is tight, precise, and smooth. He uses a raking light source from the left effectively to illuminate the figure, objects, wall, and especially the folds and geometric shapes of the doctor's brilliant white coat.

At the portrait ceremony Dr. Rubin acknowledged those professional and family members to whom he is indebted, including several of his children who chose medicine as a career: Daniel and Raphael who are pathologists (Raphael at Thomas Jefferson University), Jonathan who is a radiologist, and Rebecca who is married to a neurosurgeon. Dr. Emanuel Rubin closed his remarks with a quotation from the seventeenth-century French playwright Molière, "There is no reward so delightful, no pleasure so exquisite as having one's work known and acclaimed by those whose applause confers honor."

Russell Recchion was born in Coraopolis, a small town near Pittsburgh, Pennsylvania in 1954. He attended a program for artistically gifted children at the Carnegie Institute, and then studied at the Art Institute of Pittsburgh (1972-75). For the next few years he worked as an illustrator designing magazine covers and corporate annual reports.

He decided to switch to fine arts, and came to Philadelphia in 1978 to study at the Pennsylvania Academy of the Fine Arts. He graduated in 1982 and won the coveted Cadwalader Landscape Prize. While in school he developed outstanding techniques as a figure painter and received several commissions for portraits through local art galleries. Inspired by the city's longstanding tradition of portraiture, he decided to remain in Philadelphia to pursue this field.

Russell Recchion's sitters have included John Connelly, past president of the Crown, Cork and Seal Company, Joel Bloom, president of the Franklin Institute, and chief executive officers of Philadelphia banks, hospitals, insurance companies, and law firms.

Recchion has exhibited at galleries and art centers in the Philadelphia area, the Union League Club of Chicago, and the Spoleto Arts Festival in Charleston, South Carolina. He also exhibits frequently in Indiana where he maintains a home and where his wife is a professor of economics and city planning. In recent years he has divided his time between painting portraits in Philadelphia and documenting rural landscapes and farmlands in Indiana. In 1996 he won the Best of Show in Traditional Painting at the annual Hoosier Salon in Indianapolis.

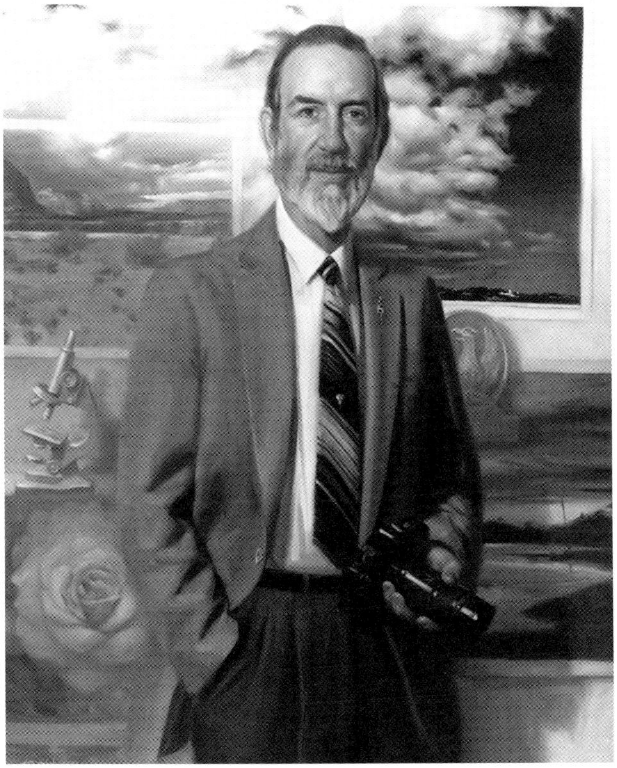

Portrait of Ronald P. Jensh

RONALD PAUL JENSH, Ph.D. (b. 1938)
By Ned Bittinger (b. 1951)

Oil on canvas
1994
39 1/2 x 31 1/2 in.

Signed and dated lower left: "Bittinger/'94"

Given by JMC class of 1994
Accession number: 1994+e.P.01

Dr. Ronald P. Jensh is a professor of pathology, anatomy, and cell biology and associate professor of pediatrics at Jefferson. His research has focused on the prevention of birth defects.

"Ron" Jensh was born in 1938 in New York City and received his undergraduate (1960) and master's (1962) degrees from Bucknell University in Lewisburg, Pennsylvania. He earned his doctor of philosophy degree from Jefferson Medical College in 1966 in anatomy, embryology, and teratology. Dr. Jensh has spent his entire career at Jefferson as a full-time faculty member, serving in several different departments since 1966.

He has been professor in the department of pathology, anatomy, and cellular biology since 1994, and has been section chief of microscopic anatomy since 1988. He has been associate professor of pediatrics since 1991, and was associate professor of radiology from 1974 to 1991.

Dr. Jensh was graduate advisor to the graduate training program (1968-82) and codirector of the predoctoral/postdoctoral training program (1971-82). As chairman of the curriculum committee (1987-93) he led a group of faculty members to modify and modernize the curriculum. Jensh was a recipient of the Christian R. and Mary F. Lindback Foundation Award for Distinguished Teaching (1973), the distinguished alumnus award of the College of Graduate Studies (1985), and the Burlington Northern Foundation Faculty Achievement Award (1989).

Dr. Ronald Jensh's early investigations concentrated on the teratogenic action of trypan blue and the causes of fetal growth retardation. Interested in scientific technique, he developed a method for photographing immunodiffusion plates, a method for rapidly preparing embryos and visualizing their bone structures, and also developed a special cage for radiation studies. He made important contributions in quantifying neural behavioral evaluations in animal studies. He was involved with an extended series of reproductive toxicity studies dealing with ionizing radiation, microwave radiation, and ultrasound.

On the national scene Dr. Jensh has been president of the Behavioral Teratology Society and a grant evaluator for the March of Dimes Birth Defects Foundation and for the radiation study section of the National Institutes of Health. He has been a consultant to companies ranging from the Ortho Research Foundation to the Mobil Oil Corporation. He has been a reviewer for the *Journal of the American College of Toxicology*, *Science*, and the *International Journal of Radiation Biology*. In 1997 he received the Bucknell University Alumni Association Award for Outstanding Achievement in a Chosen Profession.

At the portrait presentation speakers praised Dr. Jensh's warmth, dedication to teaching, and remarkable capacity for compassion. Because the scientist and educator has candidly shared aspects of his personal history to others, almost all participants made oblique or direct references to Dr. Jensh's recovery from four major heart attacks as a young man, triple bypass surgery, and a heart transplant in 1992. He is admired for his courage and faith in taking measures to promote a healthy lifestyle.

Dr. Ronald P. Jensh spoke movingly about his three inner ideals in responding to life's adversities and opportunities:

> Childhood—Never forget the child in each of us... As a child each day was an adventure...You always woke up...to see what the day would bring, and an afternoon lasted forever... Remember the spring days, the smells, the colors, the anticipation? Life needs to be a spring day for all of us...Remembering can brighten the mental rainy days and bring spring to our thoughts.
>
> Miracles—What is a miracle?...Is the beginning of life any the less miraculous because we know how a sperm and egg fuse to become a new individual?...Is the brain any the less miraculous because we are becoming more knowledgeable about how neurons interact, how neurotransmitters are used, and the powers of endorphins to affect our bodies?...A resounding no! If anything the sense of the miraculous is enhanced by our knowledge...If we take time to look, listen, and learn, we become changed every day and that becomes a miracle...
>
> Mirrors—I am a mirror, you are a mirror...We bring to this life a piece that is uniquely ourselves, the genetics, if you will, but that combines with all the experience we have as we proceed through life and encounter each scene of our own personal theatrical play...Like the fun house mirrors set opposite each other we reflect and reflect over and over again and become a miracle...You have done something for me today which I will never forget and my own personal mirror will forever be changed because of it, as will your own personal plays.

In his portrait by Ned Bittinger, Dr. Ron Jensh is shown two-thirds length and life-sized, standing in a frontal position. He holds a camera in his left hand, while his right hand is placed in his trouser pocket. His lanky physique and long, thin face are accentuated by his pointed gray beard. He gazes straight ahead with an earnest and reflective expression. He wears a white shirt, blue blazer, dark gray slacks and a diagonal striped necktie. The loosely brushed surface has a verve and dash that nonetheless captures the living presence of the figure.

He poses in front of a display of his own photographs and other objects. The objects include a brass microscope and a phoenix plaque mounted on a base with the letters "ENIX" visible, alluding to the portrait sitter's medical specialty and to his physical and emotional "rebirth." Photographic subjects reflect his myriad interests in nature: a closeup of a pink rose, a sunset, a western landscape, and billowing clouds. A serious photographer, Jensh has exhibited widely and won national awards.

Portraitist, muralist, and illustrator Ned Bittinger was born in 1951 and presently resides in Sperryville, Virginia. He earned a bachelor of fine arts degree from Denison University in Granville, Ohio in 1974 and a master's of fine arts from George Washington University in 1982. He won the David Lloyd Kreeger Award at George Washington University in 1981 and the Hayes Freedman Purchase Prize of the Kreeger Awards Competition in 1982.

Bittinger taught drawing and etching briefly at the National Collection of Fine Arts in Washington, D.C. He studied portraiture with Daniel Greene and John Howard Sanden in 1983, and has conducted workshops in Washington, and nearby Maryland and Virginia until the present.

His large scale commissions include murals for the Montgomery County Public Schools in Bethesda, Maryland and a "broker" series for Cushman Wakefield in Washington. He was also commissioned to provide illustrations for children's books for *Scholastic* magazine, and a series of benefactor portraits for Gettysburg College in Pennsylvania.

Ned Bittinger was awarded a grant by the Washington, D.C. Commission on the Arts and Humanities in 1986, and was selected as one of fifty artists by the Washington/Moscow Art Exchange in 1991. As winner in a national competition sponsored by *American Artist* magazine, he was honored with an exhibition at the Grand Central Galleries in New York in 1985.

In 1994 and 1995 Ned Bittinger was commissioned by the U.S. State Department to paint portraits of former secretaries of state Lawrence Eagleburger and James A. Baker II. Among his other portrait subjects are Dr. and Mrs. Henry Kissinger, Shirley MacLaine, Dr. Lloyd Elliott, president of George Washington University, and General Gordon H. Sullivan, Chief of Staff of the U.S. Army.

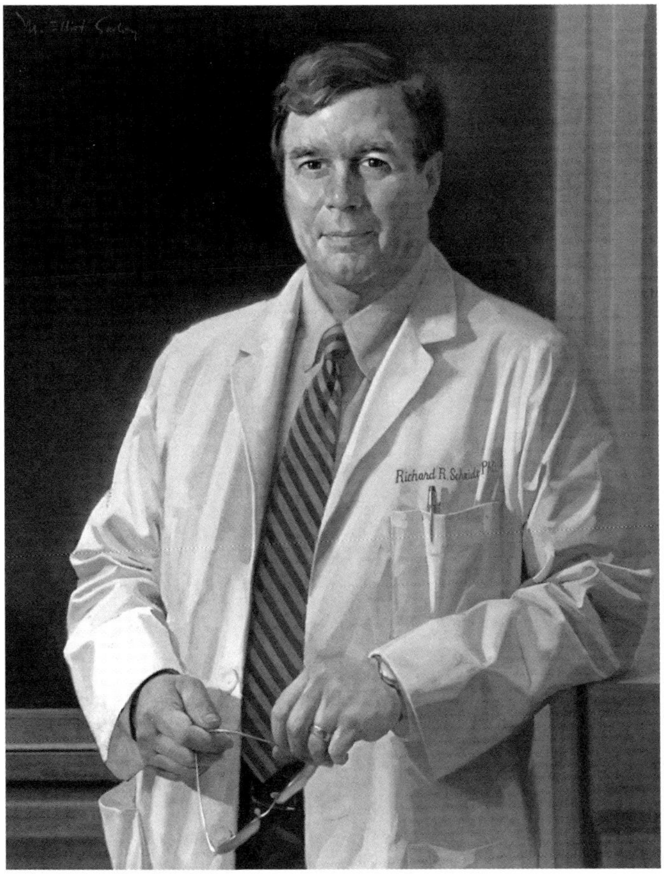

Portrait of Richard R. Schmidt

RICHARD RALPH SCHMIDT, Ph.D. (b. 1944)
By Mark Elliot Skolsky (b. 1957)

Oil on canvas
1996
34 1/4 x 27 1/4 in.

Signed upper left: "M. Elliot Skolsky"

Given by JMC class of 1996
Accession number: 1996+e.P.01

Dr. Richard R. Schmidt is professor of pathology, anatomy, and cell biology at Jefferson Medical College and vice chairman of the department. He joined the faculty in 1974 and has been an outstanding educator.

Richard Schmidt was born in 1944 in Milwaukee, Wisconsin and reared in a small town in Montana, the son of a chiropractor. He received his bachelor's degree in 1968 from the University of Wisconsin in Madison, followed by three years of postgraduate studies in zoology and then his Ph.D. degree in anatomy from the Medical College of Wisconsin in Milwaukee in 1974.

That same year Dr. Schmidt joined the Jefferson faculty as instructor in anatomy. He worked his way through the academic ranks to full professor of pathology, anatomy, and cell biology in 1994, and vice chair of the department. He was appointed the division chief of human gross anatomy in 1987, and was chairman of the departmental graduate committee from 1985 to 1990.

Dr. Schmidt's teaching responsibilities also include: lecturer and course director of principles of teratology, teacher of advanced dissection to senior students, lecturer and laboratory instructor in medical histology, and lecturer in the molecular basis of development. He has also served as a thesis and research director for doctoral students and a preceptor for medical student summer fellows.

Dr. Schmidt's research interests are in the fields of arachidonic acid metabolism and fetal thymocyte development, clinical anatomy, and the development of computerized learning programs in medical education. He is an advocate of computer-based and animated dissection instruction.

Schmidt is coauthor of *Human Anatomy* (with E. Marshall Johnson, Eldra P. Solomon, and P. William Davis, 1985). He has been a reviewer for *Teratology*, *Journal of Environmental Pathology and Toxicology*, *Journal of the American College of Toxicology*, *Journal of Immunology*, and *Life Sciences*.

In 1990 Dr. Richard R. Schmidt received the Christian R. and Mary F. Lindback Award for Distinguished Teaching in the Basic Sciences. That same year he was guest of honor at Jefferson's annual Black and Blue Ball, in recognition of his outstanding teaching and dedication. In 1998 he won the Dean's Award for Distinguished Teaching in a Basic Science.

Dr. Richard Schmidt's portrait was presented by the class of 1996 and was painted by Mark E. Skolsky. He is depicted half length and life-sized, standing in a classroom in front of a blackboard. His left arm leans on a lectern, and he holds his glasses by the temple pieces. The expression on his round-shaped, ruddy face is warm and accessible, almost smiling. He wears a blue shirt, maroon and mustard striped necktie, and a white doctor's coat. His name is embroidered above the coat pocket which holds a pen.

Skolsky's lush, smoothly brushed, sculptural style makes effective use of highlights and shadows to create a strong figural presence of the figure. The curving lines of the subject's necktie and coat suggest the rounded volumes of his body. The pinkish glow of the white coat's deep folds harmonizes with the warm tones of the sitter's complexion and the wooden architectural moldings.

Student speakers at the portrait ceremony expressed appreciation of Dr. Richard Schmidt's accessibility, tireless dedication, sense of humor, and an excitement and fervor about teaching anatomy that "still shines through" after more than twenty years. A speaker mentioned that Dr. Schmidt met his wife, the former Dulcie Bausch, in 1980 when she was a technician in biochemistry at Jefferson. She is the daughter of Richard D. Bausch, M.D., a Jefferson alumnus of 1942.

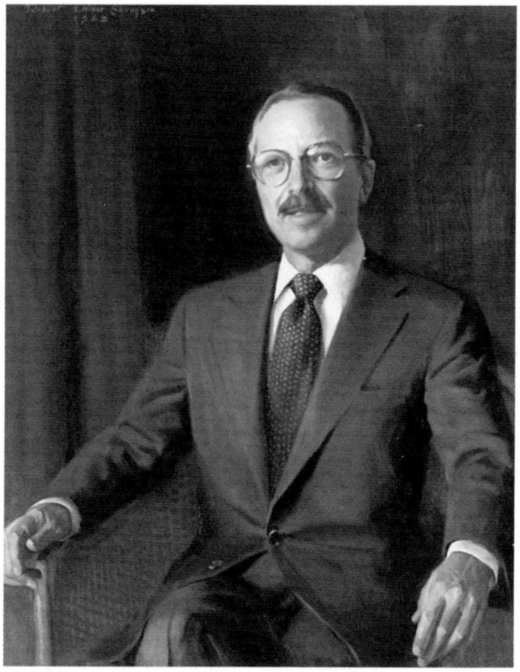

Portrait of John R. Shea

JOHN RAYMOND SHEA, Ph.D. (b. 1938)
By Robert Oliver Skemp (1910-84)

Oil on canvas
1983
36 x 30 in.

Signed and dated upper left: "Robert Oliver Skemp/1983"

Given by JMC class of 1983
Accession number: 1983+e.P.07

Dr. John R. Shea is an associate professor of pathology, anatomy, and cell biology and an associate professor of orthopaedic surgery at Jefferson Medical College. His teaching has been marked by dedication to his subject and compassion and understanding for his students.

John Raymond Michael Shea was born in 1938, a native of Burlington, Vermont. He received his undergraduate degree in biology at the Rensselaer Polytechnic Institute in Troy, New York (1960), followed by a master of science degree in anatomy (1962) and a Ph.D. degree in anatomy (1965) earned at McGill University. He acquired another master of science degree, in engineering (biomechanics), at the University of Surrey in Guildford, England (1975).

After receiving his Ph.D. at McGill Dr. John Shea stayed briefly as a lecturer in anatomy, and then in 1967 joined the Jefferson faculty as instructor in anatomy. He was appointed assistant professor of anatomy in 1968 and associate professor in 1974, and served as head of the division of gross anatomy from 1975 to 1980. Early on he was encouraged by anatomy chairman Andrew J. Ramsay, Ph.D. to excel in teaching.

Dr. Shea achieved his goals to raise the level of scholarship in anatomy lecturing, improve the quality of examinations, and improve the faculty's skill in dissection. Honored repeatedly by students for his efforts, he received the Mellon Faculty Award for faculty improvement in teaching 1968 to 1971. He won the Christian R. and Mary F. Lindback Award for Distinguished Teaching in 1970, the Phi Chi Outstanding Professor of the Year Award in 1971 and 1972, and the Phi Alpha Sigma Outstanding Teaching Award in 1980.

As head of anatomy graduate programs (1972 to 1974) he designed a leaflet to attract students that was so effective that it won a silver medal for excellence in design by Neographis. In the fall of 1974 he took a sabbatical leave at the University of Surrey to pursue his interest in the application of mechanical principles to biological systems; he participated in a collaborative program with engineers to devise learning and practical aids for children afflicted with cerebral palsy. He was elected a member of the Anatomical Society of Great Britain and Ireland in 1974.

Shea served as chairman of Jefferson's committee on student affairs in 1984. He has also been a consultant to the instructional programs of the American College of Orthopaedic Surgeons, the teaching laboratories of the College of Medicine and Dentistry of New Jersey, and product development at Wyeth Laboratories.

A man of diverse interests, Dr. Shea is an erudite scholar and lecturer on the history of medical books and the history of printing. He is also keenly interested in British pottery and the ethnographic art of Native Americans and North Africans.

Robert O. Skemp's portrait of Dr. John R. Shea, the portrait honoree of the class of 1983, is the last of eleven Jefferson professors depicted by the artist. The subject is shown two-thirds length, slightly smaller than life-sized. He is seated in a rattan armchair, facing slightly left with his head turned to look toward the viewer. His lips are slightly parted and his expression is warm and approachable. He is wearing a white shirt, maroon necktie with a small gold pattern, and a gray suit.

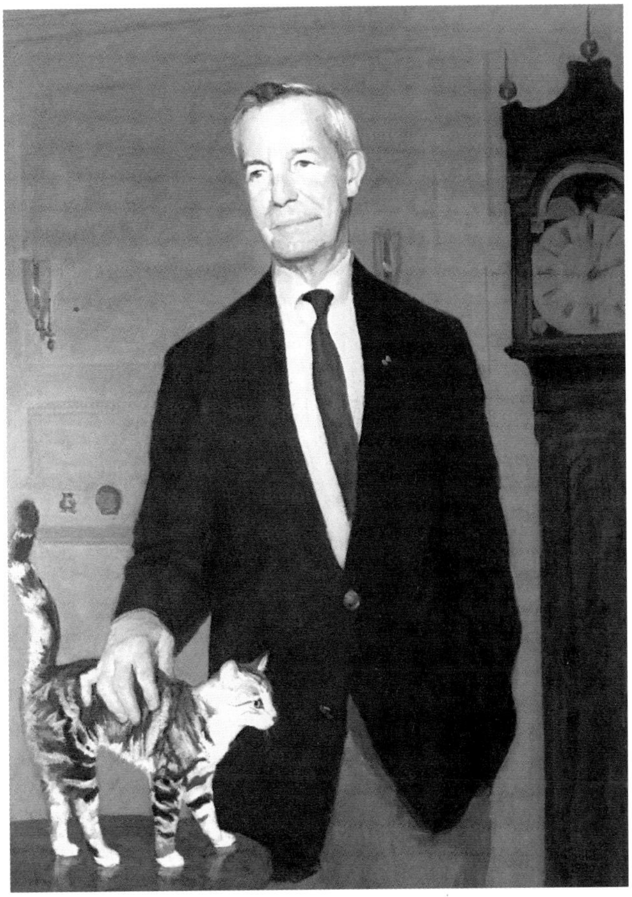

Portrait of Russell W. Schaedler

RUSSELL WILLIAM SCHAEDLER, M.D. (b. 1927)
By Paul DuSold (b. 1963)

Oil on canvas
1990
38 1/2 x 28 1/2 in.

Signed and dated lower right: "DuSold/1990"
Exhibitions: Philadelphia, *Portrait: The Art of Image*, rededication of the Morani Gallery, Medical College of Pennsylvania, 1994; Wayne, Pennsylvania, *Paul DuSold: Contemporary Traditionist Portraits*, Wayne Art Center, 1998

Given in 1990 by friends and colleagues
Accession number: 1990+e.P.08

Dr. Russell W. Schaedler was the Plimpton-Pugh Professor of Microbiology and Immunology, and served as chairman of the department from 1968 until 1991. He has taught continuously at Jefferson for three decades.

Russell Schaedler was born in 1927 in Hatfield, Pennsylvania and graduated from Ursinus College in Collegeville, Pennsylvania (1949) and Jefferson Medical

College (1953). His college career was interrupted by military service as a medical corpsman, and he finished college on the G.I. Bill. To help meet tuition expenses he worked in chemistry and biology laboratories in undergraduate school and as a basal metabolism rate technician at the Jefferson Medical College Hospital.

After his internship at Jefferson he joined the Rockefeller Institute for Medical Research (later Rockefeller University) as an assistant, and was assistant physician at the institute's hospital. By 1957 he advanced to assistant professor and resident associate physician at the institute, and in 1962 he was promoted to physician and associate professor.

Dr. Schaedler worked closely with the distinguished microbiologist René J. Dubos, Ph.D., and they were coauthors of forty papers resulting from their investigations in nutrition, infection, and especially in gastrointestinal microecology. Dr. Schaedler developed a laboratory medium known as "Schaedler's agar," used for the isolation and identification of anaerobes. His work describing the microbial flora of the mouse led to the "Schaedler cocktail," a group of indigenous organisms of the mouse used to associate germ-free animals for breeding colonies, a technique used by most American commercial breeders.[11] He has lectured worldwide on microbial flora.

Dr. Russell Schaedler joined the Jefferson Medical College faculty as professor and chairman of the department of microbiology in 1968, succeeding Dr. Kenneth Goodner. He was the first to hold the Plimpton-Pugh Professorship of Microbiology, established in 1985 by V. Watson Pugh, M.D. (a Jefferson alumnus of 1953) and his wife, Frances Plimpton Pugh, in memory of their parents.

The period soon after Dr. Schaedler's arrival was a pivotal time of change at Jefferson, and he played an important role in the college's reorganization. He was very committed to the education of medical and graduate students, and actively promoted the careers of young faculty members. He recruited a strong faculty after the department's move to new facilities in Jefferson Alumni Hall in 1969. The graduate program greatly increased in size, and the department also created a new master's program in clinical microbiology. Schaedler was one of the first to enlist members of different departments to work together on gastrointestinal investigations. Upon his official retirement in 1996 he was named the Plimpton-Pugh Professor Emeritus of Microbiology and Immunology, but students still continue to benefit from his part-time teaching.

At Dr. Schaedler's portrait presentation ceremony Dr. Robert J. Mandle commented on the legacy of a good teacher beyond his likeness in a portrait:

> Students regard Russell Schaedler as a real teacher, a stern taskmaster. He has principles, has standards, and he is not afraid to enforce the standards, he has a backbone when difficult decisions have to be made...Graduate and medical students have received much more than the facts of microbiology. They have shared and maybe even accepted his philosophy about scholarship, his love for microorganisms and the infectious process. This is a wonderful legacy and indeed a form of immortality.

Dr. Schaedler has served as a consultant to the National Institutes of Health and was twice chairman of its bacteriology and mycology study section. He was an associate member of the Enteric Commission of the Armed Forces Epidemiology Board from 1967 to 1972, and a board member of the New York Tuberculosis and Health Association from 1965 to 1969. He has served on the editorial boards of the *Journal of Bacteriology* and of the *Journal of Infection and Immunity*.

At Jefferson Dr. Schaedler has been a member of the board of directors of the Cardeza Foundation since 1972. He succeeded Dr. Mandle as chairman of the university art committee in 1986, and at Schaedler's portrait ceremony, President Lewis W. Bluemle Jr., M.D. praised his loyal stewardship of the "symbols of our heritage." Bluemle also complimented his improved landscaping of the overgrown Jefferson Alumni Hall atria. Dr. Schaedler has used his knowledge of plants to create terraced landscaping on his property in the Pocono Mountains, where he also restored an old farmhouse and built a three story barn.

The portrait of Dr. Russell Schaedler by Paul DuSold was presented by friends and colleagues in 1990. The physician is shown two-thirds length and slightly smaller than life-sized, standing informally with his left hand in his trouser pocket. His body is frontal and his head is turned and tilted slightly, looking off to the left as though in conversation. His expression is friendly, and his wide mouth seems to be suppressing a smile. He is wearing his customary attire: blue shirt, navy blue blazer with the President's Club lapel pin, gray slacks, and a dark blue necktie.

Dr. Schaedler's declaration about what a faculty portrait can be is reflected in the painting's unique domestic setting and attributes. With the explanation "Everybody presumes I can use a microscope," Dr. Schaedler has eschewed the usual medical setting in favor of the personal backdrop of his own parlor. Details of his Philadelphia Society Hill townhouse include a pale green panelled fireplace wall, glass sconces with red candles and brass fittings, an antique Sheraton tall case clock, and a tilt-top side table.

The subject's right hand strokes a gray and white striped tiger cat standing on the round table. The inclusion of "Bonk" the cat demonstrates both Schaedler's affection for his pet, and his admiration for Thomas Eakins's portrait of Dr. Benjamin H. Rand in which the professor strokes a cat that has just jumped up on his desk.

Portrait of Harry L. Smith Jr.

HARRY LOGAN SMITH Jr., Ph.D. (b. 1930)
By Dean L. Paules (b. 1931)

Oil on canvas
1988
40 x 32 in.

Signed and dated lower left: "Paules/3-88"

Given by JMC class of 1988
Accession number: 1988+e.P.01

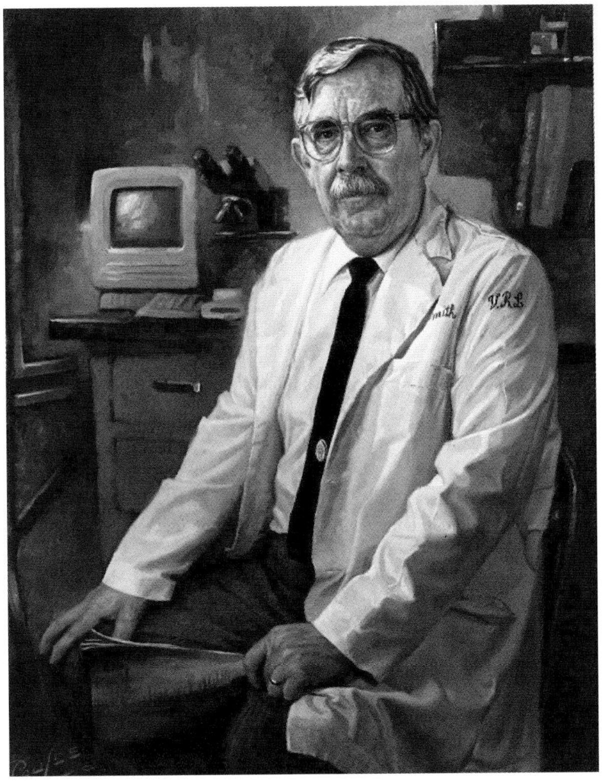

Dr. Harry Logan Smith Jr., professor of microbiology, is another alumnus who spent his entire academic career at Jefferson. He is an internationally known authority on the pathogenesis and serodiagnosis of cholera and related diarrheal diseases.

Harry L. Smith was born in 1930 and is a native of Philadelphia. After obtaining his undergraduate degree at Temple University (1952), he received his graduate education in microbiology at Jefferson Medical College: a master of science degree (1954) and doctor of philosophy degree (1957). He received his doctorate under the tutelage of Dr. Kenneth Goodner, chair of microbiology.

The invitation to Dr. Smith to join the Jefferson faculty as instructor was one of the first and most durable appointments by Dr. Goodner. Smith became interested in his mentor's study of *Vibrio* organisms and the epidemiology of cholera, and he made major contributions to public health. He received a Career Development Award from the National Institutes of Health.

Dr. Smith gained extensive field experience in gathering samples for serotyping the various organisms. He studied cholera epidemics in Thailand in 1959 and in the Philippines in 1961. He was a member of a Southeast Asian Treaty Organization cholera research team in Bangladesh in 1962 and 1969. In 1965 he studied infantile diarrhea in San José, Costa Rica. The following year he was a consultant with the Cholera Control Team of the World Health Organization in Nepal, India, and Afghanistan.

A *Vibrio* Reference Laboratory was established in 1969 at Jefferson with grant support by the United States/Japan Cooperative Scientific Program of the National Institutes of Health. Dr. Smith's collection of *Vibrio* strains and serotypes was used for reference throughout the world. He was a major contributor at a series of United States/Japan meetings on cholera, and at the Nobel-Cholera Symposium in Stockholm, Sweden in 1978.

Dr. Smith had advanced to associate professor in 1964 and full professor in 1974. For several years he was responsible for the teaching of parasitology. Smith was among the earliest Jefferson professors to use the computer as a teaching tool, and helped to develop a program for computer-simulated cases to teach the diagnosis of infectious diseases. He was a founder of the alumni association of the College of Graduate Studies, and served as president of Sigma Xi. When Dr. Smith retired in 1995 he was named emeritus professor of microbiology and immunology.

Dr. Harry L. Smith's portrait by Dean Paules was presented by the class of 1988. He is depicted two-thirds length and life-sized, seated in his office or laboratory. His head turns to gaze intently toward the spectator. His full, lined face is highlighted by wavy gray hair and mustache, and thick, dark eyebrows. He wears a white lab coat over a white shirt, black necktie with scrimshaw tie pin, and gray trousers. Embroidered on the coat are the initials "V. R. L." for Vibrio Reference Laboratory, and the last four letters of his name.

The microbiologist sits at a blue metal desk in a room crammed with objects used in his research and teaching: microscope, computer, books, and lecture notes held in his left hand. He has said that he wanted to be remembered in his lab coat because he admired the portrait of Dr. J. Earl Thomas who is so attired. His portrait was the first to include a computer. His scrimshaw tie tack is engraved with a *Giardia Lamblia*, his favorite microorganism. Dr. Smith has not only described it as "the only protozoan that looks back at you when you look at it under the microscope," but he is also famous for doing an impersonation of it.

In his response at the portrait ceremony Dr. Smith said he wished that students, "the most important thing," could have been present in his painting, as in *The Gross Clinic*. The gifted teacher, who cared about his students both in and out of the classroom, humorously counseled them:

> Your responsibility is to maintain your good name, my good name, and the good name of the institution... When you come back and look at this portrait, I only ask, are you doing the best you can in everything you are doing? You had better answer yes!

Ties to Thomas Jefferson University run deep in the Smith family. His sons Kenneth and David graduated from the medical school in 1979 and 1984, respectively, and his brother Robert is an alumnus of 1956. His daughter Diane is a 1985 graduate in physical therapy from the College of Allied Health Sciences, and another daughter Stacey worked as a nurse at the Jefferson Hospital.

Portrait of Arthur Allen

ARTHUR ALLEN, Ph.D. (b. 1928)
By Alden MacMaster Wicks (1914-87)

Oil on canvas
1979
36 x 30 in.

Signed and dated lower right: "Wicks '79"

Given by JMC class of 1979
Accession number: 1979+e.P.01

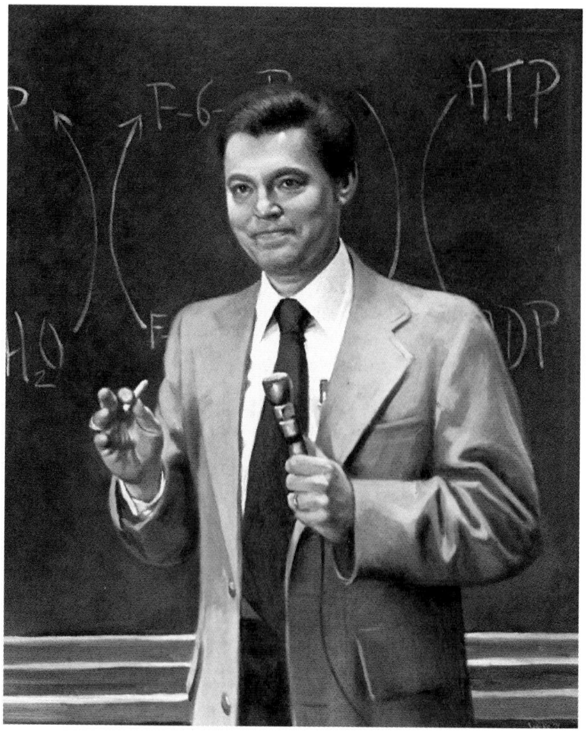

Dr. Arthur Allen is a professor of biochemistry and molecular pharmacology at Jefferson. He has been a faculty member for three decades, and has received several awards for his dedication to teaching.

Arthur Allen was born in Philadelphia in 1928 and educated at Temple University: bachelor's degree in chemistry (1950), master's degree in biochemistry (1953), and a doctor of philosophy degree in biochemistry (1956). After earning his doctorate he served as chief of the division of chemistry and toxicology of the First U.S. Army Medical Laboratory in New York.

Dr. Allen joined the Jefferson faculty in 1958 as assistant professor of biochemistry and subsequently rose in the ranks to become associate professor in 1965 and professor of biochemistry in 1983. He held positions concurrently at Temple University as lecturer in chemistry (1960-67) and adjunct associate professor of chemistry at Temple's evening school (1967-69).

Allen has served on numerous academic and university committees at Jefferson, and was chair of the subcommittee on academic leave, and chair of the subcommittee on the preclinical curriculum. He is a member of the American Association for the Advancement of Science.

Throughout his tenure Dr. Allen has been recognized as an outstanding teacher by undergraduate and graduate students. He received the Christian R. and Mary F. Lindback Award for Distinguished Teaching in 1971, and was the first recipient of the Dean's Award for Distinguished Teaching in a Basic Science in 1995. In 1994 he was elected to honorary life membership in the College of Graduate Studies alumni association.

When Dr. Allen first arrived at Jefferson he was involved in both research and teaching, but in the early 1970s made a conscious decision to concentrate on teaching and administrative work because he enjoyed the close contact with students. Sometimes referred to as "the sugar and fat man" for his special interest in carbohydrate and lipid metabolism, Allen is admired by students for his warmth and interest, shown by his remembering all their names.

The class of 1979 chose Dr. Arthur Allen as its portrait honoree. Alden M. Wicks depicted the professor half length and slightly smaller than life-sized. He is shown teaching in a lecture room, a portrayal very similar to that of Dr. Wolfgang Vogel. Allen is turned slightly left, standing in front of the blackboard and holding a microphone and a piece of chalk. His expression is animated as his blue eyes "connect" with the unseen students, and his tightly closed lips seem to be repressing a smile. His thick auburn hair is complemented by his attire: a white shirt, camel's hair jacket, brown necktie, and brown slacks.

Dr. Allen has just written formulas for key reactions in carbohydrate metabolism on the board. In a profile in the 1979 yearbook, the professor was playfully asked about his "indecipherable handwriting" and about the quantity of chalk he used during lectures. He replied that extensive writing and illustrating on the blackboard help him to pace his lectures, and enable students to keep up with the flow of information.

Allen appears both energized and relaxed in the familiar classroom setting. He has always tried to counter the perception of impersonal medical training by his enthusiastic and solicitous manner in both the lecture room and laboratory.

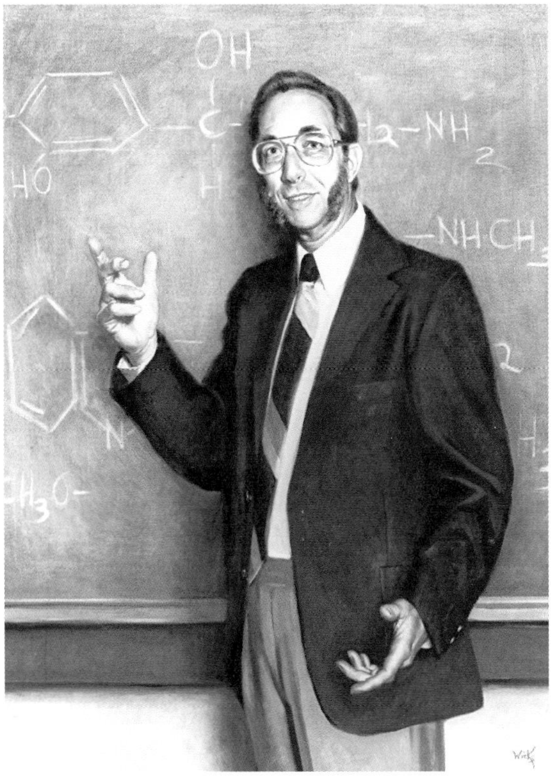

Portrait of Wolfgang H. Vogel

WOLFGANG HELLMUT VOGEL, Ph.D. (b. 1930)
By Alden MacMaster Wicks

Oil on canvas
1982
40 x 30 in.

Signed lower right: "Wicks"

Given by JMC class of 1982
Accession number: 1982+e.P.05

Dr. Wolfgang H. Vogel is a professor of biochemistry and molecular pharmacology with a secondary appointment as professor of psychiatry and human behavior at Jefferson.

Wolfgang Vogel was born in 1930, a native of Dresden, Germany. He studied for his undergraduate degree at the Universities of Bonn and Tübingen, and earned a master's degree in physical chemistry (1956) and a doctor of philosophy degree in organic chemistry (1958) at the Institute of Technology in Stuttgart. He was a postdoctoral fellow the following year in biochemistry at the Upstate Medical Center, State University of New York in Syracuse, after which he worked for two years as a chemist/physiologist at the Farbwerke Hoechst AG in Frankfurt.

Dr. Vogel's distinguished career in the United States was accomplished only after a long and arduous struggle after World War II, or as described on an award in his office: "The phoenix of Dresden becomes the eagle of Jefferson."[12] It took the utmost ingenuity to achieve his original goal of becoming a biochemist.

Wolfgang Vogel had spent the war years in Dresden, site of the Allied bombardment in 1945. Although his home was spared, the local high school was almost demolished and students subsequently attended only to receive their homework assignments. Vogel was not allowed to go to the local university because his father, a small businessman, was considered a capitalist. So Vogel made secret trips from Communist-controlled East Germany to West Berlin in order to apply to West German universities by "borrowing" the address of friends there. When accepted at the University of Bonn he obtained a passport without risking reprisals on his parents by bribing a passport clerk with two pounds of fresh butter (worth one hundred dollars on the black market).

Tuition was waived when he passed an entrance examination at the superior level. A free meal ticket was provided, but the impecunious student was forced to share cramped lodgings in a tiny, windowless room in an abandoned bunker below four hundred feet of rocks (at three dollars a month). He transferred to the University of Tübingen two years later to earn his undergraduate degree, and then completed his graduate work in Stuttgart.

It was his passion for tennis that launched the next unlikely stage of his career. At a mixed doubles match it was suggested by his tennis partner that he pursue a postdoctoral fellowship in Syracuse, New York where her brother was looking for a postdoctoral fellow as assistant. He embarked for America by steamer, determined to master the English language by learning vocabulary page-by-page from Aldous Huxley's *Brave New World*. A temporary visa necessitated his return to Germany after a year, but he was able to emigrate permanently to the United States with his new wife in 1961.

They moved to Chicago where Dr. Vogel accepted a position as research assistant and instructor, working with a professor he had known at Syracuse and who had relocated to the University of Illinois College of Medicine. The professor had switched to pharmacology, so Dr. Vogel learned a new field which he soon came to prefer. To further his knowledge he spent a year as a visiting research associate at the National Heart Institute of the National Institutes of Health. Upon his return he was promoted to assistant professor of pharmacology and research associate at Illinois.

Another Syracuse acquaintance recommended him for associate professor of pharmacology at Jefferson, and he joined the faculty there in the fall of 1967. His prior research career had not prepared him for delivering formal lectures before 220 students and he was apprehensive about his English proficiency, but he developed a love for teaching and an enthusiasm and knack for presenting difficult material, often spiced with jokes or funny aphorisms. His special rapport with students earned him the Christian R. and Mary F. Lindback Award for Distinguished Teaching in 1972. He was chosen Parents Day speaker consistently, and named the Best Teacher of the Year in 1994.

In 1974 he was promoted to professor of pharmacology, and in 1977 earned a secondary appointment as professor in the department of psychiatry and human behavior. He was vice chairman of Jefferson's pharmacology department from 1985 to 1991 and acting chairman from 1986 to 1991. In 1992 he served as interim chairman of the Institute of Pharmacology at the University of Marburg, Germany.

Professor Vogel's research and teaching interests lie in the chemistry and pharmacology of stress, psychopharmacology, neurochemistry, and biological psychiatry. An area of special interest is the discovery of five methoxytryptamine, a chemical in the brain that might be proven to cause schizophrenia or other mental illnesses. He has contributed more than 160 articles to the medical literature, and served on the editorial boards of *Contemporary Drug Problems* and *Neuropsychobiology*.

Since his arrival at Jefferson Dr. Wolfgang Vogel has been an active participant in college and university affairs. He was chairman of the department committee on graduate student training from 1969 to 1976, and has guided the degree programs of a large number of doctoral students and postdoctoral fellows. He also chaired the department committee on medical education and the committee for continuing evaluation of the code of professional conduct.

Vogel was elected a member of the American Association for the Advancement of Science and was president of the local chapter from 1974 to 1976. He has been a consultant to drug education programs in Pennsylvania and New Jersey. In 1975 he won the U.S. Senior Scientist Award from the Federal Republic of Germany.

Dr. Wolfgang Vogel was selected as senior portrait honoree by the class of 1982, and was depicted lecturing in a classroom by Alden M. Wicks. The professor is shown two-thirds length and slightly smaller than life-sized, turning away from the gray chalkboard. He faces his unseen students with an engaging expression, highlighted by his smiling mouth, blue-gray eyes gazing alertly through aviator-style glasses, and bushy, handlebar sideburns. His right hand gestures toward the chemical structures of three neurotransmitters he has just written on the board: norepinephrine, epinephrine, and serotonin. He is wearing a blue shirt, diagonally blue and gray striped necktie, navy blue blazer, and gray trousers.

In an emotional response at the portrait ceremonies, Dr. Vogel recounted an incident from his youth when he visited the University of Vienna and admired the busts and portraits of great professors, dreaming that one day his portrait might also hang on the walls of an academic institution. He continued,

> However, these gentle flames of youthful hope were soon extinguished by the gales of life's reality, and the moment of wishful thinking was soon forgotten—or so I had thought, until...the class of 1982 informed me that they had chosen me as their subject...producing a storm in my subconscious, and a flood of all kinds of neurotransmitters in my brain. All of a sudden, I once again saw myself standing in Vienna, looking at the portraits of the great scholars...[my portrait] will stimulate me to work harder and to come closer to the true art of teaching.

---

1. Frederick B. Wagner Jr., M.D., *Thomas Jefferson University: Tradition and Heritage* (Philadelphia: Lea & Febiger, 1989), 846.
2. For a complete description of the building and its research activities, see Malcolm Clendenin, "A Research Building for Building Research," *Jefferson Medical College Alumni Bulletin* 40 (summer 1991): 28-34.
3. John J. Gartland, M.D., "Jefferson's Longitudinal Study: A Landmark Research Effort," *Jefferson Medical College Alumni Bulletin* 42 (fall 1992): 4.
4. "A Student's Choice," *Jefferson Medical College Alumni Bulletin* 35 (summer 1986): 4.
5. Wagner, 455-56.
6. Robert L. Brent, M.D., Ph.D., "Growth and Maturation of the Pediatrics Department," *Jefferson Medical College Alumni Bulletin* 40 (spring 1991): 2-9.
7. Two other husband and wife portraits in the Jefferson collection painted by the same artist are: Jacob Eichholtz's portraits of Dr. John Eberle (1827) and Mrs. Eberle (1831); and Samuel B. Waugh's portraits of Dr. Samuel D. Gross (1874) and Mrs. Gross (1872).

   Two examples of husband and wife portraits painted by different artists are: Dr. Edward L. Bauer's (Cameron Burnside, 1945) and Mrs. Bauer's (M. Slesina, ca. 1982); and Percival E. Foerderer's (Sir Gerald F. Kelly, 1959) and Mrs. Foerderer's (Gerald L. Brockhurst, 1950).
8. Wagner, 615-16.
9. "Jefferson Pioneers Treatment to Recover Brain after Stroke," *Jefferson Medical College Alumni Bulletin* 44 (Sept. 1995): 17.
10. Mary Blitzer Field, "Medical Ethics," *Jefferson Medical College Alumni Bulletin* 36 (winter 1987): 7.
11. Cynthia J. T. Clendenin, "Tuning the Microcosm: Friends Honor a Microbiologist of Many Talents," *Jefferson Medical College Alumni Bulletin* 39 (summer 1990): 18.
12. "Profile," *Jefferson Medical College Alumni Bulletin* 33 (fall 1983): 7-8.

Opposite: *Athena/Minerva*

Nonmedical Art Objects

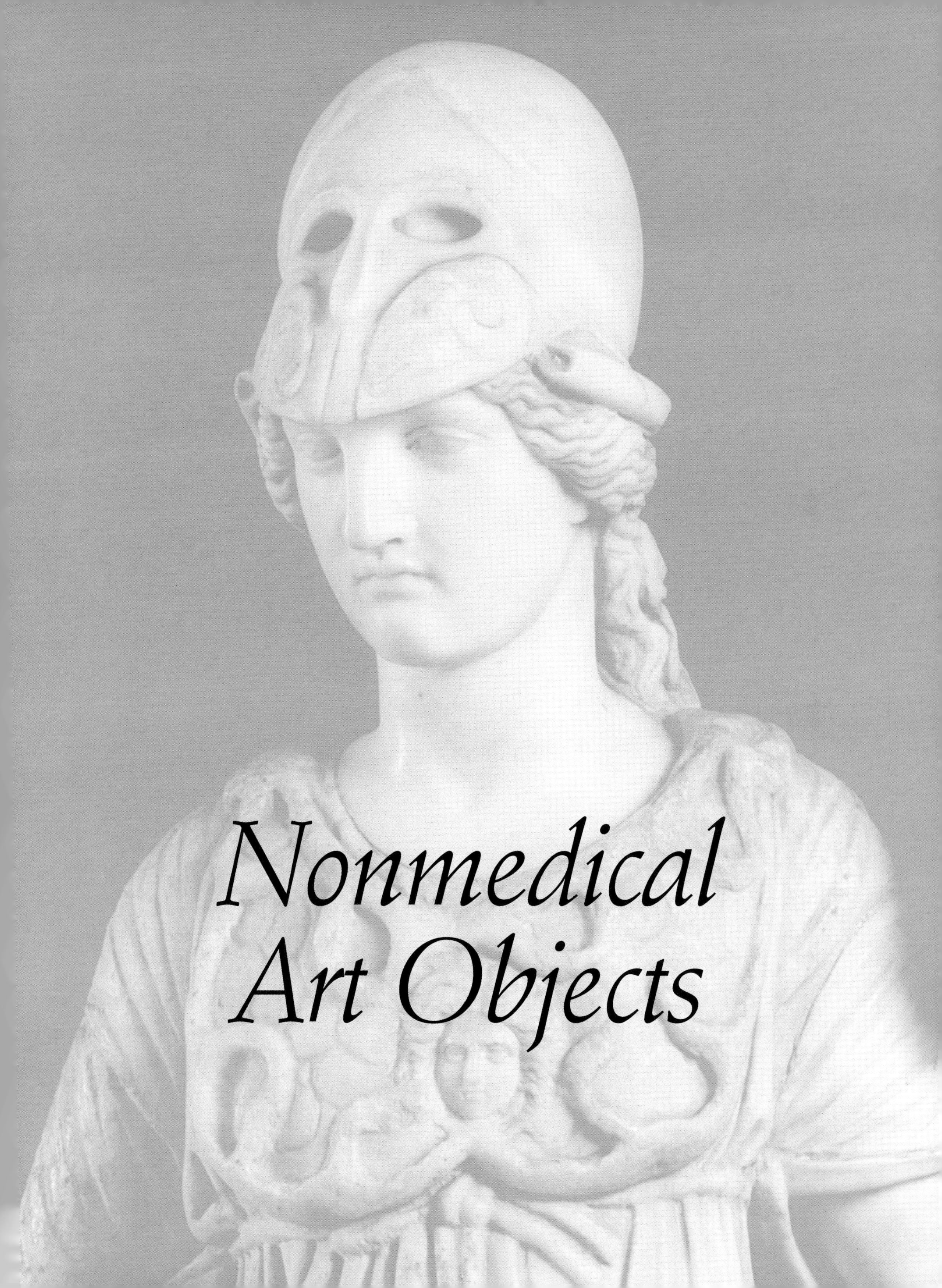

CHAPTER 11

Nonmedical Art Objects

The Thomas Jefferson University art collection includes several dozen objects not specifically related to its medical mission. Most of these art works, however, were donated by students, faculty, alumni, or trustees. Many have already been treated in the context of faculty portraits or architecture in the preceding chronological narrative, such as the statues of *Athena* and *Spinario*.

The most numerous category of nonmedical objects is portraits, and those of Thomas Jefferson predominate. The president's image is ubiquitous, especially a stylized profile head incorporated into the official logotype found on letterheads, signage, and advertising. The art collection has received three original sculptures and three replicas of paintings of Jefferson, as well as original prints and objects in other media. None of these images was created during the president's lifetime.

Thomas Jefferson as a Scientist

Thomas Jefferson had no role in the founding of Jefferson Medical College, though it bears his name, nor did he ever donate money, books, or other objects. As discussed above, the college awarded its first diplomas in 1826, two years after its charter had been granted as the Medical Department of Jefferson College in Canonsburg, Pennsylvania. Thomas Jefferson died in 1826.

However, the namesake proved to be an appropriate one, as Jefferson's activities in science, medicine, and medical education are well documented.[1] A man of the Enlightenment, he was well versed in science and experimentation and the classical world of antiquity. He contributed to the disciplines of botany, geology, agriculture, ethnology, chemistry, astronomy, meteorology, and paleontology, as well as architecture, landscape planning, and exploration. Concurrent with his term as the vice president of the United States he was president of the American Philosophical Society, the Philadelphia institution considered the headquarters of the Enlightenment in the United States.

Jefferson took a dim view of much contemporary unscientific medical therapy, believing instead that observation and experimentation are indispensable to any scientific inquiry and that any method of therapy should have practical or applied value. As an example, he supported and popularized vaccination in the United States after personally reviewing Edward Jenner's experimental and clinical data.

In 1779 he proposed and organized a medical curriculum at William and Mary College. Although this school was soon disbanded, in 1819 he established the state-supported University of Virginia at Charlottesville. Seeking the finest available physician to organize and implement a medical school there in 1825, Jefferson recruited Dr. Robley Dunglison of London as professor of anatomy and medicine. Now Jefferson could put into practice his principles concerning the training of physicians and the medical curriculum: that students should receive a thorough background of scientific medical knowledge before proceeding with clinical instruction.

Dr. Dunglison became the connecting link between President Thomas Jefferson and Jefferson Medical College. As discussed in chapter one, he was the president's personal physician and tended him during his final illness. Dunglison joined the faculty at Jefferson Medical College in 1836 and remained for the rest of his career.

Sculpted Portraits of Thomas Jefferson

Not surprisingly, Thomas Jefferson sat for life portraits by several notable sculptors and the renowned painters Charles Willson Peale, Gilbert Stuart, and Rembrandt Peale, among others. Another famous depiction of Jefferson is a profile watercolor and chalk drawing by Charles-Balthazar-Julien Fevret de Saint-Mémin, made with the help of a physiognatrace.[2]

The most enduring visual image of Thomas Jefferson and the most commonly used source for later portraits is the life portrait by the French sculptor Jean-Antoine Houdon (1741-1828). Houdon's marble bust was created in 1789, and a plaster version was exhibited at the Paris Salon that year.

Since 1934 the marble bust has been located at the Museum of Fine Arts, Boston. Two plaster replicas entered the collections of the American Philosophical Society in 1819 and the New York Historical Society in 1839. There were also contemporary commercial copies in *biscuit de Sèvres* by the Manufacture de Sèvres, as well as contemporary engraved replicas and copies in other media. Houdon's image of Jefferson has been on display in various media in public and private collections ever since its first appearance.

The marble surface of Houdon's sculpture is crisply carved, and the various textures of skin, hair, and costume are beautifully rendered. The subject is depicted bust length with his head turned slightly, and he gazes into the distance with a serious and thoughtful expression. His thick and wavy hair, deepset eyes, angular jaw, wide mouth, jutting chin, and long hair tied back in a bow have become familiar features over two centuries.

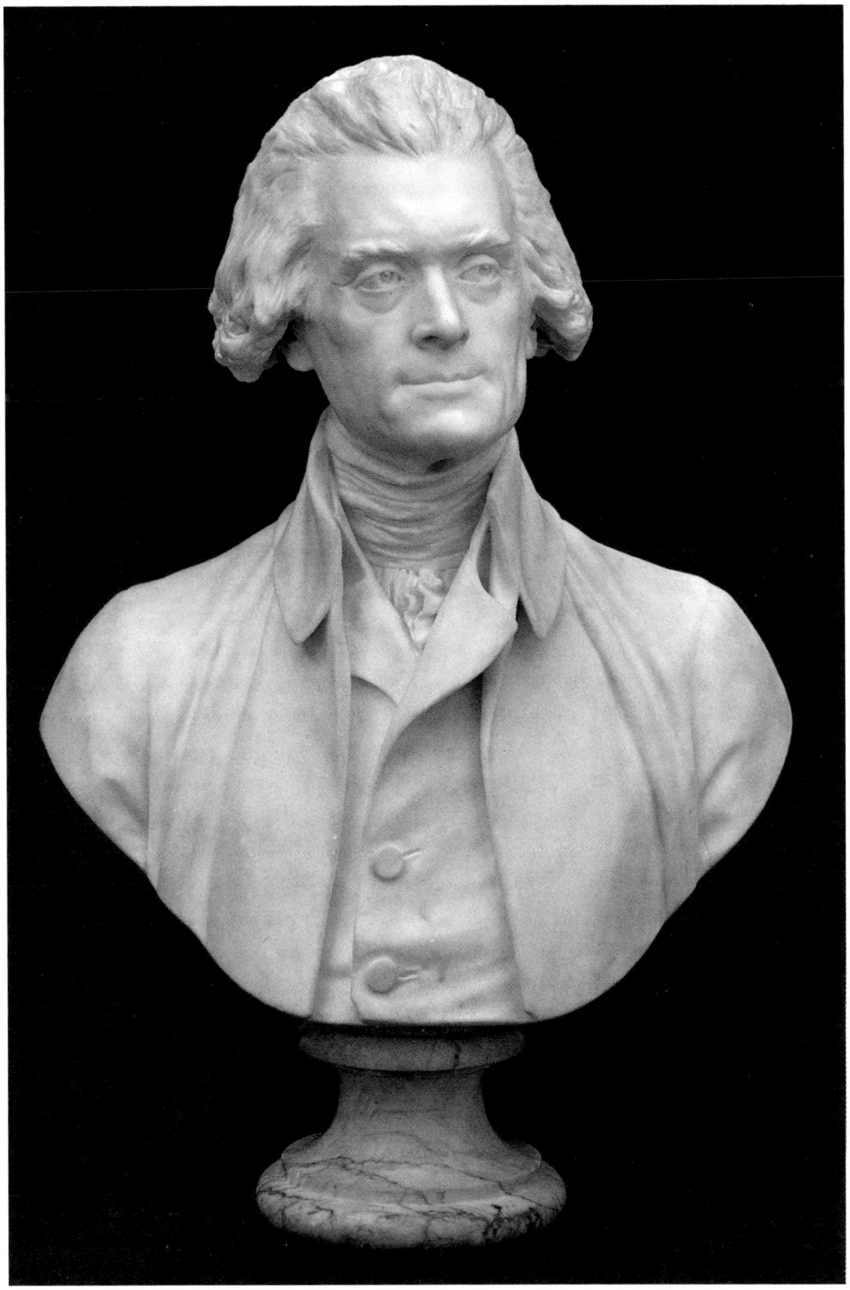

Portrait of Thomas Jefferson (1743-1826) by Jean-Antoine Houdon, marble, 1789, 27 1/5 x 19 1/5 x 10 2/5 in. (Museum of Fine Arts, Boston, George Nixon Black Fund, photograph by the museum)

Portrait of Thomas Jefferson

THOMAS JEFFERSON
By Lloyd Lillie (b. 1932)
Bronze

Cast 1987 after 1975 original
74 3/4 x 29 1/2 x 17 1/2 in.

Signed and dated top of base: "c LILLIE 1975/'87"

Given in 1987 by the Foundation of John P. McGovern, M.D.
Accession number: 1987+e.S.01

When Lloyd Lillie, a twentieth-century Boston sculptor, was commissioned to create a statue of Thomas Jefferson for the entrance to the Museum of Westward Expansion under the Gateway Arch in St. Louis in 1975, he researched Jefferson's life thoroughly and familiarized himself with all the extant sculptures and paintings of the president. He most admired the Houdon bust, because unlike many idealized neoclassical depictions, "it is a specific person."[3]

It was through his promotion of the Louisiana Purchase that the country acquired a large portion of its western lands. St. Louis, "the Gateway to the West," stands where the Missouri River empties into the Mississippi, so his image was a fitting choice for the museum there.

Lillie's bronze statue of Jefferson is full length and life-sized. The subject stands in an informal posture with weight on his left leg and left arm akimbo. His head is turned sharply, and he looks over his right shoulder with a thoughtful and optimistic expression. His long hair is tied back with a bow, and his familiar features include high cheekbones, square and jutting jaw, and large wideset eyes. His everyday apparel consists of a round-collared shirt and cravat, open jacket, breeches, long stockings, and buckled shoes.

The statue's integral base is only four inches high and there is no additional pedestal. The monument is meant to be seen at eye level, and evokes an approachable man of the people, not an aloof scholar or heroic public dignitary. The outdoor light bounces off the sculpture's rough-hewn texture and uneven surface and adds to the energy and animation of the portrayal.

Lillie said in a letter to the author that he depicted Jefferson at the time he assumed the presidency in 1801 and though it might be surprising that he looks so youthful at the age of fifty-eight, "rest assured that all the portraits done of him show that same quality" and "even his death mask portrays a man much younger than his eighty-three years."

Ironically, the attempt to place a commemorative statue of Thomas Jefferson on the Thomas Jefferson University campus provoked a tempest in a teapot. Because the university considered Thomas Jefferson a "man of vision" who symbolized its mission, and because the northeast corner of Eleventh and Walnut Streets was considered the "gateway" to its campus, it proposed to situate the statue of Jefferson in a mini-garden there in compliance with the One Percent Fine Arts Program for the Medical Office Building on the opposite corner.

However, the Fine Arts Committee of the Redevelopment Authority rejected the statue on the grounds that a commemorative portrait was "inappropriate" and "not in the true spirit of the program," and could lead to other such "advertising" portraits, e.g. portraits of Abraham Lincoln in front of every Lincoln National Bank. The controversy was widely reported locally and elsewhere, including the *Wall Street Journal* of January 28, 1987 which headlined an article, "What? A Thomas Jefferson Statue at Jefferson University? Absurd!"

The university used its own initiative to install a statue of Thomas Jefferson in another location. But Walter Erlebacher, the original choice for sculptor, had withdrawn from the project in frustration over interminable delays in the negotiations. Then the university learned that Lloyd Lillie had made a cast of his Jefferson statue for the University of Virginia in 1978. It was most gratifying that he agreed to authorize a second and final cast of his famous work for Thomas Jefferson University in 1987.

The project was underwritten by the Foundation of John P. McGovern, M.D., a professor, researcher, and director of an allergy clinic in Houston. Also a medical historian, McGovern became acquainted with Thomas Jefferson University through Dr. Frederick B. Wagner Jr.

Next to Alexander Calder's statue of Dr. Samuel D. Gross, Lillie's sculpture of Thomas Jefferson is the most important memorial statue in the university's collection. It is located in a brick niche in the west atrium of Jefferson Alumni Hall. In recognition of its symbolic value, a small replica of the sculpture is now given to the annual recipient of the Jefferson Cornerstone Award.

Lloyd Lillie was born in Washington, D.C. in 1932. He studied at the Corcoran School of Art in Washington where he won the first prize in drawing in 1956, and at the Skowhegan School of Painting and Sculpture in Maine where he twice won the purchase prize in sculpture. In 1959 he graduated from the School of the Boston Museum of Fine Arts where he won the Boit Prize in sculpture and the Clarissa Bartlett traveling

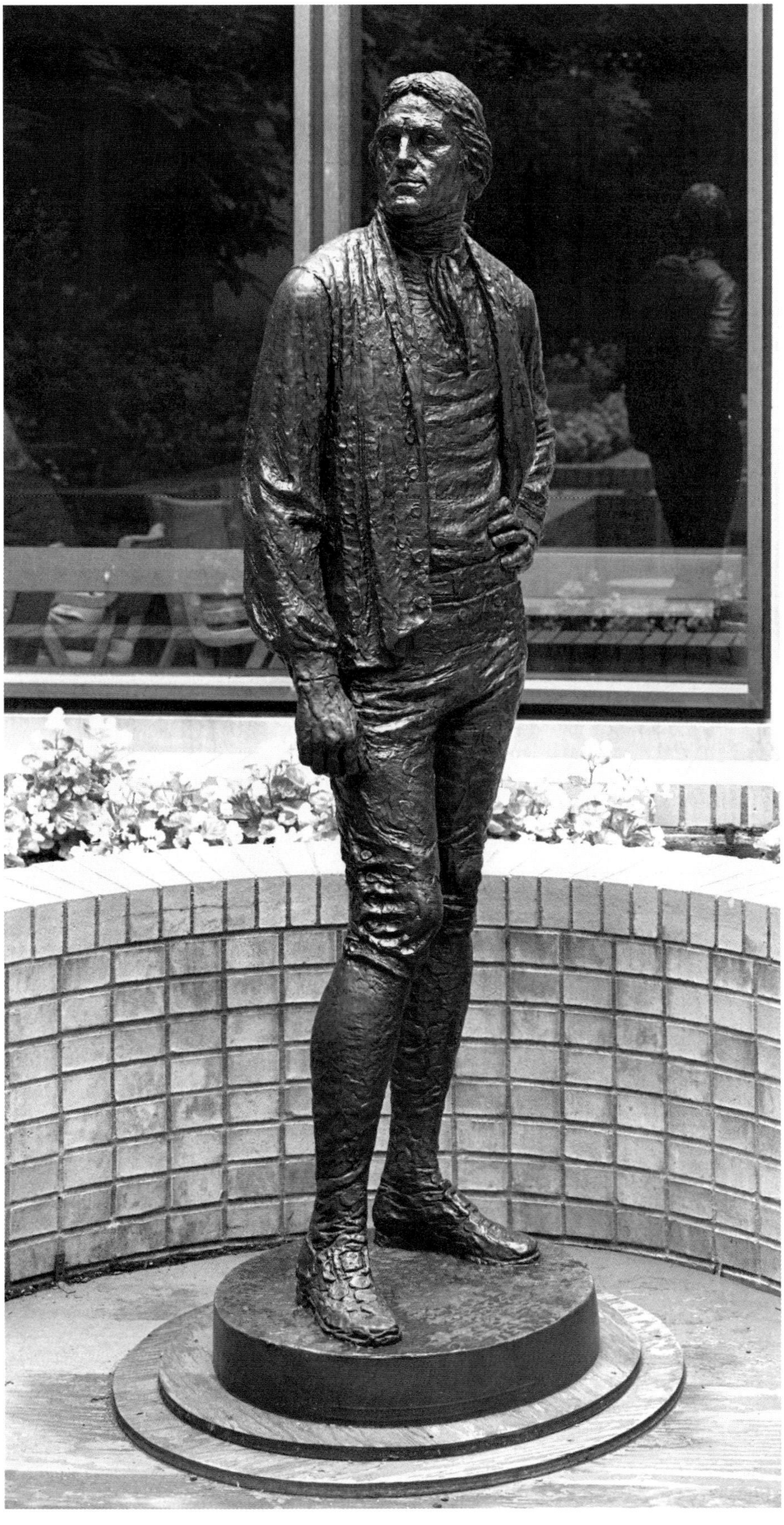

scholarship. He studied abroad at the Accademia di Belle Arti in Florence the following year. His statue of Thomas Jefferson, with its "hip-shot" pose, arm at the ready, very large hands, and searching gaze, recalls Michelangelo's statue of David at the Accademia, also a symbol of liberty.

Lillie has been a member of the sculpture faculty at Boston University since 1961 and was made full professor in 1974. He has exhibited widely and received numerous one-man shows throughout the Massachusetts area. He won the first prize in sculpture at the 1963 Boston Arts Festival and the Governor's Design Awards for Curley Park in Boston in 1986. He is represented in the collections of American embassies in North Yemen and Saudi Arabia.

Among Lillie's public commissions are designs for a medal for the Boston University Centennial Celebration and the NBA Coach of the Year Award, three *Seafarers* for the James Center in Richmond, and a relief sculpture for the Russian Bishop's House at the National Park Service in Anchorage. Some notable portrait subjects include Andrew Carnegie and Joseph Pulitzer for the American Museum of Immigration in New York, Booker T. Washington for his birthplace in Hardy, Virginia, Mayor James M. Curley for Boston, and Mayor Thomas D'Alesandro Jr. for Baltimore.

Portrait of Thomas Jefferson

THOMAS JEFFERSON
H. Daniel Webster (1880-1912)

Bronze
1907
19 3/4 x 15 x 11 in.

Signed and dated under right shoulder: "1907/H. DAN. WEBSTER/COPYRIGHT 1907 SC." Inscriptions: "JEFFERSON" on center of integral base; "First bust cast from Artist's Model/For/Jefferson Medical College/Philadelphia, Penn/A gift in memory of/Abraham Coles, A.M., M.D., Ph.D., LL.D./Class of 1835/from his son/J. Ackerman Coles, A.B., A.M., M.D., LL.D." on front of pedestal; "TIFFANY & CO." on side of pedestal

Given between 1907 and 1920 by J. Ackerman Coles, M.D. in memory of his father, Abraham Coles, M.D. (JMC 1835)
Accession number: 1907-1920.S.01

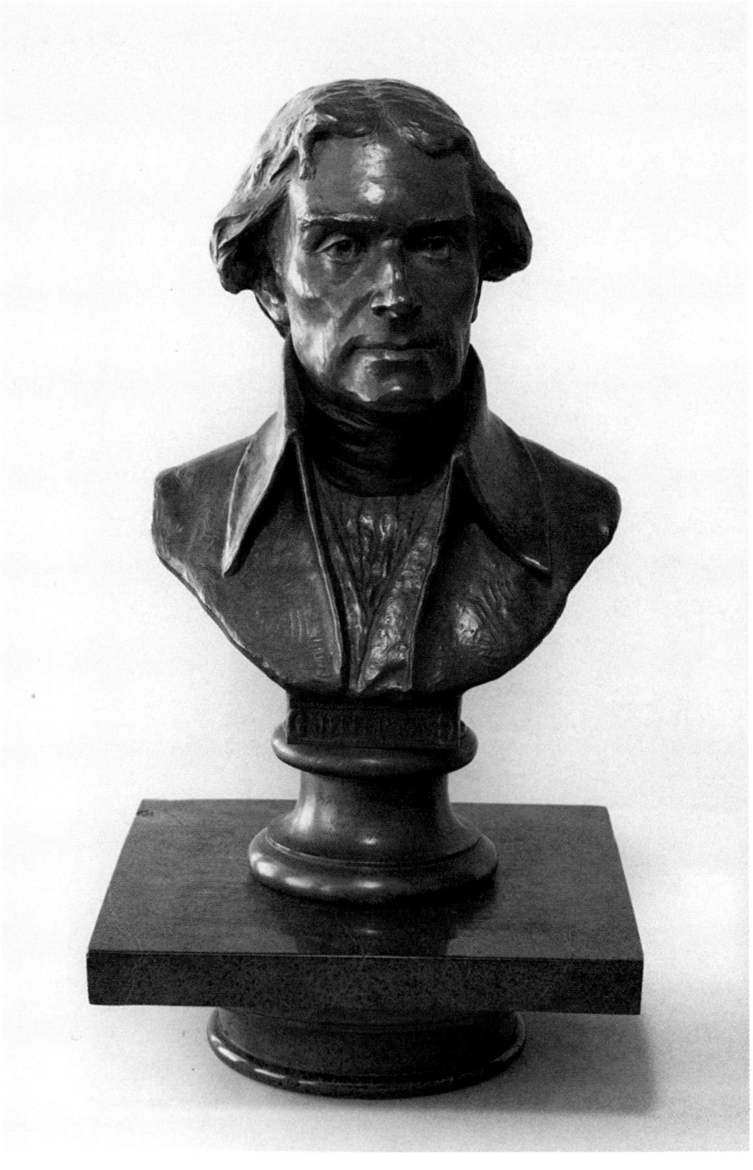

The earliest sculpture of Thomas Jefferson in the university's collection is a bronze bust carved by H. Daniel Webster in 1907. It was given by Dr. J. Ackerman Coles in memory of his father, Dr. Abraham Coles, an alumnus in the class of 1835, but the donation date was unrecorded. A period photograph by William H. Rau documents that it was at Jefferson by 1920.

The facial features in Webster's sculpture clearly derive from Houdon's depiction, although the hairstyle is adapted from a different source. In Webster's hands the carving is less incisive, the features more generalized, and the expression more neutral than in Houdon's portrait.

H. Daniel Webster was born in Frankville, Iowa in 1880 and studied at the Art Students League in New York. He is represented by a bronze *Minute Man* in Saugatuck, Connecticut, a marble statue of General W. H. Beadle in the State Capitol at Pierre, South Dakota, and bronze doors for the American National Bank Building in Austin, Texas.

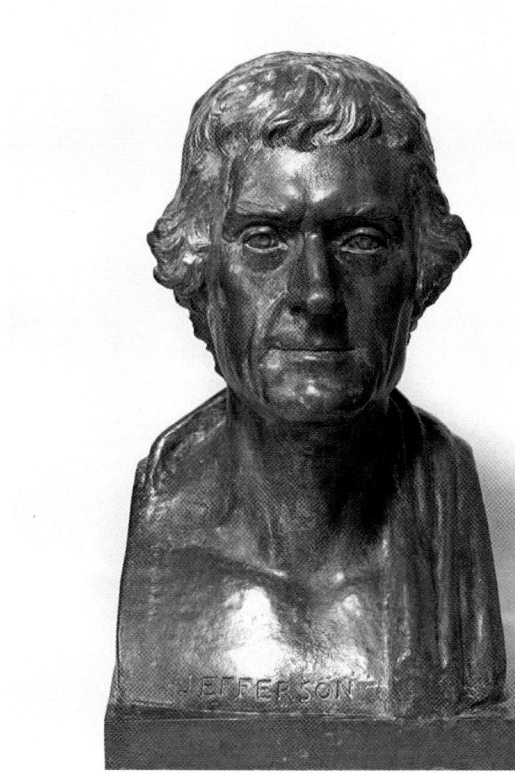

Portrait of Thomas Jefferson

THOMAS JEFFERSON
By Rudulph Evans (1878-1960)

Bronze
Cast in 1974 after original dated late 1930s-early 1940s
23 1/2 x 14 x 15 in.

Signed on side of right shoulder: "R/EVANS"
Inscription: "JEFFERSON" on bottom of chest

Given in 1974 by William W. Bodine Jr., TJU board chairman, and Mrs. Bodine; they purchased it from John F. Platt, grandson of the sculptor
Accession number: 1974+e.S.01

The sesquicentennial celebration of Jefferson Medical College and attendant fund-raising activities in 1974 provided the impetus for acquiring a third sculpture of Thomas Jefferson. The bronze bust was a donation from William W. Bodine Jr. who served as president and chairman of the board of Thomas Jefferson University.

The provenance of the piece is directly associated with one of the most heroic and familiar commemorative sculptures in America created by internationally renowned sculptor Rudulph Evans. He had been commissioned to create a statue of Thomas Jefferson to stand under the domed ceiling of the Jefferson Memorial on the east bank of the Tidal Basin in Washington, D.C. A plaster model of the nineteen-foot statue was dedicated by President Franklin D. Roosevelt on April 13, 1943, the two-hundredth anniversary of Jefferson's birth. That plaster original was replaced by the permanent bronze work in 1947.

In 1973 John F. Platt, a grandson of Rudulph Evans

and a suburban Philadelphia interior designer, offered Thomas Jefferson University a bust of Thomas Jefferson, one of two preparatory clay studies for the monument in Washington that the sculptor had been made in the late 1930s or early 1940s. When agreement was reached Mr. Platt arranged to have the original clay study cast into bronze. Among the attendees at the dedication of the Rudulph Evans bust of Jefferson at the university in June 1975 were John Platt and his wife, and Platt's mother, Mrs. Joseph B. Platt, daughter of the sculptor. She was especially pleased to see the first Evans sculpture placed in a Philadelphia building.

John Platt said that he had posed for the original statue in the Jefferson Memorial because of his similarity in height and build to the president. The larger than life-sized bust by Evans slightly exaggerates the subject's familiar visage with his thick, curly hair and chiseled features, but approximates the appearance of the Houdon version. The intensity of Jefferson's riveting gaze and tightly pursed lips is matched by the strength of his thick neck and muscular chest. Folds of classical drapery flow behind his neck and over his left shoulder, adding curved forms to the flicker of light over the sculpture's lively surface.

Rudulph Evans was born in 1878 in Washington, D.C., to a family descended from Colonial Virginia and Pennsylvania forbears, and he spent his boyhood in Warren County, Virginia. He began his sculpture studies at the Corcoran School of Art in Washington, and then briefly at the Art Students League in New York. He went to Paris in 1897 for further study at the Académie Julian, the École des Beaux-Arts, and privately with Auguste Rodin.

Evans established a successful career in Europe where he was best known for his classical nudes. After his *Golden Hour* won a bronze medal at the Paris Salon of 1914 the sculptor was entertained by the president of France, and the work was purchased by the French government for the Luxembourg Museum. Later the French made him a chevalier of the Legion of Honor. When his *Eve's Daughter* was exhibited in Rome he received felicitations from King Victor Emmanuel of Italy, and was subsequently decorated with the Order of the Crown of Italy.

Evans maintained studios abroad and in New York and Washington, and exhibited his work in many leading cities on both sides of the Atlantic. He was an academician of the National Academy of Design, an honorable fellow of the National Sculpture Society, and a member of the National Institute of Arts and Letters. He won the Elizabeth N. Watrous Gold Medal at the National Academy of Design in 1919.

Rudulph Evans is best known in this country for portrait busts and commemorative monuments. Among his other public works in Washington are the portraits of General Simón Bolívar dedicated by President Taft at the Bureau of American Republics, and William Jennings Bryan commissioned by the State of Nebraska for the U.S. Capitol. He created portraits of John Greenleaf Whittier, Henry Wadsworth Longfellow, Grover Cleveland, and Bernard Baruch for the Hall of Fame in New York, General Robert E. Lee for the Capitol at Richmond, as well as *Maiden with Swans* for a fountain at the home of John D. Rockefeller in Pocantico Hills, New York.

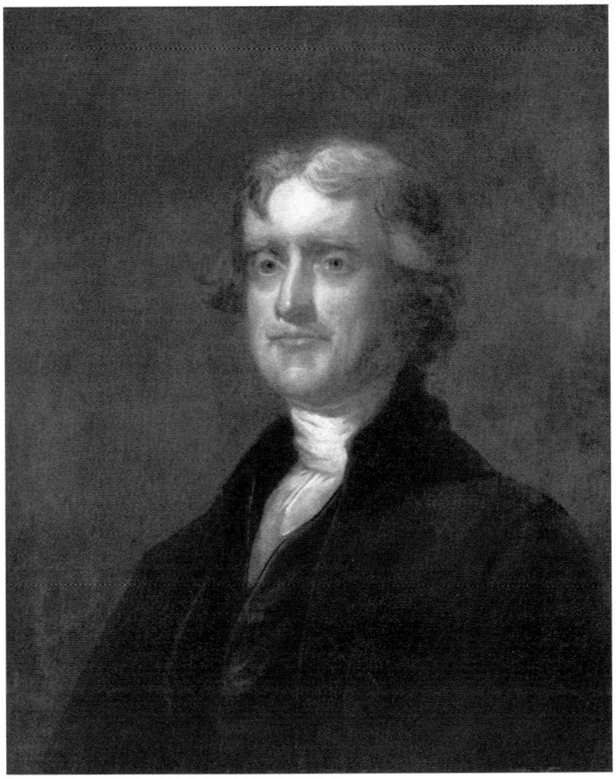

Portrait of Thomas Jefferson

THOMAS JEFFERSON
By unknown artist, after Gilbert Stuart (1755-1828)

Oil on canvas
1848-70
30 1/4 x 25 1/4 in.

Given in 1932 by Natalie Snyder of Canonsburg, Pennsylvania, whose family had received it from the Memorial Hall Committee of Jefferson College
Accession number: 1932+e.P.02

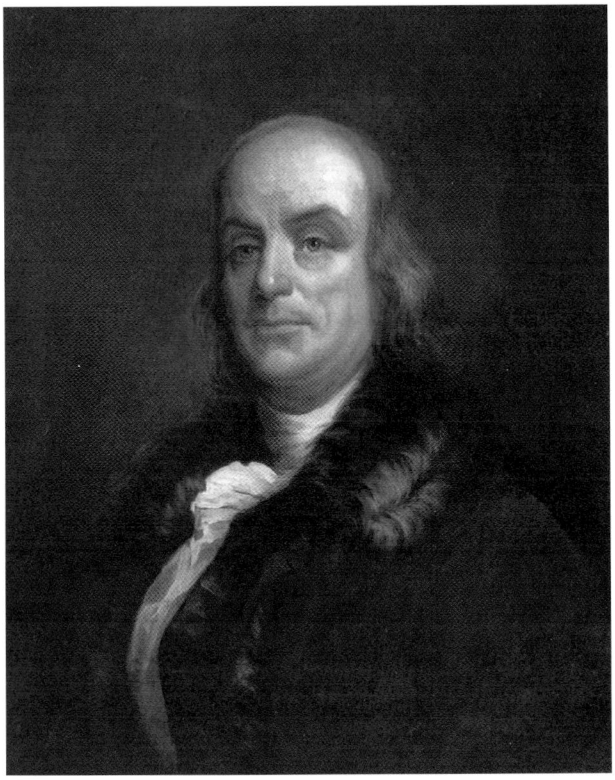

Portrait of Benjamin Franklin

BENJAMIN FRANKLIN (1706-90)
By unknown artist, after Joseph Siffred Duplessis (1751-1831)

Oil on canvas
1848-70
30 1/4 x 25 1/4

Given in 1932 by Natalie Snyder of Canonsburg, Pennsylvania, whose family had received it from the Memorial Hall Committee of Jefferson College
Accession number: 1932+e.P.01

In 1932 the art collection acquired portraits of Thomas Jefferson and Benjamin Franklin that shared a mysterious history. The convoluted provenance of the related portraits harkens back to Jefferson College.

Benjamin Franklin, like Thomas Jefferson, had almost unlimited curiosity and knowledge about the natural world. He, too, made significant contributions to science, medicine, and education. Although Franklin was not the first to conclude that lightning was an electrical phenomenon, in 1751 he was the first to publish experimental proof of the phenomenon. His interest in meteorology led him to the discovery that summer northeast storms on the eastern seaboard begin first in the southwest. Among his inventions were the Pennsylvania Fireplace (later known as the Franklin Stove), the whale oil candle, and the ventilated street lamp.[4]

In 1727 Franklin formed a group of his colleagues into the Junto, a "club for mutual improvement," out of whose efforts grew a number of public institutions. The first was Philadelphia's public library, followed by the City Watch, a local fire brigade, the American Philosophical Society, the Academy (from which rose the University of Pennsylvania), and a city hospital (Pennsylvania Hospital).

Imagine my excitement, shortly after assuming my position at Thomas Jefferson University, upon learning that the art collection included portraits of Benjamin Franklin and Thomas Jefferson donated by the illustrious subjects themselves. Imagine my perplexity, upon first viewing the paintings, that they appeared mid-nineteenth-century stylistically, yet Franklin had died in 1790 and Jefferson in 1826.[5]

My research on the paintings was launched by reading the article "Jefferson Portraits: History and Enigma" by J. Douglas Corwin, M.D. (JMC 1935) and his son James H. Corwin II, M.D. (JMC 1956) in the *Jefferson Medical College Alumni Bulletin* of winter 1974. The Drs. Corwin began by tracing the early history of Jefferson College. Because of "dire financial straits" Jefferson College in Canonsburg, Pennsylvania merged with Washington College in Washington, Pennsylvania in 1865. When two separate campuses proved impractical the institutions consolidated, and Washington and Jefferson College removed to Washington in 1869.

As the basis for the early history of the Franklin and Jefferson portraits, the Drs. Corwin turned to Helen Turnbull Waite Coleman's *Banners in the Wilderness: Early Years of Washington and Jefferson College* (1956), the main source on this topic. She wrote that Thomas Jefferson sent his portrait and some books to Jefferson College around 1802. She also said that "there is a tradition" that Benjamin Franklin also sent books together with his portrait around 1790.

Nothing in the art historical literature substantiates Coleman's claim that either Franklin or Jefferson donated an original portrait or a copy to Jefferson College or that either one even owned an oil copy by any artist. Historians of American art recognize immediately that both paintings in Thomas Jefferson University's collection are copies after celebrated portraits, and realize the artist could have been familiar with the originals from numerous painted and engraved copies.

The original source for the Jefferson copy is a portrait by Gilbert Stuart painted in 1805 (the "Edgehill Portrait" now owned jointly by the National Portrait Gallery and Monticello), so obviously the President could not have donated a copy in 1802; he did not even receive the original until 1821. The original Franklin portrait was painted in Paris in 1778 by French artist Joseph Siffred Duplessis, and it was owned by French aristocrats and never by Franklin himself. It was purchased in 1919 by an American who left it by bequest to the Metropolitan Museum of Art in 1931. Furthermore, the university's portrait of Franklin is in reverse, suggesting a copy from an engraving of the original, such as the 1778 print by Juste Chevillet (1729-90).[6]

Both portraits in the Jefferson collection are bust length and slightly larger than life-sized. The figures are turned slightly to the left and gaze out toward the observer. Benjamin Franklin's brown coat is notable for its fur collar. Thomas Jefferson wears a black coat with standup lapels. Neither portrait retains the exact dimensions of its original source. An early description of the Franklin portrait mentions his plum-colored coat. Both paintings have had extensive overpainting in the backgrounds and blotchy repair in the faces and costumes, so the original color might have been changed or else deteriorated.

Helen Coleman asserts that the Jefferson and Franklin portraits hung at Jefferson College until 1865. Because of a "civil disturbance" by citizens of Canonsburg when their cherished college left town, the portraits were removed and "stored in the attic of the old Roberts house on Central Avenue in Canonsburg from the time of the Union...until the 1930s."

Enter James H. Corwin, M.D., a Jefferson alumnus of 1903 and father and grandfather of the authors of the *Bulletin* article. He was a practitioner in Washington, Pennsylvania and a history buff. The article says that after hearing rumors that the two portraits were still extant in 1925, Dr. James H. Corwin finally traced them to the home of Natalie Snyder, an elderly spinster. After unsuccessful early attempts to secure these works for Jefferson Medical College, he enlisted the aid of Ross V.

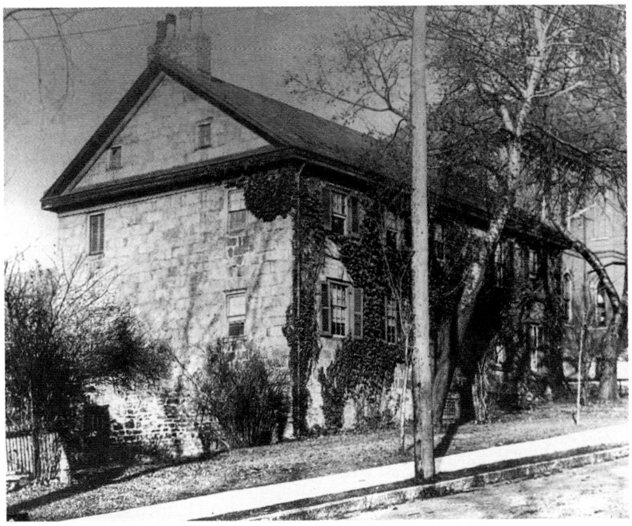

The House of Natalie Snyder, Canonsburg, Pennsylvania

Patterson, M.D., Jefferson's dean.

By 1929-30 Drs. Corwin and Patterson were competing for the art works with the President of Washington and Jefferson College who wanted to obtain the works for *his* institution. Finally Miss Snyder responded favorably to the gentler and more persuasive appeals of the Jefferson Medical College petitioners. By 1932 the portraits had been restored, framed, and relocated to the Jefferson Medical College's library in Philadelphia.

To prove my supposition that the portraits could not have been painted before the mid-nineteenth century, I pursued technical analysis with the assistance of several specialists.

The painting conservator at the Pennsylvania Academy of the Fine Arts, Mark Bockrath, determined that the commercial, linen twill canvas and wooden stretcher supports were of the same type on both paintings and were consistent with nineteenth-century artistic practice. Ultraviolet and infrared examination failed to reveal any hidden artist's signature. This is consistent with the custom that copyists seldom sign their works.

Stylistic similarities led Bockrath to conclude that both paintings were made by the same copyist at approximately the same time: the palette is identical, especially the use of broken oranges and deep transparent reds; the flesh tones have the same shadows and highlights, with the same juxtaposition of pinks and grays; the eyes are constructed similarly, especially the heavy upper lids and circular lower lids; the hair is thinly painted, with a minimum of strokes and some scratching out; a thin, umber tone underlays both figures; and the white neck linen is similarly painted and highlighted.

Bockrath agreed with my opinion that Helen Coleman's assertions about the dates were much too early. He suggested a mid-nineteenth-century range.

A prior conservator at the Pennsylvania Academy, Joseph Amarotico, had relined these portraits in 1982, so the backs of the canvases could not be examined for clues. Fortunately, his photographs of the backs of both original canvases yielded an important finding: each had an identical stencil insignia. Though very faint, the logo showed the name and part of the address of a "colourman," G. Rowney and Company of London, a manufacturer who prepared canvases for sale at art supply shops.

I located an English scholar of nineteenth-century art materials who compared our stencil with various other Rowney and Company samples. She determined by the precise wording of the firm's name and the street location that our canvases could not have been manufactured before 1848. Since the company also exported its wares to America, the origin of the canvas is not a significant factor in identifying the artist.

In August 1989 I visited Washington and Canonsburg, Pennsylvania and consulted with Douglas T. Corwin, M.D., a Jefferson alumnus of 1959, and a resident of Washington. He is the son of Dr. James Douglas Corwin, brother of Dr. James H. Corwin II, and father of Dr. Douglas T. Corwin Jr. of the class of 1993.

Dr. and Mrs. Corwin drove me to the Washington and Jefferson College campus where I discovered in the archives several early manuscript versions of Coleman's history of Jefferson College. The first version was considerably less dogmatic than the final book, saying, "We have no documented account of Jefferson's gifts [his portrait and books], but the legend has always persisted at Canonsburg." She also wrote, "Franklin died in 1790. The future academy at Canonsburg was not even dedicated until July, 1791,—but somehow we had the portrait."

Dr. Corwin kindly referred me to James T. Herron, V.M.D., a Canonsburg veterinarian and leading member of the Jefferson College Historical Society. He explained that rivalry between the towns of Canonsburg and Washington was so intense that the merger was fought all the way to the United States Supreme Court. In 1869 the court ruled the union complete and that all property of Jefferson College should be transferred to Washington and Jefferson College.

Dr. Herron provided me with newspaper reports about some indignant Canonsburg citizens who had taken matters into their own hands around 1869 and "rescued" a collection of books and furnishings. Initially Dr. Herron speculated that the portraits of Jefferson and Franklin must have been included in this cache, although not specifically mentioned. These items had belonged to the Franklin Literary Society at Jefferson College, a group chartered in 1848 and incorporated separately from the college, with its own quarters in Memorial Hall.

There is a primary source that supports this theory, at least in part. In the Washington and Jefferson archives is a diary of one Boyd Crumrine, written in 1861 when he was a student at Jefferson College. In describing the quarters of the Franklin Literary Society, he singles out a Brussels carpet, elegant armchairs, damask curtains, wallpaper with full-sized statues of the Muses, a clock, chandelier, and finally, "a fine large oil painting of Franklin over the head of the President, and another similar one of Jefferson at his right hand."

But recently Dr. Herron discovered an article from the *Canonsburg Notes* of 1894 or 1895. It says, "There is yet in the college building a very fine painting of Thomas Jefferson, presented by him to the college after the charter was secured and the college named after him, and also one of Benjamin Franklin, which for years hung on the walls of the Franklin Literary Society."

The article in *Canonsburg Notes* is referring to the work of the Jefferson Memorial Hall Committee formed in the 1890s by alumni to house the relics of the Franklin Literary Society rooms. (This committee was succeeded by the Jefferson College Historical Society which in 1974 utilized much of the old woodwork, fixtures, books, and other historical materials to recreate the Franklin Society's rooms in another location.)

To date historians have *assumed* that the portraits received from Natalie Snyder are the same as those referred to in the Coleman book, the Crumrine diary, and the newspaper article. Technical research has shown that our portraits cannot possibly be as described in the Coleman book. Unless new documentation appears, we will never know if there ever were such paintings, now lost, or if these are copies of such paintings.

Possibly the two portraits were commissioned by, or donated to, the Franklin Literary Society between 1848 and 1869 and are those mentioned in the Crumrine diary, and spirited to the home of Jefferson College professor Henry Snyder in 1869. Or possibly the portraits stayed intact with the library and furnishings of the Literary Society until the 1890s when the Jefferson Memorial Hall Committee was formed, and then came under the protection of the professor's daughter, Natalie Snyder, a committee member. Less likely is the possibility that they actually stayed in the committee's museum until the property was taken over by the local school district in 1912 and went to the Snyder home then.

Yet another scenario is suggested by the *Canonsburg Rural Notes* of July 7, 1881 reporting that in 1869 "unlawful piracy" included capturing such items as books, furniture, statuary, bronzes, medals, ornaments, carpets and "numerous other things." Perhaps a private citizen stole the paintings and subsequently sold or returned them. A final possibility is that Jefferson College owned more than one set of portraits of the Founding Fathers, not uncommon for public institutions.

All we know for sure is that our portraits were created after 1848, and that Drs. Corwin and Patterson received them in 1932 from Natalie Snyder. Unless new documentation surfaces, we will probably never know the true story. The portraits were installed in 1932 in the main reading room of the Jefferson Medical College library. In recent years they have hung in the university president's office.

Several decades later the art collection received replicas of two other painted portraits of Thomas Jefferson. In 1969 Katherine S. Ferg was commissioned by Thomas Jefferson University to copy the Charles Willson Peale portrait of 1791 (owned by Independence National Historical Park). In 1978 Molly Guion donated her copy of Rembrandt Peale's portrait of 1805 (New York Historical Society).

Indian Peace Medal of Thomas Jefferson

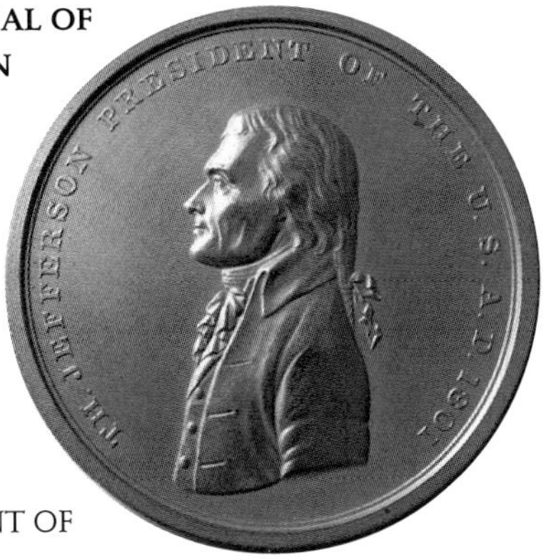

INDIAN PEACE MEDAL OF THOMAS JEFFERSON (OBVERSE)
Designed by John Reich (1768-1833)

Copper
Reissue of 1801 original
3 in. diameter

Inscription: "TH. JEFFERSON PRESIDENT OF THE U.S. A.D. 1801"

Given after 1900 by unknown donor
Accession number: 1900+f.M.01

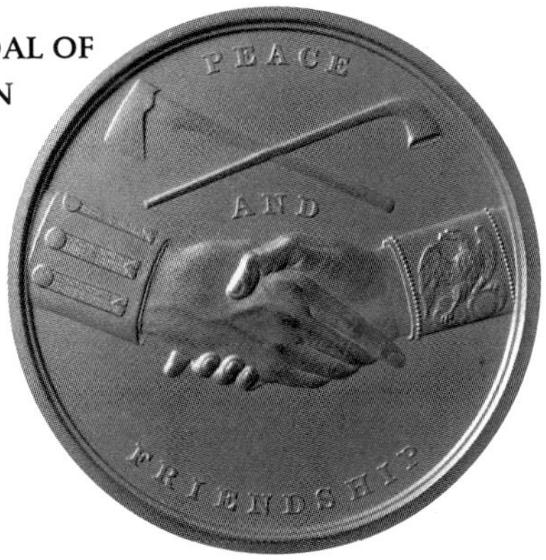

INDIAN PEACE MEDAL OF THOMAS JEFFERSON (REVERSE)

Inscription: "PEACE/AND/FRIENDSHIP"

The Indian peace medal originated as a prerevolutionary token presented by British, French, and Spanish governments to friendly Indian chiefs.[7] The medals bore the monarch's portrait on one side and his coat of arms on the other, and were used to help establish authority over the tribes and to symbolize friendship between the Europeans and the Native Americans. They were highly prized as status symbols, both for their decorative qualities and for the honor of possessing a likeness of the Great White Father.

After the war the new Federal government found it necessary to continue the practice, and began to produce new Indian peace medals as an integral feature of Indian policy, especially with regard to the government's claim of legal right to its western territories. Large numbers of the medals were distributed by military officers and Indian commissioners at the signing of treaties and visits of important chiefs to the national capital. They were also distributed by Indian agents to their charges on the frontier. Meriwether Lewis and William Clark took a supply of medals on their expedition to the Pacific, and handed them out to selected chiefs and warriors during impressive ceremonies.

The Indian peace medals were first regularized during the Jefferson administration and were created by the United States Mint in Philadelphia in 1801. They were struck in copper, pewter, and silver in diameters of two, three, and four inches. (The medals of George Washington and John Adams were issued later to complete the presidential series.)

The Indian peace medal bearing the profile of Thomas Jefferson on the obverse was the first to show a current American president in the tradition of European monarchs. Instead of a royal coat of arms, the reverse shows two hands clasped in amity, confirmed by the inscription "Peace and Friendship." The braided cuff of an American military uniform on the left has three stripes and buttons, and the wrist on the right shows a wide band ornamented with an eagle, a type worn by Indian chiefs. A peace pipe crossed with a tomahawk above the hands completes the design.

The source for the medal's profile head of Thomas Jefferson is the sculpture by Houdon. Most scholars agree that the medal was designed by John Reich, a German engraver born in Bavaria in 1768. He settled in Philadelphia in 1800 hoping for gainful employment, and was frequently employed by Robert Scot, chief engraver at the U.S. Mint. John Reich is also credited with designing Jefferson's inaugural medal in 1802. He was a founder of the Society of Artists organized in Philadelphia in 1810. Reich worked in Philadelphia until about 1813, and died in Albany, New York in 1833.

Judging from the pristine condition of the medal at Thomas Jefferson University, it is in all probability a later reissue. The Indian peace medal of 1801 was the basis for the representation of Thomas Jefferson on the American nickel first issued in 1938.

Portrait of Thomas Jefferson

THOMAS JEFFERSON
By Albert Rosenthal (1863-1939)

Lithograph
1921
Image size: 23 1/2 x 17 1/2 in.
Sheet size: 27 1/2 x 21 1/2 in.

Signed and dated center right: "Albert Rosenthal Litho/after Terra Cotta by Houdon/Copyright, 1921"
Facsimile signature below image
Inscription in pencil lower right: "To my Friend Isaac Hayes[?]/from Albert Rosenthal/Compliments and Regards/July 4, 1931[?]"

Given in 1972 by Mrs. Michael Foley, past president of TJU Hospital women's board
Accession number: 1972+e.Pr.01

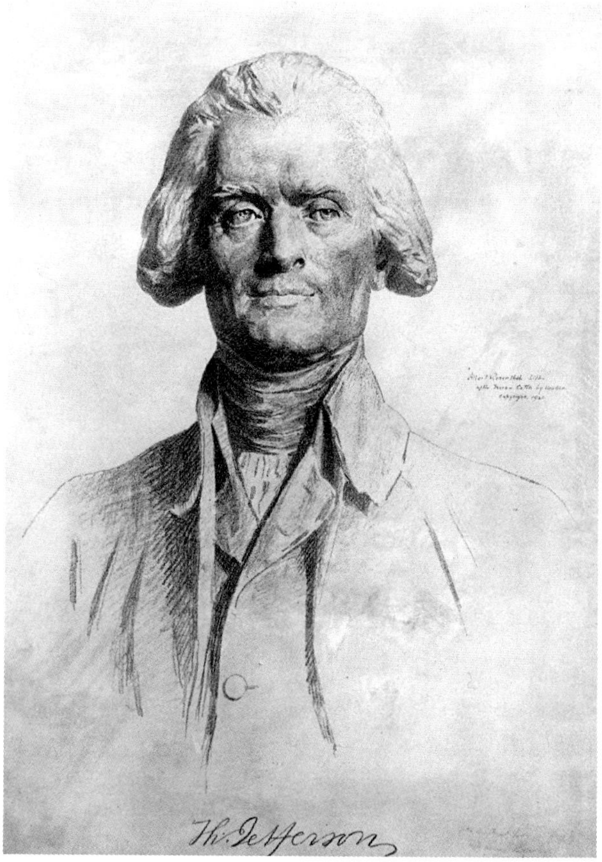

A lithographic portrait of Thomas Jefferson was created by Albert Rosenthal in 1921, and the artist stated on the print that Houdon's terra cotta (plaster?) bust was his direct source. An inscription in pencil below the image (significantly dated July 4, 1931) sends Rosenthal's compliments and regards to a friend.

Albert Rosenthal's skilled draftsmanship has produced a subtle, three dimensional, illusionistic head on the flat surface of the paper. Jefferson's face sparkles with contrasts of light and shade, as though reproducing the effects of light on Houdon's original work. The Jefferson collection includes an identical Rosenthal lithograph of Jefferson inscribed to J. Walter Rosenberg and dated May 29, 1928.

Albert Rosenthal was a painter, etcher, and lithographer born in Philadelphia in 1863. His first teacher was his father, Max Rosenthal, a Polish immigrant and noted mezzotint portrait artist. The son continued his studies at the Pennsylvania Academy of the Fine Arts, and then abroad at the École des Beaux-Arts in Paris and also in Munich. Upon his return to Philadelphia he established a career in portraiture.

Albert Rosenthal collaborated with his father on a series of five hundred portraits of prominent early Americans in etchings, mezzotints, and lithographs. Among the younger Rosenthal's national awards were bronze medals at the St. Louis Exposition in 1904 and the Panama-Pacific Exposition in San Francisco in 1915. He is represented by portraits in numerous private collections and museums throughout the country.

The art collection also received an engraved portrait of Thomas Jefferson by Alfred Bryan Hall made in 1887. Hall's print is one of the few known reproductions of a lost portrait of Jefferson made by Mather Brown in 1786.

Jefferson Medical College Plaque

JEFFERSON MEDICAL COLLEGE PLAQUE
By unknown artist

Plaster
1903
14 in. diameter

Inscription: "JEFFERSON MEDICAL COLLEGE OF PHILADELPHIA/FOUNDED 1826"
Inscription on beveled edge of costume: "COPYRIGHT 1903"

Probably commissioned in 1903 by JMC
Accession number: 1903+e.S.01

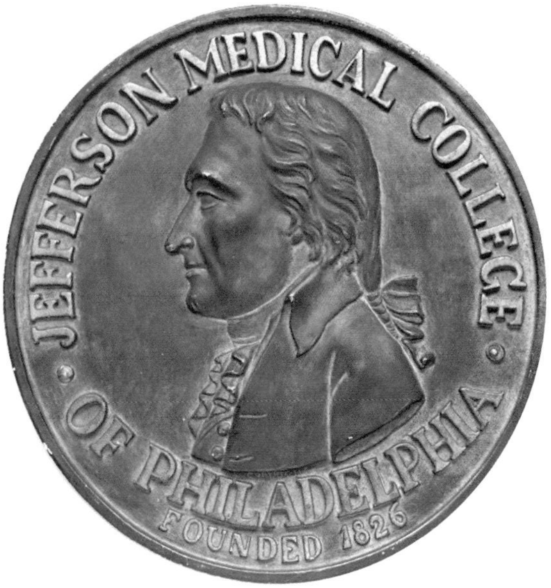

The portrait of Thomas Jefferson on a plaster medallic plaque ordered by the college in 1903 ultimately derives from Houdon's elegant marble bust of Thomas Jefferson, by way of the Indian peace medal. The plaque is the earliest nonarchitectural artifact yet found of the Jefferson head as an institutional symbol. A photograph in the archival collection shows the plaque hanging in an administrator's office in the 1898 College Building (replaced in 1931 by the Curtis Building).

However, the Jefferson portrait on the plaque shows a reduction in style and understanding of the earlier sculpture and medal. The large lettering of the plaque crowds the image. The subject looks humble rather than confident because of the downward tilt of his head and the shallow relief carving of his features. Compared to the medal the president's brow is weak, his eyes are blank, his nose is elongated, and his chin recedes. Interestingly, the year of founding of Jefferson Medical College is incorrectly given as 1826 (when diplomas were first awarded), rather than 1824.

Thomas Jefferson University Presidential Badge

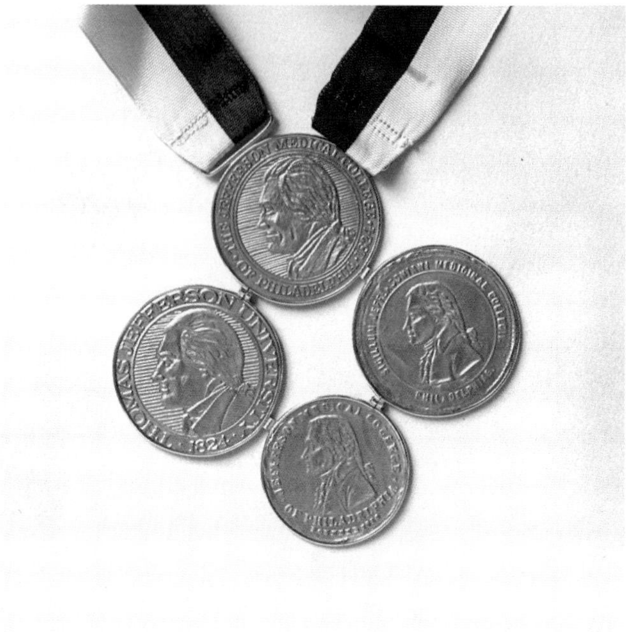

THOMAS JEFFERSON UNIVERSITY PRESIDENTIAL BADGE
By Straub for Medallic Art Co.

Gold, ribbon
1977
4 7/8 in. diameter

Signed reverse of bottom medal: "Straub 1-10 12K"
Inscription top medal: "THE JEFFERSON MEDICAL COLLEGE OF PHILADELPHIA 1824"; inscription left medal: "THOMAS JEFFERSON UNIVERSITY 1824"; inscription right medal: "SIGILLUM JEFFERSONIANI MEDICINAE COLLEGII PHILADELPHIAE"; inscription lower medal: "JEFFERSON MEDICAL COLLEGE OF PHILADELPHIA FOUNDED 1826"

Ordered in 1977 by TJU
Accession number: 1977+e.DA.01

In striking contrast to the Jefferson Medical College plaque is an imposing gold presidential badge made for the university in 1977 by the Medallic Art Company. It consists of four linked gold medals hung from blue and black ribbon (the college colors). The four profile portraits show a history of the Thomas Jefferson head as the university logo.

The medal on the bottom resembles the plaster plaque of 1903. The medal on the right with its Latin inscription looks like a bronze medal issued by the alumni association of Jefferson Medical College in 1970 in honor of its centennial. A bronze Dean's Medal which was issued in 1989 combines elements of the third medal on the left and the most recent, sleek, fourth medal on top of the presidential badge.

An Eclectic Group of Other Nonmedical Portraits

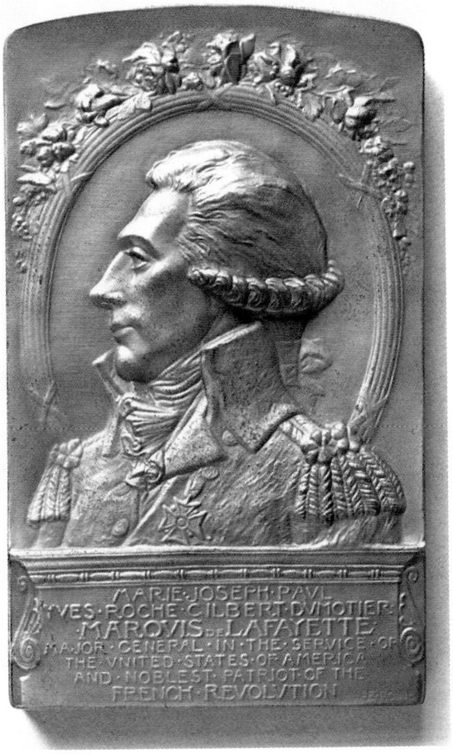

Portrait of the Marquis de Lafayette

(See color plate)

MARIE-JOSEPH-PAUL-YVES-ROCH-GILBERT du MOTIER, MARQUIS de LAFAYETTE (1757-1834) (OBVERSE)
By Jules Edouard Roine (1857-1916)

Bronze medal
1911
4 1/2 x 2 3/4 in.

Signed lower right: "J. E. ROINE"
Inscription: "MARIE JOSEPH PAUL/YVES ROCHE [*sic*] GILBERT DU MOTIER/MARQUIS DE LAFAYETTE/MAJOR GENERAL IN THE SERVICE OF/THE UNITED STATES OF AMERICA/AND NOBLEST PATRIOT OF THE/FRENCH REVOLUTION"

Given before 1946 by Robert Pierson Regester, M.D.
(JMC 1916)
Accession number: 1946+b.M.03

MARQUIS de LAFAYETTE (REVERSE)

Inscription: "AD PERPETUAM REI/MEMORIAM/MCMXI"

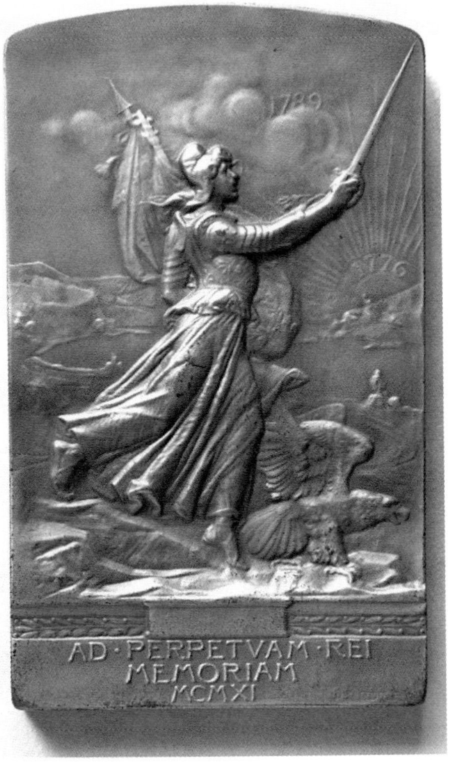

The Marquis de Lafayette played a significant role during both the American and French Revolutions, and was called the "Hero of Two Worlds." Lafayette was highly regarded by Benjamin Franklin and Thomas Jefferson, and his bust by Jean-Antoine Houdon was included in Jefferson's collection at Monticello along with other Houdon busts of Franklin, George Washington, and John Paul Jones.

The French aristocrat was appointed a major general by the colonists against the British. He fought with distinction at the Battle of Brandywine in 1777, and conducted a masterly retreat from Barren Hill in 1778. He helped persuade the French government to send a six-thousand-man expeditionary army to aid the colonists. Commanding an army in Virginia in 1780, he forced Lord Charles Cornwallis to retreat across Virginia and then entrapped him at Yorktown. A French fleet joined with several American armies in the siege and Cornwallis surrendered a few months later.

The political fortunes of the Marquis de Lafayette rose to the heights, fell precipitously, and rose again during the period of the French Revolution and its aftermath, but he remained consistently popular in the United States. He was honored with a posthumous bronze medal struck in 1911. It was designed and carved by Jules E. Roine, a French-born sculptor working in New York. It is not known who commissioned the medal.

The obverse shows a bust-length portrait of Lafayette in a profile view. He wears a wig with ear-length curls, and is attired in an elaborate military uniform with epaulets and a decoration. Encircling his head is a leafy branch mounted on fasces (a bundle of wooden rods symbolizing unity or justice). An English inscription noting his deeds in America and France is written on the plinth below the figure.

The reverse shows Liberty wearing armor, raising her sword and striding across a rocky landscape with an eagle beneath her feet. The dates of the French and American Revolutions emanate from the clouds and the sun, respectively.

Portrait of a Soldier

(See color plate)

PORTRAIT OF A SOLDIER
By Susan Macdowell Eakins
(1851-1938)

Oil on canvas
1917
30 x 25 in.

Signed and dated lower right: "S. M. Eakins 1917"
Exhibition: Philadelphia, *Susan Macdowell Eakins*, Pennsylvania Academy of the Fine Arts, May 4-June 10, 1973

On long-term loan since 1993 from the French Benevolent Society of Philadelphia
Accession number: 1993+e.P.03

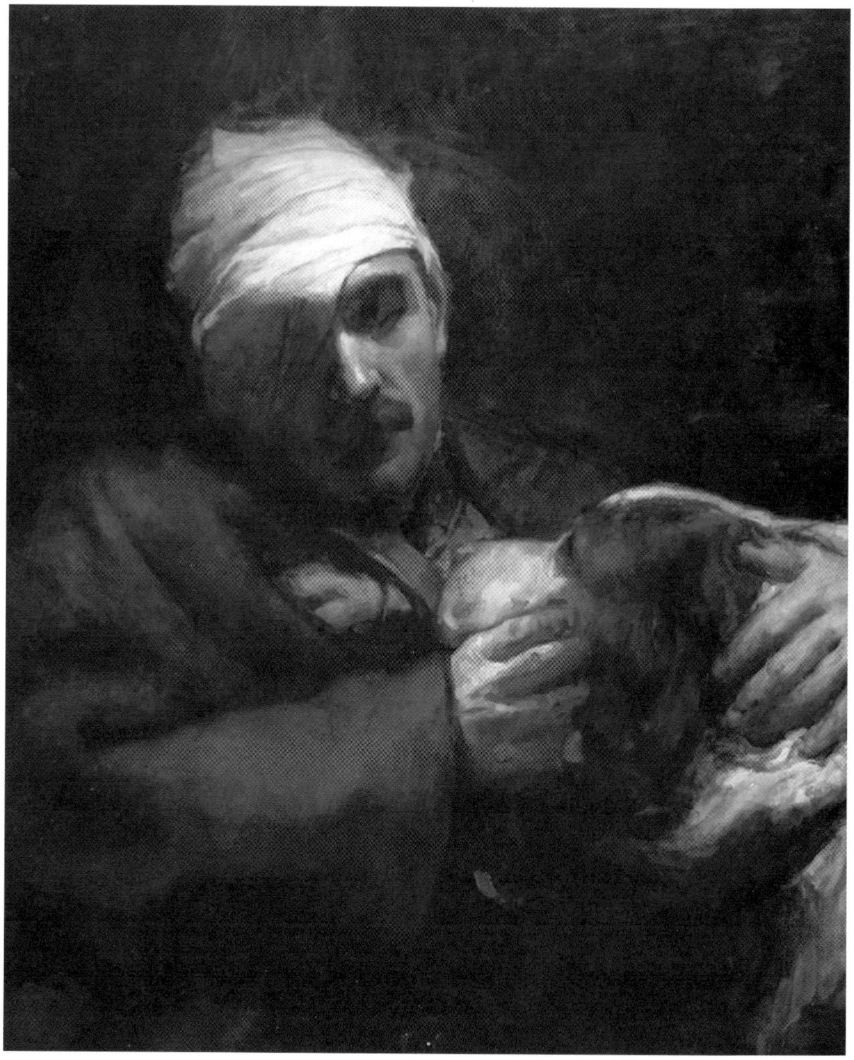

In 1993 Susan M. Eakins's *Portrait of a Soldier* was generously placed on indefinite loan to Thomas Jefferson University by the French Benevolent Society of Philadelphia. It is on view in the anteroom of the Eakins Gallery near the work of Thomas Eakins, the artist's husband. The portrait was painted in 1917 and donated by the artist that same year to the society.

Susan Eakins was inspired to paint *Portrait of a Soldier*

by a photograph accompanying an article in a French magazine, *L'Illustration* (May 5, 1917), about Julien Lemordant, a famous French artist and heroic World War I soldier. He had been wounded nine times, the last time at point blank range when a bullet struck his left temple and exited under his right eye. He was roused from unconsciousness by an enemy soldier verifying the number of dead troops. Though blind and seemingly dying, he was transferred with other prisoners and German wounded to a fortress in Bavaria, and then to a camp with appallingly harsh conditions. Finally a medical commission took pity on him and sent him to Switzerland to recuperate.

Lemordant finally returned to his atelier in Paris twenty-five months after his departure. The article describes an exhibition of the artist's paintings organized by his faithful friends and admirers including the President of the Republic, to pay homage to the pacifist turned heroic soldier. Compassionate friends reflected sadly, "All his life was in his eyes."

The portrait shows the wounded soldier with his head and right eye bandaged. He tightly embraces a setter dog which looks mournfully up at him. He wears a dark brown coat with full sleeves and a blue scarf. The poses and the patient's costume replicate almost exactly the magazine photograph presumably taken when the hero was recovering in Switzerland.

Even without knowing the pathetic details of the subject's war experiences, the viewer can sense the youthful figure's vulnerability from his gentle communication with the dog, from his morose facial expression and slouching posture, from the murky, dark background, and from the highlights on the stark white bandages contrasted dramatically with the deep shadows on the right side of his face. The magazine article encourages the reader to pray for the final resolution of the artist's sufferings and sacrifices, concluding, "The miracles of science are more numerous each day. Let us hope."

Susan Macdowell Eakins is best remembered today as Thomas Eakins's devoted wife whose first concern was promoting her husband's art, but she was an accomplished artist in her own right and continued to paint intermittently during their marriage. She was gifted in both watercolor and oil painting, and was one of the earliest Philadelphia artists to experiment with photography.

Susan Macdowell was born in 1851, the daughter of a distinguished Philadelphia engraver. She enrolled at the Pennsylvania Academy of the Fine Arts from 1876 to 1882 and was a leader among the women students. At Academy annual exhibitions Macdowell was the first recipient of the Mary Smith Prize for the best painting by a Philadelphia woman in 1879, and one of two winners of the Charles Toppan Prize for the best student work in 1882. Among her seven entries in the 1879 annual was *Anatomical Lecture at the Academy: Dr. Keen on the Facial Muscles*, depicting William Williams Keen Jr., M.D., later famed as a Jefferson neurosurgeon.

Her attention to draftsmanship, the solid rendering of the figure, and a penetrating interpretation of character show the influence of her primary teacher, Thomas Eakins. He considered her "the best woman painter in America, and that he would rather have her opinion on his work than anyone's."[8]

The two artists were married in January 1884 and resided in rented lodgings at 1330 Chestnut Street. After two and one-half years they moved to Eakins's comfortable family home at 1729 Mount Vernon Street in the Fairmount section of Philadelphia, where they lived with Benjamin Eakins, the artist's father. Although the couple had no children, the household was very lively and contained a menagerie of dogs, cats, monkeys, and other animals. Susan Eakins extended hospitality to family, students, and a wide circle of friends who often enjoyed impromptu musicales at the Eakins home.

Susan Eakins provided a steadfast and sensitive support for her husband, an often controversial public figure. She answered his correspondence and supervised the packing and shipping of his paintings to and from exhibitions. After his death in 1916 Susan Eakins worked untiringly with several devoted disciples to enhance Thomas Eakins's future prestige by placing dozens of his unsold works in prominent museums and galleries, especially the Philadelphia Museum of Art.

In the years following his death she became less retiring and was more actively engaged in the art scene until her eighty-sixth year. In 1936 she helped to organize an exhibition at the Philadelphia Art Club of twenty of her own works, along with paintings by her husband, her sister, Elizabeth Macdowell Kenton, and three followers of Thomas Eakins. She died two years later.

The first solo exhibition of her work, a retrospective in 1973 at the Pennsylvania Academy of the Fine Arts, included *Portrait of a Soldier*. An exhibition of works by Susan Eakins, her husband, her sister, and Samuel Murray was organized at the North Cross School in Roanoke, Virginia in 1977.

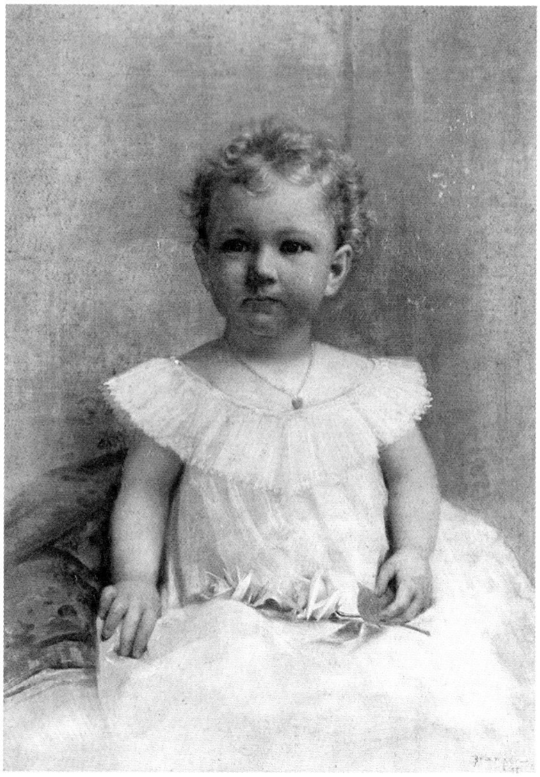

Portrait of Katharine A. Howell

KATHARINE ASHMAN HOWELL (1893-1989)
By Lloyd Branson (1861-1925)

Oil on canvas
1895
28 x 22 in.

Signed and dated lower right: "L BRANSON/'95"

Given in 1990 by bequest of the subject
Accession number: 1990+e.P.03

Thomas Jefferson University received a generous bequest and two paintings in 1990 from Katharine Ashman Howell. Although she was never directly involved with the university as a patient or volunteer, it turned out that the benefactress did have ties to Jefferson.

The donor's great-grandfather, James Veech, was an 1827 graduate of the parent institution, Jefferson College in Canonsburg, Pennsylvania. Among the many physicians in her family, at least one, John Dawson Sturgeon Jr., M.D., was a graduate of Jefferson Medical College in the class of 1920. The bequest was used to create the Katharine A. Howell Scholarship Fund.

According to her attorney, the donor's eighteenth-century forbears lived in Gloucester County, New Jersey and Fayette County, Pennsylvania. Katharine Ashman Howell was born in 1893 in Knoxville, Tennessee, the daughter of a mining engineer who "went where the work was." Katharine, an only child, was reared in Denver, Colorado where she graduated from high school. Never married, she resided in many different parts of the country and customarily spent the winters on the West Coast when she wasn't traveling. She lived parsimoniously, invested judiciously, and accumulated a sizable fortune. She died at the age of ninety-six in Santa Monica, California.

Katharine Ashman Howell was depicted in 1895 by Lloyd Branson, a painter from Knoxville who won medals at the Atlanta Exposition in 1885 and the Appalachian Exposition in Knoxville in 1910. The sitter is shown as a plump child of about two years, three-quarters length and life-sized, propped up against a pillow. She looks slightly to the left while fingering two pink, long-stemmed roses on her lap.

Her round face has appealing large blue eyes, fat cheeks, and a small mouth, all crowned by a halo of blond curls. She wears a white dress with a wide, lacy yoke that forms capped sleeves. A heart-shaped locket hangs from a delicate chain around her neck. The background colors are pale beige and mauve, in harmony with the overall delicacy of the picture.

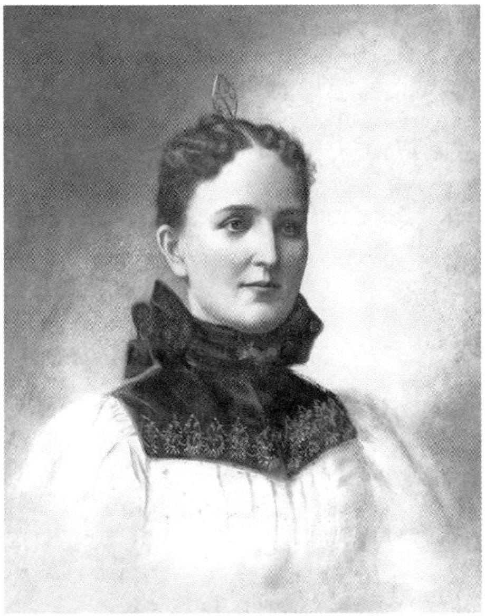

Portrait of Katharine A. V. Howell

KATHARINE ASHMAN VEECH HOWELL (ca. 1870-1920s)
By unknown artist

Pastel on canvas
1900-10
27 x 22 in.

Given in 1990 by bequest of Katharine Ashman Howell, daughter of the subject
Accession number: 1990+e.P.04

A pastel portrait of Katharine A. V. Howell, the mother of Katharine A. Howell, was probably painted in the first decade of the twentieth century, judging by her appearance. An indecipherable artist's signature at the top left includes the letters "...tzen..."

The subject is shown bust length. Her center-parted, dark brown hair is worn in tight curls framing her face, and crowned by a bronze hair ornament. Her lovely features include soulful brown eyes, high cheek bones, a Grecian nose, rosy lips, and a square jaw. Her pink gown has a dark blue velvet yoke decorated with gold stitchery, attached to a large bow tied at the sides under her chin. The varying tones of the umber atmospheric background cast the left side of her face in shadow, emphasizing her angular features and adding to her reserved and enigmatic expression.

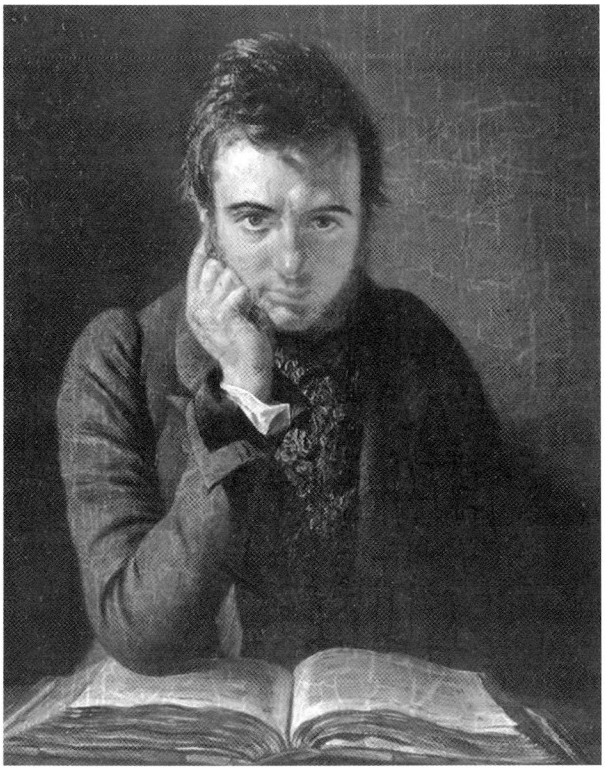

Portrait of a Scholar

PORTRAIT OF A SCHOLAR
By unknown artist

Oil on wood panel
Before 1910
9 5/8 x 7 3/4 in.

Given in 1996 by Dr. Joseph Sataloff, professor of otolaryngology, and Mrs. Sataloff
Accession number: 1996+e.P.13

Over the course of many years Dr. and Mrs. Joseph Sataloff have donated paintings, prints, and a few decorative objects to Thomas Jefferson University. An otolaryngologist, Dr. Sataloff is an expert in occupational hearing loss and the conservation of hearing.

One of the most appealing figural works is a small oil portrait of an unknown scholar. It appears stylistically to be late-nineteenth-century. The unidentified painter's command of anatomy and rendering of different textures suggest training at a professional European art academy.

The scholar is shown half length, seated behind a table on whose surface lies an open book. The figure's left elbow rests on the book, and his head leans on his hand in a philosopher's melancholy pose. Though he gazes straight ahead, his eyes are unfocused and seemingly preoccupied with inner thoughts.

The youthful man's brown hair is thick and tousled, his blue eyes large, his lips full, and his coloring ruddy. His brown coat is lined in black and a foulard silk scarf covers his shirt front. The pages of the thick book are well worn. The atmospheric background is dark green. Puzzling notations on the back of the wooden panel include a gallery number, the date 1910, and the initials "P. L."

Money Changer of Cairo

MONEY CHANGER OF CAIRO
By William James Müller (1812-45)

Oil on canvas
1838-41
28 x 37 in.

Exhibition: Birmingham, England, *Loan Collection of Paintings in Oils and Watercolours by W. J. Müller*, City Museum and Art Gallery, 1896

Given in 1996 by Dr. Joseph Sataloff, professor of otolaryngology, and Mrs. Sataloff
Accession number: 1996+e.P.18

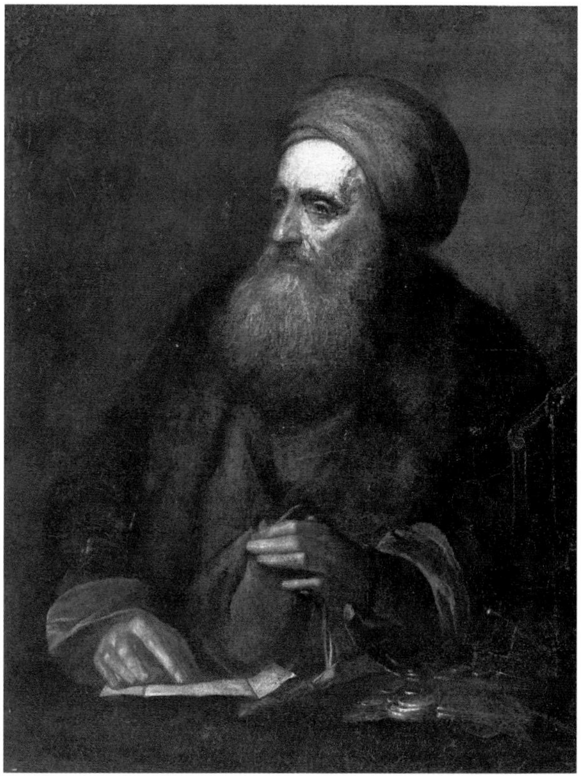

Another of several portraits donated by Dr. and Mrs. Sataloff is identified by artist and title on the rear of the canvas. *The Money Changer of Cairo* was painted in the mid-nineteenth century by the English-born artist William James Müller.

The picture's dramatic contrast of light and shade resembles seventeenth-century Dutch and Spanish portraits. Brilliant highlights on the money changer's forehead, cheeks and nose illuminate his face against the prevailing dark greenish-gray, shadowy background. He is attired in a green turban and dark brown robe.

The figure of the money changer is a Middle Eastern type almost to the point of caricature with his olive complexion, hair, and eyes, long, hook nose, thick lips, and full gray beard and mustache. He is shown half-length behind a table. His right hand points to a document, and his left hand holds some kind of fabric. Coins and a brass scale gleam quietly on the right side of the table.

Müller was born in 1812 in Bristol, England, the son of a Prussian refugee who became curator of the Bristol Museum and married an Englishwoman. Young Müller was apprenticed to Bristol artist James Baker Pyne (1800-70) for two years, and his first pictures were of his hometown and the surrounding countryside. He traveled through East Anglia and Wales and was a founder of the Bristol Sketching Club.

In 1834-35 he traveled to Switzerland, Germany, and Italy after which he had some financial success with oil paintings of continental scenes. In 1838 he sought out more exotic locales in Egypt and Greece, and was particularly impressed with colorful bazaars in Cairo and the ancient ruins along the Nile. Upon his return he moved to London and worked on this subject matter for about three years, exhibiting pictures at the Royal Academy, the British Institution, and the Society of British Artists.

Further travel took Müller to northern France in 1840,

on commission to gather material for a publication of architecture in the age of Francis I; and an expedition to the site of ancient Lycia in Asia Minor in 1843. These journeys provided the stimulus for some of his finest drawings and watercolors.

William James Müller died of heart disease at the age of thirty-three in 1845. A memorial exhibition of oil paintings, watercolors, and drawings was held at the City Art Gallery in Bristol in 1962 in commemoration of the 150th anniversary of his birth. An earlier retrospective occurred at the City Museum and Art Gallery of Birmingham in 1896. In 1984-85 the Tate Gallery of London held an exhibition featuring Müller's drawings, many of which had been donated by the widow of a former mayor of Bristol.

Group Scenes

Cavaliers in Battle

CAVALIERS IN BATTLE
Attributed to Dirk Stoop (ca. 1618-81)

Oil on wood panel
1650-75
16 x 23 1/4 in.

Given in 1994 by Dr. Joseph Sataloff, professor of otolaryngology, and Mrs. Sataloff
Accession number: 1994+e.P.02

One of the earliest paintings now in the Jefferson collection is a lively scene of cavaliers fighting on horseback, tentatively attributed to the Dutch artist Dirk Stoop.

A heated battle scene takes place under a broad blue sky with pink and gray clouds and pairs and trios of tiny birds. In the center foreground an armored soldier on a white rearing horse crosses swords with his foe. To the

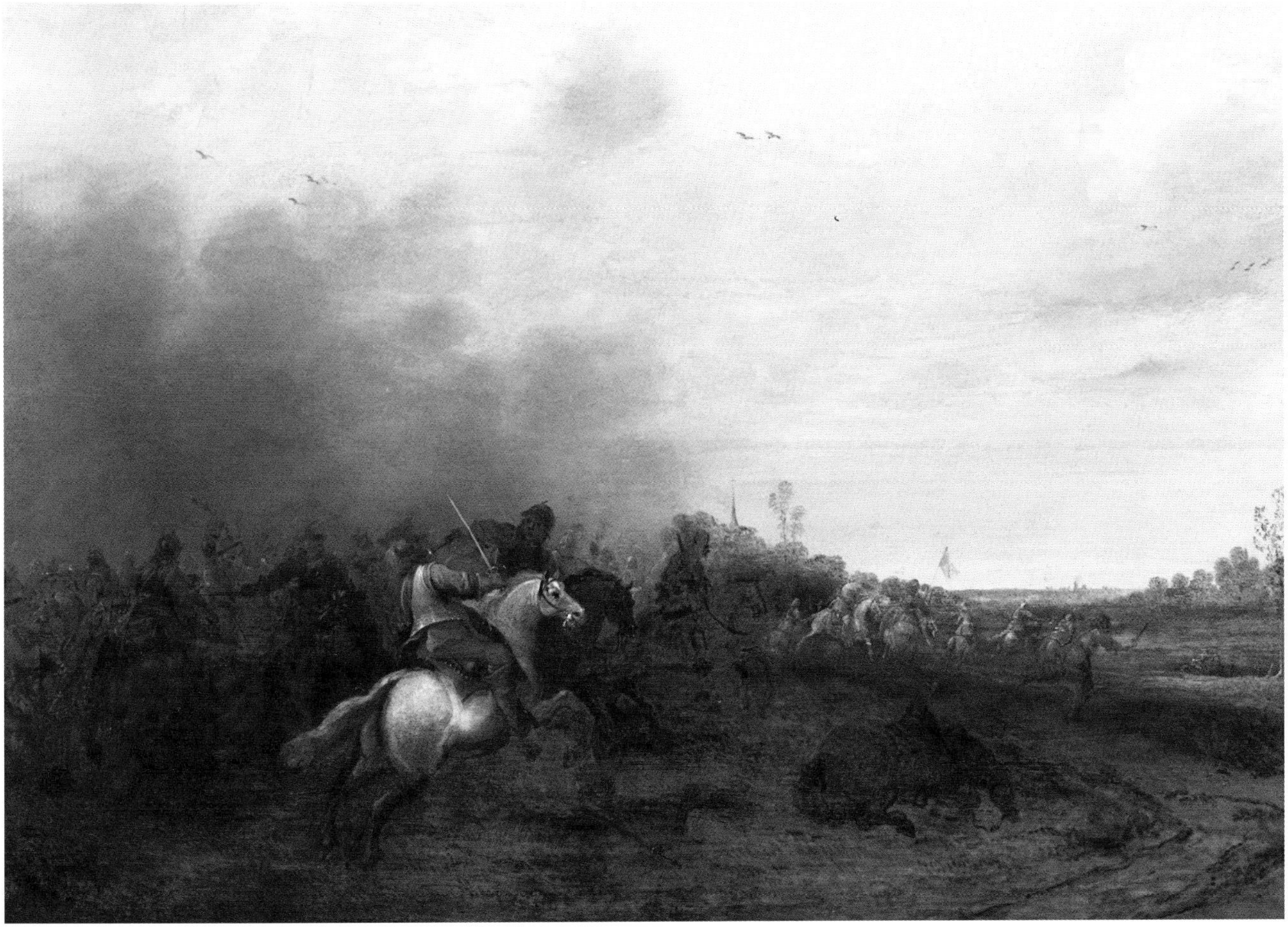

right a horse lies dying on the ground. In the middle ground a chaotic battle takes place on the left, and groups of mounted horsemen take flight on the right. On the horizon are details of the local community: feathery trees, flat plains, and a steepled church. Touches of bright red and blue further enliven the frenetic scene.

Dirk Stoop was born in Utrecht about 1618. He was in the painters' guild in Utrecht in 1638 and in Lisbon in 1662. He accompanied Princess Catherine of Bragança (wife of Charles II) to England, and returned to Utrecht in 1678. He was widely known as a painter of battle scenes and engagements of the cavalry, and as an engraver of portraits, military scenes, and vignettes from *Aesop's Fables*.

Crowd at the Cattleman

CROWD AT THE CATTLEMAN
By Humbert L. Howard (1915-90)

Watercolor, gouache, crayon, pastel on paper
Before 1974
27 1/2 x 35 in.

Signed center right: "Humbert Howard"

Given in 1974 by Ludwig E. Schlitt, M.D., pediatric resident (1958-60) at TJU Hospital
Accession number: 1974+e.P.02

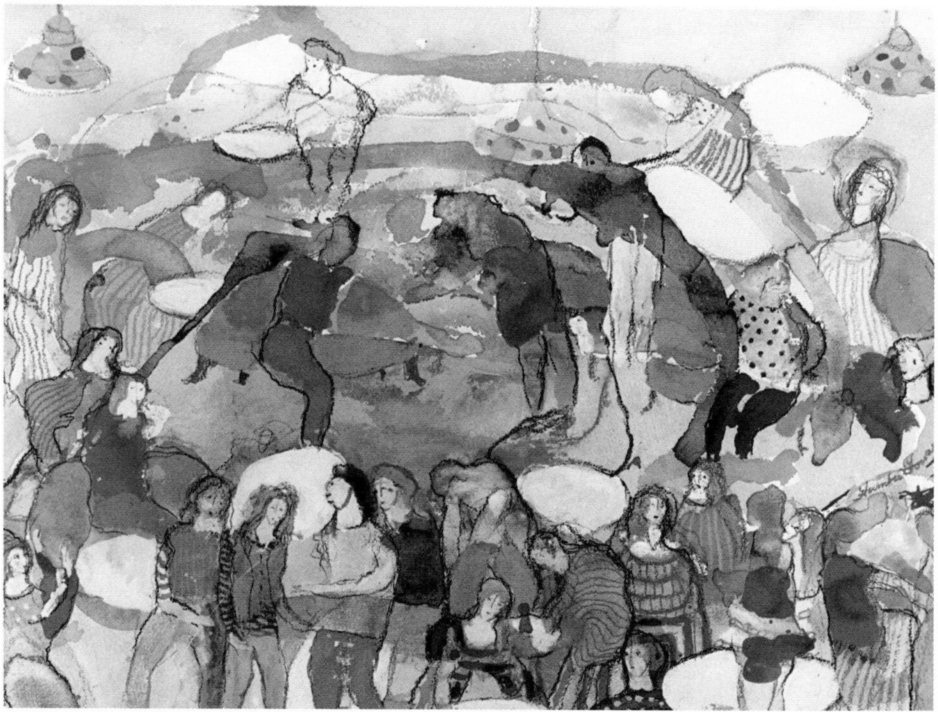

The milling about of figures in a semiabstract pleasure scene by Philadelphia artist Humbert Howard seems almost as chaotic as the painting of cavaliers attributed to Dirk Stoop. Howard's mixed media, *Crowd at the Cattleman,* depicts a New York nightclub full of revelers.

Concentric circles of casually attired young people radiate out from the central blue dance floor. On the periphery are round tables with white cloths below three chandeliers. A few foreground figures face the observer as though extending an invitation to join the dancers and onlookers. Delicate black lines emphasize contours of bodies and facial features. The bright primary colors of the costumes include patterns of stripes and polka dots. The background wall is bright yellow.

Humbert Howard's personal imagery reflects an interest in modernist styles combined with themes of human interaction. A postal worker by day and artist from the late afternoon on, Humbert Howard became one of Philadelphia's best known modern painters.

He was born in Philadelphia in 1915 and won a football scholarship to Howard University. He transferred to the University of Pennsylvania to be closer to his ill mother, and soon joined the Works Progress Administration in Philadelphia as painter and ceramicist. One of his landscapes was exhibited at the 1939 New York World's Fair.

In 1940 Humbert Howard was appointed promotional chairman of the exhibition committee of the Pyramid Club, an African-American social organization of black professionals, educators, and businessmen. Howard began to organize its annual painting exhibitions, with an interracial cross section of artists from Philadelphia, New York, and Washington. The next year he left the WPA to join the U.S. Postal Service where his delivery route allowed him to visit local art clubs. He retired from the Post Office in the mid-1970s to devote himself full-time to painting.

Howard's first solo exhibition was at the Temple University library in 1947. In 1950 his still life was purchased from the Pennsylvania Academy of the Fine Arts annual exhibition. In 1959 he left the Pyramid Club and began studies at the Barnes Foundation and three years later began studying aesthetic philosophy at the University of Pennsylvania. During the 1960s he taught painting at the Cheltenham Art Center and the Allens Lane Art Center.

Between 1968 and 1985 he won several prizes and awards: the Pearl and Lloyd Van Sciver Memorial Prize for Painting at the Woodmere Art Museum; two honorary degrees and silver medals from the International Academy of Arts and Letters in Rome; the Andrew Wyeth Prize from the Urban League of Philadelphia; the Philadelphia Water Color Prize; and the inaugural Heritage Award of the mid-Manhattan branch of the NAACP.

Humbert Howard had solo exhibitions at galleries in Philadelphia and southern New Jersey, as well as the Howard University Gallery of Art in 1959 and the Gloucester County College in Sewell, New Jersey in 1978. Six years after his death in 1990, a retrospective was held at the Levy Gallery of the Moore College of Art and Design in Philadelphia.

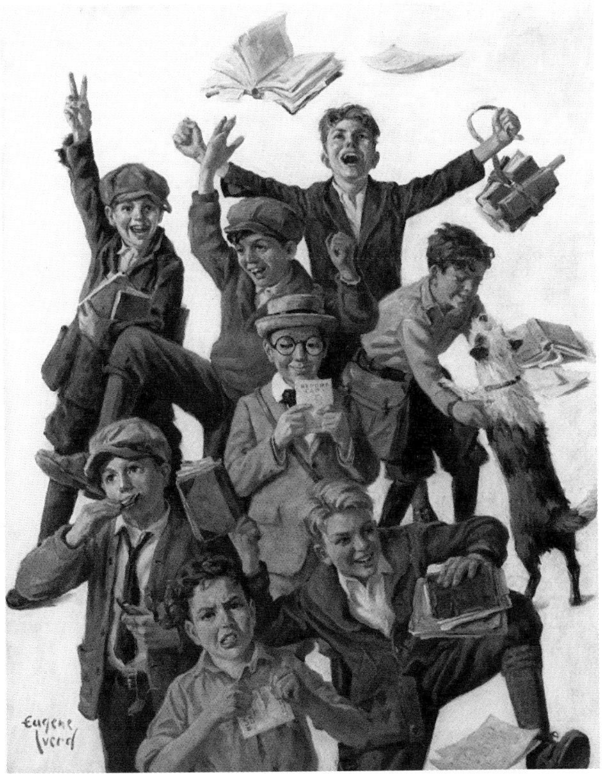

School is Out for the Summer

SCHOOL IS OUT FOR THE SUMMER
By Eugene Iverd (1893-1938)

Oil on canvas
1925-35
42 1/4 x 33 1/4 in.

Signed lower left: "Eugene/Iverd"

Given before 1950 by Joan Lorimer to Children's Heart Hospital which became Children's Rehabilitation Hospital, since 1970 administered by TJU
Accession number: CR1950+b.P.01

Generous donors made numerous gifts of fine art and decorative arts to the original Children's Heart Hospital, and some of these objects still remain at the Ford Road Campus. (See chapter nine for information about the hospital and its affiliation with Jefferson.)

Two oil paintings of children's subjects by the well known illustrator Eugene Iverd were donated by Joan Lorimer, a dedicated volunteer at Children's Heart Hospital. A winter 1965 hospital newsletter said that the paintings, *School is Out for the Summer* and *Snowball Fight,* were the original versions made by Iverd for *Saturday Evening Post* covers. They probably date to the late 1920s or 1930s.

School is Out for the Summer is a group of (mostly) joyous boys celebrating the end of the school year. Surrounding a bespectacled boy wearing a neatly pressed suit and porkpie hat, are others with loosened shirt collars or ties, and wearing sweaters or jackets, knickers, and peaked caps. Some hold books by a leather strap or in a shoulder bag, and some swing or throw books and school papers into the air. One embraces his dog, another plays his harmonica. The "goody-goody" boy in the center regards his report card with a smug expression, while the boy in front of the pack grimaces angrily while tearing up his report card.

Interestingly, all participants face front and the group rises vertically, isolated against a pale gray background with no evident horizon line. The boys' stereotypical tousled hair, toothy grins, pink cheeks, and brightly colored and disheveled clothing add strength and energy to the boisterous celebration.

Eugene Iverd was born in 1893 in St. Paul, Minnesota. He studied at the St. Paul Institute of Art and at the Pennsylvania Academy of the Fine Arts. He was a painter and illustrator who created cover designs and illustrations for *The Saturday Evening Post, American Magazine,* and other publications. He lived in Erie, Pennsylvania.

Over the Stile

OVER THE STILE
By Myles Birket Foster (1825-99)

Watercolor on paper
Ca. 1860-70
6 1/2 x 5 1/8 in.

Signed lower left: "B. F."

Given in 1996 by Dr. Joseph Sataloff, professor of otolaryngology, and Mrs. Sataloff
Accession number: 1996+e.P.14

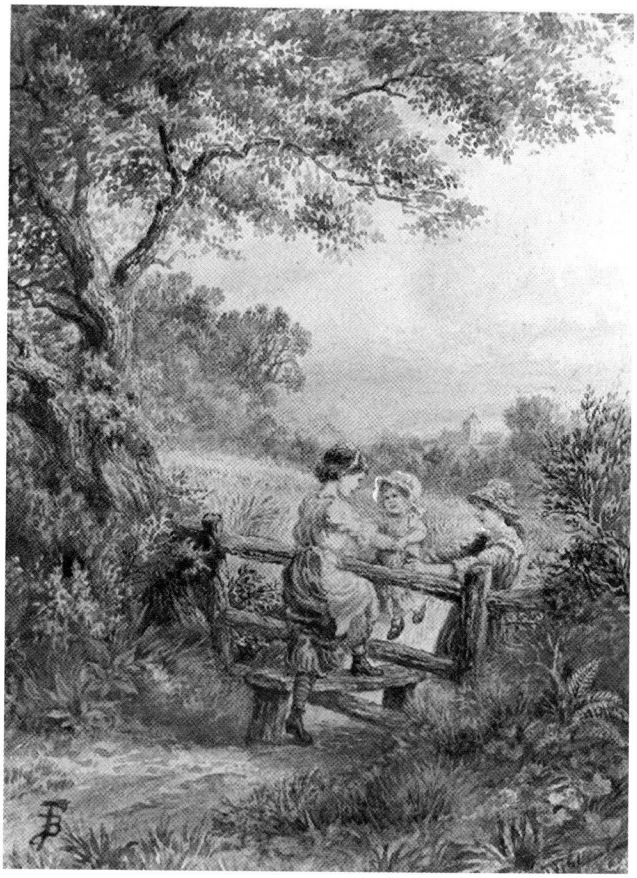

A different kind of relationship between children is depicted in a tiny watercolor by (Myles) Birket Foster, compared with the paintings of Eugene Iverd. Foster shows children quietly at play in a bucolic landscape. Although Foster too was an illustrator and painter, his delicate and airy touch contrasts starkly with Iverd's broadly painted, brightly colored, effusive style.

Foster's delicate and lyrical watercolor is typical of his small country scenes featuring exquisite details of landscape, architecture, and figures, all in pastel shades. *Over the Stile* shows a girl lifting a baby over a gate to another girl waiting on the other side. The sweetly innocent children are dressed in high button shoes and stockings, dresses with aprons, and bonnets. The figures, abundant foliage, and distant house are rendered in precise detail.

Birket Foster was born in 1825 in Tynemouth, England, the son of a timber and bottling merchant.[9] From his very earliest days at Quaker boarding schools he showed an aptitude for drawing landscapes, and at age sixteen he convinced his father to allow him to become an apprentice to a local wood engraver and publisher.

Work by Foster was included in some issues of *Punch* magazine and *The Illustrated London News* in the early 1840s. Many of these were picturesque landscapes and genre scenes of farmers at work and play made on sketching trips through the English and Scottish countryside. By the time he had completed his seven-year apprenticeship in 1847 he was well on his way to becoming one of the most popular and prolific illustrators of his time. He was noted for his illustrations of poetry, especially Henry W. Longfellow's *Evangeline: A Tale of Acadie* and Sir Walter Scott's *Lady of the Lake*, among many others.

Foster went on sketching tours of the Continent in the 1850s, and he revisited Venice several times in the late 1860s. By the late 1850s he tired of illustration and began to master the laborious art of watercolor. He exhibited with the Royal Society of Painters in Water-Colours every year between 1860 and 1899, and was made an associate of the society in 1860 and a full member in 1862. He also exhibited regularly at the Royal Academy of Arts.

Although Birket Foster garnered consistently good reviews in *The Art Journal*, some other contemporary critics thought that the children in his pictures were too pretty and graceful, and did not look like true rustics. Actually his own children posed for many of his compositions, and art scholars today think he deliberately chose to see the pleasant and picturesque side of life, realizing nostalgically that traditional English country life was threatened by increasing industrialization.

Members of the Art Union, a society for promoting the fine arts, received chromolithographs after the paintings of Foster. Examples of his work can be found in many British museums and castle collections, and in America at the Yale Center for British Art and the Henry E. Huntington Library and Art Gallery in San Marino, California. A special loan exhibition honoring the centenary of his birth was held at the Laing Art Gallery in Newcastle upon Tyne in 1925.

Decorative Arts

Tall Case Clock

TALL CASE CLOCK
Works by Herschede Co. of Ohio

Mahogany
1910-30
92 x 28 1/2 x 18 in.

Given before 1932 by anonymous donor to Children's Heart Hospital, which became Children's Rehabilitation Hospital, since 1970 administered by TJU
Accession number: CR1932+b.DA.01

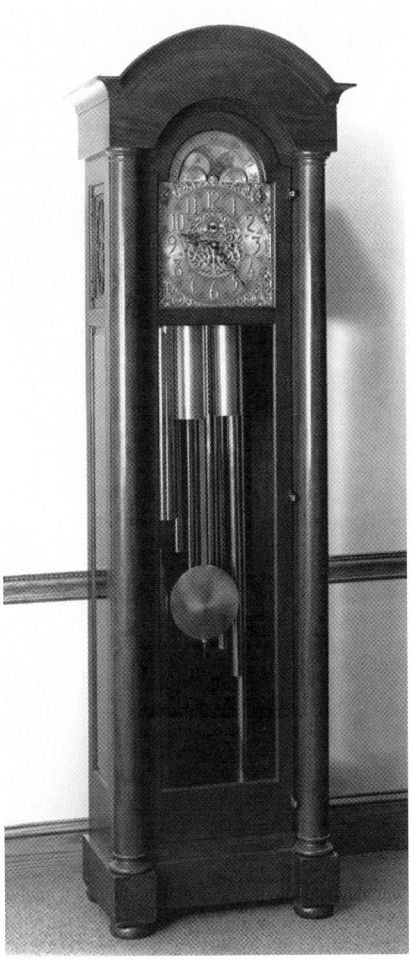

Among donations of decorative arts at the Children's Rehabilitation Hospital is a mahogany, tall case, tubular chime clock with works by the Herschede Company of Ohio. It was given to the hospital by an anonymous donor sometime before 1932. Another handsome work is a walnut partners' desk made about 1890-1920 and bequeathed by one of the hospital's founders, Dr. Joseph Sailer.

The clock has adorned the hospital's boardroom for decades. Its case is a standard American type made about 1910-30 to resemble early-eighteenth-century cases. The clock works contain a full octave, musical movement with gong; chromed tubular chimes; and a brass dial fitted with a steel chapter ring of brass Arabic numerals surrounded and centered by brass scroll work, with a seconds dial and dials for chime silent and chime selection. A painted moon phase movement is above. A twin-paneled beveled glass door exposes the chimes, brass cylinder weights, and glass pendulum.

Freestanding, tapered, round columns on the front of the clock support a plain, domical cornice. The attractively restrained case is raised on plain base moldings on bun feet.

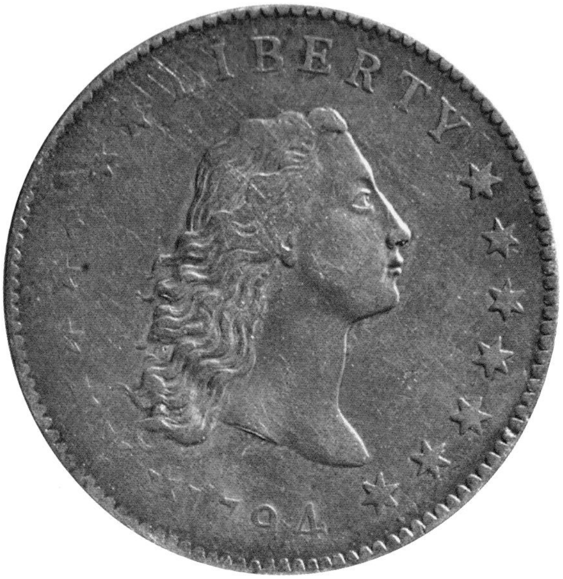

U.S. Liberty Silver Dollar

U.S. LIBERTY DOLLAR (OBVERSE)
Silver

Engraved by John Scot
1794
1 1/2 in. diameter

Inscription: "LIBERTY 1794"

Given by William K. Jenson, M.D. (JMC 1953)
Accession numbers of collection: 1997+e.M.01-15

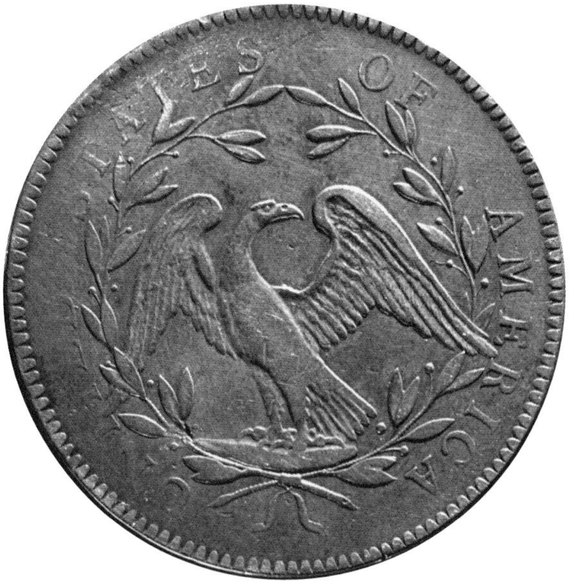

U.S. LIBERTY DOLLAR (REVERSE)

Inscription: "UNITED STATES OF AMERICA"

Jefferson alumnus William K. Jenson, M.D. donated a collection of fifteen rare American coins to the university's art collection in 1997. The set consists of the earliest silver dollars made in America, dating from 1794 to 1803. They were struck only at the Philadelphia mint, and the series terminated with a special coin in 1804.[10]

All feature a type of liberty image on the obverse. The rarest silver dollar in Dr. Jenson's collection is the earliest, because the entire mintage was only 1,758 pieces. Today only between 120 and 150 silver dollars with the date 1794 are thought to survive. It is believed that mint engraver John Scot cut the dies for this coin. He was inspired by the 1793 large Liberty Cap cent, which in turn was inspired by the Libertas Americana medal produced in France the previous decade to commemorate victories over the British.

The obverse is the Flowing Hair Liberty type. The neoclassical profile head of Miss Liberty faces right, and her streaming and rippled tresses fall to her shoulders. Along the curved periphery are eight stars to the left and seven stars to the right. The reverse is a Small Eagle type featuring a rather delicate bird with wings spread and perched on a rock, surrounded by a laurel wreath. Along the edge of the coin is an inscription reading "HUNDRED CENTS ONE DOLLAR OR UNIT," with ornaments as spacers between the words.

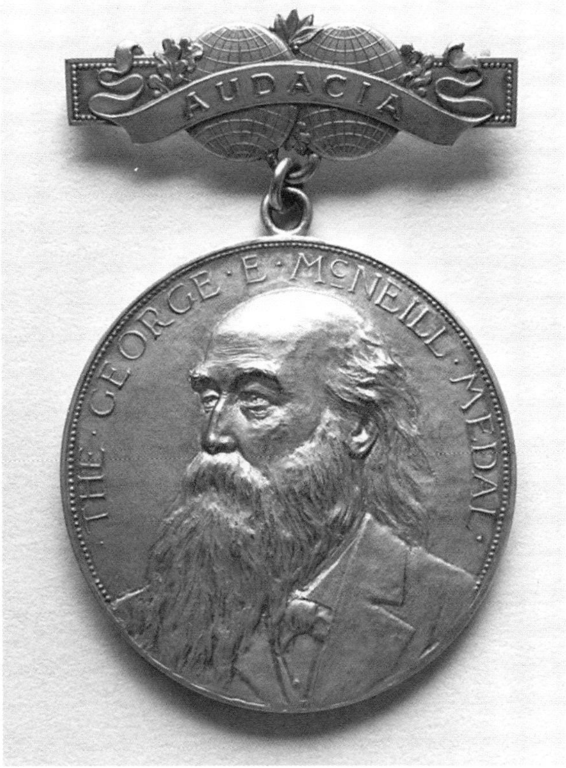

George E. McNeill Medal Awarded to James A. Hamma

GEORGE E. McNEILL MEDAL AWARDED TO JAMES ARCHIBALD HAMMA, M.D. (OBVERSE)
By Tiffany & Co.

Gold
Medal: 1 7/8 in. diameter
Pin: 1/2 x 1 7/8 in.

Inscription on medal: "THE GEORGE E. MCNEILL MEDAL"
Inscription on pin: "AUDACIA"

Given after 1953, probably by family of Dr. James A. Hamma
Accession number: 1953+f.M.01

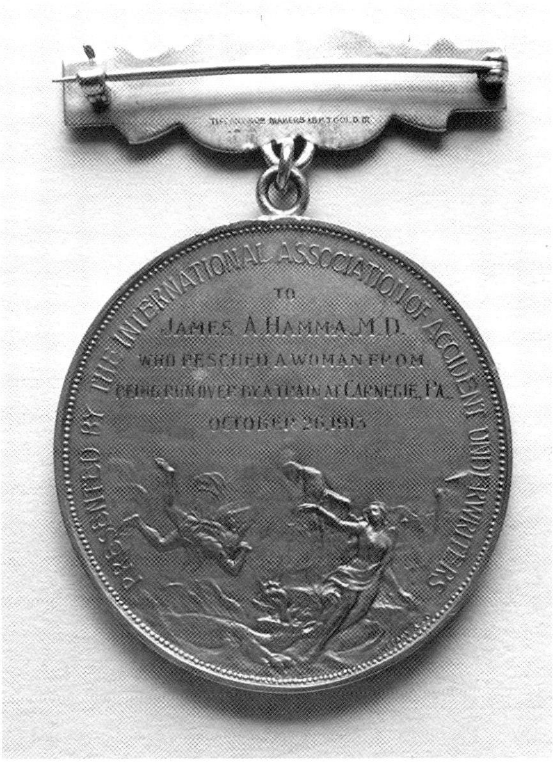

McNEILL MEDAL (REVERSE)

Pin signed: "TIFFANY & CO. MAKERS 18K GOLD"
Inscriptions: "PRESENTED BY THE INTERNATIONAL ASSOCIATION OF ACCIDENT UNDERWRITERS," surrounding "TO/JAMES A. HAMMA, M.D./WHO RESCUED A WOMAN FROM/BEING RUN OVER BY A TRAIN AT CARNEGIE, PA./OCTOBER 26, 1913"

James A. Hamma, M.D. (1877-1953), a Jefferson Medical College graduate of the class of 1897, practiced general medicine in Carnegie, Pennsylvania. In 1913 he achieved national acclaim for risking his own life to rescue a stranger. In recognition for his heroic deed he was awarded both the George E. McNeill Award and the Carnegie Hero Fund Award. Both medals were later donated to Jefferson Medical College.

According to a news report of 1913 Hamma had just crossed frost-covered train tracks in Carnegie when he heard a cry and saw that a woman had slipped and fallen between the rails. The report continued,

A few score yards distant came thundering a special through train, and in one glance the Doctor saw that the woman was doomed unless...In one bound he had reached her side and had picked her up; but the train was upon them, and it seemed that both must perish. With rare presence of mind he threw her across his shoulder and himself fell backwards, his legs across the rail but held sufficiently high for some part of the engine to touch them and swing them around out of danger...Dr. Hamma had risked his life to save the life of a stranger.

The George E. McNeill Award was given to Dr. Hamma at the fifth annual convention of the International Association of Casualty and Surety Underwriters on August 24, 1915. The obverse of the gold medal made by the Tiffany Company has a bust-length portrait of George E. McNeill. The full-bearded, long-haired gentleman is shown in two-thirds view. Inscribed on the pin is the Latin word "Audacia" (meaning daring or courage). The reverse features a devotional image of St. George, the legendary warrior saint and martyr, rescuing a sacrificial maiden from a fearsome dragon. The accompanying inscription describes Dr. Hamma's heroic feat.

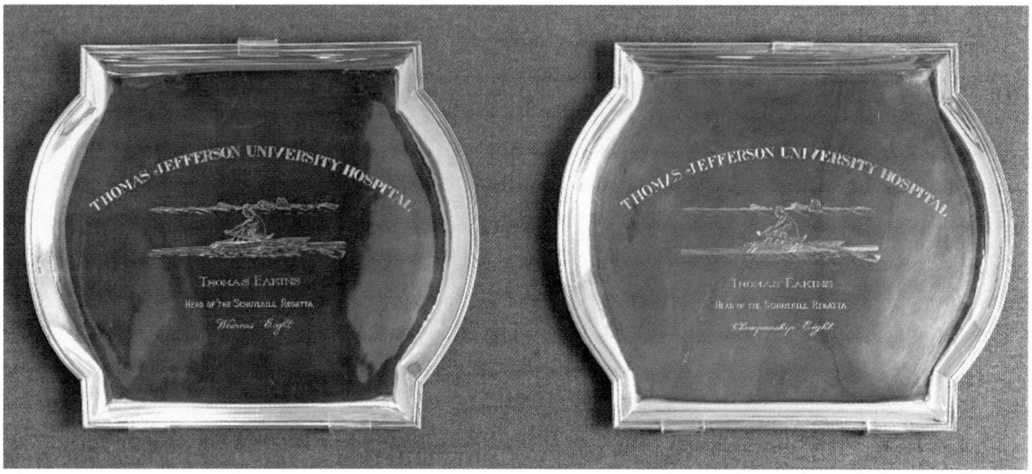

Eakins Head of the Schuylkill Regatta Trophies

EAKINS HEAD OF THE SCHUYLKILL REGATTA TROPHIES
By Schroth for J. E. Caldwell Co.

Silver
1985
Each 11 1/2 x 14 in.

Inscription left: "THOMAS JEFFERSON UNIVERSITY HOSPITAL/THOMAS EAKINS/HEAD OF THE SCHUYLKILL REGATTA/Women's eight"; right: "THOMAS JEFFERSON UNIVERSITY HOSPITAL/THOMAS EAKINS/HEAD OF THE SCHUYLKILL REGATTA/Championship Eight"
Stamped on back: "Schroth HANDMADE STERLING 41 FOR J. E. CALDWELL CO. D"

Ordered in 1985 by TJU
Accession numbers: 1985+e.DA.01-02

Between 1985 and 1990 the Eakins Head of the Schuylkill Regatta silver plates were trophies in a race cosponsored by Thomas Jefferson University Hospital. The regatta was named in memory of Thomas Eakins, whose paintings of scullers on Philadelphia's rivers reflected the popularity of the sport in late-nineteenth-century America.[11]

By 1858 Philadelphia already had nine boat clubs that promoted and regulated amateur rowing competitions. It was an egalitarian sport that included women's regattas. Among the professional rowers the brothers John and Barney Biglin were the crowds' favorites in singles and pairs rowing in the 1860s and 1870s.

The trays are in cartouche form with bowed sides, and straight corners, and a molded edge. The central image is an engraving after a watercolor made in 1873 by Thomas Eakins, *John Biglin in a Single Scull* (Metropolitan Museum of Art). The rower is seen in profile against the New Jersey shoreline of the Delaware River.

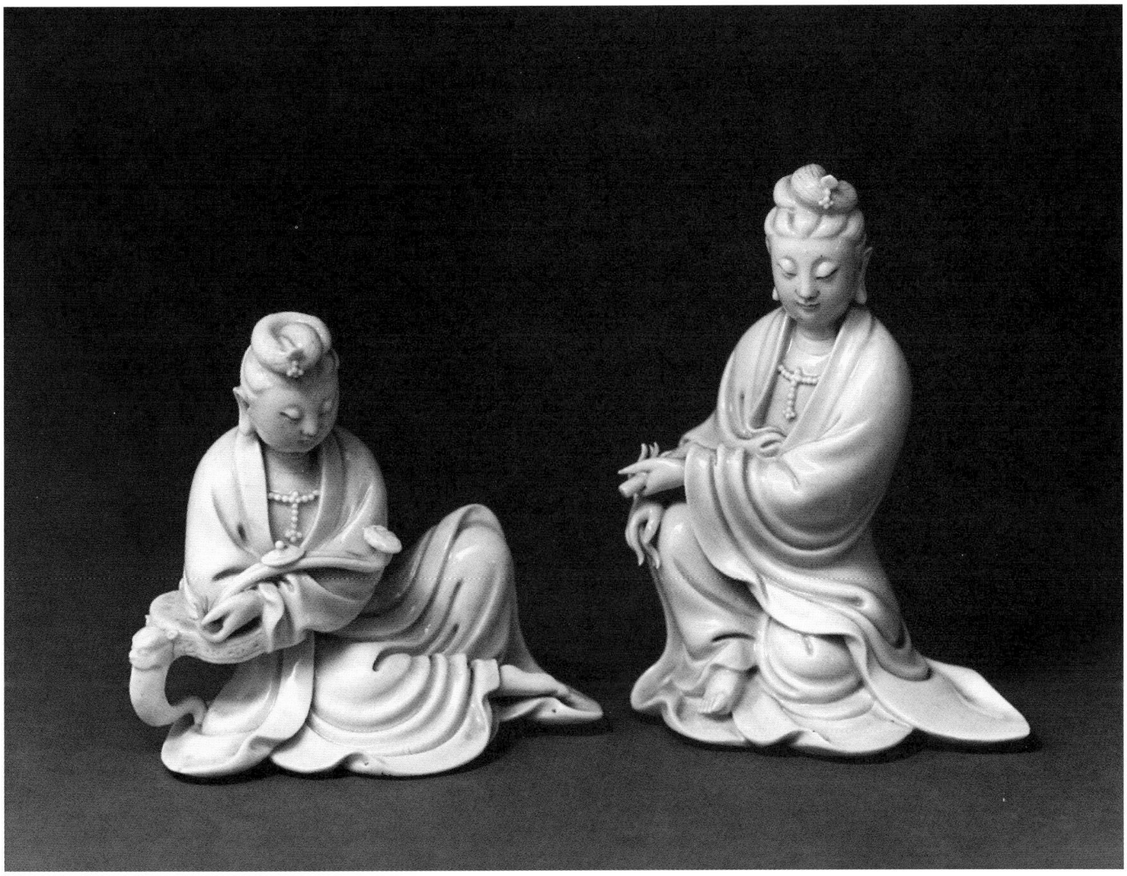

Chinese Figurines of Guanyin

CHINESE FIGURINES OF GUANYIN
By He Chaochun

Porcelain
1662-1722
Left: 5 7/8 x 4 3/8 x 2 5/8 in.
Right: 4 5/8 x 4 3/4 x 2 1/2 in.

Given in 1947 by En Shui Tai, M.D. (JMC 1928): one figure to Jefferson Medical College, the other to Haverford College; both now on long-term loan to Philadelphia Museum of Art
Accession numbers at TJU: 1947+e.DA.01a-01b
Accession numbers at PMA: 9-1947-1a&b, 2a&b
Photograph courtesy of Philadelphia Museum of Art

Like Dr. James A. Hamma, Dr. En Shui Tai was a Jefferson Medical College alumnus who displayed heroism, but of a vastly different type. Dr. Tai had to overcome military and political obstacles to practice his profession under incredibly difficult conditions in Hong Kong during World War II. In gratitude for his education in America (he graduated from Haverford College in 1924 and Jefferson Medical College in 1928), Dr. En Shui Tai presented each school with a traditional Chinese figure of Guanyin, the deity of mercy, in 1947.

Jefferson board of trustees minutes of May 19, 1947 state that the figures "represent the only remaining valuables left him after the destruction of his property in World War II." Dr. Tai did not specify which object was designated for which school. In order to keep the group intact, Haverford and Jefferson agreed to place the Guanyins on long-term loan to the Philadelphia Museum of Art. The figures are not a set, but were made during the same period by the same potter.

In 1946 correspondence with Mrs. Melrose Weed, executive secretary of the alumni association, Dr. Tai described the personal and professional hardships he had endured during the war:

> I was at Lai Chi Kok Hospital when war broke out in Dec. 1941. What little we brought from Canton was lost there. During Japanese occupation, I continued my work at Lai Chi Kok. It was then used as an Infectious Diseases Hospital. Cholera was the principal disease handled from 1942 to 1944.
>
> Our hospital was near to the Standard-Vacuum Oil

Co. Lai Chi Kok Ware House. It was subjected to heavy Allied bombing in Aug. 1944, and we escaped death in less than 300 feet away...God spared my family and myself. The whole locality was set on fire by that bombing...The fire continued for over twelve days until all the stored oil was exhausted. Even the direction of the wind did not change, otherwise, our hospital would have been destroyed. In this way God spared even our shabby worldly treasures of clothing and food...

Since Oct. 1, 1945 I was put in charge of the Tung Wah Eastern Hospital (230 beds) as the Medical Superintendent. Three other medical officers assist me. There are twenty graduate nurses and forty pupil nurses... Chief diseases handled are Tuberculosis (medical and surgical), Malaria, Beriberi, Pellagra (and other nutritional diseases), and some cases of Venereal Diseases.

Much of the equipment was lost during their [the Japanese] occupation...I had to reequipe [*sic*] it with the help of the Hong Kong Government and the British Red Cross.

High cost of living everywhere is the cause of our present misery. I am able only in earning 1/4 of our expenses. The only comfort now is that no more fear of bombing.

However, it is my earnest hope to revisit America in 1948. May God help me to accomplish it. If so I shall attend the 20th Anniversary Reunion of our class.

Dr. Tai enclosed a snapshot of his family including his children Paulina, Bonita, George Marshall, Amy McCrae, and Thomas McCrae, surely named for professor Thomas McCrae, M.D. Further correspondence shows that he fulfilled his dream of attending the reunion.

The Qing Dynasty, white porcelain ("blanc de chine") figurines of Guanyin were created in the Kangxi era (1662-1722). They were made at the Dehua kilns of Fujian Province, bearing the marks of He Chaochun, the younger brother of the more celebrated potter, He Chaozong. Guanyin is the popular bodhisattva (deity) of compassion, the protectress of the household, and patron goddess of mothers, fishermen, and domestic things. Such figures were used in shrines, on scholars' tables, and in households.

Most works made in the Dehua kilns have devotional character and were used for religious purposes. White is the color of mourning in China. Both figures are seated in the Lalitasana ("royal ease") position, with one knee raised and the other lowered, and one foot tucked under the body. They both look demurely downward with heads inclined. The earlier Indian name for this deity is Avalokitesvara, meaning "god looking down."

The figure which sits more erectly holds a scroll in her left hand. Her flowing robe is open to expose a beaded necklace with pendant, and her hair is characteristically coiled and fixed with a small jewel and a hairpin in the form of a ruyi scepter (S-shaped scepter held by statesmen). The other figure reclines on her elbow upon a table raised on a zoomorphic (fantastic beast) cabriole leg. She holds a large ruyi scepter with stylized cloud forms. Her necklace and hairstyle are similar to the first figure's. Curving lines predominate in features, attributes, and drapery.

Decorative Arts from the Louis G. Kareha Collection

DECORATIVE ARTS FROM THE KAREHA COLLECTION

Jade, quartz, coral, horn, lapis lazuli, teak

Given in 1995 by Louis G. Kareha, M.D. (JMC 1943)

Accession numbers of collection: 1995+e.DA.01-68

Another alumnus, Louis G. Kareha, M.D. of the class of 1943, was also a generous benefactor to the Jefferson art collection. In 1995 he presented his cherished collection of sixty-eight decorative arts objects, mainly of Asian origin. Dr. Kareha practiced general medicine in Abington, Pennsylvania for almost half a century before retiring to Florida in 1992 when he began to collect oriental art.

The majority of objects are Chinese jades, and other Chinese pieces made of metal, wood, cork, lapis lazuli, coral, horn, and serpentine. The eclectic group also includes a forty-one-inch carved elephant ivory tusk, a set of Russian lacquer plates, a polychromed metal figure of "Dream Girl" by Erté, and several pictures of American Indian subjects. Included in the gift are a rosewood and two teak display cabinets.

All works are modern except two jade axe heads and a jade "Happy Boy on Water Buffalo" (both shown in the photograph). Although jade is prized around the world, it has been most closely identified with Chinese civilization for more than five thousand years. Worked into ritual objects and ornaments, jade was considered the link between earth and heaven and the bridge from life to immortality, a symbol of protection, health, and strength.

The city of Hotan was the source of Asia's jade from prehistoric times until the late eighteenth century. Hotan jade is of the nephrite type, a silicate of calcium and magnesium, harder than most steel and the toughest (a measure of resistance to breaking) of all rocks, and occurring in a variety of colors depending on trace elements. Nephrite is relatively rare today, and ninety percent of the modern jade market consists of objects made of Burmese jadeite carved in Hong Kong. Jadeite is a silicate of sodium and aluminum even harder than nephrite but more brittle. Best known is the brilliant green "imperial jade" associated with jewelry, but jadeite also comes in paler greens, lavender, black, white, blue, yellow, and red.

Jade is too hard and close-textured to be carved, but is rather cut, ground, and polished by craftsmen who have passed on their skills from generation to generation. Art objects are made from a single block of jade, even those that are delicately incised, intricately pierced, or in extremely high relief.

The photograph shows objects that are Chinese and made of jadeite except where noted below. On the top row are, from left to right: a lavender, green, and white plaque with imperial horses; two rose quartz recumbent water buffalos; and a lavender, green, and white plaque with imperial horses.

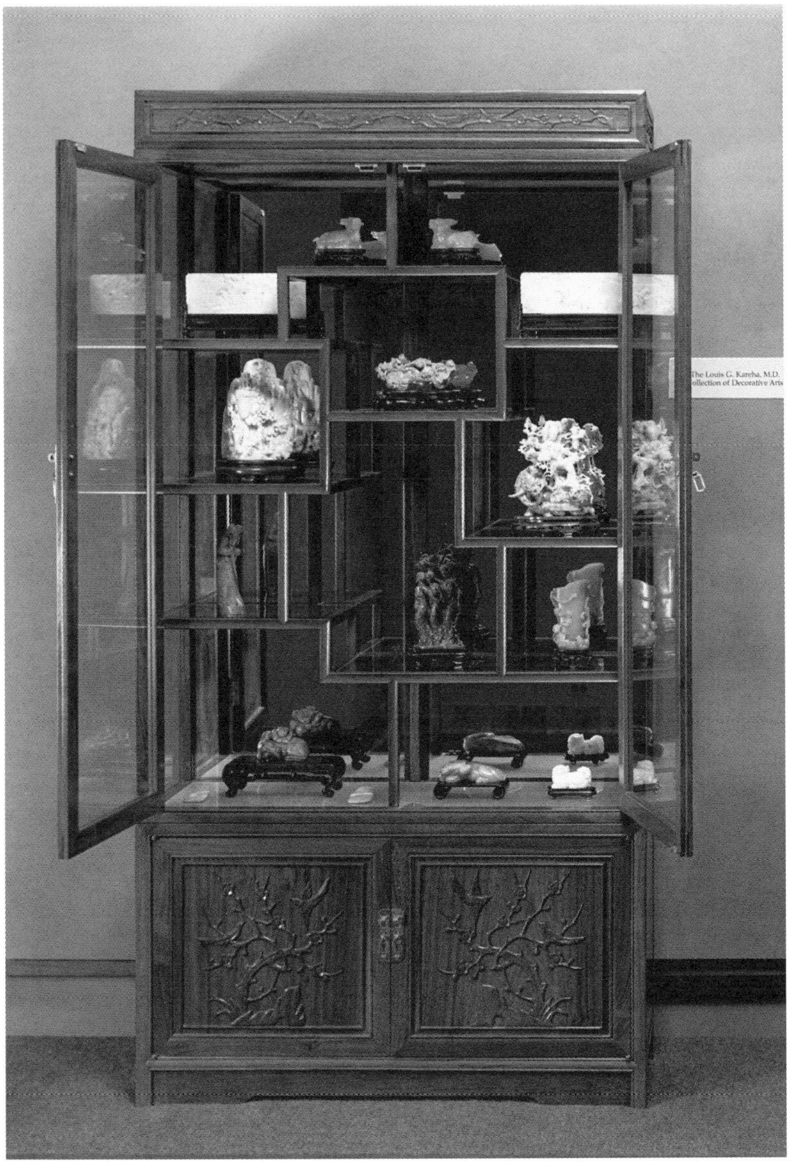

Those on the second row are: a lavender and green "Isle of Blest Immortals" carving of deities, disciples, pagoda, and trees; a coral monkey climbing on the vines of a double gourd; and an intricately carved lavender Guanyin holding a ruyi scepter and seated on a dark green kneeling elephant, surrounded by three small children floating in cloud forms.

Objects on the third row include: a rhinoceros horn figurine of Shou-Lai, god of longevity, holding a cane and cup; a Russian lapis lazuli carving of the Three Graces in front of a pedestal surmounted by two playful putti; and a green vase with beasts, clouds, and waves.

On the bottom row are: two pre-Ming dynasty axe heads flanking a pre-Ming dynasty green and rust colored "Happy Boy on Water Buffalo"; a "mutton-fat" and yellow recumbent water buffalo; and a "mutton-fat" and rust Fo Dog (lionlike guardian) watching a cub.

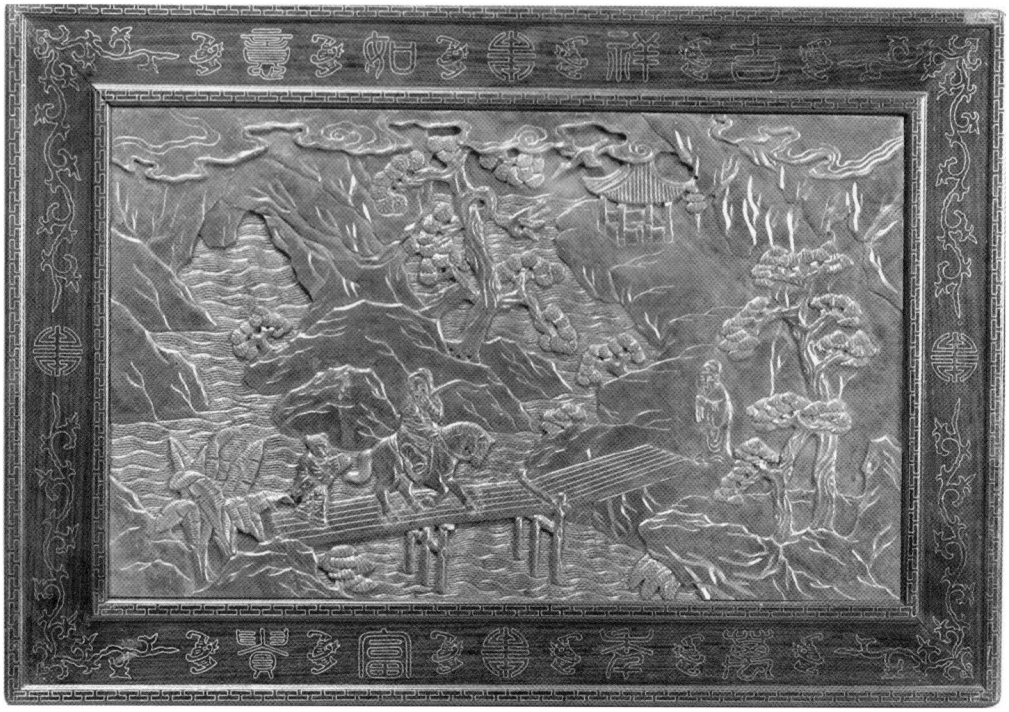

Table Screen

TABLE SCREEN

Jade, teak, silver
Twentieth century
27 1/2 x 32 1/2 x 11 in.
(see above)

One of the most spectacular pieces in the Kareha collection is a thirty-two-inch-wide, jade table screen. The mottled green screen is delicately carved with a mounted warrior followed by a servant crossing a river on a dock on stilts, heading toward the shore where a venerable, wise man waits. His pagoda-like shrine is at the top of the mountain. The figures are surrounded by stylized wavy water, foliage, pine trees, clouds, and hills. The screen rests in a teak frame inlaid with silver wire to embellish the wood with vines and calligraphy.

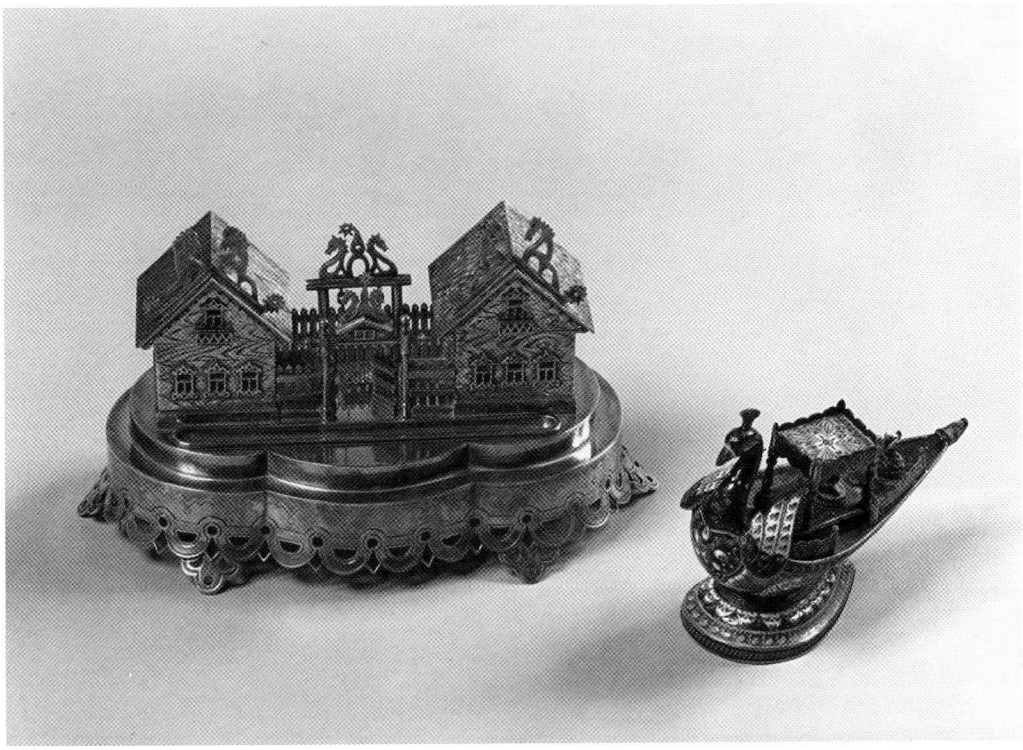

Selections from the Dr. and Mrs. Robert T. Sataloff Collection of Decorative Arts

SELECTIONS FROM THE SATALOFF COLLECTION

Silver inkstand, ca. 1890
Enamel-over-silver boat, nineteenth century

Collection given between 1995 and 1997 by Robert T. Sataloff, M.D. (JMC 1975), professor of otolaryngology, and Mrs. Sataloff

Accession numbers of collection: 1995+e.DA.69-92, 1996+e.DA.03-12, and 1997+e.DA.01-25

Robert T. Sataloff, M.D., professor of otolaryngology at Thomas Jefferson University, has made generous donations of diverse metal decorative arts from his collection between 1995 and 1997. Included are European, Russian, and Asian objects and jewelry ranging in age from medieval to early-twentieth-century.

Dr. Sataloff is a Jefferson alumnus of the class of 1975 and the son of Dr. and Mrs. Joseph Sataloff (see above). The younger Sataloff has combined his medical and musical interests in unique ways to benefit both his patients and the university's cultural life. A trained baritone and choral conductor, he helped to establish voice as a subspecialty in otolaryngology, and developed a voice center that trains otolaryngology residents and fellows from around the world.

In 1970 he founded the Jefferson choir which he has conducted uninterruptedly except while away for his residency. This choir admits all members of the Jefferson community who want to sing, without audition. In 1980 he founded the smaller and more select Chamber Singers.

The photograph includes two small but exceptional objects from the Robert Sataloff collection. On the left is a Russian, silver inkstand of architectural design thought to be made by Okurlukov about 1890. The unusual design features two roofed buildings containing inkwells which flank a central fenced courtyard with a tall entrance gate decorated with dragons. The whole construction rests on an incised and pierced stand, eight and one-half inches long in all.

The other object is a nineteenth-century, enamel-over-silver boat from Jaipur, India. It measures only five and three-eighths inches long. The brightly decorated and patterned boat is in the shape of a peacock resting on a teardrop-shaped base. The interior has a figure with an attendant beneath a high canopy with decoration that augments the overall geometric design.

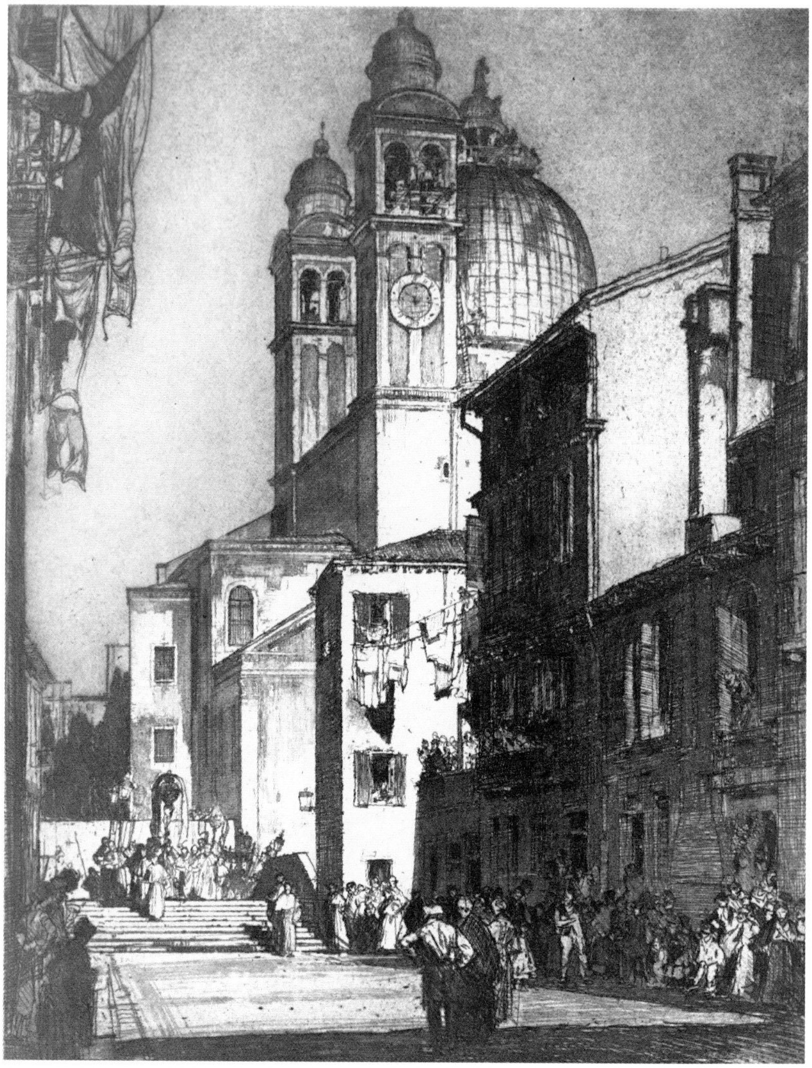

Santa Maria della Salute, Venice

SANTA MARIA DELLA SALUTE, VENICE
By Sir Frank Brangwyn (1867-1956)

Etching
1907
Image size: 21 3/4 x 17 3/8 in.
Sheet size: 31 1/2 x 26 3/4 in.

Signed lower right below image: "Frank Brangwyn"

Given in 1996 by Howard L. Field, M.D., clinical professor of psychiatry and human behavior, who had received it from Robert E. Jones, M.D., professor of psychiatry and human behavior

Accession number: 1996+e.Pr.01

Sir Frank Brangwyn was a celebrated English painter, muralist, designer, and printmaker. He did not begin to experiment with etching until 1900, originally as a relaxation while on holidays. From early on he employed a large zinc plate, rather than the more commonly used copper plate. He produced more than three hundred etchings in the first two decades of the twentieth century.

Recurring subjects are architectural landmarks, rivers and bridges, and industrial scenes. Brangwyn's expressive works combine descriptive linear draftsmanship with dramatic tonal qualities of light and shade.

A typical etching is *Santa Maria della Salute, Venice,* depicting a view from the street dominated by the famous domed church with twin towers. Clusters of people on the street and in balconies observe a solemn procession descending the church steps. Fluttering laundry on clotheslines strung between buildings on the left animates the scene. Light floods the church and the procession, while the foreground buildings and observers are in deep shadow. Variants of Brangwyn's depictions of Santa Maria della Salute won the gold medal at Venice's International Exhibition in 1907 and the Grand Prix at Milan's International Exhibition in 1908.

The Jefferson collection received three other Brangwyn etchings from Dr. Howard L. Field in 1996. *Cannon Street Station, Exterior* shows commuters descending steps from a smoky railroad station bridge and workers shoveling coal on the London quay; *Old Bridge, Albi* is a view under a Roman arched bridge toward buildings lining the river bank and distant bridges; and *House of the Poet, Elizabeth Barrett Browning, Venice* depicts festive passengers in gondolas approaching the English poet's stone palazzo, decorated with waving banners.

Of Welsh extraction, Frank Brangwyn was born in Bruges in 1867. His father was a church architect who moved the family to London in 1875. The son received little formal education but showed an aptitude for drawing. He was employed from 1882 to 1884 in the workshop of William Morris (1834-1896), the multitalented designer, poet, and originator of the Arts and Crafts Movement.

In the 1890s Brangwyn traveled through Europe, the Near East, and South Africa where he found enough subjects for a lifetime of picture making. Around 1900 Brangwyn's closeness to Morris and to designer and architect Arthur H. Mackmurdo (1851-1942) launched him into a brief but meteoric career designing jewelry and decorative objects, even whole rooms, in the international Art Nouveau style, an outgrowth of the Arts and Crafts movement.

Brangwyn was a prolific artist most widely known for his large scale murals depicting the labors of the working class. Notable commissions were for Skinners' Hall, the Royal Exchange, and Lloyd's Register, all in London; Christ's Hospital in Horsham, and the Guildhall in Swansea. He received commissions in America for the Panama-Pacific Exposition in San Francisco, the Missouri State Capitol, the Court House in Cleveland, and Rockefeller Center.

Brangwyn was elected to the Royal Academy in 1919. In 1924 a large exhibition of his work was opened by Prime Minister Ramsay MacDonald. He was knighted in 1941. The Royal Academy awarded him the unprecedented honor of a retrospective during his own lifetime in 1952. Bruges made him an honorary citizen in thanks for the gift of a large collection of his work to be housed in a special museum. Another Brangwyn museum was established in Orange, France. His work is represented in major painting and print collections worldwide.

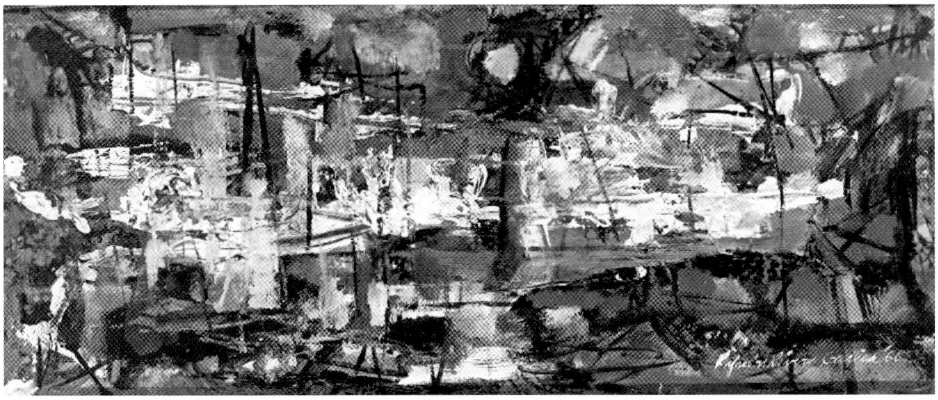

Landscape I: Puerto Rico

LANDSCAPE I: PUERTO RICO
By Rafael Rivera García (b. 1929)

Oil on wood
1960
14 1/2 x 36 in.

Signed and dated lower right: "Rafael Rivera García '60"

Given in 1990 by Lola Saska Tilden, member TJU Hospital women's board
Accession number: 1990+e.P.06

Landscape I: Puerto Rico, an abstract oil by Rafael Rivera García, was donated to Jefferson in 1990 by Lola Saska Tilden, daughter of August Saska, M.D., an alumnus of the class of 1917.

The background of the thickly painted, colorful abstraction is painted in overlapping shapes in red, green, rust, brown, yellow, black, and white. Superimposed are black vertical lines suggesting trees or masts of sailboats rising from an aquamarine shape in the center foreground. A note on the back of the painting suggests that the overall shape represents the geographical configuration of the island.

Rafael Rivera García is a native New Yorker born in 1929. After studying at the High School of Music and Art, his education continued at Columbia University, the Pratt Institute, the Institute of Contemporary Art in Boston, the University of Florida in Gainesville, and the University of Miami. In Puerto Rico he also attended the Political Institute in San Germán.

Associated with the department of fine arts at the University of Puerto Rico, Rivera García's posts have been as assistant director of the museum, director of the laboratory of industrial design, and director of the exhibition gallery of the extension division. He is a member of the Academy of Arts and Sciences of Puerto Rico, and was a founder of the Grupo Borinquen Twelve.

The painter has exhibited widely in galleries and museums in Puerto Rico, Guatemala, New York, Cleveland, Detroit, and Miami. In 1969 he had a solo show at the Museum of the University of Puerto Rico.

Pueblo

PUEBLO
By Gino Hollander (b. 1924)

Acrylic on canvas
1984
47 x 70 1/2 in.

Signed and dated lower right: "Gino Hollander 84"

Given in 1986 by Dr. and Mrs. Allen Cohen in memory of Eric Ivan Cohen
Accession number: 1986+e.P.03

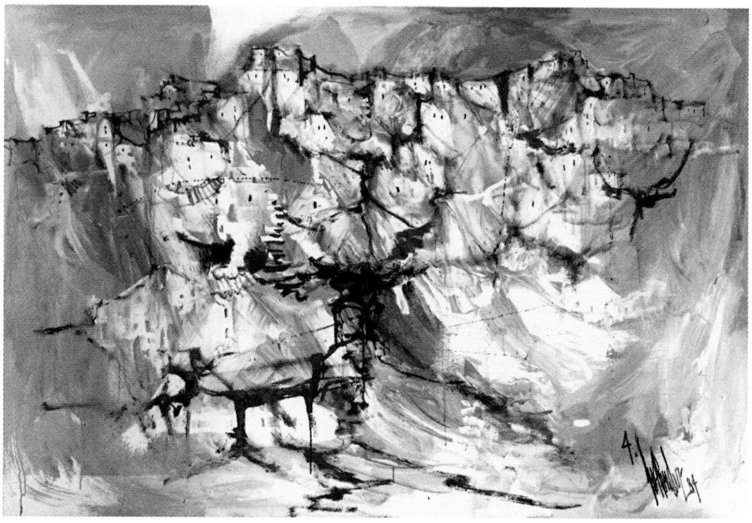

Pueblo by Gino Hollander was donated in 1986 by Dr. and Mrs. Allen Cohen. It too is a gestural, abstract, oil painting, though with more references to nature than Rafael Rivera García's *Landscape I: Puerto Rico.*

The background colors are more muted in keeping with southwest American arid land: white, yellow, tan, orange, and pale blue. Superimposed are black lines in a calligraphic suggestion of small stone or adobe dwellings built in terraces hugging an overhanging cliff. The buildings are punctuated by numerous small windows. The strong yellow and white colors suggest blinding heat and light.

Gino Hollander was born in New York in 1924 and educated at Rutgers and Hobart Universities. He has had frequent one-person shows throughout Europe and the United States. His works are found in the collections of New York University, the 92nd Street Y, and Sloan-Kettering and Columbia Presbyterian Hospitals, all in New York; and at Cornell University, the Dallas Opera and Dallas/Fort Worth Airport, Boys Town U.S.A., and the University of Minnesota.

Gino Hollander has made his home in southern Spain since the early 1960s. European institutions that have acquired his work include the Tate Gallery in London and the Museo de Bellas Artes in Spain.

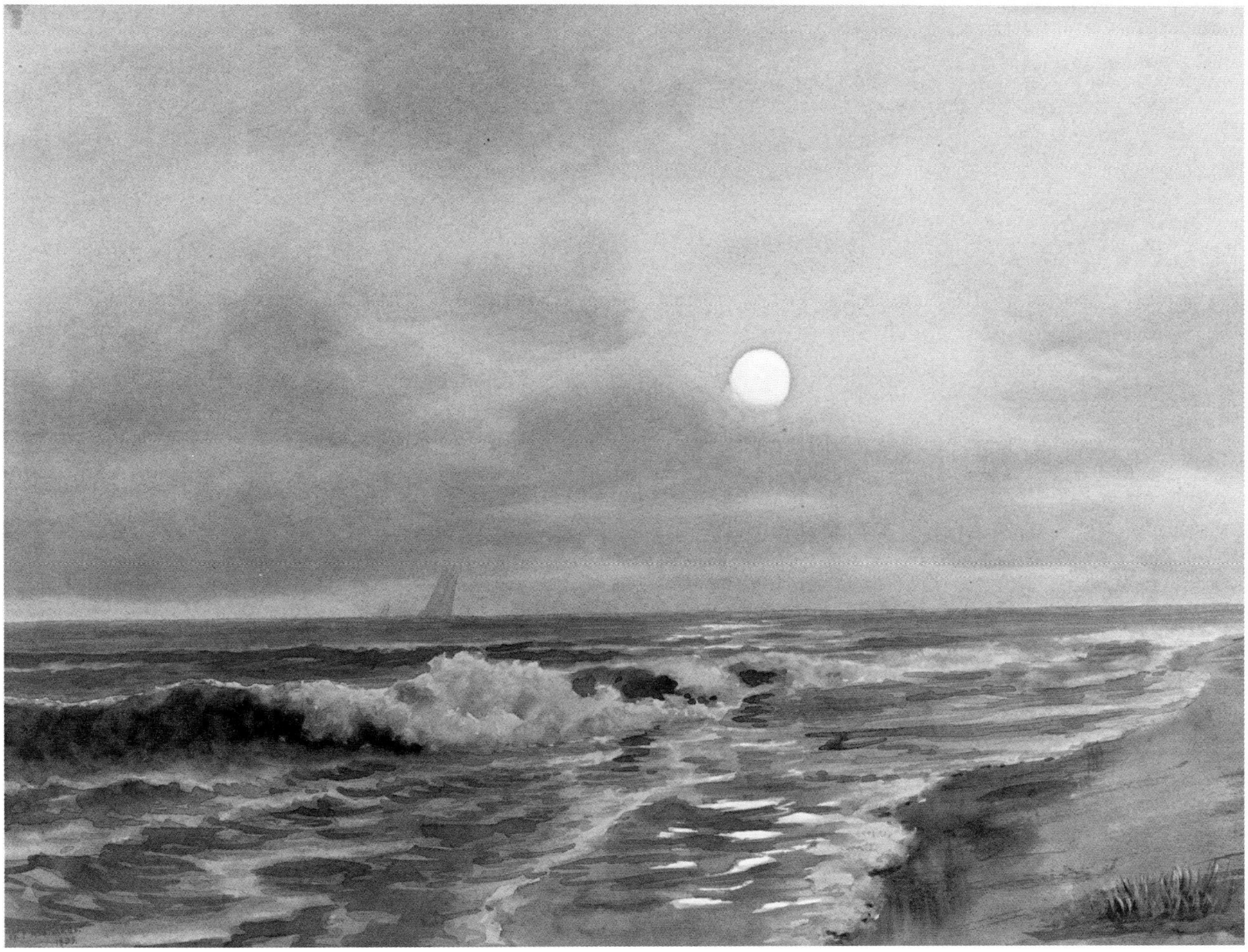

Moonlit Marine

MOONLIT MARINE
By William Trost Richards (1833-1905)

Watercolor on paper
1895
10 1/4 x 14 1/4 in.

Signed and dated lower left: "W. T. RICHARDS/1895"

Given in 1996 by Dr. Joseph Sataloff, professor of otolaryngology, and Mrs. Sataloff
Accession number: 1996+e.P.07

A lovely watercolor of waves breaking close to an irregular shoreline on a moonlit night was painted by William Trost Richards, an American nineteenth-century landscape painter. He was celebrated on both sides of the Atlantic for his paintings of the sea. Richards was noted for his careful observations of the motion of water and the effects of weather.

The cloud-filled sky occupies almost two-thirds of the painting, adding an expansiveness that belies the small dimensions of the picture. The almost full moon emerging from the clouds creates an eerie and poetic light reflecting on the water below. Behind the highest foamy crest can be seen two shadowy sailboats on the distant horizon. There is no other hint of human activity.

The tonalist, modulated colors of ivory and grayish umber above are repeated below with the addition of soft greens in the water and shore. One can almost hear the churning waves in the middle distance and the lapping water approaching the land in the foreground.

William Trost Richards was born in 1833 in Philadelphia. He made a living at the age of seventeen by designing ornamental gas fixtures for a local chandelier manufacturer, while studying art in the evening with German-born portrait and landscape painter Paul Weber (1823-1916). In 1855 Richards left for Europe to study and travel for a year, and then returned to Philadelphia.

By 1863 his mastery of the landscape genre was so

advanced that he was elected an academician at the National Academy of Design at the age of thirty. That same year he was invited to join the Society for the Advancement of Truth in Art, an American Pre-Raphaelite group, based on his botanical and geological study of nature. His paintings featured minutely detailed landscapes of the Adirondacks and other American and European picturesque locations.

On the return from another trip to Europe in 1867 he was so fascinated with the experience of a violent storm at sea, that he resolved to concentrate on marine painting as a subject. He spent the next few summers observing coastal scenes along the Atlantic seaboard, and in 1875 bought a summer home in Newport, Rhode Island. His primary subject in watercolor became the Northeast coast from New Jersey to Maine, especially the area around Newport and Jamestown. His marine subject matter introduced a new painterly style with less emphasis on detail, and looser brush strokes, broader treatment of form, and a reduced palette.

In 1878 he began a two-year visit to England where he produced oils and watercolors of scenes along the coasts of Devon, Cornwall, and Dorset that were exhibited at the Royal Academy of London and the Paris Exposition. In 1882 he built a home and studio overlooking the Narragansett Bay and Newport. He also purchased a farm in Chester County, Pennsylvania which inspired him with its wooded hills, winding streams, and fields. Oil sketches of this rural area were the foundation for more monumental oil paintings.

Richards showed regularly at the National Academy of Design, the American Water Color Society, the Pennsylvania Academy of the Fine Arts, and the Royal Academy of London. Among his awards were bronze medals at the 1876 Centennial Exposition and the Paris Exposition of 1889. The Pennsylvania Academy of the Fine Arts awarded him the Temple Silver Medal in 1885 and the Gold Medal of Honor in 1905.

Lakefront

LAKEFRONT
By Marguerite Thompson Zorach (1887-1968)

Watercolor on paper
1947
6 x 8 1/2 in.

Signed and dated lower right: "M. Zorach/'47"

Given in 1994 by Dr. Joseph Sataloff, professor of otolaryngology, and Mrs. Sataloff
Accession number: 1994+e.P.03

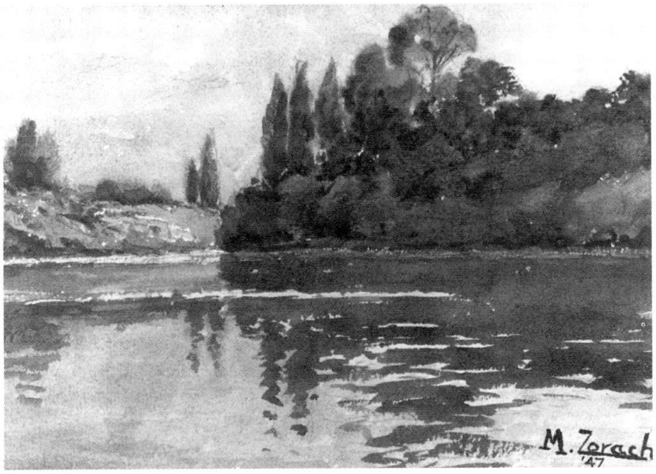

Marguerite T. Zorach was a multifaceted painter in oil and watercolor, a textile designer, printmaker, and illustrator. Her approach to landscape is generalized and her style is modernist.

Zorach's depiction uses rich, opaque colors to describe the large forms of trees and shrubbery at the edge of a lake. Deep greens, yellows, and browns of the foliage are reflected in paler and more transparent colors in the streaky water. An overcast sky of pinks, blues, and violets color the water, alternating with reflections of foliage. A few traces of uncolored white paper serve as highlights in the effervescent and sparkling scene.

Born Marguerite Thompson in Santa Rosa, California in 1887, she was reared in Fresno where her father was an attorney for the Napa vineyards. She was about to start her freshman year at Stanford University in 1908 when she was invited to study art in Europe by an aunt who paid her expenses. She spent four years in Paris studying first at the traditional École de la Grande Chaumière and then at the more avant-garde school, La Pallette, where she met her future husband, William Zorach (1887-1966). Both artists were influenced by the bold colors and shocking distortions of Fauvist and Cubist art.

Thompson traveled in the Middle East and Asia before returning to the United States. The couple was married in 1913 in New York. They exhibited and socialized with avant-garde artists in Greenwich Village and Provincetown, Massachusetts. Although sculptor William Zorach's career eventually eclipsed that of his wife, in the early years they were considered of equal importance, and exhibited jointly in museums and galleries in New York, Cleveland, Dayton, San Francisco, and Maine.

Marguerite Thompson Zorach was the only woman to be included in the landmark Forum Show at the Anderson Galleries in New York in 1916. In 1925 she became the founder and first president of the New York Society of Women Artists which sponsored lively and controversial exhibitions of modernist paintings. Her work in the last decades of her career became more representational and traditional.

Marguerite Zorach's paintings were accepted at other important exhibitions, including the Société des Artistes Indépendants and the Salon d'Automne in Paris in 1911, the New York Armory exhibition in 1913, and several times with the Society of Independent Artists in New York. She was honored with solo shows at galleries in Los Angeles and New York, Colby College in Waterville, Maine, the California Palace of the Legion of Honor, and the National Collection of Fine Arts in Washington, D.C.

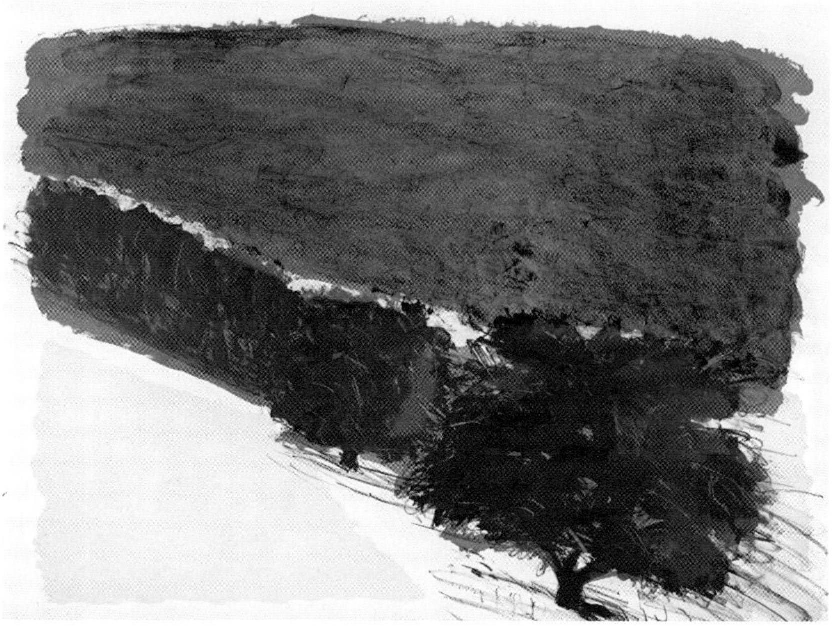

Untitled (Landscape)

UNTITLED (LANDSCAPE)
By Wolf Kahn (b. 1927)

Colored lithograph
1969
Image size: 20 3/4 x 28 in.
Sheet size: 22 1/8 x 29 3/4 in.

Signed lower center: "W. Kahn/1969"
Edition number lower left: "XXXVIII/L"

Given in 1991 by Dr. and Mrs. Gilbert W. Palley
Accession number: 1991+e.Pr.02

Dr. and Mrs. Gilbert W. Palley, employers of a grateful Jefferson patient, presented a diverse group of prints to Thomas Jefferson University in 1991. Among the works is an untitled colored lithograph by contemporary printmaker and painter Wolf Kahn.

Kahn's modernist approach to landscape is attentive to expressive brush work, abstract forms, and color that evolved from brilliantly rich to lyrically subtle. Jefferson's untitled lithograph of 1969 features a wide diagonal band of greenish-black trees, solidly rendered and almost coalescing. Above is a large, menacing, dark gray triangle suggestive of looming storm clouds. A pale yellow triangle in the lower left corner is a smaller mirror image of the upper triangle. All forms have irregular and tattered edges.

Wolf Kahn was born in 1927 in Stuttgart, Germany. He emigrated to the United States in 1940 and graduated from the High School of Music and Art in New York. After serving in the navy during the war, he studied painting with the famous painter, color theorist, and teacher Hans Hofmann (1880-1966) and became his assistant. He also studied with the modernist artist Stuart Davis (1894-1964) at the New School for Social Research. Kahn graduated from the University of Chicago in 1951 and was honored with a Fulbright scholarship and a Guggenheim fellowship. He has taught at the University of California at Berkeley, and was artist-in-residence at Dartmouth College.

Wolf Kahn has traveled extensively and painted landscapes in Mexico, Italy, Greece, Kenya, and Egypt. He resides in New York, but since 1968 has spent the summers on a farm in Brattleboro, Vermont with his wife, the painter Emily Mason.

Kahn won the Art Award from the American Academy and Institute of Arts and Letters in 1979, was elected a member of the academy in 1984, and has served as its vice president for art. He became an academician of the National Academy of Design in 1980, and was appointed to the New York City Art Commission in 1993.

Wolf Kahn has had solo exhibitions at prominent museums and galleries throughout the country, and almost annually at the Grace Borgenicht Gallery in New York since 1956. His work is included in corporate and museum collections throughout the country. He has been the subject of numerous articles and reviews and the monograph *Wolf Kahn, Landscape Painter* (1981) by Martica Sawin.

The World Is So Wonderful—and I Sob!

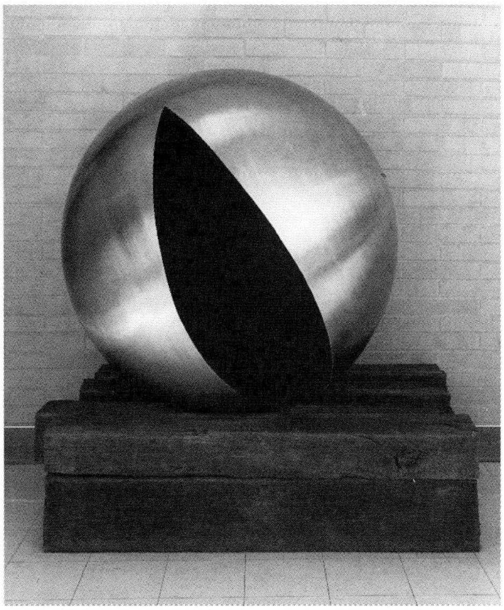

THE WORLD IS SO WONDERFUL—AND I SOB!
By Gladys Noble Wagner (1907-87)

Stainless steel, enamel, wood
Before 1982
56 1/2 x 56 x 43 1/2 in.

Signed on back right of railroad tie: "G. NOBLE WAGNER/THE WORLD IS SO WONDERFUL/—AND I SOB!"
Exhibition: Philadelphia, *Sculpture '82*, Franklin Plaza and the International Garden of Franklin Town, 1982

Given in 1982 on long-term loan by the artist, through the efforts of Lola Saska Tilden, member TJU Hospital women's board and daughter of August Saska, M.D. (JMC 1917)
Accession number: 1982+e.S.01L

The World Is So Wonderful—and I Sob! is a geometric, abstract sculpture made by Philadelphia artist Gladys Noble Wagner. It is constructed of polished stainless steel, enamel paint, and railroad ties.

The main component is a machine-milled, metal sphere, forty-two inches in diameter. It has a reflective, silvery external surface and is painted royal blue inside. A diagonal crescent-shaped hole carved into the front allows a view inside the interior's dark blue void. Because the negative space of the opening is cut on a slant, the huge round form seems to be tilting off balance. But the sphere rests firmly on rows of irregularly sized, old, rough-hewn railroad ties, two rows high and four rows deep.

The high sheen and thinness of the aluminum surface of the construction contrast with the dull, gouged surface and thickness of the recycled wooden base. The contrasts of old and new materials, smooth and rough surfaces, and positive and negative spaces are surely metaphors for the enigmatic and emotional title of the construction.

G. Noble Wagner was a native Philadelphian born in 1907. She plunged into studying art only after her five children were in school, and received bachelor's and master's degrees in fine arts from the Tyler School of Art of Temple University.

Wagner has exhibited her large-scale, geometric sculptures, paintings, and prints in solo shows at the Philadelphia Art Alliance, Franklin and Marshall College, Lehigh University, the University City Science Center in Philadelphia, and galleries in Philadelphia, Washington, New York, Chicago, and Atlanta. She won alumni awards from Tyler (1968 and 1979) and from Temple University (1970). Her work is in many private and corporate collections, as well as the Philadelphia Museum of Art and the Albright-Knox Museum in Buffalo.

G. Noble Wagner was a cofounder of the Cheltenham Art Center in 1940 and founder of the Cheltenham Playhouse, both in suburban Philadelphia. She was director of education at the art center for many years, and also instructor in art education at Temple University. She established the Aegean School of Fine Arts in Paros, Greece as a branch of the Cheltenham Art Center.

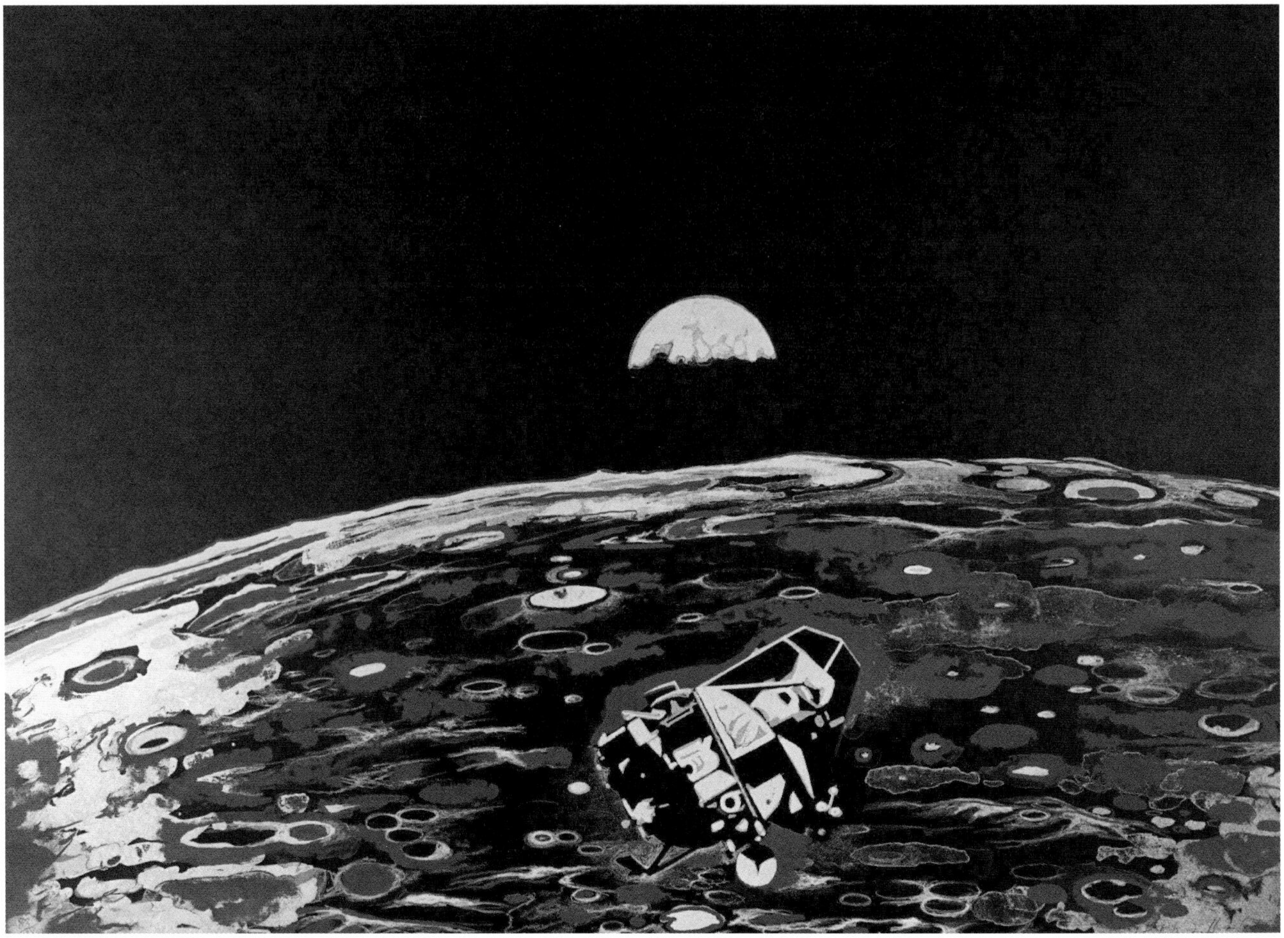

Moon Shot (Number Four)

MOON SHOT (NUMBER FOUR)
By Lowell Blair Nesbitt (1933-93)

Colored lithograph on black paper
1969
Image size: 14 3/4 x 29 3/4 in.
Sheet size: 22 x 29 7/8 in.

Signed and dated lower right: "L. Nesbitt-'69"
Edition number lower left: "83/98"

Given in 1991 by Dr. and Mrs. Gilbert W. Palley
Accession numbers of entire series: 1991+e.Pr.04-11

Among the works donated by Dr. and Mrs. Gilbert W. Palley is a series entitled *Moon Shot* by Lowell B. Nesbitt. He is one among many distinguished artists employed by NASA's art program, and is represented in the official art collection at the visitors center at the Kennedy Space Center in Florida.[12]

Nesbitt's 1969 *Moon Shot* series is comprised of eight silver and gray-toned lithographs on black paper depicting the flight of Apollo Eleven. At exactly 9:32 a.m. on July 16, 1969 the crew of Apollo Eleven, astronauts Neil A. Armstrong, Michael Collins, and Edward E. Aldrin Jr., were sent to the moon by a Saturn Five launch vehicle from Cape Kennedy, Florida. Armstrong and Aldrin descended to the moon surface on July 20 declaring, "Houston, Tranquility Base here. The *Eagle* has landed!" People the world over witnessed these events on television and will always remember Neil Armstrong saying, "That's one small step for a man, one giant leap for mankind."

The crew fulfilled President John F. Kennedy's mandate by becoming the first men to set foot on the moon and to take steps in an alien world. During their extravehicular activity they took soil and rock samples and also set up three instrument systems for collecting scientific data about solar winds, seismic activity, and the motions of the earth and moon. After two and one-half hours of working in the "magnificent desolation" of the lunar surface and planting a metallic American flag, on July 21 Armstrong and Aldrin rejoined Collins in the Command Module circling the moon. The astronauts splashed down in the Pacific Ocean and recovery was made at 12:50 p.m. on July 24, 1969.

Nesbitt's Apollo Eleven series of eight colored lithographs begins with a print consisting of quotations by astronauts Stafford, Lovell, Borman, Schweickart, Aldrin, and Armstrong written in silver script. The seven views of the lunar surface that follow were taken after historic photographs made by the astronauts; they feature long-range and then closeup views of the moon's craters and valleys. The first view (number two in the series) shows the moon viewed from the Apollo spacecraft during its approach. Number three shows the moon viewed from Apollo as the spacecraft prepares to go into lunar orbit.

Number four is pictured here, showing *Eagle*, the Lunar Excursion Module (LEM) approaching *Columbia*, the Command Module, for docking. Both spacecraft orbit the moon, and the earth can be seen 235,000 miles away in the black sky. The next image shows the moon's crater looming into view as the LEM descends to the lunar surface. Number six is the lunar landing area showing Rover tracks after the LEM left the surface for the rendezvous with Apollo. This is followed by a view of craters and Rover tracks from the LEM. The final image is of an astronaut's footprint sunk into the powdery surface of the lunar soil.[13]

Jefferson Medical College is proud to be the alma mater of astronaut James P. Bagian, M.D., who graduated with the class of 1977. After acceptance into the space program Dr. Bagian received training as a flight surgeon and took a residency in anesthesiology. In March 1989 he flew aboard the spaceship *Discovery*, carrying into space a bronze Jefferson medallion later presented to President Lewis W. Bluemle Jr., M.D.

Lowell B. Nesbitt was a well known painter, sculptor, and printmaker. Born in Baltimore in 1933, he was a graduate of Tyler School of Fine Arts at Temple University, and also attended the Royal College of Art in London where he worked in stained glass and etching.

Starting in the 1960s he adopted the photo-realist style of sharply defined edges and accentuated detail in clearly recognizable forms. The *Moon Shot* lithographs exemplify Nesbitt's artistic technique and inclination to work in series, making variations on a theme. Other recurring subjects include closeup views of flowers, groupings of fruits and vegetables, studio interiors, bridges, and facades of nineteenth-century cast iron buildings in the SoHo area of New York City. In 1980 the U.S. Postal Service issued four stamps based on his floral paintings.

Lowell B. Nesbitt had one-man exhibitions in museums and galleries in the United States, Europe, and the Far East, and is represented in numerous public and corporate collections including the Philadelphia Museum of Art, the Museum of Modern Art, the National Gallery of Art, the Art Institute of Chicago, and in Paris at the Beaubourg Museum and the Bibliothèque Nationale.

---

1. Lawrence H. Cohn, M.D., "Contributions of Thomas Jefferson to American Medicine," *American Journal of Surgery* 138 (Aug. 1979): 286-92. See references for additional sources on Jefferson's medical and scientific contributions.
2. For portraits of Thomas Jefferson see: Alfred L. Bush, *The Life Portraits of Thomas Jefferson* (Charlottesville: Thomas Jefferson Memorial Foundation, 1987); William Howard Adams, ed., *The Eye of Thomas Jefferson* (Washington, D.C.: National Gallery of Art, 1976); Noble E. Cunningham Jr., *The Image of Thomas Jefferson in the Public Eye: Portraits for the People 1800-1809* (Charlottesville: University Press of Virginia, 1981); and Fiske Kimball, "The Life Portraits of Jefferson and their Replicas," *Proceedings of the American Philosophical Society* 88 (Dec. 1944): 497-534.
3. Tom Scanlon, "Sculptor Tells How: The Making of a President," *Boston Federal Times*, May 10, 1976, 16-17.
4. For biographical information see: Ronald W. Clark, *Benjamin Franklin: A Biography* (New York: Random House, 1983), 61-91; and Esmond Wright, *Franklin of Philadelphia* (Cambridge, Mass.: Belknap Press of Harvard University Press, 1986), 56-72.
5. The results of my research using primary and secondary sources related to the Franklin and Jefferson portraits first appeared in "Acquiring Our Portraits of Franklin and Jefferson: Contributions of the Corwin Family," *Jefferson Medical College Alumni Bulletin* 41 (fall 1991): 14-15.
6. Charles Coleman Sellers, *Benjamin Franklin in Portraiture* (New Haven: Yale University Press, 1962), 247-49.
7. For information on Indian peace medals see: Adams, 78; Cunningham, 71-78; and Kenneth M. Failor and Eleonora Hayden, *Medals of the United States Mint*, rev. ed. (Washington, D.C.: U.S. Government Printing Office, 1972), 285-88.
8. Lloyd Goodrich, *Thomas Eakins*, 2 vols. (Cambridge, Mass.: Harvard University Press for the National Gallery of Art, Washington, D.C., 1982), 1:223. This opinion was noted in an interview on May 21, 1931 between Goodrich and Weda Cook (Mrs. Stanley) Addicks, a friend and portrait subject of Thomas Eakins.
9. For biography of Foster, see: Jan Reynolds, *Birket Foster* (London: B. T. Batsford Ltd., 1984).
10. A good source for information and references on American coinage is Q. David Bowers, *A Buyer's Guide to Silver Dollars and Trade Dollars of the United States*, 2d ed. (Wolfeboro, N.H.: Bowers and Merena Galleries, 1997).
11. For information on Eakins's rowing pictures and the sport in America see: Helen A. Cooper, *Thomas Eakins: The Rowing Pictures* (New Haven: Yale University Press, 1996).
12. Among other artists employed by NASA are Robert Rauschenberg, Norman Rockwell, James Wyeth, George Weymouth, John McCoy II, Peter Hurd, Lamar Dodd, and Wilson Hurley.
13. I am indebted to Robert Schulman, Director, NASA Art Program, for the technical descriptions of Nesbitt's prints.

Opposite: Skeleton from Albinus's *Tabulae sceleti...*

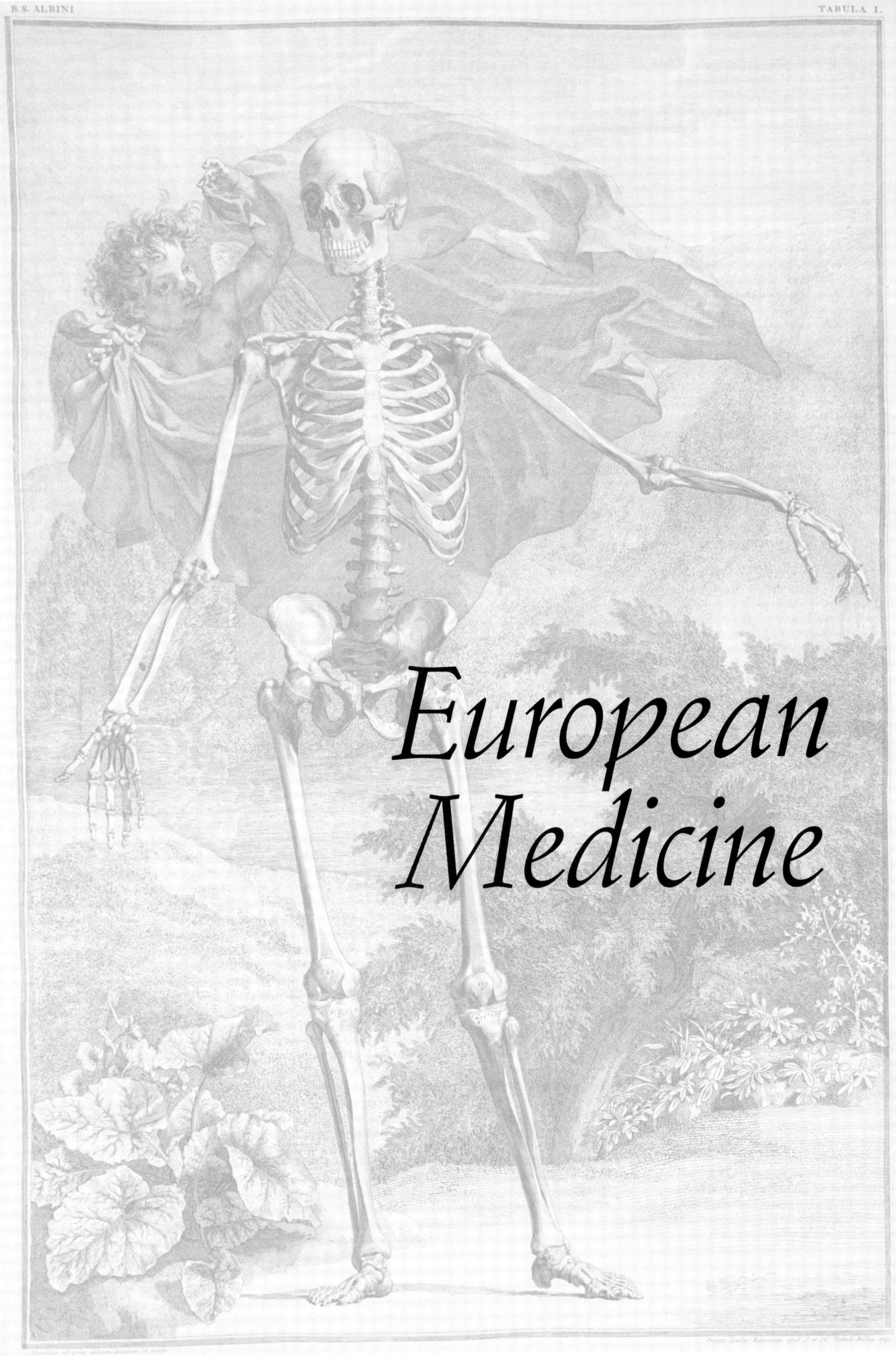

European Medicine

CHAPTER 12

European Medicine and Its Practitioners

This final chapter turns to European objects in the collection. Early Jefferson publications reveal the faculty's indebtedness to its professional forbears across the sea. Dr. Samuel D. Gross was among many who penned biographies of outstanding European physicians. And artistic influence, as well as medical, flowed in both directions across the Atlantic.

Over the years the Jefferson art collection has been enriched with objects that depict European clinical and instructional scenes, portraits and other works associated with famous practitioners, and rare anatomical and obstetrical books.

Surgical, Medical, and Instructional Group Scenes

Ambroise Paré Applying a Ligature on the Arteries after an Amputation for the First Time

AMBROISE PARÉ APPLYING A LIGATURE
By Manceau & Testard, after painting by Louis Nicolas Matout (1811-88)

Engraving, mezzotint, etching stretched onto canvas
After 1864
Image size: 20 1/4 x 37 3/4 in.
Plate size: 24 1/2 x 41 in.
Sheet size: 26 x 43 in.

Inscriptions on plate below image: "PEINT PAR L. MATOUT" and "GRAVÉ PAR MANCEAU & TESTARD" above "AMBROISE PARÉ"

Given 1911-31 by Eugene P. Bernardy, M.D.
Accession number: 1911-1931.Pr.01

The sixteenth-century French military and civilian surgeon Ambroise Paré (1509/10-90) played an important role in propelling European surgery into the modern era. Although he began his career as a common apprentice to a barber-surgeon, Paré eventually achieved great celebrity and rose to serve French royalty.

Ambroise Paré was born in Laval, France, the son of a cabinetmaker. After a meager formal education he was apprenticed to various barber-surgeons in Laval. About 1532 he went to Paris to complete his indentured education at the Hôtel Dieu. There he assisted a surgeon, attended lectures, and did some dissecting. About 1536 he entered the French military service, and in 1541 he became a master barber surgeon and was admitted to the guild of barber-surgeons.

Paré served intermittently as an army field surgeon for the next three decades, and was respected for treating the wounded of both sides during the Wars of Religion. He also engaged in a flourishing civilian practice in Paris and at court. He was honored to be chief surgeon to four French monarchs: Henry II, Francis II, Charles IX, and Henry III, receiving from the last the title "Councilor to His Majesty."

Paré is credited with modernizing Renaissance surgery both by example and by his writings which were translated into many foreign languages. His reputation was so great that he was admitted (albeit grudgingly) to the College of Saint Côme in 1554, in spite of the fact that he wrote his books and delivered his lectures in the French vernacular instead of Latin, the language employed by most educated professionals.

He reported in his first treatise of 1545 that gunshot wounds were not in themselves poisonous and did not require cautery. His military experience taught him that during amputations and wound treatment it was more effective to ligate the blood vessels to suppress hemorrhage rather than the more customary technique of cauterizing with boiling oil. He devised a kind of hemostat, the "crow's beak," used to grasp the vessels to be ligated, as described in his *Dix livres de la chirurgie* (1564). Another treatise dealing with surgical anatomy including obstetrics was published in 1549. He also wrote a popular synopsis of Andreas Vesalius's *Fabrica* (see below) in 1561. His collected works, *Les oeuvres*, were published in 1575.

Paré invented several surgical instruments, designed prostheses for limbs, and improved the hernia band. He also performed the first exarticulation of an elbow joint, described fracture at the neck of the femur, suggested syphilis as a cause for aneurysm, and did reimplantation of teeth and the restoration of missing teeth.

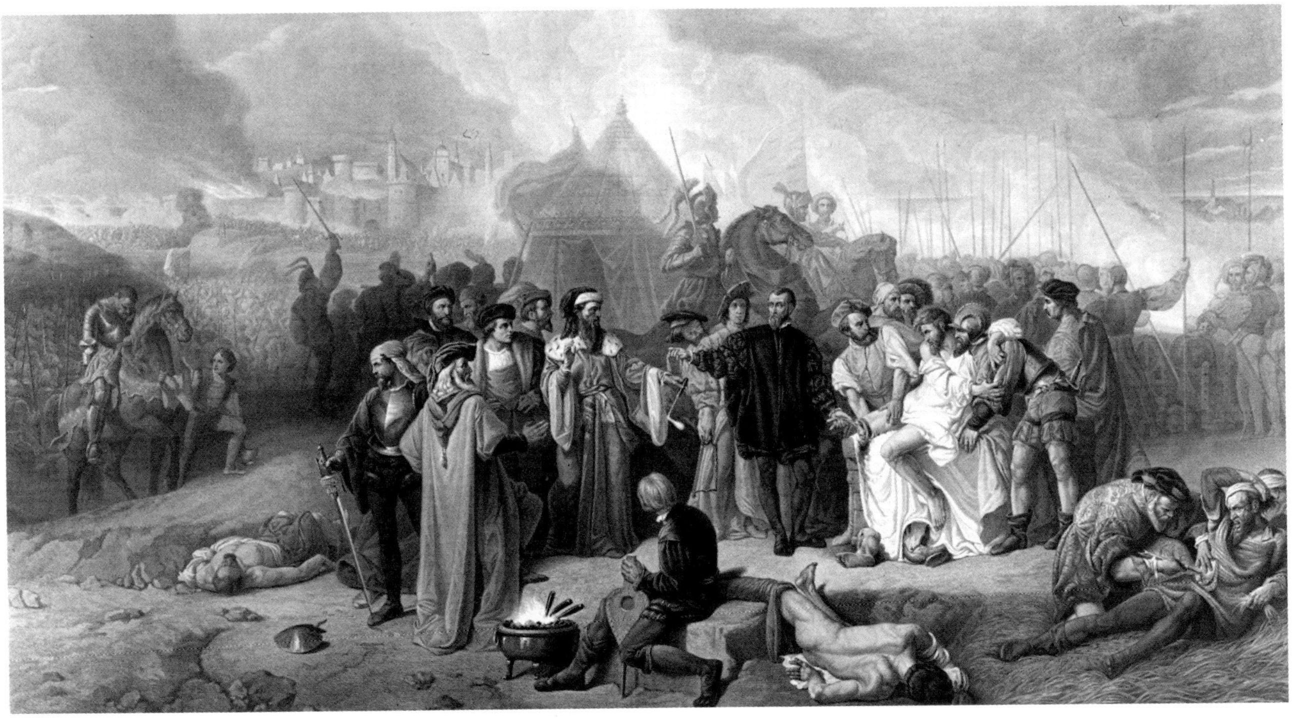

The battlefield print of Ambroise Paré ligating vessels is a copy by Manceau and Testard after a famous painting by French artist Louis N. Matout. His large mural was commissioned for installation in the grand amphitheater of the École de Médecine in Paris in 1864. It was the central panel of a three-part display about significant achievements by French surgeons.[1] Matout is best remembered today for mural decorations of chapels in French hospitals and churches.

The scene shows Ambroise Paré as a field surgeon, the central figure dressed in a short black coat and tights. He is about to ligate the arteries of a wounded soldier who is held down in his chair by two assistant surgeons. The amputated leg of this ill-fated warrior lies on the ground. Paré displays the ligature with an outstretched arm, and points disdainfully toward a brazier heating irons for cauterization, indicating his renunciation of the old technique. At the same time a disapproving group of onlookers is led by another physician, dressed in an ermine-trimmed robe and cap, showing a cauterizing iron in rebuttal of Paré's new technique.

Other wounded men and corpses sprawl in the foreground of the frenetic scene. Flanking a tent in the middle ground are soldiers on horseback and others on the ground brandishing swords and lances. A fortified castle in the distance can be seen through the smoky haze.

Dr. Samuel D. Gross praised Paré's ligature technique as "his greatest service," contrasting it with the ineffective method of cautery, and empathizing with Paré's professional tribulations:[2]

> For ages the only remedy for arresting hemorrhage was the actual cautery, or a piece of heated iron applied directly to the orifice of the bleeding vessel...The result of this practice was that the great majority of those who were subjected to it perished from secondary hemorrhage...If the artery was large, the unfortunate patient generally died soon after the accident, from the inability of the blood to form a sufficiently strong and opposing clot. In many cases the bleeding recurred from time to time until the system was completely drained of blood. The operation was not only painful, but excessively alarming, so that many persons would almost prefer death to submitting to its cruel requirements. When a limb was amputated, the custom for a long time was to plunge the stump in boiling oil or pitch...
>
> But...Opposition met him [Paré] in every quarter. Many of his most influential contemporaries became turbulent and furious in their denunciations, and Paré...suffered for awhile in his practice...
>
> The result of all this malice and opposition was that few of his contemporaries or immediate successors adopted the practice, which, consequently, soon fell into total neglect...
>
> Of the value of the ligature in suppressing hemorrhage, it would be folly at the present day to speak, when its claims are so universally established.

Anatomy Lesson of Dr. Tulp

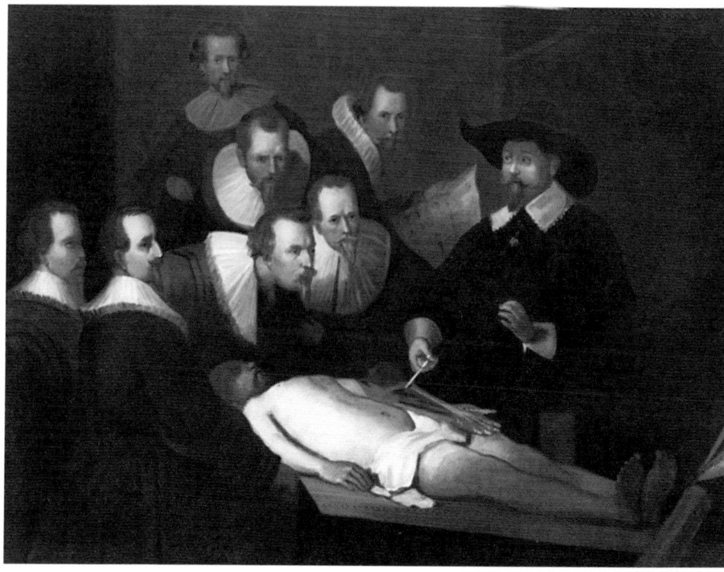

ANATOMY LESSON OF DR. TULP
By unknown artist, after painting by Rembrandt van Rijn (1606-69)

Oil on canvas
Before 1911
36 1/4 x 48 1/4 in.

Given about 1911, probably by Daniel Baugh
Accession number: 1911+c.P.01

Dr. Nicolaas (sometimes Nicolaes) Tulp (1593-1674) is best remembered today as the protagonist in Rembrandt's celebrated *Anatomy Lesson of Dr. Tulp* (Mauritshuis, The Hague). The painting was commissioned by the surgeons' guild in Amsterdam in 1632.

Dr. Tulp was well known among contemporaries for his interest in the pathological changes in the internal organs produced by disease. His *Observationum medicarum libri tres* (1641) included autopsy reports and drawings of diseased organs. The first pharmacopoeia in the Netherlands was compiled at his suggestion.

Nicolaas Tulp was born in 1593 in Amsterdam, the son of a wealthy merchant. He matriculated at the University of Leiden in 1611 and obtained his medical degree there in 1614. He was appointed praelector of anatomy in 1628 and was charged with teaching the surgeons of Amsterdam and illustrating his lectures with public dissections (though he was neither an anatomist nor surgeon). Tulp was also prominent in civic life as a member of the town council, mayor, and curator of the Athenaeum.

The surgeons' guild was among many social and professional groups which commissioned group portraits of their members in seventeenth-century Netherlands. Rembrandt's picture is among several anatomy lessons executed after dissection was legalized.

The painting shows Dr. Nicolaas Tulp demonstrating a dissection of the forearm of a cadaver to Amsterdam's guild of surgeons. An anatomical folio used for instruction is next to the feet of the modestly draped cadaver. The names of the seven surgeons gathered around the table are listed on the paper held by the figure closest to Dr. Tulp. Some scholars feel that the names were subsequently altered so that they no longer identify the actual personages in the painting. Other scholars have long disputed the accuracy of the anatomy displayed. Also in question are whether the setting is imaginary or real, and whether the demonstration was private or public.

The Jefferson copy is of historic interest, though much diminished in emotional intensity, details of costume and architecture, and chiaroscuro effect compared with the original work by Rembrandt. It appears to have been painted in the late nineteenth or early twentieth century. A photograph of 1912 shows the painting hanging in the museum of the Baugh Institute of Anatomy, and today it still hangs in the departmental offices. Copies of Rembrandt's instructional scene original proliferated in the nineteenth century. A version at the College of Physicians of Philadelphia was painted by Dutch artist Wilhelmus H. P. J. de Zwart (1862/67-1931) in 1887.

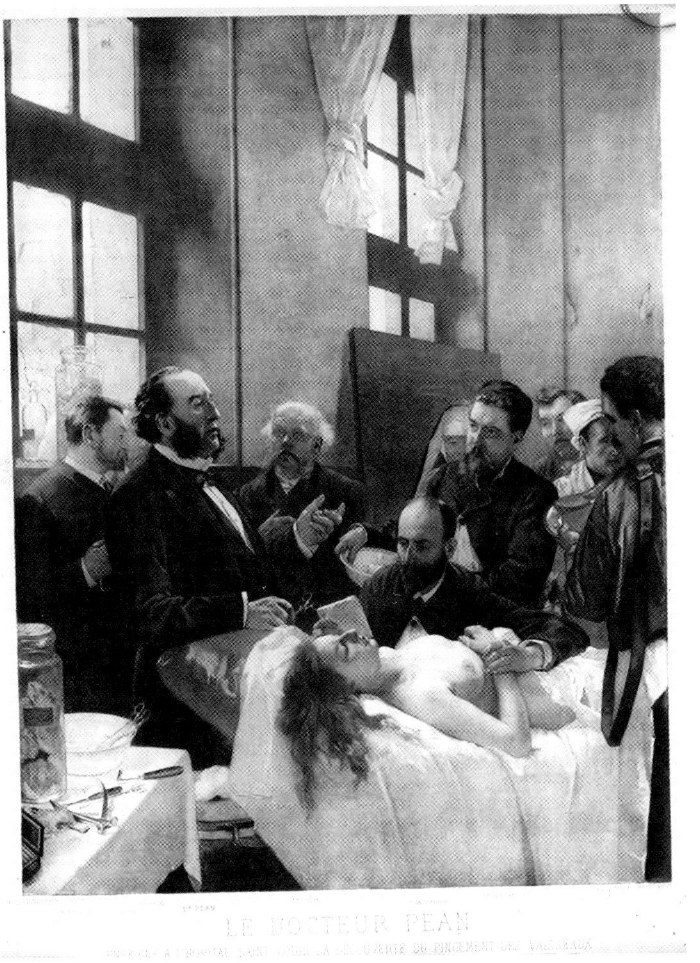

Doctor Péan Teaching His Discovery of the Clamping of Vessels at the St. Louis Hospital

DOCTOR PÉAN TEACHING HIS DISCOVERY
By Schwartzweber, after painting by Henri Gervex (1852-1929)

Photogravure
After 1887
Image size: 19 1/2 x 15 in.
Sheet size (sight size): 21 1/2 x 17 1/2 in.

Inscriptions below image: "PEINT PAR H. GERVEX" and "PHOTOGRAVURE SCHWARTZWEBER" above participants "DR BROCHIN DR COLIN DR AUBEAU DR LARIVE/DR PÉAN DR ZACHARIAN/M. MATHIEU Const^{r} d'appareils" above title "LE DOCTEUR PÉAN/ENSEIGNE À L'HÔPITAL SAINT-LOUIS SA DÉCOUVERTE DU PINCEMENT DES VAISSEAUX"

Given after 1900 by unknown donor
Accession number: 1900+f.Pr.27

A famous painting of Dr. Jules Péan by the celebrated academic artist Henri Gervex was the source for Schwartzweber's photogravure. The original work (Musée d'Orsay, Paris) was painted in 1887 and exhibited at the Paris Salon that year.

Jules Émile Péan (1830-98) was one of the most important French gynecologists of his day. A native of Chateaudun, he received his medical degree in Paris in 1860. Following several hospital appointments, he organized the Hôpital International.

Known as a skilled technical surgeon, he performed the first pylorectomy for carcinoma in 1879 (though unsuccessfully). In 1886 he described the technique of *morcellement* for removing a tumor of the uterus by crushing off little bits at a time. In 1895 he was the first to operate on diverticula of the bladder. He also devised "Péan's position" for operating, in which the patient lies on a low table and the surgeon is seated on a high chair placed between the patient's legs.

This picture shows the French gynecologist about to perform a radical mastectomy for cancer of the breast. Notably, the setting is a ward at the St. Louis Hospital in Paris, and not a clinical amphitheater as in Eakins's paintings of Drs. Samuel D. Gross and D. Hayes Agnew. Péan is standing at the head of the table about to demonstrate to his assistants the simple hemostat he invented ("Péan's forceps") to prevent hemorrhage.

The surgeons are massed around a beautiful, bare-breasted, unconscious patient whose long hair flows over the pillow. Some look at Péan while others gaze at the patient. The partial view of a nun standing in the rear may be included for the sake of probity. Dr. Péan is inexplicably garbed in formal dinner attire.

Henri Gervex was a frequent prizewinner at the Paris salons, a chevalier of the Legion of Honor, and a member of the Institute. His highly polished figural paintings often had overtones of erotic titillation, as demonstrated here.

Scholars know that Thomas Eakins was aware of Rembrandt's *Anatomy Lesson of Dr. Tulp* when he planned *The Gross Clinic*, and it is thought that Gervex was familiar with Eakins's painting of Dr. Gross. In turn, Eakins probably took into consideration Gervex's painting of Dr. Péan when he depicted Dr. Agnew performing the same operation in 1889.

Theodor Billroth Operating in the Auditorium of the General Hospital, Vienna

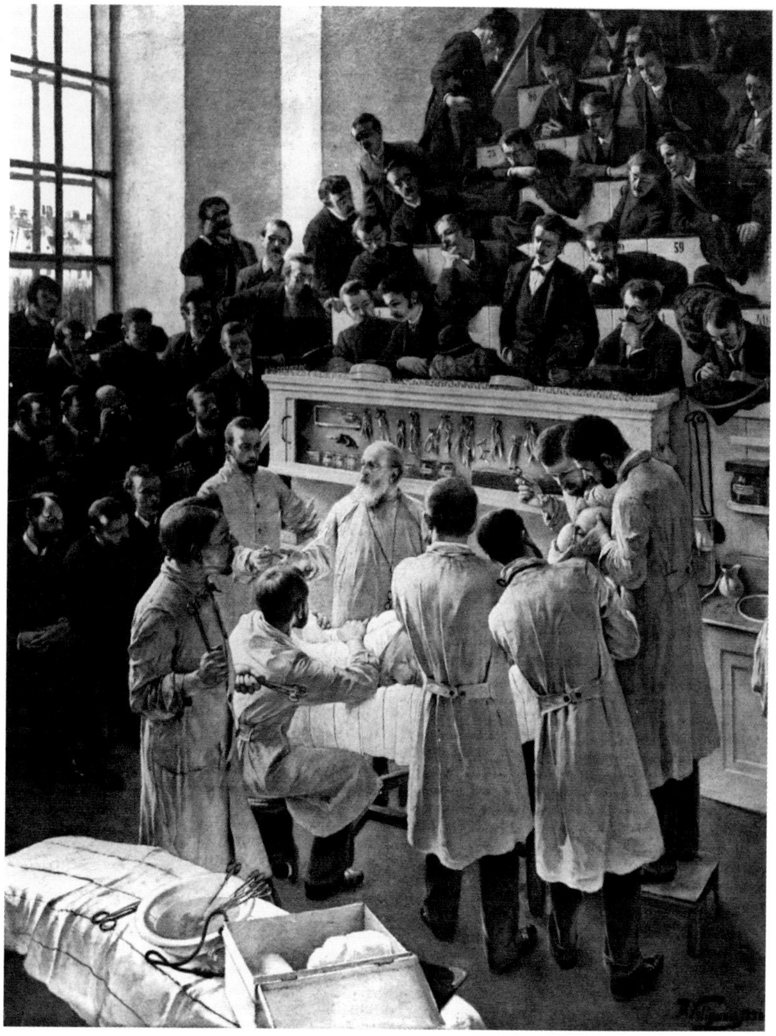

THEODOR BILLROTH OPERATING
By Dr. E. Albert & Co., after painting by A. F. Seligmann

Photogravure
After 1890
Image size: 18 1/2 x 14 1/2 in.
Sheet size: 22 3/4 x 15 1/2 in.

Painting signed and dated lower right: "A. Seligmann 1890"
Inscriptions below image: "A. F. Seligmann pinx." and "Druck & Verlag/von D^r^. E. Albert & C°." above identification of participants with drawings of heads: "Dr Boettcher Dr Billroth Dr V. Eiselsberg Dr O. Winter/Dr Heidenthaler Dr Müller Dr Salzer Dr L. v. Dittel" above title: "BILLROTH'SCHER HÖRSAAL IM WIENER ALLGEM. KRANKENHAUSE"

Given after 1900 by unknown donor
Accession number: 1900+f.Pr.09

The original oil painting and source for the photogravure of Theodor Billroth operating in the general hospital at the University of Vienna was painted by A. F. Seligmann in 1890. The picture is located at the Österreichische Galerie, Vienna.

The outstanding pioneer of visceral surgery, Theodor Billroth (1829-94) was born on the island of Rügen, the son of a clergyman. He studied medicine at Greifswald, Göttingen, and Berlin where he received his degree in 1852. After postgraduate studies in Vienna he accepted an assistant's post at the surgical clinic under Bernhard von Langenbeck in Berlin in 1856, and was named instructor in surgery and pathological anatomy.

In 1860 Billroth became professor of surgery and director of a surgical hospital and clinic in Zurich where he remained until 1867 when he moved to Vienna. He was named professor of surgery and director of the surgical clinic at the University of Vienna and practiced there until his death. His clinic attracted thousands of European and American students, and Billroth is often credited with training the next generation of leaders in the field of surgery worldwide.

Because of his interest in infection and the healing of wounds, Billroth was the first to use temperature measurement in postoperative care. He reported on the first resection of the esophagus in 1872, the first total laryngectomy in 1873, and the first resection of the pylorus for cancer with anastomoses of stomach and duodenum in 1882. He was among the first European surgeons to introduce antisepsis.

His best-remembered textbook is the monumental *Die allgemeine chirurgische Pathologie und Therapie in fünfzig Vorlesungen* (1863). Billroth was a member of the Academy of Sciences in Vienna, an honorary member of numerous other scientific societies, and recipient of sixteen high decorations.

One feels sure that A. F. Seligmann was familiar with Thomas Eakins's depictions of the clinics of Drs. Gross and Agnew, and Gervex's painting of Dr. Péan, at least in reproduction. The elements of renowned doctor in the auditorium or amphitheater discussing the procedure while presiding over an operation, training his assistants, and surrounded by an attentive audience are now familiar. According to the artist's notes the patient was an old man on whom Billroth was performing a neurotomy for trigeminal neuralgia.[3]

The artist even included a self-portrait, the observer in the first row on the far right (positioned like Thomas Eakins in *The Gross Clinic*). Another observer is the Duke of Bavaria on the far left, a regular attendee at Billroth's clinics. Even though the physicians are wearing operating gowns and the instruments have been sterilized, the audience is alarmingly close for maintaining sterile operating conditions.

The Thomas Jefferson University art collection also includes a two-schilling silver coin issued by the Austrian government on the centenary of Theodor Billroth's birth in 1929.

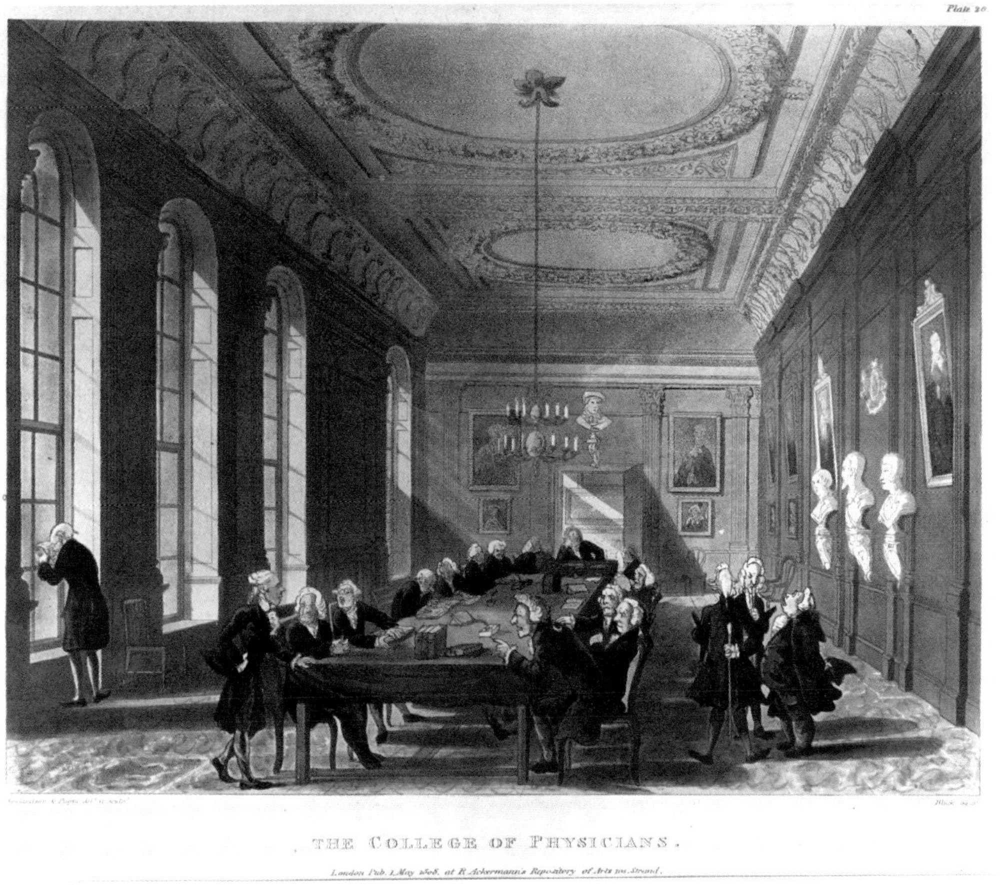

The College of Physicians

THE COLLEGE OF PHYSICIANS
By Thomas Rowlandson (1756-1827) and Augustus Charles Pugin (1762-1832), with aquatint by J. Bluck (active 1791-1819)

Colored etching, aquatint
1808

Image size: 7 3/4 x 10 1/8 in.
Plate size (sight size): 8 7/8 x 10 7/8 in.

Inscriptions below image: "Rowlandson & Pugin, del^{t} et sculp^{t}" and "Bluck, aqua^{t}"; title and publisher "THE COLLEGE OF PHYSICIANS./London Pub. 1, May 1808, at R. Ackermann's Repository of Arts 101. Strand."

Given in 1977 by Frederick B. Wagner Jr., M.D., who received it in 1955 from Mrs. Thomas A. Shallow, widow of owner
Accession number: 1977+e.Pr.01

At first glance this image of London's College of Physicians would not appear to be a depiction of medical education. The bewigged gentlemen seated around a cloth-covered table are upstaged by the vast, well appointed room with its carved ceiling and cove decorations, tall arched windows, and painted and sculpted portrait busts on the panelled walls.

The college was a social club that provided library facilities for study and research, and also maintained control over admission to the profession by the granting of licenses. Thus the young man standing in the left foreground is a student receiving an oral examination by those at the head of the table. The others are uninvolved and talk among themselves. One elderly physician uses the light from the window to illuminate a paper.

The text accompanying the etching relates an amusing anecdote about the candidate's interrogation:

> "Now, sir, in a case of desperate fever, the patient wanting relief by perspiration, how would you act?" "Why, sir," answered the student, "I should give etc. etc." "Well, sir, if that did not operate, what would you do then?" "Why, sir, I should have recourse to etc. etc." "But if that did not produce the desired effect, what remedy have you left?" "Gentlemen," said the worried student..."if all these should fail, I would direct the patient be brought here for examination; and I should despair of success by any other means, if this failed to produce relief by perspiration."[4]

The caricature was among 104 images by Thomas Rowlandson and Augustus C. Pugin for *The Microcosm of London* (1808-11), an immense, three volume publication with over a hundred thousand prints illustrating the activities and customs of a great city. It was published by Rudolph Ackermann, a German immigrant who opened an establishment called the Repository of the Arts in the Strand. This etching of the College of Physicians was one of many collaborations between Pugin, a French emigré architectural draftsman who supplied the architecture and backgrounds, and Rowlandson, an English artist who drew the figures.

Although Rowlandson was a Royal Academy-trained painter, he lost interest in "high" art in favor of social commentary. He is best remembered for his hundreds of satirical etchings, many of which dealt with medical themes such as *Doctor Syntax* and *English Dance of Death*.

The Jefferson art collection acquired another Rowlandson and Pugin print, *Middlesex Hospital, London*, also from *The Microcosm of London*. It shows the ward of London's first lying-in hospital, founded for the relief of pregnant wives of the industrious poor.

Cholera Epidemic of 1865 in Paris

CHOLERA EPIDEMIC OF 1865 IN PARIS (OBVERSE)
Designed by Eugène Laurent and carved by Alfred Borrel

Bronze medal
3 in. diameter
1866

Signed on ledge obverse and reverse: "E. LAURENT SCULP." and "A. BORREL INCIS."
Inscription on obverse: "CARITAS AVGVSTA/FIDES SPES" and "VISITE DE L'EMPEREUR NAPOLÉON III À L'HÔTEL-DIEU ÉPIDÉMIE DE MDCCCLXV"
Inscription on reverse: "CARITAS AVGVSTA/MISERORVM/SOROR" and "VISITE DE L'IMPÉRATRICE EUGÉNIE À L'HOSPICE BEAUJON ÉPIDÉMIE DE MDCCCLXV"

Given in 1940 by bequest of Pascal Brooke Bland, M.D., former chair of obstetrics
Accession number: 1940+e.M.06

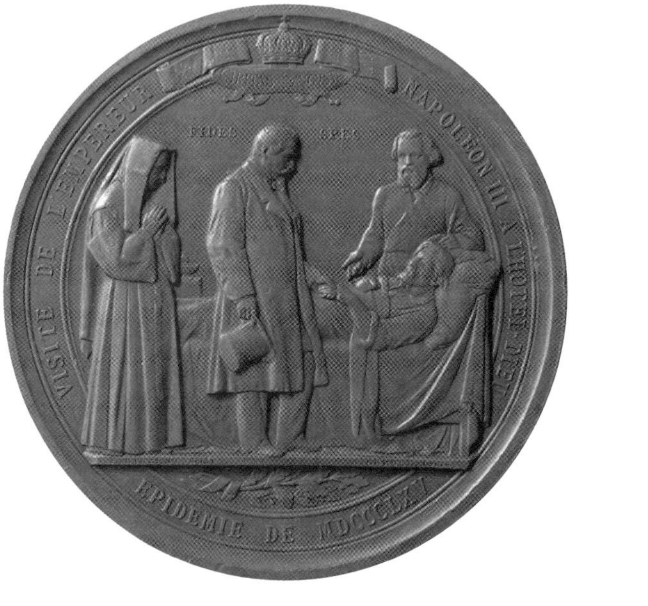

Asiatic cholera, which had been pandemic in the Far East, invaded western Europe for the first time significantly in the years between 1826 and 1837. The dread disease struck again during the following three decades. Tokens of the outbreaks were issued as amulets worn to ward off the disease, and as medals or prizes honoring those who provided outstanding aid to patients.

A large bronze medal was struck in 1866 in honor of the visits of Emperor Napoléon III and Empress Eugénie to Parisian hospitals during the cholera epidemic of 1865. The emperor visited the Hôtel Dieu, the largest hospital with a thousand beds. The empress visited the Hôpital Beaujon which had five hundred beds.

The medal was designed by Eugène Laurent and carved by Alfred Borrel. It is in high relief with deep, clear incision of the inscriptions. There is a sculptural emphasis on details of costumes, especially the deep folds in garments and bed linens. Facial features are differentiated among the characters.

The obverse, shown here, depicts the emperor wearing an overcoat and carrying his top hat standing at the bedside of an elderly male patient and grasping his hand. Flanking the central figures are a doctor gesturing toward the patient and a Sister of Charity with hands clasped in prayer. Above the emperor's head is a scroll inscribed "CARITAS AUGUSTA" and surmounted by a crown. Below the ground line are sprays of oak and laurel bound with ribbon.

The reverse shows the empress wearing a bonnet and cloak bending over the bed of a female patient and grasping her hand. Flanking them are two Sisters of Charity, one gesturing toward the patient, the other with hands folded.

Portraits

Synthesizers of Medical Knowledge

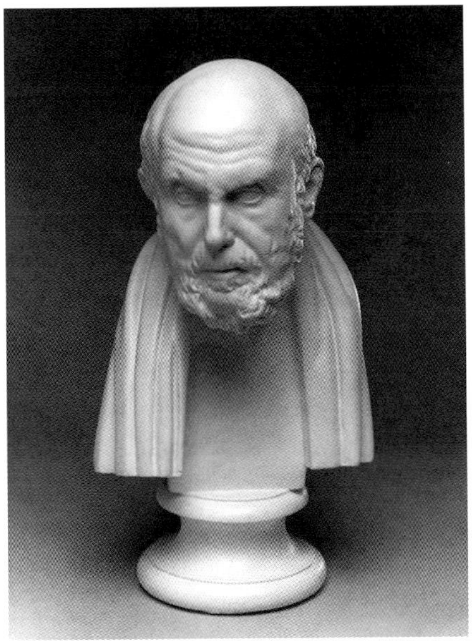

Portrait of Hippocrates

HIPPOCRATES (ca. 460-ca. 370 B.C.)
By unknown artist for Caproni Casts

Plaster
Before 1930
22 1/2 x 12 x 10 5/8 in.

Inscription below neck on rear: "ipocrate"
Inscription on rear plaque: "A. Caproni—& Bro./Caproni Casts/Boston"

Given before 1930 by unknown donor
Accession number: 1930+b.S.01

Despite fantastic legends about the achievements of Hippocrates, most scholars of the history of medicine agree that he did actually exist and was the most celebrated physician of ancient Greece. He is considered the founder of scientific medicine and has come to be seen as embodying the ideal physician.

An ancient biographer said that Hippocrates was born about 460 B.C. on the island of Cos, off the coast of Asia Minor, and died about 370 B.C. in Thessaly. He was a member of the guild of Aesclepiadae (sons of Aesculapius) and received his medical education at the famous temple of Aesculapius at Cos. Although many legends and myths have grown up about his life, very little is known in fact except that he was an itinerant practitioner, as was customary then.

Hippocrates was also a teacher and author. Writings attributed to him were compiled under the title *Hippocratic Collection*, but the work probably included treatises and books by many different authors from Cos and elsewhere.

Subjects included in the collection are: anatomy, physiology, general pathology, therapy, diagnosis, prognosis, surgery (most thoroughly on fractures and dislocations, wounds, hemorrhage, cauterization, and operations to treat tumors, fistulas, ulcers, and hemorrhoids), gynecology and obstetrics, mental illness (especially modern in assigning the brain as the organ of thought and sensation, and discussions of epilepsy, delirium tremens, depression, anxiety, and origin of dreams), and ethics (exceptional discussion of physicians' behavior, appearance, and inner life).[5]

The Hippocratic Oath, to which medical students for centuries have sworn allegiance in either its original form or with modifications, is the most widely known document associated with Hippocrates. Yet because of inconsistencies with the *Hippocratic Collection*, scholars think it unlikely that the oath originated with Hippocrates or was even composed during his lifetime.

Jefferson's plaster bust of Hippocrates is close in style and concept to a Roman marble copy of a Greek bronze original. That work was formerly thought to be a portrait of Hippocrates, but is now considered another Greek physician, Chrysippos (British Museum, London). There is a similar bust supposedly of Hippocrates in the Uffizi Gallery, Florence. Other ancient sculptures and coins with the image of Hippocrates survive, but none is contemporaneous with the physician, so his actual appearance is unknown.

In the Jefferson bust, the subject's thoughtful expression is intensified by his bald head, knitted brows and forehead wrinkles, deepset eyes, and slightly parted lips. Folds of a toga are draped over his narrow shoulders; the anatomy of his chest is not described. The bust was acquired before 1930, and a second plaster bust of Hippocrates entered the collection at a later date.

Portrait of Samuel C. F. Hahnemann

SAMUEL CHRISTIAN FRIEDRICH HAHNEMANN, M.D. (1755-1843)
By unknown artist

Engraving, etching, stipple
1850-1900
Image size: 4 1/4 x 3 1/2 in.
Plate size: 6 5/8 x 4 1/4 in.
Sheet size: 9 1/2 x 6 in.

Inscription above image: "Meyer's Conv. Lex N. 371"
Inscriptions below image: "Dr S. HAHNEMANN"/"Inst. Bibl. excudit"

Given in 1940 by bequest of Pascal Brooke Bland, M.D.
Accession number: 1940+e.Pr.03

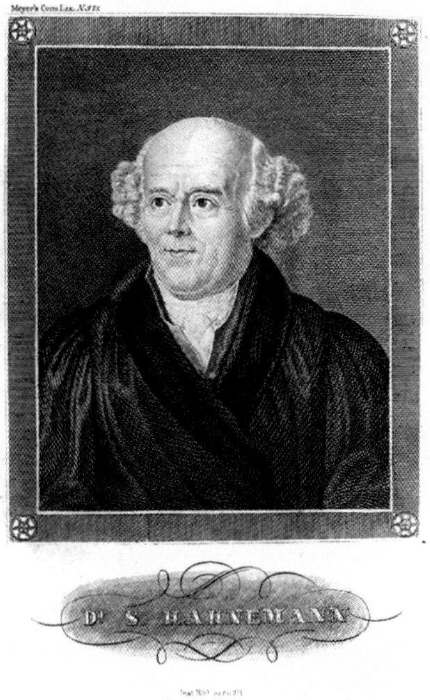

Dr. Samuel C. F. Hahnemann was a German physician and founder of the discipline of homeopathy, one of several isolated, theoretical medical systems of the nineteenth century.

Samuel Hahnemann was born in 1755 in Meissen, the son of a porcelain painter. He took his medical degree at the University of Erlangen in 1779, and practiced medicine in several towns including Dresden and Leipzig. In his early years he published papers on the uncertainty of contemporary drug treatments.

In 1796 he published his first paper setting forth his views on drugs which later formed the basis of homeopathy, a system created around the turn of the century. His findings were more fully described in *Organon der rationellen Heilkunde* (1810), with the motto *Similia sim-*

ilibus curantur (likes cure likes).

Hahnemann taught that substances or drugs that provoke reactions in healthy persons can be used to mitigate similar responses that are symptoms of disease ("the law of similars"); and that the effectiveness of the drug was in inverse proportion to the size of the dose ("the law of infinitesimals"), i.e., the more a substance is diluted, the more potent it becomes. He also believed in the abolition of bloodletting, purging, and emesis as cure-alls.

In 1812 Hahnemann was appointed to the faculty at the University of Leipzig where he taught his theory, but was forced to resign by public furor after the death of an Austrian prince under his care. While living in Köthen from 1821 to 1835 his fame grew and his publications flourished through successive editions.

Disciples spread his theories throughout Europe and America. In 1844 the American Institute of Homeopathy was founded despite strong protest from the American Medical Association. The Homeopathic Medical College of Pennsylvania was opened in Philadelphia in 1848. After several mergers and changes of location the institution was renamed Hahnemann Medical College in 1869. In 1885 it merged with Homeopathic Medical Hospital of Philadelphia to become Hahnemann Medical College and Hospital. The last homeopathic course requirement was eliminated in 1945 and no degrees in homeopathy have been granted since 1950.

Today only three states have specific licensing boards for homeopathic physicians, although several thousand other health care professionals incorporate elements of homeopathy in their practices. Millions of dollars of homeopathic remedies are sold annually over the counter.[6]

The delicately rendered, etched portrait of Hahnemann in the Jefferson collection was cut out of one of several encyclopedias of German knowledge published in the last half of the nineteenth century. Entitled *Meyer's Konversations-Lexikon*, these encyclopedias were published by the Bibliographisches Institut in Leipzig. The author was Hermann Julius Meyer (1826-1909).

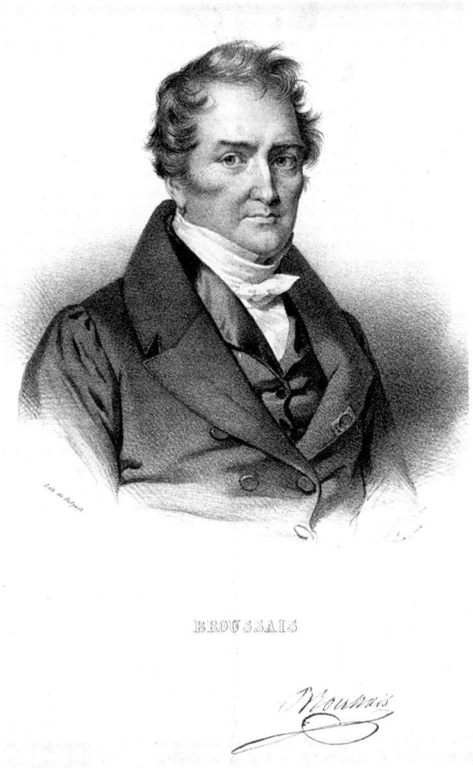

Portrait of François-J.-V. Broussais

FRANÇOIS-JOSEPH-VICTOR BROUSSAIS (1772-1838)
By M (?)

Lithograph
1825-35
Image size: 6 3/4 x 6 1/2 in.
Sheet size: 13 3/4 x 10 3/4 in.

Signed below image on right: "M"
Inscriptions below image: "Lith. de Delpech." and "BROUSSAIS" above facsimile signature of subject

Given after 1900 by unknown donor
Accession number: 1900+f.Pr.05

François-J.-V. Broussais was born in 1772 in St. Malo, France, the son of a country practitioner. He was a propounder of the doctrine of physiological medicine, and carried on a polemic against the dominant medical ideas of his time differentiating and describing diseases according to their clinical course and anatomical seat.

His early medical studies were at the Hôtel Dieu of St. Malo and at the École de Chirurgie Navale at Brest. He shipped out as a naval surgeon and then received his doctor's degree in Paris in 1802. After medical school he served as an army surgeon during Napoléon's campaigns, and later was appointed assistant professor at a military hospital in Paris. Through government influence he was appointed professor of general pathology at the Faculté de Médecine in Paris, a seat in the Académie des Sciences Morales et Politiques, the rank of inspector general in the Service de Santé Militaire, and a commander of the Legion of Honor.

Broussais's book, *Histoire des phlegmasies ou inflammations chroniques* (1808), put forward some very original ideas. His theory of "physiological medicine" was that life depends upon irritation, especially heat which excites the chemical processes in the body. Disease depends upon localized irritation of some organ. Further, he believed that nature had no healing power, so active measures of diet and bleeding were necessary to abort disease. A weakening regime featured depriving the patient of food and leeching him all over his body, as many as thirty to fifty leeches at once. His theory of irritation was taken up by some doctors in Germany and England before being generally discredited by the medical profession.

The elegantly rendered bust-length portrait of François Broussais was published by the Delpech lithograph shop in Paris. The artist is identified only by the initial "M." The subject's angular features, steady gaze, and military decoration give him a confident, almost tough demeanor, in contrast to his tasselled curls which lend him a softer and romantic look.

Anatomists and Surgeons

Although it has been long been understood that one must dissect the human body to understand the patterns and relationships of its structures, this was not always the case. Around 300 B.C. human and animal dissection was practiced in Alexandria, Egypt, and the study of anatomy flourished until Egypt was absorbed into the Roman Empire around the end of the first century B.C. The Romans passed legal sanctions to protect the dead against defilement and anatomists reverted to the dissection of animals.[7]

In the second century A.D. Claudius Galen of Pergamon wrote two great anatomical works, *On Anatomical Procedure* and *On the Uses of the Parts of the Body of Man*, based mainly on the work of the *Hippocratic Collection* and Aristotle. Galen experimented with various species of animals, especially apes, to make inferences about human anatomy.

Following Galen's death his word remained the authority, although sometimes in corrupted form, and further anatomical inquiry ceased in western Europe during the Middle Ages. However, the most important documents of Greek medicine had been translated into Arabic, and intellectual leadership passed to Islamic scholars in Asia Minor, Persia, North Africa, and Spain from about the eighth to the thirteenth centuries. Many Arabic manuscripts and Latin translations of Greek manuscripts found their way to European monasteries. Between 1100 and 1350 the center of learning shifted to Europe as fifteen universities were established in Italy, attracting students from all over the continent.[8]

Modern scholars differ on some important issues in the complex history of dissection by physicians and artists during the late Middle Ages and early Renaissance, but do agree that gradually the practice was legalized by the church and the state. A medical faculty existed at Bologna as early as the mid-twelfth century, and postmortem examination evolved into anatomical study by the beginning of the fourteenth century. The *Anathomia* (1316) of Mondino de' Luzzi, which still relied on ancient authorities, served as the practical manual of dissection for the next two centuries. The significant contribution of Andreas Vesalius, the great sixteenth-century anatomist, was to trust only observations made from his own dissection of the human body.

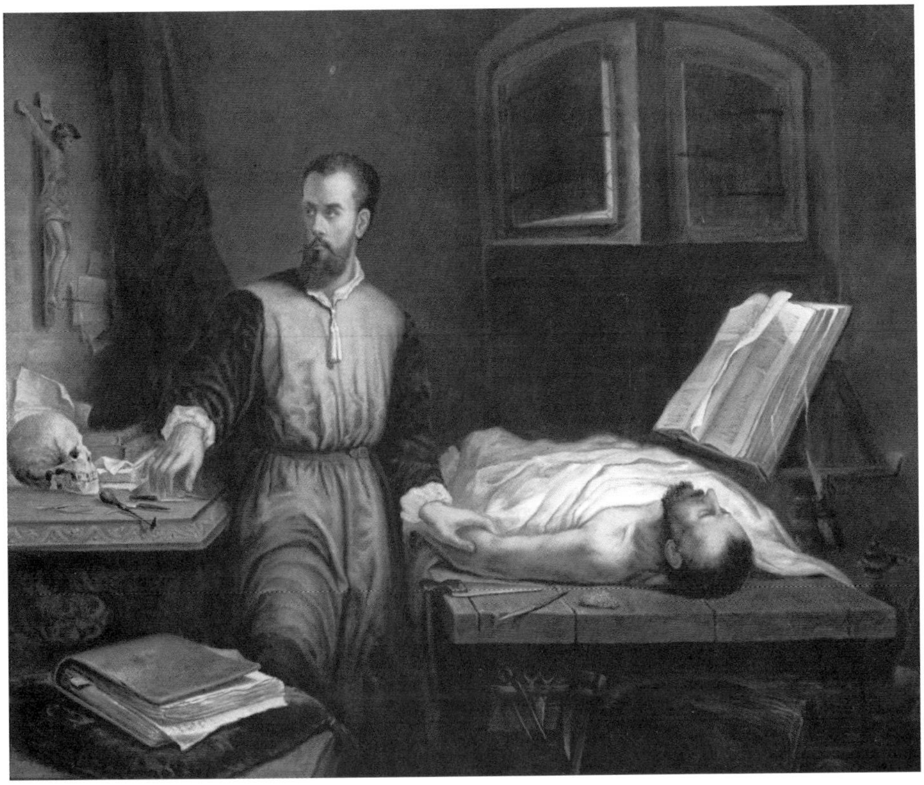

Andreas Vesalius Dissecting

ANDREAS VESALIUS DISSECTING
By unknown artist, after painting by Edouard-Jean-Conrad Hamman (1819-88)

Oil on canvas
1850-1925
25 x 30 in.

Given in 1940 by Mrs. Alexius McGlannan, daughter of an unidentified Jefferson alumnus of the class of 1869
Accession number: 1940+e.P.02

Andreas Vesalius (1514-64) was born in Brussels to a family of notable physicians. His great-great-grandfather was a professor in the medical school at Louvain, his great-grandfather was physician to the city of Brussels, his grandfather attended Emperor Maximilian I, and his father served Emperor Charles V as court apothecary.

After attending universities in Louvain, Vesalius studied medicine at the University of Paris from 1533 to 1536. Even though he witnessed only a few dissections, his interest in anatomy was already established. The invasion of Provence by Charles V forced Vesalius to return to Louvain where he finished his baccalaureate degree in 1537. While there he reconstructed a skeleton from the corpse of an executed man, and on another occasion astonished fellow students and faculty by conducting an authorized anatomical demonstration, the first in that city in eighteen years.

Vesalius continued his studies at the hospital in Venice. In 1537 he was granted a medical degree by the University of Padua, a dependent city of Venice. He was immediately appointed professor of surgery, a post that also bore the responsibility of teaching anatomy. Like most contemporary anatomists he lectured from the chair (reading from the anatomical volumes of Galen), but unlike them he performed his own dissections. He also introduced the use of illustrations to clarify his discussions, another startling novelty that attracted huge crowds.

In 1538 Vesalius published his first work, *Tabulae anatomicae sex*, consisting of six sketches of the vascular system and the skeleton. His next publications were *Institutionum anatomicarum secundum Galeni sententiam* (1538), a synopsis of the views of Galen, and *Epistola docens venam* (1539), a letter supporting the classical technique of venesection. Next he contributed three revisions of chapters to a monumental edition of the complete works of Galen: *Opera Galeni* (1541-42).

Ironically, even while working on the latter book Vesalius was preparing his own original, anatomical treatise freeing him from Galenic authority: *De humani corporis fabrica libri septem* (1543). This important work demonstrated that much of Galen's human anatomy was inaccurate because it was based on the study of animals only. Vesalius believed ardently that human anatomy could be learned only by dissection and investigation of the human body.

Although the initial reception to *Fabrica* was largely unfavorable, today it is considered by many scholars the greatest single contribution to anatomical knowledge. The work was also an exquisite and unified blend of scholarly text, innovative illustrations, and typography. Although the book was replete with errors, Vesalius made so many new discoveries that widespread fame earned him the epithet, "Father of Modern Anatomy." A condensed and less expensive version entitled *De humani corporis fabrica librorum epitome* appeared the same year.

After lecturing at the universities of Padua, Bologna, and Pisa Vesalius returned to the practice of medicine and was appointed court physician to Charles V at Speyer. A revised folio edition of *Fabrica* was dedicated to Charles in 1555. After the emperor's abdication in 1556, Vesalius joined the court of his son Philip II of Spain. His last work, *Anatomicarum Gabrielis Fallopii observationum examen*, was published posthumously in 1564.

The oil painting of Andreas Vesalius in Jefferson's art collection is a copy after a well known depiction of 1848 by Edouard-Jean-Conrad Hamman, a Belgian portrait and history painter. Hamman's portrait was originally owned by a private collector in Rotterdam, so the copyist of the Jefferson portrait probably worked after painted or engraved copies.

The painting shows Vesalius alone in a murky room performing a dissection. All windows are tightly shuttered except one in the top left corner that is slightly ajar, allowing in light that causes a raking, spotlighted effect. The anatomist looks imploringly toward a crucifix hanging on the wall, affirming his own piety and perhaps seeking inspiration or blessing for his work.

He wears a blue robe with maroon velvet sleeves and a white ruffled shirt. His left hand rests on the arm of a male cadaver partially covered by a sheet. The body is shown in foreshortened perspective with its head toward the viewer. The anatomist's right hand reaches toward instruments on the table which also holds books and a skull. Folio volumes of anatomy rest on a bookstand and on nearby tables. Additional instruments are on the planked wood dissection table.

The Jefferson library has acquired several rare copies of *Fabrica* (images discussed below), and a silver medal issued in commemoration of a statue of Vesalius erected in Brussels in 1847.

Portrait of William Harvey

WILLIAM HARVEY (1578-1657)
By Horatio Stone, M.D. (1808/10-75)

Marble
1869
29 5/8 x 16 7/8 x 13 3/8 in.

Signed and dated on back: "HORATIO STONE/FAC. ROME.1869"
Inscription on front of base: "HARVEY"

Given in 1899 by J. Ackerman Coles, M.D. and Emilie S. Coles, in memory of their father, Abraham Coles, M.D. (JMC 1835)
Accession number: 1899+e.S.01

William Harvey, the discoverer and quantifier of the circulatory system, is another towering figure in the history of anatomy. The Jefferson art collection contains several portraits of Harvey, including a sculpture by Horatio Stone, prints by Jacobus Houbraken and Charles A. Waltner, and an anonymous seventeenth-century oil painting.

William Harvey was born in 1578 in Folkestone, Kent, England, the son of a landowning family. After graduating from Caius College, Cambridge, he earned a medical degree from the University of Padua in 1602, where an influential teacher was the anatomist Girolamo Fabrici (1533/37-1619), discoverer of valves in the veins.

Harvey established a private practice in London, and was appointed fellow of the Royal College of Physicians and physician to St. Bartholomew's Hospital where he remained from 1609 to 1643. In 1615 he was made the Lumleian Lecturer of the Royal College of Physicians, requiring an annual discourse and demonstration of anatomy. His reputation soared and he was named court physician to King James I and then to Charles I. When Civil War broke out in 1642 Harvey followed the court to Oxford and was appointed principal of Merton College there. When rebels reconquered the town in 1646 Harvey quit the royal service and retired.

His greatest work, *Exercitatio anatomica de motu cordis et sanguinis in animalibus* (1628), established the continuous recirculation of the blood. By direct observation he demonstrated that the heart acts as a muscular pump that propels the blood away from the heart via the arteries and returns it to the heart via the veins, in a continuous motion. Many contemporary physicians at first opposed his ideas because they contradicted the beliefs of Aristotle and Galen. Harvey's interest in reproduction led to a publication that became a foundation of modern embryology, *Exercitationes de generatione animalium* (1651).

The over-life-sized marble bust of William Harvey was sculpted by Horatio Stone in 1869. The vigorous conception is idealized and heroic. The subject looks down with furrowed brow and a quizzical expression. His face is broadly angular and his neck quite massive. The predominant feature is the extraordinarily thick and curly hair, beard, and mustache. However, the imposing depiction does not accord with Harvey's appearance as described by a contemporary:

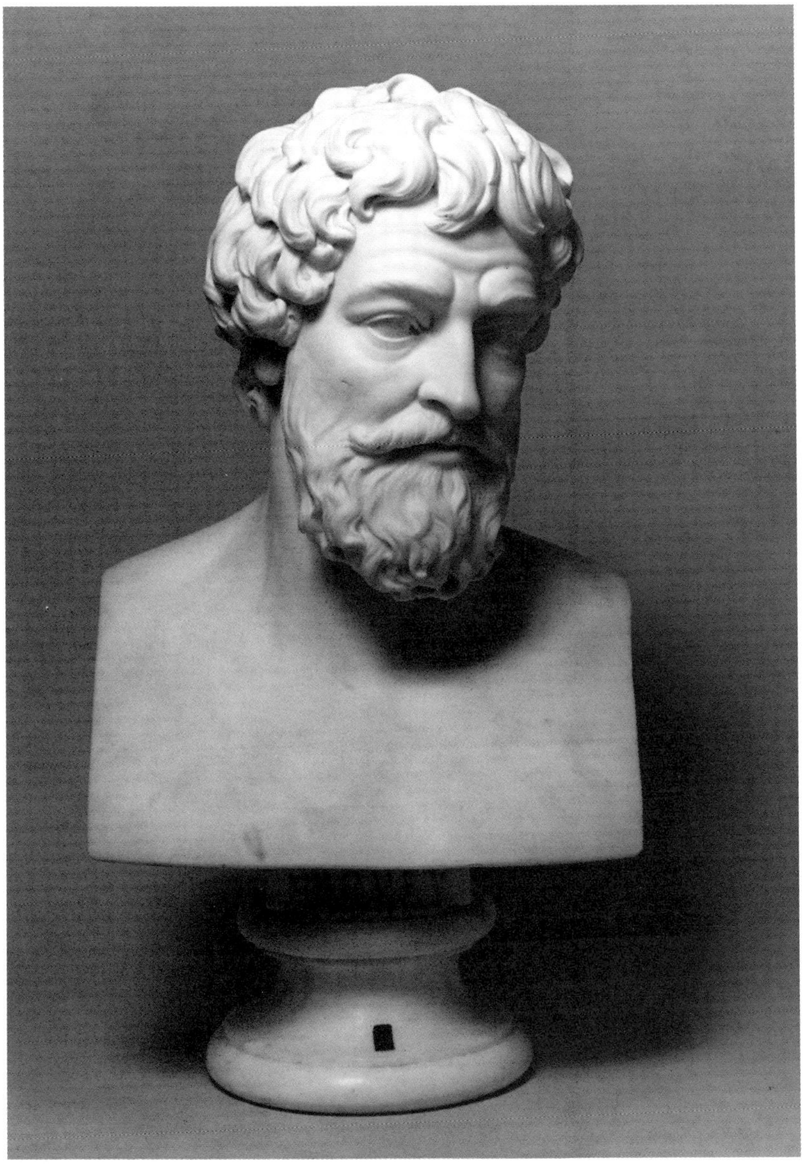

> He was not tall, but of the lowest stature, round faced, olivaster complexion; little eie, round, very black, full of spirit; his haire was black as a raven, but quite white 20 years before he died...He was...very cholerique.[9]

Horatio Stone was born in 1808 in Jackson, New York. Originally trained as a physician, he practiced from 1841 to 1847. He began sculpting professionally in 1848 and made two study trips to Italy. He moved to Washington, D.C. where he was a founder and president of the Washington Union Art Association, and was instrumental in the establishment of the National Gallery of Art and the short-lived Federal Art Commission. His marble statues and busts of Alexander Hamilton, John Hancock, Edward Dickinson Baker, Thomas Jefferson, Thomas Benton, and Chief Justice Roger B. Taney can be seen in the Capitol and the Supreme Court Building.

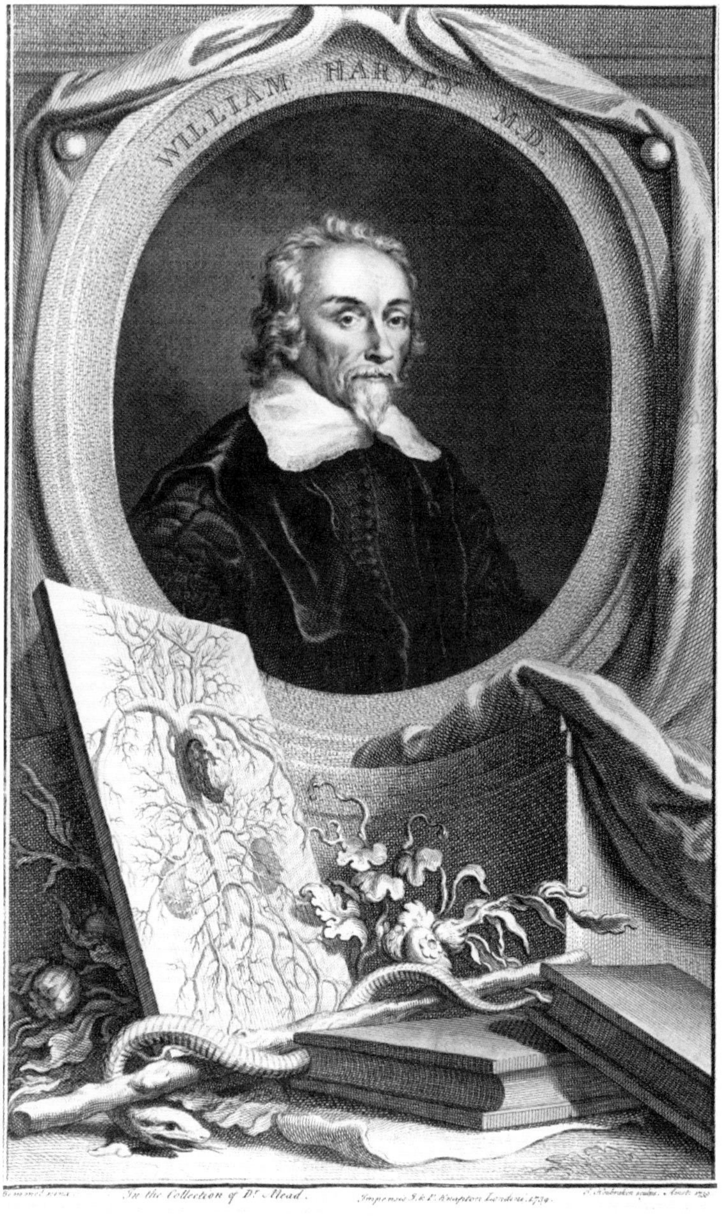

Portrait of William Harvey

(See color plate)

WILLIAM HARVEY
By Jacobus Houbraken (1698-1780), after painting by Wilhelm von Bemmel (1630-1708)

Hand-colored engraving
1739
Image size: 14 x 8 3/4 in.
Plate size: 14 1/2 x 9 1/4 in.
Sheet size: 18 1/2 x 12 3/4 in.

Inscription on frame of image: "WILLIAM HARVEY M.D."
Signed and dated lower right: "J. Houbraken Sculps. Amst. 1739"
Inscriptions below: "Bemmel pinx.," "In the Collection of Dr Mead.," and "Impensis J. & P. Knapton Londini, 1739."

Given after 1900 by unknown donor
Accession number: 1900+f.Pr.07

This large and rare print of William Harvey is an engraving with hand-applied watercolor by the Dutch artist Jacobus Houbraken. The source for the image is an oil painting of Harvey by another Dutch artist, Wilhelm von Bemmel (at the Hunterian Collection, University of Glasgow).

In the upper half of the image William Harvey is shown in an oval frame in front of a stone column covered with pink drapery. In the print he faces the opposite direction from the painting (a print is a reversed image of the engraved plate, and printmakers frequently do not trouble to reverse the image a second time).

Compared with Horatio Stone's sculpture of Harvey, the subject's cheeks are hollower, his chin more pointed, and his hair flatter and more sparse. His costume is maroon and blue with a broad, white collar. Below the framed portrait is a large diagram of the heart and blood vessels, flanked by foliage and pomegranates above a caduceus and two pink and blue books.

Bemmel's oil portrait was in the possession of Dr. Richard Mead (1673-1754) for many years. Mead was a physician and eminent scholar who amassed a library of ten thousand books in addition to vast numbers of paintings, sculptures, prints, and medals. He allowed the painting to be copied by Houbraken for his famous engraving. After Mead's death the painting was supposedly acquired for Dr. John Hunter.[10]

Portrait of John Hunter

JOHN HUNTER (1728-93)
By William Sharp (1749-1824), after painting by Sir Joshua Reynolds (1723-92)

Engraving, etching
1788
Image size: 16 3/4 x 13 3/8 in.
Sheet size: 21 5/8 x 17 1/2 in.

Signature lower right below image: "Willm Sharp sculp^{t}" Inscriptions: "Sir Joshua Reynolds pinx^{t}/JOHN HUNTER/London, Publifhed 1st Jany 1788, by Wm Sharp, N° 8,/Charles Street, Midd^{x} Hofpital: B. B. Evans, corner of the Old Jewry, Cheapfide,/& W. Skelton, N° 23 Hay Market."

Given in 1970 by Dr. J. Woodrow Savacool (JMC 1938), clinical associate professor of medicine, and Mrs. Savacool
Accession number: 1970+e.Pr.01

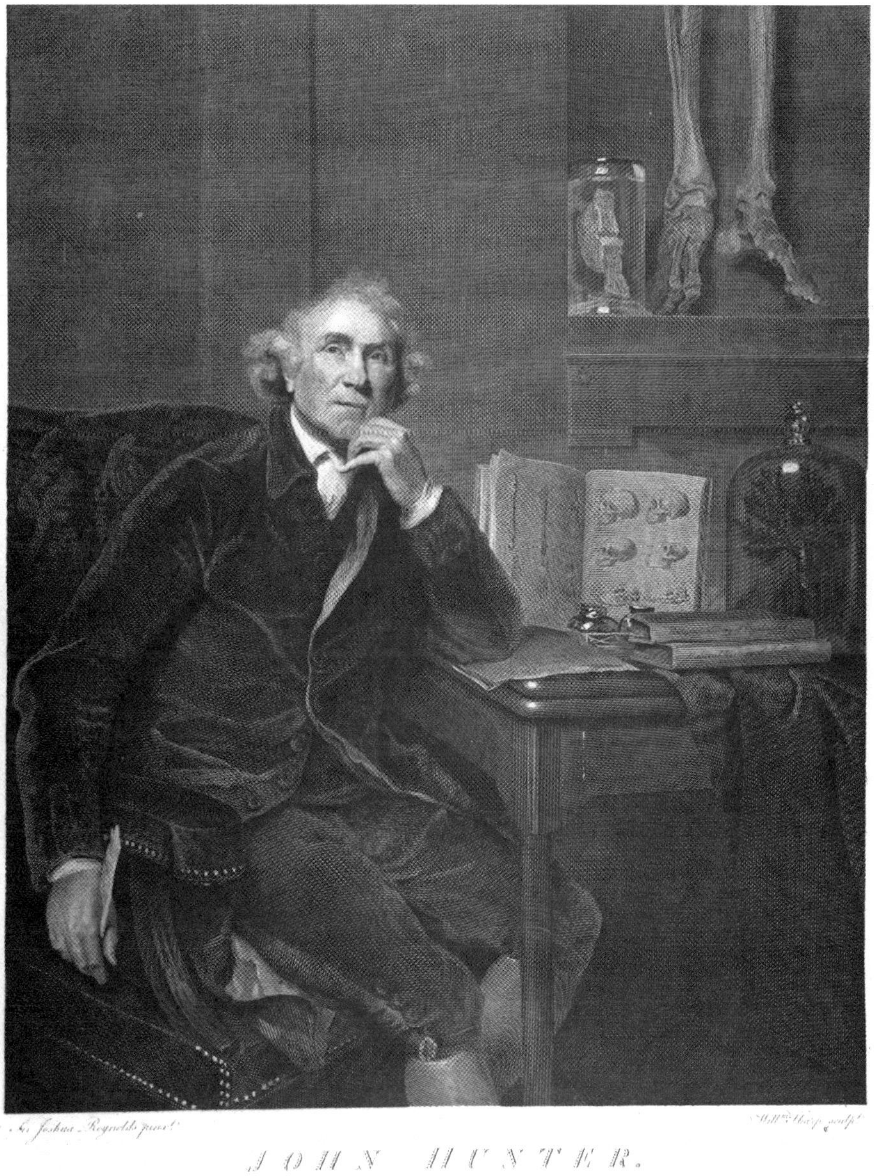

Dr. John Hunter was a celebrated eighteenth-century British surgeon credited with putting operative surgery on a solid scientific basis, grounded in his extensive knowledge of anatomy and pathology. Dr. Samuel D. Gross praised Hunter as the "grandest figure in the history of our profession," and "a philosopher whose mental grasp embraced the whole range of nature's works, from the most humble structure to the most complex and the most lofty."[11]

John Hunter was born on a small farm near Glasgow, Scotland and studied anatomy and surgery with his older brother, William, and later at hospitals in London. Especially interested in comparative anatomy, John Hunter made thousands of anatomical preparations of animals of every sort. After serving for two years as an army surgeon during the Seven Years War, he began the private practice of surgery in London and opened his own anatomical school.

He became a leading surgeon in the city, was appointed to St. George's Hospital, and elected to the Royal Society. His treatises on treatment of gunshot wounds, the natural history of human teeth, venereal disease, and his operation for popliteal aneurysm were very influential. He discovered that when an obstruction occurs in the arteries collateral vessels are developed. Many of his American and European pupils became famous in their own right, such as Drs. John Morgan, Philip Syng Physick, Astley Cooper, William Ship-pen, and Edward Jenner.

As Hunter's famed collection of more than thirteen thousand anatomical, zoological, and pathological specimens grew and more space was needed, he purchased two large homes in Leicester Square and converted the whole property into laboratories, lecture rooms, museum, and printing shops, as well as living quarters. After his death the collection was transferred to the Royal College of Surgeons where each year since the Hunterian Oration is presented.

The painter Sir Joshua Reynolds was a neighbor who finally was able to persuade Hunter to sit for his portrait in 1786. One day the reluctant subject fell into a reverie and the artist seized the opportunity to portray him while lost in thought among some of his prized possessions.[12] Seated at a table with pen in hand, Hunter has paused for a moment in his work. On the crowded tabletop are an open folio of his comparative anatomy drawings, closed volumes of *Natural History of Vegetables* and *Natural History of Fossils*, and a bell jar with an injected bronchial tree. Above is a niche containing the skeletal legs of the Irish giant, Charles Bryne.

William Sharp was one of the most accomplished eighteenth-century English engravers. He was best known for his reproductions of portraits and history paintings by old masters and contemporary artists. Although elected an honorary member of the Imperial Academy at Vienna and of the Royal Academy of Munich, Sharp refused numerous invitations to work on the Continent.

Portrait of Samuel T. von Soemmerring

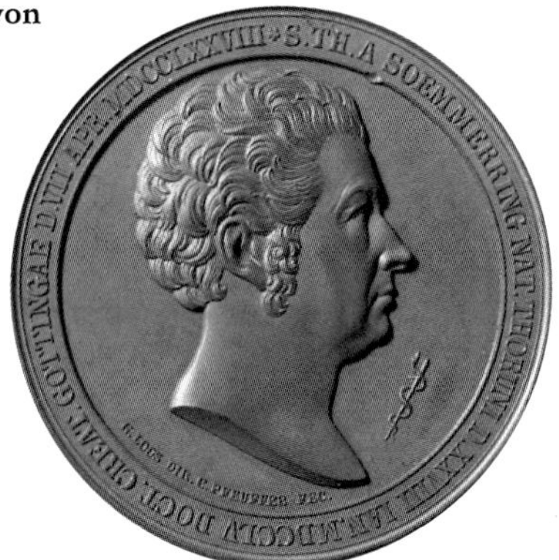

SAMUEL THOMAS von SOEMMERRING (1755-1830)
By Christoph Karl Pfeuffer

Bronze medal
1828
2 in. diameter

Signed below neck: "G. LOOS DIR. C. PFEUFFER FEC."
Inscription on obverse: "S. TH. A SOEMMERRING NAT. THORUNI D. XXVIII IAN. MDCCLV DOCT. CREAT. GOTTINGAE D. VII APR. MDCCLXXVIII"
Inscription on reverse: "ANATOMICORUM PRINCIPI ANIMAE ORGANA QUI APERUIT ARTIS VIRIQUE CULTORES. D. VII. APR. MDCCCXXVIII"

Given in 1940 by bequest of Pascal Brooke Bland, M.D.
Accession number: 1940+e.M.08

Dr. Samuel T. von Soemmerring was among the most famous German anatomists of the early nineteenth century. His publications had lasting influence in part because of his choice of exceptional engravers, such as Christian Koeck, to illustrate his works with remarkable accuracy and artistry.

The son of the municipal physician of Thorn, Poland, Soemmerring was born in 1755 and received his medical degree from the University of Göttingen in 1778. He was influenced by pupils of the great anatomist Albinus while pursuing further study in England, the Netherlands, and Scotland.

In 1779 Soemmerring became professor of anatomy and surgery at the Collegium Carolinum in Cassel, and in 1784 professor of anatomy and physiology at the University of Mainz. In 1797 he established himself as a physician at Frankfurt-on-Main, and then moved to Munich in 1805. Soemmerring was a member of the Bavarian Academy of Sciences, and even published on the electric telegraph. He became a privy councillor, and in 1808 was named a knight of the Order of the Civil Service of the Bavarian Crown and was granted personal nobility. He returned to Frankfurt in 1820 and practiced medicine there until his death in 1830.

Soemmerring was particularly interested in the anatomy of the brain and the sympathetic nervous system. His principal work is *Vom Baue des menschlichen Körpers* (1791-96). He was also admired for a series of monographs on the organs of the senses.

The bronze medal of Soemmerring by Christoph Karl Pfeuffer was struck at the Loos die-sinking establishment in 1828, commemorating the fiftieth anniversary of the subject's doctorate from the University of Göttingen. The obverse features a profile bust of the subject facing right above a caduceus, and the reverse shows the base of the brain, medulla, and cerebellum.

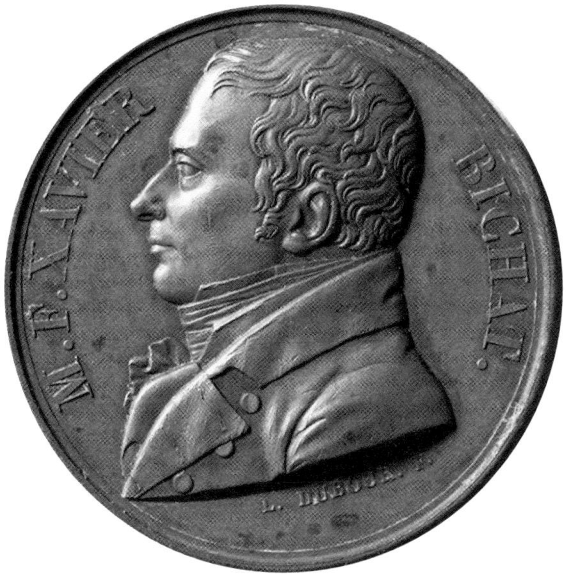

Portrait of M.-F.-X. Bichat

MARIE-FRANÇOIS-XAVIER BICHAT (1771-1802)
By L. Dubour

Bronze medal
1826
3 in. diameter

Signed below bust on obverse: "L. DUBOUR. F."
Inscription on obverse: "M. F. XAVIER BICHAT."
Inscriptions on reverse: "NÉ/À THOIRETTE/EN M.DCC.LXXI./MORT/EN M.DCCC.II/GALERIE METALLIQUE/DES GRANDS HOMMES FRANÇAIS./1826."

Given in 1940 by bequest of Pascal Brooke Bland, M.D.
Accession number: 1940+e.M.02

Although M.-F.-X. Bichat died prematurely at the age of thirty, he is considered by many scholars the creator of descriptive anatomy.

Bichat was born in Thoirette in 1771, the son of a country doctor. After studying anatomy and surgery at the Hôtel Dieu in Lyons, Bichat moved to Paris where he studied with Pierre Joseph Desault (1744-95), a distinguished surgeon who took a liking to the gifted young man, invited him to live in his home, and made him editor of the *Journal de chirurgie*. In 1800 Bichat became physician at the Hôtel Dieu and gave private lectures and demonstrations in anatomy and physiology.

He was famous for three works published between 1799 and 1801, *Recherches physiologiques sur la vie et la mort, Traité des membranes*, and *Anatomie générale*, in which he studied the structure of tissues in their normal and pathological conditions. He recognized twenty-one different membranes (tissues making up the organs), differing in their textures and properties. He taught that pathology must be based not upon the topography of organs but upon the structure of the membranes. His error was to assign a specific vital property to each tissue, a now obsolete theory.

The bronze medal of Bichat was made by L. Dubour for the Galerie Metallique des Grands Hommes Français. The obverse shows a profile bust of the subject facing left. His features, wavy hair, and details of costume are finely rendered in high relief.

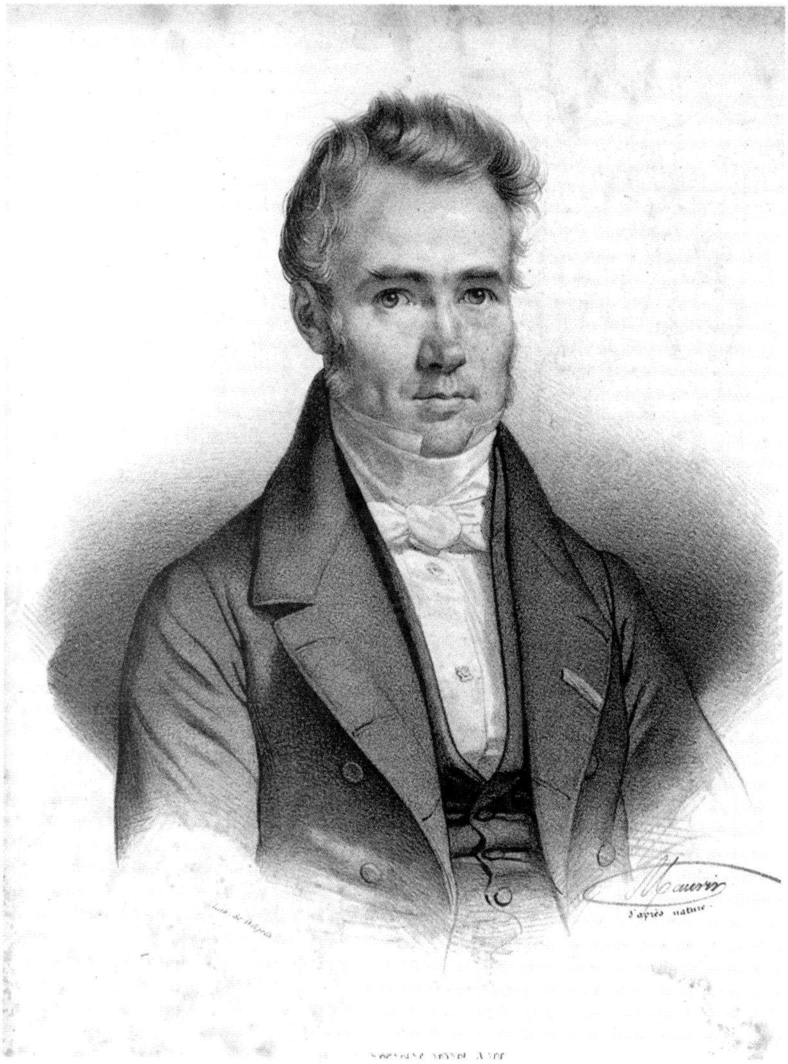

Portrait of Alfred-A.-L.-M. Velpeau

ALFRED-ARMAND-LOUIS-MARIE VELPEAU (1795-1867)
By Maurir

Lithograph
1830-40
Image size: 7 1/8 x 6 3/4 in.
Sheet size: 13 3/4 x 10 3/4 in.

Signed right center: "Maurir/d'après nature."
Inscriptions: "Lith de Delpech" followed by "VELPEAU" and facsimile signature

Given after 1900 by unknown donor
Accession number: 1900+f.Pr.20

Alfred-A.-L.-M. Velpeau was a French surgeon best known for his contributions to the literature of surgical anatomy and operative surgery.

Velpeau was born in 1795 in Breche, the son of a village blacksmith. After initially apprenticing with his father he decided to study medicine instead, first in Tours, and then in Paris where he received his degree from the Faculté de Médecine in 1823. In 1828 he was named surgeon to the Hôpital St. Antoine, in 1830 to La Pitié, and in 1834 to La Charité. He was chair of clinical surgery at the Paris Faculté from 1834 until his death in 1867.

Velpeau's best-known publications are *Traité d'anatomie chirurgicale* (1823), the first detailed work on surgical anatomy; *Nouveaux éléments de médecine opératoire* (1832), the most comprehensive French work on operative surgery; and *Traité des maladies du sein et de la région marraire* (1854), the most important work to date on tumors of the breast.

The bust-length image of Velpeau was done from life by Maurir for the Delpech lithograph shop. The subject's youth shines in his smooth skin, wide-eyed gaze, dimpled cheeks, curly hair, and dapper costume.

Portrait of Ernst von Bergmann

ERNST von BERGMANN (1836-1907)
By Torff

Bronze medal
1913
2 3/8 in. diameter

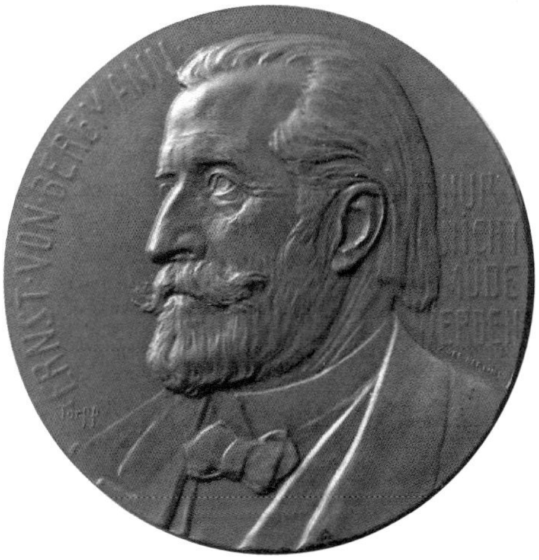

Signed on lower left above subject's shoulder: "Torff"
Inscription on obverse: "ERNST VON BERGMANN NUR/NICHT/MÜDE/ERDEN/AWES BERLIN 13"
Inscription on reverse: "DEM GROSSEN CHIRURGEN/UND LEHRER DEMRASTLOSEN FÖRDERER/ÄRZTLICHEN WISSENS UND KÖNNENS/DEM UNERMÜDLICHEN HELFER/IM DIENSTEDER MENSCHHEIT/1836-1907/GEWID VOM/ZENTRAL/KOMITE FUR/DAS ARZTL/FORTBIL/DUNG/WESEN IN/PREUSSEN"

Given in 1940 by bequest of Pascal Brooke Bland, M.D.
Accession number: 1940+e.M.01

Ernst von Bergmann was a German surgeon known for his contributions to cranial surgery and to surgical pathology.

Bergmann was born in 1836 in Riga, Latvia and graduated from the University of Dorpat in 1860. During the wars of 1866 and 1870-71, he served with the medical corps in field ambulances and hospitals. After the Franco-Prussian War ended in 1871 he was professor of surgery at Dorpat until 1878 when he was called to the chair of surgery at the University of Würzburg. In 1882 he moved to the University of Berlin where he remained for the rest of his career.

Bergmann wrote on the surgical treatment of cerebral diseases, fatty embolism, surgery of the joints, ligation of the femoral vein, and diseases of the lymphatic glands. He is the author of the classic work, *Chirurgische Behandlung der Hirnkrankheiten* (1888). In 1886 he advocated steam sterilization of instruments and dressings, and in 1891 he introduced aseptic methods to the practice of surgery.

The bronze medal of Bergmann was made in 1913 by Torff for the Central Committee for Medical Education in Prussia. He is shown in a three-quarters view facing left. The artist has paid particular attention to the subject's facial wrinkles around his eyes and forehead and thick strands of luxuriant hair, mustache, and beard.

Portrait of Johann A. J. Büttner

JOHANN ARNOLD JOSEF BÜTTNER (1766/68-1844) (OBVERSE)
By Henri François Brandt

Bronze medal
1835
1 7/8 in. diameter

Signed obverse and reverse: "BRANDT F."
Inscription: "I^{O}. AR^{N}. IOS. BUETTNER EQ. INTER SUPREMOS MED. MILIT. PRAEFECTOS SECUNDVS/MEDICI CASTRENSES BORUSS. D."

Given in 1940 by bequest of Pascal Brooke Bland, M.D.
Accession number: 1940+e.M.04

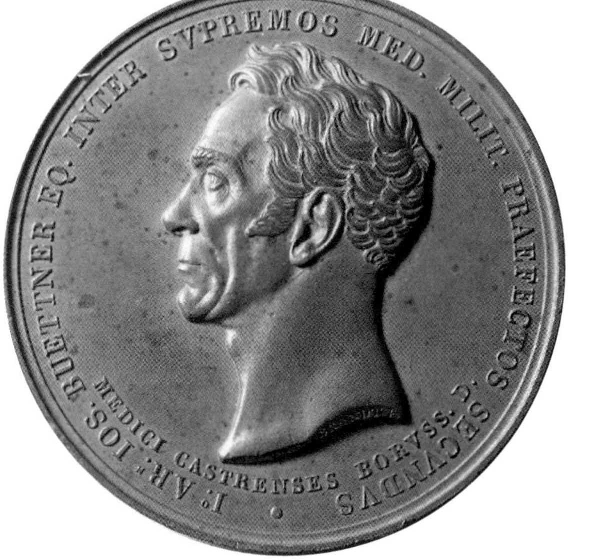

JOHANN ARNOLD JOSEF BÜTTNER (REVERSE)

Dated below image: "D. XV. OCTOB./MDCCCXXXV"
Inscription: "IN MEMORIAM SOLLEMN. X LUSTR. OFF. EXACT."

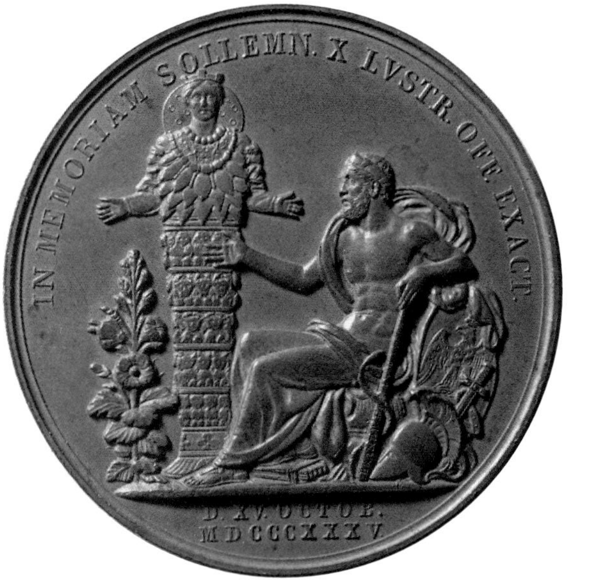

In addition to the battle scene of Ambroise Paré applying ligatures discussed above, the Jefferson collection also includes portraits of two other European military physicians: Johann Büttner and Dominique Larrey.

Johann Büttner was a native of Halberstad. He spent almost his entire career as a military surgeon in the service of the Prussian army. He rose steadily from company surgeon in 1785 to chief of the medical service in 1828. He died in Berlin in 1844.

The bronze medal made by Henri François Brandt was struck in celebration of Büttner's fiftieth year of military service. The carving of this small object is unusually sharp and clear.

The obverse is a well executed portrait with stylized, wavy hair that recalls heads of Roman emperors. The finely detailed reverse features a semi-draped, profile figure of Aesculapius seated next to a trophy arrangement that includes a caduceus, helmet, sword, and shield emblazoned with a spread eagle. He points toward a statue of Artemis, the pre-Greek earth goddess later known as Diana, whose function it was to watch over wildlife. Her haloed and crowned, columnar figure is elaborately decorated with jewelry and a costume featuring vertical stacks of primitive animals. A tall flowering plant rises up toward her outstretched right arm.

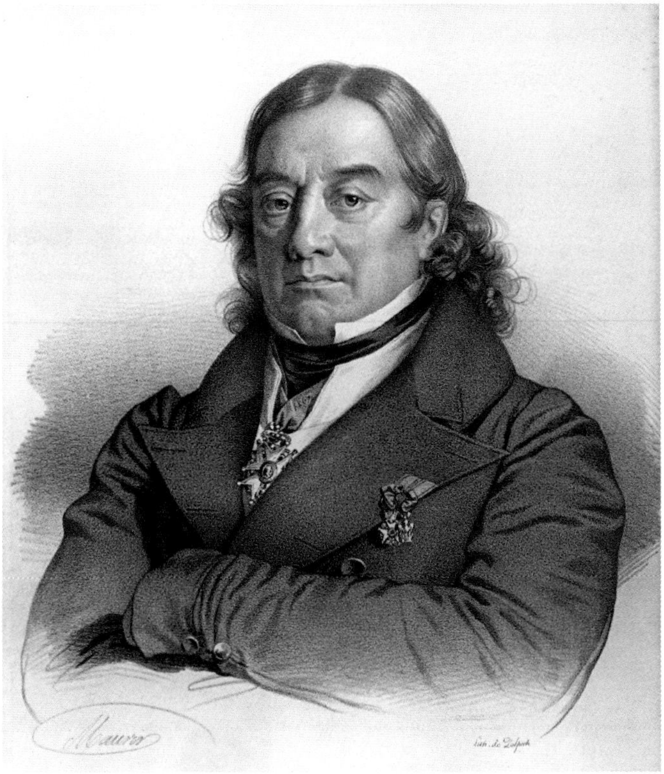

Portrait of Baron Dominique Larrey

BARON DOMINIQUE-JEAN LARREY (1766-1842)
By Maurir

Lithograph
After 1807
Image size: 9 1/4 x 9 1/4 in.
Sheet size: 13 1/4 x 10 in.

Signed lower left: "Maurir"
Inscriptions: "Lith. de Delpech/LARREY"

Given in 1940 by bequest of Pascal Brooke Bland, M.D.
Accession number: 1940+e.Pr.26

Baron Dominique-Jean Larrey was considered "the greatest military surgeon that ever lived" by many medical writers, including the Jefferson surgeon Dr. John Chalmers DaCosta.[13] Larrey's innovations included the introduction of field hospitals, ambulance service, and first aid to the wounded right on the battlefield.

Larrey was born in 1766 to a poor family in the French village of Beaudeau. He began his medical studies in Toulouse with an uncle who was a surgeon, and studied further at the College of Esquile. After passing examinations in Paris and Brest he was appointed chief surgeon on a war vessel, thus launching his military career.

Later as surgeon-in-chief of the Grand Army he took part in almost all of Napoléon's campaigns in Europe, Russia, Egypt, and finally at Waterloo. Larrey was admired by his comrades-in-arms for his good nature, courage, and compassion dealing with the wounded under battlefield conditions. Larrey's title of Baron of the Empire was bestowed by Napoléon, and in his will the emperor referred to Larrey as the "most virtuous man I have ever known" and left him a bequest.

It is reported that Larrey performed as many as two hundred amputations in twenty-four hours at Borodino. He was the inventor of the "flying ambulance" which provided first aid to the wounded immediately, not after a battle was finished. He was appointed a professor at the École de Médecine Militaire at Val-de-Grâce. His most enduring literary work is the four-volume *Memoires de chirurgie militaire et campagnes* (1812-17).

In 1802 Larrey was the first to note the contagiousness of trachoma, in 1803 he became one of the first to amputate at the hip joint, and in 1812 he published the first description of trench foot. Larrey's prodigious medical reputation saved his life after the fall of Napoléon, and in 1820 he was named a member of the newly founded Académie de Médecine.

The unidealized portrait bust of Larrey was made by Maurir for the Delpech lithograph shop. The depiction emphasizes the subject's bulky facial contours and resolute expression. His long, wispy hair is smooth on top and curled below. The ornate, star-shaped medal hanging from a ribbon around his neck is dated 1807.

Portrait of Edward Jenner

EDWARD JENNER (1749-1823)
By Edward Scriven (1775-1841) after mezzotint by John Raphael Smith (1752-1812) derived from his own oil portrait

Engraving, etching, stipple
Before 1841
Image size: 5 x 4 1/4 in.
Sheet size: 10 3/8 x 6 3/4 in.

Signed lower center: "Engraved by E. Scriven."
Inscriptions: "JENNER"; "From a Print engraved and coloured by J. R. Smith/in the pofsefsion of the late John Ring Esqr/Under the Superintendance of the Society for the Diffusion/of Useful Knowledge/London. Published by Charles Knight, Ludgate Street."

Given after 1900 by unknown donor
Accession number: 1900+f.Pr.14

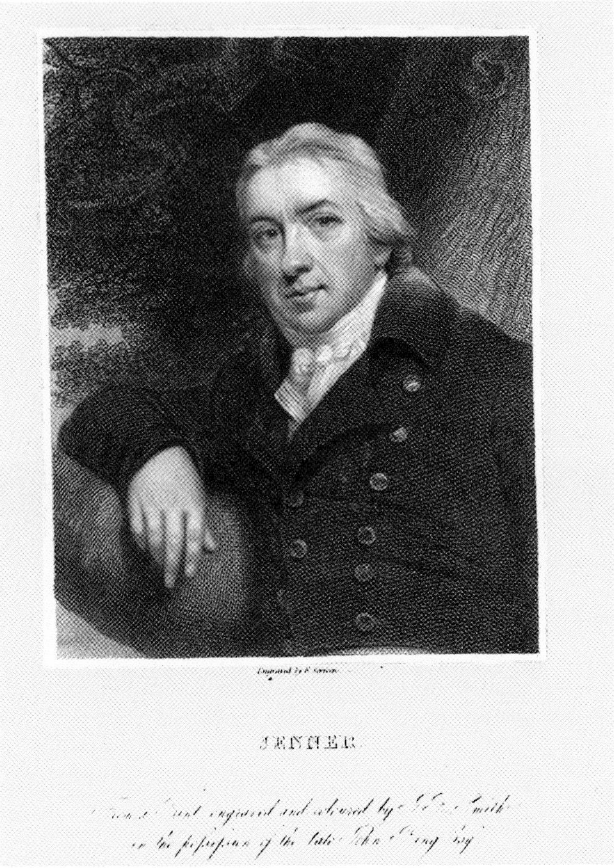

Edward Jenner was the renowned English physician and naturalist who discovered smallpox vaccination.

The son of a vicar, Jenner was born in 1749 in the small market town of Berkeley in Gloucestershire. In 1761 he began an apprenticeship with a local surgeon, with whom he worked until 1770 when he became a house pupil of John Hunter in London, studying surgery and anatomy. After his training he returned to Berkeley to become a country doctor.

Early in his practice he was asked to inoculate persons against smallpox with matter from smallpox pustules, thus giving them a mild case of the disease in order to confer immunity. He considered this relatively new practice a dangerous technique that often led to death and spread the disease further.

For many years Jenner observed that those who had suffered from what Jenner called "true cowpox," a relatively mild disease, remained immune to the ravages of smallpox. In May 1796 an outbreak of cowpox occurred and Jenner inoculated an eight-year-old boy with matter taken from the pustules of a milkmaid suffering from cowpox, and the boy recovered speedily. Later that summer Jenner twice inoculated the boy with smallpox and there was no reaction. Jenner concluded that an attack of cowpox rendered the patient immune against smallpox, and that cowpox lymph was the ideal virus for inoculation.

Jenner submitted an account of his observations to the Royal Society, but his theory was ridiculed. Undismayed, he continued his experiments and in 1798 published a booklet entitled *An Inquiry into the Causes and Effects of the Variolae Vaccinae.* Although it was coolly received at first, other scientists endeavored to repeat his experiments and soon his method was accepted and the practice became widespread throughout Europe and America. Later when it was discovered that immunity could be renewed by a repetition of the inoculation, smallpox became a preventible disease.

Edward Jenner spent the rest of his life promulgating his discovery and assisting in supplying dried lymph to the far corners of the world. By 1802 the British Parliament showed the nation's gratitude by awarding the physician ten thousand pounds, and in 1807 twice that amount. In 1803 the Royal Jennerian Society was founded in London to promote vaccination, and in 1813 Jenner was awarded an honorary medical degree from Oxford University.

The portrait of Jenner is by Edward Scriven. The English engraver supplied copies of famous paintings to publishers of illustrated books, and was the official engraver to the Prince of Wales. The source for this image was an oil portrait of Jenner painted by John Raphael Smith in 1802, and the artist's own mezzotint replica. Smith was an English engraver and miniaturist.

The original painting featured a background view of Berkeley fields with cows and a milkmaid. Scriven's small engraving is limited to the figure, shown half length and leaning with his right arm against a tree branch.

The Jefferson archival collection also includes a silver medal by Anton Guillemard commemorating the smallpox vaccination. It was struck at Prague in 1803 for the Smallpox Commission of Bohemia.

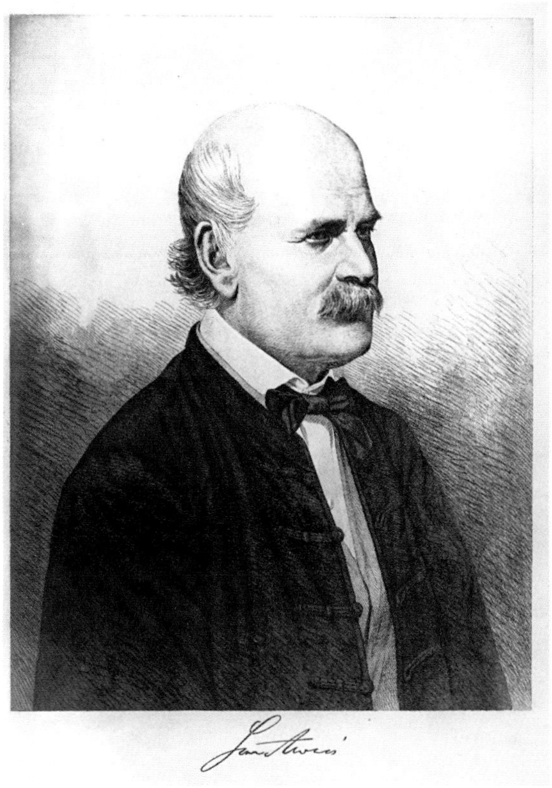

Portrait of Ignaz P. Semmelweis

IGNAZ PHILIPP SEMMELWEIS (1818-65)
By unknown artist

Etching, aquatint mounted on board
1855-65
Image size: 19 1/2 x 15 in.
Board size: 26 x 19 1/4 in.

Inscription: facsimile signature of the subject

Given after 1900 by unknown donor
Accession number: 1900+f.Pr.11

Ignaz Philipp Semmelweis was a Hungarian physician credited with the discovery of the etiology and prevention of puerperal fever. Prophylactic handwashings made him a pioneer in antisepsis during the prebacterial era.

Semmelweis was born in 1818 in Buda, Hungary, the son of a prosperous shopkeeper. He studied medicine first in Pest and then received his medical degree in 1844 from the Second Vienna Medical School. After graduation he completed a master's degree in practical midwifery and also received surgical training.

In 1846 he became an assistant at the First Obstetrical Clinic of the Vienna General Hospital where the maternal and neonatal mortality rate from puerperal fever was higher than thirteen percent. This clinic was used for the instruction of medical students. Curiously, at the same hospital's Second Obstetrical Clinic run by midwives, the mortality rate was only about two percent. The latter clinic was the teaching service for midwives. Semmelweis eventually realized that puerperal fever was not due to "epidemic constitution" as then thought.

He observed that women who were delivered rapidly before an examination had taken place never sickened, while those who had arduous labors and frequent examinations were almost certain to die from the disease; further, that the death rate was lower during hospital vacation periods and comparatively rare in rural districts. He eventually realized that infection originated from the hands of the examining physicians and students who had just conducted autopsies. There was an immediate decline in mortality when Semmelweis insisted that all physicians must disinfect their hands with chlorine water between autopsy work and pelvic examinations. By 1848 Semmelweis widened his prophylaxis treatment to include all instruments used with patients in labor.

Far from achieving approbation for his ideas, this led to a long-lasting controversy among obstetricians. There was no chance of promotion for Semmelweis in Vienna so he returned to Pest and took charge of the maternity ward at St. Rochus Hospital. In 1855 he was appointed to the chair of theoretical and practical midwifery at the university. He did not publish his theory until 1861, in *Die Aetiologie, der Begriff und die Prophylaxis des Kindbettfiebers*.

Semmelweis's ideas were not generally accepted until after his death when Louis Pasteur and Joseph Lister furnished indisputable proof. In fact the brilliant and sensitive Semmelweis was broken by the indifference of his colleagues, and was committed to an asylum in Vienna where he died soon after in 1865.

This half-length depiction of Ignaz Semmelweis by an unknown artist is a three-quarters view at a large scale. His deepset eyes look pensively into the distance. The baldness of his head is offset by thick eyebrows and bushy mustache. His collarless coat with frog closures is probably characteristic of local attire.

Portrait of Louis Pasteur

LOUIS PASTEUR (1822-95)
By Albert Rosenthal (1863-1939), after a tintype

Lithograph
1925
Image size: 19 x 15 in.
Sheet size: 22 1/2 x 18 in.

Signed and dated center right: "Lith. by Albert Rosenthal/after Photo tintype/Copyrg[t.] 1925"
Inscription in pencil lower right: "To: Dept. Preventive Medicine/& Bacteriology/Jefferson Medical College/Phila./ Albert Rosenthal-/2/12/27" above facsimile signature

Given in 1927 by the artist
Accession number: 1927+e.Pr.01

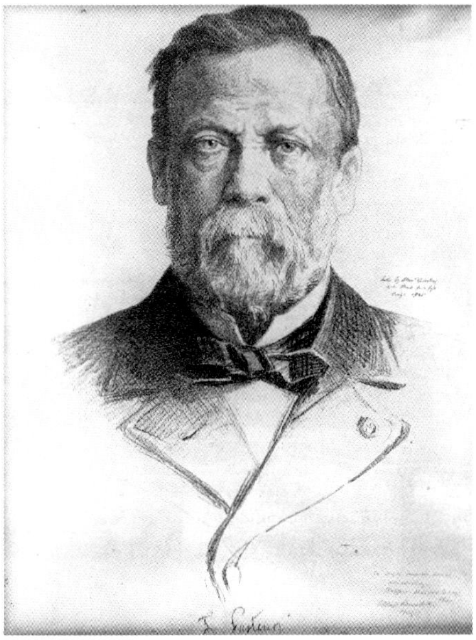

Louis Pasteur was one of the founders of bacteriology. Although not a physician, he has been called the Father of Preventive Medicine.

A tanner's son, Louis Pasteur was born in 1822 in Dôle, Burgundy and reared in Arbois. He received his bachelor's degree in letters (1840) and science (1842) from the Collège Royal de Besançon, and a doctorate in physics and chemistry at the École Normale in Paris (1847).

After serving briefly as professor of chemistry in Strasbourg, Pasteur was professor of chemistry and dean of the faculty of sciences in Lille, director of scientific studies at the École Normale, professor of chemistry at the Sorbonne, and finally, director of the Institut Pasteur in Paris.

Pasteur's landmark work on fermentation, *Études sur le vinaigre: sa fabrication, ses maladies, moyens de les prévenir; nouvelles observations sur la conservation des vins par la chaleur* (1868), showed how wine was spoiled by microbes and that microbes could be destroyed by heat. His process for the preservation of wine by sterilizing procedures came to be called "pasteurization."

Pasteur also discredited the idea of "spontaneous generation" of microbes thought to spoil milk and butter. He discovered that the bacteria of putrefaction were anaerobic, thriving only in the absence of free oxygen, while other microorganisms were aerobic. His experiments showed that the microorganisms of decomposition in wine and milk were the causes and not the consequences of the changes, and that they derived from the external environment.

Pasteur rescued the French silkgrowing industry by identifying two diseases of caterpillars, and showed the way to breed healthy stock by weeding out infected eggs and removing the source of infection in the food. He also prepared vaccines against fowl cholera, anthrax, swine erysipelas, and rabies.

Pasteur devoted the last two decades of his life to the study of the germ theory of disease. By 1888 funds were collected from donors around the world, largely due to his fame for the treatment of rabies, for the Institut Pasteur, established in Paris to study the causes, prevention, and treatment of infectious diseases.

Louis Pasteur received numerous awards from the French Legion of Honor, including the Grand Cross in 1881. Other major honors were the Grand Prize Medal of the Exposition Universelle of 1867, membership and the Copley Medal of the Royal Society, commander of the Imperial Order of the Rose in Brazil, Grand Cordon of the Order of Isabella the Catholic, and membership in the Académie de Médecine and the Académie Française.

In 1892 a grand jubilee celebration in his honor was held at the Sorbonne where the frail and aging scientist entered the proceedings on the arm of the president of the Third Republic. In 1895 Pasteur was accorded a state funeral at Nôtre Dame Cathedral with full military honors, followed by interment at the Institut.

Albert Rosenthal's head-and-shoulders depiction of Louis Pasteur is rendered in the artist's customary lively, three dimensional style. Rosenthal presented the lithograph of Pasteur to Jefferson's department of preventive medicine in 1927.

In addition to the Albert Rosenthal portrait, the Jefferson art collection has other images of Louis Pasteur: a small bronze sculpture by Théodore Rivière, given by bequest of Pascal Brooke Bland, M.D. in 1940, an oil painting (now in poor condition) by Rudolphe F. Budabin, presented by members of Jefferson's Pasteur Society in 1953, and a reproduction of a famous *Vanity Fair* lithograph of 1887.

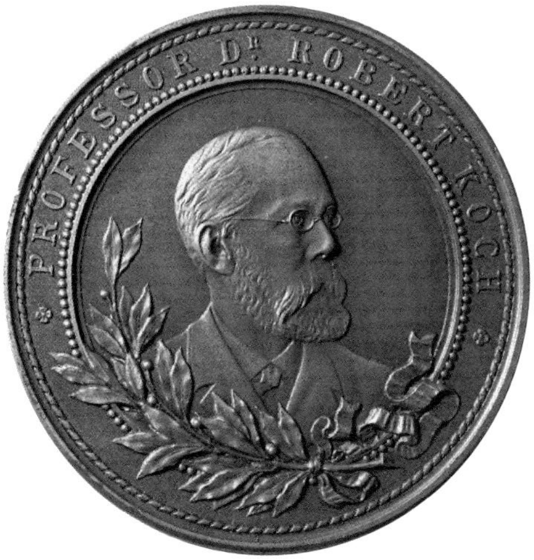

Portrait of Robert Koch

ROBERT KOCH (1843-1910)
By Wilhelm Mayer

Bronze medal
1908
1 15/16 in. diameter

Signed on reverse left center: "W. M."
Inscription on obverse: "PROFESSOR DR ROBERT KOCH"
Inscription on reverse: "UT SEMENTEM FECERIS, ITA METES"

Given in 1940 by bequest of Pascal Brooke Bland, M.D.
Accession number: 1940+e.M.07

Dr. Robert Koch was a German physician who revolutionized the discipline of bacteriology with his discoveries and techniques. He influenced authorities in many countries to introduce public health legislation based on the microbial origin of various infections.

Robert Koch was born in 1843 in Klausthal, Hannover, the son of a mining official. He earned his medical degree at the University of Göttingen in 1866 with the highest distinction. A flourishing general practice in Rakwitz was interrupted by service in the Franco-Prussian War. In 1872 he became the district physician at Wollstein where he also established a rudimentary laboratory for conducting microscopic studies.

In 1876 he announced that he had worked out the complete life history of the anthrax bacillus that caused the disease, and his meticulous work was published that year and confirmed by Louis Pasteur. Koch set forth the methods by which an investigator should work with bacteria, and demonstrated that a particular bacillus always causes a particular disease. His publication *Untersuchungen über die Aetiologie der Wundinfektionskrankheiten* (1878) described the bacteriology of six different kinds of wound infections.

When Koch was appointed advisor to the Imperial Board of Health in Berlin in 1880 he was provided with better equipped laboratories. He developed the methodology of steam sterilization by dry heat instead of chemical substances, and advocated nutrient gelatin as a solid medium. In 1882 he announced that he had discovered the tubercle bacillus by special culture and staining methods, and that tuberculosis was not a chronic disorder of nutrition as had been supposed. One disappointing result was Koch's isolation of a tuberculin which he maintained in 1890 would check the growth of tubercle bacillus; the remedy failed to live up to his hopes.

In 1885 Koch was appointed professor of hygiene and director of the Hygienic Institute at the University of Berlin. He resigned in 1891 to become chief of the Institute for Infectious Diseases. This research facility was established in his honor and attracted scientists from around the world.

Throughout his career Koch traveled widely to campaign against pestilences. In 1883 as a member of the German Cholera Commission he visited India and Egypt and discovered the cholera vibrio and its transmission by water, food, and clothing. In Hindustan he showed that bubonic plague was transmitted to humans by the rat-flea. He devised a method of inoculation against rinderpest in South Africa. He also made valuable studies of Texas fever, sleeping sickness, malaria, and blackwater fever.

When Robert Koch retired from the institute in 1904, disciples and admirers presented a Festschrift in his honor, the government established an annual honorarium of ten thousand marks, and the Kaiser awarded him the Order of Wilhelm. He received the Nobel Prize in 1905. The following year he received the Prussian Order Pour le Mérite, and was made a member of the Prussian Academy of Sciences with the title of *Excellenz*.

In 1908 proposals to establish the Robert Koch Foundation to combat tuberculosis were approved, and among the most generous benefactors were the Kaiser and Andrew Carnegie. That same year Koch was honored by Berlin physicians and received the first Robert Koch Medal, established to commemorate the greatest living physicians.

The small bronze medal by Wilhelm Mayer shows a head-and-shoulders portrait of Robert Koch. The bearded physician is wearing spectacles and looking off to the right. A branch of laurel leaves tied with a ribbon follows the curve of the medal below. The reverse of the medal features an open book, a diploma, a skull, and a caduceus from which the snake is drinking from a cup, and a Latin motto: "As you sow, so shall you reap."

Portrait of Wilhelm C. Roentgen

WILHELM CONRAD ROENTGEN (1845-1923)
By Walter Schatalow

Oil on canvas
1965
30 x 25 in.

Signed lower right: "W. S."
Inscription on rear of canvas: "Walter Schatalow/1965"

Given in 1983 by the artist in memory of Bernard L. Feuerstein
Accession number: 1983+e.P.09

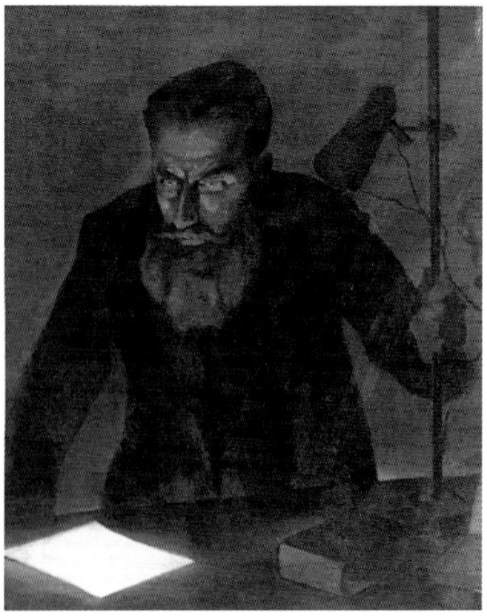

Wilhelm Conrad Roentgen, a German physicist, was the discoverer of a new kind of rays to which his name was given in his native land: Roentgenstrahlen, known elsewhere as X-rays.

The son of a cloth manufacturer and merchant, Roentgen was born in 1845 in Lennep, Germany and moved to Holland as a young child. After spending two and one-half years at the Utrecht Technical School, he received his diploma as a mechanical engineer in 1868 and doctorate a year later from the Federal Polytechnical College at Zurich.

After working as a laboratory assistant and teaching physics in Strasbourg and Hohenheim Roentgen was awarded the post of chair of physics at the University of Giessen, in Hesse (1879-88). Then he accepted the offer of the Royal University of Würzburg to be professor of physics and director of the Physical Institute, and was made rector of the university in 1894. He assumed his final post in 1900 as chair of physics and director of the Physical Institute at Munich.

Roentgen published fifty-eight important papers, most in *Annalen der Physik und Chemie,* but his celebrity rests mainly on two pieces of work. In 1888 he demonstrated quantitatively the electromagnetic theory of James C. Maxwell: that there will be a magnetic field in a dielectric such as a glass plate whenever the electric field changes. This effect was named the Roentgen current in his honor.

In 1895 Roentgen made his momentous discovery of X-rays, bringing him international fame. He had turned his attention to the phenomena of the unexpected ease with which electric current passed through a vacuum, and that the glass wall of the vacuum tube emptied of air glowed with a greenish-yellow or blue fluorescence. He found that the cathodes, negative electrodes, welded in the glass tube, through which the current entered, radiated particles which bore the current through the vacuum to the positive electrode, the anode, causing the fluorescence.

In six weeks of concentrated work, he discovered properties of the new rays: they travel in straight lines, cannot be refracted or reflected, are not deviated by a magnet, and can travel about two meters in air. He discovered their penetrating properties and produced images of objects inside a closed door, a box, a book, and the chamber of a shotgun. Finally, when he held his hand behind the screen he could see the outlines of his own fingers.

His famous pamphlet *Eine neue Art von Strahlen* (1896) caused a sensation. Notwithstanding the attention, Roentgen steadfastly refused to patent his discovery and resisted all offers of commercial exploitation in the fields of medical diagnosis and the testing of materials.

The resulting publicity afforded him many honors. In 1896 after Roentgen demonstrated the effects of X-rays to the Kaiser and his court, he was immediately awarded the Prussian Order of the Crown, Second Class. He received an honorary doctor of medicine degree from the University of Würzburg and medals from the Royal Society of London and Columbia University. He was made an honorary citizen of Lennep, and a statue of him was erected on the Potsdam Bridge in Berlin. In 1901 he won the first Nobel Prize for physics, and a medal was struck in his honor.

The painting of Roentgen by Walter Schatalow shows the physicist at work in his laboratory, standing behind a table with his apparatus activating a fluorescent screen and causing it to glow. There is a reddish glow behind the table. Schatalow's overly theatrical depiction of the notably reticent scientist is unfortunately diabolical-looking, but his facial features and luxuriant beard closely resemble contemporary photographs.

Rare Medical Books

The Thomas Jefferson University library contains over four thousand rare books related to the history of medicine and natural science. The most generous donor of historic medical books was Pascal Brooke Bland, M.D., the former chair of obstetrics, whose holdings on anatomy and obstetrics and midwifery were especially noteworthy.

In many cases the text and accompanying illustrations were collaborative efforts between physicians and artists, producing landmark publications of lasting scientific and aesthetic importance. Several of the artists employed to illustrate texts were also well known as master printmakers and painters.

The following selections merely hint at the quality and range of the collection, with works dating from 1483 to 1788. Chronological comparisons will be made of images in the following categories: title pages and frontispieces, health and hygiene, midwifery, and anatomy. Most of the earliest learned works were printed in Latin, but because titles could run on for many lines, the common abridged titles are used. Some rare books in the Jefferson collection are later publications, not the first edition of the work. With two exceptions, all the images illustrated remain intact in their original books.

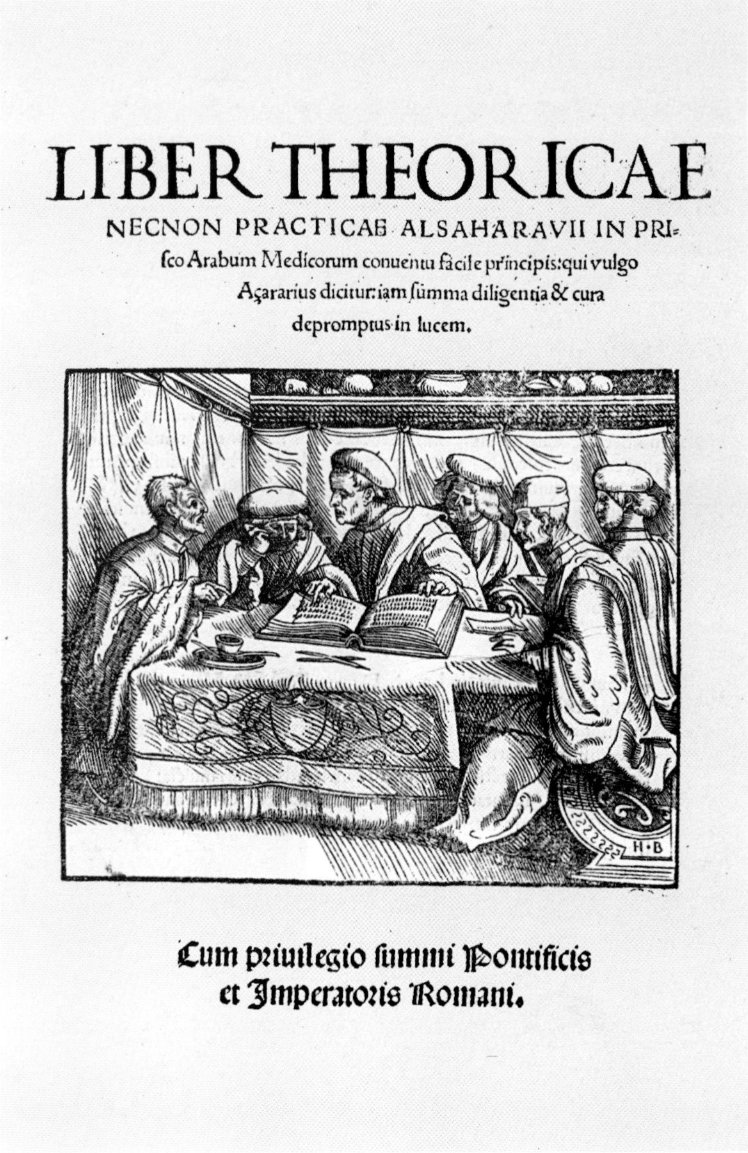
LIBER THEORICAE
NECNON PRACTICAE ALSAHARAVII IN PRI-
ſco Arabum Medicorum conuentu fácile príncipis:qui vulgo
Açararius dicitur:iam ſumma diligentia & cura
depromptus in lucem.

Cum priuilegio ſummi Pontificis
et Imperatoris Romani.

Title Page: Physicians in Discussion

PHYSICIANS IN DISCUSSION
By Hans Burgkmair the Elder (1473-1531)

Woodcut printed in black and red
Image size: 4 5/8 x 5 5/8 in.
Page size: 12 1/8 x 8 1/4 in.

Signed lower right: "H. B."

From Albucacis, *Liber theoricae necnon practicae Alsaharavii...* (Augsburg: S. Grim & M. Wirsung, 1519)

Given in 1940 by bequest of Pascal Brooke Bland, M.D.
Accession number: 1940+e.Pr.07

A common type of illustration for title pages and frontispieces depicts a group of physicians in discussion. Examples in the Jefferson collection are books by Albucacis and Albertus Magnus published in the sixteenth century.

Albucacis (also called Alsaharavius, or Abu-L-Qasim) was a Moorish physician working in Cordova, Spain in the late tenth and early eleventh centuries. He is the author of a great medicochirurgical treatise, *Altasrif* ("*Collection*"), of which only the surgical part survives today. Adapted largely from the work of Paul of Aegina, it was the leading textbook on surgery in the Middle Ages, and included descriptions of cautery, lithotomy, amputations, wound treatment, fractures, and dislocations.

Hans Burgkmair's image of doctors in discussion was used to illustrate several books, but it appeared first as the title page in Albucacis's *Liber theoricae*, published in 1519. It shows a group of six anonymous doctors wearing robes seated at a table intently discussing the merits of an open book. The leaders appear to be the three figures leaning forward and gesturing. If attire designates rank, then the physician at the far left must be presiding because his gown is the only one trimmed in fur.

A native of Augsburg, Hans Burgkmair was one of several artists employed to record the personal lives of the court of Maximilian I, the Holy Roman Emperor. In addition to hundreds of woodcuts depicting the court, Burgkmair also received commissions for oil paintings of religious scenes, landscapes, and portraits. During his travels to Italy Burgkmair absorbed many new artistic ideas and helped to introduce elements of the southern Renaissance style to Germany.

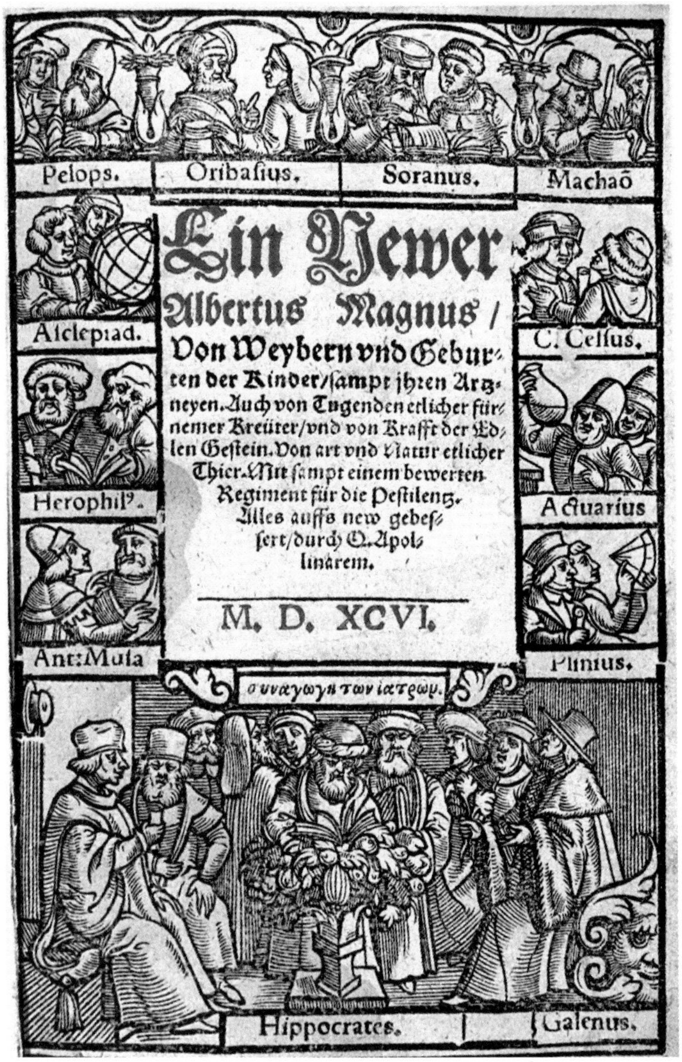

Title Page: Physicians in Discussion

PHYSICIANS IN DISCUSSION
By unknown artist

Woodcut printed in black and red
Image size: 6 3/4 x 4 3/8 in.
Page size: 7 3/8 x 5 1/2 in.

From Albertus Magnus, *Ein newer Albertus Magnus...* (Augsburg: Michael Manger, 1596)

Given in 1940 by bequest of Pascal Brooke Bland, M.D.
Accession number: 1940+e.Pr.04

The physicians depicted on the Albucacis title page are anonymous and differentiated mainly by costume and age. Title pages of some subsequent books feature physicians identified by name. In the case of *Ein newer Albertus Magnus* the generalized images are not intended to be actual likenesses.

Albertus Magnus (1193/1200-80) was a Dominican monk and naturalist, and an important philosopher who reintroduced Aristotle and Arabic science to German universities. In the physical sciences he wrote on mathematics, mechanics, sound, astronomy, and the structure of matter. He also wrote on botany and the evolution of plants and on the embryology of animals. Some scholars think that spurious medical books were attributed to Albertus Magnus or published under his name to assure a wide circulation.

The title page of *Ein newer Albertus Magnus* features bust-length portraits of physicians and scholars at the top: one mythical, ten ancient, and one medieval, each identified by name and accompanied by a companion, and many using medical props. Below is a group of full-length figures of doctors with only Hippocrates and Galen mentioned by name, but all involved in earnest discussions.

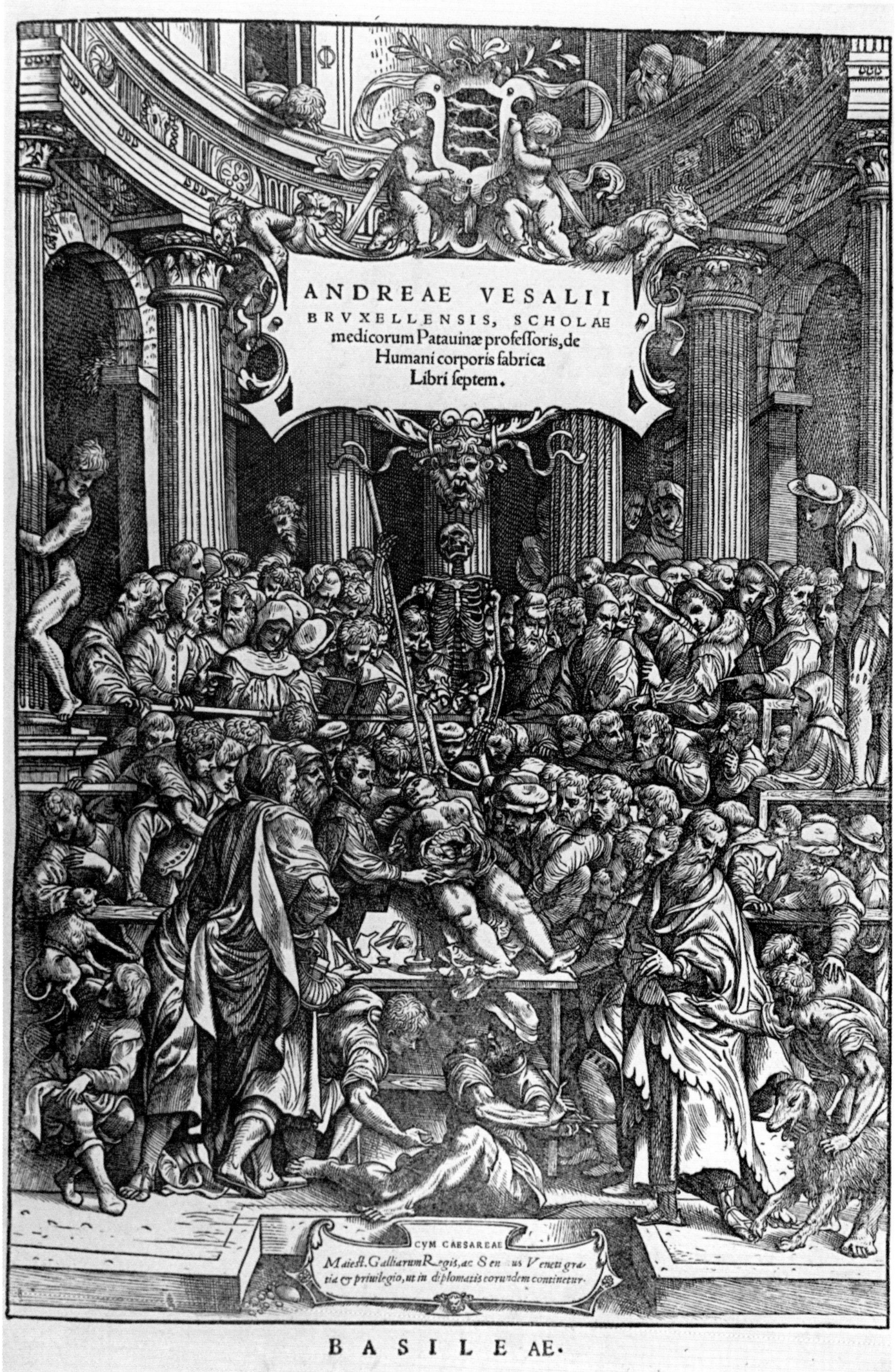
ANDREAE VESALII
BRVXELLENSIS, SCHOLAE
medicorum Patauinæ professoris, de
Humani corporis fabrica
Libri septem.
CVM CAESAREAE
Maiest. Galliarum Regis, ac S en us Veneti gra-
tia & priuilegio, ut in diplomatis eorundem continetur.
BASILEAE.

Title Page: Andreas Vesalius Dissecting

ANDREAS VESALIUS DISSECTING
Attributed to Jan Stephan van Calcar (ca. 1499-1546/50)

Woodcut
Image size: 13 7/8 x 9 3/4 in.
Page size: 16 x 11 in.

From Andreas Vesalius, *De humani corporis fabrica libri septem* (Basle: Joannis Oporini, 1543)

Given in 1977 by Robert L. Phillips, M.D. (JMC 1952)
Accession number: 1977+e.Pr.04

Over the centuries many anatomical atlases featured an illustration of the author or another experienced scholar teaching anatomy.

When Mondino de' Luzzi's *Anathomia* was republished as one of several treatises in Johannes de Ketham's *Fasciculus medicinae*, a dissection scene was included in the 1493 Italian edition. It was thought originally to depict Mondino himself seated in an elevated pulpit-like chair, the cathedra, from which he read or lectured to the students. Below, men of lower rank included an *ostensor* who used a pointer to show the area of incision and give directions, and a *demonstrator*, often a barber-surgeon, who performed the dissection.

A more recent scholarly view of this dissection illustration is that it depicts consecutive events collapsed into a single image, and that actually physicians performed all three tasks.[14] This view contradicts the visual implication of the illustration, but it is known, in fact, that Mondino and some other predecessors of Vesalius did perform dissections themselves.

Painters and sculptors were also taking an interest in the accurate representation of the human form by the mid-fifteenth century, and some applied Leon Battista Alberti's (1404-72) principle of how to get the right proportions and construction: visualize the bony insides, attach muscles and tendons, cover with flesh and skin, and finally add clothes. Artists studied anatomy in life-drawing groups and observed dissections, and by the mid-sixteenth century Florentine artists themselves were performing dissections routinely.[15] The surviving anatomical drawings of Leonardo da Vinci (1452-1519), for example, surpassed medical illustration of his own time, but his plans for a comprehensive book on anatomy never were completed.

One of the most famous images in all of medical art is the dissection title page of Vesalius's *Fabrica*. Art and medical scholars have not entirely resolved the question of the identity of the artist or artists who drew the remarkable title page and innovative dissected skeletons and muscle figures, but most credit Jan Stephan (or Joannes Stephanus) van Calcar, a Flemish artist who had been a pupil of Titian in Venice (see below). The woodcut illustrations were made under Vesalius's close supervision in Venice, a great center of printing, but he preferred to publish with the firm of Joannis Oporini in Basle. Vesalius accompanied the woodblocks on the trip over the Alps by donkey train to Basle.

The title page of *Fabrica* embodies Vesalius's views expounded in the preface, in which he staunchly defends the anatomist-surgeon as *the* authority on human anatomy, and urges that the "barbaric butchers" currently assigned the role of dissector be replaced by knowledgeable anatomists like himself.[16] Vesalius has descended from the chair to conduct the dissection himself without the aid of a book. (His likeness resembles the famous portrait in the frontispiece of the first and second editions of *Fabrica*.) An articulated skeleton with a staff is situated where the reader formerly sat. Assistants are relegated to places under the table to prepare instruments rather than help with the dissection.

The professor stands in the center of a huge crowd, both dissecting and expounding on a female cadaver lying on a table. Onlookers include students, physicians, city and university officials, representatives of the church, the general public, and figures in classical garb. A chained monkey and a dog (used in Galen's research) are now symbolically pushed to the lower left and right borders of the scene. A nude figure clinging to a column on the left suggests the importance of surface anatomy.[17]

The scene of Vesalius dissecting takes place in an imaginary Renaissance-style, outdoor amphitheater. In this period, however, it was customary for a temporary wooden structure to be erected to accommodate the crowds who witnessed the public dissections. Permanent anatomical theaters were not constructed until the late sixteenth century.

The Latin words that appear in the cartouche proclaim the author and title, in translation: "Andreas Vesalius of Brussels, professor in the medical school at Padua, *Seven Books on the Structure of the Human Body*." Above the cartouche two putti support the family heraldic device of three weasels *courant*, emblematic of the town of Wesel on the Rhine from which Vesalius's forbears came and a play on the vernacular version of his name, Wessels.[18]

Title Page: Johannes Riolan Dissecting

JOHANNES RIOLAN DISSECTING
By Reinier van Persyn
(ca. 1614-ca. 1668)

Engraving, etching, stipple
Image size: 6 1/2 x 4 1/4 in.
Page size: 6 3/4 x 4 3/8 in.

Signed lower left below image: "R. A. Persyn, Sculp."
From Johannes Riolan the Younger, *Encheiridium anatomicum et pathologicum...* (Leiden: Adriani Wyngaerden, 1649)

Given after 1900 by unknown donor
Accession number: 1900+f.Pr.03

The title page of Johannes Riolan the Younger's *Encheiridium* also includes an illustration of the author dissecting. Instead of being surrounded by a vast crowd in an imaginary amphitheater as in the Vesalius title page, Riolan performs an abdominal dissection in a shallow space accompanied by physicians identified as Johann Vesling, Albert Kuyper, Guy Patin, and A. Valcob, to whom the volume is dedicated. His companions, however, seem oblivious to the dissection and stare into space.

On the platform above is a cabinet displaying the anatomist's instruments, and flanked by male and female figures holding the caduceus. Above is a coat of arms with a skull. Numerous birds and a dog accompany the allegorical figures. As on the Vesalius title page, the dissecting scene covers the entire page. The illustrator was Reinier van Persyn, a Dutch painter and engraver.

Johannes Riolan the Younger (1580-1657) was chair of anatomy and botany at the University of Paris and chair of medicine at the Collège Royal. He also became the principal physician to the queen mother, Marie de Médicis. His *Encheiridium* (first published 1648) included a systematic presentation of both morbid and normal anatomy.

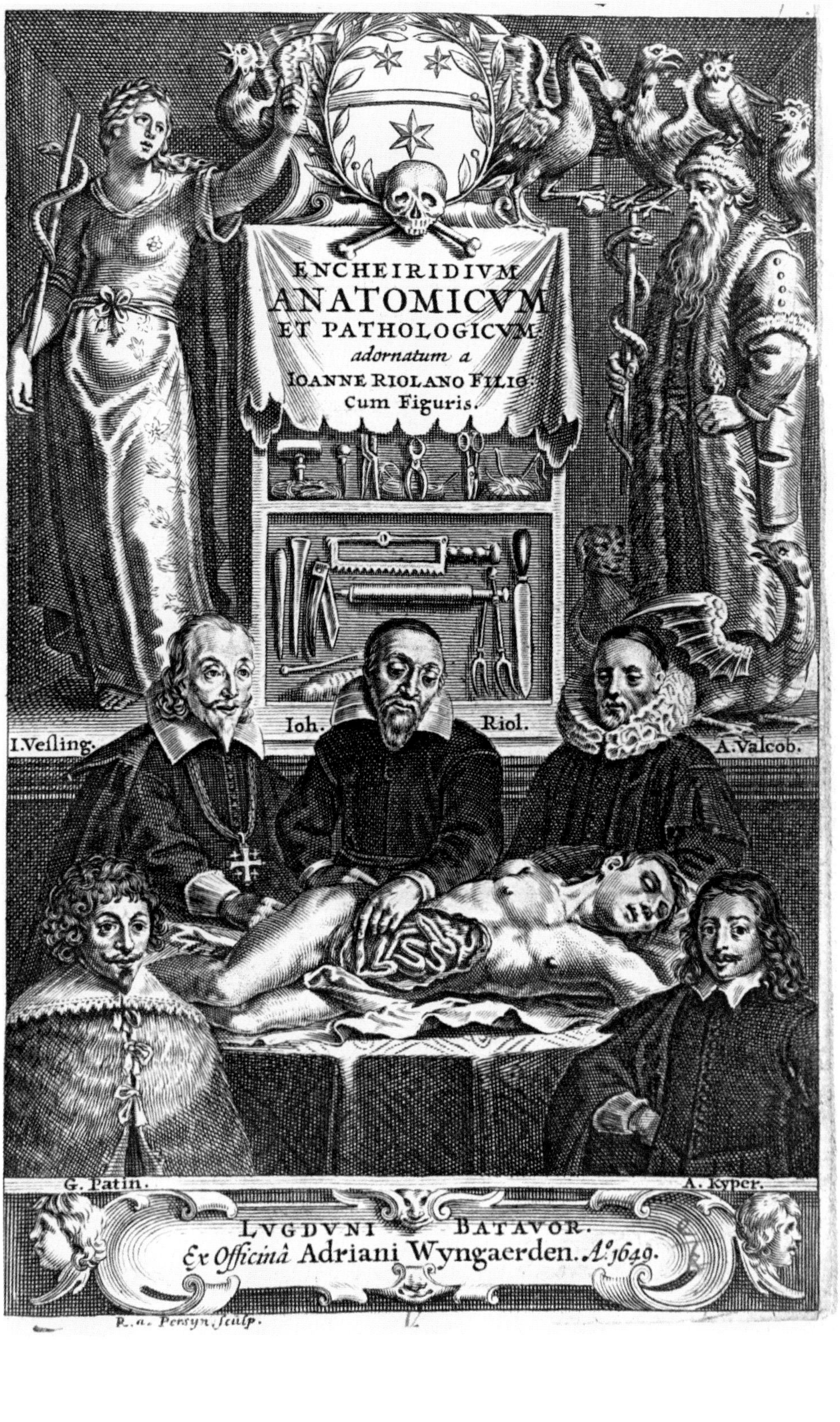
ENCHEIRIDIVM
ANATOMICVM
ET PATHOLOGICVM
adornatum a
IOANNE RIOLANO FILIO.
Cum Figuris.
I. Vesling.
Ioh. Riol.
A. Valcob.
G. Patin.
A. Kyper.
LVGDVNI BATAVOR.
Ex Officinâ Adriani Wyngaerden. A°. 1649.
R. a. Persyn, sculp.

Title Page: Bartholomaeus Eustachius Dissecting

BARTHOLOMAEUS EUSTACHIUS DISSECTING
By Petrus Leo Ghezzius (1674-1755)

Engraving; page printed in black and red
Image size: 4 x 6 in.
Plate size: 4 1/4 x 6 3/8 in.
Page size: 15 1/4 x 9 1/2 in.

From Bartholomaeus Eustachius, *Tabulae anatomicae clarissimi viri Bartholomaei Eustachii quas è tenebris tandem vindicatas* (Amsterdam: Rudolphus & Gerardus Wetstenios, 1722)

Given in 1940 by bequest of Pascal Brooke Bland, M.D.
Accession number: 1940+e.Pr.13

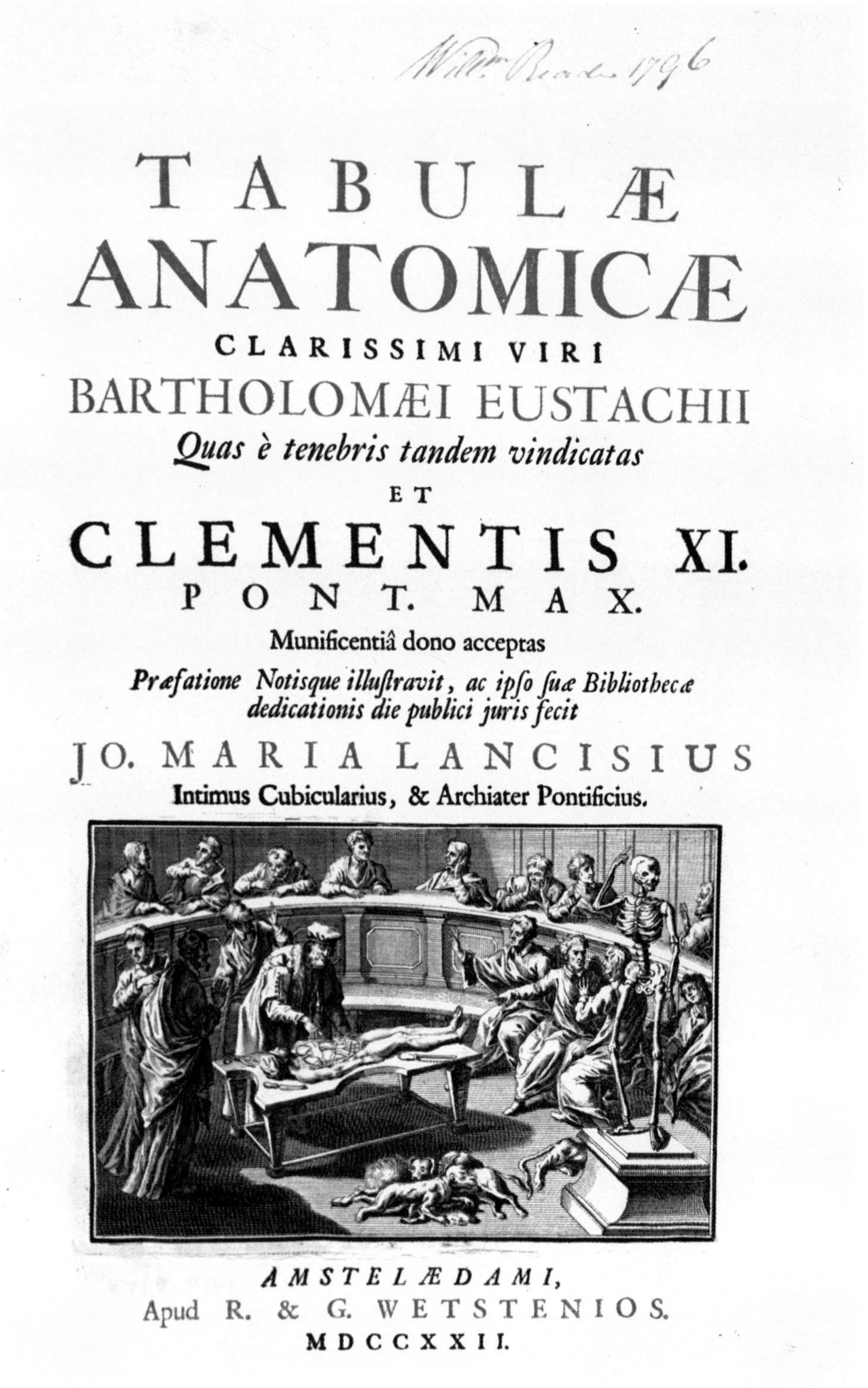

TABULÆ ANATOMICÆ
CLARISSIMI VIRI
BARTHOLOMÆI EUSTACHII
Quas è tenebris tandem vindicatas
ET
CLEMENTIS XI.
PONT. MAX.
Munificentiâ dono acceptas
Præfatione Notisque illustravit, ac ipso suæ Bibliothecæ dedicationis die publici juris fecit
JO. MARIA LANCISIUS
Intimus Cubicularius, & Archiater Pontificius.

AMSTELÆDAMI,
Apud R. & G. WETSTENIOS.
MDCCXXII.

In the *Tabulae anatomicae* (first published 1714) of Bartholomaeus Eustachius (died 1574), the dissection scene on the title page is reduced to a small rectangle in the lower half.

The author is shown dissecting the superficial muscles of a cadaver in a lecture room with curved walls. Assistants below and students above engage in animated conversation, pointedly ignoring the dissection, unlike the enthralled observers in the Vesalius title page. A skeleton standing upright on a pedestal also gestures as if included in the conversation. A group of dogs lie on the ground in front of the table. The illustrator of the title page is identified in some editions as Petrus Leo Ghezzius, a Roman artist known for satiric drawings.

Eustachius was physician to the Duke of Urbino, and then to the duke's brother, Giulio Cardinal della Rovere, whom Eustachius followed to Rome in 1549. He was appointed professor of anatomy at the Collegia della Sapienza in Rome. As an anatomist he was best known for new observations on the kidney, teeth, and ear.

While in Rome he prepared a series of forty-seven anatomical illustrations with the help of artist Pier Matteo Pini, and they were engraved by Giulio de' Musi. Only eight engravings were ever published in his lifetime and the remainder seemingly disappeared. The drawings were rediscovered in the early eighteenth century in the possession of a descendant of Pini. They were purchased by Pope Clement XI who presented them to his own physician, Giovanni Maria Lancisi, successor to Eustachius at the Sapienza. Lancisi published the entire series with his own commentary in 1714.[19]

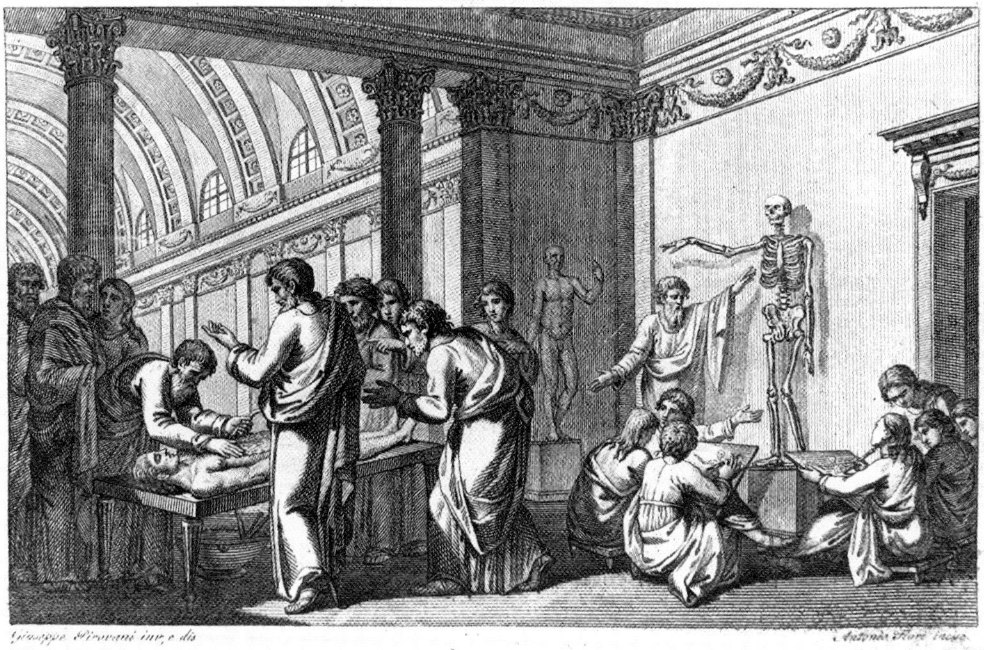

Detail from Title Page: Dissection Scene

DISSECTION SCENE

Engraving
Image size: 4 5/8 x 7 5/8 in.
Plate size: 5 1/4 x 8 in.
Page size: 17 1/8 x 11 1/2 in.

Signed below image: "Giuseppe Pirovani inv. e dis." and "Antonio Fiori incise"
From Pietro Berrettini (Pietro da Cortona), *Tabulae anatomicae ex archetypis egregii pictoris Petri Berrettini Cortonensis...* (Rome: Venantio Monaldini, 1788)

Given in 1940 by bequest of Pascal Brooke Bland, M.D.
Accession number: 1940+e.Pr.28

The final title page with an illustration of a dissection is from *Tabulae anatomicae* (first published 1741) by Pietro Berrettini (1596-1669). He was better known as Pietro da Cortona in the art world and celebrated as a painter and architect of the High Baroque.

Pietro produced about twenty anatomical drawings during his formative years in Rome. The drawings were apparently made around 1618 from dissections carried out at the Santo Spirito Hospital in Rome by an unknown anatomist.[20] As with Eustachius's work, Pietro Berrettini's muscle drawings were not published until long after his death.

Pietro's drawings were acquired by Sir William Hamilton, the archaeologist and diplomat who was British ambassador to the King of Naples. Hamilton presented the drawings as a gift to Dr. William Hunter (1718-83) and they were included in the anatomist's bequest to the University of Glasgow. The anatomical drawings were used to prepare engravings first published in 1741, more than a century after they were made.

The title page with dissection in the 1788 edition in the Jefferson collection is different from the original edition of 1741. The later illustration combines elements of the Vesalius title page with its classical architecture, and of the Eustachius title page with its small numbers of onlookers who wear classical garb. Of the four examples, the Pietro vignette has the clearest articulation of architecture and the most coherent organization of activities: one group of elders observes a dissection and another group of young students draw from a standing skeleton whose anatomy is being demonstrated by a teacher. For good measure a classical sculpture of a nude male figure is depicted in a posture similar to that of the skeleton. The scene was designed by Giuseppe Pirovani, and Antonio Fiori engraved the plate.

Frontispiece: Portrait of Antoni van Leeuwenhoek

ANTONI van LEEUWENHOEK (1632-1723)
By Abraham de Blois (active 1679-1720) after painting by Johannes Verkolje the Elder (1650-93)

Engraving
Image size: 6 x 5 3/8 in.
Plate size: 7 x 5 5/8 in.
Page size: 7 7/8 x 6 in.

Signed below image: "J. Verkolje pinx." and "A. de Blois fec."
From Antoni van Leeuwenhoek, *Arcana naturae detecta...* (Delft: Henricum à Krooneveld, 1695), bound with *Continuatio arcanorum naturae detectorum...* (Delft: Henricum à Krooneveld, 1697)

Given in 1940 by bequest of Pascal Brooke Bland, M.D.
Accession number: 1940+e.Pr.15

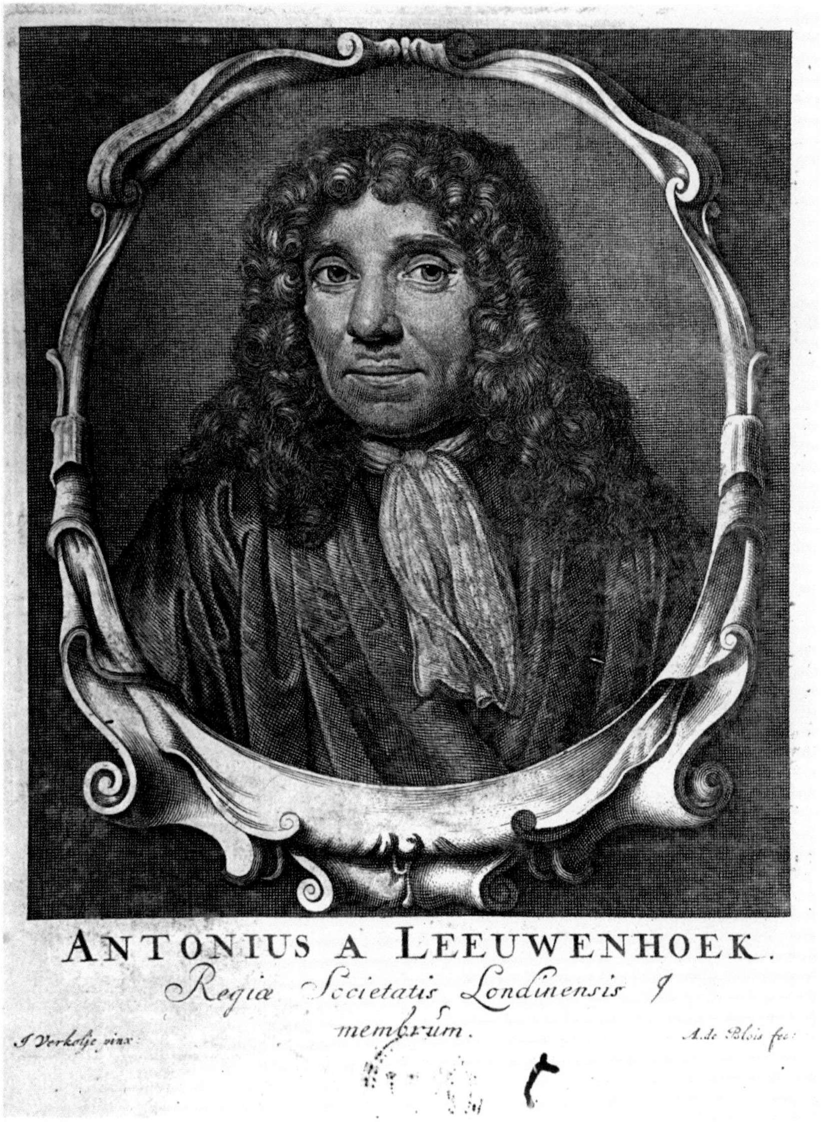

Another frequent choice of illustration for title pages and frontispieces is a portrait of the author, sometimes accompanied by allegorical, mythological, or historical figures.

A startlingly individualistic portrait is found in the frontispiece of Antoni van Leeuwenhoek's *Arcana naturae detecta* and *Continuatio arcanorum naturae detectorum* (two books bound together). The author is depicted bust length and set into a round, ornately carved frame. The scientist's stout and fleshy face is crowned by a long, flowing, curly peruke. He looks out confidently above an inscription proudly noting his membership in the Royal Society of London.

The engraver is Abraham de Blois who worked in Delft and Amsterdam. The image is after an original painting of 1686 by Johannes Verkolje the Elder (Rijksmuseum, Amsterdam). Verkolje was a Dutch painter and engraver who settled in Delft in 1672 and served several times as dean of the artists' guild there between 1678 and 1688.

Van Leeuwenhoek never attended a university and spent his career as a civil servant in Delft. His scientific life did not begin until his late thirties when he constructed his first simple microscopes or magnifying glasses. He ground most of the lenses himself for his collection of almost 250 microscopes.

Relatively isolated from academic circles, the Dutch naturalist avoided speculation and concentrated on direct observation. He devoted his time to the microscopic investigation of organic and inorganic structures and recognized the true nature of microorganisms. He was the first to describe spermatozoa and the first to see protozoa under the microscope; he gave the first complete account of red blood corpuscles; he discovered the striped character of voluntary muscles, and the structure of the crystalline lens. His thorough work confirmed Marcello Malpighi's discovery of the capillary circulation of the blood through the arteries and veins.

Many of van Leeuwenhoek's discoveries were published in the *Philosophical Transactions* of the Royal Society of London, and he was elected a fellow of that prestigious group in 1680. He was awarded a silver medal from the Louvain College of Professors, and received a pension from the city of Delft which made him special awards upon the publication of his books.

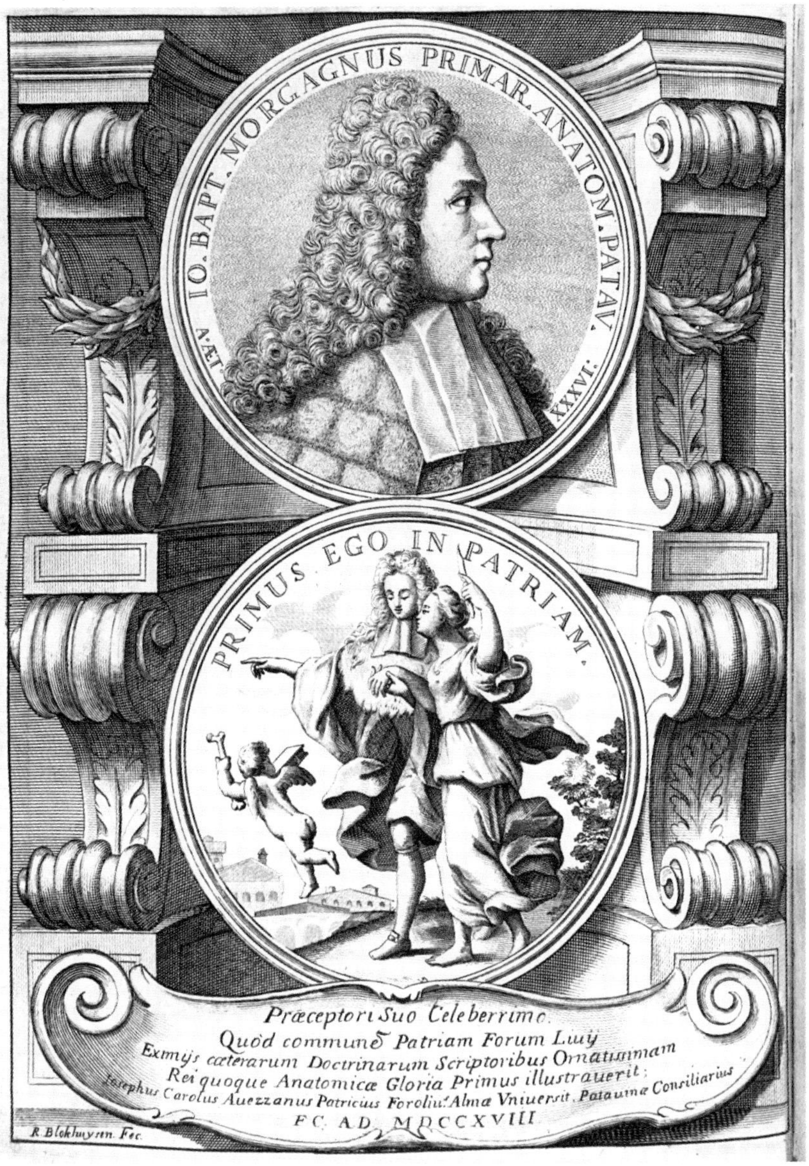

Frontispiece: Portrait of Giovanni Battista Morgagni

GIOVANNI BATTISTA MORGAGNI (1682-1771)
By R. Blokhuysen

Engraving, etching
Image size: 9 1/8 x 6 1/2 in.
Plate size: 9 3/8 x 6 7/8 in.
Page size: 9 7/8 x 7 3/4 in.

Signed lower left below image: "R. Blokhuysen Fec."
From Giovanni Battista Morgagni, *Adversaria anatomica prima* (Lyons: Johannem Arnoldum Langerak, 1718)

Given in 1940 by bequest of Pascal Brooke Bland, M.D.
Accession number: 1940+e.Pr.19

Giovanni Battista Morgagni's *Adversaria anatomica prima* features a frontispiece created by R. Blokhuysen with a double portrait and an allegorical figure.

The format is two circular framed images in an architectural setting.

Above is a profile portrait of Morgagni wearing a peruke and fur-collared academic gown. The inscription names him "the primary anatomist of Patavium" (now Padua), and states that the subject was aged thirty-six at the time of the portrait.

Below is the full length figure of Morgagni dressed as above, leading an allegorical female figure holding a knife. They are preceded by an angel with a bone and a book. The physician literally points the way down the path, and the inscription overhead says, "I am first in the country."

Morgagni was an Italian physician who took degrees in medicine and philosophy at the University of Bologna in 1701. He was admitted to the Accademia degli Inquieti in 1699 and became its head in 1704, paving the way for its incorporation into the Istituto delle Scienze in 1714. The modestly titled *Adversaria anatomica prima* (translated as "notes" or "memorandum" on anatomy) includes several new anatomical discoveries including the glands of the trachea, the male urethra, and the female genitals.

Morgagni assumed the second chair of theoretical medicine at the University of Padua in 1711, and then the first chair of anatomy in 1715, holding the latter post until his death. Recognizing the connection between external signs of diseases and anatomical changes, Morgagni is regarded as the founder of pathological anatomy. He described aortic insufficiency, mitral stenosis, and angina pectoris, and gave a classic description of heart block. At age eighty in 1761 he published his life's work *De sedibus et causis morborum*, five books concerning the seat and causes of disease anatomically studied.

Title Page: Portrait of Ulyssis Aldrovandi with Historical Personages

ULYSSIS ALDROVANDI WITH HISTORICAL PERSONAGES
By unknown artist

Engraving
Image size: 14 x 9 3/8 in.
Plate size: 14 x 9 3/8 in.
Page size: 14 x 9 1/2 in.

From Ulyssis Aldrovandi, *Ornithologiae: hoc est de avibus historiae libri XII* (Bologna: Franciscum de Franciscis Senensem, 1599)

Given in 1940 by bequest of Pascal Brooke Bland, M.D.
Accession number: 1940+e.Pr.08

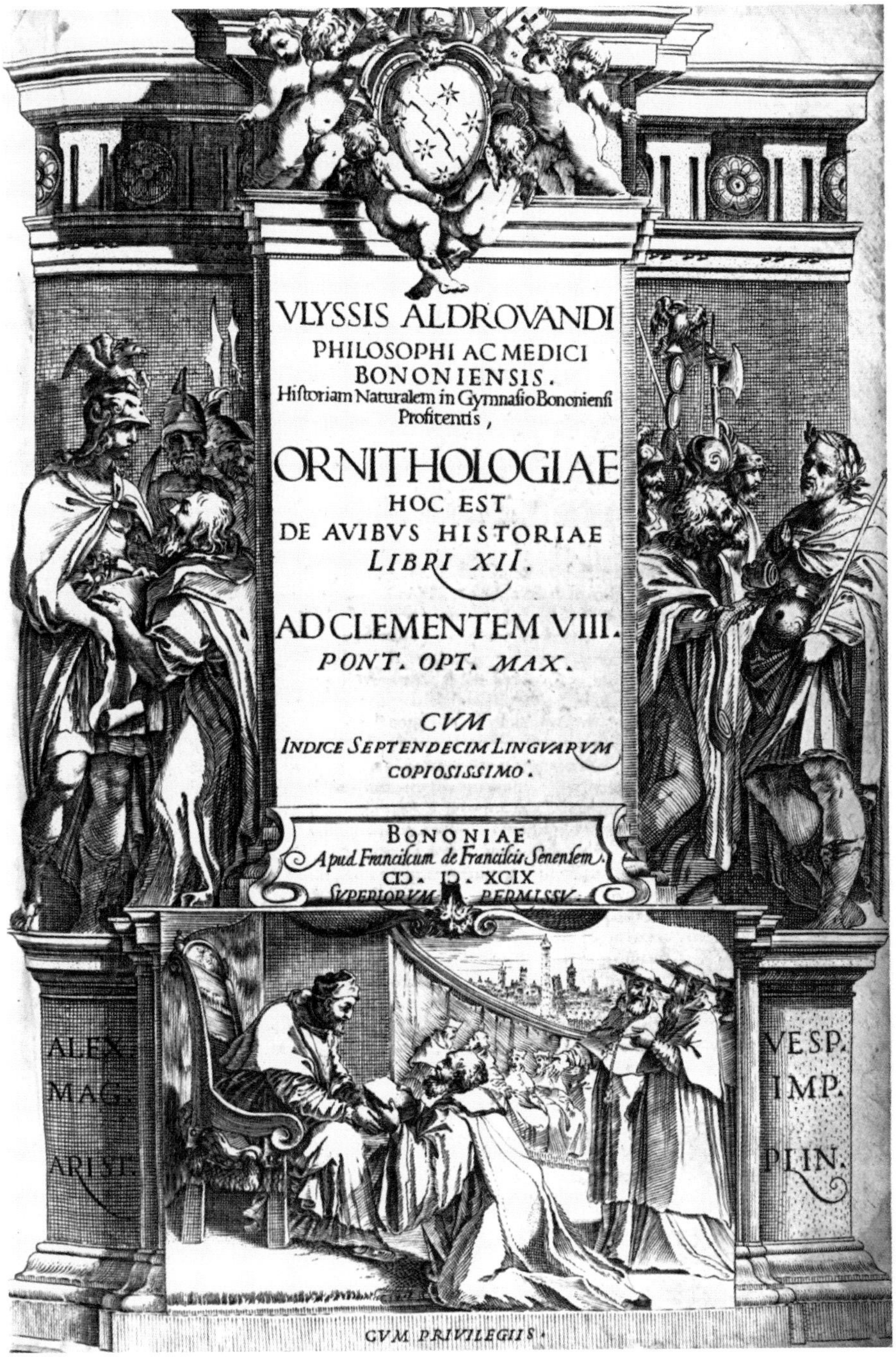

The title page in Aldrovandi's *Ornithologiae* (1599) combines the author with historical personages, in three separate vignettes in an architectural setting.

The central scene below shows Aldrovandi in an academic gown kneeling at the feet of Pope Clement VIII and presenting him with a copy of his book, as cardinals look on approvingly. Ancient intellectual predecessors are Aristotle presenting a scroll to Alexander the Great on the left, and Pliny presenting his scroll to Emperor Vespasian on the right. Crowning the scene is a group of putti supporting a coat of arms.

Ulyssis Aldrovandi (1522/24-1605/07) was an Italian physician and naturalist. He received his medical degree at the University of Bologna in 1553 and became professor and chair of the field called natural sciences today, including plants, animals, and minerals. He established a botanical garden and prepared an official pharmacopoeia. Aldrovandi bequeathed to the city his museum, library, and manuscripts of his unpublished works. His complete works on animals were published in thirteen volumes between 1599 and 1648.

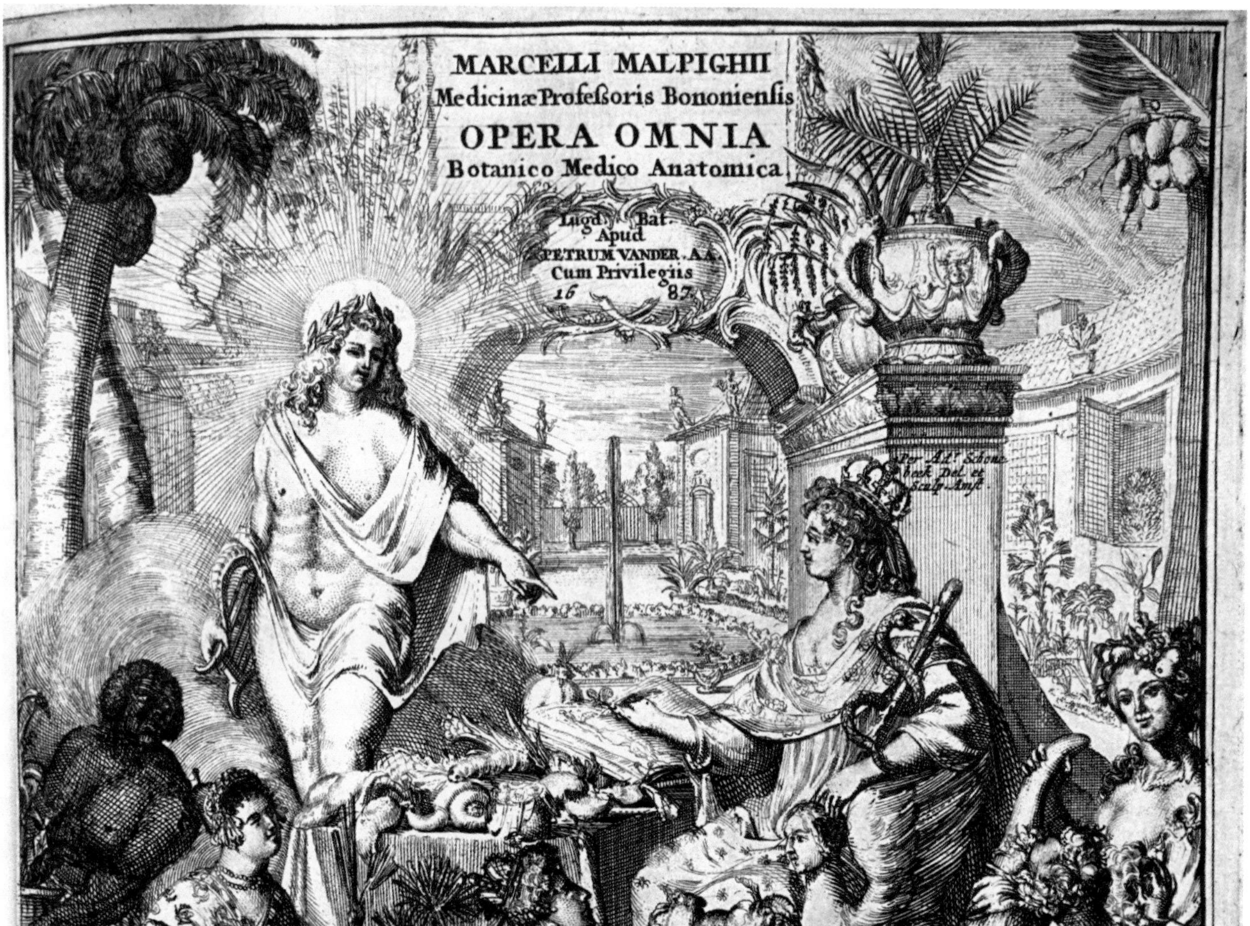
MARCELLI MALPIGHII
Medicinæ Profeßoris Bononienſis
OPERA OMNIA
Botanico Medico Anatomica
Lugd. Bat.
Apud
PETRUM VANDER. AA.
Cum Privilegiis
16 87.

Frontispiece: Mythological and Allegorical Figures

MYTHOLOGICAL AND ALLEGORICAL FIGURES
By Adriaen Schonebeek (ca. 1658-1714)

Engraving, etching
Image size: 7 7/8 x 6 1/4 in.
Plate size: 8 1/4 x 6 5/8 in.
Page size: 9 1/4 x 7 1/2 in.

Signed center right on pier: "Per Ad^{r}. Schonebeek Del. et Sculp. Amst."
From Marcello Malpighi, *Opera omnia, seu, thesaurus locupletissimus botanico-medico-anatomicus...* (Leiden: Petrum vander Aa, 1687)

Given in 1940 by bequest of Pascal Brooke Bland, M.D.
Accession number: 1940+e.Pr.16

The frontispiece of Marcello Malpighi's *Opera omnia* is a unified but complex scene set in a lush garden and populated by allegorical and mythological figures.

At the center is a Muse-like figure who is dressed in a robe and crown and holds a caduceus. This goddess of creative inspiration is seated at a table sketching or writing in a book. At her side is a sphinx, the repository of arcane wisdom.

Pointing to the author is Apollo, a semidraped figure wearing laurel leaves and carrying his lyre. A sun radiates behind his head. He is the embodiment of the rational side of man's nature and the patron of the Muses. Several female figures offer up cornucopias of fruits and vegetables to the author. Below a satyr and a river god complete the mythological cast of characters.

Adriaen Schonebeek, the designer and engraver of the scene, was born in Amsterdam about 1658. He was invited to Russia by Czar Peter I and became head of the Engraving Chamber in Moscow. He died in Russia in 1714.

Marcello Malpighi (1628-94) was an Italian physician and naturalist who was considered the founder of histology. He graduated in medicine and philosophy from the University of Bologna in 1653. He taught at universities in Pisa and Messina before returning to teach practical medicine at Bologna in 1666. In 1691 he accepted the appointment as personal physician to Pope Innocent XII.

Malpighi was the first to apply the newly invented microscope to anatomical research, and his early great observations were describing the structure of the pulmonary parenchyma and the importance of capillaries in circulation of the blood. He was famed in biology for his work on the anatomy of the silkworm, the morphology of plants, and the embryology of the chick, and in medicine for the histology and physiology of the glands and viscera, and the sensory receptors of the tongue.

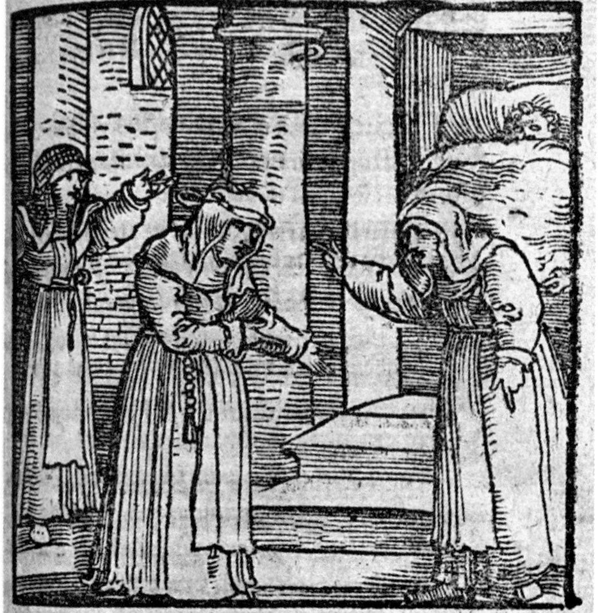

BONA VALETVDINE. 235

PHlegma dabit uires modicas, latoſq;
que breueſq;,
Phlegma facit pingueis, ſanguis reddit
mediocres,
Ocia non ſtudio tradunt, ſed corpora
ſomno.
Senſus hebes, tardus motus, pigritia, ſo
mnus,
Hic ſomnolentus, piger, & ſputamine
plenus.

g 3

Regimen Sanitatis Salernitanum: The Phlegmatic Temperament

THE PHLEGMATIC TEMPERAMENT
By unknown artist

Woodcut
Image size: 2 3/4 x 2 3/4 in.
Page size: 6 x 3 1/2 in.

From *Regimen sanitatis Salernitanum: conservandae sanitatis praecepta saluberrima...Arnoldi Villanovani...* (Frankfurt: Heirs of Christian Egenolphi, 1559)

Given in 1929 by Samuel P. Scott, benefactor of the JMC library
Accession number: 1929+e.Pr.01

Many practical treatises on health and hygiene were based on ancient and medieval beliefs. The *Regimen sanitatis Salernitanum* was the most popular medical book in Europe for many centuries after it was written about the year 1100.[21]

Tradition says it was ordered by Robert, Duke of Normandy, a Crusader who stopped at the medical school of Salerno to have an ulcerous wound treated. Arising from a Benedictine monastery this medical school and hospital had been founded in the Middle Ages, and propounded the ideas of ancient authorities such as Hippocrates and Galen. The early faculty consisted of Christian, Moslem, and Jewish scholars working harmoniously together.

The small treatise went through an extraordinary number of manuscript copies, and after the invention of printing almost three hundred other editions in numerous translations. The first printed edition was made in 1480, and the copy in the Jefferson library dates from 1559. The original text was a didactic poem written in Latin hexameter verse about the general principles and some practical rules of health and hygiene. The lack of one dominant style points to the work of many authors.

The *Regimen* taught that the constitutive elements of the human body were earth, water, air, and fire, closely corresponding to the four humors: melancholy, phlegm, blood, and choler, respectively. Good health resulted from a balance and equilibrium of the humors, and bad health was the result of a disturbed equilibrium. By means of a proper diet, rest, medicinal herbs, phlebotomy, and a cheerful disposition, equilibrium and good health could be regained.

Arnold of Villanova (1235/40-1311/12) was a Spanish

scholar of medicine, philosophy, physics, astrology, alchemy, and Greek and Arabic. He served Peter III, Alfonso III, and James II as a diplomat for the state of Aragon. He taught and practiced medicine in Montpellier and elsewhere, and is credited with the introduction of tinctures into the pharmacopeia. Arnold's commentary of corrections and amendments to the *Regimen*, written about 1290 to 1300 when he was professor of medicine in Montpellier, appears in the edition of 1480 and in the Jefferson copy.

A woodcut illustrating the phlegmatic temperament is found in the section on humors and temperaments. The drawing shows three women gesticulating and arguing among themselves, presumably over the humor of the man lolling under the billowy bedcovers. Relevant verses in an English edition published in 1575 explain the characteristics of the phlegmatic person:

> The Flegmatique are most of no great growth,
> Inclining to be rather fat and square:
> Given much unto their ease, to rest and sloth,
> Content in knowledge to take little share,
> To put themselves to any paine most loth.
> So dead their spirits, so dull their sences are:
> Still either sitting, like to folke that dreame,
> Or else still spitting, to avoid the flegme:
> One qualitie doth yet these harmes repaire,
> That for the most part Flegmatique are faire.[22]

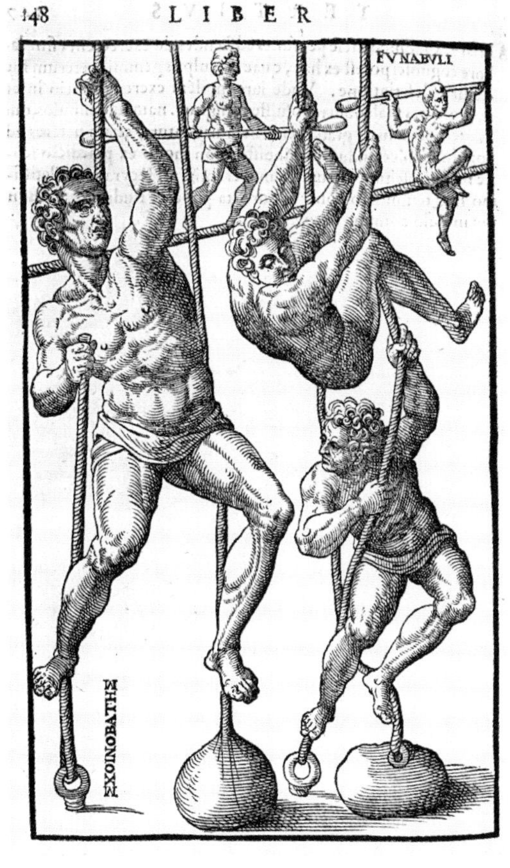

De Arte Gymnastica: Men Climbing Ropes

MEN CLIMBING ROPES
By unknown artist

Woodcut
Image size: 6 5/8 x 4 in.
Page size: 9 x 6 1/8 in.

From Hieronymus Mercurialis, *De arte gymnastica libri sex...* (Venice: Juntas, 1573)

Given in 1940 by bequest of Pascal Brooke Bland, M.D.
Accession number: 1940+e.Pr.17

Hieronymus Mercurialis's treatise, *De arte gymnastica*, was the first illustrated work on the fundamentals of medical gymnastics, and was based on the writings of classical authors. Physicians going back to Hippocrates recommended conservative prophylactic methods such as medical gymnastics as beneficial to health.

Hieronymus Mercurialis (1530-1606) was a humanist scholar, translator, and physician who served the papal court in Rome. He also wrote the first systematic treatise on skin diseases, and was among the first to publish on diseases of children and on mania.

The woodcut illustrations scattered throughout *De arte gymnastica* depict male (and a few female) figures engaged in strenuous activities: bathing, wrestling, boxing, hurling the discus and javelin, swinging, dancing, playing ball games, running and leaping, lifting weights, and climbing ropes. Some of the scenes have architectural backgrounds.

This illustration of rope climbers is a closeup view of three male figures clad in loincloths hoisting themselves up ropes that are weighted to the ground. The curly-haired athletes display overdeveloped muscles and large heads. In the background are two figures labeled "rope dancers," negotiating a tight rope with the aid of long balance poles.

Birthing Scenes and Midwifery

The occupation of midwifery has existed since ancient times but its reputation has waxed and waned over the centuries.[23] In antiquity childbirth was supervised by midwives whose knowledge and personal character were considered relatively high. Training for midwives was instituted by Hippocrates in the fifth century B.C. In the second century A.D., under Roman domination, Soranus of Ephesos wrote the first treatise on obstetrics, and this work remained the standard for over a millennium. Artifacts show that midwifery was also a recognized female occupation in ancient Egypt, India, and China.

The famous medieval medical schools were silent on midwifery because physicians were excluded from the practice by custom, modesty, and orders of the church. The practice of midwifery sank to the status of a handicraft and fell into unskilled hands, just competent enough to assist a normal birth.

The pregnant woman was then viewed as the bearer of a new life that must be baptized so that the new soul could enter the Christian community. During unsuccessful births the church ordered Caesarian section so that the child's soul could be saved by baptism, but many midwives balked at the difficult procedure. They fell into greater disrepute and were sometimes considered witches in league with Satan to kill the "fruit," so that the innocent babe would be robbed of the sacrament.

The first modern manual for midwives, *Der swangern Frawen und Hebammen Rosegarten*, was written by Eucharius Roesslin (died 1526) in 1513 at the behest of the Duchess of Brunswick. Basically a synopsis of earlier writings, especially Soranus, the manual was translated into many foreign languages and was a best-seller for two hundred years.

Conditions changed for the better in the beginning of the sixteenth century when anatomical research began to be conducted, and anatomists and barber-surgeons such as Ambroise Paré rediscovered the ancient use of the "foothold" for difficult deliveries. At the same time some wellborn ladies took up the profession of midwifery, and the birthing chair was gradually abandoned for the labor bed so that the birthing procedure was exposed to view. In the seventeenth century male midwives became the fashion, surgeons known as *accoucheurs* also gave obstetrical aid, and governmental regulation of midwives became increasingly widespread in western Europe. In the early eighteenth century academic courses of instruction for midwives were instituted at many European medical schools or hospitals. Midwifery has always existed in the United States, and is in particular resurgency today.

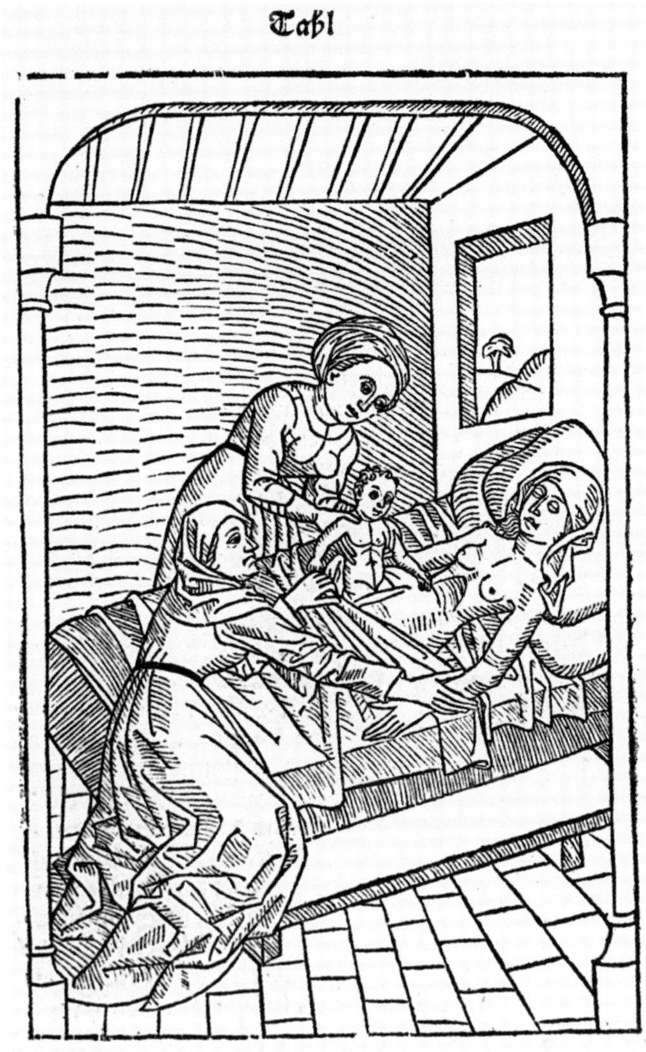

The Birth of Antichrist

THE BIRTH OF ANTICHRIST
By unknown artist

Woodcut
Image size: 7 1/2 x 5 in.
Page size: 10 3/4 x 7 1/2 in.

From *Seelenwurzgarten* (Ulm: Conrad Dinckmut, 1483)

Given in 1940 by bequest of Pascal Brooke Bland, M.D.
Accession number: 1940+e.Pr.01

The Birth of Antichrist is the oldest book illustration in the Jefferson collection. Though this image of a Caesarian section delivery was probably mistaken by Dr. Pascal B. Bland for an illustration from a medical treatise, it is actually a page removed from a German religious tract of 1483, the *Seelenwurzgarten* ("Souls' Herb Garden"). The rare woodcut is one of the oldest images of Caesarian birth in all of medical art.

There are various etymological explanations for the legend of Julius Caesar's birth by Caesarian section, but scholars today almost uniformly deny that he was born by this process, and the term itself was not used until the end of the sixteenth century.[24] In ancient times abdominal delivery was practiced only on dead or dying parturients and it is known that Caesar's mother survived his birth by many years.[25] When Caesarian section began to be performed on living women in the late sixteenth or early seventeenth century, doctors attended the patients.

The earliest images of the birth of Antichrist by Caesarian section appeared in Germany at the end of the fifteenth century. Antichrist, the enemy of Christ, was believed to take the form of a human being in whom Satan dwelt bodily. Legends vary, but most say that Antichrist was born by Caesarian section of a defiled woman, and some say through incest.

In the woodcut illustration the birth takes place in a small bedchamber. A view out the window shows a palm tree. The mother lies motionless with her eyes closed and her head propped up on pillows. She is undressed except for a headdress. A midwife holds her left arm and draws the bedcovers back, while an attendant lifts the baby by the shoulders out of a slit in the mother's abdomen. In the accompanying text the mother is condemned in harsh terms and her death in childbirth may be seen as punishment for her sins.

The *Seelenwurzgarten* image of the birth of Antichrist by Caesarian section is an example of the more "obstetrical" version of the procedure.[26] Another type is the "Satanic" version in which devils stand ready to receive the Antichrist at the moment of his birth. Sometimes an angel receives the mother's soul, a tiny figure emerging from her mouth, indicating that she will be saved and was a victim of incest. The mother is usually shown clothed and the Antichrist is pulled out through a cut in her garment over the Caesarian incision.

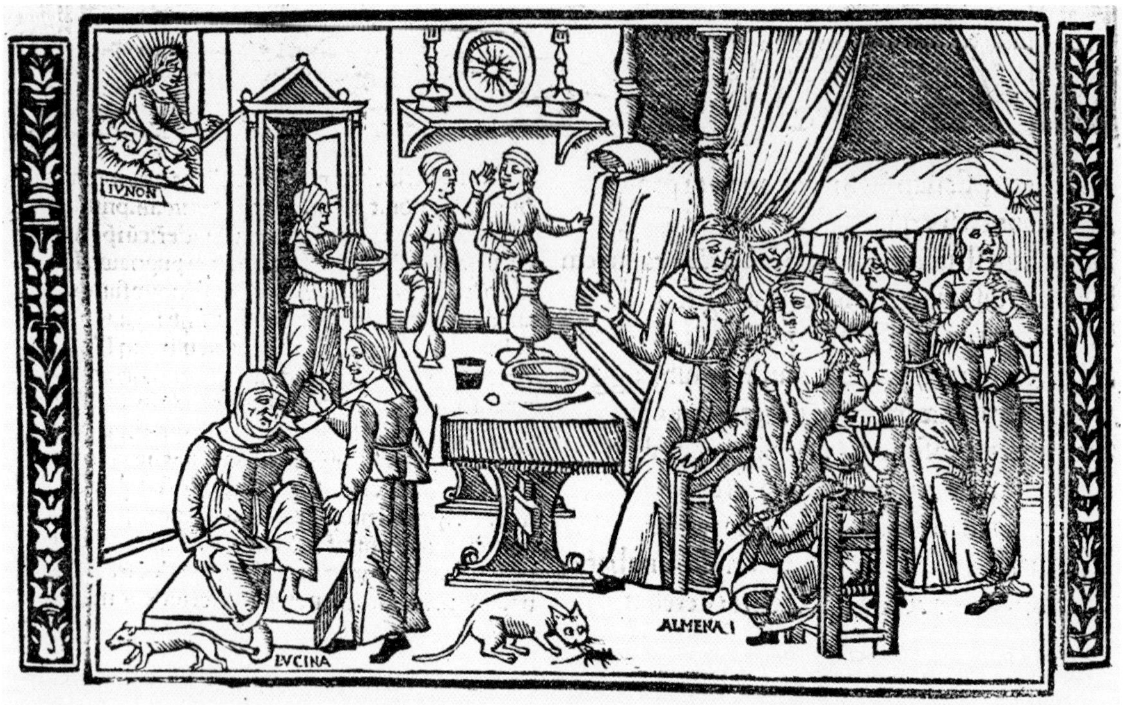

The Story of Hercules's Birth

THE STORY OF HERCULES'S BIRTH
By unknown artist

Woodcut
Image size: 3 3/4 x 6 3/8 in.
Page size: 12 x 8 1/2 in.

From Publius Ovidius Naso [Ovid], *P. Ovidii metamorphosis...* (Venice: Leonardo Lauredano, 1517)

Given in 1940 by bequest of Pascal Brooke Bland, M.D.
Accession number: 1940+e.Pr.20

In early images of vaginal birth, it can be seen that modesty was so deep-rooted that not even the midwives could see the actual birth. Illustrations of delivering women show them dressed in full-length skirts seated on the birthing chair. The midwife conducts the delivery by reaching under the folds of the mother's skirts.

The Story of Hercules's Birth is an illustration from the *Metamorphoses* of Ovid (43 B.C.-17/18 A.D.), in an edition published in Venice in 1517. The Roman author's collection of Greek and Roman stories involving changes of shape is a storehouse of mythology that has inspired poets, dramatists, painters, and sculptors ever since.

The birth of Hercules occurs in book nine of *Metamorphoses* and features an array of contentious characters. Hercules was the son of a mortal woman, Alcmena, fathered by Jupiter during the absence of Alcmena's husband Amphitryon. This act aroused the jealousy of Juno, sister and wife of Jupiter and the special protectress of women, who particularly watched over marriage and childbirth. Lucina was a minor deity who made the child see the light of day.

In the illustration Alcmena is identified as the woman seated on the birthing chair, with a midwife reaching under her skirt and assistants offering comfort and prayer. Others identified by name are Lucina who sits on a platform and Juno who peers through the window. On the table are a knife, pitcher, glass, and basin. Other participants in the crowded room prepare the feast and the canopied bed. A cat eyes a mouse in the center foreground and another strolls by the Lucina figure.

Part of the accompanying verse explains the complicated, behind-the-scenes narrative. Alcmena says,

> May the gods favor you, and shorten your labor
> When the time comes to call on Ilithyia,
> Helper of travail, and no friend of mine
> Since Juno was my enemy. I remember
> When my son's birth was near, the weight in the womb
> So heavy anyone would know the father
> Must have been Jove, and even in speaking of it
> Today, I feel once more the pangs of labor.
> Seven days, seven nights, I suffered, sick and weary,
> Raised arms to Heaven, crying for Lucina,
> With her two goddess-midwives, to come help me,
> And she did come, but with a mind corrupted
> By Juno's hate. She heard my groans, and watched me;
> Sitting there by that altar near the doorway,

She crossed her knees, and laced her hands together,
And spoke constricting charms, I pushed and struggled,
Cursed Jove's ingratitude, wanted to die,
Screamed so that even stones were moved to pity,
And other mothers came to try to help me,
Prayed, urged me to keep trying. One of them,
Galanthis, yellow-haired, one of my servants,
A good devoted girl (I loved her for it)
Saw there was something wrong, and knew that Juno
Was working mischief. In and out the doorway
Galanthis went and came, and saw the goddess
Sitting there on the altar, the crossed knees,
The hands laced tight together, and she spoke:
"Whoever you are, congratulate my lady!
Her son is born, her prayer is heard." The goddess
Leaped up, at that, and loosed her hands, and I
Was likewise loosed of my burden, and Galanthis
Broke out in laughter, but the angry goddess
Grabbed her, still laughing, yanked her by the hair,
Made forelegs of her arms, and would not let her
Rise from the ground. She kept her golden color
Though now in different shape, the little weasel
Who haunts my house, still busy in devotion,
And, so the story goes, since her mouth helped me
Give birth by telling lies, through her own mouth
Her young are born.[27]

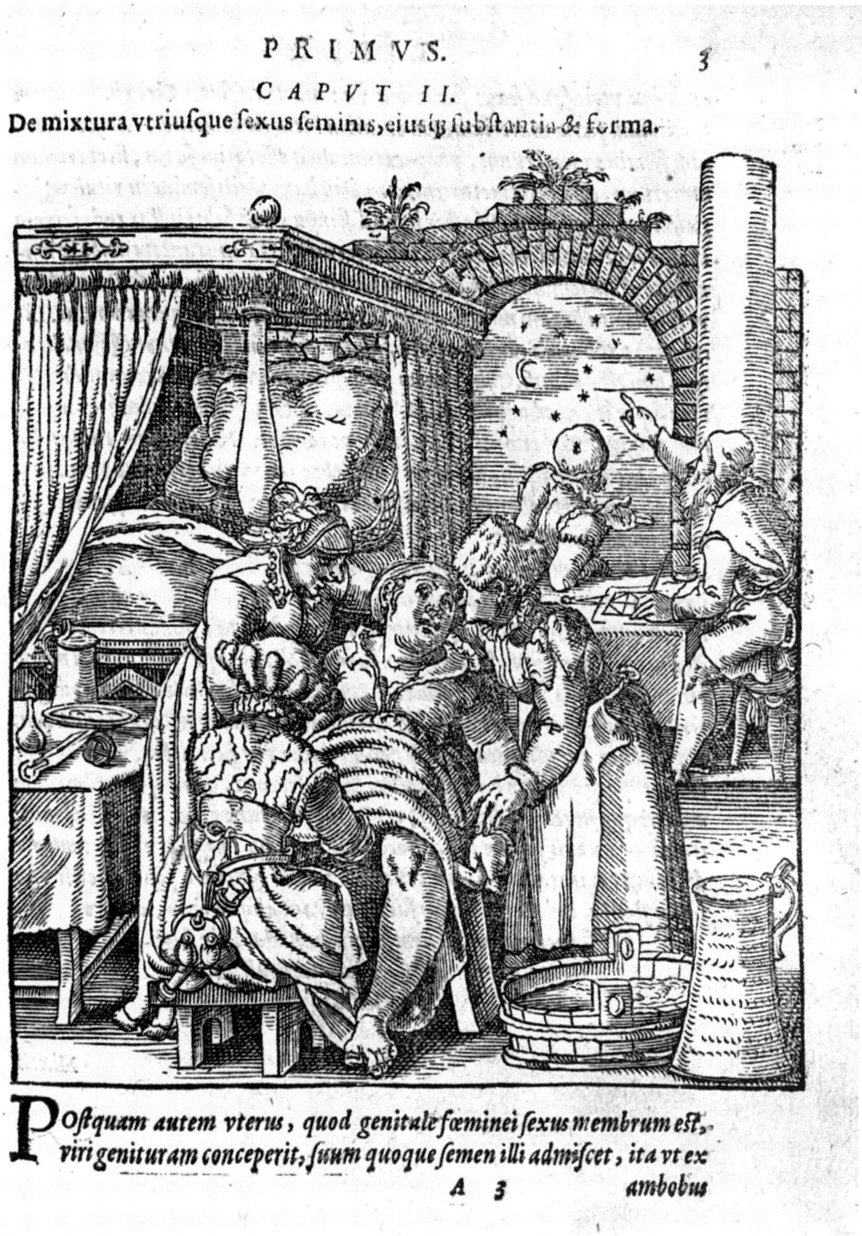
PRIMVS. 3

CAPVT II.

De mixtura vtriusque sexus seminis, eiusq; substantia & forma.

Postquam autem vterus, quod genitale fœminei sexus membrum est, viri genituram conceperit, suum quoque semen illi admiscet, ita vt ex

A 3 ambobus

Childbirth

CHILDBIRTH
By Jost Amman (1539-91)

Woodcut
Image size: 5 x 4 1/4 in.
Page size: 7 5/8 x 5 5/8 in.

From Jakob Rueff, *De conceptu et generatione hominis...* (Frankfurt: Sigismundi Feyerabendius, 1587)

Given in 1940 by bequest of Pascal Brooke Bland, M.D.
Accession number: 1940+e.Pr.21

The woodcuts illustrating Jakob Rueff's *De conceptu et generatione hominis* (1587) are the work of Jost Amman. The first edition of Rueff's famous manual on obstetrical practices was published in 1554 and contained illustrations by a different artist.

Jakob Rueff (ca. 1500-58) was the city physician and professor of medicine at the University of Zurich. Jost Amman (1539-91), a native of Zurich, was a prolific illustrator of medical and other books, primarily for publishing houses in Nuremburg and Frankfurt.

The actual birthing process depicted in *Childbirth* is typical of sixteenth-century images of this subject. A fully dressed mother grips the sides of her birthing chair, attended by a midwife aiding in the delivery along with her assistants. Nearby is a pitcher and a wooden tub for washing the newborn infant. On the table are scissors and string for cutting the cord, a flask, and a stein and plate for the postpartum repast. Adjacent is the canopied bed to which she will retire after the birth.

An unusual element in this depiction is the addition of two astrologers gazing out the window with their backs to the scene. They are studying the moon and stars in preparation for plotting the newborn's horoscope. During the Renaissance, even men of science took astrology into account.

Moments Following Childbirth

MOMENTS FOLLOWING CHILDBIRTH
By Jost Amman

Woodcut
Image size: 3 x 3 5/8 in.
Page size: 7 5/8 x 5 5/8 in.

From Jakob Rueff, *De conceptu* (as above)
Accession number: 1940+e.Pr.22

In Jost Amman's drawing of *Moments Following Childbirth* in Jakob Rueff's *De conceptu*, the new mother lies propped up in a canopied bed as two servants bring her food and drink. In the foreground one attendant bathes the newborn baby in a metal tub and another waits to receive the baby with a towel. Nearby an older child squeezes a doll and rocks the cradle. The domestic scene also includes a dog scampering across the floor with a bone, and revelers at a table enjoying a meal. In the rear room another servant is seen stirring a pot in the smoking fireplace.

QVINTVS. 34

LIBER QVINTVS.

DE MOLA ALIISQVE FALSIS *vteri tumoribus, simulq́; de abortibus & monstris diuersis, nec non de conceptus signis varijs.*

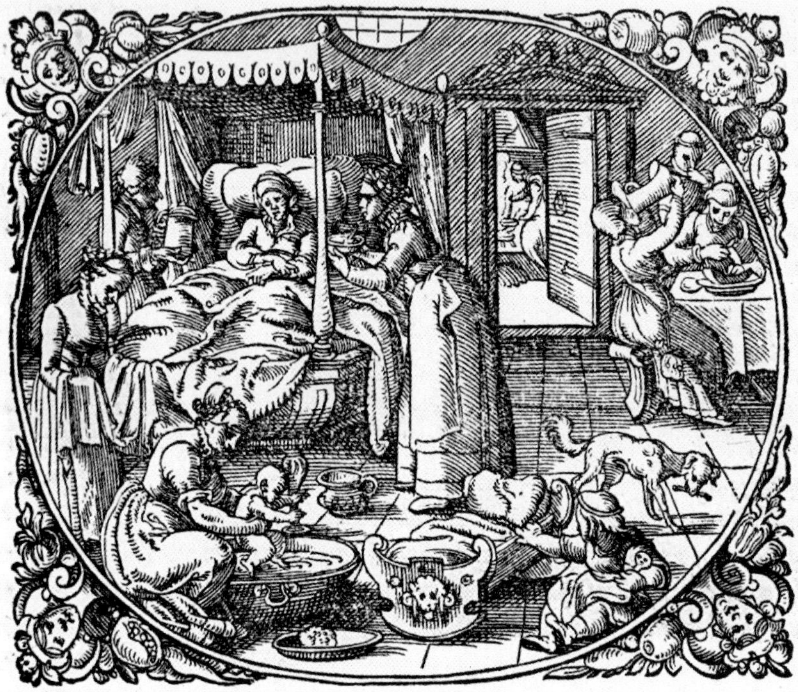

CAPVT I.

De mola, cæterisq; falsò creditis conceptibus.

QVotquot vnquam de mola scripserunt, hanc imprægnationem esse falsam dixerunt, quæ si quando ad partum veniat, informis carnis frusti similitudine prodeat. Hanc nonnulli à molon, quod rotundum Græcis sonare dicunt, eo quod ipsius quoq; forma rotunda sit, vel à Persico moli vocabulo, quod illis informe quiddam vel rudem massam significat, dictam volunt. Mola quid sit.

I 2

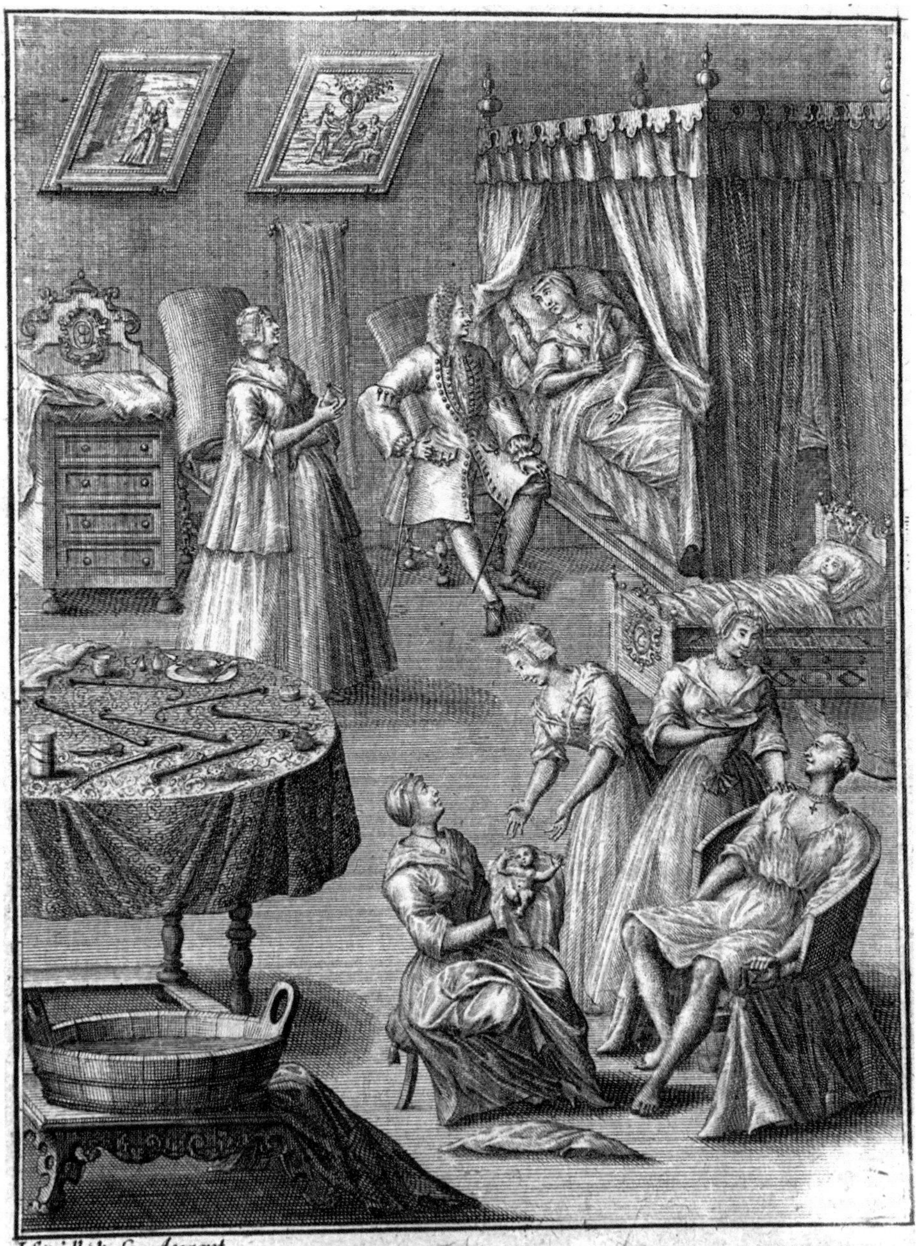

I. Stridbeck fec: Argent:

Moments Following Childbirth

MOMENTS FOLLOWING CHILDBIRTH
By Johann Stridbeck (active late seventeenth-early eighteenth century)

Engraving, etching, stipple
Ca. 1700
Image size: 7 1/4 x 5 1/2 in.
Page size: 7 5/8 x 5 3/4 in.

Signed below image lower left: "I. Stridbeck fec: Argent:"

Given in 1940 by bequest of Pascal Brooke Bland, M.D.
Accession number: 1940+e.Pr.02

Moments Following Childbirth is an engraved illustration from an unidentified, German medical or religious book, or perhaps from an aristocratic *Hausbuch* (housekeeping book). A print dealer's note attached to the sheet identifies the work as a German engraving of about 1700.

The work is signed "I. Stridbeck fec: Argent:" and his monogram, "I S," can be seen on the footboard of the cradle and on the crest of the chest of drawers. If the date of 1700 is correct, the artist could either be Johann Stridbeck I (1641-1716), a German designer and engraver, or his son and pupil, Johann Stridbeck II (1665-1714).

Judging from the sumptuous contemporary costumes, jewelry, and furniture, this image with its consecutive scenes depicts the home of a patrician family. In the foreground the mother is still seated on her birthing chair grasping the handholds. The chair's rounded back and pleated skirt resemble the chair illustrated in Rueff's *De conceptu*. She looks eagerly toward a servant who brings her nourishment. The midwife is about to hand the newborn baby to an assistant who will bathe it. A wooden tub of water rests on a low, carved table.

A large, round table with embroidered cloth is laden with various hooked instruments and scissors, a bowl, and cups. In the middle ground the baby has been swathed in blankets and lies in its cradle. The headboard of the cradle is carved with an angel. In the background the mother rests in her canopied bed and converses with her bewigged husband who is seated in a chair.

Of special interest are the religious symbols in this otherwise conventional, domestic setting. The new mother and two of her caretakers wear necklaces with crosses. Framed pictures on the wall clearly depict scenes of the Visitation and the Temptation. The Temptation had been included in some earlier sixteenth-century obstetrical books including Rueff's *De conceptu*, which showed an image of Adam and Eve with the tree of knowledge represented as a skeleton. This picture occurs at the beginning of Rueff's treatise, suggesting deep, Christian, moralistic connotations.

The Visitation is a joyful event in which the youthful Mary who had just conceived, embraces her elderly cousin Elizabeth who had become pregnant after a lifetime of barrenness. In the Temptation Adam and Eve flank the tree of knowledge of good and evil in the Garden of Eden. Eve was persuaded by the serpent to eat of the fruit of the forbidden tree, and having offered it to Adam, they received sexual knowledge and covered themselves. After the Temptation and the Expulsion from Paradise, it was decreed that Adam should earn his bread by the sweat of his brow and Eve should endure painful childbearing and subjection to man. Therefore, conception and childbirth can be associated with seduction, the Fall of Man, and suffering and death during childbirth, due to Eve's curiosity and disobedience.[28]

Anatomy

During the Renaissance anatomical research resulted in a new understanding of the structure of the human body. Scientists formed partnerships with artists to publish anatomical atlases based on their direct observations and shared concern for conveying their knowledge. The collaboration was mutually beneficial: the anatomist-surgeon who wrote the text did not have the graphic skills to record his findings accurately or artistically; the artist chosen to provide the illustrations did not himself have sufficient training in dissection or understanding of the various anatomical elements and systems. Art scholars have shown that the anatomical illustrations reflected the conventions of contemporary style and iconography.

The following selections do not attempt an exhaustive survey of anatomical illustration, but rather are highlights from the Jefferson library's extensive collection which includes landmark books from most of the important European medical centers dating from the Renaissance period. It is beyond the scope of this book to critique the accuracy of the texts and illustrations.[29]

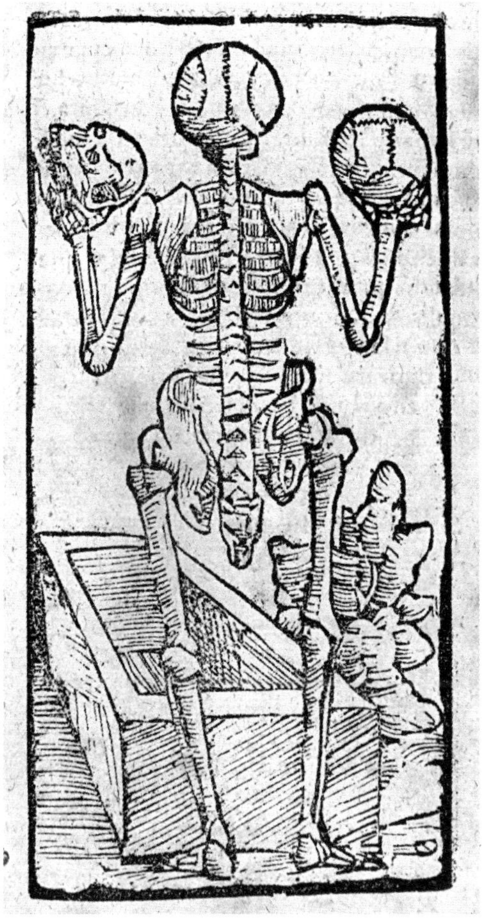

Skeleton

SKELETON
By unknown artist

Woodcut
Image size: 4 5/8 x 2 1/4 in.
Page size: 5 3/4 x 3 3/4 in.

From Jacopo Berengario da Carpi, *Isagogae breves et exactissimae in anatomiam humani corporis...* (Strasbourg: Henricus Sybold, 1530)

Given in 1940 by bequest of Pascal Brooke Bland, M.D.
Accession number: 1940+e.Pr.29

The Bolognese surgeon and anatomist Jacopo Berengario da Carpi (ca. 1460-ca. 1530) was a pioneer in anatomical illustration. His books contained the first illustrations made from nature, rather than from books or descriptions.

Berengario earned his degree at the medical school in Bologna in 1489. He also received training from his father, a surgeon in Carpi, and Aldo Manuzio, a Venetian humanist, printer, and publisher. Berengario taught surgery first in Pavia, and then in Bologna from 1502 to 1527.

His *Commentaria cum amplissimis additionibus super anatomia Mundini* (1521) was a discussion and commentary on Mondino's dissecting manual, and his *Isagogae breves* (1522) was a digest of the first book. Both were written to accompany an actual dissection. His knowledge came from dissections of hundreds of cadavers and the study of classical, Arabic, and medieval sources, providing him with the means to declare independence from the authority of Galen and Mondino. Though replete with errors, Berengario's books advanced contemporary anatomy and exerted some influence on Vesalius, Estienne, Eustachius, and other anatomists who followed.[30] Berengario pointed out that his illustrations of "muscle men" would be useful for both surgeons and artists.

His works further developed certain pictorial conventions of anatomical illustration: heroically muscled écorchés (flayed figures) drawn like living men posing in a landscape, muscle men who pull away flaps of skin, skeletons who display themselves in front of their own tombs, exuberant female figures displaying their reproductive organs, and multiple views of the same anatomical part.

The skeleton in this illustration is seen from the rear, standing with his weight on the right foot and the other foot extended. He has risen from his open tomb, and each hand displays his skull seen from a different angle.

Proportions of the Female Body

PROPORTIONS OF THE FEMALE BODY
By Albrecht Dürer (1471-1528)

Woodcut
Image size: 8 1/2 x 6 1/4 in.
Page size: 12 x 7 7/8 in.

From Albrecht Dürer, *De symmetria partium in rectis formis humanorum corporum...* (Nuremberg: Hieronymus Formschneyder representing Albrecht Dürer's widow, 1532)

Given in 1940 by bequest of Pascal Brooke Bland, M.D.

Accession number: 1940+e.Pr.25

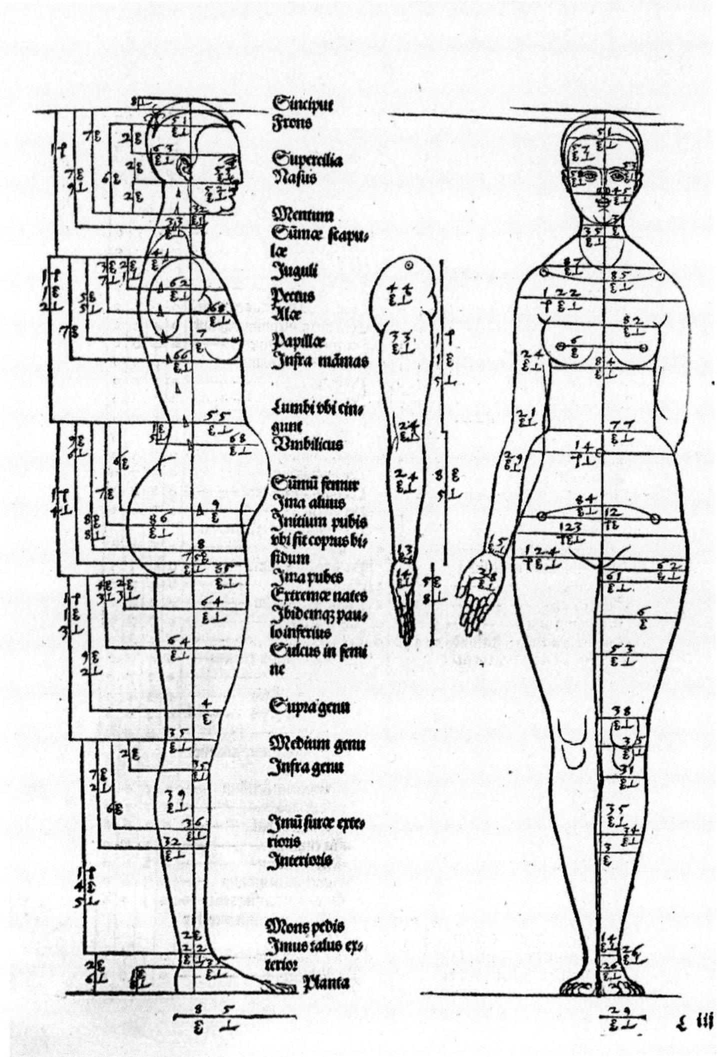

Albrecht Dürer of Nuremberg was both an exemplar of the northern artistic tradition and the first German artist to embrace the Renaissance humanism of Italy. He is probably better known today for his prodigious graphic output and scientific treatises than for his painting.

Dürer learned the art of goldsmithing from his father and studied painting, woodcutting, and copper engraving in the atelier of Michael Wolgemut. As was customary with apprentices in the artist's guild he went on his *Wanderjahre* from 1490 to 1494 traveling throughout Germany. He read about the artistic and philosophical rediscoveries of the Italian Renaissance, and travelled to Venice in 1494. He began a serious study of mathematics and art theory from ancient sources as well as from contemporaries such as Leonardo and Alberti. He visited Italy again from 1505 to 1507.

Among Dürer's panel paintings and altarpieces were portraits and religious and mythological scenes. He also participated in many decorative undertakings while working as court artist for Emperor Maximilian I. He completed many woodcut cycles on religious subjects such as the *Apocalypse, Passion, Life of the Virgin,* and an allegorical subject, *Ship of Fools.* Among his most popular single-sheet engravings were the *Prodigal Son, Adam and Eve, Knight, Death and the Devil, St. Jerome in his Study*, and *Melencolia.* His silverpoint drawings of landscape and architectural views date from a trip to the Netherlands in 1520-21.

Dürer wrote three technical books: *Underweysung der Messung mit dem Zirckel und Richtscheyt* (1525), a treatise on linear and solid geometry, astronomy, and typography; *Befestigungslehre* (1527), a treatise on fortifications and architecture; and *Vier Bücher von menschlicher Proportion* (1528), a treatise of four books on the proportions of human beings. The latter was published posthumously by his widow, but the artist had only corrected and revised the first book before his death.

Dürer used the height of the human body as the basic unit of measurement and subdivided it linearly to construct a unified artistic plan both of the figure and of the figure moving in space. His tabulation of proportions was based partly on his own observations and partly on the canons of the Italian theorists, especially Leonardo. Dürer's work allowed for modifications, and he held that an artist is free to select his own canon. Because he eventually developed multiple canons for different body types, "Dürer himself acknowledged that his studies were basically scientific in nature and of little practical value for the artist."[31]

The Jefferson edition of Dürer's book on symmetry and proportion was published in 1532 and contains the first two of the original four books. This illustration shows a female figure seen from the front and the side. The artist has indicated the distance between individual parts and between sections of the body. The length of the head is approximately one-seventh of the total height of the female body.

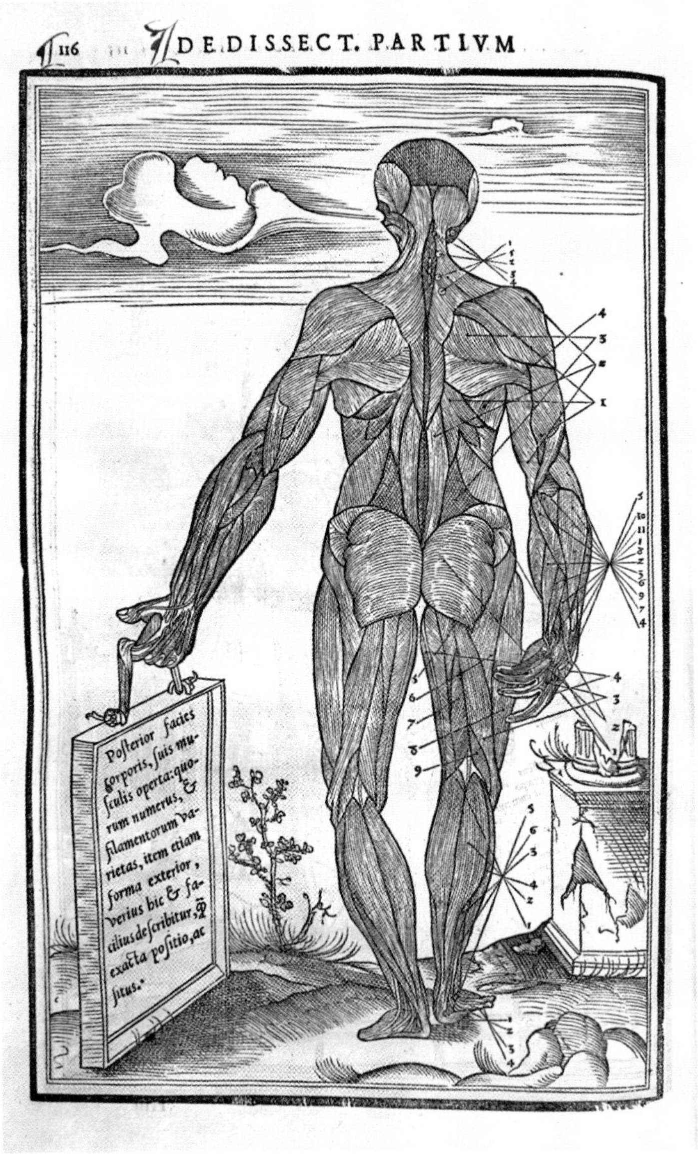

Muscle Man

MUSCLE MAN
By unknown artist

Woodcut
Image size: 10 5/8 x 7 in.
Page Size: 15 3/8 x 10 in.

From Charles Estienne, *De dissectione partium corporis humani libri tres...* (Paris: Simonem Colinaeum, 1545)

Given in 1940 by bequest of Pascal Brooke Bland, M.D. who had received it from Arno C. Voigt, M.D. (JMC 1901)

Accession number: 1940+e.Pr.11

Although Charles Estienne's *De dissectione partium corporis humani libri tres* was published in 1545, two years after Vesalius's *Fabrica,* its preparation dated back to 1530. Therefore, Estienne's innovative work should be considered another pre-Vesalian effort to use drawings effectively as illustrations of the text. However, it will be seen that Estienne's work lacks the intellectual and artistic coherence of Vesalius.

Charles Estienne (1504/05-64) was a member of a famous Parisian family of printers and publishers. He studied classical literature at the University of Padua and became interested in botany, horticulture, and medicine while in Italy (1530-34). Upon his return to Paris he took extracurricular courses in medicine and anatomy at the Collège de Tréguier. In the mid-1530s he published several treatises on natural science, as well as a short *Anatomia* (1536) of which no copies survive.

Estienne received his medical degree from the Faculté de Médecine in Paris in 1542, and taught anatomy there from 1544 to 1547. During this period his *De dissectione* manual was published, and a few years later a treatise on diet and classification of foods. He then gave up medicine to manage the family printing business. Though many books were successful, Estienne was a poor businessman, fell heavily in debt, and was accused of squandering his family's inheritance. He died in prison where he had spent the last four years of his life.

The earliest woodcut of Estienne's *De dissectione* is dated 1530, and the plates were completed and the text two-thirds printed by 1539. However publication was delayed because of professional difficulties with his collaborator, the surgeon Estienne de la Rivière (Stephanus Riverius; died 1569), who had probably done some dissection and helped with the plates. The lawsuit was settled in favor of Estienne de la Rivière and the title page credits both men. The work was published by Simon de Colines, the firm of Charles Estienne's stepfather, first in Latin (1545) and then in French (1546).

Although the text is still largely dependent on Galen and anatomical errors abound, Estienne is credited with many original anatomical observations. Among his innovative methods are the illustration of dissection in serial progression, description of the total human body (muscles, bones, organs, venous and arterial systems, nerves, glands, and joints), method of illustrating internal organs as cutout sections, directions for mounting a skeleton, setting the figures in a fully developed panoramic landscape, and a comprehensive index.[32]

The book's typography, paper, and presentation exemplify the high standards of sixteenth-century French publishing. The illustrations were once attributed to François (Jean) Jollat (active 1502-50) because his monogram occurs on three drawings, but it is unknown if he was involved with the remainder, or even if he was the designer or engraver. Furthermore, because the illustrations are of inconsistent quality and usefulness, ranging from elegant to crude, some scholars suggest the participation of more than one artist. The best illustrations are superb examples of French Mannerist style.[33]

Book One depicts standing male figures in sequential degrees of dissection showing the muscle layers, nerves, and skeletons. The écorché muscle man shown here is a stiff and awkward figure with unconvincing proportions. He holds the handle of a stone tablet with an inscription describing the musculature. The figure stands in a rudimentary landscape next to a plinth with a broken column base. His head is literally in the schematically rendered clouds.

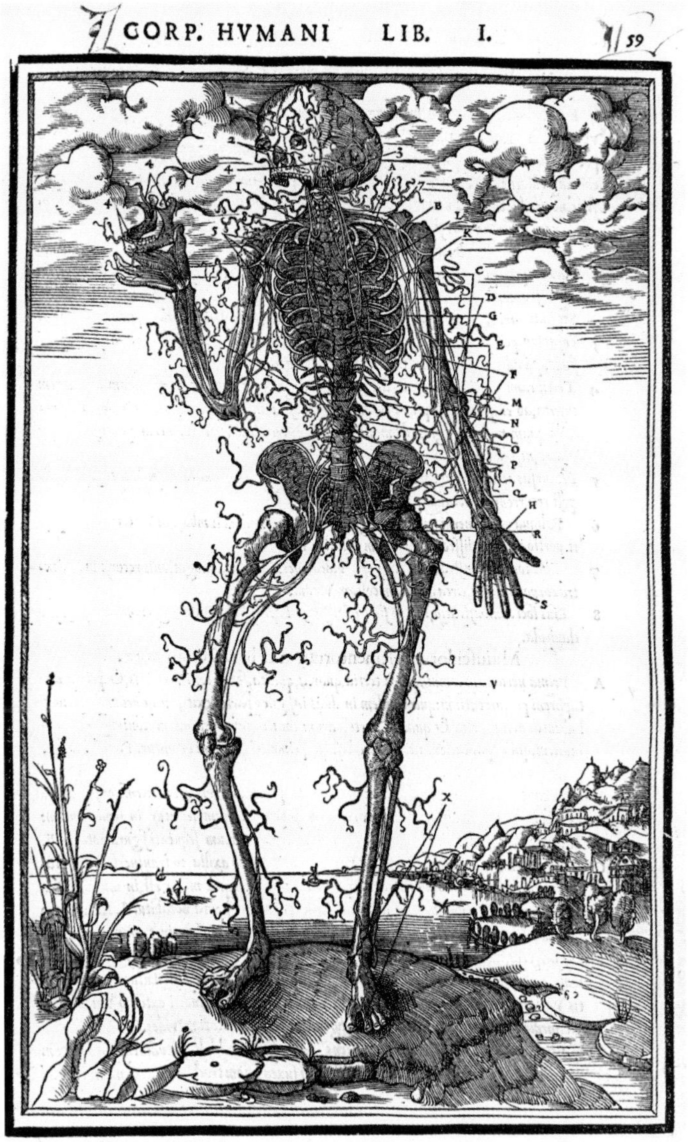

Nerve Man Skeleton

NERVE MAN SKELETON
By unknown artist

Woodcut
Image size: 10 3/4 x 6 7/8 in.
Page size: 15 3/8 x 10 in.

From Charles Estienne, *De dissectione* (as above)
Accession number: 1940+e.Pr.10

The nerve man skeleton of Book One shows the nerves emanating from a skeleton in a novel combination. The skeleton is shown from the front, displaying his mandible in his right hand. The distal portions of the nerves are decoratively coiled like curling ribbon. The jaunty figure is elevated on a hillock overlooking plants, a river with boats, a village on a hillside, and a cloud-filled sky. The skeleton's stance and the display of his own body part recall the skeleton of Berengario.

The landscape element behind the skeleton nerve man is much more skillful and developed than that behind the muscle man. The Estienne illustrations show a considerable advance over both the anatomy and rudimentary outdoor settings of Berengario.

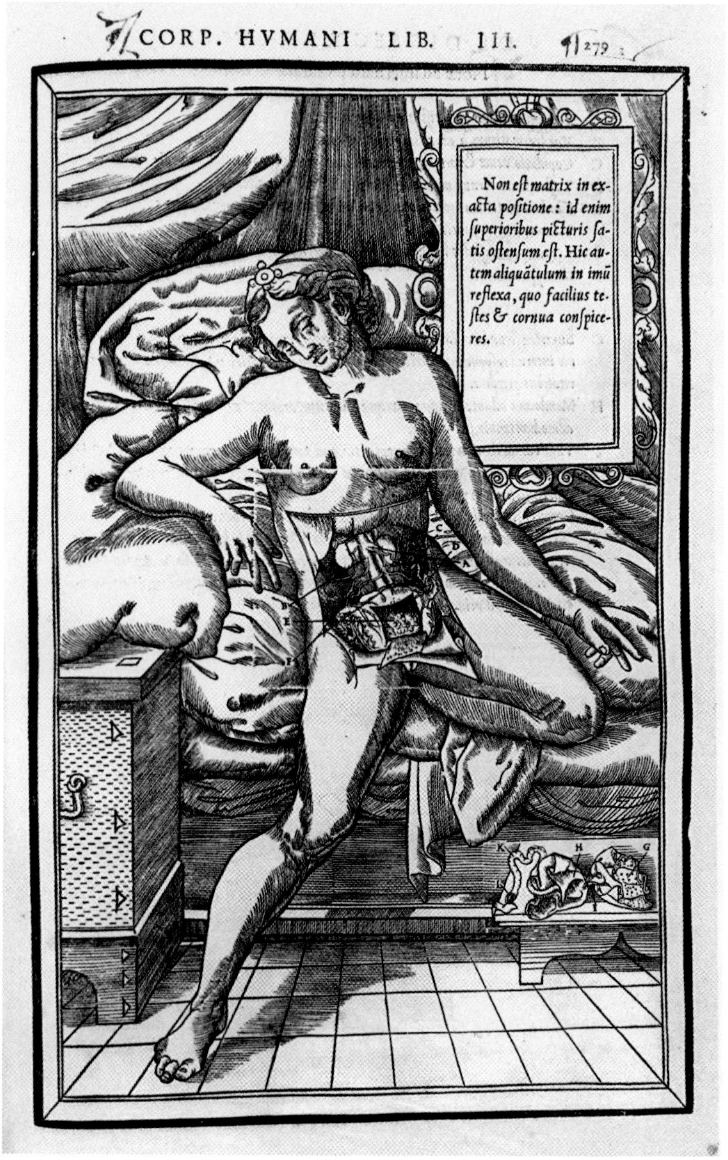

Pelvic Organs of the Female

PELVIC ORGANS OF THE FEMALE
By unknown artist

Woodcut
Image size: 10 3/4 x 6 7/8 in.
Page size: 15 3/8 x 10 in.

From Charles Estienne, *De dissectione* (as above)
Accession number: 1940+e.Pr.12

Book Two of Charles Estienne's *De dissectione* features series of successive dissections of the brain, the abdomen, and the neck. The depictions of men in contorted, almost writhing postures are typical of the Mannerist style. Book Three deals with the reproductive organs and contains a manual of practical anatomical procedures.

Berengario's earlier illustration of a female figure on a chair with the skin pulled back to display her reproductive organs has been transformed by Estienne into a fanciful, almost erotic depiction of excess and suggestion in his illustration of the pelvic organs of the female. Scholars have shown that the exaggerated poses derive from an earlier series of prints called "The Loves of the Gods," engraved after drawings by the Mannerist artists Rosso Fiorentino (1494-1540) and Perino del Vaga (1500/01-47).[34]

In the example shown here the female anatomical figure braces herself with one extended leg, as she sprawls on a billowing mound of bedclothes. Her other leg is tucked under her body. Her turbaned head rests on pillows and her eyes are closed. The fancy French interior also includes the bed's canopy, a table, footstool, and tiled floor.

One notices the outline of a small square around the dissected female organs and their associated letters. These "plugs" appear in many of the female figures and some of the male figures, and were cut separately and then set into the main block for printing. It is not known if the plugs were intended originally for another publication, or less likely, were to be replaced later with more up-to-date dissections. In the figures with plugs the dissected areas of the illustration are relatively small and indistinct compared with the rest of the nude figure and elaborate settings, whether domestic interiors or outdoor landscapes.

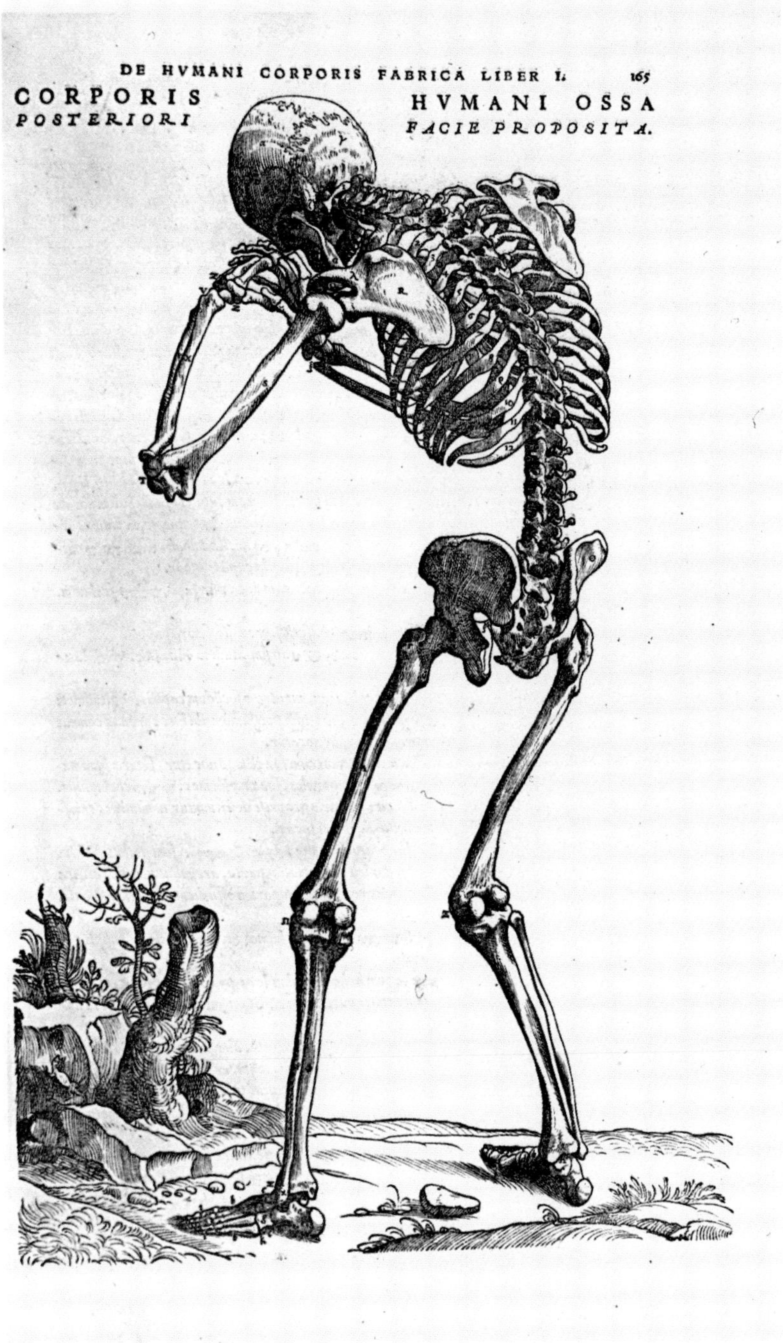

Skeleton

SKELETON
Attributed to Jan Stephan van Calcar
(ca. 1499-1546/50)

Woodcut
Image size: 13 x 8 1/8 in.
Page size: 16 x 11 in.

From Andreas Vesalius, *De humani corporis fabrica libri septem* (Basle: Joannis Oporini, 1543)

Given in 1977 by Robert L. Phillips, M.D. (JMC 1952)
Accession number: 1977+e.Pr.07

The *De humani corporis fabrica* of Andreas Vesalius (1514-64) was published in Basle in 1543. It was organized into seven books and contained over 250 woodcut illustrations of superb quality. The figures' astonishingly lifelike poses set into a naturalistic landscape with architectural elements lend the series a mysterious and dramatic narrative that goes beyond the objective depiction of the dissection. The book's integrated collaboration between physician, designer, woodcutter, and printer/publisher has been a source of admiration and influence for four and one-half centuries.

The most famous figures are the three mourning skeletons of Book One and the fourteen flayed muscle men of Book Two. The illustrations of veins and arteries in Book Three include only two full-length figures. Book Four treats the brain and cerebellum, spinal nerves, and spinal cord; Book Five the abdominal cavity, viscera, and reproductive organs; Book Six the thoracic cavity, heart, and lungs; and Book Seven the cranium, olfactory organs, and eye.

Vesalius provided each illustration with a legend called the index of characters denoting the various structures exposed. In some cases Vesalius made new discoveries and corrected in the text errors that appeared in the illustrations. His last addition was a system of cross references that further integrated the text with the illustrations.

The second edition of *Fabrica* was published in 1555 and was even more sumptuous with larger type and heavier paper. Redundancies in the text were removed and some corrections made. The most valuable addition was an extension of Vesalius's physiological experiments.

There is no doubt about the illustrators of Vesalius's prior anatomical work of 1538, *Tabulae sex*: three by Vesalius himself and three by Jan Stephan van Calcar, and it is known that the artist paid for the publication. However, attribution of the designer of *Fabrica's* illustrations has never been satisfactorily settled, though Calcar has been most consistently named. Some scholars have attributed the work to Titian (1488-90-1576), the great Venetian artist and Calcar's teacher, and others see the hand of more than one unidentified artist involved. A final issue is the belief of many scholars that the landscape panoramas were drawn by a different artist than the figures: probably Domenico Campagnola (ca.1500-64), a landscape draftsman thought to have been in Titian's studio.[35]

The three skeleton figures in Book One are dynamic and limber, unlike the previous representations of static, articulated skeletons. Vesalius was the first to join the bones together artificially, strung like beads on long wires bent to set the skeleton in the desired attitude.[36]

Though reduced to bone with no overlying structure, the skeleton men still can retain an upright pose. The first figure is in an anterior view, represented as a grave digger resting the weight of his body on his spade. The second skeleton is turned profile to the right. He stands cross legged with hands placed on a skull on top of a plinth, a vignette often compared to Hamlet soliloquizing on the skull of Yorick.

The third skeleton, shown here in a posterior aspect, is bent over at the waist. His head rests on wringing hands as though mourning or weeping. He overlooks a simple but symbolic landscape: two gnarled trees cut off bluntly at the trunk, with a few slender limbs trying to survive.

Though Vesalius's plates show some errors of proportion, his skeleton figures are extremely advanced in both science and artistry compared with the full-length skeleton of Berengario da Carpi, produced only twenty years earlier.

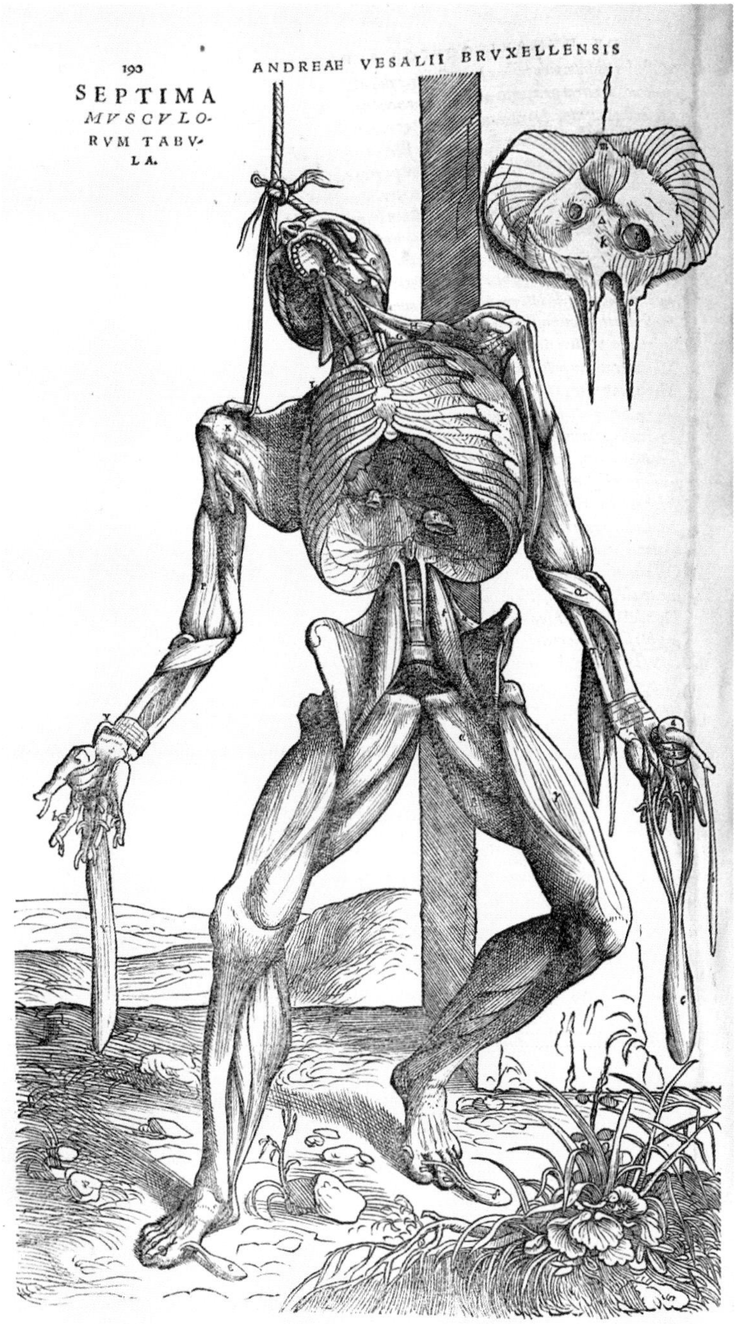

Seventh Plate of Muscles

MUSCLE MAN
Attributed to Jan Stephan van Calcar

Woodcut
Image size: 13 1/4 x 8 in.
Page size: 16 x 11 in.

From Andreas Vesalius, *Fabrica* (as above)
Accession number: 1977+e.Pr.05

Book Two contains a total of fourteen muscle men in two series. The first series has eight figures all in the anterior aspect except the second. Figures in the other series of six are in the posterior aspect. With minor exceptions both series show a continuous progression of dissection from superficial to deeper structures, revealed by the removal of overlaying tissues.

In four plates of Book One the deep fascia is cut away to reveal the superficial arrangement of muscles to physicians. In the text accompanying the first plate, Vesalius commented that these plates "display a total view of the scheme of muscles such as only painters and sculptors are wont to consider."[37] Most of the muscle men are shown in motion to illustrate the function of the muscles and help to clarify the relationships of parts.

In the seventh plate of muscles in the first series, shown here, the cadaver has been eviscerated and the collapsed figure is displayed with his head pulled back by a noose to better show the deep muscles of the neck. His legs are still somewhat self-supporting. His diaphragm hangs on the adjacent wall (as though this imaginary architectural element were really there). This position effectively shows where the diaphragm is pierced by the vena cava, aorta, and esophagus. The figure's arms are outstretched with flaps of skin hanging down.

Vesalius described his procedure of preparing the muscle men using ropes and pulleys:

> Usually when administering the dissection of a man, I draw a strong chord under the lower jaw and through each jugal bone to the vertex of the head, confined as by a noose, and either more toward the forehead or the occiput according as I had it in mind to suspend the cadaver either with the head erect or depressed. I placed the longer end of the noose across a pulley fixed to a beam of the room, and by that I drew the suspended corpse now higher now lower, taking care that it might be turned in every direction according to the requirement of the task.[38]

Ninth Plate of Muscles

MUSCLE MAN
Attributed to Jan Stephan van Calcar

Woodcut
Image size: 13 1/2 x 8 in.
Page size: 16 x 11 in.

From Andreas Vesalius, *Fabrica* (as above)
Accession number: 1977+e.Pr.06

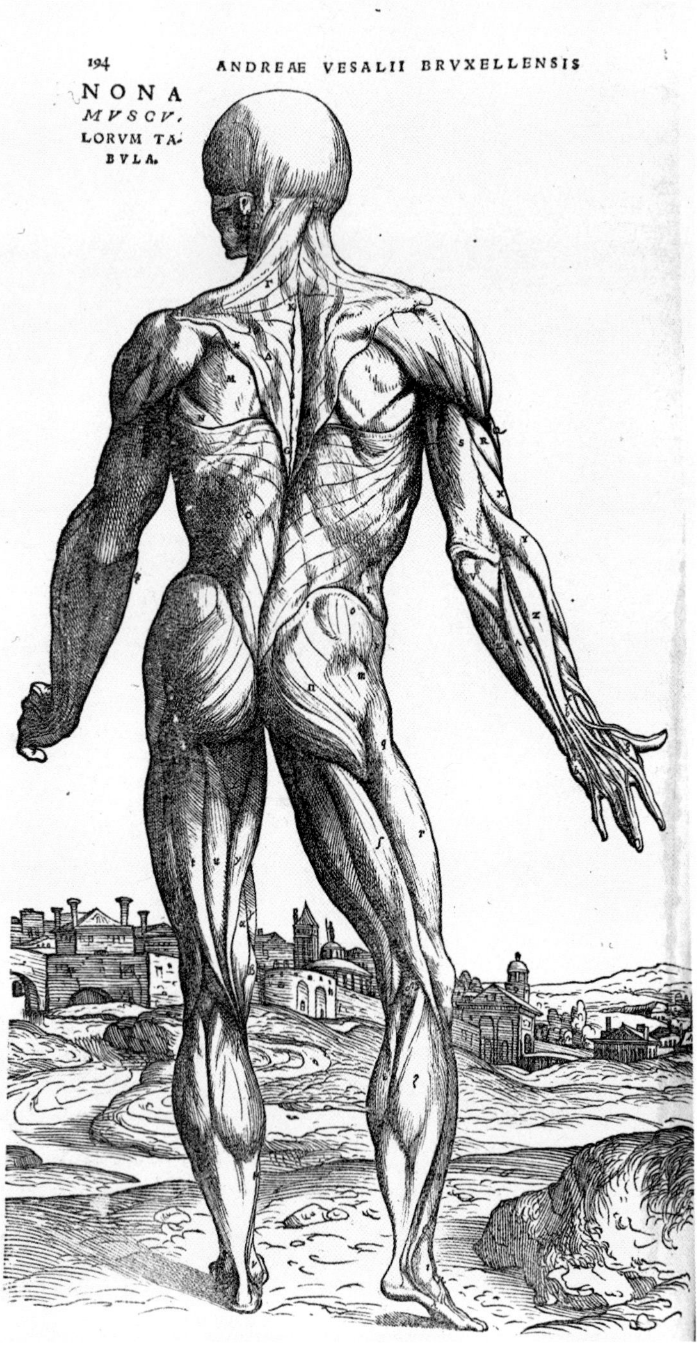

All six figures in the second series of Book Two stand without support. The écorché figure in the ninth plate of muscles, shown here, is the first illustration of the second series and the first muscle man shown from a posterior aspect. The fleshy membrane has been dissected as in plates one and two. The transverse ligaments of the forearm are dissected as in plate three, because they had already been clearly shown in the first and second plates.

The figure appears to be strolling and gesturing through a naturalistic landscape that has been extended to show a winding river and buildings clinging to the rolling hillside of a nearby village. Additional landscape elements in other plates in this series include Roman ruins and obelisks.

Compared with Estienne's stiff and flattened écorché set in a rudimentary landscape, Vesalius's figure is strong, confident, and dynamic and seems at one with the picturesque landscape. Vesalius's compositions are dramatic and the figures graceful, and he never resorted to interior domestic settings like the cluttered and overstuffed interiors of Estienne.

Scholars have long noted that the landscape backgrounds of the muscle men in Book Two can be joined to form two continuous panoramic friezes in the eight figures of the first series and the six figures of the second series. Yet to do this the figures have to be rearranged, roughly in reverse of the expected sequential order: with the most dissected figure first and the least dissected figure last, opposite to their order in the published *Fabrica*.

As a solution to this vexing problem it was recently hypothesized that the backgrounds were made in long drawings separately from the figures; the landscapes were cut into pieces and copied directly onto the plates of the individual figures by the woodcutter, without tracing them on the plates; and that they were, in fact, reversed images of the original drawings, due to the reversal in the printing process. When the plates are photographically reversed as mirror images, then the muscle men traverse the continuous landscape in the same order as the book itself, except that the first and second plates have been reordered.[39]

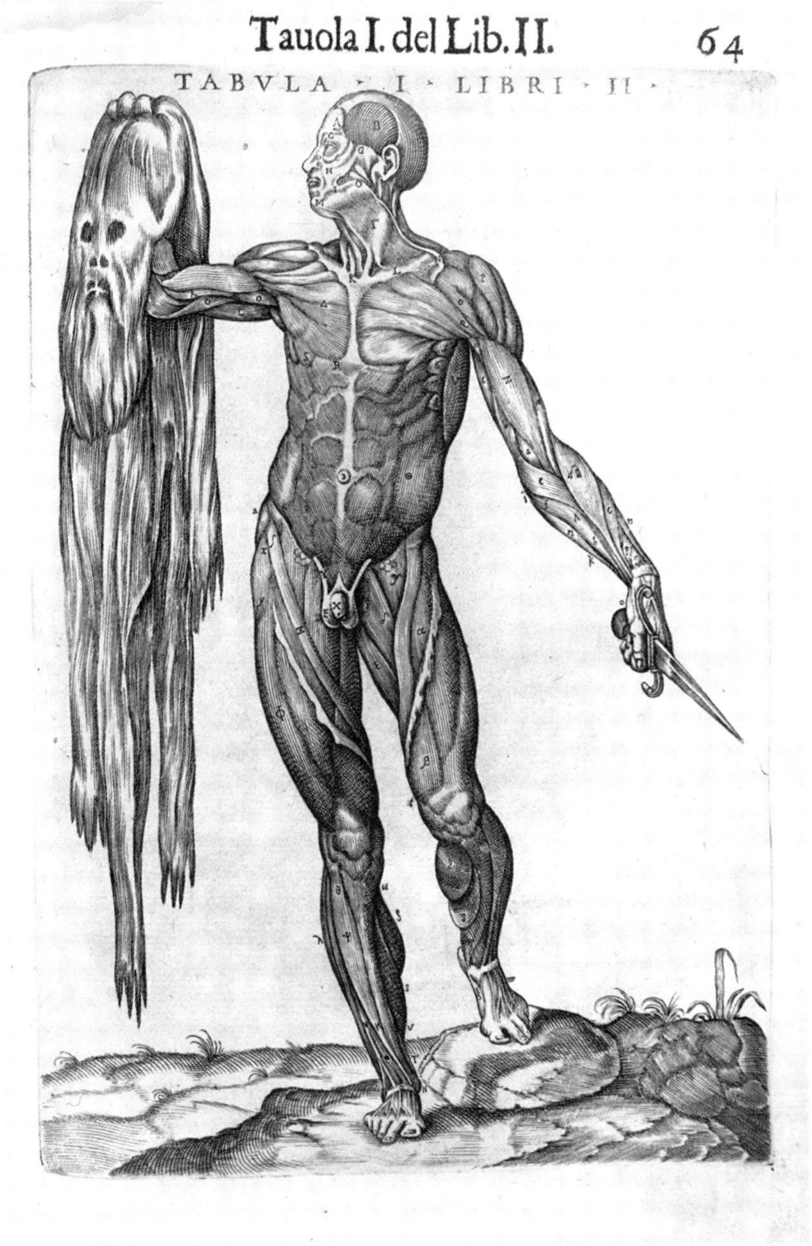

Muscle Man

MUSCLE MAN
Attributed to Gaspar Becerra
(ca. 1520-70)

Engraving
Image size: 8 1/2 x 6 in.
Page size: 11 x 7 1/2 in.

From Juan de Valverde, *La anatomia del corpo umano...* (Venice: Giunti, 1586)

Given in 1940 by bequest of Pascal Brooke Bland, M.D.
Accession number: 1940+e.Pr.27

In the century after its publication, Vesalius's *Fabrica* remained the standard in illustrated anatomical texts. However, new requirements in format, costs, language, usage, and specific needs arose, and because it was considered prohibitive to start anew, many authors issued new books based on the Vesalius text and illustrations. Most authors acknowledged their debt to Vesalius, while a few actually plagiarized him.[40]

In 1556, thirteen years after the publication of *Fabrica*, a new book on human anatomy was published in Rome by the Spaniard Juan de Valverde de Amusco (1520/25-87/88). His *Historia de la composición del cuerpo humano* was smaller in size and length, less costly, and less scholarly than Vesalius's work, and was written in vernacular Spanish. If Valverde's more succinct account was found wanting, then his readers were referred to the *Fabrica*, for he had retained the original Vesalian lettering.

The success of the Valverde book was due largely to the copperplate engravings most of which were derived from the original woodcuts in the Vesalius book. His book was translated into Italian, Latin, and Dutch and appeared in almost a dozen editions. Valverde made some significant corrections and additions to the Vesalius text, in particular the nature of the cardiac septum.

Valverde forthrightly acknowledged his debt to Vesalius,

> Although it seemed to some of my friends that I should make new illustrations without using those of Vesalius, I did not do so, in order to avoid the confusion that could follow, not knowing clearly in what I agree or in what I disagree with him, and because his illustrations are so well done it would look like envy or malignity not to take advantage of them.[41]

Although Valverde praised Vesalius, the Italian pathfinder was resentful and critical, saying, "Valverde, who never put his hand to a dissection and is ignorant of medicine as well as of the primary disciples, undertook to expound our art in the Spanish language only for the sake of shameful profit."[42] Actually, Valverde had considerable education and success, though no medical degree.

He was born about 1525 in Palencia, Spain and graduated in humanities and philosophy from Valladolid University. He received anatomical training in Padua under Vesalius's successor, Realdo Colombo, and became Colombo's assistant in Pisa in 1544 and then in Rome in 1548. Valverde became personal physician to Cardinal Juan Alvarez de Toledo, the general inquisitor in Rome to whom he dedicated his anatomy text. Valverde taught anatomy at the hospital of Santo Spirito. His earlier book of hygiene, diet, and behavior, *De animi et corporis sanitate tuenda libellus*, was issued in 1552.

Most scholars agree that Valverde's artist for the *Anatomia* was probably Gaspar Becerra (ca. 1520-70), a Spaniard. The book made numerous changes to the Vesalian images, although the "corrections" were not always accurate. Valverde's text also used about fifteen illustrations that did not appear in Vesalius, though some appear to be composites derived from the original.

One composite image of an écorché is the illustration shown here. It is an anterior view of a muscle man regarding his own flayed skin which is raised to eye level with his right hand. The distorted image of his bearded face hangs down pathetically. The figure holds a dagger in his lowered left hand, although that instrument could not have been used in a dissection. His weight is on the front foot, and the back foot is poised on toes on a rock.

Gasparo Becerra was born in Baeza, Andalusia about 1520, and was a well known painter, sculptor, and architect. During a visit to Rome he studied under Michelangelo and assisted him at the Vatican. Becerra returned to Spain in 1556 and executed some frescoes for Philip II and became painter to the court in 1563. He was very interested in the study of anatomy and produced two anatomical statues. He died in Madrid in 1570.[43]

Scholars have noted that the source for Becerra's image of the flayed man is the figure of St. Bartholomew in Michelangelo's *Last Judgment* in the Sistine Chapel, unveiled in 1541. He is shown holding his skin in one hand and the instrument of his martyrdom, the curved knife, in his other hand. The features of the tortured face in the flayed skin are those of Michelangelo himself. Additional sources in classical mythology available to Becerra were images of Apollo flaying the satyr Marsyas and Hercules flaying the lion. Marsyas was a powerful symbol for artists, because he was flayed for daring to compete artistically with Apollo, a god.

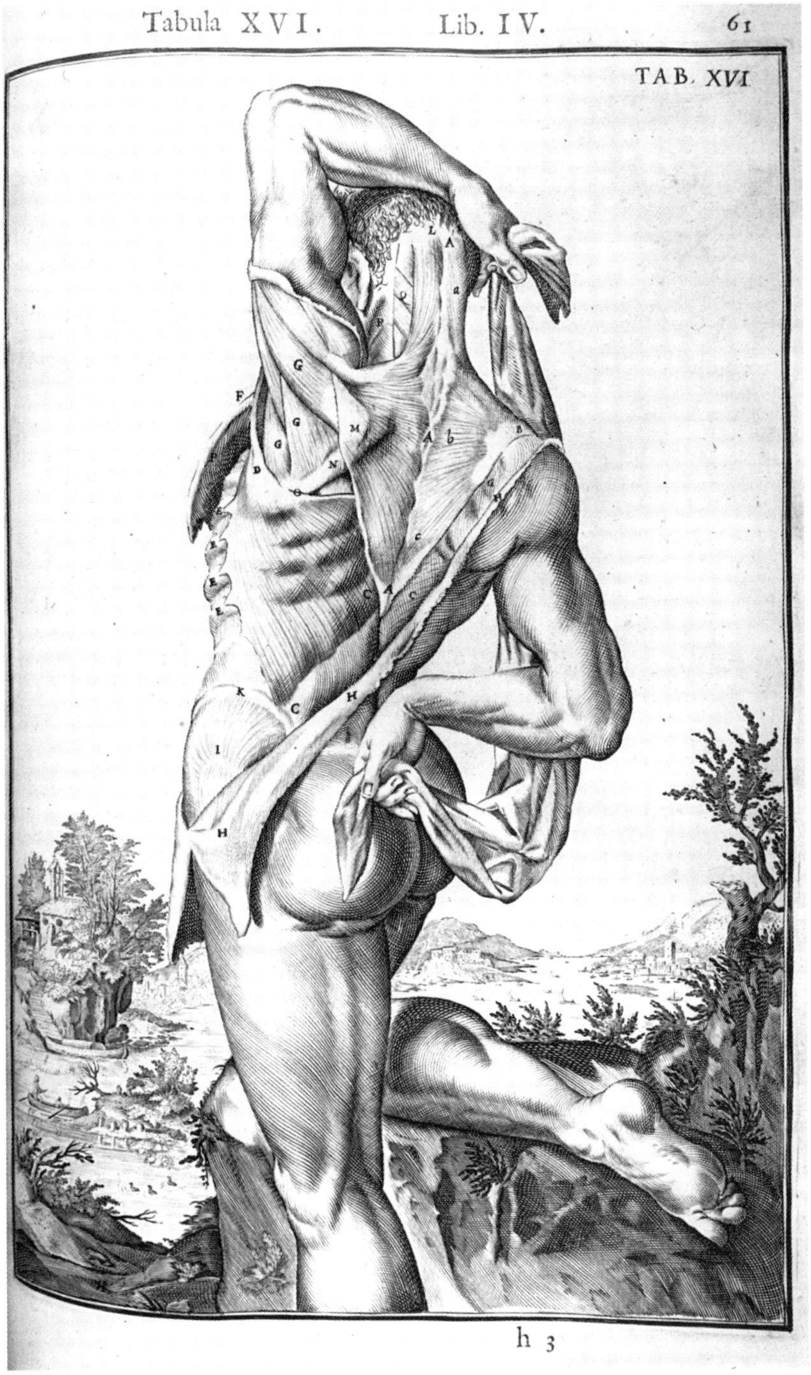

Muscle Man

MUSCLE MAN
By unknown artist

Engraving
Image size: 13 3/8 x 8 1/2 in.
Plate size: 13 1/2 x 8 5/8 in.
Page size: 15 1/4 x 10 in.

From Adriaan van den Spieghel, *...Opera quae extant, omnia,* edited by Johannes Antonides van der Linden (Amsterdam: Johannem Blaeu, 1645)

Given in 1940 by bequest of Pascal Brooke Bland, M.D.
Accession number: 1940+e.Pr.24

Seventeenth-century anatomy illustration took the conventions of previous centuries to new and exaggerated heights, especially details of the figures' poses, hairstyle, action, and landscape. The illustrations in a publication of Adriaan van den Spieghel's complete works embody this new Baroque style: several of the coquettish female figures with elaborate and flowing hairdos are situated out-of-doors; a male figure is shown spread-eagled on his back grasping an improbably bent tree limb.

Adriaan van den Spieghel (1578-1625) was born in Belgium, the son and grandson of surgeons. He studied at the universities in Louvain and Leiden, and later at Padua under Girolamo Fabrici (1533/37-1619) and Giulio Casserio (1552/61-1616), both celebrated teachers of anatomy: Fabrici on embryology and comparative anatomy, and Casserio on the anatomy of the sense organs.

In 1606 Spieghel was appointed ordinary physician to the students at the Natio Germanica in Padua, and assisted Fabrici in his private practice. In 1612 he left Italy for Germany and was appointed *medicus primarius* of Bohemia. In December 1616 he succeeded his teachers as professor of anatomy at Padua, and by the following January had performed a public dissection in the famous anatomical theater at Padua erected by Fabrici. Spieghel was elected Knight of St. Mark in 1623, two years before his death.

Spieghel's most important manuscript, *De humani corporis fabrica*, was not published until 1627, two years after his death. In his will he had entrusted the editing of his book to Daniel Rindfleisch (known as Bucretius), a young physician and associate. Since Spieghel had not provided illustrations, Bucretius obtained seventy-seven copperplates that Casserio had had made and added twenty more. It is not known why Casserio had never issued the series of engravings on successive stages of dissection, although he worked on the project for almost two decades.

The fame and success of Spieghel's book were owing largely to these drawings. The authorship of the drawings is under some dispute, most scholars favoring an Italian artist, Odoardo Fialetti (1573-1638), but another ascribing the work to an unidentified northern artist perhaps familiar with engravings by Hendrik Goltzius (1558-1617).[44] In any case, the techniques of both designer and engraver are quite distinctive and show a virtuosity and elegance of line not possible in the woodcut process.

The 1645 edition in Jefferson's collection is two volumes bound in one. In addition to the complete works of Spieghel it also includes works by others including Casserio and William Harvey.

The drawing shown here is one of the Casserio illustrations, and the dissection is unusual for not being along the midline. It features the superficial musculature of the left side of the neck, shoulder, and back, in particular the scapular region.

The partially flayed figure is shown in a twisted pose from the back. His right leg kneels on a flattened section of rock outcropping. Both arms are bent at the elbow, one twisted behind his back and the other over his head. The curving length of material held between his hands representing his flayed skin is depicted like folds of drapery. It serves to accentuate the extreme flexed action of the posture.

The muscle man rises up dramatically over a tranquil landscape. The figure and nearby rock and foliage are shaded from darks to lights, while the distant view of meandering river, village, and faraway mountains is pale. Vignettes of contemporary life on the river include men in a rowboat, sailboats, and ducks. Another rowboat is docked next to a flight of steps leading up to a church.

Whereas the energetic but dignified Vesalius écorché seen from the rear seems at one with the landscape, the Spieghel figure dominates the landscape and his athletic pose seems frivolous in comparison. In contrast to both, in Estienne's illustration of a flattened écorché holding a stone tablet, the stylized landscape elements appear almost like an afterthought.

Skeleton

SKELETON
By Jan Wandelaar (1690-1759)

Engraving
Image size: 21 3/4 x 14 3/4 in.
Plate size: 22 1/2 x 15 1/4 in.
Page size: 27 x 19 1/2 in.

Inscriptions below image: lower left, "J. Wandelaar ad ipsum Sceletum delineavit et incidit" and lower right, "Prostat Leidae Batavorum apud J. et H. Verbeek, Bibliop. 1740"
From Bernhard Siegfried Albinus, *Tabulae sceleti et musculorum corporis humani* (Leiden: Joannem & Hermannum Verbeek, 1747)

Given in 1940 by bequest of Pascal Brooke Bland, M.D.
Accession number: 1940+e.Pr.30

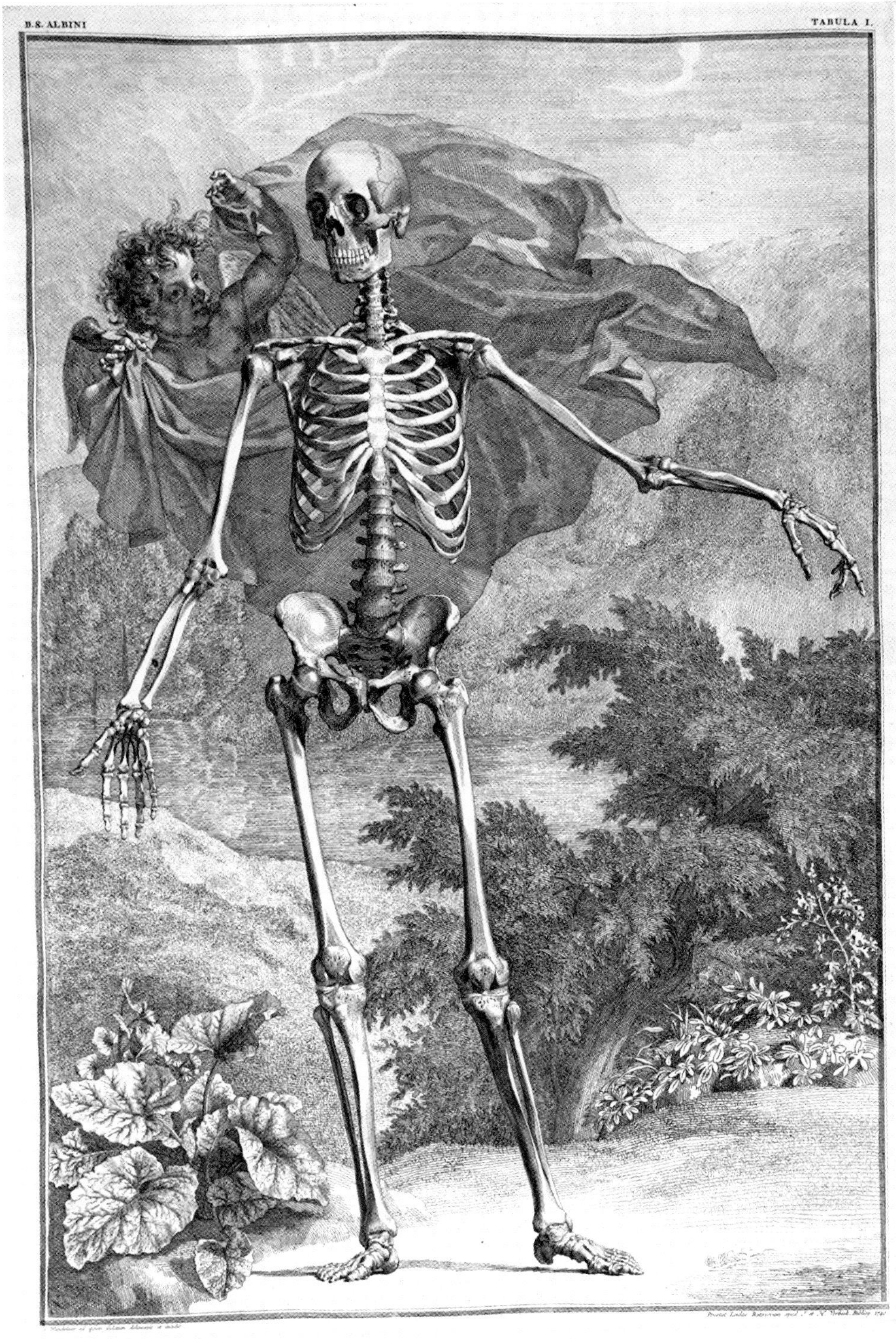

With the publications of Bernard Siegfried Albinus, anatomical illustration reached new heights of scientific and artistic excellence not seen since Vesalius two centuries earlier. So as not to disturb the beauty of his anatomical figures in their lush backgrounds, Albinus provided outline diagrams of each skeleton and muscle man with references on the opposing page.

The professional and personal relationship between Albinus and his artist, Jan Wandelaar, was unusually close, and the artist even lived in Albinus's house for the last twenty years of his life. In his preface to *Tabulae sceleti et musculorum corporis humani* Albinus spoke, perhaps with a touch of hubris, about their interdependence:

> I have not only studied the correctness of the figures, but likewise the neatness and elegancy of them. For this end I employed an artist very skillful both in drawing and engraving...For a great many years bypast, he has worked for very few besides myself; and for these last ten (most part of which he has been wholly employed in these tables) almost for me only. He both drew and engraved them under my direction. I endeavoured to make him understand as well as possible what was to be drawn, and I was constantly with him, to direct him how everything was to be done, assisting him in the drawing, and correcting what was drawn. And thus he was instructed, directed, and as entirely ruled by me, as if he was a tool in my hands, and I made the figures myself.[45]

Bernhard Siegfried Albinus was born in 1697 at Frankfurt an der Oder where his father was a professor of medicine and physician to Elector Friedrich Wilhelm von Brandenburg. The family name, originally Weiss von Weissenlöw, had been Latinized into Albinus by a great-grand-uncle.

When Albinus was age five his father was called to the University of Leiden to become professor of theoretical and practical medicine. The boy was considered a prodigy, and at age twelve began to study medicine at the university under Hermann Boerhaave (1668-1738) and the anatomists Govard Bidloo (1649-1713) and Johannes J. Rau (1668-1719). Leiden was then considered a world center for the study of medicine.

Albinus also studied anatomy and botany briefly in Paris before being recalled to Leiden to substitute for the ailing Rau. He received his medical degree in 1719 and two years later at age twenty-four was appointed professor of anatomy and surgery. He remained a resident of Leiden until his death in 1770.

Albinus's life was devoted to scholarship and he amassed a library of two thousand volumes of medical, literary, and philosophical works and a museum of specimens. In 1734 he issued a new edition of James Douglas's bibliography of anatomy. In connection with Boerhaave he edited a number of earlier medical writers including Eustachius, Fabrici, Harvey, and Vesalius and provided them with new engraved plates.

Around 1725 Albinus developed an ambitious plan to publish his own large scale engravings that would surpass any previous illustrations, including those of the celebrated authors he had edited. His methods were so painstaking that the first completed folio volume on muscles and the skeleton did not appear until 1747. Subsequent volumes comprised plates on the pregnant uterus (1748-51), bones (1753), and one plate on the thoracic duct, intercostal arteries, and azygous vein (1757). Projected series on the viscera and vessels never were completed. The whole endeavor was so enormous that in 1745 Albinus asked to be relieved of his main teaching duties. His youngest brother Frederick was appointed professor of anatomy and surgery in his place, while Bernhard became professor of medicine.

Albinus devised an innovative system that would dispense with inaccuracies he observed in other anatomists' drawings which progressed from skin to superficial muscles, to deeper muscles, down to the skeleton. He started with the skeleton as the fixed point of reference and then added the muscles, a plan recommended by Leon Battista Alberti and actually used by Eustachius. He compared the method with architects laying down a foundation.

Albinus strove for continuity among the figures, and in a long preface he described his techniques. In preparing the bones of the skeleton he encountered a problem with damage to cartilage and ligaments which no longer fit as before when rejoined. His solution was to prepare a fresh skeleton for this purpose leaving the ligaments, tendons, and cartilages attached. Since it took three months to prepare the skeleton, he prevented drying out and putrefaction by pouring water into the joints and sprinkling the whole with vinegar. With cords, weights, pulleys, and wedges he meticulously stood the skeleton in a position that was constantly compared with the pose of a thin model of the same size as the skeleton.[46]

His "homo perfectus" was a fully grown male about age twenty-five, well proportioned and of middle stature, with signs of strength and suppleness. This "average man" which he regarded as perfect was computed from a large sample of cadavers. The ideal man was inherent to his natural philosophy that the "structure and function of human, animal, and vegetable individuals were determined by a vital force in accordance with invariable laws." His ideas about a natural striving for perfection were applied to his goal of depicting the perfect man without distortion.[47]

To ensure accurate, measured drawings of correct proportions, he devised a system of two grids made with small cords. The first one with larger squares was placed directly in front of the skeleton through which the artist could observe the whole figure through a peephole at a distance of forty Rhenish feet. To fill in details a second grid with squares one-tenth the size was positioned four Rhenish feet in front of the first grid. When the grids were lined up properly the artist could verify the accuracy of various parts by means of lines and intersections.

The figures were drawn first on large sheets of paper, squared to the same size as the grids directly in front of the skeleton. These drawings were reduced and refined into folio size sheets ruled with proportionately smaller squares. Etched plates for publication were made from the latter.

The atlas contained three skeletal plates and nine plates of muscles. The skeletons are shown standing in posterior and anterior views, and walking from a profile view. Having spent thirteen years illustrating the skeletal figures, Albinus then passed on to the muscle men. He said that he dissected the muscles carefully in order to observe their positions, connection, figure, thickness, and substance. He preserved muscle specimens in a "proper liquor" before adding them to the skeleton.[48]

The Dutch artist Jan Wandelaar was already experienced in anatomical illustration before joining with Albinus. He was a portrait and landscape painter and engraver who had studied with Jakob Folkema (1692-1767), Gérard de Lairesse (1640-1711), and Willem van der Gouwen. Wandelaar had done some scientific illustrations for the anatomists Friederich Ruysch (1638-1731) and Arent Cant (1695-1723) before moving from Amsterdam to near Leiden in 1723. After Wandelaar's only son died in childhood, he went to live in Albinus's house from about 1746. The productive collaboration between Albinus and Wandelaar ended with the artist's death in 1759.

Wandelaar's idea of "ornaments" of animals and architecture added into the landscape backgrounds were to fill up the empty spaces in the plates, and to create harmony of light and shade. He said that if an observer looks at the figures through a hollow hand (cupped), they appear to be stepping out of the picture and give the illusion of three dimensions. Albinus explained Wandelaar's ideas further,

> He maintained that...he would preserve the proper light of the pictures, for if the space around the picture and between the parts should be white, the light of the pictures would suffer. He said that this means would insure that nothing would be harsh. The ornaments in the pictures of the skeleton are lighter than in the pictures of the muscles, corresponding to the lightness of the skeleton, the solidity of the muscles—they are lighter directly around the pictures and more conspicuous in the more distant places, as expediency demands.[49]

Each of the twelve skeleton and muscle man plates were signed by Wandelaar as artist and engraver. There were a total of eighty plates in *Tabulae sceleti et musculorum corporis humani.*

The anterior view of the skeleton is the first of three in outdoor settings. His arms are extended away from his body with a gesture that is almost welcoming. The foliage of trees and shrubbery, the river, and the river bank behind the figure are exquisitely rendered in delicate detail. Billowing drapery held by a tousled-hair, winged putto forms a circular cloud behind the skeleton. Perhaps the angelic infant will accompany the skeleton to his tomb, seen in the background of the next skeletal image.

Outermost Order of Muscles

MUSCLE MAN
By Jan Wandelaar

Engraving
Image size: 21 1/2 x 15 in.
Plate size: 22 x 15 1/2 in.
Page size: 27 x 19 1/2 in.

From Bernhard Siegfried Albinus, *Tabulae sceleti* (as above)
Accession number: 1940+e.Pr.05

The écorché illustrated here is one of three displaying the most superficial layer of muscles. Each has a different setting.

The figure seems to be meditating on the features of the lush landscape. Trees, rocks, brook, waterfalls, and cliffs envelop him closely with only one small opening at the top for a view of the clouds and distant mountains. Details of foliage and geology are as precisely rendered as the figure. Compared with the mannered, almost tortured figures which dominate the landscapes in Spieghel's book, Albinus's serene figures are more effectively integrated into their surroundings.

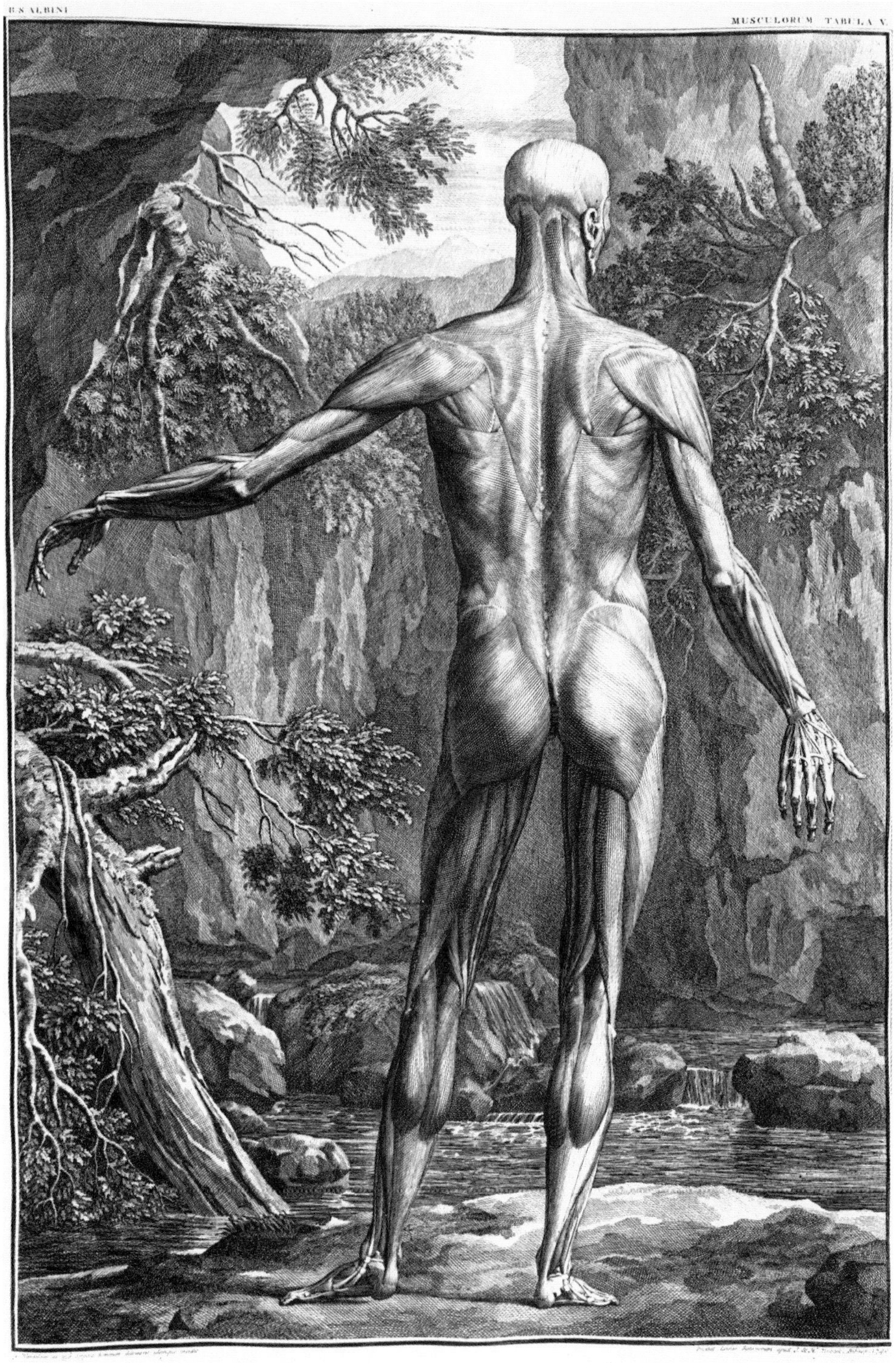

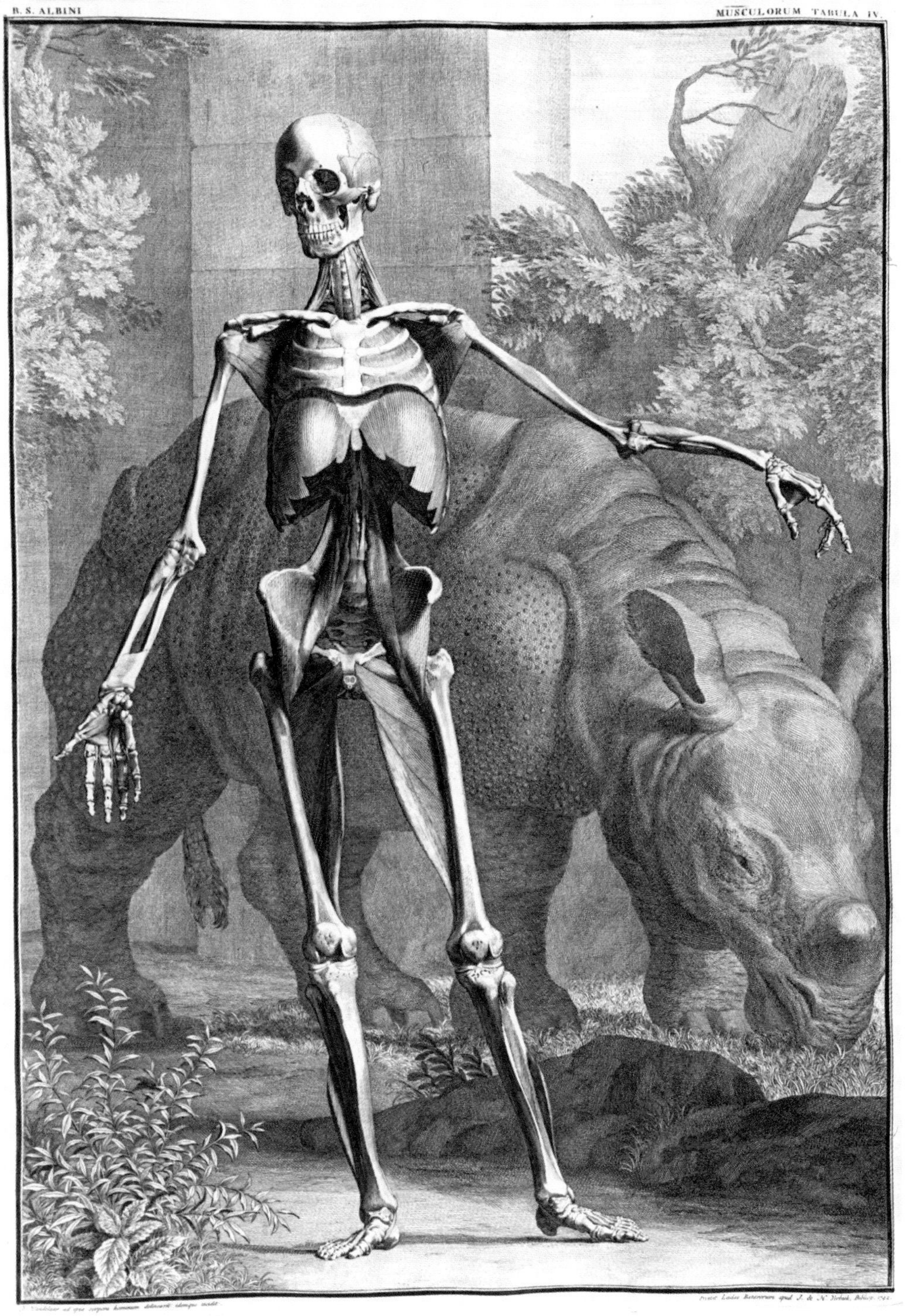

Fourth Order of Muscles

MUSCLE MAN
By Jan Wandelaar

Engraving
Image size:
21 1/2 x 15 1/4 in.
Plate size:
22 x 15 3/4 in.
Page size:
27 x 19 1/2 in.

From Bernhard Siegfried Albinus, *Tabulae sceleti* (as above)
Accession number:
1940+e.Pr.06

In the *Fourth Order of Muscles* the figure is dissected to the deepest muscular layer. The muscles that remain hold the bones together in the neck, upper rib cage, posterior abdominal cavity, and extremities. The figure is in scale to a rhinoceros which stands in front of a stone wall in the background. The presence of this creature seems like an exotic addition to modern eyes.

Actually, there was a substantial history of depictions of the rhinoceros ever since the famous woodcut published in 1515 by Albrecht Dürer. The German artist had never seen a rhinoceros but based his drawing and woodcut on a sketch and description by a Portuguese artist who had sketched the animal from life. Numerous scientists subsequently published works with images of the rhinoceros based on the Dürer image.[50]

However, Albinus and Wandelaar supposedly saw an actual specimen in Amsterdam in 1741, and Wandelaar drew this animal *ad vivum*. The artist and physician "immediately proclaimed it to be a symbol of their atlas."[51] Drawing it reflected their fascination with recording unusual anatomical details. The rhinoceros appears in two plates of the fourth set of muscles.

Not since Vesalius two centuries earlier had any anatomy illustrations had such a profound influence on subsequent medical anatomical texts. Their appeal stems from Albinus's quantitative exactitude and tenaciousness and Wandelaar's ability to render the family of skeletal and écorché figures accurately and harmoniously integrated into an idealized private world. As expressions of the Enlightenment ideal of the perfect man Albinus's illustrations served as inspiration to countless artists and physicians.

1. For information about Matout's painting and a bibliography on the artist see Elizabeth Johns, *Thomas Eakins: The Heroism of American Life* (Princeton: Princeton University Press, 1983), 73-74, plate 43.
2. Samuel D. Gross, M.D., "A Sketch of the Life, Character, and Services of Ambrose Paré," *North American Medico-Chirurgical Review* 5 (Nov. 1861): 1068-71.
3. Ira M. Rutkow, M.D., *Surgery: An Illustrated History* (St. Louis: Mosby, 1993), 398.
4. Carl Zigrosser, *Ars Medica: A Collection of Medical Prints Presented to the Philadelphia Museum of Art by Smith Kline & French Laboratories* (Philadelphia: Philadelphia Museum of Art, 1959), 26-27.
5. Albert S. Lyons, M.D. and R. Joseph Petrucelli II, M.D., *Medicine: An Illustrated History* (New York: Harry N. Abrams, 1978, reprint 1987), 206-17.
6. "Complementary Therapies: Homeopathy," *Harvard Women's Health Watch* 4 (Jan. 1997): 2-3.
7. Bernard Schultz, *Art and Anatomy in Renaissance Italy* (Ann Arbor, Mich.: UMI Research Press, 1985), 2.
8. Mimi Cazort, Monique Kornell, and K. B. Roberts, *The Ingenious Machine of Nature: Four Centuries of Art and Anatomy* (Ottawa: National Gallery of Canada, 1996), 12-13.
9. John Aubrey, quoted in Geoffrey Keynes, M.D., *The Portraiture of William Harvey* (London: Royal College of Surgeons of England, 1949), 8.
10. Keynes, 11-15, 32-34.
11. Gross, "John Hunter and his Pupils," *The College and Clinical Record* (Jefferson Medical College) 2 (Jan. 15, 1881): 15.
12. Sherwin B. Nuland, M.D., *Medicine: The Art of Healing* (New York: Hugh Lauter Levin Associates, 1992), 66.
13. "Baron Larrey: A Sketch" in *Selections from the Papers and Speeches of John Chalmers DaCosta* (Philadelphia: W. B. Saunders Co., 1931), 104. Read originally by DaCosta at a meeting of the Johns Hopkins Historical Club on Feb. 12, 1906 and reprinted in the *Johns Hopkins Hospital Bulletin* of July 1906.
14. Cazort, Kornell, and Roberts, 105-06.
15. A. Hyatt Mayor, *Artists and Anatomists* (New York: The Artist's Limited Edition in association with the Metropolitan Museum of Art, 1984), 46-50.
16. Cazort, Kornell, and Roberts, 129.
17. J. B. deC. M. Saunders and Charles D. O'Malley, *The Illustrations from the Works of Andreas Vesalius of Brussels* (Cleveland: World Publishing, 1950; reprint, New York: Dover Publications, 1973), 42 (reprint edition).
18. Saunders and O'Malley, 42.
19. K. B. Roberts and J. D. Tomlinson, *The Fabric of the Body* (Oxford: Clarendon Press, 1992), 188-89.
20. Roberts and Tomlinson, 272-73.
21. See Pascal P. Parente, *The Regimen of Health of the Medical School of Salerno* (New York: Vantage Press, 1967).
22. *The School of Salernum: Regimen Sanitatis Salernitanum*, trans. Sir John Harington (London: Humphrey Milford/Oxford University Press, 1922), 138.
23. For the cultural history of midwifery see: Jean Towler and Joan Bramall, *Midwives in History and Society* (London: Croom Helm, 1986); Harold Speert, *Obstetrics and Gynecology: a History and Iconography*, 2d ed., rev. (San Francisco: Norman Publishing, 1994); Palmer Findley, *Priests of Lucina: The Story of Obstetrics* (Boston: Little, Brown & Co., 1939); and Thomas Rogers Forbes, *The Midwife and the Witch* (New Haven: Yale University Press, 1966).
24. Renate Blumenfeld-Kosinski, *Not of Woman Born: Representations of Caesarean Birth in Medieval and Renaissance Culture* (Ithaca: Cornell University Press, 1990), 142-53. For the iconography of the Birth of Antichrist, see 125-42.
25. Speert, 302.
26. Blumenfeld-Kosinski, 137-42.
27. Ovid, *Metamorphoses*, trans. Rolfe Humphries (Bloomington: Indiana University Press, 1955), 217-19.
28. This interpretation by K. B. Roberts is found in his article, "Illustrations in a Sixteenth-century Book on Obstetrics," *Canadian Bulletin of Medical History* 1 (winter 1984): 80-95.
29. For the history of anatomical illustration see: Ludwig Choulant, *History and Bibliography of Anatomic Illustration*, trans. and annotated by Mortimer Frank (New York: Hafner Publishing Co., 1962); Charles Singer, *A Short History of Anatomy from the Greeks to Harvey*, 2d ed. (New York: Dover Publications, 1957); Diane R. Karp, *Ars Medica: Art, Medicine, and the Human Condition* (Philadelphia: Philadelphia Museum of Art, 1985); Cazort, Kornell, and Roberts; and Roberts and Tomlinson.
30. Roberts and Tomlinson, 74-77.
31. James Snyder, *Northern Renaissance Art* (New York: Harry N. Abrams, 1985), 333.
32. Cazort, Kornell, and Roberts, 137-38.
33. Karp, 156; Roberts and Tomlinson, 170-71.
34. Karp, 156.
35. Saunders and O'Malley, 25-29.
36. Mayor, 109-10.
37. Saunders and O'Malley, 92.
38. Saunders and O'Malley, 29.
39. G. S. T. Cavanagh, "A New View of the Vesalian Landscape," *Medical History* 27 (Jan. 1983): 77-79.
40. Roberts and Tomlinson, 208-10.
41. Roberts and Tomlinson, 211.
42. Roberts and Tomlinson, 211.
43. For information about Becerra and other sources for the flayed man see Lola L. Szladits, "The Influence of Michelangelo on Some Anatomical Illustrations," *Journal of the History of Medicine and Allied Sciences* 9 (1954): 420-27.
44. See Karp, 163; Roberts and Tomlinson, 263; and Cazort, Kornell, and Roberts, 167-68.
45. Robert Beverly Hale and Terence Coyle, *Albinus on Anatomy*, corrected ed. (New York: Dover Publications, 1988), 18.
46. Roberts and Tomlinson, 323-24.
47. Hendrik Punt, *Bernard Siegfried Albinus (1697-1770): On 'Human Nature'* (Amsterdam: B. M. Israël, 1983), 2.
48. Roberts and Tomlinson, 325.
49. Choulant, 280.
50. F. J. Cole, "The History of Albrecht Dürer's Rhinoceros in Zoological Literature," *Science Medicine and History: Essays on the Evolution of Scientific Thought and Medical Practice Written in Honor of Charles Singer* (London: Oxford University Press, 1953), 337-56.
51. Punt, 53.

Index of Portrait Subjects

Includes art works in all media. When multiple images of the same subject are discussed sequentially, only the page number of the first is listed. Academic degrees are not listed here.

Index of Nonportraits

Includes art works in all media including architecture. When multiple images of the same subject are discussed sequentially, only the page number of the first is listed. Note that architecture is grouped together within each chapter, usually near its beginning. Book illustrations are listed by author if known, otherwise by title. For artists' names see the index of artists.

Index of Artists and Makers

Includes artists in all media including book illustration and architecture. When more than one page is given, the first is where the artist's biography will be found.

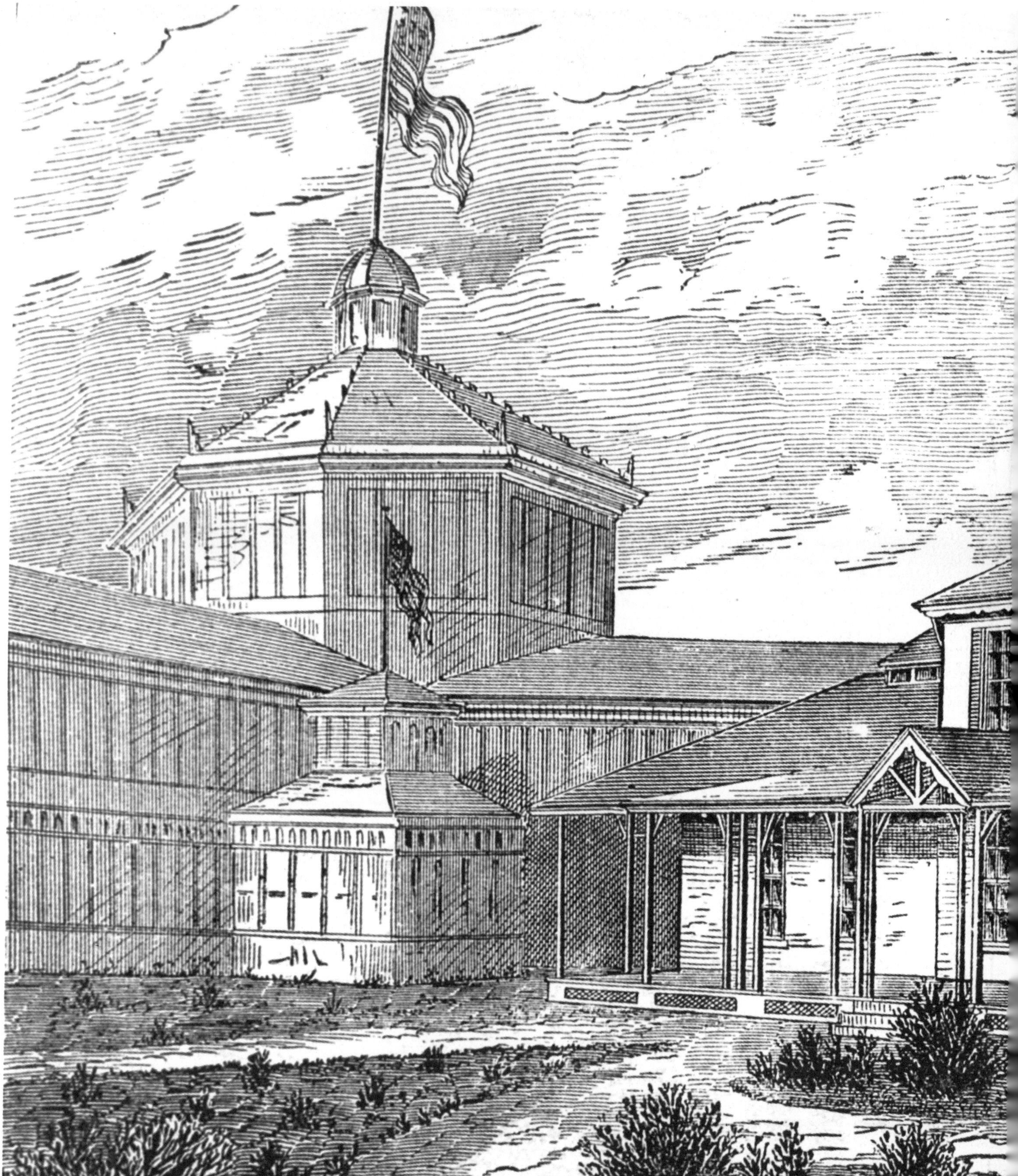

POST HOSPITAL OF T